Second Edition

Principles and Practice of Nurse Anesthesia

Second Edition

Principles and Practice of Nurse Anesthesia

Wynne R. Waugaman, CRNA, PhD
Associate Professor of Clinical Anesthesiology and Director
Department of Anesthesiology/Program of Nurse Anesthesia
School of Medicine
University of California at Los Angeles
Los Angeles, California

Scot D. Foster, CRNA, PhD
Assistant Professor of Clinical Anesthesiology/Associate Director
Department of Anesthesiology/Program of Nurse Anesthesia
School of Medicine
University of California at Los Angeles
Los Angeles, California

Benjamin M. Rigor, MD
Professor and Chairman
Department of Anesthesiology
School of Medicine
University of Louisville
Louisville, Kentucky

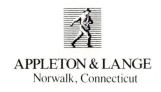

APPLETON & LANGE
Norwalk, Connecticut

Notice: The authors and the publisher of this volume have taken care to make certain that the doses of drugs and schedules of treatment are correct and compatible with the standards generally accepted at the time of publication. Nevertheless, as new information becomes available, changes in treatment and in the use of drugs become necessary. The reader is advised to carefully consult the instruction and information material included in the package insert of each drug or therapeutic agent before administration. This advice is especially important when using new or infrequently used drugs. The publisher disclams any liability, loss, injury, or damage incurred as a consequence, directly or indirectly, of the use and application of any of the contents of this volume.

Copyright © 1992 by Appleton & Lange
Simon & Schuster Business and Professional Group
Copyright © 1988 by Appleton & Lange

92 93 94 95 96 / 10 9 8 7 6 5 4 3 2 1

Prentice Hall International (UK) Limited, *London*
Prentice Hall of Australia Pty. Limited, *Sydney*
Prentice Hall Canada, Inc., *Toronto*
Prentice Hall Hispanoamericana, S.A., *Mexico*
Prentice Hall of India Private Limited, *New Delhi*
Prentice Hall of Japan, Inc., *Tokyo*
Simon & Schuster Asia Pte. Ltd., *Singapore*
Editora Prentice Hall do Brasil Ltda., *Rio de Janeiro*
Prentice Hall, *Englewood Cliffs, New Jersey*

Library of Congress Cataloging-in-Publication Data

Principles and practice of nurse anesthesia / edited by Wynne R.
    Waugaman, Scot D. Foster, Benjamin M. Rigor.—2nd ed.
        p.   cm.
      Includes bibliographical references and index.
      ISBN 0-8385-7962-0
      1. Anesthesiology.   2. Nurse anesthetists.   I. Waugaman, Wynne R.
    II. Foster, Scot Douglas.   III. Rigor, Benjamin M.
      [DNLM: 1. Nurse Anesthetists.   WY 151 P957]
    RD82.P755   1992
    617.9'6—dc20
    DNLM/DLC
    for Library of Congress   92-11074
                                                          CIP

Editor in Chief: Barbara E. Norwitz
Nursing Developmental Editor: Mark F. Wales
Production Editor: Karen W. Davis
Designer: Steven M. Byrum
Manufacturing Buyer: Alexis R. Heydt

PRINTED IN THE UNITED STATES OF AMERICA

ISBN   0-8385-7962-0

90000

9 780838 579626

*This book is dedicated to the graduate students of the UCLA Program of
Nurse Anesthesia, past, present and future, to whom we entrust the responsibility for continuing the
tradition of scholarly contribution to the profession of nurse anesthesia.*

Contents

Contributors

John Aker, CRNA, MS
Chief Nurse Anesthetist
Department of Anesthesiology
Research Medical Center
Kansas City, Kansas

Gerald David Allen, MB, FFARCS
Professor
Departments of Anesthesiology and Oral Surgery
Schools of Medicine and Dentistry
University of California at Los Angeles
Los Angeles, California

Marianne Bankert
Historian and Consultant
American Association of Nurse Anesthetists
Park Ridge, Illinois

Hollis E. Bivens, BA, MD
Professor and Chairman
Department of Anesthesiology
University of Texas/M D Anderson Cancer Center
Houston, Texas

Norman H. Blass, MD
Professor of Anesthesia and Obstetrics and Gynecology
Director of Obstetric Anesthesia
Medical College of Virginia
Richmond, Virginia

Nancy Bruton-Maree, CRNA, MS
Program Director, Raleigh School of Nurse Anesthesia
Raleigh, North Carolina
and
Visiting Professor
School of Nursing
University of North Carolina at Greensboro
Greensboro, North Carolina

Eddie Bowie
Director
Education and Quality Assurance
Department of Anesthesia and Critical Care
Pritzker School of Medicine
University of Chicago
Chicago, Illinois

Lida Inge Swafford Dahm, MD, FAAP
Director of Anesthesiology
Angleton-Danbury General Hospital
Angleton, Texas
and
Clinical Assistant Professor
Departments of Anesthesiology and Pediatrics
Baylor College of Medicine
Texas Medical Center
Houston, Texas

Michael P. Dosch, CRNA, MS
Instructor and Assistant Director
Program in Nurse Anesthesia
University of Detroit Mercy/St. Joseph Mercy Hospital
Pontiac, Michigan

Colonel Cecil B. Drain, CRNA, PhD, FAAN
Program Director and Adjunct Professor
US Army/Texas Wesleyan University
Program in Anesthesia Nursing, Phase I
Army Medical Department Center and School
Fort Sam Houston, Texas

Margaret Faut-Callahan, CRNA, DNSc, FAAN
Associate Chairperson, Associate Professor
Surgical Nursing and Program Director
Nurse Anesthesia Program
College of Nursing
Rush University
Chicago, Illinois

Linda S. Finander, CRNA, MS
Assistant Clinical Professor
Department of Anesthesiology/Program of Nurse
  Anesthesia
School of Medicine
University of California at Los Angeles
Los Angeles, California

Scot D. Foster, CRNA, PhD
Assistant Professor of Clinical Anesthesiology/Associate
  Director
Department of Anesthesiology/Program of Nurse
  Anesthesia
School of Medicine
University of California at Los Angeles
Los Angeles, California

Francis R. Gerbasi, CRNA, PhD
Assistant Professor and Director
Anesthesia Program
University of Michigan/Flint
Flint, Michigan

Michele E. Gold, CRNA, PhD
Clinical and Didactic Instructor
Department of Anesthesiology/Program of Nurse
  Anesthesia
School of Medicine
University of California at Los Angeles
Los Angeles, California

Dana Lynn Grogan, CRNA, MS
Assistant Clinical Professor
Department of Anesthesiology/Program of Nurse
  Anesthesia
School of Medicine
University of California at Los Angeles
Los Angeles, California

Thomas J. Grogan, MD
Assistant Clinical Professor
Department of Surgery, Division of Orthopedics
School of Medicine
University of California at Los Angeles
Los Angeles, California

Ira P. Gunn, MLN, CRNA, FAAN
Consultant, Nurse Anesthesia Affairs
Executive Director, Texas Association of Nurse Anesthetists
El Paso, Texas

Everard R. Hicks, CRNA, MEd
Professor Emeritus
Anesthesia for Nurses Educational Department
College of Health Related Professions
Medical College of South Carolina
Charleston, South Carolina

Don R. Hirschman, CRNA, BA
Private Practice
Outpatient Ophthalmic Anesthesia
Long Beach, California

Lesa J. Hirschman, CRNA, MS
Private Practice
Outpatient Ophthalmic Anesthesia
Long Beach, California

Linda M. Huffman, CRNA, BA
Anesthesia Technology Consultant
Healthcare Training Associates, Ltd.
San Antonio, Texas

Lorraine M. Jordan, CRNA, MS
Director of Education and Research
American Association of Nurse Anesthetists
Park Ridge, Illinois

Kathleen C. Koerbacher, CRNA, MA
Director of Anesthesia
Harris Methodist Hospital Fort Worth
Fort Worth, Texas

Leo A. Le Bel, CRNA, MEd, JD
Director
Nurse Anesthesia Program
Southern Connecticut State University/Bridgeport Hospital
Bridgeport, Connecticut

Carol Boetger Mann, CRNA, MS
Assistant Clinical Professor
Department of Anesthesiology/Program of Nurse
  Anesthesia
School of Medicine
University of California at Los Angeles
Los Angeles, California

Cathy Mastropietro, CRNA, MEd
Project Manager
Department of Education and Research
American Association of Nurse Anesthetists
Park Ridge, Illinois

Charles H. Moore, CRNA, MS, PhD
Assistant Professor of Nurse Anesthesia
Departments of Nurse Anesthesia and Anesthesiology
School of Allied Health Professions
Medical College of Virginia
Richmond, Virginia

Jeanette F. Peter, CRNA, MAEd
Assistant Clinical Professor
Department of Anesthesiology/Program of Nurse
  Anesthesia
School of Medicine
University of California at Los Angeles
Los Angeles, California

M. Regina B. Puno, MD
Assistant Professor
Department of Anesthesiology
School of Medicine
University of Louisville
Louisville, Kentucky

Joseph T. Rando, CRNA, MN
Associate Professor and Director
Program in Nurse Anesthesia
School of Nursing
University of Texas
Houston, Texas

J. L. Reeves-Viets, MD
Clinical Associate Professor
Department of Anesthesiology
Baylor College of Medicine
Houston, Texas

Leslie Rendell-Baker
Professor of Anesthesiology
Department of Anesthesiology
Loma Linda University School of Medicine
Loma Linda, California

Benjamin M. Rigor, MD
Professor and Chairman
Department of Anesthesiology
School of Medicine
University of Louisville
Louisville, Kentucky

Timothy D. Saye, MD
Assistant Professor in Residence
Department of Anesthesiology
School of Medicine
University of California at Los Angeles
Los Angeles, California

Barbara Shwiry, CRNA, BA
Clinical and Didactic Instructor
Program of Nurse Anesthesia
Department of Anesthesiology/Program of Nurse
   Anesthesia
School of Medicine
University of California at Los Angeles
Los Angeles, California

Janet S. Simpson, CRNA, JD
Holbrook, Heaven and Fay, PA
Kansas City, Kansas

Jonathan H. Skerman, BDSc, MScD, DSc
Professor of Anesthesia and Obstetrics and Gynecology
Director of Obstetric Anesthesia
School of Medicine in Shreveport
Louisiana State University Medical Center
Shreveport, Louisiana

Bruce Skolnick, MD, PhD
Senior Resident in Anesthesiology
Department of Anesthesiology
School of Medicine
University of California at Los Angeles
Los Angeles, California

Jeanne F. Slack, CRNA, DNSc
Assistant Professor and Associate Chairperson
Maternal Child Nursing
College of Nursing
Rush University
Chicago, Illinois

Michael D. Stanton-Hicks, MB, BS, Drmed, FCAnaesth
Director, Pain Management Center
Cleveland Clinic Foundation
Cleveland, Ohio

D. E. Supkis, Jr, MD
Clinical Assistant Professor
Department of Anesthesiology
University of Texas/M D Anderson Cancer Center
Houston, Texas

Doris J. Tanaka, CRNA, MS
Director and Adjunct Assistant Professor
Anesthesia Services and Program in Nurse Anesthesia
University of Detroit Mercy/Henry Ford Hospital
Detroit, Michigan

Ceil E. Vercellino, CRNA, MS
Assistant Clinical Professor and Director of Clinical Services
Department of Anesthesiology/Program of Nurse
   Anesthesia
University of California at Los Angeles
Los Angeles, California

Susan A. Ward, DPhil
Professor
Departments of Anesthesiology and Physiology
School of Medicine
University of California at Los Angeles
Los Angeles, California

Wynne R. Waugaman, CRNA, PhD
Associate Professor of Clinical Anesthesiology and Director
Department of Anesthesiology/Program of Nurse
   Anesthesia
School of Medicine
University of California at Los Angeles
Los Angeles, California

Marian Waterhouse, CRNA, MEd
Colonel, U.S. Army Nurse Corps (Ret.)
Former Director, U.S. Army Anesthesiology Program of
   Instruction for Army Nurse Corps Officers
San Antonio, Texas

Joel M. Weaver, DDS, PhD
Associate Professor of Anesthesiology
Colleges of Dentistry and Medicine
The Ohio State University
Columbus, Ohio

Laura Wong, CRNA, MS
Chief Nurse Anesthetist
Kapiolani Medical Center
Honolulu, Hawaii

Karen L. Zaglaniczny, CRNA, PhD
Assistant Professor and Education Coordinator
Program of Nurse Anesthesia
Wayne State University/Detroit Receiving Hospital
Detroit, Michigan

Christine S. Zambricki, CRNA, MS
Director of Anesthesia Services/PACU
William Beaumont Hospital
Royal Oak, Michigan
and
Director, Nurse Anesthesia Track
School of Nursing
Oakland University
Rochester, Michigan

Lieutenant Colonel Gary D. Zarr, CRNA, MS
Adjunct Assistant Professor of Health Science
US Army/Texas Wesleyan University
Program in Anesthesia Nursing, Phase I
Army Medical Department Center and School
Fort Sam Houston, Texas

Acknowledgments

In developing the second edition of *Principles and Practice of Nurse Anesthesia*, we were fortunate to retain a number of authors who participated in the first edition and recruit twenty-four new authors to provide their subject expertise. The identification of subject experts by the editors and the expertise and dedication of these contributors continue to be the heart of this project. Without the continued interest, support, and participation of these individuals, this revised edition would not have come to fruition.

We would like to give special thanks to Mark F. Wales, our Nursing Developmental Editor from Appleton & Lange, whose stylistic contribution to this edition has improved it immeasurably. His patience, guidance, encouragement, and professionalism provided the critical ingredients necessary to help us achieve our goals. We also wish to thank Pat Bensinger for her assistance with editing. Finally, we wish to thank our families, friends, and colleagues for their patience and support.

Wynne R. Waugaman
Scot D. Foster
Benjamin M. Rigor

Preface

The editors and contributors are pleased to introduce the second edition of *Principles and Practice of Nurse Anesthesia*. The textbook has been substantially modified from the first edition, largely to incorporate recent advances in equipment technologies, changed practice patterns, and new pharmacologic drugs and agents, as well as to give attention to the evolving standards of patient care.

With few exceptions, every chapter of this book has undergone substantial update and rewrite with a focus toward comprehensiveness and application of theoretical principles to clinical practice. The format of the book is changed to incorporate a new organizational structure that more closely approximates the anesthesia process and planning for case management. Major sections of the book now include Foundations, Perioperative Considerations, Applied Physiology, Applied Pharmacology, Anesthesia and the Subspecialties, and Special Problems in Anesthesia and Critical Care.

There are eight new chapters in the book including Documentation of Anesthesia Care, The Anesthesia Machine, Environmental Safety, Preoperative Medication and Techniques of Induction and Maintenance, Anesthesia for General and Genitourinary Surgery, Anesthesia for Orthopedic Surgery, Anesthesia for Organ Transplantation, and Pain Management. The chapter on Quality Assurance has been eliminated as it is covered extensively in other nurse anesthesia related texts. Many chapters such as Periopera-

tive Monitoring, Anesthesia for Plastic Surgery and the Thermally Injured Patient, and Pharmacologic Principles of Inhalation Anesthesia have been significantly broadened to accommodate rapidly expanding technologies and additions to the pharmacologic armamentarium of the anesthetist. Also introduced is an expanded version of the Legal Aspects of Anesthesia, which includes the study of ethical decision-making. A special effort has been made to enhance the content by utilization of more illustrations as well as to reference the text with the most updated information available. However, in some instances, the editors have chosen to reproduce classic illustrations depicting the text.

This text is designed primarily for the student of anesthesia who seeks a comprehensive and germane discussion of the basic and advanced principles of anesthesia practice. The editors also feel that the text will serve as a meaningful reference for those CRNAs who have already established their professional careers. The editors of *Principles and Practice of Nurse Anesthesia* have garnered the expertise of clinicians and educators in nurse anesthesia, anesthesiology, and other academic or professional disciplines to emphasize the importance of collaboration within our specialty. Above all, this second edition continues to serve as an example of how CRNAs can and should assume the responsibilities for the education of future nurse anesthetists through production of their own educational materials.

Preface to the First Edition

While there is evidence that nurses were involved in administering anesthesia dating back to the American Civil War and the Franco-Prussian War in Europe, this clinical nursing specialty became formalized during the first two decades of the twentieth century. The history of this specialty demonstrates the dedication of nurse anesthetists to the advancement of the art and science of anesthesia through their involvement in pioneering new anesthetic techniques and working with physicians and engineers to develop new and better equipment. One of the major purposes for these nursing pioneers to come together and found the American Association of Nurse Anesthetists in 1931 was to share their knowledge and develop standards for high quality education for nurses entering this specialty. Their commitment and dedication to this purpose has served as an inspiration throughout the years to succeeding generations of nurse anesthetists.

This book represents no less of a milestone in the history of nurse anesthesia than did many of the individual accomplishments of persons such as Alice Magaw, Agatha Hodgins, Helen Lamb, Hilda Salomon, Olive Berger, and others too numerous to mention. It is the first, multiauthored, comprehensive anesthesia textbook written principally by CRNAs for nurse anesthesia students and their CRNA colleagues. These CRNA authors have been joined by some basic scientists and physicians who have been directly involved in nurse anesthesia education and/or their practice. The contributors to this book have distilled the essence of the basic sciences and meshed them with concepts from the clinical and behavioral sciences in a manner which allows the learner to unify diverse knowledge components into a specific anesthesia care plan to meet the needs of an individual patient. As such, this book primarily deals with anesthesia practice, its concepts and its reality. In addition, the book addresses the environment within which anesthesia is practiced and the necessary management styles, programs, and resources to assess and assure the quality of anesthesia services.

While anesthesia practice is a dynamic, constantly changing field, this textbook provides those basic fundamentals that serve as a sound foundation for future growth and development in this field. It also may serve as a reference book for nurses in other specialties who care for the anesthetized patient. And finally, it will also be of interest to those nurses who have yet to decide upon a nursing specialty, allowing them to become more knowledgeable about this field, its educational requirements, and the clinical demands placed upon CRNAs.

The authors have kept faith with nurse anesthetist pioneers in accepting responsibility for putting something back into the specialty, rather than merely taking from those who were our predecessors. This book should serve as an incentive for other CRNA authors to undertake the writing of other needed texts or reference books from which we all can benefit.

John F. Garde, CRNA, MS

Second Edition

Principles and Practice of Nurse Anesthesia

History of Nurse Anesthesia

Marianne Bankert

"History is more than a narrative—it is a political stake. . . . History is . . . a place of struggle in itself."

Christine Delphy

The program of study for nurse anesthesia students is extremely challenging, and students may well be expected to ask, Why study history? The answer is that every profession has a culture, consisting of its values, norms, and symbols. Its history, or collective memory, is part of that culture. A profession's shared understanding of the past illuminates present experience and significantly affects decisions shaping the future. Because the contribution of the nurse to anesthesia has been virtually ignored in the literature of the field, students will not routinely acquire a sense of that achievement in the education process. It is therefore especially important that nurse anesthesia students, tomorrow's decision makers, make an effort to familiarize themselves with the impressive history of their profession.

IN SEARCH OF THE INVISIBLE PROVIDERS

The centennial of William T. G. Morton's successful demonstration of surgical anesthesia at Massachusetts General Hospital on October 16, 1946, was marked by the publication of several historical studies. A characteristic of these works was the absence of any substantial and affirmative mention of nurse anesthetists. In part to redress this situation, *The History of Anesthesia With Emphasis on the Nurse Specialist,* sponsored by the American Association of Nurse Anesthetists, was published in 1953. In her preface to that book, Virginia S. Thatcher explained, "If the place of the nurse as an anesthetist receives special emphasis in this history, it is because she has been derogated or ignored."

Yet, 35 years later, even though they annually administer approximately half of the anesthetics in this country, a national news publication could still headline nurse anesthetists as "the best kept secret in medicine."[1]

It was timely, then, for the American Association of Nurse Anesthetists (AANA) to commission a new historical study of the profession of nurse anesthesia. When I began that work in 1985, I was, of course, aware in a general sense that the nurse contribution to anesthesia had continued to go largely uncredited. Yet, like any researcher setting out on the quest for the grail of increased understanding, the discoveries and insights that would occur along this journey could not have been known to me at the start.

There were surprises.

Surgical anesthesia is a field born in the United States in the mid-19th century. Surgeon John Collins Warren, whose patient, Gilbert Abbott, was anesthetized by Morton on that momentous day in Boston, reflected 2 years later on the significance of the event:

> A new era has opened on the operating surgeon. His visitations on the most delicate parts are performed, not only without the agonizing screams he has been accustomed to hear, but sometimes in a state of perfect insensibility, and occasionally, even with an expression of pleasure on the part of the patient. . . . Unrestrained and free as God's own sunshine, [anesthesia] has gone forth to cheer and gladden the earth; it will awaken the gratitude of the present, and all coming generations. The student, who from distant lands or in distant ages, may visit this spot, will view it with increased interest, as he remembers that *here was first demonstrated one of the most glorious truths of science.* [1848][2]

Ironically, anesthesia, the gift to suffering humanity that silenced the screams of surgical patients, was no great gift to those who participated in its actualization. There was instant and bitter controversy over credit for the "discovery." Morton, his health broken from his bitter struggle to establish his claim, died "in the wildest state of excitement," probably from a stroke, at the age of 48.[3] Charles T. Jackson, the chemist who consulted with both Morton and Horace Wells on the properties of ether and nitrous oxide, became increasingly obsessed with his claim, not only for the anesthesia breakthrough but also for other scientific discoveries, and spent the last years of his life in a hospital for the insane. Wells, who had failed in his 1844 public demonstration of nitrous oxide, fell into despair and committed suicide in 1848, in a cell where he had been jailed for throwing acid on the clothing of a prostitute. At his graveside, his widow reportedly said: "My husband's great gift, which he devoted to the service of mankind, proved a curse to himself and to his family."[4] Crawford W. Long of Georgia used ether in his medical practice in 1842 but published results only after the 1846 events in Boston. Sadly, he therefore lost the honor he might have won.

Credit for the anesthesia breakthrough is a subject that continues to stir passion among devoted partisans of various claimants. Later in the century, as surgery developed and the need for professional anesthetists became clear, there would arise another controversy equally long-lived, and often bitter: Who should administer anesthetics? Anesthesia, by that time, *was* recognized as serious business but one that lacked medical status. It was the surgeon who captained the ship and collected the large fees. There was no financial incentive for a person holding a medical license to assume the work. Surgeons, to advance their specialty, needed reliable, competent, professional anesthetists. They found their answer: *nurses.* Thus, the earliest professional clinical nursing specialty was called into being (Fig. 1–1).

And, in its origins, this decision *was* economic and gender based. It would be decades before the terms *physician* and *nurse* were not synonymous with *male* and *female,* respectively.

Apart from the few physicians who had a genuine intellectual interest in anesthesia, it would take years for the economics of anesthesia to make it an attractive area for their colleagues if, at first, only as a supplemental source of income. As this change in attitude developed, it was necessary for physician anesthetists to establish their "claim" to a field of practice they had earlier rejected. To achieve this end, the accomplishments of nurse anesthetists had to be denied or denigrated or ignored.

It was the process by which a rival and less monied group (in this case, nurses) is rendered historically "invisible" that became the most intriguing part of the study of this discipline. Reminiscent of George Orwell's Ministry of Truth, a myth is launched of the early superiority of British anesthetists—a land, so the story goes, which was never so foolish as to allow nurses to administer anesthetics; the national association of physician anesthetists backdates its founding from 1936 to 1905; a new word "anesthesiologist"

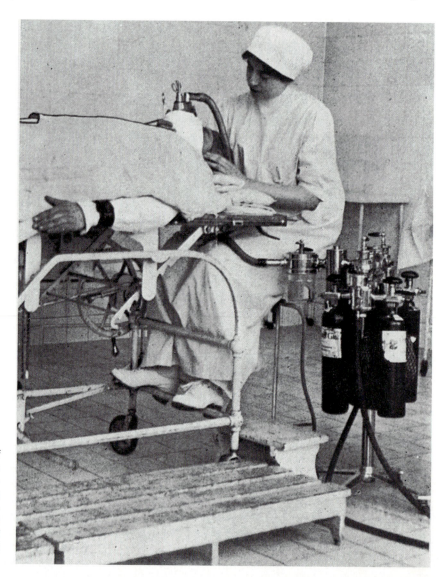

Figure 1–1. Agatha C. Hodgins, founder of what has come to be called the American Association of Nurse Anesthetists, demonstrates nitrous oxide–oxygen anesthesia with the Teter apparatus, along with watchful care. Photographs accompanied her chapter on the subject in the 1914 edition of *Anoci Association* by GW Crile and WE Lower. (*Courtesy AANA.*)

is coined in the 1930s to distinguish the work of physician anesthetists from nurse anesthetists; "historical" studies are published with titles like *The Genesis of Contemporary Anesthesiology,* as though nothing of significance occurred in the field until the 1920s when physician anesthetists began to be effectively organized. It must be noted, however, that the decision by the Anesthesia History Association to include presentations on the contributions of nurse anesthetists in its recent Third International Symposium for the History of Anesthesia (Atlanta, March 1992) may signal a welcome change in the way the history of the field is approached.

Retrieving many of those contributions was the special joy this author found in writing *Watchful Care, a History of America's Nurse Anesthetists,* as well as in subsequent studies. It is my hope that this work will stimulate and encourage CRNAs to continue, or begin, to retrieve the history of their profession. Perhaps it will be the history of a particular school or geographic area, perhaps the history of a significant individual. Perhaps, also, a greater number of those nurse anesthetists who have themselves been participants in and witnesses to history-making events will be moved to record them. This retrieval of past accomplishments is not a luxury. There is no doubt that it is the strong, even heroic, legacy of past nurse anesthetists that allows present practitioners to contend successfully with current challenges.

What follows are highlights from that ongoing body of work chosen to introduce the student nurse anesthetist to some of the achievements of pioneering nurse anesthetists, to give some sense of the evolving relationship between nurse anesthetists and the nursing profession, to discuss discrimination encountered by male nurse anesthetists, and to recognize the contribution of nurse anesthetists to the military services. Finally, in an introduction to the rapidly developing International Federation of Nurse Anesthetists, there is a suggestion of the future and its exciting possibilities.

ALICE MAGAW: "THE MOTHER OF ANESTHESIA"

The Sisters of St. Francis established St. Mary's Hospital, Rochester, Minnesota, in 1889 on the condition that Dr. William Worrell Mayo take charge of it. It would soon become a gathering place for those interested in learning techniques from its brilliant surgeons. Visitors would also see "peerless" administration of anesthetics at the hands of Alice Magaw and other nurse anesthetists of Mayo Clinic.

What was initially a matter of necessity for the Mayos became a matter of choice: "In the first place . . . they had no interns. And when the interns came, the brothers decided that a nurse was better suited to the task because she was more likely to keep her mind strictly on it, whereas the intern was naturally more interested in what the surgeon was doing."[5] The Clinic's first nurse anesthetists were two Rochester sisters, Dinah and Edith Graham, both graduates of the School of Nursing at the Women's Hospital in Chicago. Dinah's tenure was brief; Edith continued until her marriage to Charles H. Mayo in 1893. Her friend, Alice Magaw (1860–1928), another Rochester girl who graduated from the Women's Hospital in Chicago, succeeded her. So brilliant was her work that, as Mayo biographer Helen

Clapesattle has noted, she "won more widespread notice than that of any other member of the Rochester group apart from the brothers."[5]

As a nurse, Magaw could not be a member of a medical society. Her first talks were occasioned by invitations from the Olmsted County Medical Society; they were then published in state medical journals. "Observations in Anesthesia," a report on over 3000 cases, was published in the *Northwestern Lancet* in 1899. It was Magaw's first publication. In her 1906 paper, "A Review of Over Fourteen Thousand Surgical Anesthesias," Magaw emphasized that other anesthetic techniques had been tried but were found to be less satisfactory than the "open method" of ether:

> We have tried almost all methods advocated that seemed at all reasonable, such as nitrous oxide gas as a preliminary to ether (this method was used in one thousand cases), a mixture of scopolamine and morphine as a preliminary to ether in 73 cases, also chloroform and ether, and have found them to be very unsatisfactory, if not harmful, and have returned to ether "drop method" each time, which method we have used for over ten years.[6]

Medical people came from around the country and the world to observe the technique of Mayo's nurse anesthetists. An Iowa doctor said of their expertise and influence: "Many of us have had the pleasure and privilege of seeing that peerless anesthetist, Alice Magaw, and also Miss [Florence] Henderson, who anesthetizes for Dr. Charles Mayo, 'talk their patients to sleep,' and we have been charmed and instructed by the manner in which these ladies do their work. The lessons they have taught and are teaching practitioners have been carried far and wide and practiced by men throughout Iowa and many other states."[7]

The international reputation of the Mayo nurse anesthetists is reflected in a British report: "Notes on the Administration of Anaesthetics in America, With Special Reference to the Practice at the Mayo Clinic." This paper was presented by Mrs. Francis Dickinson-Berry, MD, to the Section on Anaesthetics of the Royal Society of Medicine, in 1912, and is of special interest because it is a commonplace in histories of anesthesia written from the physician's point of view that anesthesia practice in Britain, where it was limited to physicians, was superior to that in the United States with its nurse anesthetists. Dickinson-Berry's paper and the subsequent discussion make clear that some British physician anesthetists felt they had things to learn from the Mayo nurse anesthetists:

> I now come to what was one of the main objects of my tour in America, the visit to Rochester, Minnesota. Like most people, I had heard and read much of the excellence of the anaesthetics at the Mayo Clinic. In the last paper I read on the subject before leaving England the writer was inclined to attribute this partly to an inborn faculty for administering anaesthetics on the part of women, and partly to the aid of hypnotic suggestion. I was therefore very glad to have the opportunity of seeing them myself.[8]

Dickinson-Berry and her colleagues described the "open ether method in America," and agreed that it was different from that practiced in Britain:

The essential feature of the open ether method in America was the absolutely continuous administration; a drop on the mask every two seconds was the rate. In fact, at Rochester it was called the "drop method." In this country the anaesthetist would often pour 2 dr. or 3 dr. on the mask, then stop for a few minutes and then pour a few more drachms on the mask. This was not open ether as practised in America.[8]

"Ether by the open method with the skill exhibited at Rochester," said Dickinson-Berry, "requires much practice."[8]

In what is, in effect, another chapter in the chauvinistic "Great Trans-Atlantic Debate" over the relative merits of ether versus chloroform anesthesia—with the former the general favorite in the United States and the latter preferred in Britain—*the safety of the lightness of the ether anesthesia of the Mayo nurse anesthetists* became the center of the British physician anesthetist discussion. In her various papers, Magaw had noted that chloroform, though an easier anesthetic from the viewpoint of the surgeon and anesthetist (herself included), was not safer for the patient: "For the sake of the patient my preference is for ether; for myself, I would say, like most anaesthetizers, that I would prefer giving chloroform, as we escape things that naturally follow the use of ether."[9] After Dickinson-Berry's report on her visit to Mayo Clinic, the President of the Section of Anaesthetics reflected:

The most striking difference [between British and American anesthetic practice] appeared to him to be the slighter degree of narcosis which was considered necessary in America. The description of the return in stomach cases almost to consciousness, which the surgeon not only permitted but desired, showed what a difference there was in the practice of the two countries. *Evidently in the States safety was the first consideration.* [emphasis added]

Another respondent observed:

The most important conclusion from the paper . . . was that in the United States light anaesthesia was adopted *because of its safety.* The belief in England that deep anaesthesia prevented shock was dying out, but it had been the greatest handicap, and had caused more accidents in this country than anything else.[8] [emphasis added]

The conclusion drawn by another discussant is "the reason the Americans had been so successful was that they had learned from us, while we, on our part, had not learned anything like so much from them."[8]

This recognition of the nurse anesthetist's contribution to the creation of the field, with the emphasis on patient care, is not found in physician-oriented histories of American practice. Rather, these studies trace positive developments to a physician origin. It is therefore all the more important to note the title Dr. Charles H. Mayo bestowed on Alice Magaw: "Mother of Anesthesia."[10]

NURSE ANESTHETIST SERVICE IN THE GREAT WAR

World War I was the first time the army and navy trained nurses as anesthetists for war service. American nurse anes-

thetists risked their lives at the front in volunteer service, establishing an enviable record and winning the admiration of some of the most celebrated surgeons and medical practitioners in the Western world. One of the most distinguished of these was Sophie Gran Winton (1887–1989).

A graduate of Swedish Hospital, Minneapolis, Minnesota, Winton trained as an anesthetist at the urging of hospital administrator Gustaf W. Olson. She already had 5 years of experience and a record of more than 10,000 cases without a fatality when she joined the Army Nurse Corps (through the Red Cross) because "it was the patriotic thing to do" (from an interview with M. Bankert, June 1986). Winton and nine other nurses from Minneapolis Hospital Unit No. 26 were assigned to Mobile Hospital No. 1 in the Chateau-Thierry area in France with the pioneering physician anesthetist James T. Gwathmey. She later reported to her former mentor, Olson, that she

gave anesthetics from the first of June [1918] to November after the Armistice. How many anesthetics I gave during the World War, I cannot determine, except that when the big drives were on, lasting from a week to ten days, I averaged twenty-five to thirty a day. The first three months I gave chloroform entirely, after which a ruling came that we were to use ether because there had been too many deaths from chloroform in inexperienced hands. Many a night I had to pour ether or chloroform on my finger to determine the amount I was giving, because we had no lights except the surgeon had a searchlight for his work, so the only sign I had to go by was respiration.[11]

Elsewhere, she recalled that "during the drives, patients came in so fast that all the surgeons could do was to remove bullets and shrapnel, stop hemorrhages and put iodoform packs in the wound and bandage it. As soon as they were through operating on one patient, I would have to have the next patient anesthetized."[12] She frequently gave anesthesia as shells fell close to the hospital. All the nurses in Winton's unit were awarded the Croix de Guerre. She herself was also awarded six overseas service bars as well as honors from the Overseas Nurses Association, the American Legion, and the Veterans of Foreign Wars. (It is important to note that Winton and her fellow nurses who served in this war, though serving in military organizations, came under the auspices of the Red Cross. They did not receive full military rank nor the pay and allowances equal to male military personnel. Nor did they receive veterans' compensation.)

There was also Anne Penland, the only anesthetist with the New York Presbyterian Hospital Unit (Base Hospital No. 2) and the first official nurse anesthetist on the British Front. In her diary, she described the bombing of casualty clearing stations:

We saw things, heard things, and went through them, but they were not such things as anybody but the Germans might have termed warfare. Imagine deliberately bombing a camp of wounded, and I don't mean one camp but as many as they could locate. Miss [Beatrice] MacDonald's camp was the first one and it came like a bolt from the heavens; of course, before this nobody had paid a great deal of attention to the Boche planes going over us, as we foolishly gave them credit for letting us alone and attacking soldiers' camps around us. These three camps were attacked or bombed three nights in succession, and you have heard how, fortunately, Major [William] Durrach was not in his tent, as it was blown to bits.[13]

Unfortunately, nurse MacDonald lost an eye from a shrapnel wound.

Penland's own expertise in anesthesia contributed to the British decision to train their own nurses in the work; she was later decorated by the British government. This change in British policy is significant, indicating another instance of the influence of America's nurse anesthetists. As the history of the Pennsylvania Hospital Unit (Base Hospital No. 10) recorded,

> Throughout the British Army anesthetics had hitherto only been administered by doctors and when shortly after our arrival our women began their work they were greatly astonished. The skill and care which was displayed soon caused their amazement to yield to admiration. The idea was soon adopted by the British authorities, and in the early spring of 1918 classes were formed of British nurses who received instruction at our hospital and at several others, and before the end of the war a number of British nursing sisters were performing the duties in various hospitals throughout the BEF.[7]

Years later, Dr. George Crile would observe that "if the Great War had gone another year, the British army would have adopted the nurse anesthetists right in the middle of the war."[14] But, as Daryl Pearce has ably shown in her study of the professional anesthetist in Britain, a British nurse anesthetist "might (barely) be acceptable in times of war but definitely not in peace-time."[15] Though the Royal College of Nursing took the position in 1919 that the British

nurses should be given "a chance for success" in anesthesia, the field had from the beginning remained within the province of the British physician. Though the administration of anesthetics in Britain depended heavily on the "occasional" physician anesthetist and though, just as in the United States, it would be a struggle to secure recognition of anesthesia as a full medical specialty, the British physician was not disposed to surrender ground to the nurse "technician," a term of derogation that would figure significantly in the debate within the United States.

AFFIRMING THE "NURSE" IN NURSE ANESTHETIST

Perhaps the greatest irony in the history of American anesthesia professions is that *both* nurse and physician practitioners had to struggle, sometimes with others and sometimes with themselves, to find an identity within the health care structure. Physicians fought to gain acceptance by their colleagues, to win recognition that theirs was a legitimate medical specialty. Nurses struggled with self-definition before accepting themselves as a clinical specialty within nursing. Agatha Hodgins's own anger with nursing for not responding to her vision left the nurse anesthetists a legacy of alienation from the larger group (Fig. 1–2). It was somewhat portentous, then, that the May 1946 issue of the *Journal of the American Association of Nurse Anesthetists*, which contained a lengthy obituary for Hodgins, also published a panel discussion titled, "The Nurse Anesthetist's Plans for Tomorrow's Responsibilities." The latter contained observations from a director of nursing education that did, indeed,

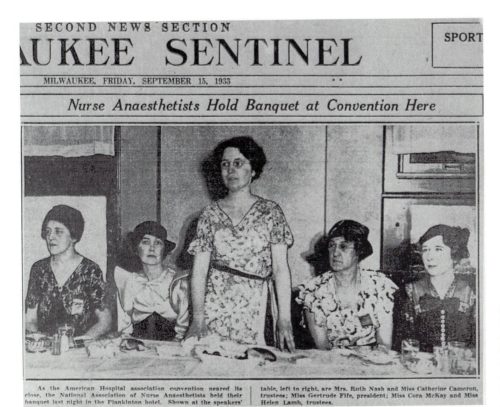

SECOND NEWS SECTION

...UKEE SENTINEL

SPORT

MILWAUKEE, FRIDAY, SEPTEMBER 15, 1933

Nurse Anaesthetists Hold Banquet at Convention Here

As the American Hospital association convention neared its close, the National Association of Nurse Anesthetists held their banquet last night in the Plankinton hotel. Shown at the speakers' table, left to right, are Mrs. Ruth Nash and Miss Catherine Cameron, trustees; Miss Gertrude Fife, president; Miss Cora McKay and Miss Helen Lamb, trustees.

Figure 1–2. The first annual meeting of Hodgins's National Association of Nurse Anesthetists was front-page news in 1933. The meeting was held in Milwaukee, in conjunction with the American Hospital Association. (*Courtesy AANA.*)

signal the future relationship of nurse anesthetists with nursing.

Madeline McConnell first reminded her nurse anesthetist audience that "it is nursing's educational requirements [that] form the basis of your professional standing." She then affirmed: "The American Nurses' Association is interested in the nurse anesthetists as a field of specialization. We watch with interest and with a certain amount of pride your development. We wish you great success and we feel, too, that the Nurses' Association, per se, has a responsibility to see that applicants come to you soundly prepared and, likewise, we are interested in the sound development of the field."[16] These are words Hodgins had wanted to hear in 1909. Nursing was catching up with its first clinical specialty.

The rapprochement took more time, however. All of nursing was going through a reorganization, but the resultant new structures of 1952 (a revamped American Nurses' Association and a National League for Nursing built on the retained charter of the National League for Nursing Education) disappointed nurse anesthetists and some others, because there was no representation for clinical nursing specialties. Thus, nurse anesthetists faced what AANA charter member Verna Rice called "doom by domination"[17] from both nursing and medicine. They could only continue on a rather solitary path.

Nursing leader Janet Geister (who was executive director of the American Nurses' Association in 1932, when Hodgins made her unsuccessful request for affiliation) reflected on the major failure of nursing's reorganization effort in a 1958 address to the AANA. "We must walk together," Geister said, but the 1952 plan "did not recognize the rise of specialist groups, a substantial part of the nursing force, whose internal affairs demand a larger degree of self-government than can be provided within a parent association." She called for unity:

> . . . the kind of unity in which the specialist groups can participate freely, yet retain control over internal affairs. It's the kind of unity that can consolidate for the common good the competence, judgment and good will within nursing. It can be achieved without costly, wearying discussions of framework and bylaws. Its cost is not in dollars, but in new thinking—and if we will, we can have it tomorrow.[18]

The kind of organization Geister envisioned did not come "tomorrow," but in 1973, with the formation of what came to be called the "National Federation for Specialty Nursing Organizations," of which the American Association of Nurse Anesthetists was a founding member. A loose affiliate of specialty nursing organizations and the American Nurses' Association, the Federation seeks to achieve greater coordination in areas of mutual interest (e.g., continuing education, expanding role of the nurse, licensure and legal aspects of practice, certification, payment for services). Membership is open to nursing organizations that are national in scope, governed by elected bodies, have bylaws defining purposes and functions for improvement of health care, and have a body of knowledge and skill in a defined area of clinical practice. The nurse anesthetists at last had a structure for collegial identity and with the potential for effective action.

Geister also noted that, because nursing is such intensive work, the tendency can be to emphasize *action* rather than *reflection*, with resultant difficulties. She said, "This preoccupation with *doing* has blurred our understanding of some of the *whys* of our doing—and when we make major moves without such understanding we build up trouble."[18]

In the AANA, it has been the work of Ira Gunn, CRNA, that has provided valuable historical and philosophical contexts in which to consider issues confronting nurse anesthetists. For example, in 1968, in a paper titled "Current Nursing Issues and Their Implications for the Preparation of Nurse Anesthetists," she alerted members to the need for putting an end to the "orphan" image of nurse anesthetists. Declaring "The nurse anesthetist must establish her identity somewhere if she is to have a progressive future," Gunn asked, "In reality, where do we belong?" She then reflected:

> I believe that basic nursing is a prerequisite to anesthesia as we administer it. The opportunities for and knowledge gained from the study of physiological changes in patients during the [nursing] course are indispensable in the preparation of alert, knowledgeable, safe anesthetists. I believe that the attitudes of compassion, protection, and support of patients fostered in schools of nursing are essential ingredients to the development of responsible, safe anesthetists. I believe that anatomy, physiology and chemistry taught during the course have the potential of an excellent base on which to build our broader and greater knowledge of the human body and its function, as it relates to anesthesia.[19]

In the coming years, Gunn's work would continue to reflect this thinking, defining the nurse anesthetist as the first of a "new breed of nurse, the nurse functioning in an expanded, extended role, before her role in most other specialties was dreamed of, or formalized."[20]

MALE NURSE ANESTHETISTS

Even though some male religious communities (most notably, the Alexian Brothers) have had a centuries-old commitment to nursing, males have had to overcome considerable resistance before being accepted into secular nursing. The AANA was no exception. The admission of males to membership was long resisted.

In her first presidential report (1936), Hilda Salomon called for "some definite action . . . regarding the acceptance of male anesthetists."[21] In the course of her first term, the application of a registered graduate male nurse had been denied by the trustees. Subsequent efforts to change Association bylaws in 1937, 1942, and 1945 were also unsuccessful. Not until 1947 were men permitted to join. A recently discovered memo in the AANA Archives (now being arranged and prepared for research) reflects some of the debate surrounding this question (and adds another perspective to the discussion of the role of gender in the economics of anesthesia). On April 18, 1947, Ruth Bergman, Chairman of the AANA Membership Committee, wrote to fellow committee members "Re: Acceptance of male nurse anesthetists as members in the A.A.N.N. [sic]":

> Here are some of the facts about male nurse anesthetists:
>   At least four approved schools of anesthesia accept male nurses as students.

That at least twelve have graduated from these schools.
That many are on the waiting list to be admitted.
Many have applied for admission to our assn.
Many are writing in to our executive office asking for information concerning our assn.

If these approved schools are willing to admit male nurses as students should we not also permit them to join our organization. That their acceptance should depend on their qualifications and preparation and not on sex.

Male anesthetists can contribute much to our organization. As members it might affect our salaries as some may be married with families to support and must be paid accordingly. Since the general public tend [sic] to regard womens [sic] work as unimportant our profession might gain prestige with both sexes in it.

Many opportunities for male anesthetists such as prisons, mental hospitals, camps, etc.

Have you any further comments for or against male nurse anesthetists?

Please give your opinion.

According to Miriam Shupp, the change in the bylaws was quietly made by her in the midst of members' concern over who would be eligible to take the qualifying examination ("any *person* who"). "Of course Hilda [Salomon] was delighted, because she had been yelling about that for years, that it wasn't fair" (in an interview with Ruth Satterfield, CRNA, AANA Archives, undated).

A similar barrier existed in the Army Nurse Corps. It was only in 1955 that the Bolton Bill, H.R. 911, provided for the commissioning of male nurses in the Armed Forces. The first male commissioned was nurse anesthetist Edward L. T. Lyon (Fig. 1–3). By this time there were 308 males in the AANA, and, on the occasion of Lt. Lyon's commission, it was observed with some satisfaction in the *AANA NewsBulletin* that

> Although in the minority, the men members have already evidenced a strong interest in the advancement of the association's work and have made valuable contributions as directors of schools of anesthesia for nurses, as instructors in these schools, and as officers of state and regional affiliates. In addition, several are serving on national committees.[22]

In 1972, John F. Garde was elected President of the AANA, the first male (and youngest) CRNA to hold that position. He has been followed by CRNAs Ronald F. Caulk (1977–1978), Jimmy N. Kerley (1979–1980), Patrick M. Downey (1983–1984), Richard G. Ouellette (1985–1986 and 1989–1990—the first president to be elected to a second term after leaving office), David R. Fletcher (1990–1991), and, currently, Scott Gray (1991–1992).

VIETNAM

In 1961, the *AANA NewsBulletin* noted the trend in the U.S. Army toward increasing the number of male anesthetists. Dubbed "Ethernauts," the first all-male class to complete the year-long course in anesthesiology for nurses at Walter

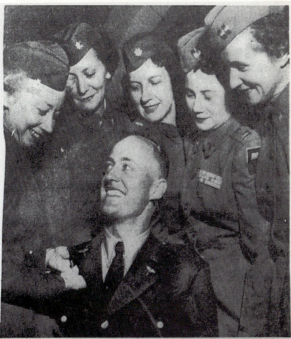

Figure 1–3. Nurse anesthetist Edward L. T. Lyon was the first male nurse to receive a commission in the Army Nurse Corps. The year was 1955. At the time there were 308 males in the AANA. (*Courtesy AANA.*)

Reed General Hospital, Washington, DC, graduated in May of that year. Letterman General Hospital School of Anesthesia, San Francisco, then graduated an all-male class. The increased training also reflected a greater military need, as involvement in Vietnam deepened.

The role of male nurses in that conflict was unique. As Dr. Richard Redman, RN, has noted, it was

> the first war in American history in which professional nurses were drafted as nurses for military service. While nurses have always been involved in U.S. military activities, they had served as volunteers, never as conscripts. That tradition was

broken when a special call was issued by the Department of Defense to meet increased requirements for military personnel during escalation of the Vietnam war. Interestingly, nurses who were women were specifically excluded.[23]

Special Call Number 38 produced a total of 151 nurses.[24]

Nurse anesthetists in Vietnam had a special role to play in the approaches to the treatment of the severely wounded. They served on helicopter missions, providing emergency first aid and resuscitation techniques to casualties, many of whom formerly would have died before or during evacuation. On arrival at the surgical facility, it was often the nurse anesthetist who became the director of initial or continued resuscitation procedures.

The Vietnam experience of CRNAs has been recorded in both novel and memoir form. In a fictionalized biography, *Forever Sad the Hearts*, Patricia L. Walsh has described her 14 months of service as a volunteer nurse anesthetist in a civilian hospital established by the U.S. Agency for International Development.[25] The experience of a male nurse anesthetist has been recorded in a letter dated July 6, 1988, by David R. Fletcher, AANA president, 1990–1991. He has recalled in part:

I entered the service in 1964 as an Operating Room Nurse and during my first assignment requested and was sent to the Flight Nurse Course in 1965; I received my flight nurse wings upon completion of that course. In 1967, I was accepted and sent to the Nurse Anesthesia Residency Program at Wilford Hall Medical Center, and graduated as an anesthetist in July, 1967. Nine months after graduation from anesthesia school I received my orders to Da Nang Air Base and the 903rd Aeromedical Evacuation Squadron (AMES) as a flight nurse. The detachment at Da Nang had seven nurses (two anesthetists and five general duty) and thirty-two technicians. We were responsible for the evacuation of patients in the I corps of northern Southern Vietnam. . . .

At times we were called to evacuate patients from areas close to the battle area and would be under fire while loading patients. There were times when the aircraft was hit by ground fire, and I guess by luck no one was hurt or hit.

A day's work was often sixteen to eighteen hours. Some days you would start at noon with an assigned mission and follow the set mission and end when the mission ended. Other days you were on call and did emergency flights when a call came. This type of flight might be to a provincial hospital or it might be a critical patient who needed care at a special hospital. Or it might be a battle that was occurring and they needed patients transported to hospitals. We had a standing rule to transport all individuals no matter their condition because they had no chance in the field and their only hope was at a larger medical facility.

Nurse anesthetists also contributed to patient care in the Vietnam experience through the development of new field equipment. Army Colonel, Ret., John A. Jenicek noted that anesthesia equipment had not been changed in the field units since World War II. The Cuban incident briefly mobilized the equipment and fleetingly exposed its antiquity and inadequacy; however, the field chests were closed again before any significant changes were made, although many were actually initiated based on communications received from nurse anesthetists on the scene.[26] By July 1967 a new field anesthesia machine was standardized and in place in all active hospital units in Vietnam. The new machine, smaller and lighter than the 1939 model, had an increased carbon dioxide-absorbing canister, and could supply ether, nitrous oxide, cyclopropane, methoxyflurane, halothane, and oxygen or air for anesthesia as needed. A new field chest was also in place, one that could provide the anesthetist with about 3 days' worth of supplies. The Army nurse anesthetists made significant contributions to the design of this unit.

Nurse anesthetists were also among those who made the ultimate sacrifice. Of the 10 nurses who lost their lives in the Vietnam conflict, 2 were male, both nurse anesthetists: First Lieutenant Kenneth R. Shoemaker, Jr., CRNA, and First Lieutenant Jerome Edwin Olmsted, CRNA. Both were assigned to the 67th Evacuation Hospital at Qui Nhon, and were killed in the crash of a C-47 transport plane carrying wounded from Pleiku to Qui Nhon. Their names are inscribed on the Vietnam Veterans Memorial Wall in Washington, DC.

THE INTERNATIONAL FEDERATION OF NURSE ANESTHETISTS

It is interesting to recall that, in 1931, Agatha Cobourg Hodgins, a Canadian by birth, originally founded the International Association of Nurse Anesthetists at University-Lakeside Hospital, Cleveland, Ohio. In her attempt to bring the new organization into an affiliation with the American Nurses' Association, she soon changed its name to the National Association of Nurse Anesthetists. (In 1939, it became the American Association of Nurse Anesthetists.) However, it was not until 1978, with the emergence of the International Federation of Nurse Anesthetists, that Hodgins's original vision of an "international" organization became a reality.

Because of a lack of evidence, it is only possible to speculate why Hodgins initially planned an "international" organization. Perhaps her experience in France in 1914–1915 was a factor. She was then part of George Washington Crile's Lakeside Unit at the American Ambulance Hospital. In Crile's words, "We literally introduced gas–oxygen anesthesia into war surgery and into England and France."[27] Hodgins responded to many requests to teach their methods to British and French anesthetists. Perhaps she was influenced by the action of her nemesis (and that of all nurse anesthetists), Francis H. McMechan, MD. In 1925, the pioneering physician anesthetist changed the name of his National Anesthesia Research Society to the International Anesthesia Research Society. In any case, the severe heart attack Hodgins suffered on January 1, 1933, limited her involvement in the development of her young organization.

The AANA Archives contain evidence of sporadic international contacts among nurse anesthetists. For example, in 1949, Venny Snellman, Director of Nursing Education for the State Medical Board, Helsinki, Finland, wrote to AANA Executive Director Florence McQuillen, CRNA:

May I ask for information regarding your special field? In Finland nurses have been, are and will be giving anesthetics. There is so far only one doctor-anesthetist in the whole country and though there is a hope that several will be trained and appointed in the near future, the actual giving of anesthetics will be in the hands of nurses. We are therefore most anxious to get a key person trained.

Similarly, in 1950, Alena Paleckova of Prague, Czechoslovakia, wrote:

> I am a nurse with a diploma from a two-years school for nurses at Prague. I am very much interested in anesthesiology and I am working at a residency of anesthesiology at a great hospital. [The] leading physician of this residency, L. Spinadel, M.D., who is a member of American Association of Anesthetists, is my teacher. He hopes I shall be well trained for independent work as a nurse-anesthetist very soon. This specialty for nurses is not yet established in Czechoslovakia and I hope to be the first nurse-anesthetist in my country.

Though many nurse anesthetists from other countries did come to study in the United States, and though many American nurse anesthetists taught abroad (for example, Helen Vos, CRNA, AANA president, 1965–1966, served as director of the anesthesia program at United Christian Hospital in Lahore, Pakistan), there were obstacles to extensive cooperation. During the McCarthyite 1950s, for example, the AANA Board of Directors (beleaguered for decades by hostile physician anesthetists) expressed a fear of being lured into a communist enterprise, and the 1951 retirement plans of the eminent American nurse anesthetist Helen Lamb to demonstrate Foregger equipment in Switzerland were thwarted by the anti-nurse anesthetist sentiments of a French physician.

A new era in international relationships among nurse anesthetists began in 1978.

That year two European nurse anesthetists attended the AANA annual meeting in Detroit. One of them, Hermi Lohnert of Switzerland, inquired of President Ronald F. Caulk, CRNA, whether the Association would be willing to support an international symposium for nurse anesthetists. Caulk noted, "Of course, the AANA agreed" (in a letter from R. F. Caulk, November 3, 1988).

In 1985, the First International Symposium was held in Lucerne, Switzerland. Approximately 250 nurse anesthetists from 11 countries attended. In 1988, the Second International Congress of Nurse Anesthetists was held in Amsterdam; it was attended by 511 nurse anesthetists from 16 countries. Interest in an international organization was widespread, and a planning meeting was held in Switzerland in September 1988. There resulted agreement on a name, the International Federation of Nurse Anesthetists, as well as objectives and functions of the new group.

Seven objectives were developed and agreed on:

1. To promote cooperation between nurse anesthetists internationally.
2. To develop and promote educational standards in the field of nurse anesthesia.
3. To develop and promote standards of practice in the field of nurse anesthesia.
4. To promote opportunities for continuing education in anesthesia.
5. To assist nurse anesthetists' associations to improve the standards of nurse anesthesia and the competence of nurse anesthetists.
6. To promote the recognition of nurse anesthesia.
7. To establish and maintain effective cooperation between nurse anesthetists, anesthesiologists, and other members of the medical profession, as well as hospitals and agencies representing a community of interest in nurse anesthesia.

Five functions were adopted:

1. To promote continual high quality of patient care.
2. To serve as the authoritative voice of nurse anesthetists and nurse anesthesia internationally.
3. To provide a means of communication among nurse anesthetists throughout the world.
4. To promote the independence of the nurse anesthetist as a professional specialist in nursing.
5. To advance the art and science of anesthesiology. [letter from R. F. Caulk, November 3, 1988]

The International Federation of Nurse Anesthetists (IFNA) was formally established in Teufen, Switzerland, on June 9, 1989. The 11 charter members were Austria, Federal Republic of Germany, Finland, France, Iceland, Korea, Norway, Sweden, Switzerland, United States of America, and Yugoslavia. IFNA's headquarters were located in St. Gallen, Switzerland.

Attendance at each world congress has more than doubled. The Third International Congress of Nurse Anesthetists, held in Oslo, Norway (June 1991), was attended by 1100 nurse anesthetists representing 25 countries. Addressing the gathering, IFNA President Ronald F. Caulk, CRNA, United States, observed ironically, "Twenty years ago, nurse anesthetists in the United States were still being told by physicians that theirs was the only country that had nurse anesthetists!" The Fourth Congress will take place in Paris, France, in 1994, with an anticipated attendance of more than 2000.

This international organization of nurse specialists has the potential to be of great significance for worldwide improvement of anesthesia care. Moreover, it represents the real maturity of the profession: secure in itself, and turned to the world.

"THINKING IN TIME": THE USES OF HISTORY FOR NURSE ANESTHETISTS

In 1988, two Harvard professors, Richard E. Neustadt and Ernest R. May, were named as the first recipients of a $150,000 Grawemeyer Award for Ideas Improving World Order. What was their valuable insight? A variation on Georges Santayana's familiar theme: "Those who cannot remember the past are condemned to repeat it." In their study, *Thinking in Time: The Uses of History for Decision Makers*,[28] Neustadt and May argue that contemporary political leaders would profit by drawing on the past when dealing with the world's problems. Such attention, they suggest, might have rewritten some "horror stories" in recent American history, including Truman's failure to unite Korea, Kennedy's blunder in the Bay of Pigs, and Johnson's misunderstanding of Vietnam. What is true for U.S. government leaders is surely no less true for those who aspire to leadership in the nurse anesthetist profession. Wise decisions, taking into account the profession's history, are essential because the risk is absolute: nothing less than continued professional existence.

Fortunately for today's nurse anesthetists, the history of the profession *has* been "a living heritage." For example, a reading of AANA presidential reports over the years reveals that such leaders typically have encouraged members to meet current challenges in part by recalling the achievement and commitment of the profession's pioneers. Another example of the valuing of past experience can be found in the AANA's recent report of the National Commission on Nurse Anesthesia Education. After an Executive Summary, it presents "A Brief Historical Context of Nurse Anesthesia Education," noting that "a historical context is essential to understanding" the current situation.[29]

As mentioned earlier, it has notably been the work of Ira Gunn, CRNA, that has set discussions of issues confronting nurse anesthetists in illuminating historical contexts. It seems especially appropriate, therefore, to close this chapter with her eloquent reflection on how crucial to CRNAs is a knowledge of their history:

> Without a knowledge of our professional history, we are deprived of the justifiable pride we can take in the outstanding contributions of past nurse anesthetists: the remarkable quality of the anesthesia services they provided under primitive conditions; their significant contributions to the development of the art, science and early technology of anesthesia as well as the anesthesia procedures associated with open chest and even cardiac surgery; and their capability for meeting almost insurmountable challenges in the practice and its environment. It can teach us what it takes of individuals and of the collective body to make the system work for CRNAs even when the opposition is formidable and, most notably, to make needed changes. And, it affords us examples to emulate and imbues us with confidence, for we, too, with the same commitment to the profession and to the quality of our services, have no reason to fear the future or its challenges.[30]

This paper is a compilation of previously unpublished material as well as selections from the author's *Watchful Care, a History of America's Nurse Anesthetists* (New York: Continuum Books; 1989) and "A Living Heritage" (*CRNA Forum.* 1990;6:2–18) (used with permission). For a clinical history of anesthesia, see Calverley RK. Anesthesia as a Specialty: Past, Present, and Future. In: Barash PG, Cullen BF, Stoelting RK, eds. *Clinical Anesthesia.* Philadelphia: JB Lippincott; 1989:3–33. The student is also referred to the Bibliographic Note in *Watchful Care.*

REFERENCES

1. Gavzer B. What this medical battle could cost you. *Parade Magazine.* 1988;8:10–11.
2. Cited in Robinson V. *Victory over pain.* New York: Henry Schuman; 1946:128.
3. Raper HR. *Man against pain: The epic of anesthesia.* New York: Prentice-Hall; 1945:179.
4. Cited in Fulop-Miller R. *Triumph over pain.* Indianapolis, IN: Bobbs-Merrill; 1938:182.
5. Clapesattle H. *The doctors Mayo.* Minneapolis, MN: University of Minnesota Press; 1941:429, 427.
6. Magaw A. A review of over fourteen thousand surgical anesthesias. Reprinted in *BNANA.* 1939;7:63.
7. Littig LW. Anesthesia fatalities in Iowa. *Trans West Surg Gynecol Soc* 1907;17:133. Cited in Thatcher VS. *History of anesthesia, with emphasis on the nurse specialist.* Philadelphia: JB Lippincott; 1953:61, 100.
8. Dickinson-Berry FM. Notes on the administration of anaesthetics in America, with special reference to the practice at the Mayo Clinic. *Proc R Soc Med* 1912–1913;6(pt 1, Section on Anaesthetics, Dec. 6, 1912):15–16, 25, 20, 21, 24.
9. Magaw A. Observations on 1092 cases of anesthesia from Jan. 1, 1899 to Jan. 1, 1900. *St. Paul Med J.* 1900;2:309.
10. Hunt VC. The present-day sphere of the nurse anesthetist. *BAANA.* 1941;19:321.
11. Quoted in Olson GW. The nurse anesthetist: Past, present and future. *BAANA.* 1940;8:298.
12. Winton SG. The war years. *AANA News Bull.* 1984;38:6.
13. Penland A. Quoted in Lee E. *History of the School of Nursing of the Presbyterian Hospital.* New York: GP Putnam's Sons; 1942:106–107.
14. Crile GW. Greetings. *BNANA.* 1936;4:184.
15. Pearce D. *Specialization in medicine: An art or a science? The status of anaesthetics.* London: The Wellcome Institute for the History of Medicine; 1988. Thesis.
16. McConnell M. The director of nursing education. *AANA J.* 1946;14:42.
17. Rice VM. Nurse anesthetists and the ANA. *AANA J.* 1951;19:62–64.
18. Geister J. We must walk together. *AANA J.* 1959;27:123, 120.
19. Gunn IP. Current nursing issues and their implications for the preparation of nurse anesthetists. *AANA J.* 1968;35:416–417.
20. Gunn IP. Preparing today's nurse anesthetists to meet contemporary needs: A philosophic and pragmatic approach. *AANA J.* 1974;42:33.
21. Salomon H, CRNA. President's report. *BNANA.* 1936;4:186.
22. Army Reserve commissions now open to male nurses. *AANA News Bull.* 1955;9:9. It should be noted that Frank T. Maziarski, CRNA, MS, Seattle, WA, quickly followed Lyon as the second male nurse commissioned in the Army Nurse Corps.
23. Redman R. The nurse and the draft in the Vietnam War. *Bull Am Assoc Hist Nurs.* Winter 1986.
24. Gurney C. The nurse and the draft. *Bull Am Assoc Hist Nurs.* Spring–Summer 1986.
25. Walsh PL. *Forever sad the hearts.* New York: Avon Books; 1982.
26. Jenicek JA. Viet Nam—New challenge for the army nurse anesthetist. *JAANA.* 1967;35:349.
27. Crile GW. *George Crile, an autobiography.* Crile G, ed. Philadelphia: JB Lippincott; 1947:I, 199.
28. Neustadt RE, May ER. *Thinking in time: The uses of history for decision makers.* New York: Free Press; 1986.
29. *National Commission on Nurse Anesthesia Education.* A brief historical context of nurse anesthesia education. Park Ridge, IL: American Association of Nurse Anesthetists; 1990:6–10.
30. Gunn IP. Notes from the Editor. *CRNA Forum.* 1990;6:20.

Legal and Ethical Aspects of Nurse Anesthesia Practice

*Janet S. Simpson and
Scot D. Foster*

The practice of any nursing specialty requires that the practitioners have a comprehensive understanding of the legal and ethical tenets that underlie and delimit their scope of authority, practice rights, and responsibilities. This section of text is designed to acquaint student nurse anesthetists with the range of issues that will ultimately impact on the manner and methods of their clinical practice. Included in the section on legal issues are (1) a review of the precedence for the practice of anesthesia by nurses, (2) an overview of the American legal system as it relates to practice, (3) the basis of court decisions as derived from legislation, statutes, and constitutional and common law, (4) a guide to understanding complex issues of medical malpractice, and (5) an analysis of areas of recurring malpractice liability.

Within the past decade, there has been a renewed emphasis on the responsibility all health care practitioners have for making professional ethical decisions as well as assisting patients in making choices for themselves and their families. The author reviews reasons leading to this renewed emphasis on ethical decision making by health care practitioners and describes how to identify ethical questions, frame ethical statements, assess personal values, and apply them in a systematic method to validate personal ethical decisions.

LEGAL ASPECTS OF NURSE ANESTHESIA PRACTICE

Determining the Scope of Anesthesia Practice for CRNAs

The basic licensure that allows a nurse to practice nurse anesthesia is the Registered Nursing License. This license must be obtained and maintained in effect at all times that one is delivering anesthesia services to patients in a given state. Penalties can be levied for failure to comply with state licensure requirements and may vary with the type of infraction or relative to specifics of the regulations promulgated by a particular state. Penalties may include censure,

license restriction, or criminal charges. Obviously, such proceedings are serious and require that one attend to the basic requirement of maintaining a valid nursing license.

Some states, such as California, require state certification to practice as a CRNA, in addition to the basic RN license. This recognition may come in the form of legal authority (certification) to use the name Certified Registered Nurse Anesthetist or, in other states, is referred to as an ARNP, Advanced Registered Nurse Practitioner certificate. These requirements and titles vary from state to state. Some states require special certification by law; others have this recognition available on a voluntary basis. It should be clearly understood, however, that these special certifications, if required or available, are often *in addition to* certification or recertification as a CRNA by the Council on Certification, which is associated with the American Association of Nurse Anesthetists. The reason for this situation is that states maintain the right and obligation to accept or promulgate standards and license requirements above and beyond those of a professional organization and, therefore, reserve the right to establish licensing and certification requirements of their own for any health care provider practicing within their state. As a result, states may formulate their own particular requirements or accept those of the AANA (most commonly) as sufficient recognition for the authority to practice. Through this type of requirement, the state demonstrates its interest in assuring citizens that only qualified health care providers are delivering anesthesia services. Again, it is incumbent on the CRNA to determine these locality differences when seeking authority to practice.

Although most states have requirements relative to who can and cannot administer anesthesia within state boundaries, not all states have specific statutes or regulations that mandate licensure or certification for the practice of anesthesia. Consequently, on a theoretical basis, any registered nurse or physician can practice anesthesia; however, it is becoming increasingly difficult to do that because of practice or payment restrictions imposed from other external agencies such as the Joint Commission for the Accreditation of Hospitals/Organizations and the Health Care Finance Administration, which administers the federal

Medicare program. Also, it should be understood that membership in the American Association of Nurse Anesthetists is a voluntary action on the part of the practitioner. Membership cannot be required by law and does not constitute automatic certification or licensure. Certification or recertification by the respective AANA-associated council may or may not automatically sanction practice rights within a particular state. Each state where a nurse anesthetist contemplates providing services should be investigated through that state's licensing board for a full explanation of requirements and limitations of licensure.

The scope of practice for a nurse anesthetist will vary from state to state. Although usually determined by local hospital policy and practices, the CRNA scope of practice may be affected by regulations within the state's Nurse Practice Act, licensure of other health care providers in the state, common law or case law, and traditional practice patterns. The Nurse Practice Act may describe the type of anesthesia services that can be provided by a nurse anesthetist in significant detail. In other states, authority to practice is defined in very global terms, usually with the effect of much greater latitudes in practice patterns. Acts may also describe the relationship that the state expects to exist between the nurse anesthetist and the individual performing the diagnostic or surgical procedure (surgeon). For instance, if direct supervision by a physician is required, that would likely be detailed in the Act. If a consulting relationship is anticipated, that likewise may be described in the Nurse Practice Act.

Licensure of other health care providers in the state and the Acts that regulate them may also guide the anesthetist in areas of acceptable practice. A physician's practice may be defined in the statutes with an admonition that anyone performing these activities without physician licensure may be subject to penalties. Therefore, by exclusion, the anesthetist can determine that a part of the scope of practice for nurse anesthetists, although not clearly delegated to the CRNA provider, may be within the domain of acceptable practice, yet have no applicability to CRNAs practicing in a neighboring state. On the contrary, a completely different section of a state's laws may spell out the relationship between health care providers, including physicians and nurse anesthetists. For instance, in Kansas, state law specifically mentions and defines health care providers, including both the nurse anesthetist and physician. In addition, Kansas has statutorily stated that one health care provider is not responsible for the actions of another, and if a physician surgeon becomes involved in decisions surrounding the anesthetic, he or she will be held accountable for those judgments.[1] If, however, all aspects of the anesthetic are managed by the nurse anesthetist, the physician surgeon escapes legal liability for the negligent acts of the nurse anesthetist.

Even absent definitive statutory direction on the subject, a state's courts can establish limitations on practice. As will be addressed in further detail within the text, courts' opinions may mold the scope of practice. As an example, before enactment of the statute in Kansas that holds each health care provider responsible for his or her own acts, the Kansas Supreme Court had taken a different view of the relationship between nurse anesthetists and physicians and

even a different view of the relationship among physicians. In *Voss v. Bridwell*, a surgeon was held accountable for the actions of a resident anesthesiologist even though that resident was under the direct supervision of a faculty anesthesiologist.[2] Similarly, in *McCullough v. Bethany Medical Center*, the Kansas Supreme Court indicated that a physician had a duty to supervise the practice of a nurse anesthetist.[3] Fortunately for the scope of practice of nurse anesthetists, this line of cases was interrupted by the 1986 reform statute referenced earlier.

Traditional practice patterns also affect the scope of practice. If an institution requires a team approach to the delivery of anesthesia services, that is, a nurse anesthetist and anesthesiologist, these traditional practice patterns affect the anesthetist's ability to establish an autonomous practice within that framework and therefore some CRNAs may view this as a limitation to their practice. Of course, examples of the reverse, where the scope of practice is enlarged because of traditional practice patterns, also exist. (*Note*: For a complete history of the legal precedence for CRNA practice, please refer to Bankert M. *Watchful care, a history of Americas' nurse anesthetists*. New York: Continuum Books; 1989.)

Overview of the American Legal System

The American legal system is designed to resolve disputes and solve problems. Inherent in most situations are at least two views or two sides to any question. Therefore, the American legal system is designed to accommodate multiple parties and provide a forum for airing views and receiving a relatively predictable result.

Any claim of medical negligence filed with a court of original jurisdiction is a civil action. Civil, in this context, means the plaintiff is seeking compensation for a perceived injury, that is, money damages. The other broad category of actions are criminal in nature, wherein the penalties may include incarceration as well as money penalties. Criminal actions are not the subject of this discussion.

Medical negligence, or medical malpractice as it is often termed, is only one of many civil actions entertained by our courts. Other examples of civil lawsuits include claims of trespass, contract actions, probate matters, boundary disputes, and other forms of personal injury. The plaintiff may ask the court to order another party to act in a certain manner and to compensate with money damages.

If a dispute arises in a case of medical negligence, the plaintiff files suit in the court of original jurisdiction. This is the first rung of the ladder of courts that could ultimately become involved in deciding the case. It is the court that will hear the facts, determine questions of law, and guide a jury through trial and deliberations or enter a ruling deciding the case if a jury is not requested. The name for this court varies from state to state. In some states it is called the District Court and in some states, the Circuit Court. In all instances, this court guides the lawsuit through its discovery phase and through trial. Discovery is the phase of the action when each party, through his or her attorney, investigates the facts, claims, and assertions that seem pertinent. Discovery parameters are generally quite broad. Anything that could possibly lead to information that could be relevant at trial is subject to inspection, absent a specific rule protecting that information from disclosure.

For instance, as a defendant in a medical negligence lawsuit, you may be questioned regarding your relatives in the county where the case will be tried. Although this may seem an invasion of personal privacy, such information could become relevant if a jury panel is selected with the intent to select individuals with no knowledge of the parties or facts of the case. Discovery generally encompasses obtaining the plaintiff's medical records, consulting or deposing fact witnesses who have knowledge of the events complained of, deposing both plaintiff and defendant, and obtaining expert opinions to support and refute the relative positions of the parties. Viewing this process strictly from a defense standpoint, your attorney will direct energy toward reviewing the plaintiff's medical records accumulated before and after the incident in question. A literature review will generally be conducted to find support for your actions in sound, medically recognized journals and texts. Expert witnesses will be retained to testify that the treatment provided was within the appropriate standard of care. Other experts may be retained to review the patient's medical condition and offer opinions regarding long-term prognosis or alternative theories on how the injury may have occurred. Most state courts follow the Federal Rules of Civil Procedure, which call for a relatively free exchange of information between plaintiff and defendant, through counsel. After discovery is completed, the issues to be taken before the court and jury are finalized. The lawsuit is now ready for trial. As the plaintiff has the burden of persuading the jury that the claims are true, the court system allows the plaintiff to go first in all presentations. The plaintiff's attorney makes an opening statement and is followed by the defense attorney. The plaintiff's attorney calls witnesses to support his or her client's claims and each witness may be cross-examined by defense counsel. Once the plaintiff has put forth all the evidence and witnesses allowed by the court, considered by the plaintiff to be important for his or her case, the defendant may proceed with witnesses and evidence. At the conclusion of the defendant's case and only with the court's permission, the plaintiff may call rebuttal witnesses to refute portions of the defendant's evidence. The attorneys then give their closing arguments. The plaintiff's attorney speaks first and is followed by the defense attorney. If the plaintiff's attorney requests, a part of the allotted argument time may be saved until after the defense attorney has concluded. In this way, the plaintiff has the first word throughout the trial and the last word to the jury in argument.

If the losing party is dissatisfied with the trial court's rulings during the pretrial period or during the trial itself, that party can perfect an appeal. All states have an intermediate appellate court and a supreme court or court of last recourse. The appellate court can confirm the trial court's rulings and the jury's decision. Alternatively, the appellate court can overturn the entire process and send the case back for a second trial. If this occurs, instructions in the form of the Court's opinion are generally issued to guide the trial court in conducting the second trial. An appeal to the intermediate appellate court is a matter of right for the losing party. The appellate court makes its decision based on the trial court record and legal briefs submitted by counsel for each side. Generally, oral arguments from the attorneys are also entertained by the appellate court. The attorneys present their respective arguments and answer questions appellate judges may pose. No testimony from witnesses or new evidence is received by the appellate court. Its decisions generally regard questions of law rather than fact. An appeal to the state's supreme court is not a matter of right. Rather, the supreme court determines if an ambiguous point of law could be clarified or altered by its review, if a new statute should be tested for validity, or if other circumstances merit the court's attention. The time required for the entire appellate process varies dramatically from state to state. Some states conclude appellate review within 18 months of presentation of the case. Others require as long as 5 years.

The federal court system is organized in the same manner as described above. There are 89 trial courts, called U.S. District Courts, in the 50 states. The 90th and 91st trial courts are found in the District of Columbia and Puerto Rico. Appeals taken from the U.S. District Courts are handled by 12 circuits called the U.S. Courts of Appeals. A very limited number of cases are ultimately reviewed by the Supreme Court of the United States.[4]

Legislation, Interpretation of Statutes, and Constitutional and Common Law

Court decisions are based on a variety of sources. Past law recited as court opinions, statutes, and rights ensured by state and national constitutions are all taken into account when a trial judge or appellate court considers a given dispute. A statute, sometimes referred to as legislation, sets laws to govern our actions. By contrast, a constitution is a set of principles by which a government body, state or federal, governs itself. Statutes create new areas of law, fill gaps in present law, and change court-determined or common law.

Courts review statutory law. They interpret a statute and apply it to specific factual circumstances raised in lawsuits. They expand the statute and apply it to other subjects not originally contemplated by the legislature. Courts also test the statute to see if it will stand constitutional challenge. Tort reform refers to change in our system of redressing civil wrongs such as medical negligence. In cases of constitutional challenge of tort reform legislation, three questions have generally been raised. The first is the right to a trial by jury. For instance, any time the legislature limits the amount of money that can be awarded for a given injury, the question arises as to whether or not a plaintiff's right to have his or her claim determined totally by a jury of peers has been invaded. The second question raised is the right of due process. This generally means an individual's right to reparation for injury, ordered by a court of competent jurisdiction, in due course of procedure and after a fair hearing.[5] This is the precise system to which we have been referring in describing our American judicial system. The third constitutional question raised deals with the rights and immunities of citizens. All individuals possess equal and inalienable rights, including life, liberty, and the pursuit of happiness. Tort reform draws into question whether the plaintiff patient and defendant health care provider are treated equally under the law.

Common law is a tradition that the United States shares with most other English-speaking countries. It is a body of law that was developed in England and spread to countries that England ruled or settled. Historically, common law was unwritten law as compared with written or statutory law. Common law is now memorialized in opinions written by appellate courts of the various state and federal systems. Common law is sometimes called case law, as the opinions describe the manner and rationale for a court's decision on a given disputed circumstance, hence on a case.

The legislature can modify common law claims and remedies. This occurs when an interest or injustice arises that requires rebalancing the legal scales. As an example, common law has generally allowed juries to award damages to an injured plaintiff without limit; however, the increased cost and availability of malpractice insurance, such as occurred in the late 1970s, led to tort reform measures that capped the total amount of money recoverable for noneconomic damages in a few states. In analyzing a constitutional challenge, the appellate courts generally held that something must be given to the plaintiff in exchange for limiting the recovery, a *quid pro quo*. This item given in exchange was often the assurance for citizens that malpractice insurance would be available for recovery in the event a claim of medical negligence was proven. The plaintiff gives up the chance of an unlimited noneconomic jury award in exchange for an assurance that the health care provider will have malpractice insurance from which to collect an award. An adequate substitute remedy must be provided for the common law right that is infringed or abolished.[5]

Understanding Medical Malpractice

Definitions and Anatomy of a Negligence Action. In a case of medical negligence, the plaintiff has the burden of establishing four elements to prevail: duty, breach, causation, and damages.[6]

Duty. The plaintiff must establish that a *duty* flows from the defendant to the plaintiff. If the defendant undertakes the treatment of a person, a duty arises to use and exercise the degree of skill and proficiency that is commonly exercised by an ordinary, skillful, careful, and prudent health care provider engaged in a similar area of practice. Most states require that standard-of-care evidence take into consideration the same or similar circumstances that exist in a given factual setting. This prevents the small rural hospital and provider from being held to precisely the same criteria expected of a tertiary care, urban hospital and provider. The disparity between resources available in such varied institutions and settings should be considered; however, a basic minimum level of functioning is required to satisfy the criteria. In cases of alleged anesthetist negligence, it is generally easy to show that a duty flows from the anesthetist to the patient plaintiff. If an anesthetist provides care to a patient, the duty to comply with the appropriate standard of care exists.

Breach. The plaintiff must prove that a *breach* of the appropriate standard of care has occurred. By far the most com-

mon method of establishing this element is through expert testimony. The subject matter in medical negligence actions is often complex and beyond the general knowledge of the average lay juror, absent assistance through expert testimony.

Four areas should be considered when developing expert testimony. First, the facts in existence at the time of the incident are to be considered by the jury, rather than facts revealed by subsequent developments in a patient's course of care and treatment or subsequent developments in medical technology. Standard-of-care testimony should be couched in terms of information and technology available to the anesthetist at the time each specific action in the course of care is undertaken. Second, the standard of care of the profession as a whole is to be considered, rather than that of one member of the profession. An expert witness should establish that he or she is knowledgeable regarding a variety of practice settings and courses of practice rather than one particular setting where that expert may practice. Third, members of the health care profession are entitled to exercise judgment and discretion in treating patients. No presumption of negligence is made by reason of an adverse result following medical treatment. Fourth, although varying from state to state, an expert generally must express his or her opinion in terms of "very likely," "more likely than not," and so on. This testimony is commonly delivered in terms of greater than 50 percent likelihood, or "tipping the scales of justice." It is not sufficient for a medical expert to use conjecture or surmise in criticizing another health care provider.

In addition to expert testimony as a method to establish the standard of care, a plaintiff may inform the jury regarding policies and procedures of the institution that guide a provider's conduct. The standard of care can also be established by using guidelines or standards adopted by a professional organization such as AANA or ASA (American Society of Anesthesiologists) by statutes and regulations in effect in the given state, and, in some instances, by prior case law that has been reported on the subject in question.

Occasionally, the allegation of negligence involves conduct that may be within the common knowledge of jurors. If the court agrees as a matter of law that the subject is within the common knowledge of individuals, a plaintiff may be allowed to proceed without expert testimony to establish a standard of care. An example of a common knowledge exception could include a patient being dropped during transfer from a gurney to the operating room table. Common knowledge of the jury could allow its members to consider whether or not such an incident could arise, absent negligence.

Causation. The anesthetist or other health care provider can be responsible for medical negligence only if the negligent act *caused* (causation) injury and harm. The plaintiff must introduce evidence that affords the jury a reasonable basis to conclude that it is more likely than not that the defendant's conduct caused or contributed to cause the injury now complained of. Again, proof of causation cannot rest on conjecture. The mere possibility of such causation is generally not enough to sustain the plaintiff's burden of proof in this regard. Expert medical testimony is generally necessary to establish the causal link between the alleged

negligent act or omission and the injury resulting to the patient. A variety of experts may be called on to establish or refute this allegation, depending on the nature of the injury, for example, neurologists, pathologists, perinatologists.

Damages. The plaintiff must also prove the nature and extent of the injury and *damages* claimed. Evidence of this element may be provided by the plaintiff in terms of medical expenses, lost wages, and other economic losses; pain, suffering, and disfigurement associated with the injury; and loss of services to the injured party's spouse that he or she would otherwise routinely supply. In cases of significant or catastrophic economic damage, expert witnesses are often employed by the parties to describe or refute the future anticipated economic needs of the plaintiff, present value of the same, and prognosis for total or partial recovery from the injury.

Role of Tort Reform in Medical Malpractice

In the latter half of the 1970s, several legal trends became apparent. First, medical costs were increasing at an alarming rate. Predominant issues involved medical negligence, their consequent claims, professional liability insurance availability and rates, and jury verdicts. A few states were keenly aware of an impending crisis and legislatures took action. In 1975 and 1976, Indiana, Nebraska, and Kansas established Stabilization Funds to pay awards for settlements or verdicts greater than $100,000 and to ensure the availability of professional liability insurance to health care providers. Tennessee abolished the collateral source rule and placed limits on contingency fees in 1976.

Over the next 10 years, the number of claims of medical negligence continued to increase. As would be expected, premiums also increased dramatically as did settlements and amounts of jury awards. Between 1986 and 1990, another flurry of legislation made its way through committees, public hearings, and the houses of most state legislatures. The basic theories of tort reform, in addition to those mentioned, can be categorized into several areas.[7-9] Subsequent to the establishment of these statutory changes, the courts began to test each provision to determine exactly how it would be enforced and whether it could stand constitutional challenge.

1. Many states placed limits on the dollar amount recoverable for noneconomic losses. Alabama set a limit of $500,000; Alaska, $500,000; Colorado, $250,000; Maryland, $350,000; and Minnesota, $400,000.
2. The collateral source rule, which prevents juries from knowing of outside sources of benefits, that is, Medicare, Medicaid, and third-party insurance payments, was abolished in many states.
3. Joint and several liability among defendants, which makes one defendant obligated to pay any or all of the jury verdict entered against the group of defendants, was abolished or modified.
4. Statutes of limitations were decreased, particularly with regard to minors' claims.
5. Schedules were imposed allowing periodic payments of large verdicts, generally setting a specific dollar threshold or allowing court discretion.
6. Medical malpractice pretrial screening panels were established to evaluate claims before suit. The results of these panels are generally nonbinding, but admissible if a suit ensues.
7. Sanctions, including attorney fees and court costs, were established for filing frivolous lawsuits. Limitations were placed on contingency fees, that is, the percentage a plaintiff's attorney collects from the total settlement or jury award. Either sliding scales were established or such decisions were left to the court's decision. Limits were also placed on punitive damage awards, usually to limit dollar recovery.
8. Limits were set on prejudgment interest.

The process of litigation within the court system varies in speed throughout the country, taking from 1 to 6 years to reach a jury. Appeals may consume another 18 months to 5 years. Consequently, the cost incurred in this process is substantial.

Generally recognized problems and occasional failure of the tort reform effort center around specific constitutional arguments: the Seventh Amendment, right to trial by jury; Fifth Amendment, right of due process; and Fourteenth Amendment, rights and immunities of citizens, are usually pled. Many legislatures are also hindered by provisions within their own state constitutions.

Still, success in a limited form is apparent. Availability of professional liability insurance has improved in states with recent legislation. The rate of rise of liability insurance premiums has slowed and, in some instances, premiums have declined. The number of lawsuits being filed has decreased, at least for the moment; however, it is difficult to assess the impact on the dollar amount of jury awards. Across the country, there are frequent awards in excess of $5 million. It is also difficult to assess the specific effect of legislation as oftentimes awards are reported in total, absent the application of the tort reform measure; that is, the jury awards total damages and the court applies the noneconomic damage cap, thereby reducing the collectible verdict.

Actual statistics that can unequivocally be tied to a provision of tort reform legislation are difficult to locate. Only educated projections are possible. Risk management and self-policing of the health care professions may have the largest impact. Although not specifically part of tort reform, such changes in the health care professions ensure delivery of an improved quality of care to patients. Improved quality of care translates into fewer adverse outcomes and fewer lawsuits.

Legislatures will continue to deal with the problem for another 2 to 3 years. As the courts find infirmities in statutes and their application, lawmakers will modify the provisions to pass appellate court muster, affecting jury awards and collectible verdicts favorably. Evidence of collateral sources will allow a jury to informatively consider the true nature of medical expenses incurred, both past and future. Benefits of social assistance programs may be raised for the jury's consideration. Old and stale claims will be prohibited as the statute of limitations contracts. Most importantly, the public will continue to be educated regarding the financial limitations of our medical system to compensate an individual for an adverse medical outcome.

Role of a Health Care Provider Defendant in a Medical Negligence Action

Assume for a moment the dreaded has come true. You, as an anesthetist, have been named as a defendant in a medical negligence lawsuit. Consider what you can expect during the course of litigation and how you can assist in presenting a favorable case.

An attorney is retained by your malpractice insurance carrier to represent you in the action. Generally, medical negligence defense attorneys have specialized in this area and work extensively with health care providers and medical issues. That is the first expectation you should have in meeting with your counsel. It is ill advised to pressure your insurance carrier to appoint an attorney friend as counsel in your case. Someone who routinely handles domestic or estate matters would ill serve your purpose in defending a medical negligence action.

In spite of considerable expertise in the area of medical negligence defense, many attorneys need assistance with interpretation of the anesthetic record. The complex form involving multiple symbols, graphs, and references from one part of the form to another represents a confusing maze for some counsel. You therefore need to assist your attorney in providing an interpretation of each and every mark on the anesthetic record. You should also assist your counsel by describing the normal routine practice involved in handling an anesthetic such as the one in litigation. Assuming your anesthetic record is exemplary, there are still events and observations that go unrecorded. Providing your counsel with details of the day-to-day management of the anesthesia department and of given cases provides additional insight when dealing with the facts of the particular case. If your counsel is unfamiliar with anesthesia equipment in general, it would be helpful to provide him or her with a tour of the operating setting and an explanation of the function of all monitors available. You will also want to describe for your counsel the lines of interaction and general means of communication existing between the operating staff, recovery staff, and any and all physicians associated with the surgery and anesthetic. *Do not discuss the case with anyone other than your counsel.*

Your counsel will need to retain one or more expert witnesses to testify on your behalf, in both the area of standard of care and the area of causation. You should therefore communicate with your counsel and assist him or her in identifying individuals with particular expertise in the area in question. All contact of potential expert witnesses should be handled by your counsel to protect the confidential nature of those discussions.

At some point, either in a deposition or in live testimony at trial, you will be asked to explain to persons other than your attorney the events surrounding the anesthetic and injury of which the plaintiff complains. Allow time for extensive consultation with your counsel to apprise yourself of the types of questions that will be asked and the plaintiff's emphasis in pursuing the claim. *There is no substitute for an in-depth knowledge and understanding of the patient's condition, the anesthetic record, all drugs and equipment used, and the chart in general.* Spend whatever time is necessary to fully acquaint yourself with the chart, including significant laboratory values and other studies performed. If the patient suffers from chronic disease processes, those may well be important from an anesthetic standpoint. Any and all anticipated complications of the anesthetic, given the type of surgery and risks the patient presents preoperatively, should be well in mind and thoroughly considered before testimony is provided. Further, each and every medication administered preoperatively, intraoperatively, and postoperatively should be a part of your working knowledge, and play a justifiable role in the anesthetic plan.

It is not always possible, but certainly beneficial, for your counsel to consult with potential expert witnesses prior to your deposition testimony. An unbiased professional may have explanations you have not considered regarding causes of the untoward event. As a defendant, you are entitled to attend any and all court hearings and depositions during the course of your litigation. Your participation is helpful in that you can assist counsel with technical details in an on-the-spot manner.

At some point in the litigation, it will become apparent that the plaintiff is seeking a certain sum of money. Settlement discussions are routinely undertaken. To fully evaluate a medical negligence case, the defense must understand the plaintiff's position. From an insurance company's viewpoint, minor claims may be more expensive to handle and process through litigation than to settle. From your standpoint as an anesthetist, settlement of claims may depend on the amount of insurance coverage you maintain, your relationship within the scheme of multiple defendants, whether or not you are the primary insured on a policy, and a variety of other factors. As a defendant, you have a right to be involved in settlement negotiations. You may not have an absolute right to decline settlement. As a rule, however, insurance companies are interested in the defendant's perspective and wishes regarding settlement or trial of an action. Open discussions with your counsel throughout the course of the litigation will assist in avoiding surprises and miscommunication where settlement is concerned.

Assuming your case goes to trial, you should anticipate a personal appearance for the entire trial. The defense must present the jury with a concerned and interested defendant. Depositions of all professional individuals and key fact witnesses who will testify in the trial should be reviewed prior to trial. You can assist counsel in technical aspects of the defense only if you are aware of experts' and other defendants' positions regarding standard of care and elements of causation involved in the case. You may also be able to suggest demonstrative aids to assist the jury in understanding the concepts at issue.

Role of CRNAs in Analyzing Areas of Recurring Liability

The American Society of Anesthesiologists Committee on Professional Liability gained access to and reviewed closed files from 1985 through 1989 of various medical malpractice insurance companies.[10] One thousand five hundred forty-one cases were examined to determine the frequency of specific negative outcomes. After analysis of those cases, the most prevalent negative outcomes included death, 565 cases; nerve damage, 227 cases; and brain damage, 188 cases. To further examine precipitating factors in these negative outcomes, the cause of injury was examined. Problems associated with managing the respiratory system were the predominant factors, totaling 34 percent of total adverse outcomes.[11] This category of problems was further defined as follows. Inadequate ventilation, inadequate oxygenation, or both accounted for 13 percent of complications including 139 deaths. Of this 13 percent, 42 percent were associated with inadequate monitoring and 13 percent with personnel problems. Esophageal intubations accounted for 6 percent of the negative outcomes, including 76 deaths. In 59 of the 94 cases in which this was the precipitating factor, bilateral breath sounds had been noted by the anesthetist. Difficult intubations accounted for an additional 6 percent of the adverse outcomes, including 40 deaths, and airway obstruction accounted for 2 percent of total adverse outcomes. Bronchospasm accounted for an additional 2 percent, aspiration for 2 percent, premature extubation for 1 percent, inadvertent extubation for 1 percent, and inadequate inspired oxygen concentrations for 1 percent. All of these respiratory management problems together constitute 34 percent of the negative outcomes studied. Another study performed by PHICO Insurance Company of Mechanicsburg, Pennsylvania, examined 239 anesthesia incidents from a group of 2388 surgery and recovery room claims for the period July 1, 1985, through June 30, 1990. The description of cause suggested intubation and extubation as a combined cause for 38.1 percent, or 91, of the adverse outcomes. An improper technique in managing patient care accounted for 19.2 percent adverse patient reactions for 15.1 percent, positioning for 10 percent, monitoring errors during and after the procedure for 6.3 percent, improper intravenous technique for 3.3 percent, anesthetic overdose for 2.1 percent, undetected equipment malfunction for 1.7 percent, misadministered medication for 1.3 percent, and miscellaneous incidents for 2.9 percent. It should be noted that the statistics contained in this section include claims as well as lawsuits. Occasionally, claims can be settled with a patient prior to costly litigation and involvement of counsel.

In light of the statistics presented, it is of value to examine factors that have been studied and determined to play a role in the claims. Improved monitoring could have prevented complications in 31 percent (445) of 1437 claims. In a separate study, an end-tidal CO_2 monitor might have prevented the complication in 15, or 3 percent, of the cases. A pulse oximeter, if used appropriately, may have prevented the complications associated with 196, or 41 percent, of the cases. The combination of an end-tidal CO_2 monitor and pulse oximeter could have prevented the complications found in 239 of the cases, or 49 percent of the adverse outcomes. Other monitors, as a group, may have prevented the complications in 34, or 7 percent, of the cases.

In addition to improved monitoring simply preventing the adverse outcome, it has been determined that injuries are more severe in cases where better monitoring probably would have made a difference. Problems are identified by the anesthetist much later without appropriate monitors and there is less time to react within the smaller window of opportunity to correct the problem. Also, in cases where monitoring was judged to have an impact, the claims payout was 7.5 times higher to dispose of the claim when compared with an alternative case using improved monitoring. This factor stands for one simple proposition. It is much easier to defend a case should there be a negative outcome, if data collected by monitoring techniques are available to document the patient's condition throughout the anesthetic and recovery period. In the cases referenced in this discussion, the median payout without additional monitors was $225,000, compared with a median payout of $30,000 in cases with more extensive monitoring.

Anesthetists are often held responsible for injuries occurring in the recovery room, even though the anesthetist may not be in direct attendance. Of 84 recovery room claims studied, it was determined that better monitoring would likely have prevented a mishap in 39 percent of those claims. The best monitor for continuous use in the recovery room is the pulse oximeter. It has been suggested that in cases where monitoring would likely have made a difference in a recovering patient and such monitors were not employed, the median payout was $325,000, versus $17,500 as a median payout in adverse outcomes where additional monitoring was used.[12] From a defense standpoint, it is difficult to approach a jury in a recovery room injury case. Laypersons have a perception that adverse events usually occur in the operating room as they view that area as the most critical. The recovery room is generally viewed as a highly intensive environment where nursing contact is one-to-one or one-to-two and recovery is viewed as a period of stabilization after surgery has been successfully completed. Lay juries are often less inclined to accept an adverse outcome from the recovery room, as compared with the operating room.

Some states have gone so far as to mandate routine use of pulse oximeters and end-tidal CO_2 monitors. New York and New Jersey are examples of states with such legislation as of 1989. As a profession, anesthetists should not rely on legislatures to mandate and control the standard of care. This should be an area where the anesthetist takes the lead in setting the standard.

Informed Consent. Anyone providing health care to a patient may be liable for failure to obtain an informed consent prior to undertaking the act of care when the patient is mentally and physically able to consult regarding his or her condition and the procedure is not an emergency. A patient signs a general consent form allowing nurses, technicians, and others to touch her or him and perform routine measures such as drawing blood, obtaining urine samples, and checking vital signs. A surgeon obtains a detailed and specific consent form authorizing surgery. The anesthetist often is found between these two zones in that the routine form signed by the patient on admission to the hospital does not mention the possibility of an anesthetic or its effects. The specific form authorizing surgery makes a vague reference to anesthesia in most circumstances, but likewise does not address specific risks associated with the procedure. Every anesthetist should consider developing an informed consent form and presenting it to each patient for signature following an explanation of risks that may be encountered during the course of the anesthetic. An informed consent form should include the items listed in Table 2–1.

A health care provider is generally not required to dis-

TABLE 2–1. ESSENTIAL ELEMENTS OF AN INFORMED CONSENT FORM

1. A statement identifying the type of anesthetic to be undertaken, e.g., general oral endotracheal anesthetic
2. A statement confirming that risks were discussed with the patient
3. A list of the risks discussed with every patient
4. A blank for additional risks or alternatives of treatment that apply specifically to this patient's case and the discussion undertaken with the patient
5. A statement that the patient understands the information and voluntarily consents to the anesthetic
6. A statement extending consent to anyone in the anesthesia department
7. Signatures of the patient, witness, and anesthetist
8. The date and time for each signature

close every conceivable result no matter how remote; rather, he or she is bound to disclose only those risks that a reasonable practitioner would also disclose in the same or similar circumstances. The frequency of occurrence and extent of danger are factors generally considered when advising a patient of possible risks. Once again, expert testimony is routinely provided to describe, for the jury's benefit, the risks involved in a procedure and the standard within the profession regarding delivery of information to a patient on a given subject. An anesthetist should not rely on a physician surgeon to explain the risks of the anesthetic to a patient.

Lines of Responsibility

An anesthetist should always plan to be held accountable for his or her conduct and judgments involving patient care. This accountability varies considerably from state to state in terms of the liability of interrelationships between physicians who may be functioning as supervising anesthesiologists or surgeons, the institution involved, nurses, and the anesthetist. Common law applied in some states today and in all states in the past simply held that the hospital was responsible for the conduct of everyone performing within its walls and the surgeon was responsible for all events occurring in the operating suite. A refinement of this proposition resulted in respondeat superior and vicarious liability rulings from the courts. *Respondeat superior* literally means "let the master answer." The master is liable in certain cases for wrongful acts and omissions of his or her servant. Vicarious liability means an individual or party bears responsibility for the acts of another based on some relationship. The relationship is often one of employer/employee or one of assumed or apparent authority of one party over the second. In applying these theories, the court and jury are asked to examine the relationship between the hospital, physician, anesthetist, and nurse, and make a determination of lines of responsibility based on those roles.

More recent trends take into account the technical knowledge required of a surgeon, anesthetist, or nurse. They also take into account the specific obligations of a facility providing care to a patient, as in providing adequate numbers of trained nurses, properly functioning equip-

ment, and so forth. Juries are then directed to evaluate the performance of a given health care provider and determine whether or not that performance complies with the appropriate standard of care. Each health care provider is held accountable only for her or his role or area of responsibility with the patient.

Documentation

An integral component of performing within appropriate standards of care includes documenting said performance.[13] Not only does the anesthesia record provide ready reference during the case to show a trend of the patient's reaction to medications and the surgical procedure, it can provide a basis for pursuing and defending a claim of medical negligence. Lawsuits are often filed years after the incident in question. An anesthetist may or may not remember a given patient or the procedure involved. An anesthetist certainly will not remember vital signs obtained on a minute-by-minute basis and medications delivered to the patient unless they are recorded precisely, accurately, and completely.

An anesthetist must chart all monitors used during a procedure. In addition to noting that certain monitors are used, the anesthetist must report chronologically an interpretation of the data provided from those monitors. This points out the attention given by the anesthetist to the monitor and an awareness of the patient's condition at any given moment. Calculations performed in advance of the procedure and during the procedure are helpful information in reconstructing an anesthetist's thought processes at a much later time. As an example, if total blood volume is calculated and the general habit of the anesthetist includes considering blood replacement once 20 percent of the volume is lost and that procedure is not followed, a brief explanation of the rationale should be included. Also, running estimates of data that cannot be precisely measured should be included on the anesthesia record. These estimates could include intravenous fluid administered, urine output, and estimated blood loss. Also, if techniques vary from case to case in evaluating a patient's condition, the precise technique used should be noted on the record. As an example, some practitioners use weighing sponges to estimate blood loss; others use an "eyeball" approach. Specific activities of the surgeon or anesthesiologist that affect the anesthetist's thought processes and plan in providing the anesthetic, that is, change of patient's position and decision to hold transfusion until the recovery period, should be noted on the anesthetic record.

An anesthetist can provide an exemplary anesthetic, affording the patient every safeguard available, with an untoward result. Unless an anesthetic record provides a detailed assessment of the course, it could prove difficult to support the anesthetist's position.

Conclusion

Anesthesia is a high-risk specialty area that can present with severe injuries when a complication or untoward event arises. For this and other reasons, medical malpractice awards have generally increased, some to astronomic levels.

An anesthetist's safest course of action lies in an acute awareness of national standards of care, a patient's individual circumstances, and an in-depth knowledge of the specialty area that can be applied at a moment's notice to a given factual circumstance. Documentation of the course of treatment and the patient's responses provides support for the anesthetist's care and judgment when an untoward event occurs and a third party seeks to investigate the appropriateness of care and cause of injury. Advanced monitoring techniques are readily available and provide little element of risk or invasion to the patient. Providing full information to the patient allows informed consent regarding choices, procedures, and potential outcome.

The courts and legislatures have, over the years, recognized the increasing autonomy of health care providers in various specialties. In addition, limitations on the amount of recovery have been set in place to curtail extreme plaintiff verdicts and stabilize the health care market. As a whole, we are only beginning to see results from tort reform. An individual anesthetist defendant can make a significant difference in the outcome of a claim simply by practicing anesthesia in a careful manner commensurate with the appropriate standards of care and, then, by participating to the fullest extent in the defense of a lawsuit should that situation arise.

ETHICS IN ANESTHESIA PRACTICE*

Among the many professional responsibilities the CRNA owes to patients, those that involve ethical decisions will perhaps emerge as some of the most complex, difficult, and time consuming to handle, certainly in relation to the daily "clinical" decisions for which we have been well prepared educationally. Yet, ethical decisions remain as challenges that the nurse anesthetist will undoubtedly face and become instrumental in solving. It is the intent of this author to examine, from a very practical perspective, the nature of ethical decision making in the health care setting, including discussion of the types of ethical decisions common in the field and the role of CRNAs in making decisions, framing ethical questions, and presenting methods for validating personal ethical decisions. The balance of the chapter deals with the study of ethics in human subject research and professional publication.

Moral philosophy is perhaps one of the oldest academic disciplines known to humans, the early and most traditional study of which was attributed to Plato, Aristotle, and Socrates. Throughout the centuries, philosophers have sought to define more clearly the process of moral reasoning, refine ethical debate, and describe moral philosophies intended to guide human thought and action as to what

behaviors constitute right and wrong behavior. Loosely defined, moral reasoning is the study of the "rightness or wrongness" of any particular action. The study of ethics differs somewhat as defined by Brody; ethics is the study of *rational processes* for determining the best course of action in the face of conflicting choices.[14] In other words, a person may act morally in that they attempt to do or act on what is "right," yet that person is not acting ethically until he or she has put this moral decision to the test of a systematic and rational method of analysis, in an attempt to validate the decision.

In fairness to the reader and the general integrity of the discipline, one would be remiss not to mention the fact that there are many different types of moral philosophy, that is, a conceptual framework of principles from which a person can determine morally appropriate actions. Although this text elaborates on a third, distinct, and much more contemporary model, the two most frequently cited are from the utilitarian and deontological theorists. Utilitarianism, as proposed in the writings of David Hume and John Stuart Mill, suggests that the worth of actions is determined by their consequences. A common feature of these theories is that duty and right conduct are subordinated to what is good, for right and duty are defined in terms of goods or that which produces goods.[15] Often, these types of theories are called consequentialist or teleological (ends based). Deontological theories (duty based), such as those of Immanuel Kant, are classically opposite the utilitarian approach. They suggest that the concept of duty is independent of the concept of good. Right actions cannot always be based entirely on the consequences of action.

Range of Ethical Responsibilities for the CRNA

Before proceeding further, it might be beneficial to describe why the study of ethics is so important for the CRNA— why, often, the nurse anesthetist is thrust into an unwilling position as the primary provider who can and will be expected to fully participate in ethical problem solving. Whether we are comfortable or not with this new responsibility, it would be helpful to appreciate the circumstances that have drawn us into this situation.

Today, virtually every public information medium is addressing a myriad of ethical problems facing society. Among the most pressing for resolution seem to be the issues of abortion, active euthanasia, and distribution of scarce health care resources; but beyond those are countless others. These issues are exceptionally complex, perhaps so much so that they seem to defy solution. Nevertheless, society continues to awkwardly seek consensus relative to the values it places on issues of human rights to human life, the quality of life, and the rights and obligations of choice, access, and equity. Seemingly most of these issues emerge from the health care field or are significantly influenced by the medical and nursing disciplines. Why then has the domain of ethical considerations come so clearly to the center stage of health care over the past several decades?

The reason is on one hand incredibly simple and on the other hand vastly complicated; in short, our rapidly changing world offers more choices of action for any particular situation than it ever has before in the existence of

---

* The predominate philosophic basis for this section is borrowed from the writings of Dr. H. Brody, author of *Ethical Decisions in Medicine*. After a thorough review of the literature in this area, Dr. Brody's text stands alone in its contribution to the study of ethics because of its unique application to the health care provider and general readability. The author fully acknowledges Dr. Brody's insightful analysis of the process of ethical decision making throughout this narration, in addition to those areas of the text that were directly cited.

humankind. As long as the number of choices or options increases, so do the number of consequences spawned of those choices. Therein lies the study of ethical questions to which we refer later. As long as our choices necessitate consequence, we are obliged to evaluate those consequences according to the values we hold. That is, we are obliged to determine the "rightness or wrongness" of our actions on the basis of a personal value system we seek to develop congruent to the universal values of society. For a health care worker to become effective in solving ethical dilemmas or validating ethical decisions, he or she must exercise "ethical behavior," that is, engage in a systematic analysis of personal values.

Examples of the choices alluded to in the previous discussion abound in health care, of which follows a very brief and woefully incomplete list. Primary among them is advancing technology that has allowed people to live longer and more functional lives, in some cases necessitating choices between who may or may not receive a valued therapy because of its cost or availability to particular age groups or social strata. Advances in biogenetics will soon offer a dizzying array of alternatives in selection of genetic traits of offspring. There are now groups publicly practicing active euthanasia, professing the right to die with dignity. Allied to these examples are those that do not directly involve clinical decisions, but are nevertheless an integral part of the health care professional's responsibility including ethical issues that derive from conflicting employment relationships, institutional codes of conduct that limit basic rights and prerogatives, and, of course, problems related to scientific fraud and securing of patient rights in conducting experimental research. Compounding the complexity of these issues is the dramatically changed environment in which decision making occurs. No longer do patients tolerate the paternalistic nature of medical decision making. In times past, what the doctor advised or decided was dutifully followed without question. Today, a much more aggressive and informed populace demands that such decisions be left to the patient: autonomy to make decisions in one's own personal best interest, based on personal values. These emerging attitudes have forever changed the face of medicine and subsequently the decision-making power and authority of the clinical discipline. Not only has the number of choices increased dramatically, but those who participate in making the decisions have also changed.

Role of CRNAs in Ethical Decision Making

On a much more practical level, the CRNA should become aware of how the responsibility for ethical decision making becomes manifest in general clinical practice as well as in other related professional activities. Some well-known health care authorities claim that virtually every clinical decision encompasses a moral dimension if two criteria are met. First, the decision must involve real choices between possible courses of action and, second, the persons involved must place a significantly different value on each possible action or on the consequences of that action.[14] With these criteria in mind, several examples come to mind that will directly involve the CRNA.

1. A critical patient comes to surgery with a chart notation for "Do Not Resuscitate." If the patient arrests are you willing to abide by these orders? What if you choose not to follow these orders?
2. A patient suffering from acute multisystem trauma requires surgery. You discover that the patient, because of religious beliefs, will not allow you to transfuse blood products. Will you accept duty for the patient and comply with his or her request? Are you ready for the consequences?
3. An AIDS patient requires exploratory bowel surgery. Can or will you accept or refuse to provide the anesthetic on the basis of your interpretation of "life-style" issues?
4. Will you participate in abortions? Does it make a difference at what stage of pregnancy the mother is and for what reason the abortion is being performed?
5. You are seeking employment as a private contractor in a hospital where another CRNA is already employed. Will you undercut their contract? Will you notify them of impending competition for the contract?

All of these situations require an ethical stance based on a complete and thorough assessment of your value system. Each requires a clear choice to be made between several possible courses of action and each person involved will likely place a significantly different value on each possible action or consequence of that action.

What Is an Ethical Question?

Before proceeding to the actual process of ethical problem solving, it is important to be able to distinguish between what does and does not constitute an ethical question. Brody suggests that ethical questions "require judgments to which facts may contribute, but which must be decided in the end by weighing values."[14] A clear distinction should be made between the process involved in solving ethical versus clinical problems. In the arena of clinical questions, decisions can usually be made on empirical evidence or facts. Clinical judgments are then usually refined on the basis of experience gained from "clinical impression," which consequently leads to a particular decision or diagnosis. Unlike ethical decision making, the application of facts or clinical data as a means of solving ethical problems rarely, if ever, contributes to satisfactory solutions for ethical questions. Clinical data may be used to substantiate or justify a particular line of ethical thought but infrequently will the data solve the ethical problem, as an analysis of values does not become part of the process of decision making.

Formulating Ethical Statements. A preliminary step in ethical problem solving involves the translation of an ethical question into the form of an ethical statement. This process helps clarify the ethical problem by organizing it into component parts for closer scrutiny, as will be demonstrated below. Having earlier been provided some examples of ethical questions, one can now translate those questions into a statement format by using the following equation[14]:

In situation *X*, person *Y* ought to do thing *Z*

Note that this statement includes what is to be done, who is to do it, and under what conditions the statement is applicable. An ethical statement should require overt action, in other words, that some particular task be done or direction taken. A passive stance is not appropriate to an ethical statement. In addition, an ethical statement describes what "ought" to be done; implicit in the statement is the notion that one particular act has a higher intrinsic value than another. It is critical to the process of ethical problem solving that ethical statements be carefully constructed as subsequent analysis of the ethical question may involve manipulation of the variables "who, what, and under what conditions." Following are some examples of ethical statements including all criteria discussed. Remember that these statements are formulated for examination and analysis only and in final form may differ substantially from the original.

1. In all circumstances, pregnant women should have the option of abortion.
2. When providing anesthesia care in a known high-risk delivery situation, the CRNA should give all care priorities to the mother rather than the fetus.

3. During the perioperative course, CRNA should always attempt to sustain life by any means possible.

The Process of Validating Decisions. The reader should refer to Figure 2–1 to conceptualize the process of validating personal ethical decisions.[14] This paradigm requires that the problem solver make explicit his or her values and then judge their validity on the basis of estimating their continuity with any potential consequences. In other words, should any potential consequence cause the problem solver significant emotional or cognitive dissonance, the ethical stance or belief (ethical statement) may have to be revised.

Step 1. Identify the moral problem. Be certain that this is actually an ethical problem by considering the qualifying criteria discussed earlier.
Step 2. List all possible alternative choices for action. Be as exhaustive as possible.
Step 3. Make a choice of which action is preferable to you on the basis of your personal value system. It may be that this choice is based initially on your "gut" reaction, before you subject it to analysis.

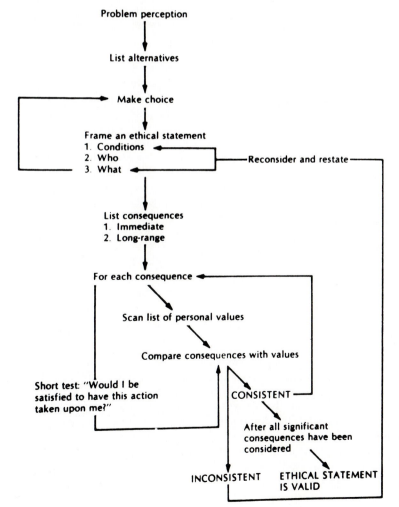

Figure 2–1. Method for ethical decision making. (*Reprinted, with permission, from Brody.*[14(p10)])

Step 4. Formulate an ethical statement. Translate your moral problem into an ethical statement containing the *X, Y,* and *Z* variables (who, what, and under what conditions).

Step 5. List all possible short- and long-range consequences of the choice you have selected.

Step 6. For each consequence, write down your personal values that relate to this situation and compare consequences with the values. If there is no inconsistency or conflict you can consider your statement ethically *valid.*

Step 7. If conflicts exist, return to your ethical statement, revise one of the three variables (*X, Y,* or *Z*), and repeat steps 4 to 6 until there is no conflict between personal values and potential consequences of your action.

Assessing the Worthiness of Values. It should be obvious by now that this paradigm will work only when the values selected for analysis have some inherent legitimacy, worthiness, or credibility. If they do not, one could perpetrate some heinous crime and justify the action on ethical grounds. There are basically three ways to determine the worthiness of values.[14] The first is by what is referred to as commonsense morality. For instance, one could not justify killing another human being on the grounds that one wanted some particular material property in his or her possession. In civil society, these types of moral imperatives are often based in law, religious teachings, or general societal traditions. A second method of authenticating the worthiness of values is by deductive reasoning. Here conclusions are drawn about a particular situation on the basis of logic and rational thought. A third method is to employ what Rawls terms *equilibrium justification.*[16] This is a process of finding the "best fit" between general moral principles and judgment regarding the appropriateness of an action. One might ask, What are these general moral principles? There are many, but among the most revered in our society and those that have withstood the test of time are the principles of autonomy, beneficence, nonmaleficence, and justice. Autonomy, as one would expect, is the freedom of a person to make her or his own choices unencumbered. Should the person not be competent to make those determinations, society has the obligation to protect the individual from exploitation. Nonmaleficence purports the notion that above all, one person should do no harm to another. Beneficence embodies the concept of preventing evil or harm, removing evil and promoting good or right conduct. Justice promotes the concept of fairness and equity, for all persons an equal share.

Ethical Decision Making in Practice

The following example is provided to demonstrate how the process of ethical decision making can be applied to clinical practice in anesthesiology. Remember the decision rendered here is only one of several decisions that could have been made in an "ethical manner." Your solution may be different, yet be ethically and morally sound.

Case Study. An elderly, critically ill female has been brought to the operating room for suspected abdominal bleeding. The chart contains DNR (do not resuscitate) orders requested by the family. On incision it is found that the bowel is infiltrated with massive metastatic disease as are other vital organs in the area. The surgeon closes and suggests that you administer a "sleep dose" of pentathol to spare the family "any more grief and anguish, not to mention more hospital bills." The patient's vital signs continue to deteriorate and death appears imminent. What action do you take?

Step 1. [Identify the ethical question.] A critically ill patient in whom death appears imminent. A suggestion has been made to institute active euthanasia.

Step 2. [List alternatives.] (1) Administer a lethal dose of pentathol. (2) Ignore surgeon and admit patient to ICU. (3) Start pharmacologic and fluid resuscitation. (4) Turn decision over to supervisory anesthesia personnel.

Step 3. [Make choice.] Start pharmacologic and fluid support.

Step 4. [Formulate ethical statement.] *In all circumstances, the CRNA should attempt to sustain life.*

Step 5. [List consequences.] (1) Anger the surgeon. (2) Lose job. (3) Anger the family for defying DNR orders. (4) Avoid legal action. (5) Increase patient costs.

Step 6. [Assess personal values.] (1) Family-generated values are primary in decision making. (2) The CRNA accepts responsibility for all personal actions and decisions. (3) The CRNA should always attempt to sustain life.

Step 7. [Assess for conflicts between personal values and potential consequences.] Everything is congruent except for the fact that the action chosen is in conflict with the family's request for DNR. As one of the values selected is family value primacy, the ethical statement will have to change.

Step 8. [Change ethical statement.] *The CRNA should attempt to sustain life to the extent it is not in violation of the patient's or family's justifiable request otherwise.*

The ethical statement can now be considered valid assuming that there are no further conflicts between values and consequences. Such decisions also need to be made in view of the universal ethical principles previously discussed. In addition, ethical decisions are not made in isolation; consequently, conflicting moral values between those parties involved in the decision may have to be re-reviewed and negotiated on the basis of the unique circumstances the situation presents.

Ethics in Human Subject Research

The protection of human subjects from the vagaries of malevolent investigators is a relatively recent phenomenon. It was not until the atrocities of Nazi Germany were exposed after World War II that a concerted international effort was mounted in this area. Initial attempts at such control were alluded to in both the Nuremberg Code and the Helsinki Agreements, but those accords left much of the enforcement responsibility for the protection of human subjects to the investigator. It was not until 1966 that the U.S. Public Health Service issued guidelines for researchers seeking grant money from public funds that dealt directly with the issues of human studies protection and established formally the Institutional Review Board (IRB), a locally constituted body charged with the responsibility for overseeing compliance with human subject policy. Inherent within those guidelines are the moral values and ethical principles by which all researchers must abide. Table 2–2 lists the federally required criteria for IRB approval of research.

Virtually all institutions of research and higher learning have available all federally mandated policies and procedures involving human subject research. Prior to engagement in any type of research, it is incumbent on the CRNA researcher to become fully apprised of these policies and procedures.

Ethics in Research Publications

Within the last decade, the awareness of issues relating to ethical behavior in research publications has become widely discussed both within the research community and the general public; unfortunately most of that recognition resulted from major press reports of the apparent increasing incidence of scientific fraud. As in any endeavor, the potential exists in human behavior to ignore moral principles or ethical analysis of particular choices or actions. The arena of scientific research has not been exempt from these temptations. As a result of these several incidences, most colleges, universities, and other institutions where research takes place have renewed efforts to monitor the conduct of researchers by instituting policies governing ethical and procedural practices to be followed during the research process. To acquaint the novice researcher with the primary ethical considerations inherent to the research process, the following issues represent the major tenets that may constitute fraudulent or otherwise unethical behavior.

Falsification of Data. Falsification of data occurs when the researcher knowingly misrepresents data either through sheer fabrication or through manipulation of existing data that may give stronger support to the researcher's hypothesis. In some cases of falsification, it has been shown that the experiments were never conducted. Falsification of data is often discovered through mechanisms of peer review, inability to replicate results, careful review of statistical analysis by a scientific colleague, or excessive publication not in porportion to the time or expertise available. It is *always* advisable that researchers keep in their possession all original raw data records.

TABLE 2–2. FEDERAL CRITERIA FOR IRB APPROVAL OF RESEARCH

1. Risks to subjects are minimized by using procedures that are consistent with sound research design and that do not unnecessarily expose subjects to risk and, whenever appropriate, by using procedures already being performed on the subjects for diagnostic or treatment purposes.

2. Risks to subjects are reasonable in relation to anticipated benefits, if any, to subjects and the importance of the knowledge that may reasonably be expected to result. In evaluating risks and benefits, the IRB should consider only those risks and benefits that may result from the research (as distinguished from risks and benefits of therapies subjects would receive even if not participating in the research). The IRB should not consider possible long-range effects of applying knowledge gained in the research (e.g., the possible effects of the research on public policy) as among those research risks that fall within the purview of its responsibility.

3. Selection of subjects is equitable. In making this assessment the IRB should take into account the purposes of the research and the setting in which the research will be conducted.

4. Informed consent will be sought from each prospective subject or the subject's legally authorized representative, in accordance with and to the extent required by (law). (See section in this chapter on informed consent. IRB consents are very similar, with the addition that the subject may withdraw from the experiment at any time without prejudice.)

5. Informed consent will be appropriately documented, in accordance with and to the extent required by (law).

6. Where appropriate, the research plan makes adequate provision for monitoring the data collected to ensure the safety of subjects.

7. Where appropriate, there are adequate provisions to protect the privacy of subjects and to maintain the confidentiality of data. Where some or all of the subjects are likely to be vulnerable to coercion or undue influence, such as persons with acute or severe physical or mental illness or persons who are economically or educationally disadvantaged, appropriate additional safeguards have been included in the study to protect the rights and welfare of these subjects.

From Department of Health and Human Services. Title 45 Code of Federal Regulations Part 46, Revised March 1983.

Plagiarism. Plagiarism is the willful replication of a significant portion of another's ideas or text on the pretense it is one's own. Unfortunately, the definitions of plagiarism and determinations as to the extent of what constitutes plagiarism vary widely. Some authors feel no culpability in borrowing from two lines of narrative to several full paragraphs of another author's work without citation or reference. Most often it is advisable for the author *always* to cite direct quotations regardless of the size of narration. Great care must be applied even when paraphrasing another's ideas or methods, except those that are already known to the community of readers to be generally accepted knowledge.

Abuse of Confidentiality. Confidentiality is abused when the researcher knowingly uses or publishes ideas of others given the understanding that the material would not be released for public consumption. It also is applicable to the release of research subjects' names or other means of identification when it was promised that such information would not be released. Also, if a CRNA serves as a reviewer for federal grants or other publications, it is unethical to release author names or institutions, especially in cases where it is used to further one's own ends or to take decided advantage of a situation.

Dishonesty in Publication. Dishonesty in publication occurs any time a researcher (1) deliberately seeks publication of material that acts to mislead the reader in substantive ways, (2) lists authors who have not contributed to the research effort in any credible way, (3) seeks publication without the permission of all authors listed, (4) attempts to publish manuscripts in several publications at one time, and (5) uses editorial reviewer comments as basis of manuscript revision and resubmits the manuscript to another journal.

Violation of Research Procedures and Protocols. Research procedures and protocols are violated when the researcher (1) abrogates responsibility to report known unethical practices of colleagues, (2) knowingly acts in violation of federal, state, or local regulations regarding research practices including policies of the IRB, and (3)

makes ineffective or destroys property of other researchers including data, supplies, and equipment.

REFERENCES

1. Kansas States Annotated 40–3403(h).
2. *Voss v. Bridwell*, 188 Kan. 643, 364 P.2d 955 (1961).
3. *McCullough v. Bethany Medical Center*, 235 Kan. 732, 683 P.2d 1258 (1984).
4. 28 U.S.C.A. §1252, 1253.
5. *Kansas Malpractice Victims' Coalition v. Bell*, 243 Kan. 333, 757 P.2d 251 (1988).
6. Black HC. *Black's law dictionary.* St. Paul, MN: West; 1979.
7. Tort reform made gains. *Independent Agent.* January 1988: 58–65.
8. Denkovich L. *State Health Notes.* 1987; 75:1–4.
9. Gordon D, Summer M. Tort reform: The state of states. *Options.* October 1987: 13–18.
10. Cheyney FW, Posner K, Caplin RA, et al. Standard of care and anesthesia liability. *JAMA.* 1989; 261:1599–1603.
11. Risk analysis: Anesthesia malpractice: An overview. ECRI, PIMCO, September 1990.
12. Zeitlin GL. Recovery room mishaps in the ASA closed claims study. *ASA News.* 1989; 53(7):28–30.
13. *Accreditation manual for hospitals, 1990.* Chicago: Joint Commission on Accreditation of Health Care Organizations; 1989.
14. Brody H. *Ethical decisions in medicine.* 2nd ed. Boston: Little, Brown; 1981:5–31.
15. Beaucamp TL, Childress JF. *Principles of biomedical ethics.* 2nd ed. London/New York: Oxford University Press; 1983:19.
16. Rawls J. *A theory of justice.* Cambridge, MA: Belknap Press; 1971:17–22.

3

Documentation of Anesthesia Care

Ira P. Gunn

That anesthesia providers are ambivalent in their attitudes concerning record keeping is reflected in the amount of space devoted in the literature to anesthesia records. Dripps et al[1] devote a chapter to the anesthesia record, as do Klein and Landers.[2] Editors of other current anesthesia textbooks address only briefly the importance of anesthesia records, without addressing the subject in detail.[3-5] Some comments about anesthesia records may be made in a historical chapter, or more often in one devoted to the medicolegal aspects of anesthesia practice. Thus, it appears that although many anesthetists understand the importance of documenting anesthesia care, they often leave learning the appropriate elements of anesthesia documentation to on-the-job training. More emphasis must be placed on adequate, accurate, and timely documentation of care provided if these records are to be considered a reliable resource for the purposes used and if they are to protect anesthesia providers from unfounded allegations of negligence.

In a study reported in 1990 involving anesthesiology residents and CRNAs, MacDonald et al[6] found that anesthesiology residents and CRNAs spent 59.1 percent of their time monitoring their patients (44.8 percent directly and 14.3 percent indirectly), and 10.9 percent of their time on record-keeping activities. The other 30.1 percent of the time was spent in other activities associated with anesthesia management, as well as idle time. The authors had performed a previous study and, comparing it with the 1990 study, found that the anesthetists had increased their direct patient monitoring activities 2.5 times. They also suggested that with the use of automated or semiautomated anesthesia record keeping, another 10 to 12 percent could possibly be reallocated to patient care. This study does not demonstrate that the amount of time spent in documentation during the period of actual anesthesia management is excessive. But neither does it address the degree of adequacy of the record keeping.

ANESTHESIA DOCUMENTATION: APPRECIATING ITS VALUE

The anesthesia record is a vital resource in making patient care decisions, trending patient responses to interventions, and evaluating care. As a document reporting care given and patient responses, it is a tool for education and research, for assessment of compliance with professional standards, and for identification of need for new or modified institutional and departmental policies. Anesthesia records are legal documents reflecting the anesthetist's professional judgments and interventions as they relate to a specific patient's requirement for care, exercised and provided within the constraints of the risks accepted within the patient's consent for the anesthesia and related procedure. The anesthesia record is also a business record and as such has been made subject to subpoena for specific legal reasons such as alleged malpractice. Further, the anesthesia record, as a reflection of the extent to which the provider complied with standards of care, is an instrument of accountability. By its nature, next to verbal reporting of patient responses to the care provided, patient care documentation serves as the most important communication function between health providers involved in the overall care of a patient. And finally, patient care documentation is a permanent record of care provided to a patient at a specific point in time.

In this chapter, anesthesia record keeping is addressed from many facets to stress its importance in our day to day practice. Although space constraints preclude elaboration and examples, the substance of this chapter has been distilled from the experiences of practitioners, educators, researchers, peer reviewers, and expert witnesses in their judgments about anesthesia records. It is also written with a view toward risk management and quality assessment.

It is important that forms, or checklists, that will be used for anesthesia record keeping be designed to serve as a check on our memory and to prompt us to appropriate actions.[7] Such a form has been designed by the American Association of Nurse Anesthetists' (AANA) Practice Committee (Fig. 3–1).[8] It is evident from its obvious detail, that the analogy between administering an anesthetic and

ANESTHESIA RECORD

				START	STOP
Procedure			Anesthesia		
Date	OR No.	Page of	Surgeon(s)	Procedure	

PRE-PROCEDURE
- ☐ Identified: ☐ ID Band ☐ Questioning
- ☐ Chart Reviewed ☐ Permit Signed
- ☐ NPO Since _____
- **Pre-anesthetic State:** ☐ Calm
- ☐ Awake ☐ Asleep
- ☐ Apprehensive ☐ Confused
- ☐ Uncooperative ☐ Unresponsive

PATIENT SAFETY
- ☐ Anes. Machine # _____ Checked
- ☐ Safety Belt On ☐ Axillary Roll
- ☐ Armboard Restraints ☐ Arms Tucked
- ☐ Pressure points checked and padded
- **☐ Eye Care:** ☐ Ointment ☐ Saline
- ☐ Taped ☐ Pads ☐ Goggles

MONITORS AND EQUIPMENT
- ☐ Steth: ☐ Precord ☐ Esoph ☐ Other
- ☐ Non-Invasive B/P: ☐ Left ☐ Right
- ☐ Continuous EKG ☐ V Lead EKG
- ☐ Pulse Oximeter ☐ Oxygen Sensor
- ☐ End Tidal CO₂ ☐ Gas Analyzer
- ☐ Temp. ☐ Nerve Stimulator
- ☐ Warming Blanket ☐ EEG ☐ Doppler
- ☐ Airway Humidifier ☐ Fluid Warmer
- ☐ NG / OG Tube ☐ Foley Catheter
- ☐ Art.Line _____
- ☐ CVP _____
- ☐ PA Line _____
- ☐ IV(s) _____
- ☐ _____

ANESTHETIC TECHNIQUE
- **General:** ☐ Pre-Oxygenation ☐ L.T.A.
- ☐ Rapid Sequence ☐ Cricoid Pressure
- ☐ Intravenous ☐ Inhalation
- ☐ Intramuscular ☐ Rectal
- **Regional:** ☐ Spinal ☐ Epidural
- ☐ Axillary ☐ Bier Block ☐ Ankle Block
- ☐ _____ ☐ Position _____
- ☐ Prep _____ ☐ Local _____
- ☐ Needle _____
- ☐ Drug(s) _____
- ☐ Dose _____ ☐ Attempts x _____
- ☐ Site _____ ☐ Level _____
- ☐ Catheter _____ ☐ See Remarks
- **Other:** ☐ M.A.C. ☐ _____

AIRWAY MANAGEMENT
- **Intubation:** ☐ Oral Tube size _____
- ☐ Stylet used ☐ Nasal ☐ Regular
- ☐ Magill's ☐ Direct ☐ RAE
- ☐ Fiber optic ☐ Blind ☐ Armored
- ☐ Blade _____ ☐ Laser
- ☐ Secured at _____ cm ☐ Endobronch.
- ☐ Attempts x _____ ☐ ET CO₂ present
- ☐ Breath sounds _____
- ☐ Uncuffed, leaks at _____ cm H₂O
- ☐ Cuffed ☐ Min. occ. pres. ☐ Air ☐ NS
- **Airway:** ☐ Oral ☐ Nasal ☐ Difficult,
- **Circuit:** ☐ Circle ☐ NRB | see Remarks
- ☐ Mask Case ☐ Nasal Cannula
- ☐ Via Tracheostomy ☐ Simple O₂ mask

RECOVERY

Location	Time
B/P	O₂ Sat.
P	R	T

- ☐ Awake ☐ Stable ☐ Nasal Oxygen
- ☐ Drowsy ☐ Unstable ☐ Mask Oxygen
- ☐ Somnolent ☐ Intubated ☐ T-piece Oxygen
- ☐ Unarousable ☐ Ventilator ☐ Oral/nasal airway

Recovery Notes

FLUID TOTALS

Crystalloid _____ EBL _____
Blood _____ Urine _____

REMARKS

TIME:

FLUIDS / AGENTS
- Oxygen (L/min)
- ☐ N₂O ☐ Air (L/min)
- (%)

TOTALS

- Urine (ml)
- EBL (ml)

MONITORS
- EKG
- % O₂ Inspired
- O₂ Saturation
- End Tidal CO₂
- Temp.: ☐ °C ☐ °F

SYMBOLS

VITAL SIGNS

Baseline Values — 200, 180, 160, 140, 120, 100, 80, 60, 40, 20
- B/P
- P
- R

Symbol	Meaning
✕	ANESTHESIA
☉	OPERATION
∨ ∧	B/P CUFF PRESSURE
⊥ ⊤	ARTERIAL LINE PRESSURE
▲	MEAN ARTERIAL PRESSURE
•	PULSE
○	SPONT. RESP
⌀	ASSISTED RESP
⊠	CONTROLLED RESP
⊤	TOURNIQUET

VENT
- Tidal Volume
- Resp. Rate
- Peak Pressure
- PEEP

Symbols for Remarks

Position

PATIENT IDENTIFICATION

Anesthesia Provider

CONTROLLED DRUGS

Drug	Issued	Used	Destroyed	Returned	Provider
					Witness

Figure 3–1. Sample anesthesia record form. (*Reprinted, with permission, from the American Association of Nurse Anesthetists.*[9(p6)])

flying an airplane has some merit, except that we have not yet found the ideal "black box" backup tape to assist us in studying objectively those cases that went wrong.

PREANESTHESIA DOCUMENTATION

Documentation of anesthesia care begins in the preanesthesia period, covers intraanesthesia care, and extends through the postanesthesia period until the patient has been declared to have recovered fully from the effects of the anesthesia management, or until one no longer has a responsibility to the patient. Preanesthesia records, often written on patient progress notes, or on special forms devised for that purpose, include (1) the recording of a patient's history and physical from the perspective of the patient's requirement for anesthesia, including the assigned physical status of the patient; (2) a brief statement concerning the anesthesia management plan that does not lock the provider into only one way for performing the anesthesia; and (3) a patient (or guardian)-signed anesthesia consent along with evidence of counseling concerning the potential risks of the planned management. Figure 3–2 is a sample preanesthesia form that may be printed on the back side of the anesthesia record.[8] Note that it also includes a small space for a postanesthesia note. Should this not be adequate for a given patient, the patient progress report is another place where postanesthesia notations may be recorded.

If no dedicated form or place on the anesthesia record for the preoperative interview and assessment exists, it is advisable to initiate the actual anesthesia record at that time, transferring any information to that record that would cue the anesthetist or any clinician who relieves the assigned anesthetist during the case to highly pertinent information. Such quick reference information might be the age and sex of the patient, hematocrit, height and weight (preferably in kilograms), and pertinent allergy, respiratory, cardiac, renal, or metabolic status that might have definite implications to anesthesia management. Consideration should be given to noting at the top of the record that a given patient is human immunodeficiency virus (HIV) positive, has other significant infections, or has a compromised immune system. The mandating of the use of universal precautions for AIDS, hepatitis B, and other infections may, in the future, make such notations somewhat obsolete. But today, they serve as good reminders that we should be especially concerned with infection control in some patients and give evidence of the steps we have taken to prevent cross-contamination as a part of our anesthesia practice. (Standard IX of the AANA Standards of Nurse Anesthesia Practice states: "Appropriate safety precautions shall be taken to minimize the risk of infection for the patient, CRNA, and other staff.")[9] The new standards on infection control published by the U.S. Center for Communicable Diseases and by the Occupational Health and Safety Agency reinforce the AANA standard.

Prior to receiving the patient in the operating room setting, any needed calculations should have been completed and checked for accuracy related to ventilation and ventilatory parameters, blood volume and fluid requirements, drug dosages, and so forth. Performing these calculations ahead of time minimizes the chances for error in the rush to get started with the anesthesia. Further, the completion of this process facilitates record keeping. Such preplanning allows the anesthetist to minimize the amount of time devoted to record keeping that may detract attention from the patient while preparing him or her for the anesthesia or during the anesthesia itself.

The basis for not writing out a finalized, detailed anesthesia management plan in the patient's record preoperatively does not negate the requirement that one must have a complete management plan, including well-thought-out alternatives, if needed. It does, however, relate to the fact that often plans cannot be fully finalized until the database is complete and a final review of the patient's status has been made immediately prior to initiating the anesthetic. Further, on occasion, the surgeon may announce, in the last moments before an anesthetic is begun, a change in the planned procedure or the surgical anesthesia requirements, necessitating changes in the plan of anesthesia management. The final decisions pertaining to the anesthetic must fall within the scope covered by the informed consent, or else such changes could present legal problems at a later date unless fully explained on your record. If the patient has been premedicated, the patient in all probability would not be considered capable of rendering an informed decision amounting to a change in the consent previously given.

Unfortunately, the cost-containment strategies imposed on hospitals and surgicenters relating to prospective pricing for diagnostic related groups has not only promoted greater use of ambulatory surgical settings, but has fostered the concept of "same-day surgical admissions" for many patients who will of necessity require a period of hospitalization before they are discharged to intermediate-care facilities or home. This further constrains the time anesthetists have for interviewing patients and preparing for the anesthesia, including record keeping, unless a successfully operated preoperative clinic can be established and used for this purpose. Often under these conditions, the anesthetist who sees the patient preoperatively is not the anesthetist who will be doing the anesthesia. This creates the potential for differing opinions as to preference and appropriateness of the anesthesia care plan for which the patient has been counseled. In these circumstances, the informed consent recorded should permit sufficient flexibility to cover the range of anesthetic management techniques that are appropriate to the patient and the surgery but identifying any to which the patient has specific objection.

Complete and accurate recording of a preanesthesia evaluation including a management plan for the anesthesia and a notation that the patient has made an informed consent as to the plan of care lends evidence to compliance with the first three AANA Standards of Nurse Anesthesia Practice. Standard I states that a thorough and complete preanesthesia assessment shall be performed; Standard II states that informed consent for the planned anesthetic intervention shall be obtained from the patient or legal guardian; and Standard III states that a patient-specific plan for anesthesia care shall be formulated.[9] It should, however, be noted in the interpretation of Standard III that it is not enough to formulate a patient-specific plan; it must also be coordinated with other appropriate health care providers.[9] Thus, documentation should include whether such coordi-

PREANESTHESIA EVALUATION

| Age | Sex M F | Height in / cm | Weight lb / kg |

Proposed Procedure

Pre-Procedure Vital Signs
B/P   P   R   T

| Previous Anesthesia / Operations | None ☐ | Current Medications | None ☐ |

| Family History of Anesthesia Complications | None ☐ | Allergies | NKDA ☐ |

AIRWAY / TEETH / HEAD & NECK

History From:
☐ Patient   ☐ Significant Other
☐ Parent / Guardian   ☐ Chart
☐ Communication / Language Problems
☐ Poor Historian

SYSTEM	WNL	COMMENTS	DIAGNOSTIC STUDIES
RESPIRATORY	☐	Tobacco Use: ☐ Yes ☐ No _____ Packs / Day for _____ Years	EKG
Asthma Productive Cough Bronchitis Recent URI COPD SOB Dyspnea Tuberculosis Orthopnea Pneumonia			Chest X-ray
CARDIOVASCULAR	☐		
Abnormanl EKG Hypertension Angina MI ASHD Murmur CHF Pacemaker Dysrhythmia Rheumatic Fever Exercise Tolerance Valvular Disease			Pulmonary Studies
HEPATO / GASTROINTESTINAL	☐	Ethanol Use: ☐ Yes ☐ No Frequency _____ "Street Drug" Use: ☐ Yes ☐ No Frequency _____	
Bowel Obtruction Cirrhosis Hepatits / Jaundice Hiatal hernia / Reflux Nausea & Vomiting Ulcers			Other
NEURO / MUSCULOSKELETAL	☐		**LABORATORY STUDIES**
Arthritis Muscle Weakness Back Problems Neuromuscular Dis. CVA / Stroke / TIAs Paralysis DJD Paresthesia Headaches / ↑ ICP Syncope Loss of Consciousness Seizures			Hgb / Hct / CBC
RENAL / ENDOCRINE	☐		Electrolytes
Diabetes Renal Failure / Dialysis Thyroid Disease Urinary Retention Urinary Tract Infection Weight Loss / Gain			Urinalysis
OTHER			
Anemia Immunosuppressed Bleeding tendencies Pregnancy Cancer Sickle Cell Dis. / Trait Chemotherapy Recent Steroids Dehydration Tranfusion History Hemophilia			Other

Problem List / Diagnoses

PHYSICAL STATUS
1
2
3
4
5
E

POSTANESTHESIA NOTE

Planned Anesthesia / Special Monitors

Signed _____ Date _____ Time _____

Pre-Anesthesia Medications Ordered

PATIENT IDENTIFICATION

| Evaluator Signature | Date

Time |

Figure 3–2. Sample preanesthesia evaluation form. (*Reprinted, with permission, from the American Association of Nurse Anesthetists.*[9(p8)])

nation was undertaken and with whom. As this may of necessity be done immediately before induction of anesthesia, a space on the preanesthesia evaluation form should permit either such a comment or a check mark indicating the accomplishment of this task.

Immediately before the anesthetist receives the patient to begin preparation for induction of anesthesia, the preanesthesia check of the anesthesia machine and other equipment should be made and documented. Such documentation demonstrates compliance with recommendations of the Food and Drug Administration, as well as with the AANA Standards of Nurse Anesthesia Care. (Standard VIII states: "Appropriate safety precautions shall be taken to minimize the risks of fire, explosion, electrical shock, and equipment malfunction."[19])

DOCUMENTATION IN THE INTRAANESTHESIA PERIOD

Documentation of the intraanesthesia period begins when the anesthetist receives the patient within the operating room suite or holding area and initiates the last-minute review of the patient record and patient questioning to complete the data and information required for finalizing the anesthesia management plan. This is the time that information such as that found in Figure 3–1 in the preprocedure and patient safety portion of the anesthesia record should be completed.

Immediately prior to induction of anesthesia, baseline data for principle monitoring modalities should be recorded, including temperature measurements particularly on the very young, the elderly, any patient presenting with an infection or who has had an elevated temperature within the past 24 hours, and those for whom hypothermia is planned as an adjunct to anesthesia. There are those who believe that because of the extent to which inadvertent hypothermia occurs in many patients, partially as a result of the temperature levels maintained in the operating rooms, the exposure of patients necessitated by the surgical preparation of skin prior to draping, the loss of heat through opened abdomens, and the flushing of body cavities with various fluids, monitoring of temperature should be a required monitoring modality and should be reflected on the anesthesia record. At the date of this writing, however, continuous temperature monitoring is not required on every case, but access to such monitors is required.[9] (It should be noted that some departmental or institutional policies may require temperature monitoring on all patients. Anesthetists place themselves in legal jeopardy if they do not comply with their own institutional policies even if they are more strict than the generally accepted national standard of care.)

The intraanesthesia period is documented most often on an anesthesia record form adopted specifically for this purpose (Fig. 3–1). This completed form is often considered "the anesthesia record," but is only the intraoperative component of the anesthesia record. As can be noted, these forms are developed in a manner to facilitate documentation, using a system of checks for indicating completion or use, symbols denoting specific measurements or position, and notations depicting drug and fluid use, ventilatory settings, and patient responses and anesthetist interventions not covered in the physiologic monitoring and other notations. Figure 3–3, an enlargement of a portion of the anesthesia form depicted in Figure 3–1, represents the symbols commonly used for denoting anesthesia and operative times (beginning and ending), measurements of monitoring modalities, and tourniquet usage.

Record Preparation for Anesthesia Induction

Although many anesthesia record forms are self-explanatory, to the novice some comments regarding the impor-

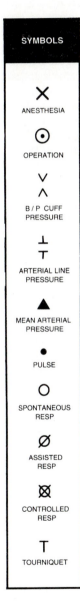

Figure 3–3. Standardized symbols frequently used on the graphic component of the anesthesia record denoting selected time and physiologic monitoring indices. (*Reprinted, with permission, from the American Association of Nurse Anesthetists.*[9(p6)])

tance of the items is warranted. On the sample anesthesia record seen in Figure 3–1, the information in the upper columnar portion of the form is exceedingly important because it demonstrates that the anesthetist has verified the identity of the patient, checked the patient record and verified the surgical procedure to be performed, re-verified the completion of both a surgical consent and an informed consent for surgery and for anesthesia, and noted the time of last oral intake. In verifying the surgical procedure, it is also important to verify and document which arm, which leg, or which side is to be operated on when appropriate. That errors have been made regarding the patient identity or appropriate informed consent is well documented in the malpractice literature.[10, 11]

It is also important to note the preanesthesia psychologic and conscious-awareness state of the patient when received in the operating room, as it may denote the adequacy of the dose and timing of the preoperative medication or a change in physiologic status. Some anesthetists prefer that the preoperative medication and time of administration be noted on the anesthesia record, if indeed it has been ordered and administered to facilitate the actual establishment of the anesthetic state. If there is no dedicated space on the anesthesia form, this may be included at the top of the remarks column. If the patient is confused, uncooperative, or unresponsive, this may warrant a comment in the remarks column if such states were not noted in the preanesthesia evaluation.

Data such as found within the Monitoring and Equipment column in our sample anesthesia record (Fig. 3–1) should be reflected on the anesthesia record in use. The location of insertion of any arterial line, central venous pressure (CVP) catheter, pulmonary artery (PA) catheter, and intravenous catheter for fluid management should be noted. In documenting the location of the catheters, the size of catheter or needle should also be noted. Although many anesthetists have in the past performed Allen tests to check collateral circulation in the hands when radial cannulation is considered, reports of studies demonstrating its unreliability in predicting arterial embolization have reduced its use and subsequent documentation.[3]

Documenting Anesthesia Induction and Maintenance

Appropriateness of the anesthesia plan is reflected by the anesthesia record and its depiction of the anesthesia technique(s) chosen, the drugs and gases used, the fluid therapy management, and the monitoring modalities used, as they all relate to the patient's psychologic and physiologic status and the surgical requirements for the anesthesia. The documentation of the implemented plan normally begins with induction and ends with emergence; however, in some emergency cases it may begin with selected resuscitation aspects of care or with a fluid preloading of the patient to accommodate a dilated vascular bed anticipated because of the anesthetic technique chosen. These interventions need documenting on either the patient progress report, the preanesthesia record, or the anesthesia record. Any alterations of the plan, resulting either from a patient's response to the

anesthesia or the medical intervention or from complications that may occur, should be evident in the ongoing documentation. A notation in the shift of anesthesia care may also be noted within the patient record.

Regardless of the anesthesia record form used in an institution, data common to those identified in the Anesthesia Technique and Airway Management columns, as well as on the graphic portion of the sample form (Fig. 3–1), should be appropriately completed at the time of induction of anesthesia and establishment of the airway and ventilatory pattern. Recorded data concerning technique, anesthesia agents, and airway establishment and maintenance are key to assessing and evaluating the anesthesia plan implemented as well as the ease or difficulty of its accomplishment.

The major portion of an anesthesia record is designed in a graphic format where provider intervention and patient measurements and responses can be recorded and related by time. Provider interventions include those of the anesthetist, the surgeon, or others that depict care given or procedures performed on the patient during the anesthesia, including patient responses to tissue or organ manipulation, blood loss, and nerve stimulation. By far, most of the interventions recorded will be those of the anesthetist, as is in the case of induction of anesthesia.

Intravenous catheters or needles inserted to provide fluids, blood, and blood products to the patient during the anesthesia should be documented on the anesthesia record as to site and size. The fluids administered—crystalloids and colloids, blood and blood products—should also be noted on the graphic form as to time started and time completed. Drawing a line between the two time notations on the graphic record where the fluid or blood is recorded indicates continuous administration. In the case of blood or blood products, the identification number of each unit administered should be recorded either on the graphic portion of the chart at the time the unit is started or in the remark column.

All drugs administered to the patient for induction should be noted as to time and dose given, route of administration, and, where appropriate, concentration of drug or gas used. In documenting the administration of inhalation gases as a part of the anesthesia and ventilation, not only should the liters-per-minute flow be documented, but a line should be drawn denoting continuous or intermittent administration. Any change in gas setting should be noted in a timely fashion so that the concentrations of the gases can be calculated and assessed. The concentrations of vaporized liquid agents delivered to the patient should be noted on the anesthesia graphic record, including the times of any changes and of completion. Should intravenous drug infusions, for example, pentothal and propofol, be administered over a period, this should be noted by a continuous line beginning at the time started and ending at the time completed. Rate of administration or dosage/time unit should also be recorded. If administration is intermittent, the record should reflect this as well.

Lack of appropriate vigilance in recognizing airway and ventilatory adequacy has been the major causation of serious brain injury or death in patients undergoing anesthesia.[12] Although there is evidence that catastrophic airway and ventilatory complications are on the decline since monitoring standards have included pulse oximetry and end-tidal carbon dioxide measurements, esophageal intubation is still a problem in anesthesia. If unidentified, esophageal intubation leads to serious brain damage or death. Thus, it is exceedingly important that placement of the endotracheal tube be verified and that verification be documented. Such documentation includes evidence of bilateral inspection of the chest for equal expansion on positive-pressure breathing, auscultation for bilateral and equal breath sounds on each side of chest, inspection of the abdomen, and auscultation of stomach at time of ventilation. Today, it is also essential to document proper placement of the endotracheal tube by monitoring end-tidal carbon dioxide. Capnography is the most advantageous monitor for alerting the anesthetist that an endotracheal tube is in the esophagus.[13] Further, assessment and documentation of oxygen saturation assist in identifying whether the endotracheal tube may be in a mainstem bronchus, rather than the trachea, compromising the patient's ventilation and oxygenation. If there is any question of adequacy of the airway, steps must be taken to correct it and those steps documented. Further, if more than one anesthesia provider checks for adequacy of tube placement, this should be documented.

Documentation of use of regional anesthetic techniques, sites of needle placement, and the drugs common to these must be recorded appropriately on the anesthesia record. Specific information regarding the make and lot of the regional kit used should be noted, including the type and size of needle and catheter as may be appropriate. The drugs used, along with their dosage and the total quantity and baricity of the solution (when appropriate), are noted. If a vasopressor is used to prevent or treat hypotension during spinal or epidural anesthesia, the drug, dosage, and route of administration must be recorded. The level and adequacy of the anesthesia should be assessed and so noted on the record. Any difficulties and complications should also be documented.

Documenting Patient Position. A variety of surgical procedures require a patient to be repositioned for surgery after anesthesia has been established and the patient stabilized. It is important to note on the anesthesia record the time of positioning, the actual position in which the patient is placed, and any physiologic changes that might have occurred as a result of the positioning. Any placement of rolls or padding to promote better ventilation and protect anatomic structures, such as the eyes and particular nerves, should also be noted on the anesthesia record. (Eye protection techniques should be noted on the anesthesia record regardless of the patient's position.)

Documenting Patient Monitoring. Documentation of continuous and periodic monitoring of important cardiovascular, respiratory, and renal physiologic indices provides the anesthetist with a continuous record of patient responses to the anesthesia and surgical interventions. Pulse and blood pressure measurements should be taken and recorded every 5 minutes, as should mean arterial pressure

when an artery is cannulated for this purpose. Pulmonary artery and/or central venous pressures or other cardiovascular indices should be recorded each time measured.

The ECG pattern should be noted on the record at various intervals and when changes occur that are not readily corrected. When noted, obvious causes for changes, such as a reflex bradycardia under light anesthesia, should be noted. If serious dysrhythmias occur and the ECG monitor is capable of making a recording, it would be well to do so until the problem is corrected. Such strips, with time coordinated with the anesthesia chart, should be preserved with the patient record.

Assessment of respiratory indices should be made on a continuous basis and recorded at 5-minute or other appropriate intervals. If the patient is on a ventilator, the ventilatory parameters should be recorded and the respiratory rate and pressures needed to achieve the fixed volume for respiratory exchange should be assessed every 5 minutes; however, if these parameters remain constant, the ventilator respiratory rate symbol with a line denoting periodic assessment and no changes can be used. It would be advantageous to record the ventilator respiratory rate symbol at least every 15 minutes even with the continuous line. If manually controlling or assisting respirations, respiratory rate should be recorded every 5 minutes using the appropriate symbol. The appropriateness of oxygen delivery through the anesthesia machine should be assessed every 5 minutes by use of an oxygen analyzer placed on the inspiratory limb of the machine and recorded as inspired oxygen concentration (FIO_2) on the graphic record. Pulse oximetry and end-tidal carbon dioxide measurements should be assessed at least every 5 minutes and, if stable, may be recorded at 15-minute intervals with a line drawn between the measurements to denote the continuous assessment. Any changes in these measurements should be recorded as they occur.

Neuromuscular blockade monitoring should be documented periodically during the course of the anesthesia when agents for this purpose are used. Further, documentation of monitors used and measurements made for some specialized surgical procedures should be included on the anesthesia record or, if computerized and recorded, printed out and attached to the record.

Urine output measurements usually will be assessed and recorded in selected patients. These measurements may be performed every 15 minutes or every hour depending on the surgery, physiologic or pathologic status of the patient, and goals for fluid management. Urine output should be recorded at least hourly unless more frequent measurements are indicated. If a gastric tube is in the stomach, total drainage and characteristics of the drainage should be recorded. Further, if peritoneal ascites or thoracic effusions are aspirated during the surgical intervention, the quantity and characteristics of these aspirates should be documented.

Estimations of blood loss should also be made and documented on the anesthesia record. Although the circulating nurse may also be recording these measurements on the forms she or he is responsible for completing, it is important that they also appear on the anesthesia record. Where documentation of such measurements is duplicated on two records, coordination between the two providers is essential to ensure they are reporting similar measurements for similar periods.

Documenting Anesthesia Emergence and Transfer of Care

Documentation of interventions performed to reverse the anesthesia process and permit patient emergence from anesthesia is also essential. Throughout this process, continued documentation of physiologic monitoring measurements is essential until the monitors are removed. Further documentation should include the times the anesthesia agents, oxygen, and compressed air are turned off; the drugs and dosages used for narcotic and muscle relaxant reversals, including the effects of the drugs; repositioning information, when required for extubation of the trachea; and notations regarding suctioning and extubation if done in the operating room. If selected monitors are to be used in transport these should be noted, as should oxygen administration if it is continued.

In transferring the patient to the care of PACU or surgical intensive care personnel, assessment of the status of the patient should be documented by both the anesthetist and the PACU or ICU nurse. Any disagreement relative to the assessment must be resolved before the anesthetist leaves and this agreement should be documented. The minimum essential components of this assessment that should be documented are the state of consciousness, the presence or absence of reflexes, the adequacy of the airway and ventilation, blood pressure and pulse measurements, skin color, and ECG pattern. Oxygen administration should be continued in the PACU or ICU and noted on the anesthesia record as being continued at the time of transfer of care from the anesthetist to the PACU or ICU nurse. A general statement should be on the record concerning the physical status of the patient at the time of transfer, giving evidence that the patient's condition permitted the transfer. A comment should be made documenting that a report concerning the patient, surgery, and anesthesia was given to the receiving nurse.

In finalizing the anesthesia record, total drug dosages and fluid administered should be quantified, totaled, and recorded, as should the fluids, by type. Total loss of blood should be estimated and recorded. Other output, urine, gastric fluids, ascites, effusions, and so on should be quantified and recorded on the anesthesia record in the appropriate spaces or within the remarks column. When the anesthesia record does not have adequate space for such recording, an alternative is to document this in an anesthesia note on the progress notes within the patient's health record.

POSTANESTHESIA EVALUATION DOCUMENTATION

If patients remain within the hospital, follow-up visits to the patient should be made to evaluate and document the patient's overall response to the anesthetic. Anesthetic or anesthetic-related complications should be documented, as should any recommendations for care and consultation. In the presence of complications, these complications should be followed up and documented at least until they have been resolved or the patient has been discharged from the facility.

Full documentation of anesthesia care during the intraanesthesia and anesthesia emergence periods, including the periods wherein transfer of care to the PACU or ICU nurse is made and the postanesthesia evaluation is completed, will provide evidence of compliance with the following Standards of Nurse Anesthesia Care:

- Standard IV: The anesthesia care plan shall be skillfully implemented and the plan of care adjusted as needed to adapt to the patient's response to the anesthetic. Vigilance shall be maintained for untoward identifiable reactions and corrective actions initiated as required.
- Standard V: The patient's physiologic condition shall be monitored consistent with both the type of anesthesia care and the specific patient needs.
- Standard VI: There shall be prompt, complete, and accurate documentation of pertinent information on the patient's record.
- Standard VII: The responsibility for the care of the patient shall be transferred to other qualified providers in a manner which assures continuity of care and patient safety.
- Standard X: Anesthesia care shall be assessed to assure its quality.[9]

OTHER ANESTHESIA CARE DOCUMENTATION CONSIDERATIONS

Although the amount of documentation discussed thus far sounds overwhelming, the fact that anesthetists have been accomplishing this, albeit some doing it better than others, lends evidence that it is not an impossible task. In fact, the study reported earlier in the chapter indicates that only about 11 percent of the time spent in administering and managing an anesthetic is devoted to documentation.[6] Some other important notations should also be incorporated on the anesthesia record.

Relief of Anesthesia Providers

Any relief of the anesthesia provider for a break, for lunch, or at the end of a shift should be noted with the name and credentials of the person providing the relief. Further, both providers should make a patient assessment and agree on the status of the patient at the time of relief and that agreement noted.

Obstetric Anesthesia Records

Although the obstetric patient presents specialized requirements for care and documentation, it should be noted that anesthesia records demonstrating appropriate monitoring should be maintained when initiating and monitoring an epidural anesthetic for pain relief during labor. Further, time of birth and sex of baby, as well as any evidence of spontaneous cry or alertness, should be recorded on the anesthesia record. Time of placental delivery should also be noted in addition to any oxytocic drugs or drips administered. It should be remembered that when an anesthetist is in attendance for a delivery, the standards for patient monitoring are the same as for a patient within surgery and evidence of such monitoring should be documented.

Consultations

Any consultations sought and given should be recorded on the anesthesia record as to the purpose of consultation, if not obvious by the chart, and the name of the consultant. The consultant may want to document his or her consultation on the patient progress report in the patient chart.

Emergency Laboratory or Blood Requirements

Emergencies may arise during the course of anesthetic management that require additional laboratory tests. Documentation of the times such tests were requested and reports were returned from the laboratory should be recorded, along with who received the reports. Should an emergency arise necessitating blood administration, and blood must be sent for type and crossmatch, the time blood is drawn for that purpose and sent to the laboratory and the time the blood was made available to the anesthetist should be recorded. Should there be excessive delays in receiving the blood, any attempts to expedite the process should be noted.

Physiologic Alterations and Needed Interventions

Any drugs administered or anesthetic agents adjusted to correct physiologic alterations or complications should be noted on the anesthesia record. If drug administration results from a requested consultation, that fact must be noted. If the reason for the use of a drug is not apparent on the graphic portion of the anesthesia record on which the monitoring indices are noted, the reason should be given in the remarks column along with any other actions taken. An example of this latter situation may be the sudden appearance of urticaria following initiation of a blood transfusion and intervention with an antihistamine drug.

Required Reporting of Unusual Occurrences

Unusual occurrences that result in patient injury or potential injury should be noted on the anesthesia record though a more detailed reporting of the event should be completed on another form designated for that purpose when appropriate. Completion of the form should be noted on the anesthesia record. Specific departmentally or institutionally required reporting concerning the progress of the anesthetic should be accomplished and documented.

Cardiopulmonary Emergencies

The American Heart Association and others involved in teaching cardiopulmonary resuscitation have recognized the problems associated with acute, emergency care and the essential nature for complete, accurate, and timely documentation during such periods of resuscitation. They have defined a role for a record keeper on the resuscitation team with no other responsibilities but to maintain a record of the actions taken and the drugs administered by care providers (by name and by time), including the patient responses during the resuscitation.

In anesthesia, and in most operating rooms, this model has not been followed although it might well be considered in anesthesia emergencies. This type of emergency, along with sudden complete respiratory obstruction, is when the patient is most vulnerable to serious brain damage and death and when the actions taken by the members of the health care team are most crucial to the outcome of such events. It is impossible for those health professionals who are actively responding to such emergencies to document the care provided in a timely fashion. Further, the stress of the situation lends itself to memory lapses about the observations made and the actions taken, including the sequencing and timing of specific observations and activities. This is also the period during which when health providers are most vulnerable to malpractice allegations.

Although some institutions do have policies that require their cardiopulmonary resuscitation team to respond to such emergencies within the operating room, concern must be given to the potential for contamination and infection, even with a successful resuscitation. Although assistance is often made available to the health care team during such emergency periods, consideration should be given to developing a group of knowledgeable people who could take over the recording function as may be needed during these emergencies within the operating or delivery room setting.

After any anesthetic catastrophic event, it is important that the anesthesia provider take the time to reassess the care management. Where needed, he or she should summarize what appeared to happen and how it was managed on a progress note if such a notation can add anything to the already existing anesthesia record. Again, it is very important that such notations not be in conflict with the anesthesia record.

Care Performed Outside the Surgical Suite

When called on to perform resuscitation, establish and intubate an airway, perform an arterial or venous cannulation, or implement a request for pain management, the anesthetist must decide to what extent these should be fully documented on the patient's progress notes or on an anesthesia record or other departmental form designed for these purposes. These interventions and the patient's responses must be documented in detail. Such recordings must indicate who is assuming the care for the patient when the anesthetist leaves.

OTHER PRECAUTIONS

Correcting Mistakes in Documentation

It is imperative that records be corrected in a manner that permits readers to see what was originally documented as well as the correction. Erasures or recopied records, when recognized, are associated in courtrooms with presumption of guilt and it can be difficult to convince a jury otherwise. Errors should be noted by a single line drawn through them and initialed, and the correction made. Recopying of records may be permissible if the record recopied is not destroyed but is attached to the recopied record along with any notations that may have necessitated the recopying. Certainly it is preferable not to do either, but at times it may be necessary.

Avoiding Conflicting Records

In the operating room or in the obstetric delivery room, circulating nurses are required to document selected aspects of their practice including some of those events that anesthetists record on their anesthesia record. It is exceedingly important that both use the same clock so that the times match. Although it may be impossible for two people with different backgrounds and experiences to view an event exactly alike, it is important that differences in such viewpoints, where crucial, be resolved, if possible, in a timely manner. Conflicting records can create problems for the entire health team involved in the care of the patient should any question of negligence of care arise.

SUMMARY AND CONCLUSIONS

Documentation of anesthesia care is an essential component of anesthesia practice. Often, the anesthesia record can be either our best defender or our worst accuser in morbidity and mortality conferences, peer and quality assessment reviews, and the courtroom. These records must be a reliable account of the care provided and patient responses if they are to be truly valuable in teaching and in research.

The increasing number of monitors used in anesthesia today has in some instances enhanced patient safety and increased documentation requirements. In the large majority of anesthesia cases, manual (hand) documentation does not provide serious impediments to patient monitoring and intervention; however, when providing anesthesia to poor-risk patients, or for the more complex surgical cases, or when serious emergencies occur, the need for documentation and intervention increases concurrently and may become problematic. In such situations, documentation must take a second seat to the care provided, leaving the provider at increased risk should patient injury result.

There are those anesthetists who believe that automated record keeping is on the horizon for anesthesia providers. Some companies have already developed automated anesthesia records to assist anesthetists in performing this task in a timely fashion; however, because of the artifacts still present in these systems, many anesthetists are fearful of such automation. When automated record keeping is used, attention must be given to identifying these artifacts and noting their cause. For instance, when monitoring end-tidal carbon dioxide, the recorder cannot distinguish between disruption of the monitor's recordings caused by removal of the monitor for intubation and that caused by a sudden ventilator disconnect; or in the case of a blood pressure measurement, the recorder cannot distinguish between

the real diastolic pressure and one precipitated by exertion of undue force on the cuff by a member of the surgical team during a measurement.

Some believe that as voice recognition and artificial intelligence circuitry are added to monitoring computers, anesthesia providers will wear headsets and dictate comments that will be time lined to coincide with the automatic recording of monitoring data. Such a scenario is totally possible, but it does prompt some questions: For what patients? In what size hospitals? And, at how much additional cost? The growing concern with health care costs as they relate to technology development and use will bring about greater study of the incorporation of such advanced technology into the care of patients. The decreasing incidence of severe morbidity and mortality related to use of current monitors may well mitigate against incorporation of such sophisticated and more costly technology for all patients. Further, we could become so entranced in our technology that we might lose sight of our patients and fail to keep in visual and tactile contact with them. Certainly there can be a middle ground where, perhaps for 80 to 90 percent of patients, assistance in documentation of care through time-lined recordings even on magnetic tape can be superimposed on the automated physiologic monitoring recorders to make this aspect of practice easier for the provider.

The anesthesia provider's essential expertise in anesthesia care documentation is in knowing what and when to document, interpreting such documentation in a manner that reflects the actual findings or events, and translating the documentation into needed care inventions. Anesthesia care must be defensible from the standpoint of quality. The anesthesia provider must be willing to be held accountable for the care provided and documented, whether this be with respect to her or his own personal values, the values of his or her profession or peers, or the courtroom. Anesthesia documentation must also be a source for identifying researchable questions and improving the care we provide tomorrow. As such, care documentation may not be one of the most pleasant components of our practice but, next to the care itself, it is the most essential.

REFERENCES

1. Dripps RD, Eckenhoff JE, Vandam LD. *Introduction to anesthesia, the principles of safe practice.* 7th ed. Philadelphia: WB Saunders; 1988.
2. Klein SL, Landers DF. *Anesthesiology, problems in primary care.* Oradell, NJ: Medical Economics Books; 1990.
3. Barash PG, Cullen BF, Stoelting RK, eds. *Clinical anesthesia.* Philadelphia: JB Lippincott; 1989.
4. Miller RD, ed. *Anesthesia.* 3rd ed. New York: Churchill Livingstone; 1990;2.
5. Stoelting RK, Miller RD. *Basics of anesthesia.* New York: Churchill Livingstone; 1984.
6. MacDonald JS, Ozwonczyk A, Gupta B. A second-time study of the anesthetist's intraoperative period. *Br J Anaesth.* 1990;64:582–585.
7. Chopra MB, Bovill JG, Spierdijk. Checklists: Aviation shows the way to safer anesthesia. *APSF Newslett.* 1991;6:26, 29.
8. American Association of Nurse Anesthetists. *Documenting the Standard of Care: The Anesthesia Record.* Park Ridge, IL: AANA; 1991.

9. American Association of Nurse Anesthetists. Standards of nurse anesthesia practice. In: *Guidelines for nurse anesthesia practice*. Park Ridge, IL: AANA; 1989.

10. Fiesta J. *The law and liability, a guide for nurses*. New York: Wiley; 1983.

11. Faden RR, Beauchamp TL, King NMP. *A history and theory of informed consent*. New York: Oxford University Press; 1986.

12. Cheney FW, Kroll, DA. Medicolegal aspects of anesthetic practice. In: Barash PG, Cullen BF, Stoelting RK, eds. *Clinical anesthesia*. Philadelphia: JB Lippincott; 1989.

13. Duberman SM, Bendixen HH. Concepts of fail-safe in anesthetic practice. In: Pierce EC Jr, Cooper JB, eds. *International anesthesiology clinics, analysis of anesthetic mishaps*. Boston: Little, Brown; 1984;22(2):149–165.

4

Metric Medical Mathematics

Marian Waterhouse

Metric medical mathematics is utilized in the application of metric equivalents to drugs and solutions. Knowledge of these calculations is essential to the nurse anesthetist for the accurate computation of drug dosages, diluents, and infusions. The mathematics of biochemistry is integral to the understanding of electrolyte balance as well as to the computation of pH. Although most vaporizers in anesthesia practice today are temperature compensated and do not require the anesthetist to perform calculations to ensure appropriate administration of volatile agents, there are still anesthesia machines in use that are 15 to 35 years old and may require a number of calculations and adjustments to deliver the anesthetic vapor accurately. This chapter will provide formulas and computation examples for numerous mathematical computations encountered in anesthesia practice.

RELATIONSHIPS OF MATHEMATICAL EQUIVALENTS

There are four common ways to express mathematical equivalents: fractions, ratios, decimals, and percent.

Changing Fractions to Ratios

A ratio is a fraction. The fraction ½ may be expressed as the ratio 1:2. A ratio of 1:2, or the fraction ½, means one of two equal parts, or $1 \div 2$.

Changing Fractions or Ratios to Decimals

A decimal is a fraction whose denominator is 10, or any power of 10, that is, 100, 1000, 10,000, and so on. The denominator of a decimal is signified by the placement of the number to the right of a decimal point. A fraction is changed to a decimal by dividing the numerator by the denominator.

$$1:2 = \tfrac{1}{2} = \tfrac{5}{10} = 5 \div 10 = 0.5$$

$$1:4 = \tfrac{1}{4} = \tfrac{25}{100} = 25 \div 100 = 0.25$$

$$1:8 = \tfrac{1}{8} = 1 \div 8 = 0.125$$

Changing Decimals to Percent

Percent means "per hundred" or "divided by 100." To change a decimal to a percent, move the decimal point two places to the right.

$$1:2 = \tfrac{1}{2} = 1 \div 2 = 0.50 = \tfrac{50}{100} = 50.0\%$$

$$1:4 = \tfrac{1}{4} = 1 \div 4 = 0.25 = \tfrac{25}{100} = 25.0\%$$

$$1:100 = \tfrac{1}{100} = 1 \div 100 = 0.01 = 1.0\%$$

$$1:8 = \tfrac{1}{8} = 1 \div 8 = 0.125 = 12.5\%$$

APPLICATION OF METRIC EQUIVALENTS TO DRUGS AND SOLUTIONS

Metric Units of Weight and Volume

Many mathematical errors made in calculating measurements of drugs and solutions occur because people do not remember that *milli-* means "thousandths" (not hundredths). To avoid such errors, it it imperative to remember the following relationships:

1 gram (g)	= 1000 milligrams (mg)
1 kilogram (kg)	= 1000 grams (g)
1 liter (L)	= 1000 milliliters (mL)
	= 1000 cubic centimeters (cc)
1 mg	= 0.001 g
1 mL or 1 cc	= 0.001 L

For the purpose of this text, 1 gram of drug dissolved in 1 milliliter of liquid solvent is a 100 percent solution. Therefore: 1 g = 1 mL, or 1 cc. All mathematics problems involving drugs and solutions can be quickly calculated if the number of milligrams per milliliter desired after dilution (or the percentage of the solution) and the total dosage (or total volume) of solution required are known.[1]

Multiplication and Division of Grams, Milligrams, Liters, and Milliliters

Multiplication and division of the units are used extensively when figuring drug problems. The units are fractions and therefore must be treated as such. Cancellation is usually possible, as illustrated here.

$$500 \text{ mg} \div 100 \text{ mg/mL} = 500 \text{ mg} \div \frac{100 \text{ mg}}{\text{mL}}$$

$$= 500 \text{ mg} \times \frac{\text{mL}}{100 \text{ mg}} = 5 \text{ mL}$$

(See the examples below.) Labeling all parts of the equations is very important so that the meaning will be clear. In any one equation, figures must all be in the same unit or measure:

- If gram is used, all weight terms must be in grams.
- If milligram is used, all weight terms must be in milligrams.
- If milliliter is used, all volume terms must be in milliliters.
- If liter is used, all volume terms must in liters.

Only when one unit can be canceled out while converting from one unit to another may both units appear in the same problem:

$$\frac{1 \text{ g}}{5 \text{ mL}} \times \frac{1000 \text{ mg}}{\text{g}} = \frac{1000 \text{ mg}}{5 \text{ mL}} = 200 \text{ mg/mL}$$

Refer to Table 4–1 when figuring Examples 1 to 10. Start each problem from the boldface type in Table 4–1.

EXAMPLE 1

Make 20 mL of a 2 percent solution from a pure (100 percent) liquid drug.

Step 1: Make a table of the mathematical equivalents for 2 percent and 100 percent, as illustrated in Table 4–1. Any one of the columns in Table 4–1 can be used to figure the grams per milliliter of a solution. For a 2 percent solution:
   a. Percent means grams per 100 mL. Therefore, a 2 percent solution has 2 g/100 mL of solution.
   b. The decimal means grams per milliliter. If there is 2 g/100 mL, there is 0.02 g/mL of solution.
   c. The ratio and the fraction also mean grams per milliliter. A 2 percent solution has 2 g/100 mL, or 1 g/50 mL. A 1:50 or 1/50th solution contains 1 g of drug in 50 mL of solution, or 0.02 g/mL.
   d. The milligram per milliliter column indicates the number of milligrams dissolved per milliliter of solution. To change grams to milligrams, multiply the decimal by 1000.

$$0.02 \text{ g/mL} \times 1000 \text{ mg/g} = 20 \text{ mg/mL}$$
$$\text{of solution}$$

TABLE 4–1. MATHEMATICAL EQUIVALENTS FOR EXAMPLES 1–10[a]

Example	Ratio (g/mL)	Fraction (g/mL)	Decimal (g/mL)	Percentage (g/100 mL)	mg/mL	g/L
1	1:1	1/1 or 100/100	1.00	**100%** = 100 g/100 mL	1000 mg/mL	1000 g/L
	1:50	1/50 or 2/100	0.02	**2%** or 2 g/100 mL	2000 mg/100 mL or 20 mg/mL	20 g/L
2,7,9				**1%** or 1 g/100 mL	1000 mg/100 mL = 10 mg/mL	
				10% or 10 g/100 mL	10,000 mg/100 mL = 100 mg/mL	
3	**1:200,000**	1/200,000			1000 mg/200,000 mL = 1 mg/200 mL = 0.005 mg/mL	
	1:1000	1/1000			1000 mg/1000 mL = 1 mg/mL = 0.1 mg/0.1 mL	
4	**1:100,000**	1/100,000	0.00001 g/mL	0.001 g/100 mL = 0.001%		
5,10			**0.25 g/5 mL** = 0.05 g/mL		250 mg/5 mL = 50 mg/mL = 25 mg/0.5 mL	
6				**2.5%** = 2.5 g/100 mL		25 g/L
7	[b]			**0.002%** = 0.002 g/100 mL	2 mg/100 mL = 0.02 mg/mL	
8	**1:4000**	1/4000			1000 mg/4000 mL = 1.0 mg/4 mL = 0.5 mg/2 mL	

[a] See text.
[b] See above for 1%.

Step 2: The problem calls for 20 mL of a 2 percent solution. Table 4–1 shows that a 2 percent solution contains 20 mg/mL.

$$20 \text{ mg/mL} \times 20 \text{ mL} = 400 \text{ mg},$$
total amount drug needed

Step 3: Table 4–1 shows that a pure (100 percent) drug contains 1 g/mL of solution, or 1000 mg/mL. A total of 400 mg of drug is needed.

$$400 \text{ mg} \div 1000 \text{ mg/mL} = 400 \text{ mg} \times \frac{\text{mL}}{1000 \text{ mg}}$$
$$= \text{\textonesuperior/}_{10} \text{ mL, or } 0.4 \text{ mL}$$

The amount of 100 percent drug needed is 0.4 mL.

Answer

Take 0.4 mL of stock 100 percent drug and add 19.6 mL of solvent; 20 mL of a 2 percent solution, containing 20 mg/mL, will have been made.

EXAMPLE 2

Make 50 mL of a 1 percent solution from a 10 percent solution.

Step 1: Use the applicable parts of Table 4–1.

$$1\% = 1\text{g/100 mL} =$$
$$1000 \text{ mg/100 mL} = 10 \text{ mg/mL}$$

$$10 \text{ mg/mL} \times 50 \text{ mL} =$$
$$500 \text{ mg, total amount drug needed}$$

Step 2:

$$10\% = 10\text{g/100 mL} = 10,000 \text{ mg/100 mL}$$
$$= 100 \text{ mg/mL}$$

Step 3:

$$500 \text{ mg} \div 100 \text{ mg/mL} = 500 \text{ mg} \times \text{mL/100 mg}$$
$$= 5 \text{ mL}$$

Answer

Take 5 mL of a 10 percent solution and add solvent to 50 mL; 50 mL of a 1 percent solution, containing 10 mg/mL, will have been made.

EXAMPLE 3

Make 20 mL of epinephrine 1:200,000. Available are 1-mL ampules of 1:1000 epinephrine and 50-mL vials of saline.

Step 1:
$$1:200,000 = 1 \text{ g/200,000 mL}$$
$$= 1000 \text{ mg/200,000 mL}$$
$$= 1 \text{ mg/200 mL}$$
$$= 0.005 \text{ mg/mL}$$

$$0.005 \text{ mg/mL} \times 20 \text{ mL} = 0.1 \text{ mg, total amount of epinephrine needed}$$

Step 2:

$$\text{Stock epinephrine 1: 1000}$$
$$= 1 \text{g/1000 mL} = 1000 \text{ mg/1000 mL}$$
$$= 1 \text{ mg/mL} = 0.1 \text{ mg/0.1 mL}$$

Answer

Add 0.1 mL of epinephrine 1:1000 to 19.9 mL of saline; 20 mL of a 1:200,000 solution of epinephrine, containing 0.005 mg/mL, will have been made.

EXAMPLE 4

What percentage is a 1:100,000 solution? Percent means g/100 mL.

$$1:100,000 = 1 \text{ g/100,000 mL} = 0.001 \text{ g/100 mL} = 0.001\%$$

EXAMPLE 5

The label on the ampule reads "0.25 g pentobarbital, 5-mL ampule." The desired dosage is 25 mg of pentobarbital to be given intravenously. How much of this ampule should be given to the patient?

$$0.25 \text{ g} = 250 \text{ mg}$$

The ampule contains 250 mg/5 mL, or 50 mg/mL.

$$25 \text{ mg} \div \frac{50 \text{ mg}}{\text{mL}} = 25 \text{ mg} \times \frac{\text{mL}}{50 \text{ mg}} = \frac{1}{2} \text{ mL}$$

Answer

Give 0.5 mL of the drug. Because there is 50 mg/mL, there is 25 mg/0.5 mL.

EXAMPLE 6

Make a 2.5 percent thiopental sodium (Pentothal) solution. Available are 5-g powdered ampules of Pentothal and 1000-mL bottles of solvent.

$$2.5\% = 2.5 \text{ g/100 mL} = 25 \text{ g/1000 mL}$$

Answer

Add 5 ampules of thiopental sodium (Pentothal), powdered 5-g ampules, to 1000 mL of solvent.

EXAMPLE 7

The patient's blood pressure is falling rapidly. An intravenous infusion of phenylephrine (Neo-Synephrine), 0.002 percent, is indicated. The drug will be added to the remaining 250 mL of an infusion already running. The phenylephrine ampule is a 1 percent solution. How much of the drug should be added to the bottle?

Step 1:

$$0.002\% = 0.002 g/100 \text{ mL} = 2 \text{ mg}/100 \text{ mL}$$
$$= 0.02 \text{ mg/mL}$$
$$0.02 \text{ mg/mL} \times 250 \text{ mL} = 5 \text{ mg phenylephrine}$$
$$\text{required}$$

Step 2:

$$1\% = 1 \text{ g}/100 \text{ mL} = 1000 \text{ mg}/100 \text{ mL}$$
$$= 10 \text{ mg/mL}$$
$$5 \text{ mg} \div 10 \text{ mg/mL} = 0.5 \text{ mL}$$

Answer

Add 0.5 mL of 1 percent phenylephrine to the 250-mL infusion; a 0.002 percent solution of phenylephrine (Neo-Synephrine) containing 0.02 mg/mL will have been made.

EXAMPLE 8

Give neostigmine (Prostigmin), 1 mg. Neostigmine, 1:4000, 2-mL ampules are available.

$$1{:}4000 = 1 g/4000 \text{ mL} = 1000 \text{ mg}/4000 \text{ mL} = 1 \text{ mg}/4 \text{ mL}$$
$$= 0.5 \text{ mg}/2 \text{ mL}$$

Answer

A neostigmine, 1:4000, 2-mL ampule contains 0.5 mg of drug. To give 1 mg of neostigmine, two 2-mL ampules of 1:4000 neostigmine (Prostigmin) should be administered.

EXAMPLE 9

If 1 mL of 1 percent tetracaine hydrochloride (Pontocaine) is added to 1 mL of 10 percent dextrose in preparation for a spinal anesthetic, what percentage and how many milligrams per milliliter will result for each drug?

Step 1: The tetracaine hydrochloride problem:

$$1\% = 1 g/100 \text{ mL} = 1000 \text{ mg}/100 \text{ mL}$$
$$= 10 \text{ mg/mL}$$

Answer

After adding 1 mL of 1 percent tetracaine hydrochloride to 1 mL of another solution, there will be 10 mg tetracaine hydrochloride/2 mL, or 5 mg/mL.

$$5 \text{ mg/mL} = 500 \text{ mg}/100 \text{ mL}$$
$$= 0.5 g/100 \text{ mL}$$
$$= 0.5\% \text{ tetracaine hydrochloride}$$
$$\text{(Pontocaine) solution}$$

Step 2: The dextrose problem:

$$10\% = 10 g/100 \text{ mL} = 10,000 \text{ mg}/100 \text{ mL}$$
$$= 100 \text{ mg/mL}$$

Answer

After adding 1 mL of 10 percent dextrose to 1 mL of another solution, there will be 100 mg dextrose/2 mL, or 50 mg/mL.

$$50 \text{ mg/mL} = 5000 \text{ mg}/100 \text{ mL} = 5 g/100 \text{ mL}$$
$$= 5\% \text{ dextrose solution}$$

EXAMPLE 10

Pentobarbital, 10 mg, is to be given to a child. Available is pentobarbital 0.25 g/5-mL ampule. How should this medication be given?

$$0.25 g/5 \text{ mL} = 250 \text{ mg}/5 \text{mL} = 50 \text{ mg/mL}$$

Dilute the drug so that it is easy to give 10 mg. A satisfactory way to do this would be to add to 1 mL (50 mg) of the pentobarbital ampule enough saline to make 10 mL. Then there would be 50 mg/10 mL, or 5 mg/mL.

Answer

To receive 10 mg of pentobarbital, the child should be given 2 mL of the pentobarbital solution diluted to 5 mg/mL.[1]

MATHEMATICS OF BIOCHEMISTRY

The reader is advised to study Chapter 5 (Principles of Chemistry and Physics in Anesthesia) with the rest of this chapter.

A study of the nature of electrolytes is fundamental to understanding the biochemistry of the living body. There are two ways molecules behave in solutions:

1. The molecules may split or dissociate to form ions. This process is known as ionization, and chemical compounds that behave in this way are known as electrolytes. Sodium chloride is an example of an electrolyte in body water. In solution, each molecule ionizes into one positive sodium ion and one negative chloride ion.

$$NaCl \rightarrow Na^+ + Cl^-$$

2. Molecules in solution that do not ionize are known as nonelectrolytes. Dextrose and urea are examples of nonelectrolytes in body water.

Gram Atomic Weights

The atomic weight of an element, expressed in grams, is called the gram atomic weight (GAW) of that element. Hydrogen is used as a standard because it has a GAW of 1 g. Note in Table 4–2 the following:

- 1 GAW of hydrogen weighs 1 g.
- 1 GAW of sodium weighs 23 g.
- 1 GAW of potassium weighs 39 g.

The combining ability of 1 GAW of sodium or potassium is identical to that of 1 GAW of hydrogen, although 1 GAW of potassium weighs 39 times as much as does 1 GAW of hydrogen, and 1 GAW of sodium weighs 23 times as much as 1 GAW of hydrogen.

Gram Molecular Weights

The molecular weight of a compound, expressed in grams, is called the gram molecular weight (GMW) of that compound. One GMW is commonly known as 1 mole, or 1 mol.[1]

Gram Equivalent Weights

The number of milligrams per milliliter of an electrolyte solution yields no information regarding its potential for maintaining electrical neutrality within the body. The *number* of ions or molecules in a solution must be counted. An equivalent weight counts the number of ions, that is, the number of positive and negative charges possessed by an element or radical. Note in Table 4–2 that 1 GAW of hydrogen weighs 1 g, the least of all the elements, and hydrogen ionizes to H^+ (it has only one positive charge). For these two reasons, hydrogen is used as the element with which all other elements are compared.

One ion of each of the other elements weighs more than one ion of hydrogen; however, the relative weight of each ion is *not* a factor involved in the *combining* ability of each ion. It is the *number of charges,* positive or negative, possessed by the individual ion (or radical) that is counted when comparing its combining ability with that of one ion of hydrogen.[1]

Definition. An equivalent weight of an element is its weight in grams that is equivalent to, or equal in combining weight to, that of 1 g of hydrogen. The gram equivalent weight (GEW) of an element (or radical) is the number of GAWs, or the *fraction* of 1 GAW of that element that exactly combines with, or replaces, 1 GAW of hydrogen.

One ion of hydrogen has the same combining ability as one ion of sodium or potassium.

$$H^+ + Cl^- \rightarrow HCl$$
$$Na^+ + Cl^- \rightarrow NaCl$$
$$K^+ + Cl^- \rightarrow KCl$$

In each of these equations, one ion of H^+, one ion of Na^+, or one ion of K^+ combines exactly with one ion of Cl^-.

1 GAW (or 1 g) H^+ + 1 GAW (or 35 g) Cl^-

$\rightarrow$ 1 GMW (or 36 g) HCl

1 GAW (or 23 g) Na^+ + 1 GAW (or 35 g) Cl^-

$\rightarrow$ 1 GMW (or 58 g) NaCl

1 GAW (or 39 g) K^+ + 1 GAW (or 35 g) Cl^-

$\rightarrow$ 1 GMW (or 74 g) KCl

These equations illustrate the meaning not only of GAW and GMW, but also of GEW. It can be seen that 1 GAW of sodium, weighing 23 g, can exactly replace 1 GAW of hydrogen, weighing 1 g. Also, 1 GAW of potassium, weighing 39 g, can exactly replace 1 GAW of hydrogen, or 1 GAW of sodium, and 1 GAW of H^+ or Na^+ or K^+ can exactly combine with 1 GAW of Cl^-. Also demonstrated is the fact that, because 1 GAW of Na^+ or 1 GAW of K^+ exactly replaces 1 GAW of H^+, the GEW of Na^+ or K^+ is the same as its respective GAW.

Elements with a Valence of 2. An element with a valence of 2 or more presents a different situation. Table 4–2 indicates that sulfur has a valence of -2. This means that one ion of sulfur can combine with two ions of H^+. Therefore, one ion of H^+ combines exactly with one-half ion of S^{2-}.

1 GAW (or 32 g) S^{2-} + 2 GAW (or 2 g) H^+

$\rightarrow$ 1 GMW (or 34 g) H_2S

The GEW of S^{2-} (or the amount of sulfur that combines with 1 GAW or 1 g of hydrogen) is equal to half its GAW. Thus

$$\text{GEW } S^{2-} = \frac{1 \text{ GAW (or 32 g) } S^{2-}}{2} = 16 \text{ g}$$

Referring to the definition of GEW, it is evident that the GEW of sulfur is the *fraction* of its GAW that combines exactly with 1 GAW (or 1 g) of H^+.

1 GEW (or 16 g) S^{2-} + 1 GEW (or 1 g) H^+

$\rightarrow$ 1 GEW (or 17 g) H_2S

1 GEW S^{2-} + 1 GEW H^+ $\rightarrow$ 1 GEW H_2S

Avogadro's Law and Number

Avogadro's Law. Avogadro's law states that 1 GMW of any compound contains the same number of molecules as 1

TABLE 4–2. COMMON GRAM ATOMIC WEIGHTS AND VALENCES

	Symbol	Gram Atomic Weight	Valence
Elements			
Bromine	Br	80	−1, −3, −5, −7
Calcium	Ca	40	+2
Carbon	C	12	+4, −4
Chlorine	Cl	35	−1
Hydrogen	H	1	+1
Iron	Fe	56	+2, +3
Magnesium	Mg	24	+2
Nitrogen	N	14	+3, +5
Oxygen	O	16	−2
Potassium	K	39	+1
Phosphorus	P	31	+3, +5
Sodium	Na	23	+1
Sulfur	S	32	−2, +4, +6
Radicals			
Ammonium	NH_4		+1
Bicarbonate	HCO_3		−1
Carbonate	CO_3		−2
Chlorate	ClO_3		−1
Hydroxyl	OH		−1
Nitrate	NO_3		−1
Phosphate	PO_4		−3
Sulfate	SO_4		−2

GMW of any other compound. Similarly 1 GAW of element contains the same number of atoms as 1 GAW of any other element.[1-3]

Avogadro's Number. Avogadro's number describes 1 GMW of any substance as containing

6.02×10^{23} (or 602,000,000,000,000,000,000,000) molecules

(see also Chapter 6).[1,2] Similarly, there are 6.02×10^{23} atoms in 1 GAW of any element. In 1 GAW or 1 GEW of hydrogen, there are 6.02×10^{23} ions. In 1 GAW or 1 GEW of chloride, there are 6.02×10^{23} ions. Therefore,

$$6.02 \times 10^{23} \text{ ions of } H^+ + 6.02 \times 10^{23} \text{ ions of } Cl^-$$

$$\rightarrow 6.02 \times 10^{23} \text{ molecules of HCl}$$

In 1 GAW of sulfur there are 6.02×10^{23} ions. In 1 GEW of S^{2-} there are 3.01×10^{23} ions.

$$1 \text{ GEW (or } 6.02 \times 10^{23} \text{ ions) } H^+$$

$$+ 1 \text{ GEW (or } 3.01 \times 10^{23} \text{ ions) } S^{2-}$$

$$\rightarrow 1 \text{ GEW (or } 3.01 \times 10^{23} \text{ molecules) } H_2S$$

Figure 4–1 shows that only 0.5 GAW of S^{2-} is needed to neutralize 1 GAW of H^+.

Milliequivalent Weights

A milliequivalent weight of an element is its weight in milligrams that is equivalent to or equal in combining weight to that of 1 mg of hydrogen.

As explained earlier, *milli* means "thousandths."

$$1000.0 \text{ mg} = 1.0 \text{ g}$$

$$1.0 \text{ mg} = 0.001 \text{ g}$$

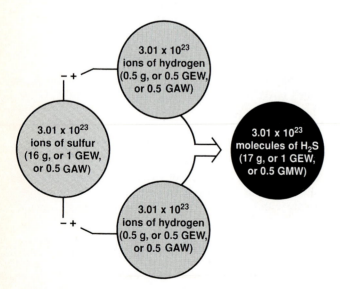

Figure 4–1. Diagram showing how 3.01×10^{23} ions of sulfur combine with 6.02×10^{23} ions of hydrogen to make 3.01×10^{23} molecules of H_2S. (*Reprinted, with permission, from Waterhouse.*[1])

1000.0 milliequivalent weights (mEq) = 1.0 equivalent weight (GEW)

$$1.0 \text{ mEq} = 0.001 \text{ GEW}$$

For NaCl,

$$1.0 \text{ GEW weighs } 58 \text{ g}$$

$$0.001 \text{ GEW weighs } 0.058 \text{ g}$$

$$1.0 \text{ mEq (weight) weighs } 0.058 \text{ g}$$

$$1.0 \text{ mEq weighs } 58.0 \text{ mg}$$

For H_2S

$$1.0 \text{ GEW weighs } 17 \text{ g}$$

$$0.001 \text{ GEW weighs } 0.017 \text{ g}$$

$$1.0 \text{ mEq (weight) weighs } 0.017 \text{ g}$$

$$1.0 \text{ mEq weighs } 17.0 \text{ mg}$$

Milliequivalents measure body concentrations of specific ions known as electrolytes. There is an optimum concentration of each electrolyte in each tissue or fluid compartment. Various laboratory tests of electrolytes are reported in milliequivalents because this is the only method by which specific laboratory results can be compared meaningfully with normal body electrolyte concentrations. In addition, electrolyte replacement therapy with drugs or intravenous fluids can be accurately determined by assessing the milliequivalent concentrations of the various body fluids.

Osmotic Pressure of Solutions

Figure 4–2 illustrates osmotic pressure, which can be defined as the pressure developed when two solutions of different concentrations of the same solute are separated by a membrane permeable to the solvent only. For example, Figure 4–2 shows that a 5 percent dextrose in water (D_5W) solution requires a certain amount of mechanical or hydrostatic pressure (illustrated by the plunger) to prevent osmosis of water from compartment B into compartment A. If there were only a 1 percent solution in the A side, just one-fifth as much pressure by the plunger would be required to prevent osmosis of water from compartment B into compartment A. Conversely, if $D_{10}W$ were in compartment A, twice as much pressure by the plunger would be required to prevent osmosis of water from compartment B into compartment A.

If compartment B were a 1 percent solution and compartment A were a 5 percent solution, and there were no plunger, water would diffuse by osmosis from compartment B into compartment A until an equilibrium was reached and the solutes on both sides of the membrane were of equal concentration.

Individual molecules and individual ions that are too large to pass through a semipermeable membrane exert osmotic pressure. The amount of osmotic pressure that one molecule of a nonionizing, nondiffusible substance exerts is the same amount of osmotic pressure as that of one molecule of any other nonionizing, nondiffusible substance.

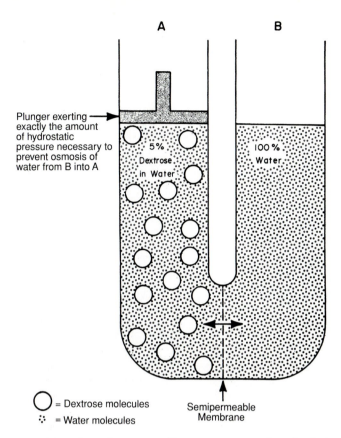

A   B

Plunger exerting
exactly the amount
of hydrostatic
pressure necessary to
prevent osmosis of
water from B into A

5%
Dextrose
in Water

100%
Water

○ = Dextrose molecules
∴ = Water molecules

Semipermeable
Membrane

Figure 4–2. Osmotic pressure. The exact amount of mechanical or hydrostatic pressure required by the plunger to stop the water from flowing from compartment B, into compartment A, through a membrane that is impermeable to dextrose molecules is known as the osmotic pressure of that solution. (*Reprinted, with permission, from Waterhouse.*[1])

EXAMPLE 11

One nonionizing protein molecule with a GMW of 70,000 g has the same osmotic effect as one molecule of dextrose with a GMW of 180 g. Each molecule of dextrose plugs a pore in the semipermeable membrane as effectively as does one molecule of protein. (Compare the weights of a golf ball and a Ping-Pong ball. If they are the same size, each can effectively plug the same hole.)

EXAMPLE 12

One ion of a nondiffusible electrolyte has the same osmotic effect as one molecule of any nonionizing, nondiffusible substance, or as one ion of any other ionizing, nondiffusible substance. One molecule of a nondiffusible, nonionizing substance or one ion of a nondiffusible electrolyte is known as one solute particle that exerts osmotic pressure.

Osmoles and Osmolarity

Osmoles. The *number* of ions or molecules in a solution must be counted if osmotic pressure is to be measured because it is the *number* of particles of solute that creates the osmotic pressure of a solution. The unit of measure for osmotic activity is the osmole (osm). An osmole equals 6.02×10^{23} particles of dissolved solute that cannot diffuse through a semipermeable membrane. These particles of solute may be a combination of several different kinds of nondiffusible ions and molecules in a given solution.

One GMW of a dissolved, nonionizing, nondiffusible solute equals 1 osm. One GMW of such a solute contains 6.02×10^{23} molecules (Avogadro's number). One GAW of an electrolyte that ionizes in solution equals 1 osm. One GAW of such a solute contains 6.02×10^{23} ions.

Osmotic pressure is calculated by adding all the nondiffusible molecules and ions in a solution. For example, one Na^+ ion, or one Ca^{2+} ion, or one dextrose molecule exerts one particle of osmotic pressure. The concentration of all the added particles of solute in a solution is generally given in osmoles per liter (osm/L) of solution.[2,3]

Osmolarity

- Osmotic pressure of 1 GAW Na^+/L = 1 osm/L.
- Osmotic pressure of 1 GAW Cl^-/L = 1 osm/L.
- Osmotic pressure of 1 GMW NaCl/L = 2 osm/L.
- Osmotic pressure of 1 GMW dextrose/L = 1 osm/L.

The osmolarity of a solution is the number of osmoles or the fraction of one osmole that is dissolved in a given unit of solvent; osmolarity is generally expressed as osmoles per liter of solvent. (It is the multiple of 6.02×10^{23} particles or the fraction of 6.02×10^{23} particles that exists in one liter of solvent.)

Relationship of Osmolarity to Osmotic Pressure

Definition of Osmotic Pressure. The osmotic pressure of a solution is that pressure in millimeters of mercury (mm Hg) that when applied to a solution will just prevent osmosis of solvent into it through a semipermeable membrane (like the plunger in Fig. 4–2).[1-3]

If, at 0C, 1 GMW or 1 GAW of any substance is dissolved in exactly 22.4 L of water, it will exert a pressure of one atmosphere (1 atm, 760 mm Hg).

Nonionizing Solutions. One GMW of any nonionizing, nondiffusible solute dissolved in 22.4 L of water at 0C has an osmotic pressure of 760 mm Hg and contains 6.02×10^{23} particles. The osmolarity of this solution is 1 GMW/22.4 L, or 1 osm/22.4 L of solvent (Avogadro's Law).

The osmotic pressure of 1 osm/22.4 L is 760 mm Hg; 760 mm Hg pressure equals 1 atm. Therefore, the osmotic pressure of 1 osm/22.4 L of solvent = 1 atm, or 760 mm Hg. If 1 osm of any solute is dissolved in 1 L of solvent, the osmotic pressure equals 22.4×760 mm Hg, which equals 17,024 mm Hg or 22.4 atm (Fig. 4–3). The solute has been concentrated 22.4 times.

Ionizing Solutions. One GMW of an ionizing, nondiffusible solute, such as NaCl, dissolved in 22.4 L of water at 0C has an osmotic pressure of 760 mm Hg $\times$ 2, which equals 1520 mm Hg, or 2 atm.

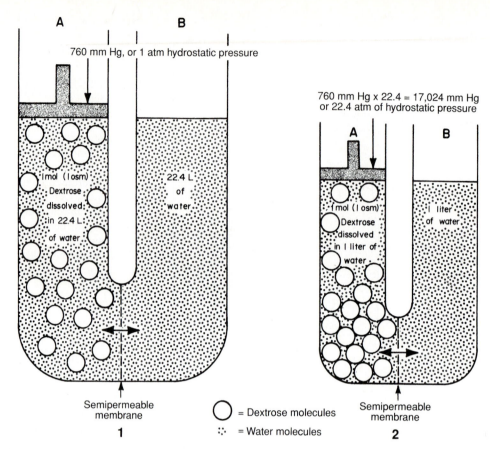

Figure 4–3. Osmotic pressure exerted by 1 GMW of dextrose dissolved in 22.4 L of water (diagram 1) and by 1 GMW of dextrose dissolved in 1 L of water (diagram 2) when compartments A and B are separated by a membrane that is impermeable to dextrose molecules. (*Reprinted, with permission, from Waterhouse.*[1])

One GMW of NaCl contains 6.02×10^{23} molecules. Each molecule ionizes into two ions. The number of particles has doubled. Therefore, 1 GMW NaCl = 2 osm, or 12.04×10^{23} particles, each of which exerts osmotic pressure.

$$2 \text{ osm dissolved in } 1 \text{ L H}_2\text{O} = 2 \times 760 \text{ mm Hg} \times 22.4$$
$$= 34,048 \text{ mm Hg or } 44.8 \text{ atm}$$

To summarize:

- 1 osm = 1 GMW nonionizing substance.
- 1 osm = 0.5 GMW ionizing monovalent substance.
- 1 osm = 0.33 GMW ionizing bivalent substance.

Osmolarity of Body Fluids at Body Temperature

The osmotic pressure of 1 GMW/22.4 L at 0C is 760 mm Hg. Absolute zero is –273C. Zero degrees centigrade is 273 degrees warmer than absolute zero. Human beings have a normal body temperature of +37C. Gay-Lussac's law states that, if the volume of a gas remains constant, the pressure varies directly with the absolute temperature, 1/273 for each degree centigrade. Solutes in solution abide by this law. At 0C, the osmotic pressure exerted by 1 osm of solute per liter of water is

$$273/273 \times 760 \text{ mm Hg} \times 22.4 \text{ L} = 17,024 \text{ mm Hg}$$

(See Fig. 4–3.)

At 37C, the osmotic pressure exerted by 1 osm solute/L of water is

$$\frac{273 + 37}{273} \times 760 \text{ mm Hg} \times 22.4 \text{ L} = 19,331 \text{ mm Hg}$$

To reduce these figures to a useful size, milliosmoles (mosm) are used. Just as 1000 mg = 1 g and 1 mg = 0.001 g, so 1000 mosm = 1 osm and 1 mosm = 0.001 osm.

At 37C the osmotic pressure of

- 1 osm of solute/L = 19,331 mm Hg.
- 1000 mosm of solute/L = 19,331 mm Hg.
- 1 mosm of solute/L = 19.3 mm Hg.

Osmotic Pressure of Body Fluids

The round figure 300 mosm/L (or 0.3 osm/L) osmotic concentration is used for convenience when discussing the osmotic pressure of body fluids (see also Chapter 18).[2] As 1 mosm/L of water creates an osmotic pressure of 19.3 mm Hg at 37C, the osmotic pressure of

$$300 \text{ mosm/L} = 19.3 \text{ mm Hg} \times 300 = 5790 \text{ mm Hg}$$

Summary

- 1 GMW (or 1 GEW) glucose (180 g) = 1 osm (does not ionize).
- 1 GMW (or 1 GEW) NaCl (58 g) = 2 osm (ionizes into two particles).

- 1 mEq Na^+ (23 mg) = 1 mosm.
- 1 mEq Cl^- (35 mg) = 1 mosm.
- 1 mEq NaCl (58 mg) = 2 mosm.
- 0.5 mEq Na^+ (11.5 mg) = 0.5 mosm.
- 0.5 mEq Cl^- (17.5 mg) = 0.5 mosm.
- 0.5 mEq NaCl (29 mg) = 1 mosm.

Therefore

$$1 \text{ mEq (or 1 mosm, or 23 mg) } Na^+$$

$$+ 1 \text{ mEq (or 1 mosm, or 35 mg) } Cl^-$$

$$\rightarrow 1 \text{ mEq (or 2 mosm, or 58 mg) NaCl}$$

- 1 GMW $CaCl_2$ (110 g) = 3 osm (ionizes into three particles).
- 1 GEW $CaCl_2$ (55 g) = 1.5 osm.
- 1 mEq $CaCl_2$ (55 mg) = 1.5 mosm.
- 1 GAW Ca^{2+} (40 g) = 1 osm.
- 1 GEW Ca^{2+} (20 g) = 0.5 osm.
- 1 mEq Ca^{2+} (20 mg) = 0.5 mosm.
- 1 mEq Cl^- (35 mg) = 1 mosm.

Therefore

$$1 \text{ mEq (or 0.5 mosm, or 20 mg) } Ca^{2+}$$

$$+ 1 \text{ mEq (or 1 mosm, or 35 mg) } Cl^-$$

$$\rightarrow 1 \text{ mEq (or 1.5 mosm, or 55 mg) } CaCl_2$$

Note:

$$1 \text{ mEq } Ca^{2+} + 1 \text{ mEq } Cl^- \rightarrow 1 \text{ mEq } CaCl_2$$

$$0.5 \text{ mosm } Ca^{2+} + 1 \text{ mosm } Cl^- \rightarrow 1.5 \text{ mosm } CaCl_2$$

Solutions

Tonicity of Solutions. Tonicity refers to the osmotic pressure of a solution relative to that of body fluids. Isotonic, isoosmotic, or physiologic solutions have an osmotic pressure similar to that of body fluids, or about 300 mosm/L. Hypertonic or hyperosmotic solutions have an osmotic pressure greater than 300 mosm/L. Hypotonic or hypoosmotic solutions have an osmotic pressure less than 300 mosm/L.[3]

Molar Solutions. A 1-molar solution of any solute contains 1 GMW, or 1 mol/L of solution. The molar concentration of a solution is the number of moles or the *fraction* of 1 mol of solute present in 1 L of solution.

One GMW of dextrose ($C_6H_{12}O_6$) weighs 180 g; 180 g/L is an 18 percent solution. (See the discussion of drugs and solutions and Table 4–1.) An 18 percent solution of dextrose in water ($D_{18}W$) is a 1 molar dextrose solution.

Osmolarity of Solutions. To calculate the osmolarity of a solution, all the solute particles in a given volume of that solution must be counted.

EXAMPLE 13

What is the osmolarity of 5.4 percent DW?

$$5.4\% \text{ DW} = 54 \text{ g of dextrose/L of solution}$$

$$1 \text{ molar DW} = 180 \text{ g/L}$$

Therefore, the molarity of

$$5.4\% \text{ DW} = \frac{54 \text{ g}}{L} \div \frac{180 \text{ g}}{mol} = \frac{54 \text{ g}}{L} \times \frac{mol}{180 \text{ g}} = \frac{0.3 \text{ mol}}{L}$$

As shown above, 1 molar dextrose = 1 osmolar dextrose; 0.3 molar dextrose = 0.3 osmolar dextrose, or 300 mosm/L, an isotonic solution.

EXAMPLE 14

What is the osmolarity of 5.4 percent dextrose in 0.87 percent NaCl? As shown in Example 13, the osmotic pressure of 5.4 percent DW is 300 mosm/L.

$$0.87\% \text{ NaCl} = 8.7 \text{ g NaCl/L}$$

$$1 \text{ molar NaCl} = 58 \text{ g/L}$$

The molarity of

$$0.87\% \text{ NaCl} = \frac{8.7 \text{ g}}{L} \div \frac{58 \text{ g}}{mol} = \frac{8.7 \text{ g}}{L} \times \frac{mol}{58 \text{ g}} = \frac{0.15 \text{ mol}}{L}$$

One molar NaCl equals 2 osmolar NaCl. Each molecule ionizes into two ions. Therefore, 0.15 molar NaCl = 0.3 osmolar NaCl, or 300 mosm/L. The osmotic pressure of 5.4 percent dextrose in 0.87 percent NaCl is

$$\begin{array}{rl} 300 & \text{mosm of dextrose/L} \\ +300 & \text{mosm of NaCl/L} \\ \hline 600 & \text{mosm/L, a hypertonic solution} \end{array}$$

Because the osmotic pressure of body fluids is about 0.3 osm/L, it is necessary to calculate the percentages of all injectable solutions to be sure that they are compatible with the body fluids.

Molar solutions are not necessarily the same as osmolar solutions:

$$1 \text{ GMW/L dextrose} = 1 \text{ osmolar solution}$$

but

$$1 \text{ GMW/L NaCl} = 2 \text{ osmolar solution}$$

Therefore,

$$0.3 \text{ molar (or 0.3 osmolar) dextrose solution} = 0.3\,(180\,g)/L$$

$$= 54\,g/L = 5.4\% \text{ DW}, \quad \text{an isotonic solution}$$

And

$$0.3 \text{ molar NaCl} = 0.6 \text{ osmolar solution,}$$
$$\text{which is hypertonic}$$

$$0.15 \text{ molar (or 0.3 osmolar) NaCl} = 0.15(58\,g/L) = 8.7\,g/L$$

$$= 0.87\% \text{ NaCl,}$$
$$\text{an isotonic solution}$$

Normal Solutions. A 1 normal solution of any solute contains 1 GEW/L of solution; a 0.5 normal solution contains 0.5 GEW/L, or 0.5 mEq/ml of solution.

One GEW of NaCl weighs 58 g; 58 g NaCl/L = 5.8 percent NaCl. A 1 molar solution of NaCl equals a 1 normal solution of NaCl.

One GEW[2] of $CaCl_2$ weighs 55 g because it is a bivalent electrolyte. Therefore, a 1 normal solution of $CaCl_2$ contains 55 g/L, or 5.5 percent $CaCl_2$.

The concentration of a 1 normal solution of $CaCl_2$ is only half that of a 1 molar $CaCl_2$ solution, which weighs 110 g. Therefore, 0.5 molar $CaCl_2$ equals 1 normal $CaCl_2$.

Avogadro's Law and Solutions. Avogadro's law states that equal volumes of solutions of equal molarity contain the same number of moles and equal numbers of molecules. Avogadro's law is illustrated in Table 4–3. The table shows that ionizing solutions such as NaCl and $CaCl_2$ contain many more particles that exert osmotic pressure than do nonionizing solutions such as glucose.

The pH Concept

The number of hydrogen ions in 1 L of a solution is called the hydrogen ion concentration per liter, commonly abbreviated [H+]. The pH scale is used to simplify the expression of astronomic numbers of hydrogen ions. Hydrogen ions must be counted because it is the *number* of free H+ in a solution that determines its acidity: the more H+ in a solution, the more acid it is. There are 6.02×10^{23} atoms in 1 GAW (or 1 GEW) of hydrogen. The abbreviation pH means power of the hydrogen ion concentration. The pH is the power to which the number 10 must be raised to find the exact number of hydrogen ions that exist in a liter of a given solution. The pH of a solution is therefore an exponent of the number 10. The pH is also a logarithm because logarithms express powers of 10. (A log is the power to which the fixed number, 10, must be raised to produce a given number.) The pH of a solution is derived by converting the value of the [H+] to a single exponent of 10 by calculating its logarithm. The logarithm, or exponent of 10, of the [H+] will always be negative because the number of hydrogen ions being counted is a fraction of 1 GEW of hydrogen, that is, a fraction of 6.02×10^{23} hydrogen ions. (The log of a fraction is always negative.) To avoid the con-

stant use of a negative number, the sign of the negative exponent is arbitrarily changed to positive and called pH (see also Chapter 6).[1, 3]

Any one of the following equations can be used to find the pH of a solution:

$$\text{pH} = -\log \text{ of the } [H^+] \tag{1}$$
$$\text{pH} = \log 1/[H^+] \tag{2}$$
$$\text{pH} = \log \text{ of the } [H^+] \text{ expressed as a positive number} \tag{3}$$

To find the [H+] of a solution when the pH is known:

$$[H^+] = 1 \times 10^{-\text{pH}} \text{ Eq of hydrogen/L} \tag{4}$$
$$[H^+] = 1/10^{\text{pH}} \text{ Eq of hydrogen/L} \tag{5}$$

To find the pH of pure water:

$$[H^+] \text{ of pure water} = 1 \times 10^{-7} \text{ Eq/L}$$
$$= 0.000\,000\,1 \text{ Eq/L}$$

Using Eq. 1,

$$\log (0.000\,000\,1) = -7$$
$$\text{pH} = -(-7)$$
$$\text{pH of water} = +7$$

Using Eq. 2,

$$\text{pH} = \log 1/0.000\,000\,1$$
$$\text{pH} = \log 10\,000\,000 = 7$$

Using Eq. 3,

$$\log (0.000\,000\,1) = -7$$
$$\text{pH of water} = +7$$

Using Eq. 4,

$$[H^+] \text{ of water} = 1 \times 10^{-7} \text{ Eq of hydrogen/L}$$
$$[H^+] \text{ of water} = 0.000\,000\,1 \text{ Eq/L}$$

TABLE 4–3. AVOGADRO'S LAW AND SOLUTIONS[a]

	1 M solutions			
NaCl				*Glucose*
1 L H_2O 1 GMW 1 mol NaCl	Volume (1 L) 1 GMW (1 mol) 58 g/L 5.8% (5.8 g/100 mL) 6.02×10^{23} molecules 12.04×10^{23} ions or particles	= = ≠ ≠ = ≠	Volume (1 L) 1 GMW (1 mol) 180 g/L 18% (18 g/100 mL) 6.02×10^{23} molecules Does not ionize	1 L H_2O 1 GMW 1 mol glucose
	0.5 M solutions			
$CaCl_2$				*Glucose*
1 L H_2O 0.5 GMW 0.5 mol $CaCl_2$	Volume (1 L) 0.5 GMW (0.5 mol) 55 g/L 5.5% 3.01×10^{23} molecules 9.03×10^{23} ions or particles	= = ≠ ≠ = ≠	Volume (1 L) 0.5 GMW (0.5 mol) 90 g/L 9.0% 3.01×10^{23} molecules Does not ionize	1 L H_2O 0.5 GMW 0.5 mol glucose

[a] Equal volumes of solutions of equal molarity contain the same number of moles (GMW) and equal numbers of molecules (Avogadro's law). Reprinted, with permission, from Waterhouse.[1]

Using Eq. 5,

$$[H^+] \text{ of water} = 1/10,000,000 \text{ Eq/L} = 0.000\ 000\ 1 \text{ Eq/L}$$

Pure water is neutral. This means that it is neither acidic nor basic. There are identical numbers of H^+ and hydroxyl ions $(OH)^-$, in pure water (Table 4–4).

$$0.000\ 000\ 1 \text{Eq } H^+ + 0.000\ 000\ 1 \text{Eq } (OH)^-$$

$$\rightarrow 0.000\ 000\ 1 \text{Eq } H(OH)$$

pH of Acids and Bases. The hydrogen ion concentration of an acid is greater than 0.000 000 1 Eq/L. Because pH is, in reality, a negative number, the pH of acids is always less than 7. A solution with more free hydrogen ions than pure water is acidic. If it has an $[H^+]$ of 8.7×10^{-6} (or 0.000 008 7) Eq/L, it has a higher $[H^+]$ than pure water. Therefore it is an acidic solution. Its pH is 5.06, a value less than 7, signifying an acid solution. Because the $[H^+]$ of a base is less than 0.000 000 1 Eq/L, the pH of a base is always more than 7. If a solution has an $[H^+]$ of 6.7×10^{-9} (or 0.000 000 006 7) Eq/L, it has a lower $[H^+]$ than pure water. It is an alkaline solution with a pH of 8.17, a value greater than 7.

Blood pH. Normal $[H^+]$ of human blood is 0.000 000 040 Eq/L, or 40 nanoequivalents (nEq)/L, or 4×10^{-8} Eq/L. To express the pH of blood, any one of the above equations may be used.

Using Eq. 1,

$$\text{pH of blood} = -(\log 0.000\ 000\ 04)$$

$$\text{pH of blood} = -(-7.4)$$

$$= +7.4$$

Using Eq. 2,

$$\text{pH of blood} = \log 1/0.000\ 000\ 04$$

$$= \log 25\ 000\ 000$$

$$\text{pH of blood} = 7.4$$

TABLE 4–4. pH SCALE ILLUSTRATING THE RELATIONSHIP BETWEEN [H⁺], pH, AND [(OH)⁻]

When: [H⁺] =	pH =	[(OH)⁻] =
1.0 GEW/L of free H⁺	0	0.000,000,000,000,01 Eq/L
0.1	1	0.000,000,000,000,1
0.01	2	0.000,000,000,001
0.001	3	0.000,000,000,01
0.000,1	4	0.000,000,000,1
0.000,01	5	0.000,000,001
0.000,001	6	0.000,000,01
0.000,000,1	7	0.000,000,1
0.000,000,04	7.4	0.000,000,25
0.000,000,01	8	0.000,001
0.000,000,001	9	0.000,01
0.000,000,000,1	10	0.000,1
0.000,000,000,01	11	0.001
0.000,000,000,001	12	0.01
0.000,000,000,000,1	13	0.1
0.000,000,000,000,01 Eq/L	14	1.0 GEW/L of free (OH)⁻

Using Eq. 3,

$$\text{pH of blood} = \log 0.000\ 000\ 04 \text{ expressed as a positive number}$$

$$= \log 0.000\ 000\ 04 = -7.4$$

$$\text{pH of blood} = +7.4$$

Equations 4 and 5 *prove* that the pH of blood is 7.4.

Using Eq. 4,

$$[H^+] \text{ of blood} = 1 \times 10^{-7.4} \text{ Eq/L} = 0.000\ 000\ 04 \text{ Eq/L}$$

Using Eq. 5,

$$[H^+] \text{ of blood} = 1/10^{7.4} \text{ Eq/L} = 1/25,118,864 \text{ Eq/L}$$

$$[H^+] \text{ of blood} = 0.000\ 000\ 04 \text{ Eq/L}$$

Because the pH of blood is greater than 7, the $[H^+]$ of blood is less than that of water, so blood is slightly alkaline.

pH of Normal Solutions of HCl. The $[H^+]$ of 1.0 normal solution of HCl is 1 Eq/L.

$$\text{pH of 1.0 normal HCl} = \log 1/1.0 = \log 1 = 0$$

$$[H^+] \text{ of 0.1 normal HCl} = 0.1 \text{ Eq/L}$$

$$\text{pH of 0.1 normal HCl} = \log 1/0.1 = \log 10 = 1$$

$$[H^+] \text{ of 0.01 normal HCl} = 0.01 \text{ Eq/L}$$

$$\text{pH of 0.01 normal HCl} = \log 1/0.01 = \log 100 = 2$$

$$[H^+] \text{ of 0.000 000 1 normal HCl} = 0.000\ 000\ 1 \text{ Eq/L}$$

$$\text{pH of 0,000\ 000\ 1 Eq/L HCl} = \log 1/0.000\ 000\ 1$$

$$= \log 10,000,000 = 7$$

Summary of pH Concept. The relationships between $[H^+]$, pH, and $[(OH)^-]$ are illustrated in Table 4–4.

1. pH is an exponent of 10 used to express the $[H^+]$. It is the log of the $[H^+]$ expressed as a positive number.
2. Table 4–4 shows that, at a pH of 7, both the $[H^+]$ and the $[(OH)^-]$ have the same value. The solution is neither acidic nor basic. It is a neutral solution.
3. A *decrease* of 1.0 on the pH scale means that the $[H^+]$ has been multiplied by 10. For example, if the pH of a solution is 4, the $[H^+]$ is 10 times greater than that of a solution with a pH of 5. If the pH of a solution is 9, the $[H^+]$ is 100 times less than that of a solution with a pH of 7.
4. The $[H^+]$ multiplied by the $[(OH)^-]$ always has 14 decimal places.

$$[H^+] \times [(OH)^-] = 1 \times 10^{-14} = 0.000\ 000\ 000\ 000\ 01$$

Application of pH to Human Life. The range of $[H^+]$ compatible with human life is extremely narrow. Table 4–5 shows that the pH range compatible with human life lies between 6.8 and 7.8, with a *normal* range of 7.35 to 7.45. Note that a solution with a pH of 6.8 contains ten times as many hydrogen ions as does a solution with a pH of 7.8.

The pH concept is widely used in science and medicine today. If the mathematics behind its use is understood, it can be very useful as a tool for interpreting blood gases,

TABLE 4–5. pH SCALE AND HUMAN LIFE

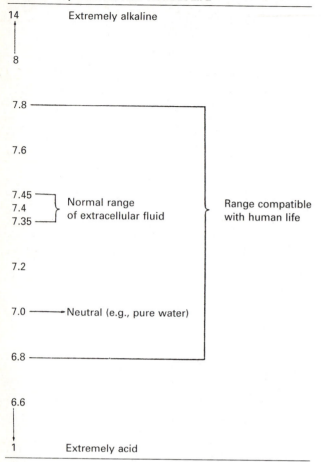

Reprinted, with permission, from Waterhouse.[1]

pulmonary function studies, respiratory care, and some laboratory or diagnostic studies. The pH must also be considered in the manufacture of drugs and of the solutions used in all fields of medicine and biologic science.[1]

ANESTHETIC VAPORIZER CALCULATIONS

A thorough mastery of the physics of gases and vapors is essential before the mathematics behind anesthetic vaporizer calculations can be understood.[4–6]

Vaporizer flowmeters are designed specifically to direct oxygen through volatile anesthetic agent vaporizers. These vaporizer flowmeters may indicate either the milliliters per minute, expressed as cubic centimeters per minute, of saturated anesthetic *vapor* that emerges *from* the vaporizer or the amount of *oxygen* flow (cc/min) *into* the vaporizer. It is imperative that the anesthetist fully understand the calculations involved for each type of flowmeter because the results are very different. The accompanying vapor pressure–temperature graph (Fig. 4–4)[6] illustrates the varying vapor pressure–temperature curves for enflurane, halothane, and isoflurane. This discussion will include examples for calculating various concentrations of these three agents when using each type of vaporizer.

Direct-Metering Vaporization (Ohio Heidbrink DM 5000 Anesthesia Machines)

Direct-metering vaporizer flowmeters are calibrated to indicate, in cubic centimeters per minute, the amount of anesthetic *vapor* that is being introduced into the patient's circuit. Part or all of the life-sustaining (diluent) oxygen is diverted into the vaporizer, picks up the vapor, and conducts it to join the total mixture of anesthetic gases. The oxygen that is diverted into the vaporizer comes out 100 percent saturated with the agent at 23C to 24C. The vaporizer is heated to ensure a stable temperature.[4,7]

The total output of the DM 5000 Ohio vaporizer is the sum of the flowmeter readings. The agent concentration is the direct ratio of the vaporized agent flow rate to the total flow rate of agent, oxygen, and other diluent gases. (See the manufacturer's literature for a discussion of computing agent concentrations at ambient temperature extremes or change in altitude.)[5] Anesthetic vaporizer percentages and flow rates can be calculated just as easily as the drugs and solutions discussed in the first section of this chapter. Use a table, such as Table 4–1, substituting a column for

$$\frac{\text{cc/min vapor flow rate}}{\text{cc/min total flow rate}}$$

in place of mg/mL.

Calculating Percentages Using a Direct-Metering Machine at 24C

EXAMPLE 15

What percentage halothane (or any volatile agent such as enflurane, isoflurane, and methoxyflurane) is being conducted to the patient when the vaporizer flow rate is 100 cc/min halothane vapor, and the diluent gas flow rates are 2500 cc/min nitrous oxide and 2500 cc/min oxygen?

Step 1: Make a table such as Table 4–1.

$$\frac{100 \text{ cc/min halothane vapor}}{5000 \text{ cc/min} + 100 \text{ cc/min, total flow}}$$

$$= \tfrac{1}{51} \text{ (the fraction) or } 1:51 \text{ (the ratio)}$$

(For practical purposes, round figures are used. This machine setting would be a 1:50 concentration. Only when very high flow rates are required would the additional gas add significantly to the total flow rate, and it should then be included in the calculations. See Example 25.)

Step 2:

$$\tfrac{1}{50} = 0.02, \quad \text{the decimal}$$

Step 3: Percent means per hundred. Thus,

$$0.02 \times 100 = 2\%$$

Answer

Two percent halothane is being conducted to the patient.

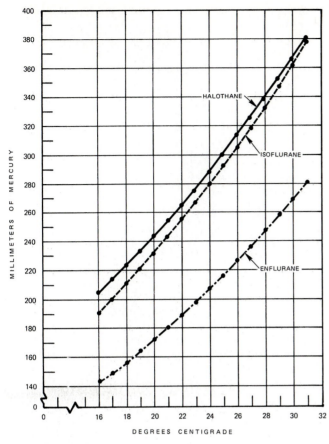

ANTOINE EQUATIONS
USED FOR GRAPH

HALOTHANE ———————

$$LOG_{10} p = 6.76799 - \frac{1043.697}{t + 218.262}$$

ISOFLURANE – – – – – – –

$$LOG_{10} p = 5.69778 - \frac{536.4589}{t + 140.991}$$

ENFLURANE –·–·–·–·–·–

$$LOG_{10} p = 6.98840 - \frac{1107.839}{t + 213.063}$$

Figure 4–4. Vapor pressure–temperature graph for enflurane, halothane, and isoflurane.

EXAMPLE 16

What percentage halothane (or any volatile agent, such as enflurane and isoflurane) is being conducted to the patient when the vaporizer flow rate is 100 cc/min halothane vapor, and the diluent gas flow rates total 6 L/min?

Step 1: Determine the ratio or fraction.

$$\frac{100 \,cc/min \,vapor}{6000 \,cc/min + 100 \,cc/min \,vapor}$$

Step 2: Reduced, the fraction is ⅟₆₀ or 0.016, the decimal.

Step 3: The percent is 0.016 × 100, or 1.6%.

Answer

Percentage halothane = 1.6.

EXAMPLE 17

What percentage halothane is being conducted to the patient when the vaporizer flow rate is 40 cc/min and the diluent gas flow rates total 4 L/min?

Step 1: The ratio or fraction is

$$\frac{40 \,cc/min \,vapor}{4000 \,cc/min + 40 \,cc/min \,vapor} = \frac{1}{100}$$

Step 2: The decimal is 0.01.

Step 3: The percent is 0.01 × 100 or 1%.

Answer

One percent halothane is being conducted to the patient.

Calculating Vaporizer Flow Rates Using a Direct-Metering Machine at 24C. It is often necessary to calculate the agent flow rate for a desired concentration and diluent flow rate.

Step 1: Convert the percentage to a decimal, as in Table 4–1.

Step 2: Multiply the decimal by the total flow rate.

EXAMPLE 18

What should the cubic centimeter-per-minute agent flow rate be when a 2 percent enflurane concentration is desired with a 5 L/min diluent flow rate?

Step 1:

$$2\% = 0.02, \text{ the decimal}$$

$$(2\% \text{ means } ^2\!/_{100} = 2 \div 100 = 0.02)$$

Step 2:

$$\text{Enflurane flow rate} = 0.02 \times 5000 \text{ cc/min}$$

$$= 100 \text{ cc/min}$$

Answer

The flow rate should be 100 cc/min.

EXAMPLE 19

What should the vaporizer flow rate be when a 1.5 percent enflurane concentration is desired with a 6 L/min diluent flow rate?

Step 1:

$$1.5\% = 0.015$$

Step 2:

$$\text{Enflurane flow rate} = 0.015 \times 6000 \text{ cc/min}$$

$$= 90 \text{ cc/min}$$

Answer

The vaporizer flow rate should be 90 cc/min.

EXAMPLE 20

What should the vaporizer flow rate be when 1 percent isoflurane concentration is desired with a 4 L/min diluent gas flow rate?

Step 1:

$$1\% = 0.01$$

Step 2:

$$\text{Isoflurane flow rate} = 0.01 \times 4000 \text{ cc/min}$$

$$= 40 \text{ cc/min}$$

Answer

The vaporizer flow rate should be 40 cc/min.

Carrier Oxygen Vaporizer Flowmeters (Classic Verni-Trol and Side-Arm Vaporizers)

There are several differences between the direct-metering vaporizer just discussed and the Ohio 2000 machine and Side-Arm Verni-Trol anesthetic vaporizer (Fig. 4–5).[5,7]

1. Some vaporizers are heated to maintain a 23C to 25C temperature; some are not heated.
2. Vaporizer flowmeters have a separate oxygen source; they do not use part of the diluent oxygen.
3. Vaporizer flowmeters indicate the amount of oxygen flowing into the vaporizer, *not* the amount of anesthetic vapor coming out of it.
4. The anesthetist must calculate the cubic centimeters per minute of actual vapor coming out of the vaporizer into the patient's circuit.

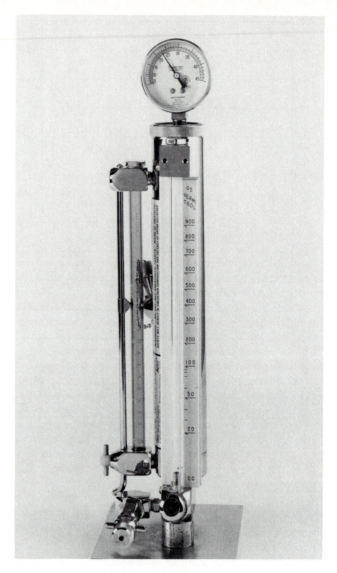

Figure 4–5. Ohio Side-Arm Verni-Trol Anesthetic Vaporizer. (*Courtesy of Anaquest, BOC, Madison, Wisconsin.*)

Calculating Percentages Using the Side-Arm or Classic Verni-Trol Machine at 24C. Refer to a vapor pressure–temperature graph for the agent in use. Assume, in the following examples, that the vaporizer temperature is about 24C. Read the vapor pressure of the agent for that temperature. This vapor pressure (VP), divided by the ambient pressure (AP) (which is 760 mm Hg at sea level) minus the vapor pressure, equals the fraction of the carrier oxygen flow rate that is pure vapor being carried into the patient's circuit. This relationship expressed as an equation is

$$\frac{\text{VP}}{\text{AP} - \text{VP}} = \begin{array}{l}\text{fraction of carrier oxygen flow rate} \\ \text{that is pure vapor carried}\end{array}$$

Halothane. The vapor pressure of halothane at 24C is 288 mm Hg (see Fig. 4–4). Thus,

$$\frac{288 \text{ mm Hg}}{760 \text{ mm Hg} - 288 \text{ mm Hg}} = \frac{288 \text{ mm Hg}}{472 \text{ mm Hg}} = 0.6$$

This equation shows that every cubic centimeter of oxygen flowing into the halothane vaporizer carries 0.6 cc of pure halothane vapor out of the vaporizer with it.

EXAMPLE 21

What percentage halothane is being conducted to the patient when the carrier oxygen flow rate through the vaporizer is 100 cc/min, and the diluent gas flow rates total 5 L/min?

Step 1: 0.6 × 100 cc/min = 60 cc/min of halothane vapor being carried by the 100 cc of oxygen. The total amount of gas emerging from the vaporizer is 100 cc of oxygen plus 60 cc of halothane vapor, or 160 cc/min.

Step 2: Once the amount of actual vapor has been established, the rest of the calculations are identical to those discussed earlier for the direct-metering vaporizers; that is, the agent concentration is the direct ratio of the agent flow rate, just calculated, to the total flow rate. Make a table to determine the fraction or ratio.

$$\frac{60 \text{ cc/min halothane vapor}}{5000 \text{ cc/min} + 100 \text{ cc/min oxygen} + 60 \text{ cc/min vapor}}$$

$$= \frac{60 \text{ cc/min}}{5160 \text{ cc/min}} = 0.0116$$

Step 3: Percent = 0.0116 × 100 = 1.16%, or about 1.2%.

Answer

The percentage halothane being conducted to the patient is about 1.2. (The same answer will be obtained if round figures are used:

$$\frac{60 \text{ cc/min}}{5000 \text{ cc/min}} = 0.012; \quad 0.012 \times 100 = 1.2\%).$$

Compare this answer with that for Example 15.

EXAMPLE 22

What percentage halothane is being conducted to the patient when the carrier oxygen flow rate through the vaporizer is 80 cc/min, and the diluent gas flow rates total 6 L/min?

Step 1: Calculate the amount of halothane vapor 80 cc of oxygen will carry at 24C.

0.6 × 80 cc = 48 cc halothane vapor carried by 80 cc of oxygen

Step 2:

$$\frac{48 \text{ cc/min}}{6000 \text{ cc/min} + 80 \text{ cc/min} + 48 \text{ cc/min}}$$

$$= \frac{48}{6128} = 0.0078$$

Step 3: Percent = 0.0078 × 100 = 0.78%, or about 0.8%.

Answer

The percentage halothane being conducted to the patient is about 0.8. (The same answer will be obtained if round figures are used: 48 cc/min ÷ 6000 cc/min = 0.008; 0.008 × 100 = 0.8%.)

EXAMPLE 23

What percentage of halothane is being conducted to the patient when the carrier oxygen flow rate through the vaporizer is 40 cc/min, and the diluent gas flow rates total 4 L/min?

Step 1: 0.6 × 40 cc = 24 cc halothane vapor carried by 40 cc of oxygen at 24C.

Step 2:

$$\frac{24 \text{ cc/min}}{4000 \text{ cc/min} + 40 \text{ cc/min} + 24 \text{ cc/min}}$$

$$= \frac{24}{4064} = 0.0059$$

Step 3: Percent = 0.0059 × 100 = 0.59%, or about 0.6%.

Compare this answer with that for Example 17.

Enflurane. The vapor pressure of enflurane at 24C is 207 mm Hg (see Fig. 4–4).

$$\frac{VP}{AP - VP} = \text{fraction of carrier oxygen flow rate that is pure vapor carried}$$

$$\frac{207 \text{ mm Hg}}{760 \text{ mm Hg} - 207 \text{ mm Hg}} \quad \frac{207}{553} = 0.37$$

Thus, every cubic centimeter of oxygen flowing into the enflurane vaporizer carries 0.37 cc of pure enflurane vapor out of the vaporizer with it.

EXAMPLE 24

What percentage enflurane is being conducted to the patient when the carrier oxygen flow rate through the vaporizer is 250 cc/min, and the diluent flow rates total 5000 cc/min?

Step 1: 0.37 × 250 cc/min = 93 cc/min enflurane vapor carried by the 250 cc of carrier oxygen. The total amount of gas emerging from the vaporizer is 250 cc/min carrier oxygen plus 93 cc/min enflurane vapor, or 343 cc/min.

Step 2: The enflurane concentration is the direct ratio of the agent flow rate to the total flow rate. The percentage of enflurane equals this direct ratio times 100.

% Enflurane

$$= \frac{93 \text{ cc/min} \times 100}{5000 \text{ cc/min} + 250 \text{ cc/min} + 93 \text{ cc/min}}$$

$$= \frac{9300 \text{ cc/min}}{5343 \text{ cc/min}}$$

$$= 1.74\%$$

Answer

The percentage enflurane being conducted to the patient is 1.74. (If round figures had been used, 9300/5000 = 1.9%.)

EXAMPLE 25

What percentage enflurane is being conducted to the patient when the carrier oxygen flow rate is 700 cc/min, and the diluent flow rates total 6000 cc/min?

> *Step 1:* 0.37×700 cc/min = 259 cc/min enflurane vapor carried by the 700 cc of carrier oxygen. The total amount of gas emerging from the vaporizer is 700 cc/min carrier oxygen plus 259 cc/min enflurane vapor, or 959 cc/min.
>
> *Step 2:*

$$\% \text{ Enflurane}$$

$$= \frac{259 \text{ cc/min} \times 100}{6000 \text{ cc/min} + 700 \text{ cc/min} + 259 \text{ cc/min}}$$

$$= \frac{25,900 \text{ cc/min}}{6,959 \text{ cc/min}}$$

$$= 3.7\%$$

Answer

The percentage enflurane being conducted to the patient is 3.7. (If round figures had been used, 25,900/6000 = 4.3%. This equation illustrates a situation where accurate calculations should be made. The difference between accurate calculations and round figures is too great to be ignored.)

Calculating Vaporizer Flow Rates for Desired Percentages, Using the Side-Arm or Classic Verni-Trol Machine at 24C

Halothane. Because, at 24C, each cubic centimeter of carrier oxygen from the Side-Arm vaporizer picks up 6/10 cc of halothane vapor, the carrier oxygen flow rate must be 10/6 times that of the vapor actually carried.

EXAMPLE 26

What should the carrier oxygen flow rate be when a 1 percent halothane concentration and a 4 L/min diluent gas flow rate are desired?

> *Step 1:*
$$1\% = 0.01$$
$$= 0.01 \times 4000 \text{ cc/min}$$
$$= 40 \text{ cc/min halothane vapor}$$
> *Step 2:*

$$\text{Carrier oxygen flow rate}$$
$$= 10/6 \times 40 \text{ cc/min halothane vapor}$$
$$= \frac{400 \text{ cc/min}}{6} = 66 \text{ cc/min}$$

Answer

The carrier oxygen flow rate should be 66 cc/min.

Proof

As each cubic centimeter of oxygen carries 0.6 cc of halothane vapor,

$$66 \text{ cc oxygen} \times 0.6 = 40 \text{ cc/min halothane vapor}$$

$$\% = \frac{40 \text{ cc halothane vapor/min} \times 100}{4000 \text{ cc/min} + 66 \text{ cc oxygen/min} + 40 \text{ cc vapor/min}}$$

$$= \frac{4000 \text{ cc/min}}{4106 \text{ cc/min}}$$

$$= 0.97\%, \text{ or about } 1\%$$

EXAMPLE 27

What should the carrier oxygen flow rate be when a 1.5 percent halothane concentration and a 6 L/min diluent gas flow rate are desired?

> *Step 1:*
$$1.5\% = 0.015$$
$$= 6000 \text{ cc/min} \times 0.015 = 90 \text{ cc/min}$$
> *Step 2:*
$$\text{Carrier oxygen flow rate} = 10/6 \times 90 \text{ cc/min}$$
$$= 150 \text{ cc/min}$$

Answer

The carrier oxygen flow rate should be 150 cc/min.

Proof

As each cubic centimeter of oxygen carries 0.6 cc of halothane vapor,

$$150 \text{ cc oxygen} \times 0.6 = 90 \text{ cc halothane vapor}$$

$$\% = \frac{90 \text{ cc halothane vapor/min} \times 100}{6000 \text{ cc/min} + 150 \text{ cc/min} + 90 \text{ cc/min}}$$

$$= \frac{9000 \text{ cc/min}}{6240 \text{ cc/min}} = 1.44\%$$

(If round figures had been used:

$$\% = \frac{9000 \text{ cc/min}}{6000 \text{ cc/min}} = 1.5\%.)$$

Enflurane. Because, at 24C, each cubic centimeter of carrier oxygen from the Side-Arm vaporizer picks up 37/100 cc of enflurane vapor, carrier oxygen flow rate must be 100/37 times that of the vapor actually carried. (See the discussion on enflurane between Examples 23 and 24.)

EXAMPLE 28

What should the carrier oxygen flow rate be when a 1.5 percent enflurane concentration is desired with a 6 L/min diluent flow rate?

Step 1:

$$1.5\% = 0.015$$

$$= 0.015 \times 6000 \text{ cc/min} = 90 \text{ cc/min}$$

Step 2:

Carrier oxygen flow rate

$$= 100 / 37 \times 90 \text{ cc/min}$$

$$= (9000 \text{ cc/min})/37 = 243 \text{ cc/min}$$

Answer

The carrier oxygen flow rate should be 243 cc/min. Compare this answer with that for Example 19.

Proof

As each cubic centimeter of oxygen carries 0.37 cc of enflurane vapor,

$$243 \text{ cc of oxygen} \times 0.37$$

$$= 90 \text{ cc of enflurane vapor}$$

$$\% = \frac{90 \text{ cc/min enflurane vapor} \times 100}{6000 \text{ cc/min} + 243 \text{ cc/min} + 90 \text{ cc/min}}$$

$$= \frac{9000 \text{ cc/min}}{6333 \text{ cc/min}} = 1.42\%, \text{ accurate answer}$$

(If round figures had been used:

$$\% = \frac{90 \text{ cc/min enflurane vapor} \times 100}{6000 \text{ cc/min}} = 1.5\%.)$$

EXAMPLE 29

What should the carrier oxygen flow rate be when a 3.5 percent enflurane concentration is desired with a 5 L/min diluent flow rate?

Step 1:

$$3.5\% = 0.035$$

$$= 0.035 \times 5000 \text{ cc/min} = 175 \text{ cc/min}$$

Step 2:

$$\text{Carrier oxygen flow rate} = \frac{100}{37} \times 175 \text{ cc/min}$$

$$= \frac{17,500 \text{ cc/min}}{37}$$

$$= 473 \text{ cc/min}$$

Answer

The carrier oxygen flow rate should be 473 cc/min.

Proof

As each cubic centimeter of oxygen carries 0.37 cc of enflurane vapor,

$$473 \text{ cc of oxygen} \times 0.37$$

$$= 175 \text{ cc of enflurane vapor}$$

% Enflurane

$$= \frac{175 \text{ cc/min enflurane vapor} \times 100}{5000 \text{ cc/min} + 473 \text{ cc/min} + 175 \text{ cc/min}}$$

$$= \frac{17,500 \text{ cc/min}}{5,648 \text{ cc/min}} = 3.1\%, \text{ accurate answer}$$

(If round figures had been used:

$$\% = \frac{175 \text{ cc/min enflurane vapor} \times 100}{5000 \text{ cc/min}} = 3.5\%.)$$

Isoflurane. The vapor pressure of isoflurane at 24C is 280 mm Hg (see Fig. 4–4).

$$\frac{280 \text{ mm Hg}}{760 \text{ mm Hg} - 280 \text{ mm Hg}} = \frac{280 \text{ mm Hg}}{480 \text{ mm Hg}} = 0.583, \text{ or } 0.6$$

This equation shows that every cubic centimeter of oxygen flowing into the isoflurane vaporizer carries about 0.6 cc of pure isoflurane vapor out of the vaporizer with it. The vapor pressure curve of isoflurane is so close to that of halothane that, for practical purposes, isoflurane calculations for the Side-Arm or classic Verni-Trol vaporizers are the same as those for halothane. Anesthetists who use other well-known agents should be able to calculate percentages and agent flow rates through various vaporizers by referring to appropriate vapor pressure–temperature graphs, such as in Fig. 4–4.

REFERENCES

1. Waterhouse M. *Practical mathematics in allied health.* Baltimore: Urban & Schwarzenberg; 1979:21–35, 65–85.
2. Guyton AC. *Textbook of medical physiology.* Philadelphia: WB Saunders; 1991:44–46.
3. Wylie WD, Churchill-Davidson HC. *A practice of anaesthesia.* Chicago: Year Book Medical; 1984:570.
4. Miller RD. *Anesthesia.* New York: Churchill Livingstone; 1990:184–194.
5. *Operation and maintenance manuals, Heidbrink series 2000 and series DM 5000.* Madison, WI: Ohio Medical Products; 1978.
6. Rogers RC, Hill GE. Equations for vapor-pressure versus temperature deviation and uses of the Antoine equation on a hand-held programmable calculator. *Br J Anaesth.* 1978;50:415–430.
7. Hill DW. *Physics applied to anesthesia.* Boston: Butterworths; 1980:260, 336–337.

Principles of Chemistry and Physics in Anesthesia

Leo A. Le Bel

Physics and chemistry help us to understand the fundamental processes by which nature operates. This chapter addresses those science concepts and principles that impact daily anesthesia practice; a sound understanding of them is required of all nurse anesthetists. The distinction between chemistry and physics often becomes blurred, because we now have a better appreciation of the fact that the two disciplines share many common processes. This frequently makes it difficult to organize concepts logically. As with the first edition, this edition tries to group related concepts and at the same time maintain a traditional approach by separating concepts primarily on their association with either physics or chemistry. The important point to remember is that many concepts are valid for both sciences.

GENERAL CONCEPTS

Every material item possessing mass and occupying space represents a form of *matter*. Matter exists in three states: gases, liquids, and solids. All matter is composed of one or more basic parts referred to as *elements* (Table 5–1). Eighty-eight elements occur naturally. Some, most radioactive substances for instance, occur only under specific conditions. Of the naturally occurring elements, most are solids, 11 are gases, and 2 are liquids. Twenty elements are commonly abundant and 15 occur in the body. Elements cannot normally be further decomposed. When two or more elements are chemically combined, the substance is referred to as a *compound*.

Mass designates the quantity of matter and is generally characterized in terms of weight units (e.g., ounces, pounds, grams). *Weight*, however, is a measure of the forces of attraction between two bodies (e.g., you and the earth or you and the moon), expressed in terms of a scale—pounds. That is, you have a different weight depending on whether you are standing on earth or on the moon. This is because the frame of reference between you and the two objects is different.

Because the masses of the earth and moon are different, your weight (mass) compared with each of them varies.

This force of attraction between two bodies is called *gravity*. It varies inversely with the square of the distance between the two objects. Gravity is a basic force in nature. Other forces we commonly observe include mechanical, electrical, and chemical energy. Force is merely one way of talking about energy.

Energy is defined as the ability to do work or ability to produce a change in matter. *Work* is performed when a force is exerted over a distance, such as moving a weight of 1 g a distance of 1 cm. Converting water to steam, a change in matter, also requires energy. Energy is thought of in two forms: *kinetic energy*, which is energy in motion, and *latent energy*, which is energy stored for later use.

Applying some form of energy to matter can result in either a physical or a chemical change. An example from anesthesia practice is the vaporization of a liquid to a gas by the application of heat. This represents a *physical change*. The state, but not the composition, of the substance is changed. In a *chemical change* a new substance is formed.

What force does depends on the form of the force (heat, gravity, etc.) and the manner in which it is applied to matter. For example, force may displace a stable object, accelerate a moving object, or change the direction (vector) of a moving object. The basic units of measurement for force are the dyne and the newton; they are defined as follows:

Dyne (dyn): Force required to move a 1 - g mass 1 cm/s.

Newton (N): Force required to move a 1 - kg mass 1 m/s.

Note that each is defined in terms of moving a mass of given weight, a given distance, in a specified unit of time. Movement over a given distance in a specified time is called *acceleration*. Thus, the general formula for force can be expressed as

$$\text{Force } (f) = \text{mass } (m) \times \text{acceleration } (a)$$

The force required to expand the lungs of an anesthetized patient can be expressed in terms of dynes, although it is

TABLE 5–1. TABLE OF ELEMENTS: INTERNATIONAL ATOMIC WEIGHTS BASED ON CARBON–12 ISOTOPE[a]

Name	Symbol	Atomic Number	Atomic Weight	Name	Symbol	Atomic Number	Atomic Weight
Actinium	Ac	89	(227)	Mendelevium	Md	101	(256)
Aluminum	Al	13	26.98154	Mercury	Hg	80	200.59
Americium	Am	95	(243)	Molybdenum	Mo	42	95.94
Antimony	Sb	51	121.75	Neodymium	Nd	60	144.24
Argon	Ar	18	39.948	Neon	Ne	10	20.179
Arsenic	As	33	74.9216	Neptunium	Np	93	237.0482
Astatine	At	85	(210)	Nickel	Ni	28	58.71
Barium	Ba	56	137.34	Niobium	Nb	41	92.9064
Berkelium	Bk	97	(247)	Nitrogen	N	7	14.0067
Beryllium	Be	4	9.0118	Nobelium	No	102	(254)
Bismuth	Bi	83	208.9804	Osmium	Os	76	190.2
Boron	B	5	10.81	Oxygen	O	8	15.9994
Bromine	Br	35	79.904	Palladium	Pd	46	106.4
Cadmium	Cd	48	112.40	Phosphorus	P	15	30.97376
Calcium	Ca	20	40.08	Platinum	Pt	78	195.09
Californium	Cf	98	(251)	Plutonium	Pu	94	(242)
Carbon	C	6	12.011	Polonium	Po	84	(210)
Cerium	Ce	58	140.12	Potassium	K	19	39.098
Cesium	Cs	55	132.9054	Praseodymium	Pr	59	140.9077
Chlorine	Cl	17	35.453	Promethium	Pm	61	(145)
Chromium	Cr	24	51.996	Protactinium	Pa	91	231.0359
Cobalt	Co	27	58.9332	Radium	Ra	88	226.0254
Copper	Cu	29	63.546	Radon	Rn	86	(222)
Curium	Cm	96	(247)	Rhenium	Re	75	186.2
Dysprosium	Dy	66	162.50	Rhodium	Rh	45	102.9055
Einsteinium	Es	99	(254)	Rubidium	Rb	37	85.4678
Erbium	Er	68	167.26	Ruthenium	Ru	44	101.07
Europium	Eu	63	151.96	Samarium	Sm	62	150.4
Fermium	Fm	100	(253)	Scandium	Sc	21	44.9559
Fluorine	F	9	18.99840	Selenium	Se	34	78.96
Francium	Fr	87	(223)	Silicon	Si	14	28.086
Gadolinium	Gd	64	157.25	Silver	Ag	47	107.868
Gallium	Ga	31	69.72	Sodium	Na	11	22.98977
Germanium	Ge	32	72.59	Strontium	Sr	38	87.62
Gold	Au	79	196.9665	Sulfur	S	16	32.06
Hafnium	Hf	72	178.49	Tantalum	Ta	73	180.9479
Hahnium	Ha	105	(260)	Technetium	Tc	43	98.9062
Helium	He	2	4.00260	Tellurium	Te	52	127.60
Holmium	Ho	67	164.9304	Terbium	Tb	65	158.9254
Hydrogen	H	1	1.0079	Thallium	Tl	81	204.37
Indium	In	49	114.82	Thorium	Th	90	232.0381
Iodine	I	53	126.9045	Thulium	Tm	69	168.9342
Iridium	Ir	77	192.22	Tin	Sn	50	118.69
Iron	Fe	26	55.847	Titanium	Ti	22	47.90
Krypton	Kr	36	83.80	Tungsten	W	74	183.85
Lanthanum	La	57	138.9055	Uranium	U	92	238.029
Lawrencium	Lr	103	(257)	Vanadium	V	23	50.9414
Lead	Pb	82	207.2	Xenon	Xe	54	131.30
Lithium	Li	3	6.941	Ytterbium	Yb	70	173.04
Lutetium	Lu	71	174.97	Yttrium	Y	39	88.9059
Magnesium	Mg	12	24.305	Zinc	Zn	30	65.38
Manganese	Mn	25	54.9380	Zirconium	Zr	40	91.22

[a] Number in parentheses is the mass number of the most stable isotope of that element.
Reprinted, with permission, from King GB, Caldwell WE, et al. College chemistry. *7th ed. Belmont, CA: Litton (division of Wadsworth); 1977.*

more common to express it as centimeters of water pressure:

$$1 \text{ cm H}_2\text{O} = (\text{approx.}) \ 980.7 \text{ dyn}$$

Therefore,

$$20 \text{ cm H}_2\text{O} = 19,614 \text{ dyn}$$

the approximate amount of force normally required to inflate adult lungs.

The concepts of mass and energy are basic to an understanding of chemistry and physics. Energy acts on mass (matter), and a change in mass involves the addition or release of energy. Indeed, mass and energy are interchangeable concepts, a truth recognized first by Albert Einstein in his formulation of the equation

$$E = mc^2$$

in which E = energy, m = mass, and c^2 = the speed of light—the acceleration point at which, it is generally believed, mass becomes nonexistent, and all is pure energy. The universe contains a finite amount of matter, and therefore the amount of energy present in the universe is also finite. Matter and energy can neither be created nor destroyed. These two concepts are referred to as the *law of conservation of mass* and the *law of conservation of energy*.

MEASUREMENT

The aforementioned dyne and newton are examples of how natural phenomena can be defined and measured. A common method for making those measurements facilitates communication between scientists and ensures that observations are made in a standardized and reproducible fashion. In 1960, the international scientific community adopted a new system for measuring physical and chemical events. It is known as the international system, or *SI system*. It was to replace the older and less precise English and metric systems, although some of their components were to be retained. Though most laboratory research done throughout the world has moved to the SI system, the American health care industry has been reluctant to adopt the system. The reasons for this are unclear although it may be related to the fact that Americans have a general aversion to change, especially when they do not see the need for it in their daily lives. In any case, the question remains as to whether information on the SI system should be retained. A review of

chemistry and physics texts in use as of 1991 at several major American universities shows that those texts continue to cover the SI system in detail. Also, our country is committed by international agreement to adopt the SI system. For these reasons, information on the system is retained in this edition. At some future time, all scientific measurements, including those in medicine, will be expressed in SI units.

The SI system (the name derives from the French, *Système International*), has seven basic units (Table 5–2). The first three (length, mass, and time) can be used to describe almost any physiochemical property of a substance. This is why the units are considered "basic." The remaining four are also basic units for electrical flow, heat, amounts, and brightness.

A major drawback to SI measurements is that they are not useful for expressing very large multiples, or very small fractions, of a basic unit. For this reason, prefixes are added to the basic SI unit to express very large or small measurements. The prefixes used (Table 5–3) are retained from prior use with the metric system. For example, the basic unit of length, the meter, can, by use of the prefixes, be expressed in either fractions or multiples:

$$1 \text{ kilometer} = 1000 \text{ meters}$$

$$1 \text{ millimeter} = 1/1000\text{th meter}$$

In addition to basic units, the SI system also uses what are termed *derived units* (Table 5–4). Generally, this indicates that the measurements will vary with prevailing conditions

TABLE 5–2. BASIC SI UNITS

Physical Quantity	Unit	Symbol
Length	meter	m
Mass	kilogram	kg
Time	second[a]	s
Electric current	ampere	A[b]
Temperature	kelvin	K[b]
Luminous intensity	candela	cd
Amount of substance	mole	mol

[a] Minute (min), hour (h), and day (d) will remain in use although they are not official SI units.
[b] These units are named after individuals; therefore symbols are capitalized.

Reprinted, with permission, from Can Anaesth Soc J *1982;29(6):652–654.*

TABLE 5–3. PREFIXES FOR SI UNITS

Factor	Name	Symbol	Factor	Name	Symbol
10^{18}	exa-	E	10^{-18}	atto-	a
10^{15}	peta-	P	10^{-15}	femto-	f
10^{12}	tera-	T	10^{-12}	pico-	p
10^{9}	giga-	G	10^{-9}	nano-	n
10^{6}	mega-	M	10^{-6}	micro-	μ
10^{3}	kilo-	k	10^{-3}	milli-	m
10^{2}	hecto-	h	10^{-2}	centi-	c
10^{1}	deca-	da	10^{-1}	deci-	d

Reprinted, with permission, from Can Anaesth Soc J *1982;29(6):652–654.*

TABLE 5–4. DERIVED SI UNITS

Quantity	SI unit	Symbol	Expression in Terms of SI-Based Units or Derived Units		
Frequency	hertz	Hz	1 Hz	=	1 cycle /s (1 c s^{-1})
Force	newton	N	1 N	=	1 kg × m/s^2 (1 kg × m s^{-2})
Work, energy, quantity of heat	joule	J	1 J	=	1 N × m
Power	watt	W	1 W	=	1 J/s (1 J s^{-1})
Quantity of electricity	coulomb	C	1 C	=	1 A × s
Electric potential, potential difference, tension, electromotive force	volt	V	1 V	=	W/A (1 W A^{-1})
Electric capacitance	farad	F	1 F	=	1 A × s/V (1 A × s V^{-1})
Electric resistance	ohm	Ω	1 Ω	=	1 V/A (V A^{-1})
Flux of magnetic induction, magnetic flux	weber	Wb	1 Wb	=	1 V × s
Magnetic flux density, magnetic induction	tesla	T	1 T	=	Wb/m^2 (1 Wb m^{-2})
Inductance	henry	H	1 H	=	1 V × s/A (1 V × s A^{-1})
Pressure	pascal	Pa	1 Pa	=	1 N/m^2 (1 N m^{-2})
				=	1 kg/m × s^2 (1 kg m^{-1} s^{-2})

The liter (10^{-3} m^3 = dm^3), though not official, will remain in use as a unit of volume, as will the dyne (dyn) as a unit of force (1 dyn = 10–5 N).
Reprinted, with permission, from Can Anaesth Soc J *1982;29(6):652–654.*

and so must be actually measured in each instance. Hence, they are measurements derived from a particular situation. As with the basic units, the prefixes in Table 5–3 can be used to express multiples or fractions of a measurement.

Table 5–5 provides factors for conversion of commonly encountered measurements in anesthesia from the older (but perhaps yet current) units to the SI system and back again. For example, if one wants to record a blood pressure reading reported as 120/80 mm Hg (1 mm Hg = 1 torr), then under the SI system this would be expressed as 16/11 kPa (kPa = kilopascal, the basic unit for measuring pressure). Converting from one reading to the other, or vice versa, requires multiplying or dividing by the conversion factor given in Table 5–5. Using the tables as a reference, the reader can convert from one unit of measure to another and back again. Tables 5–5 to 5–9 give the old and new units, and conversion factors, for most measurements encountered in medicine.

One caution must be exercised in using the prefixes in Table 5–3. It is important that the prefix be appropriate to the idea to be conveyed. Using millimeters when one really wishes to express kilometers results in a millionfold error. Such errors are certainly intolerable in both science and medicine. The same applies to the expression of numbers where the misplacement of the decimal point by one number results in a tenfold difference. Administering 0.1 mg of a potent drug is not the same as administering 0.01 mg.

STATES OF MATTER

Much of what has been discussed regarding general concepts also applies on the atomic, subatomic, and molecular levels as well as on the large scale of everyday existence. The three states of matter (gases, liquids, and solids) are distinguished by specific characteristics. Solids have volume and shape and cannot be compressed, for example, a cube of ice. Liquids have volume but no specific shape. Rather, they assume the shape of their container, for example, water. Gases have neither shape nor volume. They expand indefinitely, for example, steam.

Note that in our example we do not have three different substances (ice, water, and steam), but three different physical states of the same substance. The difference between the states is related to the activity of the molecules that make up the substance and the forces that act on it. For example, removing heat (energy) by cooling causes water molecules to draw close together, because of gravitational and other forces, and to become solidified. If additional energy is added to the water, say by the application of heat, the additional energy accelerates molecular activity and makes it easier for the molecules to overcome the forces that draw them together. As the forces are overcome, the molecules are dispersed and the water becomes steam. This same principle also applies to liquid anesthetics, which, through the addition of heat energy, are vaporized to gases that can be administered to patients. Before taking a close look at how atoms, subatomic particles, and molecules interact, two additional concepts require discussion because they have application to anesthesia practice.

TABLE 5–5. SI CONVERSION FACTORS

		Conversion Factor	
SI Unit	Old Unit	Old to SI (*Exact*)	SI to Old (*Approximate*)
kPa	mm Hg^a	0.133	7.5
kPa	1 standard atmosphere^b (approx 1 bar)	101.3	0.01
kPa	cm H$_2$O	0.0981	10.0
kPa	lb/sq in	6.89	0.145

^{a} For example, systolic blood pressure of 120 mm Hg = 16 kPa and diastolic blood pressure of 80 mm Hg = 11 kPa.
^{b} 760 mm Hg.
Reprinted, with permission, from Can Anaesth Soc J *1982;29(6):652–654.*

TABLE 5–6. BLOOD CHEMISTRY: UNITS AND CONVERSION FACTORS

Measurement	SI Unit	Old Unit	Conversion Factor Old to SI (Exact)	Conversion Factor SI to Old (Approximate)
Blood				
Acid–base				
P_{CO_2}	kPa	mm Hg	0.133	7.5
P_{O_2}	kPa	mm Hg	0.133	7.5
Standard bicarbonate	mmol/L	mEq/L	Numerically equivalent	
Base excess	mmol/L	mEq/L	Numerically equivalent	
Glucose	mmol/L	mg/100 mL	0.0555	18.0
Plasma				
Sodium	mmol/L	mEq/L	Numerically equivalent	
Potassium	mmol/L	mEq/L	Numerically equivalent	
Magnesium	mmol/L	mEq/L	0.5	2.0
Chloride	mmol/L	mEq/L	Numerically equivalent	
Phosphate (inorganic)	mmol/L	mEq/L	0.323	3.0
Creatinine	μmol/L	mg/100 mL	88.4	0.01
Urea	mmol/L	mg/100 mL	0.166	6.0
Serum				
Calcium	mmol/L	mg/100 mL	0.25	4.0
Iron	μmol/L	μg/100 mol	0.179	5.6
Bilirubin	μmol/L	mg/100 mL	17.1	0.06
Cholesterol	mmol/L	mg/100 mL	0.1259	39.0
Total proteins	g/L	g/100 mL	10.0	0.1
Albumin	g/L	g/100 mL	10.0	0.1
Globulin	g/L	g/100 mL	10.0	0.1

Reprinted, with permission, from Can Anaesth Soc J 1982;29(6):652–654.

Density shows the relationship between the weight and volume of a substance. The formula for density is

$$\text{Density} = \frac{\text{weight}}{\text{volume}}$$

In most cases, density is expressed in grams per cubic centimeter, but for gases it is expressed as grams per liter. The density of air is 1.3 g/L. Hydrogen has a density of 0.09 g/L. Therefore, hydrogen rises in air. Similarly, the density of water is 1.0 g/cc, and that of ice, 0.92 g/cc. Therefore, ice floats in water.

Specific gravity (sp gr) expresses the ratio between two densities. It does not have measuring units of its own, but is merely used to make comparisons. For example,

$$\text{Specific gravity} = \frac{\text{density of substance } X}{\text{density of water (or air)}}$$

The standard of comparison normally used is the density of water. For gases, air is the comparison standard. Specific gravity tells us how much lighter or heavier a substance is than the standard with which it is compared. Both substances must be compared under similar conditions of temperature and pressure. The concept of gravity is important to anesthesia because it tells us which gases will be heavier than room air. Nitrogen, helium, and water vapor are all lighter than air, whereas carbon dioxide and nitrous oxide are about 1.5 times heavier. Oxygen is only slightly heavier than air (sp gr = 1.1).

TABLE 5–7. BIOCHEMICAL CONTENT OF OTHER BODY FLUIDS

Measurement	SI Unit	Old Unit	Conversion Factor Old to SI (Exact)	Conversion Factor SI to Old (Approximate)
Urine	mmol/24 h	mg/24 h	0.025	40.0
Creatinine	mmol/24 h	mg/24 h	0.00884	113.0
Potassium	mmol/L	mEq/L	Numerically equivalent	
Sodium	mmol/L	mEq/L	Numerically equivalent	
Cerebrospinal fluid				
Protein	g/L	mg/100 mL	0.01	100.0
Glucose	mmol/L	mg/100 mL	0.0555	18.0

Reprinted, with permission, from Can Anaesth Soc J 1982;29(6):652–654.

TABLE 5–8. HEMATOLOGY

Measurement	SI Unit	Old Unit	Conversion Factor Old to SI (*Exact*)	SI to Old (*Approximate*)
Hemoglobin (Hb)	g/dl	g/100	Numerically equivalent	
Packed cell volume	No unit[a]	percent	0.01	100
Mean cell Hb concentration	g/dl	percent	Numerically equivalent	
Mean cell Hb	pg	μμg	Numerically equivalent	
Red cell count	cells/L	cells/mm^3	10^6	10^{-6}
White cell count	cells/L	cells/mm^3	10^6	10^{-6}
Reticulocytes	percent	percent	Numerically equivalent	
Platelets	cells/L	cells/mm^3	10^6	10^{-6}

[a] Expressed as decimal fraction, e.g., normal adult male value 0.40 to 0.54.
Reprinted, with permission, from Can Anaesth Soc J *1982;29(6):652–654.*

ATOMIC STRUCTURE OF MATTER

Elements exist as discrete atoms of specific configuration. Combining two or more atoms of the same element or two or more atoms of different elements produces a *molecule.* Many millions of molecules are required to provide enough volume for a substance to be visible because of the infinitesimal size of atoms. A single atom of an element retains all of the properties of the element, and all atoms of the same element are identically configured. Atoms of different elements differ not only in their configuration, but also in size, weight, and chemical properties.

We now know atoms are themselves made up of smaller parts. The nucleus, or central core, of the atom is made up of protons and neutrons. Circling in orbits around the nucleus are the electrons. Additional subatomic particles have been identified (e.g., positron, muon, neutrino, and pion, each with its corresponding antiparticle) but their importance lies in the field of high-energy physics, and they are not essential to understanding atomic structure as it relates to anesthesia practice. Therefore, the following discussion is limited to the proton, neutron, and electron. The three differ from each other in two respects: mass and electric charge. Hydrogen, the simplest, lightest, and most abundant element in the universe, can illustrate the basic configuration of atoms. The hydrogen ion has one proton of positive charge and a neutron with no charge that make up its nucleus. Both proton and neutron have the same mass. The electron that orbits the nucleus has a negative charge equal to the charge of the proton, but with a mass only 1/1800th that of the nucleus.

The *atomic weight* of an atom is determined by the masses of the protons and neutrons contained in its nucleus. Because protons and neutrons are equal in mass, they are each said to represent one *atomic mass unit* (amu). The electrical charge of the nucleus is determined by the number of protons. This is called the *atomic number.* As the number of protons in the nucleus is increased by one, the next heavier element is obtained. Hydrogen has one proton, helium has two protons, lithium has three protons, and so on. As protons are increased in number, the number of positive charges goes up correspondingly. To maintain electrical balance, the number of electrons must go up by the same number. In this way the atom remains electrically neutral because all positive charges are balanced by an equal number of negative charges.

As electrons travel about the nucleus, they do not all travel the same path; rather, they travel different paths (directions) in orbits of varying distance from the nucleus. In helium, for instance, the two electrons travel different paths in the same orbit, that is, at essentially the same distance from the nucleus. For other atoms with more electrons of the same orbital distance from the nucleus, the electrons travel at different angles (paths) from each other and electrons at other orbital distances do the same.

Each succeeding electron orbit is not only further in distance from the nucleus, but each orbit can contain only a specific number of electrons. Each succeeding orbit is filled, in turn, from the next innermost orbit. These orbits are also referred to as *energy levels,* as each orbit varies in the energy its electrons possess relative to electrons in the other orbits. There are actually some variations within orbits, referred to as suborbits, but for our purposes, these can be ignored. The

TABLE 5–9. pH AND H$^+$ ACTIVITY

pH	H$^+$ Activity (nmol/L)
6.80	158
6.90	126
7.00	100
7.10	79
7.20	63
7.25	56
7.30	50
7.35	45
7.40	40
7.45	36
7.50	32
7.55	28
7.60	25
7.70	20

Reprinted, with permission, from Can Anaesth Soc J *1982;29(6):652–654.*

first energy level contains a maximum of two electrons; the second can have eight, as can the third. Up to element number 20 (calcium), the two–eight–eight configuration is retained. After that, electrons move randomly between energy levels; that is, they can skip from orbit to orbit. The outermost level can contain one to eight electrons. To understand the operations of atoms, it is important to recognize that (1) the outermost energy level of an atom is most important because it is the number of electrons in this orbit that determines the chemical activity of the atom; and (2) each atom desires stability to achieve a configuration of a complete (eight-electron) outer orbit, the basis for chemical reactions between elements. This tendency for atoms to fill outer orbits with eight electrons is called the Theory of Octet. The numbers of protons and neutrons in an atom are not always equal. When the number of neutrons in the nucleus is less or greater than the number of protons, the weight of the nucleus will be different. The element retains its chemical properties because the number of protons and electrons determines these, but, because of the change in weight caused by the loss or gain of neutrons, the element will have different physical properties. Such elements are called *isotopes*. Many of the radioactive isotopes are useful diagnostic tools in medicine. It is because an element can exist as different isotopes that atomic weights cannot be given as whole numbers. Instead, the weight of an element given in a periodic table represents the balance of weights in a mixture of that element's basic and isotope atoms.

As mentioned previously, combining two or more atoms of the same or different elements produces a molecule. When atoms of different elements are combined we call the molecular substance a *compound*. Because we deal mostly with compounds rather than lone elements in anesthesia, it is often more practical to discuss molecules than atoms. Generally, a molecule of a compound is made up of atoms of several elements. By adding the atomic weights of all elements in a molecule, we obtain the compound's *molecular weight*. Sodium (Na) has an atomic weight of 22.989, and chlorine (Cl), 35.453. As an atom of each, chemically combined, produces a molecule of sodium chloride (NaCl), the molecular weight of sodium chloride is 58.442. (In reality, sodium chloride, common table salt, exists in crystal form, where each chloride is surrounded by six sodium ions, and vice versa. These concepts are dealt with later, but the example of adding atomic weights to obtain molecular weight remains valid.)

A molecule of a substance is always made up of the same number of the same atoms, in the same configuration. This is known as the *law of definite composition*. For this reason, the molecular weight of a given compound always remains the same. Because a single molecule is so small and lightweight, it is preferable to speak of a large number of them together, 1 gram's worth. This is known as the *gram molecular weight* (GMW). It is also called one mole. One mole is equal to the total of the atomic weights of each and every atom in the compound and is expressed in grams.

When speaking of atomic or molecular weights, we are really comparing the mass of one atom or molecule with that of an equal unit of carbon (C-12). Carbon-12 serves as the standard against which other elements are compared. It would take 6.02×10^{23} carbon-12 atoms to add up to 12 g of carbon. The number of atoms required to provide the gram molecular weight of any element is always 6.02×10^{23}. This is known as *Avogadro's number*. It is the basis for expression of the mole. Atomic weights of different elements must always contain the same number of atoms. Therefore, the mole is an Avogadro's number of formula units of a substance. Avogadro's number applies to molecular weights as well as atomic weights. Hence, 1 GMW of a compound always contains 6.02×10^{23} molecules.

VOLUME, PRESSURE, AND FORCES

Volume is the expanse of space occupied by a given number of atoms or molecules. One atom or molecule occupies little space, but a large collection of them can occupy enough space to enable measurement. For solids, the basic units of measurement are the cubic meter (cm^3) and the cubic centimeter (cc). For liquids and gases, volumes are measured in liters (L) and milliliters (mL). Any aggregate collection (volume) of atoms or molecules also exerts pressure. *Pressure* arises from two primary sources: from the gravitational pull on the atoms or molecules and from the energy forces that operate within the atoms themselves.

Sea-level atmospheric pressure results from the earth's gravitational pull on the atoms and molecules that make up the surrounding air. Similarly, hydrostatic pressure at ocean depths results from gravitational influences on the molecules of water. Density also plays a role in determining pressure. A column of mercury will exert more pressure than an equal volume of water because mercury is more dense. This fact makes measuring blood pressure with a mercury manometer more practical than using a water manometer. By the contraction or expansion of a given number of molecules, the density of those molecules is changed and more or less pressure is exerted. This is discussed in the section on gas laws.

The other primary factor by which atoms or molecules are able to exert pressure relates to the *kinetic theory of matter*, which states that *all matter consists of atoms or molecules in constant motion*. Therefore, pressure is also generated by the force of atoms or molecules striking a surface as they move about. An example is the pressure exerted against the walls of a cylinder containing anesthetic gases. An appreciation for the importance of the kinetic theory of matter is essential to a proper understanding of other concepts such as vaporization, temperature, and the behavior of gases. An additional concept related to the kinetic theory of matter is that of *momentum*. If two atoms of given mass travel at a certain rate, they are said to have momentum. Their masses and velocities represent a sum of energy. If they collided, and were perfectly "elastic," they would each leave the collision with the same mass and velocity or energy as they had before the collision. In reality, perfect elasticity does not exist, so atomic or molecular collisions result in a loss of momentum. The concomitant release (loss) of energy produces heat. In the SI system, pressure is measured in pascals (Pa) and perhaps someday all pressure measurements will be expressed in this fashion. For the present, pressure is measured in a number of ways. This stems from both historical and practical considerations. In anesthesia practice measurements include millimeters of mercury (also known as torr pressure), centimeters of water, pounds per square inch, and others.

Molecules have an inherent capacity to interact with each other. Four principal forces of interaction are important enough to deserve mention: adhesion, cohesion, surface tension, and van der Waals forces. *Adhesion* is the force of attraction between unlike molecules. In a liquid flowing through a glass tube, adhesive forces slow the passage of liquid molecules traveling next to the glass walls, whereas liquid molecules in the center of the fluid column travel at a faster rate. This is because of the attraction between the dissimilar molecules of the liquid and glass. The concept of adhesive force is used in anesthesia draw-over vaporizers in which liquid anesthetic is drawn onto a cloth wick by adhesion. This is called *capillary action*. Gas flowing over and through the wick causes vaporization of the liquid and allows the anesthetic to be delivered as a gas. *Cohesion*, on the other hand, is the force of attraction between like molecules. The outward bulge of water in a container filled to the brim is called a meniscus. This bulge is due to the cohesive forces of the water molecules. They gather together above the container rim where adhesive forces are working. If the water level is below the vessel rim, the meniscus is inverted, as adhesive forces are still operating and are stronger than the water's cohesive forces.

In addition to being affected by adhesion and cohesion, molecules at the surface of a liquid, the liquid–gas interface, are subject to unequal stresses. This difference in molecular forces between the air and water creates a high-force level, called *surface tension*, at the very top layer of liquid molecules. Cleaning agents, such as soaps, alter surface tension. This concept is used to improve cleaning of anesthesia equipment. Cohesive forces influence vapor pressure, boiling point, heat of vaporization, and viscosity as well as surface tension. Both adhesion and cohesion result from the electrical properties of molecules, which in turn stem from the atomic configuration of the elements that make up the molecule. This topic is discussed in more detail later.

The fourth type of intermolecular force has extensive and important applications for anesthesia practice. When molecules, because of their shape and the pattern of their electrical charges (caused by electron travel around the nuclei), are aligned in such a way that the molecule has a relatively positive end and a relatively negative end, they are said to be in a "dipole" configuration. The molecule is electrically polarized. This situation sets up the molecule to interact electrically with surrounding molecules. Though such forces operate only over a short distance, they are relatively strong, and they increase with the size of the molecule. They affect the boiling point, surface tension, and viscosity of the substance. They also affect the amount of energy (heat) required to vaporize the substance. All of these are concepts important to anesthesia practice.

Polar molecules have a higher intermolecular force than nonpolar ones. But even nonpolar molecules, if by chance improperly ordered, assume a brief polar configuration. This "induced" dipole configuration causes the surrounding molecules also to assume a dipole configuration. Adjacent atoms then begin to act synchronously rather than independently. These induced dipole configurations are termed London dispersion forces, after the German who

first theorized them. They are also called *van der Waals* forces, although this latter term is more often used to denote all types of intermolecular forces. All intermolecular forces, especially dispersion forces, greatly influence the behavior of a substance.

HEAT AND TEMPERATURE

Heat is a form of energy. The intensity of heat is indicated by temperature. As mentioned previously, physical changes in a substance are often induced by reduction or addition of heat, and temperature has important implications for the action of solids, liquids, and gases.

Temperature Scales

Scientifically, temperature is measured on the Kelvin (K) (or absolute [A]) temperature scale. More common to everyday life and anesthesia practice are the Fahrenheit (F) and Celsius or centigrade (C) scales. Converting from one scale to the other is relatively easy.

$$F = (C \times 1.8) + 32$$
$$F = [(K - 273) \times 1.8] + 32$$
$$C = (F - 32) \div 1.8$$
$$C = K - 273$$
$$K = C + 273$$
$$K = [(F - 32) \div 1.8] + 273$$

Note that conversion between Fahrenheit and Kelvin scales first required conversion to the centigrade scale. The 1.8 conversion factor results from the fact that both Fahrenheit and centigrade scales are based on the freezing point and boiling point of water. The temperature variation between these two points is divided into 100 degrees on the centigrade scale and 180 degrees on the Fahrenheit scale, or a ratio of 1.8 to 1. As the freezing point "baseline" differs by 32 degrees, this conversion factor is required to achieve comparable numerical equivalency between the two scales. The 273 conversion factor represents the difference between the 0C freezing point of water and the equivalent point on the Kelvin scale. The Kelvin scale begins at "absolute zero" (approximately −273C), that point at which, at least theoretically, all molecular motion stops.

Measurement of Heat Capacity

Although temperature scales are useful indices of the changes wrought by heat, they do not measure the amount (capacity) of heat expended in working that change. For measuring the amount of work performed by heat, other work units are used. The amount of heat required to raise the temperature of 1 g of water 1C is called the *calorie* (also known as the gram calorie or small calorie). To raise the temperature of the same 1 g of water to 5C would require five times as much heat; to raise it to 100C would require 100 times as much heat. One thousand small calories equals 1 kilocalorie. The small calorie is abbreviated to cal; the large, or kilocalorie, is abbreviated to Cal. This large caloric measurement is the one used by nutritionists when referring to the amount of calories contained in food or expended by exercise. The *British Thermal Unit,* or BTU, is the amount of heat required to raise the temperature of 1 pound of water 1 degree Fahrenheit. It is equivalent to 252 small calories.

It is also useful to be able to equate work performed by other means, such as mechanical energy, to work performed by heat. The joule is used to make such comparisons. A gram calorie is approximately equal to 4.185 joules. Other measures of work, such as the foot-pound, can be converted to joules also (1 joule = 1.355 foot-pounds of work). This makes it possible to compare work performed by various means. The amount of heat that raises the temperature of a given mass of substance at atmospheric pressure by one degree unit is called the *thermal heat capacity* of the substance. In most cases, this is expressed as calories per gram per degree centigrade. A term often confused with thermal capacity is specific heat. The *specific heat* of a substance is the ratio of the amount of heat needed to raise the temperature of one unit mass by one degree centigrade compared with the quantity of heat needed to raise the temperature of an equivalent mass of water by one degree centigrade. To obtain the amount of energy required to change *x* grams of a substance *y* degrees of temperature, multiply the total weight in grams by the number of degrees of temperature change desired and multiply again by its specific heat.

Of interest to anesthetists is the fact that gases have two specific heats: one at which the gas maintains the same volume, and one at which the gas maintains the same pressure. As will be seen later, one cannot change the volume of a gas without affecting the pressure it exerts or change the pressure without changing the volume. In general, gases have low specific heats, whereas solids and liquids have high specific heats. Inhaled cold gases must therefore depend on external sources of heat if they are to be warmed to body temperature. Also, vaporization quickly ceases as a spontaneous process in bubble vaporizers unless external heat is applied. This is because gases possess low specific heats. Water has a very high specific heat compared with most substances.

The rapidity of heat exchange between molecules varies with each substance. Substances whose molecules exchange heat readily are said to be thermally conductive. This *conduction* is one of three means by which heat may be transferred from one place to another. The other ways by which heat may be transferred are convection and radiation. *Convection* is the transfer of heat by means of air currents. The surrounding air transports and dissipates the heat absorbed from a substance to other areas. *Radiation* is the transfer of heat energy in the form of waves, usually by electromagnetic means. Microwave ovens are an example of radiation.

Gases composed of single atoms are free to travel in three paths: (1) back and forth, (2) vertically, and (3) sideways. Polyatomic gases have a greater degree of freedom; that is, the various atoms may be traveling in several directions at once. The more directions in which a given gas can travel, the more heat that will be required to raise the temperature of that gas. The heat required to raise the temperature of one mole of a gas one degree centigrade is called the *molal heat capacity,* and it increases as the number and weight of atoms in the gas molecule increase. This makes the gas less susceptible to combustion. If inert gases, especially those with high thermal capacities, are mixed with combustible gases, the mixture is less likely to become ignited. The high-thermal-capacity inert gases absorb ignition heat and therefore "cool" the mixture so that it does not readily ignite. They are therefore called *quenching agents* and are discussed in the section on Fire and Explosion Hazards in Chapter 7.

Converting a substance from the solid to liquid state or liquid to gas state, or vice versa, requires a gain or loss of additional heat or energy. These are referred to as *latent heats of vaporization, condensation, crystallization, and melting.* To convert 1 g of boiling water at 100C requires almost 540 additional calories to break the molecular forces and allow the liquid to become a gas (heat of vaporization). When cooling steam, an additional 540 cal of heat energy must be lost to allow the molecules to come close enough together for the intermolecular forces to take over and change the gas to a liquid (heat of condensation). Similarly, extra energy or heat must be extracted from a gram of water at 0C to be converted to ice (heat of crystallization), as removal of the heat allows greater action by the intermolecular forces that draw the molecules into a solid. Melting ice to water (heat of melting) requires that a similar amount of energy be added.

The contraction or expansion of molecules that accompanies a change in the state of matter is dependent on two factors: temperature and pressure. For gases with very high molecular velocities, the change to the liquid state cannot be accomplished without first cooling the gas substantially. After cooling, pressurizing the gas will force it into the liquid state. For all gases, a temperature exists above which liquefaction is impossible regardless of the amount of pressure applied. This is known as the *critical temperature.* The pressure required to cause liquefaction at the critical temperature is known as the *critical pressure.* At the critical temperature and pressure, one gram molecular weight of the gas will occupy a specific volume termed the *critical volume* and have a density termed the *critical density.* By the proper application of temperature and pressure, it is possible to store large amounts of gas as very much smaller amounts of liquid. These principles are used in the storage of bulk volumes of oxygen for hospital use.

THE PERIODIC TABLE

All chemical elements can be grouped on the basis of their similarities in properties (Table 5–10). This was first recognized by the Russian chemist Mendeleyev. He arranged the then-known elements in a chart in order of their increasing atomic weights. He noted that elements with similar properties recurred at regular intervals or "periods," and he placed these in vertical groupings. Some inconsistencies were noted and later resolved by reordering the tables on the basis of increasing atomic number. Gaps in the original chart led Mendeleyev to predict, rightly, that vacant spaces represented as yet undiscovered elements, ones whose properties he could predict on the basis of the grouping to which they belonged. Periodic tables provide the chemical symbols commonly used for each element. For each ele-

TABLE 5–10. PERIODIC TABLE OF THE ELEMENTS[a]

KEY TO CHART

Atomic Number → 50 +2 ← Oxidation States
Symbol → Sn +4
1983 Atomic Weight → 118.71
18 18 4 ← Electron Configuration

New notation
Previous IUPAC form
CAS version

PERIODIC TABLE OF THE ELEMENTS

Group 1 IA	2 IIA	3 IIIB / IIIA	4 IVB / IVA	5 VB / VA	6 VIB / VIA	7 VIIB / VIIA	8	9 VIIIA / VIII	10	11 IB	12 IIB	13 IIIB / IIIA	14 IVB / IVA	15 VB / VA	16 VIB / VIA	17 VIIB / VIIA	18 VIIIA	Orbit
1 H +1 −1 / 1.00794 / 1																	2 He 0 / 4.00260 / 2	K
3 Li +1 / 6.941 / 2-1	4 Be +2 / 9.01218 / 2-2											5 B +3 / 10.81 / 2-3	6 C +2 +4 −4 / 12.011 / 2-4	7 N +1 +2 +3 +4 +5 −2 −3 / 14.0067 / 2-5	8 O −2 / 15.9994 / 2-6	9 F −1 / 18.9984 / 2-7	10 Ne 0 / 20.179 / 2-8	K-L
11 Na +1 / 22.9898 / 2-8-1	12 Mg +2 / 24.305 / 2-8-2											13 Al +3 / 26.9815 / 2-8-3	14 Si +2 +4 −4 / 28.0855 / 2-8-4	15 P +3 +5 −3 / 30.9738 / 2-8-5	16 S +4 +6 −2 / 32.06 / 2-8-6	17 Cl +1 +5 +7 −1 / 35.453 / 2-8-7	18 Ar 0 / 39.948 / 2-8-8	K-L-M
19 K +1 / 39.0983 / -8-8-1	20 Ca +2 / 40.08 / -8-8-2	21 Sc +3 / 44.9559 / -8-9-2	22 Ti +2 +3 +4 / 47.88 / -8-10-2	23 V +2 +3 +4 +5 / 50.9415 / -8-11-2	24 Cr +2 +3 +6 / 51.996 / -8-13-1	25 Mn +2 +3 +4 +7 / 54.9380 / -8-13-2	26 Fe +2 +3 / 55.847 / -8-14-2	27 Co +2 +3 / 58.9332 / -8-15-2	28 Ni +2 +3 / 58.69 / -8-16-2	29 Cu +1 +2 / 63.546 / -8-18-1	30 Zn +2 / 65.39 / -8-18-2	31 Ga +3 / 69.72 / -8-18-3	32 Ge +2 +4 / 72.59 / -8-18-4	33 As +3 +5 −3 / 74.9216 / -8-18-5	34 Se +4 +6 −2 / 78.96 / -8-18-6	35 Br +1 +5 −1 / 79.904 / -8-18-7	36 Kr 0 / 83.80 / -8-18-8	-L-M-N
37 Rb +1 / 85.4678 / -18-8-1	38 Sr +2 / 87.62 / -18-8-2	39 Y +3 / 88.9059 / -18-9-2	40 Zr +4 / 91.224 / -18-10-2	41 Nb +3 +5 / 92.9064 / -18-12-1	42 Mo +6 / 95.94 / -18-13-1	43 Tc +4 +6 +7 / (98) / -18-13-2	44 Ru +3 / 101.07 / -18-15-1	45 Rh +3 / 102.906 / -18-16-1	46 Pd +2 +4 / 106.42 / -18-18-0	47 Ag +1 / 107.868 / -18-18-1	48 Cd +2 / 112.41 / -18-18-2	49 In +3 / 114.82 / -18-18-3	50 Sn +2 +4 / 118.71 / -18-18-4	51 Sb +3 +5 −3 / 121.75 / -18-18-5	52 Te +4 +6 −2 / 127.60 / -18-18-6	53 I +1 +5 +7 −1 / 126.905 / -18-18-7	54 Xe 0 / 131.29 / -18-18-8	-M-N-O
55 Cs +1 / 132.905 / -18-8-1	56 Ba +2 / 137.33 / -18-8-2	57* La +3 / 138.906 / -18-9-2	72 Hf +4 / 178.49 / -32-10-2	73 Ta +5 / 180.948 / -32-11-2	74 W +6 / 183.85 / -32-12-2	75 Re +4 +6 +7 / 186.207 / -32-13-2	76 Os +3 +4 / 190.2 / -32-14-2	77 Ir +3 +4 / 192.22 / -32-15-2	78 Pt +2 +4 / 195.08 / -32-16-2	79 Au +1 +3 / 196.967 / -32-18-1	80 Hg +1 +2 / 200.59 / -32-18-2	81 Tl +1 +3 / 204.383 / -32-18-3	82 Pb +2 +4 / 207.2 / -32-18-4	83 Bi +3 +5 / 208.980 / -32-18-5	84 Po +2 +4 / (209) / -32-18-6	85 At −1 / (210) / -32-18-7	86 Rn 0 / (222) / -32-18-8	-N-O-P
87 Fr +1 / (223) / -18-8-1	88 Ra +2 / 226.025 / -18-8-2	89** Ac +3 / 227.028 / -18-9-2	104 Unq +4 / (261) / -32-10-2	105 Unp / (262) / -32-11-2	106 Unh / (263) / -32-12-2	107 Uns / (262) / -32-13-2												O-P-Q

*Lanthanides

58 Ce +3 +4 / 140.12 / -20-8-2	59 Pr +3 / 140.908 / -21-8-2	60 Nd +3 / 144.24 / -22-8-2	61 Pm +3 / (145) / -23-8-2	62 Sm +2 +3 / 150.36 / -24-8-2	63 Eu +2 +3 / 151.96 / -25-8-2	64 Gd +3 / 157.25 / -25-9-2	65 Tb +3 / 158.925 / -27-8-2	66 Dy +3 / 162.50 / -28-8-2	67 Ho +3 / 164.930 / -29-8-2	68 Er +3 / 167.26 / -30-8-2	69 Tm +3 / 168.934 / -31-8-2	70 Yb +2 +3 / 173.04 / -32-8-2	71 Lu +3 / 174.967 / -32-9-2

(Orbit: N O P)

**Actinides

90 Th +4 / 232.038 / -18-10-2	91 Pa +4 +5 / 231.036 / -20-9-2	92 U +3 +4 +5 +6 / 238.029 / -21-9-2	93 Np +3 +4 +5 +6 / 237.048 / -22-9-2	94 Pu +3 +4 +5 +6 / (244) / -24-8-2	95 Am +3 +4 +5 +6 / (243) / -25-8-2	96 Cm +3 / (247) / -25-9-2	97 Bk +3 +4 / (247) / -27-8-2	98 Cf +3 / (251) / -28-8-2	99 Es +3 / (252) / -29-8-2	100 Fm +3 / (257) / -30-8-2	101 Md +2 +3 / (258) / -31-8-2	102 No +2 +3 / (259) / -32-8-2	103 Lr +3 / (260) / -32-9-2

(Orbit: O P Q)

[a] Numbers in parentheses are mass numbers of most stable isotope of that element.

Reprinted, with permission, from Weast RC, ed. CRC handbook of chemistry and physics. 71st ed. Boca Raton, FL: CRC Press: 1991–1992.

ment, two numbers are given: a whole number representing the atomic number of the element (number of nuclear protons), and a decimal number representing the element's atomic weight. Some tables also provide the arrangement of electrons according to their energy levels, for example, two–eight–eight–two. Group numbers are provided at the very top of the chart. They indicate the number of electrons in the outer shell. With this knowledge, one can predict the chemical behavior of the element. For example, elements in group I have one electron in the outermost shell, those in group VII have seven, and so forth.

In most charts metals are listed on the left, nonmetals on the right, and transition elements, which can act as either metals or nonmetals, in the middle. Therefore, as one scans the table from left to right, the elements have decreasingly fewer metallic properties and increasingly more nonmetallic properties. The families of elements, those that behave similarly both chemically and physically, are given in vertical columns. Knowing the properties of one element in the family tells you the properties of the other elements in that family, properties that depend on the number of electrons in the outer shell. Within each family, there will be variations in activity level. In general, elements on the left-hand side increase in activity as one reads down the table. The transition elements vary in activity depending on circumstances. Group VIII elements are nonreactive with the other elements. They are inert. The horizontal rows of elements are

termed *periods* because each element in the row differs in chemical properties.

All of the elements can be categorized in one of the four main classes: metals, nonmetals, transition elements, and inert gases. Metals tend to have a shiny appearance, be soft, have low melting points, and be good conductors of heat and electricity. Group IA is called the alkali metal group, and group IIA is the alkaline earth metal group. Nonmetals vary greatly in properties; most are gases, some are solids, and one is a liquid. Except for carbon, they conduct heat and electricity poorly. They tend toward dullness. Group VIIA, which contains chlorine, fluorine, bromine, iodine, and astatine, is called the *halogen* or salt-former group, because these elements are found in many salt compounds. Transition elements are able to act as either metals or nonmetals, or as acids or bases as will be discussed later. They are also termed *amphoteric* elements. Carbon is the premier example of this group. The fact that it contains four electrons in its outer orbit means that it readily loses or gains electrons in trying to achieve stability. It is for this reason that carbon is so valuable to organic chemistry. Inert gases are also known as the "rare" or "noble" gases. They are chemically inert, not reacting with any of the other elements. Except for helium, which has two electrons in its outer shell, all of the elements in this category have eight electrons in their outer shell. They are stable because their outer shell is completely filled.

Of all the elements known today, only about a dozen have special importance to the human body and anesthesia practice. These include oxygen, carbon, hydrogen, sodium, potassium, calcium, iron, phosphorus, chlorine, sulfur, and, less important, the trace elements iodine and cobalt. Knowing the information provided in a periodic table enables one to understand more easily the properties of certain elements. By being able to group like elements on the basis of their properties, one can more easily understand how chemical reactions take place.

CHEMICAL BONDING

Compounds are formed by combining and recombining the various elements, excluding those of the inert group. The joining together of elements into molecules and compounds is termed *chemical bonding*. Bonding is dependent primarily on the configuration of atoms of each involved element, especially the distribution of electrons in the outer shell. Only elements with eight electrons in their outer shells are stable; helium is an exception, being stable with two electrons. Elements with one to seven electrons in their outer shells will react, almost always in a way that helps them to become more stable, that is, by trying to achieve an eight-electron outer shell. Achieving stability requires one of two things to occur: either outer-shell electrons are lost, enabling the element to achieve eight-electron stability in the next innermost shell, or enough electrons are gained from another element to obtain the required eight-electron configuration. Therefore, elements normally having one, two, or three electrons in their outer shells tend to lose them readily, whereas elements having five, six, or seven electrons tend to take on additional electrons to achieve stability. Each of these patterns is energy efficient; that is, less energy is required to remove two electrons from an element's outer shell than would be required to add the necessary six needed for stability. Conversely, less energy is required to gain one electron for an element having seven electrons in its outer shell than would be required to lose the seven electrons.

Remember, each atom by itself is electrically neutral, proton charges balancing electron charges. In bonding chemically with other elements this electrical neutrality is lost, and the resulting particles are called *ions*. Where electrons are lost, the particle will have a positive charge because more protons than electrons are present. These ions are called *cations*. Conversely, if electrons are gained, the particle will have more negative charge. These particles are called *anions*. In all chemical reactions, it is always electrons, never protons, that are lost or gained. In becoming ions, atoms lose their original physical and chemical properties and develop new ones. For example, the poisonous gas chlorine reacts with sodium to become common table salt, sodium chloride, a solid with entirely different physical and chemical properties.

From the preceding discussion on the periodic table, it can be seen that metals, to the left of the table and having one to three electrons in their outer shells, tend to lose electrons, becoming cations in the process. The nonmetals, to the right of the chart and configured with five, six, or seven electrons in their outer shells, tend to gain electrons and become anions. Metals and nonmetals react well together, one losing and the other gaining electrons. The transfer of electrons between the two results in what is termed an *electrovalent compound*. The process is termed *ionic bonding* because each atom has, in effect, become an ion. In each case of ionic bonding, the number of electrons lost by one element is always equal to the number gained by the other element. Electrovalence means simply that a given number of electrons have been transferred to form the new compound and that the two ions thus created have opposite, and therefore mutually attracted, electrical charges (anion/cation) that enable the new compound to maintain stability. As mentioned previously, elements with four electrons in their outer shell tend to share electrons with other elements but may lose or gain them to achieve stability.

In naming ionically bonded compounds, the name of the metal is used first, followed by the name of the nonmetal modified to *-ide* to indicate that it is part of a compound. For example, combining sodium and chlorine produces sodium chlor*ide*. Most diatomic (two-atom) compounds are named in this fashion. In some cases, one of the ions cannot yield or gain the same number of electrons as the element with which it is reacted. In these cases, two or more atoms of one element may combine with one atom of the other element. In this way, electrical balance is achieved. If instead of reacting chlorine with sodium, we react it with calcium, we get calcium chloride, but the chemical formula $CaCl_2$ indicates that two chlorine atoms have been combined with one atom of calcium to achieve the necessary electrical balance. Polyatomic compounds must always be electrically balanced.

In a discussion of chemical reactions, several terms are frequently encountered: oxidation number or state, radical, valence, and covalence. The *oxidation number* denotes the electrical state of the atom: positive, negative, or neutral. A positive state exists when electrons have been given up; a negative state, when electrons have been accepted. Plus or minus signs denote the state; the number denotes the number of electrons shifted. Oxidation numbers refer only to one atom of the element in the compound. Elemental atoms, being electrically balanced and neutral, have a zero oxidation number. The algebraic sum of any compound must always equal zero. Some elements can exist in any of several states. That is why the exact number and state must be specified. Iron, for example, can exist in either a 2+ or a 3+ state. To correctly name the compound in written or spoken form, the metal of the compound is given the ending *-ous* for lower states or *-ic* for higher states. Therefore, Fe^{2+} is a fer*rous* compound, whereas Fe^{3+} is a fer*ric* compound. For elements having more than two possible oxidative states (e.g., tin [Sn]), the correct state is described by Roman numerals: tin(IV) chloride.

The term *radical* describes a group of atoms that have bonded together but act as an individual atom in chemical reactions. Radicals exhibit specific behaviors not characteristic of the atoms that constitute them. Many radicals are involved in bodily reactions and are thus important in anesthesia. These include the hydroxyl (OH), bicarbonate (HCO_3), phosphate (PO_4), ammonium (NH_4), carbonate (CO_3), sulfate (SO_4), and nitrate (NO_3) radicals. The *-ate* ending indicates a radical of higher oxidative state. An *-ite* ending is used for lower-state radicals, for example, nitrites (NO_2) and sulfites (SO_3). So radicals, too, can have different oxidative states. Radicals are often written within parentheses, a subscript indicating the number of radicals in the compound, for example, $Ca(OH)_2$. The term *valence* was originally used to denote the number of electrons in an atom's outer shell that could be shifted in chemical reactions. The term has largely been replaced by the more correct *oxidation number*. Covalence is a term that denotes the number of electron *pairs* that are shared by atoms in a compound. In covalent compounds, electrons are fully shared between the atoms; in electrovalent compounds, electrons are shared only in that one element loses electrons and the other gains them, more an exchange than a sharing. Rules for determining oxidation numbers of compounds may be found in standard chemistry texts.

WRITING CHEMICAL FORMULAS

Chemical formulas are a shorthand method of expressing the changes taking place in chemical reactions. Using symbols for each element found in periodic tables and taking into account radicals, oxidation states, and electrical balance, one can write complex reactions in a manner that precisely explains what has occurred in the reaction. The reactions are also expressed in a way that can be universally understood. Care must be taken to write equations correctly, using proper symbols. Sodium chloride and sodium chlorate are not the same compound. *Empirical formulas* indicate the proportion of each type of atom in a compound, but they do not indicate the specific number of atoms in it. Their usefulness is limited. *Chemical equations* or *formulas* are more practical. When properly written, they indicate the proper amounts and electrical balance of reactants and their end products. In equations, reactants are written to the left, products are to the right, and the direction of reaction is indicated by an arrow. Where reactions proceed in both directions, double arrows are used, each in the opposite direction, the length of each arrow indicating the relative degree to which the reaction proceeds in that direction. Virtually all chemical reactions, including those that occur within the body, involve one or more of the following: emission or absorption of heat; emission of an odor; formation of a gas or precipitate; a change in color, fluorescence, or luminescence. These are sometimes indicated in a chemical formula by symbols that help clarify what can be expected from the reaction. In all cases, either the reactants or the products are known.

Writing the equation begins by setting down each of the component elements. The next step is to write each molecule's oxidation number as a superscript and to check that their algebraic sum equals zero.

Reactants: Sodium (Na) and sulfate (SO_4)

Step 1. $Na + SO_4 \rightarrow ?$

Step 2. $Na^{1+} \ SO_4^{2-} \rightarrow ?$ Algebraic sum is not
equal to zero
$(1+) + (2-)$

Checking the equation, we find an imbalance in the oxidative states. To rectify this, a procedure analogous to obtain-

ing an arithmetic lowest common denominator is used. It simply involves crisscrossing the oxidation numbers. Superscripts may then be erased.

Step 3. $Na^{1+} (SO_4)^{2-} \rightarrow Na_2 (SO_4)$

The final step is to balance the complete equation to ensure that an equal quantity of each element is shown on both sides of the equation. This may involve trial and error to determine the proper coefficient(s) needed to balance the equation. A coefficient is the number placed in front of the chemical symbol to denote the number of molecules undergoing reaction. In this example, the coefficient 2 must be placed in front of the Na to balance the equation.

Step 4. $2Na + SO_4 \rightarrow Na_2 (SO_4)$ sodium sulfate

In this final equation, we express the idea that two atoms of sodium combine with one radical of sulfate to produce one molecule of sodium sulfate. This is but one type of chemical reaction, but the same general principles are used in writing equations for other reactions.

There are four basic types of chemical reaction: *synthesis, decomposition, single displacement,* and *double displacement.* The previous example typifies a synthesis reaction wherein simple elements are combined into a more complex compound. In a decomposition reaction, a complex substance is broken down into less complex ones. In a single displacement reaction, one element replaces another in a compound. Reacting zinc with hydrochloric acid produces zinc chloride and the release of hydrogen. The hydrogen atom in the hydrochloric acid molecule is replaced by a zinc atom. This type of reaction is also known as a substitution or replacement reaction. In a double displacement reaction, parts of two compounds are exchanged for one another. Reacting silver nitrate and sodium chloride yields silver chloride and sodium nitrate, sodium and silver having both been exchanged.

Another type of chemical reaction is *oxidation–reduction.* Atoms losing electrons are said to be oxidized. Atoms gaining electrons are said to be reduced. Such processes are essential to the chemistry of living tissues. Body energy is gained by oxidation of carbohydrates, fats, and proteins, each oxidation reaction being balanced by a reduction reaction. Chemical compounds, such as Dakin's solution and hydrogen peroxide, have antiseptic and cleaning uses because of their strong oxidizing properties.

PROPERTIES OF SOLUTIONS

Water

Water is called a universal solvent because so many substances may be dissolved in or combined with it. A large proportion of the human body is made up of water and virtually all bodily chemical reactions depend on its presence. A gain or loss of body water characterizes many disease states. Even healthy adults fasting 24 hours may lose 5 percent of their body water. Infants and children can lose twice that amount in the same period, enough water loss to produce neurologic and other symptoms. For these reasons, understanding the properties of water is important to anesthesia practice.

The density of water is considered to be 1 g/mL, and this concept will suffice for most practical applications, although it is important to realize that the density of water is dependent on temperature and, in some circumstances, pressure. As water is warmed, its volume increases and its density decreases. This is in keeping with what has previously been discussed regarding the effect of temperature on molecular action. At atmospheric pressure, cooling water contracts its volume and increases its density. But as the temperature reaches 4C, additional cooling results in volume expansion, about a 10 percent increase by the time the freezing point of 0C is reached. In winter, exposed water pipes rupture because of this volume expansion. In the same way, water-laden body cells exposed to extreme cold expand and rupture, causing the tissue damage associated with frostbite.

Water, like all liquids, is subject to certain forces and exhibits certain properties. These include *cohesion, adhesion,* and *capillary action*, all of which have been previously discussed. When water is placed in a glass capillary tube, the central portion of the water level will be drawn downward. The smaller the tube bore, the more noticeable the central downward depression. For this reason, calibrated tubes (manometers) containing aqueous solutions should be read at the bottom of the liquid depression. Along the edges of the tube, the water can be seen to rise noticeably because of adhesive forces. Adhesive forces help account for the "wetting" properties of water and other liquids. They also account for the creeping of a liquid up the sides of a tube, as when blood is drawn with a capillary tube.

With aqueous solutions, cohesive forces are usually overcome by adhesive forces; however, certain liquids have cohesive forces so strong that adhesive forces become negligible. Mercury is such a liquid. Placing mercury in a glass blood pressure manometer results in a meniscus or liquid level that is raised in the center. Such manometers should be read at the liquid's highest point.

Water can exert a vapor pressure. As with all liquids, its molecules are constantly in motion, the extent of motion being dependent on the energy they possess and whether additional energy in the form of heat is absorbed from the surrounding atmosphere. In their random motion, some molecules gather enough energy to break free from the liquid and enter the atmosphere as a vapor. The more heat applied, the greater the number of molecules released. When the molecules escape, they exert a vapor pressure. That pressure also rises with increasing temperature. When the vapor pressure of escaping molecules is high enough to displace the air above it, the water boils. At sea-level atmospheric pressure (760 torr), water boils at 100C. Below sea level, where atmospheric pressure is higher, water boils at a higher temperature. More escaping molecules are required to reach a specific vapor pressure. At high altitudes, the converse is true because atmospheric pressure is lessened. The boiling point of water is therefore dependent on the pressure exerted by the surrounding atmosphere, and vapor pressure always equals atmospheric pressure at the boiling point. As more external heat is applied to the water, the liquid's temperature remains stable. The extra energy just allows more of the molecules to escape, thereby increasing the speed of the evaporation process. Steam sterilizers,

by increasing their internal atmospheric pressure, allow water temperature to exceed 100C and thus kill bacteria that might otherwise survive that temperature.

Vaporization continually occurs at any liquid–air interface, although not rapidly. A pan of water left open to the atmosphere will eventually fully evaporate. In anesthesia vaporizers, liquid anesthetic is continually vaporized within the chamber. But because the chamber is closed, the enclosed atmosphere becomes fully saturated, a state of equilibrium is achieved, and vaporization slows. Opening the circuit allows vapor to escape into the anesthetic delivery system and vaporization again becomes a continuous process. The process is driven by heat absorbed from the room atmosphere and conducted through the metal framework of the machine to the vaporizer. High ambient temperatures allow vaporization to proceed at a faster rate. If room temperature drops, less energy or heat is conducted to the vaporizer and the process slows. For this reason thermometers that read vaporizer temperature were included on most anesthesia machines. They allowed the anesthetist to be cognizant of temperature changes that affected the concentration of the agent being administered. Today, new anesthesia machines no longer have such universal vaporizers. Rather, they use draw-over vaporizers. Draw-over vaporizers, by virtue of their internal design, allow the same concentration of agent to be delivered despite temperature fluctuation of several degrees. These are known as temperature-compensated vaporizers. For these, no thermometer is needed for the liquid anesthetic. This is because within the range of the vaporizer's operating temperatures, the delivered vapor concentration will be unaffected by the liquid's temperature. One may still see anesthetic liquid thermometers on the universal vaporizers of older machines.

Another evaporation process of concern in anesthesia practice is the continuous evaporation of body water from skin surfaces and exposed abdominal and thoracic organs. Because this evaporation is barely noticeable, such losses are termed *insensible losses*. The volume of fluid a patient may lose in this manner can be substantial and must be accounted for by the anesthetist in calculating fluid replacement. Fever substantially increases the amount of insensible fluid lost. Of less frequent concern, yet another evaporative process seen in anesthesia practice relates to those substances that have low boiling points and thus evaporate readily when applied to the skin. Ethyl chloride, a topical anesthetic, typifies such substances.

One especially important property of water relates to its molecular structure and is termed *hydrogen bonding*. Water is composed of one oxygen and two hydrogen atoms. Although a molecule of water is electrically neutral, its structure is such that the molecule assumes an asymmetric distribution. Rather than the hydrogen atoms being located to either side of the oxygen atom, they both align to one side of the oxygen, being separated by an angle of approximately 104 degrees. This configuration is assumed because it allows the hydrogens and oxygen to combine with the least expenditure of energy. It also makes one side of the molecule relatively positive, and the other side relatively negative. In other words, the molecule assumes a dipolar configuration. This configuration facilitates development of attractive forces *between* water molecules, and the hydrogen atoms of one water molecule become oriented toward the oxygen atom of another water molecule. Thus, a latticework arrangement develops. These hydrogen bonds, though weak when compared with covalent bonds, are biologically important. They account for the relative instability of complex proteins and help maintain amino acid peptide integrity for synthesis of new proteins. Because water has polarity, it is an excellent solvent for other polar molecules, such as alcohols, but not for nonpolar substances, such as oils. Hydrogen bonding helps account for many properties of water, such as its high boiling point and surface tension. Dissolving solutes in water not only produces anions, cations, undissociated molecules, or radicals, but it also changes what are termed the *colligative properties* of water. Colligative changes are alterations in physical properties wrought by disruption of water's normal structure. This disruption results in elevation of the boiling point, depression of the freezing point, lowering of the vapor pressure, and a change in osmotic pressure.

A final property of water important to anesthesia practice is its ability to combine with other elements directly to form crystalline structures known as *hydrates*. Baralyme, a mixture of barium and calcium hydroxide used in anesthesia circuits to absorb exhaled carbon dioxide, contains water as a hydrate. Hydrates always contain water in a definite proportion, the water of crystallization. Barium hydroxide in an octahydrate, containing eight water molecules in its structure. When hydrates are exposed to excessive heat, the water portion is evaporated and the remaining substance is referred to as an *anhydrate*. Hydrates that spontaneously lose their water content on exposure to air are called *efflorescent compounds*. *Hygroscopic compounds* are those that absorb water from the surrounding air. If they actually become dissolved in the absorbed water they are termed *deliquescent*. Surgical casts made from plaster of Paris (calcium sulfate) are efflorescent hydrates. When the water evaporates, the remaining anhydrate, gypsum, expands and hardens into whatever shape has been formed.

Natural water contains many impurities. If large amounts of calcium and magnesium bicarbonate are present, the water is referred to as *hard water*. Water that contains primarily sodium ions is termed *soft water*. Natural water is not pure enough for medicinal use, which requires ion-free water. Purifying water requires demineralization and distillation. Distillation involves boiling, followed by cooling and condensation of the steam. Dissolved gases are evaporated off and particulate matter is left as residue. Distilled water for injection normally undergoes triple distillation to ensure purity.

Solutions

A *solution* may be defined as a uniformly distributed, homogeneous mixture of two or more substances that can vary in proportion. Dissolving instant coffee crystals in a cup of hot water results in a solution, and solutions are one of the main ways by which the body absorbs the nutrients it needs for sustenance. Under some conditions, chemical reactions proceed more quickly in a solution. Substances dissolved in

a solution are termed *solutes*. The dissolving medium is termed the *solvent*. For a given temperature, only a limited amount of solute can be dissolved per volume of solvent. This limit is termed its *solubility*. Dissolving solids in liquids forms one type of solution. Other combinations are also possible. Gases may be dissolved in gases or liquids in other liquids. The latter type of solution is the one most often encountered and one in which the distinctions between solute and solvent become blurred. Solvents may be classed as either polar or nonpolar, based on their molecular structure. Polar solvents, like water, are excellent for dissolving ionic compounds. Nonpolar solvents are better for dissolving covalent and nonpolar compounds. Solutes placed in dissolving media become uniformly distributed. At first, the solution is *unsaturated*; that is, more solute can be dissolved without precipitating. At the point at which addition of more solute results in precipitation, the mixture is said to be *saturated*. Saturation occurs because the equilibrium point between particles going into solution and those being forced out of solution has been reached. Heating the mixture allows more solute to be added, whereas cooling it increases precipitation. Under some conditions, however, it is possible to cool a mixture without creating precipitation. The mixture is then said to be *supersaturated*. Such solutions are very unstable.

Gases in Solution

Solubility varies with the solute, nature of the solvent, and temperature. Solubility of gases in liquids, for example, in blood, is similar to that of solids dissolved in liquids, except that the amount or weight of gas dissolved per volume of blood, at constant temperature, is directly proportional to the pressure of the gas over the liquid (Henry's law). The pressure or tension of gas in solution is always equal to that of the gas above the air–liquid interface. If a mixture of gases is dissolved, each gas comes to its own equilibrium. (It is assumed that gases will not combine with the blood or solvent.) Because the number of gas molecules in solution varies directly with pressure, the *volume* of dissolved gas is independent of pressure, if temperature is constant. This is in keeping with Boyle's law, covered in more detail later. Hence, dissolved gas bubbles expand or contract as necessary to maintain equilibrium pressure with undissolved gas.

What if the temperature is changed? Increasing heat, as occurs with a rise in body temperature, displaces gases from solution. Cooling allows more gas to go into solution. So, in terms of gas solubilities in the body, solubility varies inversely with temperature. Therefore, a patient who is allowed to become hypothermic during anesthesia develops a higher relative blood concentration. The same is not true for solids dissolved in liquids, where addition of heat allows an increased amount of solute to be dissolved.

Henry's law has daily application in anesthesia practice because it accounts for gas tensions that develop between alveoli and blood and between blood and other body tissues. The potentially hazardous implication of this principle is seen with caisson disease (decompression sickness), in which a sudden decrease in atmospheric pressure causes rapid expansion of dissolved gases that then occlude small blood vessels.

Solubility Coefficients

The volume of gas dissolved or absorbed in a given volume of liquid can be measured by a variety of means. One method, in which measurements are reported under conditions of standard temperature and pressure (STP), is the Bunsen absorption coefficient. Another, the Ostwald solubility coefficient, is usually reported at the temperature and pressure of the experiment, frequently at body temperature. Other methods are also available.

Because solubility of a gas varies with the tissues in which it is dissolved, it has become common practice to speak of the relative ratios of dissolved gas between body compartments. These are termed *distribution* or *partition coefficients*. They are useful tools for comparing anesthetic agent distribution between body tissues and for predicting the clinical effects of those agents.

Although anesthetists are often concerned with solubility of gases in blood and other body tissues, there are times when they may be more concerned with the solubility of nonvolatile solutes. It then becomes important to know that addition of solute to a liquid, like coffee crystals placed in a cup of hot water, lowers the liquid's vapor pressure. This is because the solute lowers the fraction of solvent present. The decrease in vapor pressure is proportional to the concentration of solute in solution (Raoult's law).

ACIDS, BASES, AND SALTS

Earlier, in the discussion pertaining to organization of the periodic table, metals, nonmetals, and transition elements were discussed. A related and important topic is that of acid–base balance. The entire body chemistry is aimed at maintaining homeostasis by balancing acids against bases, a process termed *neutralization*. An *acid* can be any substance that separates into ions, at least one of which must be hydrogen. The other ions can be nonmetals or radicals. A hydrogen ion is really a proton. Having given up its electron, the atom therefore has a positive charge. This is why acids are said to be proton donors. In solution, they tend to attach themselves to water molecules as hydronium ions by a bond that is easily broken, releasing the hydrogen for other chemical reactions.

Acids ionize in water to form an electrolyte solution capable of conducting electricity, a property of acids. Other properties include a sour, tart taste; corrosiveness; an ability to change the colors of dyes; and an ability to react with some, but not all, metals. Acids react with metallic oxides to form a salt and water, and with carbonates and bicarbonates to produce carbonic acid. Carbonic acid, in turn, can be decomposed to carbon dioxide and water. A common reaction for acids is neutralization of bases. This, too, forms a salt and water. Acids are classed as either strong or weak depending on the extent of ionization. Some are relatively stable; others, such as carbonic acid, decompose readily. Concentrated acids are more corrosive than dilute ones. Important acids to body chemistry are the amino acids used for building proteins and lactic acid produced by metabolism within muscles. Acids are also important pharmacologically. Salicylic acid, the essential ingredient in aspirin, is a good example.

A *base* is any substance that can neutralize an acid and, in water, ionize to produce hydroxyl ions (OH). Though not producing hydroxyl ions on dissociation, carbonates and bicarbonates are also considered bases because they effectively neutralize acids. In contradistinction to acids, bases are proton acceptors. They often have greasy consistencies in solution and possess a metallic, bitter taste. Like acids, bases can be corrosive and change the color of dyes. They react with soluble salts to form an insoluble hydroxide, which precipitates. Bases can react with some metals to release hydrogen just as acids can. Two bases important to anesthesia practice are sodium bicarbonate, used to treat acute metabolic acidosis, and calcium hydroxide, important for chemical absorption of carbon dioxide from breathing circuits. Strong and weak bases are also distinguished by the extent to which they ionize in solution.

Salts are formed by neutralization reactions between acids and bases. Through such reactions, body cations and anions are kept in a narrow range of ever-changing concentrations. Salts are of three types: *normal salts*, which have no replaceable hydrogen or hydroxyl groups; *acidic salts*, which contain partly neutralized hydrogen; and *basic salts*, in which only part of the hydroxyl group has been replaced. This last group maintains the properties of both a salt and a base. Salts have physiologic importance: maintaining osmotic pressure, body tissue building, nerve and muscle functioning, and maintenance of body fluid pH.

The term *pH* indicates the concentration of hydrogen ion in the body (relative acidity or alkalinity). It is expressed as a whole number plus a decimal fraction (e.g., pH 7.54) representing the reciprocal or negative logarithm of the hydrogen ion concentration in moles per liter. A pH of 7.00 indicates neutrality, acids and bases being in balance. Readings from 7 to 14 indicate increasing alkalinity. Readings from 7 downward indicate increasing acidity. Because the numbers indicate a logarithmic change, based on powers of 10, a pH change from 6.00 to 5.00 is really a tenfold increase in the number of circulating hydrogen ions. Certain body fluids may normally be either acidic or basic (e.g., urine and gastric juices are typically quite acidic), but it is blood pH with which anesthetists are most often concerned. Blood pH is normally 7.40. A drop to 7.20 is considered severely acidotic; a blood pH below 7.00 is immediately life-threatening without treatment. When pH rises to 8.00 or higher, a similar situation ensues. Indeed, treating acute acidotic states by excessive administration of intravenous sodium bicarbonate can result in death from acute alkalosis.

If a 7.00 pH is considered neutral, why is normal blood pH 7.40? Neutrality (pH 7.00) is most ideally required at the cellular level, where all metabolic activity occurs. Blood, like urine and gastric juice, has a somewhat different normal pH; however, blood quickly reflects changes occurring at the cellular level, so pH analysis and blood gas measurements remain the best, current indicators of cellular metabolic states. In an attempt to measure cellular pH changes directly, increasing use has been made of transcutaneous analyzers. Research substantiates that this technique may be more useful for early detection of tissue acidosis or alkalosis. Cost and technical factors have limited routine employment of such devices, but as these problems are solved, transcutaneous electrode monitoring is likely to become an important aspect of anesthesia management. For additional information on pH, see Chapter 4.

A concept allied to pH, and one important to pharmacologic aspects of anesthesia practice, is that of the drug dissociation constant, pK_a. This constant expresses the pH at which a drug is dissociated so that bound and unbound ions are chemically balanced. Changes in pH increase or decrease the amount of drug available to perform a specific action. More detailed information on this concept can be found in pharmacology texts.

A last topic important to any discussion of acids and bases is that of buffers. Buffer systems are important in helping maintain normal pH, and they can neutralize either acids or bases. Most often, buffers are composed of a weak acid and the sodium or potassium salt of that acid, called the conjugate base. If a strong acid is added to any buffer pair, a weak acid and a neutral salt is produced. Buffer pairs reacting with strong alkalis form a weak alkaline salt and water.

The carbonate–bicarbonate buffer system illustrates how buffers act. Carbon dioxide produced by cellular metabolism combines with water in the blood to form carbonic acid. Being weak, carbonic acid dissociates only slightly so that few hydrogen ions are released. Those that are released leave behind a bicarbonate radical, so that both carbonic acid and bicarbonate are present in solution. As additional hydrogen is added, increasing acidosis, it combines with the bicarbonate to form additional carbonic acid. The bicarbonate has, in effect, tied up the excess hydrogen and thus reduced acidity.

If extra base had been added instead of hydrogen, it would be neutralized by the carbonic acid that is present. This removes or buffers excess hydroxyl ions so that pH is again restored. The body maintains a bicarbonate ion-to-carbonic acid ratio of 20 : 1. This is in keeping with the Henderson–Hasselbalch equation:

$$pH = pK_a + \log \frac{[HCO_3]}{[H_2CO_3]}$$

The pK_a of carbonic acid (H_2CO_3) at body temperature is 6.10, and the normal concentrations of bicarbonate and carbonic acid are 24.0 and 1.2 millimoles or a ratio of 20 : 1. Therefore,

$$pH = 6.10 + \log 20$$

$$pH = 6.10 + 1.30$$

$$pH = 7.40$$

The body's other buffers operate in a similar fashion. They include the phosphate, protein, and hemoglobin buffer systems. Regulation of acid–base status is a function of both respiratory and renal systems. Disruptions of regulation produce either acidosis or alkalosis, whose components may be respiratory, metabolic, or mixed. Although regulation or acid–base status constitutes an important aspect of anesthesia practice, the complexity of these disorders places the topic beyond the scope of the present discussion. For additional information, the reader is referred to special texts dealing exclusively with acid–base disorders.

OSMOSIS

For a gas to reach blood from the surrounding atmosphere, it has to pass through the lung's alveolar–capillary membrane. Diffusion of a dissolved substance through a semipermeable membrane is termed *osmosis*. An example occurs at the cellular level, where gases and other substances pass into and out of the cell, whose wall is, in effect, a semipermeable membrane. This diffusion or passage of substances from one side of the membrane to the other depends on the selectivity of the membrane and the relative concentrations of the substances on either side. Osmosis is an important body process, being necessary for urine formation, distribution of water to various body compartments, and maintenance of blood volume.

Membrane *permeability* refers to the ease or difficulty with which substances may pass through a membrane. In the body, membranes usually separate two aqueous compartments having different concentrations of ions and molecules. The membrane selectively allows passage of water but not of solutes. The direction of water flow is from the area of low solute concentration to the area of high concentration. The force that moves the water is *osmotic pressure*. Water movement will continue until concentrations on both sides of the membrane equilibrate. Osmosis then stops. Further loss or addition of solute will restart the osmotic process. Osmosis allows for fluid shifts between intracellular and extracellular fluid compartments. Alterations in the fluids' ionic content occur as the individual takes in more salt by ingestion or as water losses occur through urine formation. There is, therefore, a constant flux in water level and ion concentration between each compartment.

Two solutions exerting the same osmotic pressure are isotonic to each other; that is, pressure is exerted in equal but opposing directions. Physiologic intravenous solution of 0.9 percent sodium chloride in sterile water is isotonic compared with blood. Solutions containing smaller concentrations of solutes are termed *hypotonic*. Their administration causes additional water to flow into red cells, the area of higher solute concentration, causing them to swell and rupture, or hemolyze. Intravenous solutions containing more solutes or salts than blood cause red cells to lose water. This red cell shrinkage is called *crenation* or *plasmolysis*, and fluids that cause it are said to be *hypertonic*. Any two fluids separated by a semipermeable membrane can be iso-, hypo-, or hypertonic relative to one another. For additional information on solutions and osmosis, see Chapter 4.

Suspensions and Colloids

Dissolved salts in water represent a true solution, but some substances cannot dissolve in a solvent. Rather, they remain intact as fine particles. When placed in water, they give it a milky appearance. Particles are merely suspended in the solvent and such mixtures are termed *suspensions*. Between suspensions and true solutions, we have *colloids* or colloidal solutions. Colloidal solutions occur when solutes are too small to be suspended but too large to form a true solution. Colloids disrupt and disperse light (*Tyndall effect*). Particles in such a solution move about in random fashion as if colliding with invisible molecules of solvent. This zigzag motion of colloidal particles describes *Brownian movement*.

Concentrations of Solutions

The ratio of dissolved solute to volume of solvent determines solution concentration. Most often, this information is presented in terms of how many grams of solute are dissolved per 100 mL of solvent (percent solutions). A 0.9 percent physiologic saline solution contains 0.9 g of salt in each 100 mL. As mentioned earlier, the molecular weight of a compound is expressed in moles (mol). One mole of a compound dissolved in 1 L of solution results in a 1 molar solution, abbreviated 1 M. Doubling or tripling the amount of dissolved substance in the same volume makes it a 2 molar (2 M) or 3 molar (3 M) solution. The same holds true for fractions of a mole, for example, 0.3 M. A *molal* solution is identical to a molar solution except that the temperature of the solution is 4C, at which 1 L of water equals 1000 g. At other temperatures the weight of water varies slightly from the 1000 g. Molal solutions are based on the amount of solute per 1000 g.

The number of particles in a solution, not their size or weight, determines the amount of osmotic pressure generated. An ionized substance exerts more pressure than a nonionized one. This is because, in ionizing, a greater number of discreet particles are formed. The osmotic activity of a given molar solution is expressed in *osmoles* (osm). One dissolved GMW of a substance per liter is equal to 1 osm. If the substance does not ionize, molarity and osmolarity are equal. But if the substance ionizes, osmolarity equals the solution molarity multiplied by the number of ionized particles. A 1 M solution of substance that ionizes into two particles exerts 2 osm of pressure. If the substance ionizes into three particles, as does calcium chloride, a 1 M solution will exert 3 osm of pressure.

According to Avogadro's law, 1 GMW of a substance contains 6.02×10^{23} molecules. If vaporized, that substance would occupy, at STP, a volume of 22.4 L, the *gram molecular volume*. If 1 GMW of nonionizing substance is placed in a volume of 22.4 L of solution on one side of a semipermeable membrane, it would take a force of 1 atm to prevent water migration across the membrane. With a substance ionized into two particles, osmolarity would be doubled, and 2 atm of pressure would be required to prevent transmigration of water. Thus, it is possible to visualize how much pressure osmolarity actually involves; however, osmoles are too large a unit for discussion of the osmotic activities in human biology, so osmolarity of body fluids is expressed in terms of milliosmoles (mosm) per liter. A milliosmole exerts a pressure equal to 1/1000th of an osmole. Average osmolarity of body fluids is approximately 300 milliosmoles (mosm). The milliosmole should not be confused with the millimole, which is 1/1000th of a mole. Sodium, potassium, and chloride contribute the most to osmolarity of body fluids.

Normality

In discussing the concepts of molarity and osmolarity, emphasis was on GMW and the number of particles formed in dissociation. GMW per liter determined molar concentration, whereas the number of particles determined osmolarity (osmotic force). Neither of these concepts addresses the chemical activity/reactivity of the dissolved substance. The *equivalent* expresses the ability of a substance to react or combine chemically with other substances. *Equivalent weight* of a substance is the weight in grams (*gram equivalent weight* or *GEW*) that will react with 1 g of hydrogen, or 8 g of oxygen. GEW is calculated by dividing GMW by the positive oxidation number of the substance. Placing a GEW of a substance in 1 L of solution creates a 1 *normal* (N) *solution*. Doubling that amount of substance in 1 L produces a 2 normal solution; halving the amount produces a 0.5 normal solution. (*Caution*: The terms *normality* and *normal solution* as discussed here refer to definitions of chemical concepts. They should not be confused with medical use of the term *normal*, as in normal saline solution, which implies that a solution is physiologically compatible with body fluids. So-called "normal" saline is not a 1 normal solution.) In terms of chemical reactivity, one GEW of any one substance is equal in combining power to one GEW of any other substance, even though their GMWs might vary substantially. *Normality* expresses the concentration of a solution in terms of chemical reactivity.

Equivalent weights are too large to express concentrations found in body tissues, so a more useful term is used, the *milliequivalent*. One milliequivalent (mEq) is 1/1000th of an equivalent weight. This term is more useful for expressing concentration of body ions than milligrams per volume of fluid, which provides no useful information about electrical balance. When necessary, milligram percent may be converted to milliequivalents by using the formula

$$mEq = \frac{mg\% \times 10}{atomic\ weight} \times valence$$

It also is occasionally necessary to convert molarity to normality. This is accomplished by multiplying molarity by valence, because with normality we are considering the influence of positive valences. Reversing the procedure enables us to change normality to molarity. Normality divided by valence equals molarity. The relationship between milliequivalents and milliosmoles can be summarized as follows:

1. For univalent cations (e.g., sodium or potassium)

    1 mEq of cation = 1 mosm

2. For nonionizing substances (e.g., sugars)

    1 mEq = 1 mosm

3. For bivalent cations (e.g., calcium),

    (mEq ÷ valence); therefore 1 mEq of cation = 0.5 mosm

    2 mEq of cation = 1 mosm

4. For trivalent cations

    1 mEq = 0.33 mosm

    3 mEq = 1 mosm

GASES

As discussed earlier, gases are notable in that their molecules are widely dispersed. Intermolecular forces are slight compared with liquids and solids. Therefore, gases may easily be compressed. Lacking strong intermolecular attraction and possessing high velocities, gases tend to expand indefinitely. These two characteristics, compressibility and expandability, distinguish gases from liquids and solids. Gases also have a high degree of freedom or random motion, enabling them to travel large distances quickly. This accounts for our ability to detect odors at a distance. Random movement of gas molecules resembles Brownian movement in colloidal solutions. Because of random motion and high velocity, gases in a container collide with the walls of that container, exerting a pressure against it. The smaller the container is made, the more often the molecules collide. This exerts an increasing amount of pressure against container walls. Heating the container accelerates molecular motion and this, too, serves to increase the pressure exerted by the gas. The ability of gases to vary in pressure or volume as the container is changed is an important concept for understanding the gas laws that are discussed later.

Weight of a volume of gas can be expressed in several ways. It may be expressed as density: molecular weight (at STP) divided by gram molecular volume (22.4 L). But more often, we are interested in its specific gravity, that is, how much lighter or heavier it is than another gas. By convention, this is calculated by comparing the weight of a volume of the gas to the weight of an equal volume of dry air, taken to be a weight of one. Gases with a specific gravity less than one will rise in room air; those with a specific gravity greater than one will flow toward the floor. This fact is used clinically in doing gas inductions, especially for children. By using gases heavier than the atmosphere, the anesthetist can hold the mask above a child's face, yet gases will still flow down over the nose and mouth, where the child breathes them in.

Diffusion

Diffusion is the process whereby gases move from an area of high concentration to one of low concentration. Movement of oxygen from the alveoli to blood and of carbon dioxide from blood to alveoli is, in part, the result of diffusion processes. By diffusion, a volume of gas will uniformly distribute throughout a container. If two or more gases are mixed, they each will mix and distribute uniformly. How quickly the process comes to equilibration depends on the molecular weight of the gas and its temperature, diffusion occurring more rapidly with increasing temperatures. Lighter gases diffuse more rapidly than heavy ones. This principle underlies *Graham's law*, which states that the rate of gas diffusion varies inversely with the square root of its molecular weight. Therefore, in a mixture of gases A and B, where B has a molecular weight four times greater than that of A, A will diffuse twice as rapidly as B. Conversely, gas B will take twice as long to diffuse as will gas A. $(A = \sqrt{1} = 1, B = \sqrt{4} = 2.)$

As gas moves from an area of high concentration to an area of lesser concentration, a difference develops in the pressure (pressure gradient) exerted by the gas at those two sites (concentrations). At first, when the pressure gradient is large, diffusion proceeds rapidly. As concentrations and pressures become equalized, the rate of diffusion slows. This is known as *Fick's law*. Diffusion rate is proportional to the difference in partial pressures. At the start of a general anesthetic, the anesthetist uses high delivered gas concentrations and high pressures, generated by compression of the breathing bag. This accelerates the diffusion process and contributes to the patient becoming anesthetized more quickly.

The atmosphere we breathe is a mixture of gases including oxygen, nitrogen, and smaller amounts of carbon dioxide, inert gases, and water vapor. At sea level, this mixture exerts a pressure equal to 760 mm Hg (torr) or 1 atmospheric pressure (atm). Each gas contributes a portion of this total pressure, the *partial pressure*. If our atmosphere consisted of equal amounts of four gases, each would contribute 25 percent of the total pressure, or 190 torr. So the total pressure exerted by any mixture of gases is equal to the sum of all the partial pressures (*Dalton's law*). Any volatile liquid anesthetic converted into a vapor acts as a constituent gas of the mixture and adheres to the principle expressed by Dalton's law. Diffusion becomes a clinically important phenomenon when hyperbaric pressures are used. By using higher than atmospheric pressures, more oxygen can be delivered into a patient's blood.

The Gas Laws

An *ideal* gas would be one existing in a very rarefied environment where no intermolecular forces are exerted. *Boyle's law*, formulated on the basis of an ideal gas, expresses the compressibility of such gases. It states that at constant temperature, the volume of a gas varies inversely with its pressure. Therefore, multiplying the gas volume by its pressure would, for a fixed weight of gas, always equal a constant. But with *real* gases, especially at low temperatures and under high pressures, there are intermolecular forces that must be taken into account. This is why van der Waals' modification of Boyle's law has greater applicability in explaining the behavior of real gases. It takes into account forces of cohesion and the volume occupied by gas molecules. In this formulation, the reduction in pressure caused by cohesive forces is added to the molecular motion pressure. This is then multiplied by the total volume occupied by the gas less the maximum compressible volume occupied by the molecules. In this way, the pressure/volume constant more clearly expresses the behavior of real gases. At low pressures and high temperatures, however, real gases behave more like ideal gases.

Heating a gas expands it. If pressure is held constant, the amount or volume of expansion is proportional to the increase in absolute temperature. This is *Charles' law*. Cooling the gas makes the converse true also. For every degree centigrade decrease in temperature, gas volume will change by 1/273 so that at absolute zero temperature (− 273C, 0K), the gas would theoretically have no pressure or volume. The volume change expressed in Charles' law is based on changes in absolute or Kelvin temperature. That same scale is important to the formulation of *Gay-Lussac's law*, which states that when volume is kept constant, gas pressure varies directly with absolute temperature. Charles' law and Gay-Lussac's law are similar in that they both serve to explain the effect of absolute temperature changes on volume and pressure of a gas.

The foregoing gas laws have been formulated into a *general gas law*: $PV = nRT$, where pressure (P) multiplied by volume (V) is equal to the number of molecules (n) times a constant (R), which is the same for all ideal gases, times absolute temperature (T). This general gas law is useful for explaining the behavior of ideal gases. A modified version is more relevant to clinical practice when one wants to determine the effects of changes in volume, temperature, or pressure. The modified formula is

$$P_1 V_1 A_2 = P_2 V_2 A_1$$

where P_1 = initial pressure, V_1 = initial volume, A_1 = initial temperature (Kelvin), P_2 = new pressure, V_2 = new volume, and A_2 = new temperature (Kelvin). For example, if one starts with a 1000-L volume of gas at 273K (0C), which exerts a pressure of 1000 pounds per square inch (psi), and doubling the temperature ($273 \times 2 = 546$) causes a fourfold increase in pressure, what will be the new volume of gas?

$$100 \times 1000 \times 546 = x \times 4000 \times 273$$

$$54,600,000 = x \times 1,092,000$$

$$x = \frac{54,600,000}{1,092,000}$$

$$x = 50 \text{ L}$$

According to Charles' law, doubling the temperature could be expected to double the volume, making it 200 L. But, by Boyle's law, a quadrupling of pressure would decrease volume to one quarter. The net change in volume then must be one fourth of 200 or 50 L. This simple example serves to illustrate how the formula can be used to solve practical problems in the clinical setting, for example, calculating the volume of gas in a cylinder transported from a cold outdoor environment to a warm indoor one. It must be remembered, however, that temperatures must be converted to Kelvin scale and all volumes and all pressures must be in the same measurement units.

Vapor Pressures and Vaporization

Vaporization is the conversion of a volatile liquid to a gas or vapor. Within anesthesia vaporizers, the end atmospheric pressure is typically composed of carrier gas (usually oxygen) and the vaporized anesthetic. If 50 mL of vapor is produced for each 100-mL flow of oxygen into the vaporizer, then the final atmosphere consists of 150 mL exerting a total of 760 torr pressure. The partial pressure of the anesthetic is one third (50/150) of 760 torr, or 253.33 torr (the vapor pressure). This example is very close to the 243-torr vapor pressure exerted by the anesthetic halothane at 20C. When the combination of anesthetic vapor and carrier gas is added to the nitrous oxide and additional oxygen of the diluent flows, the partial pressure of the anesthetic vapor, at point of delivery to the patient, will be less than the pressure

exerted by the vapor coming out of the vaporizer. Assuming 50 percent concentrations of nitrous oxide and oxygen at a total diluent flow of 5 L, the final delivered atmosphere will consist of 2500 mL oxygen (diluent) + 2500 mL nitrous oxide (diluent) + 100 mL (carrier gas) + 50 mL of anesthetic vapor, a total of 5150 mL. As the anesthetic vapor is only 50 mL of this total, or 0.97 percent (5150 : 100% :: 50 : x), the final delivered anesthetic concentration will be 0.97 percent. It will also exert that portion of the total pressure, or $0.0097 \times 760 = 7.3$ torr. So partial pressure gradients apply to both gases and vapors. This knowledge makes rapid calculation of the amount of vapor produced, required carrier gas flow, required diluent flow, or delivered concentration very easy. They may be calculated as follows:

1. Calculation of amount of vapor being produced, with knowledge of the vapor pressure of the agent at the temperature at which vaporization is occurring:
   a. Agent vapor pressure: total pressure (760 torr*) :: x : 100%.
   b. $100\% - x\%$ = % exerted by carrier gas ($y\%$).
   c. Carrier gas milliliters (known) : $x\%$ (from step a) :: vapor milliliters : $y\%$ (from step b). (Calculate for the vapor milliliters produced.)
2. Knowing the vapor pressure of the agent at use temperature, calculate the amount of carrier gas required to produce a specific amount of vapor. Use the same calculations as in step 1, making the assumption that 100 mL of carrier gas is to be used. Then, knowing the amount of vapor being produced for each 100 mL of carrier gas, calculate the amount of carrier gas required to produce other vapor pressures:

$$\frac{100 \text{ mL carrier gas}}{\text{amount of vapor produced}} :: \frac{x \text{ (amount of carrier gas required)}}{\text{vapor amount desired}}$$

* *Note*: At other than sea level, total pressure (atmospheric pressure) will be other than 760 torr. Pressure decreases with altitude.

3. Calculate the diluent flow required to achieve a desired concentration, knowing the amount of anesthetic vapor being produced (i.e., knowing the information from steps 1 and 2, which are calculated only from the known vapor pressure of the agent). Multiply the amount of vapor being produced by 100. This tells you the amount of diluent flow required to achieve a 1 percent concentration. Halving the diluent flow doubles the concentration. Doubling the diluent flow halves the concentration. Knowing how much diluent flow is required to produce a 1 percent concentration, one can calculate the desired concentration diluent flow as

$$\frac{1\%}{\text{required diluent flow}} :: \frac{\text{desired concentration}}{(x) \text{ required diluent}}$$

$$(1\% \times 100) \qquad \qquad \text{flow}$$

4. The concentration of agent delivered can now be calculated:

$$\frac{[\text{Vapor pressure of agent} / (\text{atmospheric pressure} - \text{vapor pressure of agent})] \times \text{flow of carrier gas} \times 100^{\dagger}}{\text{total flow}}$$

For additional information on calculating delivered anesthetic concentrations, see Chapter 4.

† 100 = percent conversion to move decimal point.

Clinically, total flow is often taken to be only the diluent flow because this makes mental calculation simpler and errs on the safe side; that is, actual delivered concentration will be slightly less than the calculated delivered concentration. To be precise, total flow should include diluent flow amount, carrier gas amount, and amount of vapor produced. It must be remembered that these calculations are based on knowing the vapor pressure of the agent at the temperature at which it is being used. Changes in ambient temperature, either up or down, will vary the vapor pressure. Fortunately, the change in vapor pressure over the range of clinically used temperatures (20C to 25C) is minimal in terms of the effects on the final concentration delivered to the patient. Wide variations in temperature must, however, be accounted for.

Unless additional heat is provided, vaporization has a cooling effect, so that over time, less concentration is delivered. If additional heat is provided, vapor pressure of the agent is increased, producing a greater delivered concentration. Traditionally, anesthesia machines have been manufactured from highly conductive metals that allow heat from the ambient atmosphere to be continually drawn to the vaporizer, thus providing continued energy for vaporization. Today, most machines use temperature-compensated draw-over vaporizers to minimize the impact of temperature variations.

Depending on the vaporizer used, several other factors play a role in vaporization efficiency. The amount of contact carrier gas has with liquid anesthetic is one factor. Failure to keep a vaporizer adequately filled results in low delivered concentrations and the patient awakens, despite the fact that carrier gas flow is adequate. Rapid gas flow through a vaporizer may outpace the vaporization process and also result in low delivered concentrations, because carrier gas–liquid contact is brief. Contamination of wicks by moisture prevents mixing of volatile agents and carrier gas so no anesthetic vapor is produced. In certain equipment designs, pressure on the breathing bag creates negative pressures within the vaporizer that vacuums liquid anesthetic into the delivery circuit, a potentially hazardous occurrence. Adding baffles that prevent liquid from entering the breathing circuit is helpful in minimizing this problem. These problems emphasize that anesthetists must be thoroughly familiar with the design and operation of the vaporizers and circuits they use. Sudden malfunctions are cause for removing equipment from service until the problem is identified and remedied.

Principles engendered by the gas laws, laws of diffusion, and vaporization process have wide application in clinical settings because they help explain how gases behave. They help explain ventilation, internal and external respiration, the behavior of gases in closed body cavities, and the usefulness of therapeutic gases.

The Therapeutic Gases

Therapeutic gases find their principal medical applications in anesthesia and respiratory therapy. Some, nitrous oxide and oxygen for instance, are widely used each day. Others have more limited uses. The following discussion reviews basic properties of the more useful gaseous agents.

Oxygen. Oxygen is by far the most widely used medical gas. This colorless, tasteless, odorless gas constitutes one fifth of our atmosphere and is an essential requirement for survival because it is the primary element used by the body as an oxidant for metabolic reactions. It is transported in the body combined with hemoglobin and, to a lesser extent, in simple solution within blood. The amount in solution can be increased by hyperbaric administration. Disease states that interfere with delivery or utilization of oxygen require treatment by administration of increased oxygen levels up to 100 percent by mask, nasal catheter, or endotracheal tube. Some substances, for example, cyanide and carbon monoxide, interfere with oxygen–hemoglobin binding. Sodium nitroprusside, a hypotension-producing drug used in anesthesia, can produce such a block because it contains significant amounts of cyanide.

Oxygen occurs naturally in three isotopic forms, the most common being oxygen-16. Here, one atom combines readily with another atom to form molecular oxygen, O_2. Three atoms combine to form O_3, ozone, a constituent of the upper atmosphere that helps protect the earth from the sun's radiation. Molecular oxygen used for medicinal purposes is 98 to 99 percent pure. When cooled below its boiling point (− 183C), it becomes a light blue liquid. Further cooling to − 217C solidifies the liquid. Oxygen is a paramagnetic substance and is drawn to magnetic fields. Under proper conditions, it may form free radicals, superoxide anions, thought to be implicated in oxygen toxicity. Oxygen is highly reactive, combining with a wide range of substances. It spontaneously reacts to discolor or oxidize many metals, makes fats or oils rancid, and supports combustion of flammable substances. It also forms peroxides, H_2O_2.

Molecular oxygen has a weight of 32, a density just over 1.4 at STP, and a specific gravity of 1.105 compared with air. Its critical temperature is − 118.4C. Oxygen has a low specific heat and is readily soluble in water, about 5 mL per every 100 mL at 0C. Under normal conditions, approximately 0.3 mL of oxygen is in simple solution in each 100 mL of blood. Each gram of hemoglobin chemically combines with 1.34 mL of oxygen. The gas is commercially prepared by fractional distillation of liquefied air. Its concentration in a mixture of gases, as from anesthesia machines, can be measured by oxygen analyzers, of which there are several types. Oxygen saturation of hemoglobin can be detected by oximeters. The gas is most commonly stored as a compressed gas in green or green and white cylinders of various sizes at pressures around 2000 psi. For large-use facilities, such as hospitals, bulk liquid storage is used. As the liquid is warmed and decompressed, it converts to the gaseous form. Prolonged administration of high oxygen concentrations can produce changes in lung tissue, producing symptoms of oxygen toxicity. The exact cause is not yet known. Several mechanisms may be involved.

Nitrogen. Nitrogen, as an inert element, does not readily combine with other substances. It, too, is prepared by fractional distillation of liquid air and is odorless, colorless, and tasteless. Atomic weight is 14, but like oxygen, nitrogen exists primarily as a diatomic structure, N_2, with a molecular weight of 28, the two atoms held together by a triple bond. Nitrogen has a density of 1.205 at STP and is lighter than air, having a specific gravity of 0.967. Under appropriate conditions it can combine with hydrogen, or with oxygen, with which five oxide combinations are possible. One is nitric oxide, NO, a possible impurity of nitrous oxide gas which is used to formulate nitric acid. Nitrous oxide, another oxide, is widely used as an anesthetic. It is the only nontoxic oxide of nitrogen. Large amounts of nitrogen are in simple solution in blood and other body fluids. Introduction of anesthetic agents into the body requires displacement of nitrogen, a process termed *denitrogenation*. Under conditions of sudden atmospheric decompression, expansion of nitrogen bubbles within the body gives rise to gaseous emboli that occlude blood vessels and disrupt circulation. Treatment is by rapid recompression followed by slow decompression. Untreated, patients will develop symptoms of narcotization. Severe symptoms can produce death. Detection of nitrogen in a gas mixture is accomplished by gas chromatography or mass spectography.

Nitrogen can also be liquefied (boiling point = −196C) and used as a cooling agent, as for cryosurgery. Caution should be exercised because contact with liquid nitrogen can produce "cold burns." Freezing tissue samples for microscopic analysis is sometimes accomplished with this agent. It is also used as a compressed gas for powering various tools used in surgery. Combined with oxygen, it serves as a breathing mixture for deep-sea diving and flying, and for medicinal uses where administration of pure oxygen is contraindicated. Its low reactivity makes it useful for adjusting atmospheres where combustible materials are kept or where the chance for fires is great. It is noncombustible and is stored either in liquid form or as a compressed gas in black cylinders at a pressure of approximately 2000 psi. Compressed air, the mixture of nitrogen and oxygen used medically, is stored in yellow containers. Oxygen–nitrogen mixtures for nonmedicinal purposes are stored in black and green cylinders.

Nitrous Oxide. Nitrous oxide is the most important inorganic gas used in clinical anesthesia practice. It has a molecular weight of 44.02 and is roughly 1.5 times as heavy as air (sp gr = 1.527). Nitrous oxide is colorless but possesses a slight taste and odor. It is not considered irritating when inhaled. Its boiling point is − 89C, the critical temperature. Manufacture is by decomposition of ammonium nitrate. Nitrous oxide is stored as a liquid in blue cylinders. Cylinder pressure varies with room temperature but aver-

ages 750 to 800 psi. If moisture is present around the cylinder outlet, condensation and freezing can occur. This is no longer a common problem with modern preparation of the gas. To prevent contamination of cylinders by higher oxides of nitrogen that can cause epithelial damage to lungs, commercial production is carried out in multiple stages, which ensures purity. Nitrous oxide is relatively insoluble (blood solubility is 0.47), so that it enters and exits the body quickly and relatively unchanged. It does, however, rapidly diffuse into endotracheal tube cuffs and closed body compartments. This can be a problem during certain types of pneumoencephalograms or when patients have a bowel obstruction. Expansion of the gas generates detrimental increases in pressures. Providing analgesia requires relatively high concentrations (50 to 70 percent), and the minimum alveolar concentration (MAC) required to provide complete anesthesia would exceed 100 percent, so nitrous oxide is regarded as an incomplete anesthetic. Nitrous oxide is nonflammable but, containing oxygen, it supports combustion. Under most conditions, however, the gas is stable, neither decomposing nor polymerizing. It maintains its stability even when passed through carbon dioxide absorption canisters.

Carbon Dioxide. Carbon dioxide is an organic compound. Its main importance lies in the fact that it is the end product of the body's biochemical respiration. It also has some limited use as a respiratory stimulant. Carbon may combine with oxygen to form either carbon monoxide or carbon dioxide. The former is lethal when inhaled because it prevents oxygen from combining with hemoglobin. Carbon dioxide (CO_2) also forms a small part of our atmosphere, 0.03 percent. It combines readily with water to form carbonic acid, important in acid–base regulation. But in general, it is a stable chemical. Similar to nitrous oxide in molecular weight (44) and specific gravity (1.54), it too is easily compressed to a colorless liquid and is stored as such in gray cylinders. Carbon dioxide is absorbed and neutralized by alkalis to form carbonates or, if large amounts of CO_2 are present, bicarbonates. Having a very high molal heat capacity, carbon dioxide is an excellent quenching agent for reducing flammability of combustible mixtures or for extinguishing fires. Absorption techniques are used to detect its presence in a mixture of gases because it absorbs infrared waves. Measurement of end-expired carbon dioxide has become a more widely used clinical tool in the past few years. Carbon dioxide is also used for calibrating blood gas analysis machines. A 5 percent carbon dioxide and oxygen mixture has been used as a respiratory stimulant in the past, especially for postoperative patients. The technique has largely fallen out of use because disadvantages often outweigh possible benefits. But it may have limited application. Exhaled carbon dioxide collecting in anesthesia breathing circuits, especially circle systems, must be disposed of physically or chemically to prevent rebreathing of CO_2 and development of hypercarbia. This topic is discussed separately later.

Helium. As one of the "rare" gases, helium is an inert, stable gas. Its principal anesthesia use has been as a diluent for other gas mixtures. The second lightest known element, helium exists as a single atom (atomic number 2, molecular weight 4) and diffuses readily, almost three times faster than oxygen. It is this property that makes helium useful for patients with severe respiratory obstruction, because less respiratory effort is required to breathe a helium–oxygen mixture than a pure oxygen atmosphere. An additional advantage is that helium is only slowly absorbed from occluded alveoli, minimizing development of atelectasis. Both properties facilitate oxygen delivery to patients with respiratory obstruction from airway narrowing.

Helium is also tasteless, odorless, and colorless. It liquefies only at extremely cold temperatures, below −269C, which is almost to the absolute zero point. It is quite insoluble, about 0.87 mL/100 mL at body temperature, so that it is readily eliminated from the body when administration is discontinued. Possessing a high degree of heat conductivity, helium has in the past been used as a quenching agent to reduce flammability of explosive or flammable anesthetic mixtures. Elimination of flammable agents from anesthesia practice has eliminated the need for quenching agents, but helium used as a carrier gas for delivery of oxygen in cases of respiratory obstruction still finds limited application.

HUMIDITY

The gases just described are dry, having no moisture content of their own. When administered to patients, they exert a drying effect that may damage tissues of the respiratory system. To overcome this problem, gases may be humidified. Adding water to dry gases (humidification) is a technique often employed during long surgical cases, not only to prevent respiratory system damage but also to reduce loss of body heat and moisture. Having a GMW of 18 g, water added to an atmosphere of dry gas lightens the atmosphere because it replaces diatomic molecules, oxygen and nitrogen, which are considerably heavier. The effect is to reduce barometric or atmospheric pressure. How well saturated with moisture dry gases become depends on the temperature of the environment and the amount of water present.

Dry air entering the lungs must be humidified by the respiratory passages. At normal body temperature, this creates a stable *water vapor tension* (*partial pressure*) of about 47 torr. Even when the atmosphere is highly saturated with water, it is cooler and less saturated than alveolar air. So body heat and water are lost in heating even this air. When patients breathe gases within a closed system where carbon dioxide is absorbed chemically, the relative humidity approaches 100 percent. The patient's exhaled air, coupled with water liberated by the chemical reactions of carbon dioxide absorption, provides the moisture-building mechanism. But even then, the water gradient is from the lungs to the atmosphere, because of the temperature difference. If water particles are large enough, they are seen as a mist or fog. Clinically, humidification is provided by bubble-through vaporizers or by nebulization. Some anesthesia humidifiers electrically warm and humidify the air passing through in an attempt to minimize body water loss. Temperature monitors should then be used in the delivery circuit to prevent delivered gas from exceeding body temperature. If delivered anesthetic gases are not humidified,

large amounts of body water are lost as lungs work to moisten the incoming air by evaporation of their cellular water. Humidity may be classed as either *absolute*, the maximum saturation of a given volume of air in grams per liter possible at a given temperature, or *relative*, the saturation actually present compared with the maximum possible saturation. Relative humidity is expressed as a percentage of the possible total. Dew point is the temperature at which, if a volume of air is cooled, excess moisture precipitates out. Measurement of humidity is termed *hygrometry*. One method uses a combination of two thermometers, one attached to a capillary-action wick soaked in water which, in a dry atmosphere, evaporates quickly to cause a marked fall in temperature, and one exposed to room air. The temperature difference between the two thermometers will be small if humidity is high. A greater difference occurs when humidity is low. Other methods, including electrically operated devices, are available for measuring humidity.

Barometers are used for recording atmospheric pressures. Several types are used. One, the closed *liquid-type* manometer, consists of a long, calibrated tube placed in a pool of mercury open to atmospheric pressure. Changes in pressure are transmitted against the mercury, which rises or falls in the tube. Variations of this type include both open and closed U-tube devices. *Aneroid* types (e.g., Bourdon gauges) transmit changes in pressure exerted against a diaphragm, through levers and gears, to a needle, which registers on a calibrated scale. Similar manometers are used in a variety of anesthesia settings for measuring tank pressures, blood pressures, and other pressures.

FLOW OF FLUIDS

Both gases and liquids may be thought of as fluid in that both are capable of flow through tubes or orifices. A *tube* is defined as a pathway whose length is greater than its diameter. An *orifice* is considered to have diameter but no or negligible length. Flow through tubes or orifices occurs when a pressure differential develops on either side of the pathway, the direction of flow being from high to low pressure. *Steady flow* occurs when all molecules of fluid pass through the pathway in the same direction and at the same velocity. Flow may be one of two types: *laminar flow*, where all molecules travel a parallel path within the tube, or *turbulent flow*, where some molecules take on a nonparallel path with respect to the other molecules (eddy currents). This concept is important to anesthesia practice because more energy is required to pass fluid through a tube in which flow is turbulent. An excellent example is the turbulence created in breathing circuits by kinking tubes or use of right-angle connectors. These reduce the efficiency of gas delivery. High flows increase the velocity of the molecules and thus create turbulence. This occurs when critical flow rates are exceeded. Laminar flows are typically associated with low velocities. Velocity will vary with the cross-sectional area of the tube pathway. The volume of flow per unit of time is a function of the cross-sectional area times velocity. Volume passed by a tube per unit of time is dependent not only on cross-sectional area, but also on tube length, pressure differential, and viscosity of the fluid. These relationships are summarized by *Poiseuille's law*, which states that for laminar flow in a cylindrical tube, volume of discharge is directly proportional to pressure gradient, inversely proportional to viscosity, inversely proportional to tube length, and directly proportional to the fourth power of the radius. This means that doubling the length halves the output, requiring an increase to twice the driving pressure to maintain the same output. Halving the length doubles output, so half the driving pressure is required to maintain output per unit of time. Of greater importance in most applications is the fourth power of the radius. Doubling or halving the radius results in a 16-fold change in flow. This is because a number of changes occur including a redirection of molecular velocities. Poiseuille's law finds numerous applications in anesthesia, for example, in breathing circuits, in the size of intravenous tubing, in changes in airway size, and in blood flow through constricted vessels. For liquids in a confined pathway, *Pascal's law* applies. Pascal's law states that, for confined liquids, any applied pressure is transmitted undiminished to all parts of the liquid. This accounts for the fact that a driving pressure may be developed in a closed system (e.g., water pipes), such that when the system is opened, flow begins immediately.

Fluid flows encounter resistance because traveling molecules create friction along pathway walls. Some of the driving pressure is directed toward overcoming forces of friction. It is friction that accounts for a drop in pressure as tube length is increased, usually as the square of the rate of flow. Friction is always higher with turbulent flows. For any given liquid, at any given temperature, a point exists, known as the *critical flow rate*, beyond which flow cannot be laminar because frictional forces limit laminar flow and create turbulence. This situation is analogous to the concept of electrical resistance found in Ohm's law.

Friction arises from two sources. One was described before where molecules of the flowing fluid are impeded by contact with molecules of the container walls. The other arises as internal friction within the flowing fluid caused by molecules passing alongside other molecules. This internal friction is termed *viscosity*. Molecules flow fastest in the center of the fluid, slowest at the edges nearest the container walls. Viscosity is dependent on the nature of the substance and its temperature. Liquids generally become less viscous as temperature increases, whereas gases usually increase in viscosity. Viscosity is not related to the density of the substance. Carbon dioxide, which is heavier and denser than oxygen, nonetheless flows faster through a tube of the same size. This is because its coefficient of viscosity is lower. Mixing of gases or liquids alters viscosity. The ratio of viscosity to density of a gas does influence critical flow rate. This ratio is termed the *Reynold's number*.

When liquids flow through a tube, a side pressure is exerted against the wall of the tube. The faster the flow through the tube, the less side pressure generated against the walls. This is known as *Bernoulli's law*. If the pathway varies in cross-sectional diameter, then at the point of greatest constriction, speed of flow will be greatest and side pressure least. Conversely, at the widest point, side pressure is greatest and speed of flow the slowest.

It is Bernoulli's theory that underlies the operation of a Venturi tube. This tube consists of a constricted path along which calibrated manometers are placed, proximal and distal to the constriction. The tube is used to measure volumes and flow rates of passing fluids. Venturi found that if the tube constrictions gradually widened out in cone fashion at an angle less than 15 degrees, distal pressures and flow rates reverted to what they were proximally. For constrictions that abruptly returned to the size and shape of the proximal tubing, pressures remained below what they were proximally. By constructing a tube with a cone-shaped constriction and placing a right-angle port at the point of greatest constriction, where pressure is least, possibly even subatmospheric, it becomes possible to draw a fluid, either gas or liquid, into the main tube. There it mixes with the primary fluid for delivery to the distal opening. This device is called an injector (Fig. 5–1). The principle is used in atomizers and nebulizers for delivering drugs and aerosols or for humidifying anesthetic gases. With injectors, the ratio of aspirated fluid remains constant despite changes in primary fluid flow (the Venturi effect).

To summarize what has thus far been presented regarding fluid flow through tubes and orifices:

- Flow through tubes is dependent primarily on viscosity and is hardly affected by density.
- Flow through orifices is dependent primarily on density, viscosity playing a minor role.

The picture is, however, somewhat more complex in that orifices may be of two types, *fixed* and *variable*. In the former, the size of the opening remains fixed, so that as more gas arrives from the source, pressure builds on the proximal side. Flow rate for any gas of given density will be dependent on, and proportional to, the square root of the proximal/distal pressure differential.

With fixed orifices, the initial proximal/distal pressures will be equal, and flow rate will equal one unit of the appro-

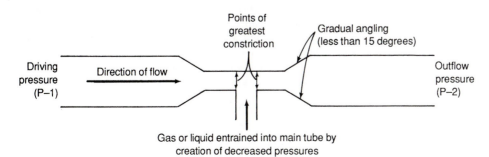

Figure 5–1. Venturi tube injector.

priate measurement, for example, L/min, mL/min. As proximal pressure is increased fourfold, flow rate doubles. Quadrupling proximal pressure again results in a fourfold flow rate increase from the initial flow rate. These changes are summarized as follows:

Proximal Pressure	Distal Flow Rate	Distal Pressure	Difference
1	1	1	1 : 1
4	$\sqrt{4} = 2$	1	4 : 1
16	$\sqrt{16} = 4$	1	16 : 1

But what happens when two different gases having dissimilar densities flow through the same fixed orifice? They develop different pressure gradients, less pressure being generated by the less dense, lighter gas. The pressure differential of two gases compared in this fashion will vary inversely with the square root of their densities. For example, hydrogen is 1/16th as dense as oxygen ($H_2 = \sqrt{MW\ 2}$, $O_2 = \sqrt{MW\ 32}$, or a ratio of 1 : 16). Taking the square root of this density difference ($\sqrt{16} = 4$) tells us that oxygen, the heavier gas, will create a fourfold pressure difference compared with hydrogen. Therefore, proximal and distal pressures for hydrogen and oxygen are always in a ratio of 1 : 4; flow rate doubles with each fourfold increase in pressure differential, but actual flow rate for oxygen will be double that of hydrogen because the net proximal–distal pressure differences for oxygen are always greater because of the density difference between the two gases.

	Proximal Pressure	Flow Rate*	Distal Pressure	Actual Flow Rate†
H_2	1	1	1	1
O_2	4	1	4	2
H_2	4	2	1	2
O_2	16	2	4	4
H_2	16	4	1	4
O_2	64	4	4	8

* Discounts density; flow rate is equal to the square root of the pressure differential only.
† Actual flow rate considering pressure differential and gas densities.

From the foregoing table:

	Proximal Pressure	Distal Pressure	Net Difference	Actual Flow Rate
H_2	4	1	3	2
O_2	16	4	12	4

If oxygen could be reduced to the same net difference as hydrogen, oxygen's actual flow rate would be 3/12ths of 4. Then, oxygen would flow only one fourth as fast: 1 L/min against hydrogen's 2 L/min.

	Proximal Pressure	Distal Pressure	Net Difference	Actual Flow Rate
H_2	4	1	3	2
O_2	4	1	3	1 (3/12ths of 4)

This demonstrates the next point about flow through fixed orifices: the flow rate per unit of time of a light, less dense gas can be accomplished through a smaller orifice than can the same flow rate for a heavy gas. Lastly, if the proximal–distal pressure difference is kept constant, flow rate will be directly related to the orifice diameter squared, a concept underlying the operation of anesthesia machine variable-orifice flowmeters. In reality, a variable-orifice flowmeter tube will be internally tapered so that when placed vertically, the tapered end is at the bottom. Within the tube, a floating bobbin (rotameter or float) moves up and down against a calibrated scale to indicate flow rate. A brief glance at the calibration scale will indicate that flow rates are not uniformly linear as one moves up or down the scale. A further comparison of flowmeters for the same gas from several machines will also reveal slight differences between supposedly similar flowmeters. This is because flowmeters must be individually calibrated against a standard, and the scale for each tube must take into account slight variations that have occurred in the manufacturing process. For this reason, broken flowmeters should have both the tube and corresponding scale replaced by another matched set. There are also wide variations, not always easily noticeable to the naked eye, between flow tubes for different gases. Each tube must take into account the density and viscosity of the gas for which it was designed. It also makes interchanging flow tubes between agents extremely hazardous because readings will no longer be accurate. Catastrophes have occurred in the past because of failure to appreciate these differences. Tapered tube/rotameter devices are known as Thorpe tubes.

Within a Thorpe tube, gas flows up from the source, around the bobbin, to the mixing manifold. The ring (annular) area around the bobbin increases as it moves up the tube because the cross-sectional area is greater (less tube tapering). The increase in annular opening is such that, relative to the length of the bobbin, more of an orifice is created. At low flows near the bottom of the tube, the ratio of bobbin length to annular opening more nearly approaches the configuration of a tube. Therefore, low gas flow is a function of viscosity, in line with Poiseuille's law. At high flows, where the opening is more of an orifice, flow rate depends on gas density. This is in keeping with Graham's law. Some flowmeters use a double taper within the tube to improve their accuracy at low flows.

With variable-orifice flowmeters, gas flow pushes the bobbin upward and gravity pulls it down. These flowmeters have an advantage over fixed-orifice meters in that the pressure difference across the orifice remains constant, and flow rate is measured against changes in the effective diameter of the orifice. This allows for all flowmeter tubes to be of approximately the same size, a mechanical advantage in machine design. Other types of flowmeters have been and are being used, but variable-orifice flowmeters are by far the most widely used. These principles have application to other types of flowmeters also.

CARBON DIOXIDE ABSORPTION

Hypercarbia and respiratory acidosis develop when the body is unable to rid itself of end products of metabolism,

or when a patient is allowed to breathe from an atmosphere high in CO_2 content. The latter situation can develop when a person rebreathes from an anesthesia circuit unless means are taken to disperse exhaled CO_2 or to remove it by chemical means. In nonbreathing anesthesia circuits, exhaled carbon dioxide is eliminated by diverting it to room atmosphere or into a scavenging device that removes it from the operating room environment. High fresh gas flows, in effect, blow the carbon dioxide out of the system.

With circuits that allow rebreathing of exhaled gases, such as a circle system, chemical removal provides a means of eliminating excess carbon dioxide. The amount chemically removed depends on whether the circuit is fully closed, allowing rebreathing of all exhaled gases, or partially closed, allowing only a fraction of exhaled gases to be rebreathed (semiclosed system). The rate of fresh gas inflow relative to production of exhaled CO_2 is also a factor.

Chemical absorption depends on the fact that carbon dioxide is a gaseous, nonmetal oxide, forming carbonic acid when in contact with water, and is capable of reacting with metal oxides. Metal oxides in contact with water form hydroxides (bases), which can neutralize acids. How effective a metal oxide will be in neutralizing acids depends on the metal's reactivity (position on the periodic table). Alkali metals are the most active. Of this group, potassium and sodium hydroxides are most commonly used. Alkaline earth metals are less reactive than alkali metals but may also be used. Of this group, barium and calcium hydroxides are used most often. As neutralization occurs, the reaction produces water and the carbonate of the metal hydroxide evolves; for example, calcium hydroxide becomes calcium carbonate. Additional exposure of the carbonate to the acid produces a bicarbonate. Sodium, potassium, calcium, and barium hydroxides can all eventually be converted to bicarbonates. Although some bicarbonate may form in CO_2 absorption canisters, complete conversion is usually not seen because canister efficiency is depleted before the conversion is complete. The canister must then be changed to maintain efficient CO_2 absorption. The carbonates formed are quite stable, decomposition occurring only under unusual conditions. As neutralization proceeds, the canister heats because of exothermic reactions produced by the hydroxides dissolving in water (heat of solution). Hydroxides have such affinity for water that they are termed *hygroscopic*; that is, they are substances that absorb, even become dissolved in, water from the surrounding environment. Yet a small amount of water is added as a film to soda lime granules to allow for ionization. The amount of water has to be controlled because too much reduces absorption efficiency.

Size, shape, and consistency of absorbent granules are important in maximizing efficiency. Granules are of a size termed 4–8 mesh because they must pass through a mesh screening having four to eight openings per inch. Because hydroxides are normally soft and easily pulverized, a small amount of silica is added to increase hardness. Granules should have a hardness number greater than 75, a number determined by agitating the granules with steel ball bearings prior to passing them through the sizing mesh. The shape of each granule, which looks like a small piece of lava rock with many indentations, maximizes the surface area available for chemical reactions.

Soda lime is composed of 4 percent sodium hydroxide, 1 percent potassium hydroxide, and 14 to 19 percent water, the balance being calcium hydroxide. This is known as the "wet" variety and is the most commonly used absorbent today. Silica may be added in small amounts to increase hardness. The amount of sodium hydroxide is limited, to prevent caking caused by hygroscopic absorption of water. Caking reduces absorption efficiency and increases resistance to gas flow within the circuit. With older forms of soda lime, a phenomenon known as "peaking" or "regeneration" occurred. After prolonged use, the soda lime efficiency would fall. Removing the canister from use allowed for some carbonate to be reconverted to soda lime. The canister could be reused with high efficiency but only for short periods. With modern canisters, peaking is of little clinical importance.

Because soda lime is used in the presence of dry gases, one might think that absorption efficiency is reduced. This is not the case, provided the moisture content for granules is high (about 14 percent). Besides water adhered to granules, additional water for chemical reactions is provided by exhaled moisture and by chemical release of hydrogen and hydroxyl ions, which combine to form water. Production of water by chemical reactions liberate heat, 13,700 cal per mole of carbon dioxide absorbed, which warms gases within the absorber. If excessive heat develops, the canister may feel warm to the touch. Excessive temperatures may have an adverse impact on patients by preventing dissipation of body heat.

Barium hydroxide granules are not as widely used. These granules differ in some respects from those of soda lime. Because barium hydroxide is an octahydrate ($Ba(OH)_2 \cdot 8H_2O$), additional water is not required. The barium hydroxide type of absorbent also contains calcium (about 80 percent) and potassium hydroxide (1 percent). It too is 4–8 mesh in size, but no hardening material is added. The water of crystallization keeps dust formation to a minimum. Heat production and additional water formation are essentially the same as with soda lime. As with soda lime, a color indicator is used to indicate expenditure of the granules; however, barium hydroxide does not regenerate to any appreciable extent.

Color indicators or dyes are added to both soda lime and barium hydroxide to indicate the extent to which absorbent has been exhausted. Those indicators are themselves either acids or bases that react to hydrogen ion concentration with a color change. With regeneration, dye color disappears. But any change in absorbent coloration indicates reduced efficiency with further use, and one should consider replacing the canister. A number of indicator dyes are used including ethyl violet, Clayton yellow, ethyl orange, mimosa Z, and phenolphthalein. Package inserts generally describe the color change to be expected from a particular brand of absorbent. Indicators are not absolutely reflective of the extent to which absorbent has been used because a number of factors may impact on dye color changes.

Absorbers used today have a dual-canister configuration. Fresh canisters come packaged in airtight containers to prevent moisture contamination prior to use. Each has a baffle at the top and bottom, which some manufacturers seal with an adhesive label. Failure to remove the label will obstruct gas flow within the absorber. Typically, modern absorbers are designed to allow a flow of gas exceeding expected tidal volumes breathed by patients. They also minimize mechanical resistance to breathing. A number of factors influence the efficiency of absorbers including the rate and pattern of ventilation, amount of carbon dioxide produced by the patient, rate of fresh gas flows used, and pattern of gas flow through the absorber. This last factor results in what is termed *channeling*. As gases pass through the canister, they take the path of least resistance. This path is usually along the sides of the canister where granules are less tightly packed. The effect is to funnel flows over the same areas of absorbent. Because of channeling, absorbent around the walls of the container is used up first, one factor responsible for rapid indicator dye changes along easily visible canister outer walls.

The chemical steps involved in carbon dioxide absorption may be summarized as follows:

1. Exhaled carbon dioxide combines with available water to form carbonic acid:

$$CO_2 + H_2O \rightarrow H_2CO_3$$

2. Carbonic acid dissociates into hydrogen and bicarbonate ions:

$$H_2CO_3 \rightarrow H^+ + HCO_3^-$$

3. The metal oxides dissociate to their respective ions. Soda lime absorbent includes sodium, calcium, and potassium hydroxides. Barium hydroxide lime includes calcium, potassium, and barium hydroxides.

Sodium	$NaOH$	$\rightarrow$	$Na^+ + OH^-$
Calcium	$Ca(OH)_2$	$\rightarrow$	$Ca^{2+} + 2\,OH^-$
Potassium	KOH	$\rightarrow$	$K^+ + OH^-$
Barium	$Ba(OH)_2 \cdot 8H_2O$	$\rightarrow$	$Ba^{2+} + 2\,OH^- + 8H_2O$

4. Hydroxides react with carbonic acid to produce carbonates:

Sodium	$2\,NaOH + H_2CO_3 \rightarrow Na_2CO_3 + 2H_2O + heat$
Calcium	$Ca(OH)_2 + H_2CO_3 \rightarrow CaCO_3 + 2H_2O + heat$
Potassium	$2\,KOH + H_2CO_3 \rightarrow K_2CO_3 + 2H_2O + heat$
Barium	Here four reactions are involved.

a. Barium hydroxide directly reacts with carbon dioxide:

$$Ba(OH)_2 \cdot 8H_2O + CO_2 \rightarrow BaCO_3 + 9H_2O + heat$$

b. Water from step a combines with carbon dioxide to form carbonic acid:

$$9H_2O + 9CO_2 \rightarrow 9H_2CO_3 + heat$$

c, d. The carbonic acid reacts with the available calcium and potassium hydroxides:

$$9H_2CO_3 + 9Ca(OH)_2 \rightarrow 9CaCO_3 + 18H_2O + heat$$

$$2KOH + H_2CO_3 \rightarrow K_2CO_3 + 2H_2O + heat$$

When regeneration reactions are allowed to occur, only sodium and potassium carbonates are reconverted to their respective hydroxides by reacting with unused calcium hydroxide. This is because both carbonates are soluble. Barium carbonate and calcium carbonate, being insoluble, cannot be reconverted to hydroxides. Two regenerative reactions are thus possible:

$$K_2CO_3 + Ca(OH)_2 \rightarrow CaCO_3 + 2KOH$$

$$Na_2CO_3 + Ca(OH)_2 \rightarrow CaCO_3 + 2NaOH$$

Regenerative reactions further deplete available calcium hydroxide and contribute to additional formation of calcium carbonate.

SOUND, OPTICS, AND IONIZING RADIATION

Sound

Sound, optics, and ionizing radiation are grouped together for two reasons. First, all of them relate more to physics than to chemistry. Second, each has only an indirect or peripheral relationship to anesthesia practice.

Sound waves are longitudinal waves created by molecular displacement within the conducting medium. They can travel through solids, liquids, or gases, the rate of conduction being fastest in solids and slowest in gas mediums. As the waves make contact with the tympanic membrane, secondary oscillations are developed that, through the auditory mechanism, are perceived as sound.

As with any wave phenomenon, the waves occur with varying frequency per unit of time. Wave frequency determines the perceived tone so that changes in frequency are detected as changes in pitch; however, pitch and frequency are not truly synonymous because pitch is a subjective interpretation. Frequency can also be expressed and measured as the number of cycles (waves) per second. The older measurement term *cycles per second* (cps) has been replaced by *hertz* (1 hertz [Hz] equals 1 cps). Doubling a given base frequency produces a *harmonic* of that frequency. Tuning forks used for testing auditory acuity are set to vibrate as harmonics of a two-cycle-per-second base, so that a fork vibrating at 512 Hz represents an eighth harmonic. Sound wave velocity in air is 1089 ft/s (331 m/s), accounting for sound's rapid dispersion. Stethoscopes used for listening to heart tones help diminish the otherwise rapid loss of those sounds. Loudness, or sound intensity, depends on the level of energy expended in generating the sound. A yell generates more loudness than a whisper of similar frequency because energy expenditure is greater. Sound intensity is measured in decibels (db). Quiet breathing produces a sound level of about 10 db, the lower threshold for audible sound. Normal conversation tone generates about 60 db, and loud noises such as clatter caused by a metal operating room tray being dropped can exceed 100 db. Levels above 120 db may cause pain. The Occupations, Safety, and Health Act sets a maximum average exposure level of 90 db. Continuous exposure to higher levels can result in hearing impairment. In addition, a number of physiologic responses to noise are known to occur. These include sleep alterations, depressed mental functioning, changes in endocrine function including glucocorticoid and catecholamine release, and cardiovascular vasoconstriction. Chronic exposure to high levels of background noise is now considered a form of nonspecific stress. As most operating rooms have highly sound-reflective walls, floors, and ceilings, anesthetists and other operating room personnel risk chronic exposure to high noise "pollution." Use of soundproofing materials within operating rooms is limited by the need for facilities that can be made bacteriostatic.

As a noise source moves toward a listener, the sound's frequency appears to change, even though the sound is being generated at a constant frequency. This difference between perceived and actual sound frequencies is known as the Doppler effect and is due to the fact that the number of sound wave fronts converging on the listener (per unit of time) increases as the noise source moves toward him or her. The Doppler principle is used in anesthesia monitoring devices able to emit sound and also receive the reflected waves. Such devices are used for blood pressure monitoring and detecting blood flow changes through the heart. Pulsations cause heart or blood vessel position to change with respect to the sensing device. The reflected sound waves change correspondingly, and this frequency change is detected by the sensor, which emits the altered tones from a built-in speaker. Such Doppler devices allow more accurate blood pressure readings and detection of heart sound changes caused by air emboli. As little as 0.5 mL of air passing through the heart can be detected in this way.

Sound waves are often thought of in terms of the frequency range perceptible to human ears, but they exist above and below that range as well. Those under normal range (below 20 Hz) are referred to as *subsonic*. Those above the range of normal hearing (about 20,000 Hz) are termed *ultrasonic*. The ultrasound range has several useful applications in medicine. Newly developed ultrasonic detectors are important as diagnostic tools. Their growing popularity stems from the fact that they can be used noninvasively. Ultrasonic waves are also used for cleaning. Often found in operating rooms, ultrasonic cleaners are highly efficient in removing tenacious debris from difficult-to-clean areas, such as removing mucus from inside a bronchoscope. They operate on the basis of a cavitation process. As sound waves are transmitted through the cleaning medium (water), pressure changes create numerous small bubbles. Rupture of the bubbles creates negative pressure, which acts as a vacuum to break up and disperse dirt or colloidal proteinaceous material.

Optics

Optics is the science concerned with the study of light. Visible light forms but a small portion of a continuum of radiant energies known as the electromagnetic spectrum. At the low end of the spectrum are electrical waves of long wavelength. Above this range we have, in order of decreasing wavelength, long and short radio waves, infrared light waves, visible light, the ultraviolet light range, x-rays, gamma rays, and cosmic rays. The nature of these radiations is controversial. Early light theories postulated a continuous waveform. Later, light was thought to be a particle, and later yet, a form of electromagnetic wave. The wave–particle controversy continued for decades, with adherents and scientific "proof" abundant on both sides. The controversy stemmed from the fact that wave theories are generally correct for explaining the behavior of light but cannot explain all its properties. For example, the photoelectric effect (electron emission from substances exposed to light) was first described by Hertz. But it was Einstein who later explained the phenomenon on the basis of light being a particle. Einstein also first postulated that light is quantified into small bundles called photons, each possessing an energy proportional to its wave frequency. Today it is generally accepted that light has a dual nature and that other electromagnetic radiations also represent *quanta* of energy. This quantum of light energy, the photon, is now assumed to be a massless particle capable of carrying energy and momentum from place to place. Light is subject to gravitational bending, but being massless, it can never itself come to rest. That is, it can never be stopped, so that it becomes impossible to ever capture (detect) a photon.

Light travels at a phenomenal speed, 2.98×10^8 km/s (about 186,000 miles per second); yet it can easily be refracted (bent) as it moves from one medium to another, as from air to water. Prism laryngoscopes use this principle. Light travels in two planes, horizontal and vertical, so it is said to be polarized, and one or the other plane may be blocked by polarized filters. If light is directed on a reflective surface at an angle, it is reflected from that surface at an equal angle. It is thus possible to concentrate light where it is needed. Fiberoptic laryngoscopes and microscopes use this principle. Shining white light through a prism separates it into individual colors or frequencies by dispersion, a property underlying the operation of spectroscopes. The candela (cd) is the SI unit of measurement for light intensity.

Lasers are a form of light energy increasingly used as a surgical tool. Atoms exposed to an energy source have their electrons forced into a higher energy state, a process called excitation. As the electron returns to its normal energy state, a photon is released. That photon may then collide with other "excited" atoms, causing release of another photon of the same frequency. This process repeats and is termed *stimulated emission*. The photons multiply as a chain reaction. If the reaction takes place inside a substance with a crystalline configuration, such as a ruby crystal, a large number of photons pass down the crystal's axis. Mirrors are used to deflect additional photons into traveling the same axis, so that as more and more photons are released, all are of the same frequency or wavelength and travel in the same direction. A partially transparent mirror allows the laser light to be emitted. As it leaves, beam intensity can be controlled and focused to allow its use as a surgical tool.

The term *laser* itself describes the process: light amplification by stimulated emission of radiation. Laser light differs from other forms of light not only in the manner by which it is produced but also in its nature. It is monochromatic, coherent, and parallel. Because each photon represents a packet of energy, concentrating the sum energies of all the photons makes lasers extremely powerful.

Besides solid lasers, such as those employing a ruby, there are also gas lasers. These have more surgical applications. Generally they use carbon dioxide, argon, or helium neon. Carbon dioxide lasers, in particular, find wide application. They deliver a beam in the infrared range (10.6 μm), which destroys tissue and coagulates blood by a thermal effect. The amount of tissue destroyed depends on its moisture content and the amount of laser energy used. Lasers have some important implications for anesthesia. The light may be reflected, so all personnel must use eyewear to protect delicate eye tissue from beam contact. Endotracheal tubes or other equipment may be damaged by the high energies of a misdirected laser beam. When used in the presence of high delivered oxygen concentrations, flash fires can occur as endotracheal tubes or other items are heated to the combustion point and fueled by the oxygen.

Ionizing Radiation

Ionizing radiation is that energy associated with substances whose atomic nuclei spontaneously decompose (radioactivity) to transmute the substance into another element. This spontaneous degeneration releases three forms of energy particles: alpha, beta, and gamma. An alpha particle is essentially the nucleus of the helium atom stripped of its electrons, leaving it with two positive charges and an atomic mass unit of 4. Beta particles are massless electrons possessing a negative charge. Gamma radiation is a nonparticle electromagnetic radiation of shorter wavelength (higher frequency) than x-rays. Radioactive elements are typically unstable isotopes, substances with altered atomic masses because of a change in neutron number within the nucleus. Cobalt-60, sodium-24, phosphorus-32, iodine-131, and radioactive iron and gold are all isotopes with useful diagnostic and therapeutic applications in medicine.

The rate at which a radioactive substance decomposes is its *half-life*, the length of time required for a given mass to be reduced by half. Half-life can vary in time from minutes to thousands of years, depending on which substance is involved. A similar term, *biologic half-life*, refers to the time required for half a given dose of radioactive isotope to be eliminated from the body.

Alpha, beta, and gamma radiations vary in both the speed at which they travel and in the amount of ionizing potential they possess. Ionization occurs as the particles interact with either the orbital electrons or the nuclei of other atoms, including those in body tissues. Alpha particles are highly ionizing but travel slowly and can be stopped by skin so that their biologic importance is limited. Beta particles have higher velocities and are more penetrating but have a lower ionizing potential. Gamma radiation travels at the speed of light and is extremely penetrating, but has the least energy. All, however, are capable of causing ionization, thereby converting other substances into ions or radicals. Proteins become altered, and genes may be changed so that cellular growth becomes abnormal. These changes produce radiation sickness, the symptoms of which vary with the dose of radiation received.

Radiation is measured in several forms. The curie (Ci) is a measure of the activity of radioactive substances. The roentgen measures exposure to x-rays or gamma radiation. But it is the rad (radiation absorbed dose) that has great biologic importance because it measures the dose absorbed by body tissues. The rem (roentgen-equivalent-man) is the amount of any absorbed radiation equivalent to one roentgen. The RBE (relative biological effectiveness) is used to compare an absorbed dose of radiation with that of cobalt-60. It is used primarily in radiation therapy to measure tissue effects of a given radiation dose.

Radiation can be detected in a variety of ways including radiation badges, dosimeters, and radiation counter devices. The maximum permissible dose (MPD) is a calculated value indicating how much radiation may be absorbed before detrimental effects are produced on important body organs (genitals, heart, blood-forming organs, etc.). How much radiation a person receives depends on a number of factors including type of radiation, length of exposure, distance from the source, previous level of exposure, and amount of shielding.

In terms of a single exposure, total absorbed dose determines the extent and severity of radiation illness produced. Less than 100 rad produces minimal biologic injury. Above this level, three recognized syndromes may occur. Up to 600 rad, patients develop a hematopoietic syndrome characterized by anemia and hemorrhage caused by suppression of blood-forming organs. With 600 to 1000 rad, a gastrointestinal syndrome occurs accompanied by symptoms of nausea, vomiting, diarrhea, fever, abdominal pain, and loss of hair. At doses exceeding 1000 rad, patients develop a central nervous system syndrome, which is inevitably fatal. Symptoms include lethargy, ataxia, and convulsions. Doses of 3000 rad or greater are usually fatal within a few hours to days.

BIBLIOGRAPHY

Adriani JA. *The chemistry and physics of anesthesia.* Springfield, IL: Charles C Thomas; 1962. (A classic work.)

Beiser A, Cummings B. *Physics.* 4th ed. Menlo Park, CA: Bubco; 1989.

Blatt FJ. *Principles of physics.* 3rd ed. Boston: Allyn & Bacon; 1989.

Dorsch JA, Dorsch SE. *Understanding anesthesia equipment.* 2nd ed. Baltimore: Williams and Wilkins; 1984.

Gillespie RJ, Humphreys DA, Baird NC, Robinson EA. *Chemistry.* 2nd ed. Boston: Allyn & Bacon; 1989.

Huheey JE. *Inorganic chemistry: Principles of structure and reactivity.* 3rd ed. New York: Harper and Row; 1986.

Meyer E. *Chemistry of hazardous materials.* 2nd ed. Englewood Cliffs, NJ: Prentice-Hall; 1989.

Oxtoby DW, Nachtrieb NH. *Principles of modern chemistry.* New York: CBS; 1986.

Principles of Organic Chemistry and Biochemistry in Anesthesia

Leo A. Le Bel

Until 1828, scientists thought the chemistry of living organisms distinct from that of inorganic substances. In that year, a German chemist named Wohler prepared urea, a supposed organic substance, from ammonium cyanate. By demonstrating that organic compounds were not dependent on bodily chemistry for their production, Wohler introduced a new branch of chemistry. Organic chemistry is devoted to the study of compounds formulated from a base of carbon atoms; the diversity of organic compounds is extensive. Drugs, petroleum products, plastics, and numerous other substances we encounter daily depend on the versatile atomic structure of the carbon atom.

THE CARBON ATOM AND THE ALKANES

Carbon has six protons and six electrons in its atomic structure. The electrons are distributed according to the theory of octet: two in the first orbit and the remaining four in the outer orbit. It is carbon's four outer electrons that give it its unique properties. Carbon shares its outer electrons with other atoms, in pairs, forming a *covalent bond*. In covalent bonding, sharing of electrons benefits each basic atom. Carbon forms such bonds with many elements, including other carbon atoms. In particular, it readily combines with hydrogen atoms having one outer-orbit electron. This provides needed stability for both atoms. By sharing carbon's electrons, hydrogen assumes the stable configuration of a helium atom. Carbon and hydrogen so readily come together that they form a whole group of distinct compounds, the hydrocarbons.

Simplest of the hydrocarbon structures is one carbon atom surrounded by four hydrogen atoms, the gas methane (CH_4).

The next most complex hydrocarbon structure is called ethane. It contains two carbon atoms that each share one electron. The remaining carbon electrons pair with hydrogen electrons (CH_3—CH_3).

After ethane comes propane. Propane has three carbon atoms linked together, hydrogen filling the remaining binding sites. In order of increasing complexity, propane is followed by the compounds listed below:

Hydrocarbon Structure	Number of Carbon Atoms
Butane	4
Pentane	5
Hexane	6
Heptane	7
Octane	8
Nonane	9
Decane	10

The list continues, but these are the more commonly encountered compounds. Note that in each case the next higher compound in the series differs from the preceding one by C—H_2. This means the number of hydrogens is always twice the number of carbon atoms plus two ($2n + 2$). For example, decane with 10 carbons contains 22 hydrogens ($2 \times 10 + 2 = 22$). In this series of straight-chain hydrocarbons, known as the alkane series, each bond is accounted for by an individual atom. The hydrocarbons of this group are therefore said to be saturated. Removing a hydrogen results in the substance becoming a radical. For example, removing a hydrogen from methane (CH_4) leaves the methyl radical (CH_3). The methyl group is often encountered in organic chemistry and biochemistry. Radicals are named by converting the *-ane* ending of the parent compound to a *-yl* ending; methane becomes methyl, propane becomes propyl, and so on. Most saturated hydrocarbons are formed from fractional distillation of petroleum products. Compounds having fewer than 5 carbon atoms are gases, those having 5 to 16 are liquids, and those containing more than 16 carbons are solids. Alkanes are not extremely active chemically, although they burn readily and react with the halogens, especially chlorine and bromine, a fact important to the development of halogenated anesthetics. When burned, straight-chain hydrocarbons form water and carbon dioxide. Because of its limited chemical reactivity, the alkane series was formerly known as the paraffin group, *paraffin* meaning "little activity." They tend to be insoluble in water, though they are soluble in weakly polar solvents, such as the ethers. Isomers may be formed from many, but not all, alkanes having three or more carbon atoms. Isomers are discussed later.

The IUPAC (Geneva) System

Organic compounds can become exceedingly complex in structure. To simplify the naming of substances, the International Union of Pure and Applied Chemistry (IUPAC) developed a system for naming organic compounds known as the Geneva system. The more common or important rules are summarized here:

1. For branched-chain alkanes, the name is based on the longest continuous (i.e., unbranched) chain of carbons in the compound. For example,

$$CH_2-CH_2$$
$$CH_2-CH-CH_2 \quad CH_3$$
$$CH_3 \quad CH_3$$

when straightened, becomes

$$CH_3-CH_2-\overset{CH_3}{\underset{}{CH}}-CH_2-CH_2-CH_2-CH_3$$
$$1 \quad 2 \quad 3 \quad 4 \quad 5 \quad 6 \quad 7$$

The longest continuous chain totals seven carbons. The compound is therefore a heptane.

2. When naming positions of chains (e.g., methyl group in the example), beginning at either end of the longest continuous chain, assign a number to each long-chain carbon so that the first branching occurs at the carbon with the lowest number. In the example, numbering from the right would put the methyl group at carbon 5. Numbering from the left puts it at carbon 3. Branching is named from the lowest-numbered carbon atom at which branching occurs (3-methylheptane). If another methyl group occurred at carbon 4, the compound would be 3,4-methylheptane.

3. The terms *primary*, *secondary*, and *tertiary* are used to differentiate different forms of the same compound. These terms can also designate the number of direct bonds to other carbon atoms. For example, a tertiary

butyl would have one carbon attached directly to three carbons of the group:

$$CH_3-\overset{CH_3}{\underset{CH_3}{C}}-$$

4. Substituents (atoms of groups) may be indicated by a prefix and a number showing their position relative to the long chain. For example, 1,3,7-dimethyl nonane indicates that two methyl groups are located on each carbon at positions 1, 3, and 7 of the longest chain.

5. When identical groups are located on the same carbon of the main chain, numbers are supplied for each group. For example, 2,2-dimethylhexane says that two methyl groups are attached to the same carbon atom. Hyphens and commas are used to organize the parts of the name of the substance. Hyphens always separate numbers from word parts, and commas separate numbers from numbers. The intent is to make the final name one word.

6. Whenever two or more different groups are attached to the chain, several ways are acceptable for organizing the name of the compound. The last portion of the compound name will be the main-chain alkane. Other parts can be ordered in terms of their increasing complexity; for example, methyl, ethyl, propyl, or they can be listed in alphabetical order.

The Geneva system has other rules, but these basics should suffice for most compounds the anesthetist is apt to encounter. Radicals formed from alkane structures are sometimes termed *alkyl*s. Besides the methyl radical, other common radicals are ethyl (C_2H_5) and propyl (C_3H_7).

In addition to straight-chain alkanes, there are also ring-structured saturated hydrocarbons. The one of most interest to anesthetists is cyclopropane (C_3H_6). These ring structures are called *cycloalkanes*.

$$\begin{array}{c} H \quad H \\ \diagdown \diagup \\ H \diagdown \overset{C}{\underset{}{}} \diagup H \\ \diagdown \overset{C-C}{\underset{\diagup \quad \diagdown}{}} \\ H \qquad H \end{array}$$

Ring structures require additional energy to maintain their configurations, and this explains their instability. Cyclopropane is explosive for this reason.

New compounds can be obtained by substituting other atoms for hydrogen in straight-chain alkanes. Substituting chlorine for a hydrogen in methane produces methyl chloride. Such substitution compounds are termed *derivatives*. Other important nonalkyl substitutes include fluorine, chlorine, bromine, iodine, and the nitro (NO_2) and amino (NH_2) groups. It is also possible to combine several organic substances into new complex molecules with new properties.

The process is known as *polymerization* and the new substance as a *polymer*.

Alkenes and Alkynes

Chemically treating saturated hydrocarbons to remove hydrogen atoms produces unsaturated hydrocarbons that contain either two or three bonds between carbons. Those containing two bonds are called alkenes, those with three bonds alkynes. Because of their unsaturated double or triple bonding, these substances tend to be chemically reactive.

Alkenes have the general formula C_nH_{2n}. The ring structures previously described, known as cycloalkanes, also have the general formula C_nH_{2n}. Alkenes and cycloalkanes have two hydrogen atoms less than alkanes. The first member of the alkane group is ethylene, and the series is sometimes called the ethylene series. Older terminology referred to them as the olefin series. The gas ethylene has been used in anesthesia, but it was never extremely popular. It does form the basis for the production of many compounds including polyethylene, from which certain types of surgical suture are made.

Alkynes have the general formula C_nH_{2n-2}. They contain one triple bond. Just as alkene compounds end their names in *-ene*, alkynes have names ending in *-yne*. The first of the series is ethyne, more commonly known as acetylene. *Dienes* and *trienes* are organic compounds that contain two or three double bonds within their structure. They are not part of the alkene series, the members of which contain only one double bond.

Isomers

Compounds having the same molecular formula but different structures are termed *isomers*. Carbon compounds facilitate isomeric structures because the carbon atom possesses the characteristic of being able to rotate its bonds about its central axis. Isomers are of two main types: structural isomers and stereoisomers. The latter is further divided into two types: optical isomers and geometric isomers. *Structural isomers* usually differ in both physical and chemical properties from one another. The straight-chain form is known as the *normal isomer*. When one methyl group is branched off the major chain, the compound is called an *isoisomer*.

Normal   Isoisomer

Stereoisomers. Stereoisomers have identical structural formulas but differ in their spatial arrangement. *Optical isomers* occur when the groups attached to the carbon atom differ from one another. This causes a bending (rotation) of light passing through the substance's vertical axis. Light polarized to the right produces a *dextro isomer*. When the light is polarized to the left, the *levo* (or sinister) *isomer* is formed. The two forms are mirror images of one another. The *dextro* and *levo* isomers are also known as enan-

tiomorphs. Where both forms are mixed, no polarization of light occurs, and the mixture is termed *racemic*.

Geometric Isomers. *Geometric isomers* are formed from compounds containing two carbon atoms joined by a double bond. The double bond locks the carbons so that no axial rotation can occur. Two forms are possible: *cis isomers* and *trans isomers*. In the *cis* isomer form, groupings are arranged on the same side of the double bond. With *trans* isomers, they are located on opposite sides of the bond. Their spatial configuration is therefore different.

Cis isomer   *Trans* isomer

Tautomerism. A variation of structural isomerism occurs when, in certain compounds, atoms are able to shift from one position to another. This ability is known as *tautomerism*. Such shifts are often found in barbiturate drug structures. Isomers thus formed are known as *tautomers*, also called *ketoenol isomers*, because one group of compounds, ketones, are often able to shift a hydrogen bond from the attached carbon. The keto form hydrogen or radical is thus shifted to the carbonyl portion of the structure, the enol form. In the following example, R represents any given radical.

Keto form   Enol form

Some compounds, notably proteins, are capable of temporarily reorganizing their shapes so that the spatial orientation of any part of the structure changes in relation to its other parts. These so-called *conformational changes* are often induced by other physical or chemical factors. Removing the causative factor allows the compound to revert to its original shape.

Class Divisions of Organic Compounds

Organic compounds are normally divided into specific classes on the basis of identifiable structural groupings. The general formula for each group provides the common configuration for the class. R is used to represent any base group or radical.

Halogen Compounds

Halogen compounds have the general formula R—X, in which X can be any halogen atom, that is, chlorine, bromine, and so on. Alkyl halogen compounds (alkyl halides) are formed by replacing one or more hydrogen atoms of an aliphatic (straight-chain) compound with a halogen. Chloroform ($CHCl_3$), though no longer used as an anesthetic, is an example. It was prepared by chlorination of methane, three hydrogen atoms being replaced by chlorine.

Also used as an organic solvent, chloroform easily decomposes in the presence of light and air to phosgene, a poisonous gas. Ethyl chloride (C_2H_5Cl), a topically applied skin anesthetic, is another halide. Yet another halogenated compound used in anesthesia was trichlorethylene. Being double bonded (unsaturated), trichlorethylene was very unstable, especially in the presence of soda lime, where it decomposed to toxic by-products (dichloracetylene, phosgene, and carbon monoxide) to produce neuritis of cranial nerves and other problems. Despite such previous difficulties, most modern inhalation anesthetics have resulted from halide conversion of aliphatic or ether compounds.

Alcohols

Alcohols are derived from hydrocarbons in which a hydrogen is replaced by an OH group (general formula: R—OH). Thus, replacing hydrogen in methane produces methyl alcohol. Similarly, ethyl alcohol is derived from ethane, propyl alcohol from propane, and so on. Alcohols have a distinctive taste, burn readily, and enter into many chemical reactions. The simpler alcohols are readily soluble in water. Alcohols are classed as *primary*, *secondary*, or *tertiary* depending on the position of the radical(s). With a primary alcohol, the OH group is attached to the carbon atom at the end of a straight chain. In secondary alcohols, two radicals are joined to the carbon atom holding the OH group. Similarly, a tertiary alcohol has three organic radicals attached to the carbon having the OH group. The following structures illustrate the differences:

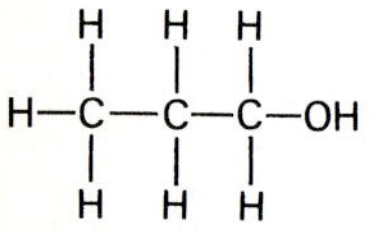

Propyl alcohol (primary) 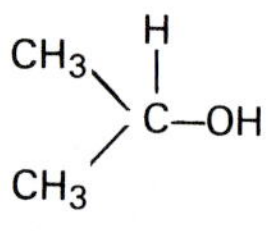   Isopropyl (secondary) 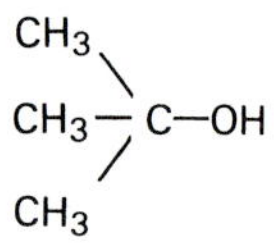   Tert-butyl alcohol (tertiary)

Although often neutral in chemical reactions, alcohols may behave as weak acids under appropriate conditions, and all are readily oxidized. When a primary alcohol is oxidized, an aldehyde is formed:

Methyl alcohol + oxygen → formaldehyde

Oxidizing a secondary alcohol produces a ketone:

Isopropyl alcohol + oxygen → acetone + water

Both aldehydes and ketones are discussed later. Oxidation of tertiary alcohols can produce a variety of compounds. Complex alcohols form the basis for such substances as glycol (ethylene glycol), commonly used as antifreeze and poisonous if taken internally. Most alcohols contain some water, but an anhydrous form is sometimes used to perform

a permanent neurolytic block in the treatment of intractable pain.

Aldehydes

Aldehydes have a functional group that give them their characteristic properties.

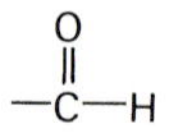

As previously mentioned, aldehydes are formed from oxidation of primary alcohols. This process involves removal of two hydrogen atoms from the hydrocarbon. The molecular oxygen that oxidizes the hydrocarbon splits, one atom of oxygen joining the two hydrogens to form water. The remaining oxygen becomes double-bonded to the carbon atom. Oxidation of hydrocarbons normally produces a new compound, in this case aldehyde, and water. Two important aldehydes encountered in medicine are formaldehyde and acetaldehyde. Both are gases at room temperature, have suffocating odors, and are strong reducing agents. Formaldehyde is used as a tissue preservative. Acetaldehyde is a breakdown product of ethyl alcohol, which forms the basis of commercial liquors. Aldehydes have a marked tendency to combine with themselves (polymerization). Acetaldehyde polymerizes to the hypnotic drug paraldehyde.

Ketones

Ketones are formed by oxidation of secondary alcohols. They have the general configuration known as the carbonyl group.

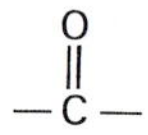

The best example is acetone. It is derived from isopropyl alcohol in the same manner as aldehydes, discussed in the preceding section. Acetone is a colorless liquid with a pleasant odor. An excellent solvent, acetone is particularly useful for removing residual adhesive tape from patients' skin. Diabetic ketoacidosis is a condition in which the body produces excessive amounts of ketones.

Organic Acids

Organic acids are hydrocarbons in which one or more hydrogens has been replaced by a carboxyl (COOH) group. The carboxyl grouping is really a combination of the carbonyl and hydroxyl groups already discussed and is characteristic of all organic acids. The hydrogen atom of the group ionizes in solution to give the compound acidic properties. Organic acids may be formed in one of two ways. They may be produced by oxidation of a primary alcohol to an aldehyde, which is further oxidized to the acid, or they may be produced by treating an organic acid salt with a strong mineral acid (e.g., sodium acetate when reacted with sulfuric acid yields acetic acid and sodium hydrosulfate). Because the hydrogen of the functional group is ionizable, it is replaceable by all metals above it in the electromotive series. As with other acids, the organic acids react with bases to form salts and water. One important organic acid is acetic acid (also known as ethanoic acid because it is derived from ethane), formed in the body by further oxidation of acetaldehyde. Organic acids are also important to the formation of body fats.

Esters

Esters are produced by the interaction of an alcohol with an acid. They are very volatile and have pleasant odors. Esters have the general formula R—COO—R. Isoamyl nitrite, used in a breakable ampule to treat angina pectoris by relaxing smooth muscles of the cardiovascular system, is an example. The drug is inhaled and enters the bloodstream where it dilates vessels and lowers blood pressure. A whole series of local anesthetic compounds are classed as esters. Most are esters of *para*-aminobenzoic acid. Tetracaine, used for subarachnoid block anesthesia, is an example of this group. Cocaine, a benzoic acid ester, is another local anesthetic. Used primarily for topical anesthesia of mucous membranes, it is also associated with a high incidence of illegal abuse. Benzoates and *para*-aminobenzoic acid are discussed later.

Ethers

Ethers are organic oxides having the general formula R—O—R. They consist of two hydrocarbon radicals joined by an atom of oxygen, which is the functional group. Diethyl (C_2H_5—O—C_2H_5) and divinyl (C_2H_3—O—C_2H_3) ethers have largely been removed from anesthesia practice because of their volatility and explosiveness. For years they were anesthetic mainstays, and even today, the public associates the practice of anesthesia with administration of ether. The explosive ethers have been replaced by halogenated, nonexplosive ones.

Methoxyflurane (2,2-dichloro-1,1-difluoroethyl methyl ether) is a pungent, sweet-smelling, potent anesthetic. Its use has diminished since the discovery that fluoride ions released during breakdown can contribute to high-output renal failure. Accumulation of the ions is both time and dose related.

Enflurane (2-chloro-1,1,2-trifluoroethyl difluoromethyl ether) is another sweet-smelling, nonflammable ether anesthetic. Still widely used, it is chemically very stable and does not require a preservative. Although it too may produce some renal dysfunction by ion accumulation during metabolism, the incidence is significantly less than with methoxyflurane.

Isoflurane (1-chloro-2,2,2-trifluoroethyl difluoromethyl ether) is the newest halogenated ether to be introduced into practice. Its properties are similar to those of enflurane, but induction and recovery periods are slightly shorter.

Halothane

Halothane (2-bromo-2-chloro-1,1,1-trifluoroethane) is another halogenated anesthetic compound, but it is *not* a halogenated ether. Halothane rightfully belongs in the class of halogenated hydrocarbons. It is a saturated compound with a pleasant odor and is still widely used despite its rare implication as a possible cause of hepatic damage. The structural formulas for the commonly used anesthetic agents are grouped together in Figure 6–1. Characteristics of the agents are listed in Table 6–1.

Amines

Amines have the general formula R—NH_2 and may be regarded as derivatives of ammonia (NH_3). The functional group is the nitrogen atom. Like alcohols, amines are also divided into primary, secondary, and tertiary forms. A primary amine has one hydrogen of ammonia replaced by an organic radical, such as a methyl or ethyl group. In secondary amines, two hydrogens are replaced by organic radicals; in tertiary amines all hydrogens are replaced by a radical. Amines confer hydrophilic properties to a molecule, making it more water soluble. They react chemically with water to form a base and with acids to form ammonium (NH_4) salts. Combined with a benzene ring structure, they become aromatic amines. Many vasopressor drugs used in anesthesia, including phenylephrine, epinephrine, and norepinephrine, have such a structure.

Quaternary Bases

Quaternary bases are formed from ammonium hydroxide (NH_4OH), the hydrogen atoms around the nitrogen being replaced by alkyl radicals. They have bacteriostatic and germicidal properties. More important to anesthesia, they form an essential part of the structure of muscle relaxants, ganglionic blocking agents, and cholinergic compounds. An example is succinylcholine:

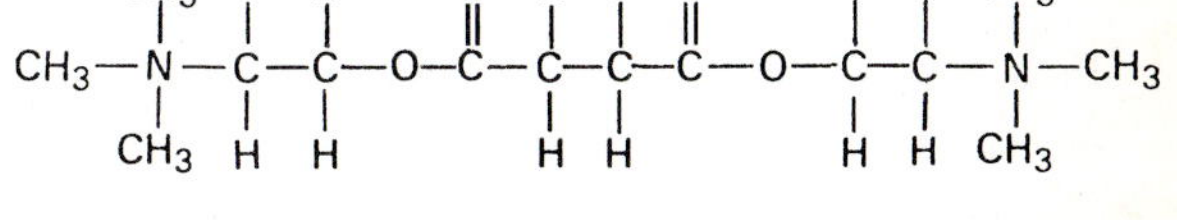

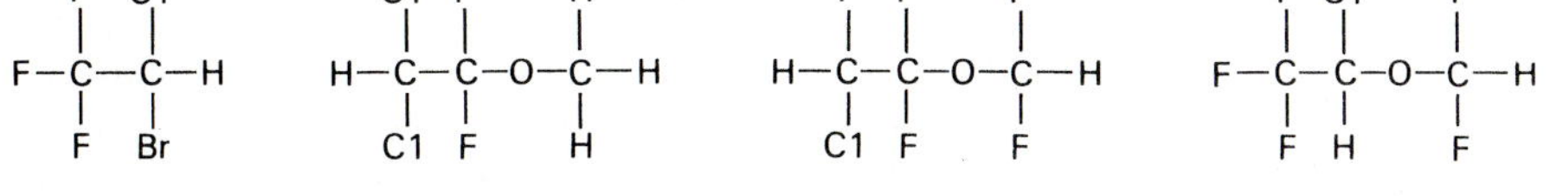

Figure 6–1. Structural formulas for commonly used anesthetic agents.

TABLE 6–1. CHEMICAL CHARACTERISTICS OF COMMONLY USED ANESTHETIC AGENTS

Characteristic	Halothane	Methoxyflurane	Enflurane	Isoflurane
Molecular weight	197.39	164.97	184.50	184.50
Boiling point (degrees C)	50.30	104.60	56.50	48.50
Specific gravity of liquid	1.86	1.40	1.51	1.50
Specific gravity of vapor	8.86	6.13	6.40	—
Vapor pressure at 20C	243.00	23.00	174.50	238.00
Minimum alveolar concentration (MAC)	0.74	0.16	1.68	1.15
Solubility coefficients				
Blood/gas	2.30	13.00	1.91	1.40
Brain/blood	2.60	1.70	1.40	2.60
Muscle/blood	3.50	1.30	1.70	4.00
Fat/blood	60.00	49.00	36.00	45.00
Oil/gas	224.00	890.00	98.50	99.00
Rubber/gas	120.00	630.00	74.00	62.00
Induction concentrations	2.0–3.0%	1.0–1.5%	3.4–4.5%	1.5–3.0%
Maintenance concentrations	0.4–1.5%	0.2–0.5%	1.5–3.0%	1.0–2.5%

Amides

Amides are characterized by the functional group

$$-\overset{\overset{\text{O}}{\|}}{\text{C}}-\text{NH}_2$$

sometimes written as —$CONH_2$. They are related to carboxylic acid. Urea, the body's end product of protein metabolism, is the best example. Amides constitute the second main group of local anesthetic compounds. Lidocaine is the most prominent example. Amines and amides are frequently confused. They may be distinguished by remembering that amines retain their hydrogen atoms intact, whereas in amides, the hydrogens surrounding the nitrogen atoms are replaced by radicals.

Amino Acids

Amino acids contain both an amino group (—NH_2) and an acid group (—COOH). Proteins are built by combining amino acids and, conversely, hydrolysis splits a protein into its constituent amino acids. The amino group can react with carboxyl groups to form acid amides. This reaction results in the liberation of water and the formation of *peptides*. Polypeptides are long chains of cojoined peptides. By these processes, amino acids can be combined and recombined into thousands of protein combinations, each differing in chemical properties. Of the approximately 20 known fundamental amino acids, 10 are essential to life. One of these, alanine, typifies the basic structure of amino acids:

$$\text{CH}_3-\underset{\underset{\text{NH}_2}{|}}{\text{CH}}-\text{COOH}$$

Because amino acids possess both an acidic group and a basic group, they act as either. This accounts for their amphoteric nature and allows them to become self-neutral-

ized. When this occurs, a dipolar ion called a *zwitterion* is formed. Self-neutralization also means that amino acid molecules are themselves electrically neutral. This facilitates their combination with other acids or bases, a trait that allows them to function as a body buffer system.

Besides amines, amides, and amino acids, other nitrogen-containing compounds are possible. Reacting alcohol with *nitrous* acid forms a nitroso group (—NO_2). Substituting *nitric* acid results in the formation of a nitro group (—NO_3). Nitroso compounds are referred to as nitrites, whereas nitro compounds form nitrates. Amyl nitrite exemplifies the former, and glycerol trinitrate (nitroglycerine) typifies the latter. Both have useful medicinal properties as coronary vasodilators.

Nitrogen-containing heterocyclic ring structures form the basis for pyrroles, pyridines, and purines. Pyrroles are one component of hemoglobin, pyridines form part of nicotinic acid and vitamin B, and purines form part of the genetically important RNA and DNA molecules. Other heterocyclic nitrogen-containing compounds are important for formulation of a number of alkaloids encountered in anesthesia practice, including morphine, codeine, cocaine, atrophine, quinine, reserpine, and LSD (lysergic acid).

Thio Compounds

Thio compounds occur when oxygen-containing organic molecules have their oxygen replaced by an atom of sulfur, the functional group. This exchange occurs readily because both oxygen and sulfur are within the same periodic group. Sulfur-containing substances are distinguished by a number of terms: thio-, sulfhydryl-, mercapto-, and sulfides. Alcohols, ethers, acids, or amides may all contain sulfur. Thiourea, condensed with malonic acid, helps form the thiobarbiturates. Widely used as anesthesia induction agents, thiobarbiturates are bitter-tasting yellow powders, whose sodium salts are highly alkaline (pH 9 to 11) and soluble in water. A number of these ultrashort-acting barbiturates are used clinically, all derived from the basic barbiturate acid (keto) structure:

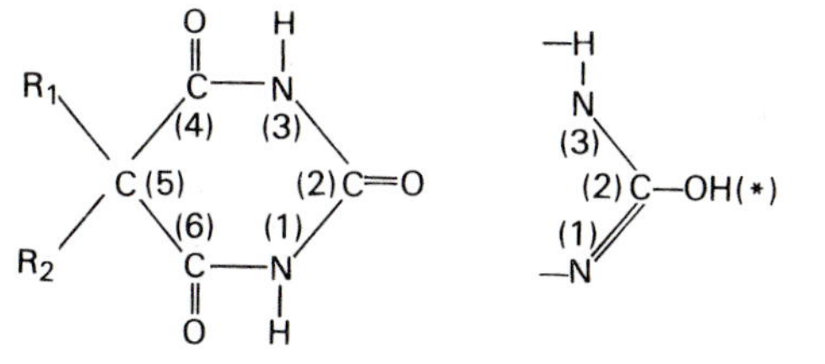

Keto form   Enol form

(*Note*: Position numbers of the ring are in parentheses.)

1. Hydrogens at (1) and (3) are referred to as imide hydrogens. They confer acidity on the compound. When one or the other or both imide hydrogens are replaced by a methyl or ethyl group, a nitrogen-substituted barbiturate is formed. Such drugs excite the central nervous system.
2. An oxygen at position (2) characterizes oxybarbiturates. Substitution of this oxygen with sulfur forms thiobarbiturates.
3. R_1 and R_2 are aliphatic compounds (one long and one short chain), which confer hypnotic potency to the compound.
4. The migrated hydrogen (*) may be substituted with an alkaline metal (e.g., sodium) to form a salt, making the drug more water soluble.

The ultrashort-acting thiobarbiturate sodium thiopental (sodium 5-ethyl-5-(1-methylbutyl)-2-thiobarbiturate) best exemplifies the structure of these compounds:

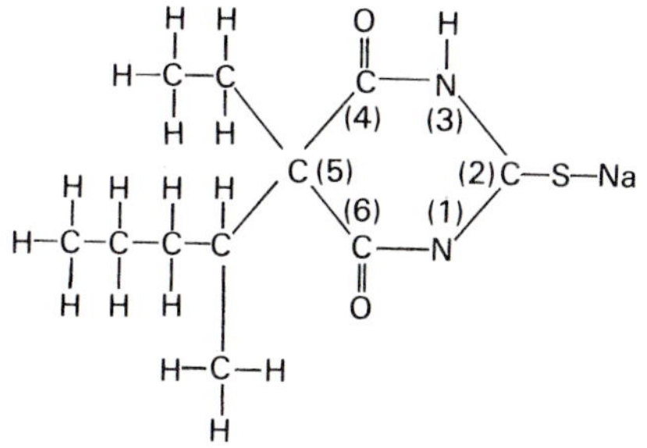

Sodium thiopental

Like other thiobarbiturates, this drug is stable in dry form but subject to decomposition when in solution. Concurrent administration with an acidic drug may cause precipitation. Thiopental is normally used in a 2.5 percent concentration prepared by adding 5 g of powder to 200 mL of diluent. The diluent may be sterile water, sodium chloride, or dextrose solution. Thiopental is the thio analog of another useful drug, pentobarbital, one of the oxybarbiturates. Although several groups of barbiturates exist, most clinically useful ones are either oxybarbiturates or thiobarbiturates.

Two other sulfur-containing groups are medicinally useful: *sulfonamides* and *sulfones*. The former are derived from sulfonic acid (SO_2OH). An acid amide member of this group, sulfanilamide ($—SO_2 NH_2$), was the first systemic antimicrobial drug to gain wide use. Sulfones have the identifying group

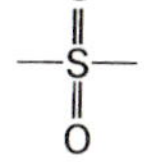

Phenolsulfonphthalein dye is a member of this group. It is used to measure the excretory ability of the renal system.

Aromatic Compounds

Aromatic hydrocarbons are formed when six carbon atoms are placed in a ring configuration containing three double bonds attached to alternate carbon atoms. Such double bonds are not the same as those in alkene structures. Rather, they represent oscillating electrons that are dispersed over the entire ring structure. This is often indicated by drawing the structure as a hexagon with an enclosed circle. Benzene (C_6H_6) is the simplest and most characteristic compound of the aromatic hydrocarbons. Its structure is

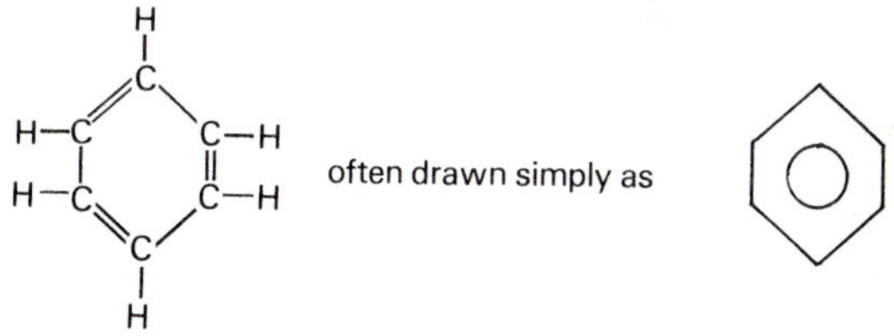

often drawn simply as

In these compounds only one hydrogen is attached to each carbon atom. New compounds are formed by replacing one or more hydrogens with radicals. If only one substitution is made, the position of the radical need not be stated; however, if two or more substitutions are made, some means of distinguishing their locations is necessary. This is done using the terms *ortho*, *meta*, and *para*. In an *ortho* isomer, the two radicals are attached to adjacent carbon atoms. With a *meta* isomer, the radicals containing carbon atoms are separated by an intervening carbon atom. The *para* isomers show two intervening carbon atoms. Generally, aromatic compounds are poorly reactive but highly flammable and volatile, their fumes often being toxic. They are also insoluble in water.

Multiple benzene rings can be joined to form *polynuclear aromatic compounds*. Two rings form naphthalene; three rings, anthracene. Another tribenzene ring, in which the third ring is moved out of the horizontal arrangement to an angled position, is called phenanthrene. It forms the basic structure for vitamin D, cholesterol, and sex hormones. Polynuclear aromatic structures are important to the formation of numerous pharmacologic preparations used in medicine. Producing these drugs usually involves converting single or polynuclear aromatic compounds to aromatic radicals. Virtually all the same radicals are possible with aromatic compounds as were possible with straight-chain hydrocarbons. Removing a hydrogen from benzene forms the phenyl radical. Radicals exist only in combination with other radicals or functional groups, never alone. A few of the more pertinent aromatic radicals are reviewed next.

Halogen aromatics are formed by substituting a halogen for a benzene hydrogen. Chlorobenzene is formed by substituting a chloride atom for one of benzene's hydrogens. A more complex structure, hexachlorophene, used as a surgical preparing solution, contains two halogenated benzene rings joined by a methylene group. Both rings also contain an —OH group, which makes them a hydroxy aromatic structure as well.

Hydroxy aromatic compounds are called *phenols*, from the combination of *phenyl* with the *ol* ending of alcohol. As the name implies, they contain both a phenyl group and a hydroxyl group. Phenol, known also as hydroxybenzene or carbolic acid, was the first widely used antiseptic solution. Though no longer used, it remains the germicide against which all others are compared.

Carboxylic acid derivatives are formed when a benzene hydrogen is replaced by a —COOH group. The simplest of these structures is benzoic acid. Aromatic esters are produced in the same manner as other esters, and a number of salicylate compounds are formed from them. The structures for hydroxy and carboxylic acid molecules can be diagrammed:

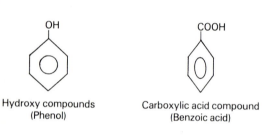

Hydroxy compounds
(Phenol)

Carboxylic acid compound
(Benzoic acid)

As previously mentioned, aromatic nitro compounds, aldehydes, ketones, amines, and amides are also possible. A number of more complex medicinal compounds (e.g., phenacetin) are drawn from these variations, and each group is formed in the same manner as already described for their nonaromatic counterparts.

Two other ring structure types are important in organic chemistry. The first is the heterocyclic compounds, such as the thiobarbiturates, which contain elements other than carbon in the main structure. The second group is the cycloalkanes, ring structures in which each carbon has two hydrogen atoms or radicals attached to each carbon. These differ from benzene in which each ring carbon has only one hydrogen attached and the entire structure shares oscillating electrons. Cyclopropane, the highly unstable and explosive anesthetic agent widely used in past years, typifies the cycloalkanes. (The terms *alicyclic compound, cyclic hydrocarbon,* and *carbocyclic* are used interchangeably with cycloalkane.)

Certain generalizations can be made regarding the relationship of hydrocarbon structures to their chemical and pharmacologic activity.

1. Volatility, flammability, and water solubility decrease as molecular weight increases; however, the higher the molecular weight, the more likely the substance will split into smaller, lighter compounds.
2. As carbon atoms are added to a saturated hydrocarbon series, pharmacologic potency usually increases and the margin of safety decreases.
3. As molecular weight increases, so too does lipid solubility and the magnitude of the oil/water distribution coefficient.
4. Potency also increases with the degree of unsaturation. Substances containing double or triple bonds are more unstable and therefore more willing to react. The more easily they react, the more potent they are likely to be.
5. Replacing hydrogen atoms with an —OH (hydroxyl) group usually decreases potency.

Most pharmacologic agents have extremely complex structures encompassing multiples of the components discussed in this section. Detailed structures of specific drugs can be obtained from pharmacology texts, but primary groupings presented here should allow identification of a drug's class and major molecular components. Understanding these enables the anesthetist to better judge the clinical effects of drugs and agents.

BIOCHEMISTRY

Biochemistry is the branch of science concerned with chemical reactions and substrates necessary to the life of biologic organisms. Biologic substrates can be loosely classed as water, carbohydrates, lipids, proteins and nucleic acids, enzymes, vitamins, and hormones. These help build cell structures for organs and systems. In turn, structure will determine function, enabling muscles to contract, nerves to conduct impulses, and so forth. In addition, substrates are involved in chemical reactions that provide the organism with energy. Bioenergetic processes allow the body systems to perform work and maintain a homeostatic environment.

The Substrates

Water. Water is the most abundant material constituting living organisms, accounting for 60 percent of total weight in human adults, 80 percent in infants. It serves as a solvent, lubricant, chemical reactant, and coolant for the body. The major portion of body water is chemically bound to cell constituents, but a smaller portion exists as "free" water, mostly in the blood and urine. The chemical properties of water make it the ideal physiologic solvent. It has a high dielectric constant ($D = 80.4$), which allows it to carry other substances as ions without allowing the substances to combine. As most nutrients and wastes that enter and leave the body do so as molecules in ionic form, water serves as a transport system. Water's high heat of vaporization (540 cal/g) and high heat capacity allow the body to dissipate or absorb large amounts of heat readily, thus maintaining body temperature within a narrow range. As a conductor of electricity, water facilitates nerve impulse transmission. Its dipolar configuration (see Chapter 5, Properties of Solutions) gives water the capacity for hydrogen bonding. This property is physiologically important because it gives appreciable structure to water and other substances such as proteins. Water is necessary for hydrolysis reactions (reaction of a salt ion with water to form an acid plus a base).

This, along with its limited ability to dissociate to H^+ and OH^- ions, allows it to play a role in acid–base balance.

Carbohydrates. Carbohydrates are another substrate. They are produced in plants by the interaction of photosynthesis and light on carbon dioxide and water. The term implies that carbon is attached to water in hydrate form. In reality, the carbon is attached to a number of separate hydrogen and hydroxyl groups. Moreover, an aldehyde or ketone group is often present because sugars are derived from polyhydric alcohols, those containing multiple OH^- groups. All have the general formula CHO, and four classes of sugars exist: monosaccharides, disaccharides, oligosaccharides, and polysaccharides. *Monosaccharides*, the simplest sugars, cannot be further hydrolyzed. They have the formula $C_nH_{2n}O_n$. Simple sugars are further classed as *trioses*, *tetroses*, *pentoses*, or *hexoses* based on the number of carbon atoms present. Each may also be an aldose or ketose depending on which functional group it contains. For example, glucose is an *aldose*, whereas fructose is a *ketose*. Carbohydrate chemical structures are often drawn in straight-chain form, but such a form cannot account for all of their chemical properties. A cyclic hemiacetyl structure suffices to explain their chemical properties, but diffraction studies using x-ray analysis show them to have a bent-ring configuration resembling a chair. For most discussion purposes, the straight-chain formulation is adequate.

D-glucose   D-fructose

Disaccharides are those sugars that, when hydrolyzed, yield two monosaccharides of either identical or dissimilar configuration. Sometimes included with the *oligosaccharides*, this class includes maltose and sucrose. Oligosaccharides yield two to six simple sugars when hydrolyzed, whereas *polysaccharides* yield more than six. Starches and dextrins are polysaccharides. Along with glycogen, they represent carbohydrates that are normally stored by the body for later use, whereas simple sugars are readily available for energy processes. Oxidation of carbohydrates produces carbon dioxide, water, and energy. This process is discussed later. As may be discernible from the two structures diagrammed earlier, carbohydrates are capable of forming isomers. (See Isomers under the Carbon Atoms and the Alkanes.) Most, but not all, biologically important sugars are *dextro* isomers. In addition, alpha and beta *anomers* occur when groups attached to the first carbon become rotated in position. Alterations in the positions of hydrogen and hydroxyl groups on carbon atom 2, 3, or 4 result in *epimers*. Galactose, for example, is an epimer of glucose, the change occurring on the fourth carbon atom.

Of the monosaccharide subclasses, several are biologically important. D-Glyceraldehyde is a triose sugar that results from oxidation of glucose. Ribose and deoxyribose, both pentoses, are important to the structure of RNA and DNA. Hexoses are the physiologically most important simple sugars. This group includes glucose, galactose, and fructose.

Glucose, always present in human blood, is the principal carbohydrate to pass into cells. Once there, it is readily oxidized for energy. Galactose, a glucose isomer, is produced from hydrolysis of milk sugar (lactose). Fructose, obtained from the same foodstuffs as glucose, is often chemically interchangeable with it.

Sucrose, lactose, and maltose are classed as disaccharides. They are isomers of one another. The first, sucrose, is table sugar. When hydrolyzed by the body enzyme sucrase, it breaks down to invert sugar, a mixture of glucose and fructose. Lactose, principal ingredient of breast milk, hydrolyzes to glucose and galactose under the influence of the enzyme lactase. Malt sugar, or maltose, is broken down by maltase to two molecules of glucose.

When a number of monosaccharides are joined together (polymerized), a polysaccharide is formed. Important members of this group are cellulose, starch, and dextrins. Cellulose constitutes the fiber portion of many foods providing the diet with bulk necessary for stimulating intestinal peristalsis. It passes through the body essentially unchanged because it cannot be hydrolyzed by body enzymes. Starch, on the other hand, can be hydrolyzed, first to dextrin, then to maltose, and finally to glucose. Dextrin is formed by partial hydrolysis of starch. Adhesive tape adheres to the skin because of its dextrin base. Spilling an iodine-based reagent such as povidone–iodine on the tape causes it to turn a blue-black color. The reaction indicates the presence of hydrolyzed starch. Starch is actually a composition of straight and branched structures (amylose and amylopectin). Glycogen resembles amylopectin, but is more branched. It is produced in the liver and stored both there and in muscle. As blood glucose level is depleted by exercise, glucose is replenished by hydrolysis of glycogen. This process helps the body maintain a constant blood sugar level of narrow range.

Polysaccharides contribute to tissue structure. The *mucopolysaccharides* or glucosaminoglycans are an example. They consist of amino sugars and uronic acids and help build skin, bones, and other tissues. One mucopolysaccharide of particular importance to anesthetists during surgery is the anticoagulant heparin. Heparin is composed of two compounds derived from glucose, glucuronic acid and glucosamine. Dextran, a plasma substitute sometimes used to treat severe hypovolemic shock, is a high-molecular-weight polysaccharide compound. *Glycoproteins* (mucoproteins) combine protein and polysaccharide structures. They contribute to the composition of mucous secretions and plasma α-globulins. The substances (isoagglutinogens) of red blood cells responsible for determining blood type and pituitary hormones (like luteinizing hormone and human chorionic gonadotropin) also have glycoproteins in their composition. Glycoproteins, along with glycolipids, contribute to the structure of cell membranes.

Sugars that can be easily oxidized by Benedict's or Fehling's solution or Tollen's reagent are known as reducing sugars. All mono- and disaccharide sugars except sucrose have this property because they contain an easily oxidized aldehyde group. The CH_2OH group in sugars can also be oxidized, either alone or with the aldehyde group. The latter produces a carboxyl group. It is also possible for the hydroxyl group to react with acids to produce esters. This occurs with phosphoric acid, the esters of which, when hydrolyzed, produce high-energy bonds for bioenergetics. Oxidation facilitates conversion of chemical energy within sugars to other forms more easily stored or used by cells to perform work.

Lipids. *Lipids* are related to fatty acids and have two distinguishing properties: (1) they are relatively insoluble in water and (2) they are easily soluble in nonpolar solvents. All are greasy to the touch and have a glistening appearance. Fats, oils, and waxes are included in the class. Having a specific gravity less than one, they float on water. Dissolving lipids in water forms an emulsion, which separates into layers on standing. Like carbohydrates, lipids are composed of carbon, oxygen, and hydrogen but may also contain nitrogen and phosphorus. Lipids are the major constituent of adipose tissue. Colorless, odorless, and tasteless, lipids perform a multiplicity of functions for the body, acting as sources of energy and as insulation and protection for organs and the body as a whole. Ingested lipids are emulsified by bile in the intestines and carried in that form to body cells.

Hydrolysis of fats produces fatty acids, which normally contain an even number of carbon atoms and have a straight-chain configuration. *Saturated fats* contain no double bonds, whereas *unsaturated fats* contain one or more such bonds. Under the Geneva system, fatty acids are named by substituting *-oic* for the final *e* in the name of the hydrocarbon containing the same number of carbon atoms. Saturated acids thus end in *anoic*, whereas unsaturated ones end in *enoic*. An eight-carbon fatty acid would be named octanoic, derived from octane. Carbon atoms are numbered from the carbon that helps form the carboxyl group. Superscripts are used with unsaturated lipids to indicate the number of carbons, number of double bonds, and their position, for example, $C^{20:1;10}$.

Lipids are classed on the basis of their solubility and their hydrolysis products. *Simple lipids* are esters formed by reacting fatty acids with alcohols. Those that contain another group in addition to the ester are termed *compound lipids*. Two specialized groups in this class are the *phospholipids*, which contain a fatty acid, alcohol, and phosphoric acid residue, and the *cerebrosides*, which contain fatty acids, carbohydrates, and nitrogen, but no phosphoric acid. Lipoproteins are also compound lipids. Derived lipids or fatty acids are formed by hydrolyzing the other groups. Glycerols, sterols, aldehydes, and ketone bodies are included in this category.

Acetic acid (vinegar, CH_3COOH) is the fatty acid forming the basis for the *saturated series* of lipids. They have the general formula $C_nH_{2n+1}COOH$. Acetic acid's structure is

$$
\begin{array}{c}
O \\
\parallel \\
C-OH \\
| \\
H-C-H \\
| \\
H
\end{array}
$$

Propionic, butyric, and caproic acids are also important saturated fatty acids. Respectively, their formulas are C_2H_5COOH, C_3H_7COOH, and $C_5H_{11}COOH$. Palmitic, stearic, and arachidic fatty acids have dietary importance, and lignoceric acid is important to the structure of brain and nervous tissues.

In addition, *unsaturated* fatty acids are classed on the basis of their degree of unsaturation. *Monounsaturated* acids have the general formula: $C_nH_{2n-3}COOH$. Oleic acid is an example of this group. It is found in nearly all fats. *Polyunsaturates* can have two or more double bonds. Linoleic, linolenic, and arachidonic acids have, respectively, two, three, and four double bonds. Prostaglandins, compounds that exert a number of physiologic effects on blood vessels, muscles, and other tissues, are derived from arachidonic acid. Unsaturated fatty acids may have a number of geometric isomers.

The alcohols in more complex lipid structures include glycerol and cholesterol. Triacylglycerols, more commonly known as *triglycerides* or neutral fats, are esters formed from glycerol and fatty acids. Hydrolysis splits the triglycerides to the alcohol and fatty acids that formed them. Neutral fats can be oxidized for energy, and most body cells except the brain can use broken-down triglycerides interchangeably with glucose for energy. Breakdown of fatty acids occurs in cell mitochondria by a process termed *beta oxidation*. The acid is first combined with coenzyme A (CoA), discussed later under Enzymes, to form a molecule known as fatty acyl-CoA. This process is energized by the degradation of adenosine triphosphate (ATP) to adenosine monophosphate (AMP) with concurrent loss of two high-energy phosphate bonds. The second step of the process involves removal of two hydrogen atoms from carbons of the fatty acyl-CoA, leaving a residual double bond. The hydrogens are joined to flavin adenine dinucleotide (FAD) and are later oxidized. The remaining double bond joins with water so that one hydrogen attaches to one carbon and a hydroxyl radical attaches to the other carbon. Next, two more hydrogen atoms are removed by nicotinamide adenine dinucleotide (NAD), which combines with one hydrogen and the hydrogen from the hydroxyl group. The two removed hydrogens are later oxidized. The process breaks the alpha and beta carbons of the compound to form a long chain and a short chain. The long chain combines with new CoA and the process is repeated from the second step onward. The short chain is really acetyl-CoA because it remains bound to the original coenzyme A that started the process. The entire process is repeated over and over again until the entire fatty acid has been converted to acetyl-CoA.

In turn, some acetyl-CoA combines with oxaloacetic acid and joins in the citric acid cycle, a process discussed later. Those molecules that do not, pair and condense to form molecules of acetoacetic acid. This acid is then converted to β-hydroxybutyric acid and lesser amounts of acetone. Small amounts of hydroxybutyric acid and acetone are always present in the blood, but their accumulation can cause a condition known as *ketosis*. Acetoacetic acid is a keto acid; it, β-hydroxybutyric acid, and acetone are known as ketone bodies. Ketosis occurs with starvation and certain diseases that derange metabolism (e.g., diabetes mellitus). Carbohydrates and proteins can also be converted to acetyl-

CoA and, in turn, can be built into triglycerides, thus adding to stored body fats.

Along with hydrolysis (reacting lipids in the presence of catalytic enzymes to produce glycerol and fatty acids), lipids may be split by *saponification*, a process that involves splitting a glyceride with a base, such as sodium hydroxide, to produce glycerol and the salt of a fatty acid. This process is not important physiologically but is used in making soaps. Volatile fatty acids often turn rancid and develop a foul odor. The process is like the one that converts lipids to body energy, that is, hydrolysis of the ester followed by oxidation to aldehydes and ketones, which are then acted on by bacteria to produce butyric acid.

The *iodine number* of a lipid substance indicates the degree of unsaturation: A high number indicates a high degree of unsaturation and vice versa. Hydrogenation is the process of adding hydrogen atoms to unsaturated lipids to produce saturated compounds.

Phospholipids include phosphatidic acid, phosphatidylglycerol, phosphatidylcholine, phosphatidylethanolamine, phosphatidylinositol, phosphatidylserine, lysophospholipids, plasmalogens, and sphingomyelins. The first is an important intermediate in triglyceride production. The second helps form cardiolipin, a phospholipid found in mitochondria. The third, phosphatidylcholine, also known as lecithin, is widely dispersed throughout the body and has both metabolic and structural functions. For example, dipalmityl lecithin is a surface-active agent responsible for alveolar surface tension; its destruction results in respiratory disease. Cephalins, formed from ethanolamine phospholipids, are similar to the lecithins. Plasmalogens also resemble lecithins and cephalins. They constitute as much as a tenth of the phospholipids found in brain and muscle. Sphingomyelins are also found in large quantities in the brain and other parts of the nervous system.

Cerebrosides, or glycolipids, contain a combination of galactose and sphingosine, derived from the amino acid serine. They are often grouped with sphingomyelins as sphingolipids. Found in large quantities in the brain and nervous system, especially in medullated nerve fibers, they are also present in the spleen and other reticuloendothelial tissues. On hydrolysis, many phospholipids produce phosphoric acid and a nitrogen-containing compound.

Steroids are often found in association with fats. All are formed from a cyclic nucleus similar to that of phenanthrene. (See The Carbon Atom and the Alkanes.) Like other compounds previously mentioned, they too are capable of forming a number of isomers. Steroids that contain at least one hydroxyl group and no carbonyl or carboxyl groups are called sterols. One, cholesterol, has been implicated in cardiovascular disease and the development of gallstones. Steroids help form a number of biologically important substances including sex hormones, vitamin D, adrenocortical hormones, and the bile acids (cholic acid). In addition, cardiac glycosides and some alkaloid drugs may also contain steroidal structures.

Lipids are insoluble in water because they contain a large number of nonpolar hydrocarbon groups. Those lipids that do contain some polar groups (e.g., sphingolipids, phospholipids, and fatty acids) may be partly soluble. At oil–water interfaces these molecules become oriented in a particular direction. Polar groups orient to the water, nonpolar groups to the lipid. Cell membranes are considered to consist of a bilayer of such polar lipids. Aggregation of these polar groups containing lipids in a highly aqueous medium causes formation of micelles, groups of molecules that orient their polar sides to the water, thus forming a ball-like arrangement. The nonpolar portion of the molecules points in toward the center of the ball. Larger micelles arrange themselves in the same manner but are usually stabilized by emulsifying agents, which help form a surface layer that separates the aqueous phase from the nonpolar ends of the molecules. In 1935, Danielli and Davson[1] proposed that cell membranes were composed of lipid bilayers sandwiched between proteins. Later, this description was modified to include protein "pores" embedded in the bilayer. Singer and Nicolson[2] proposed that the entire structure constituted a fluid mosaic capable of temporary restructuring to allow for entry of drugs and other substances. This fit well with the earlier observation of Overton[3] (circa 1900) that many compounds penetrated cells on the basis of their lipid solubility rather than molecular size. Current thinking postulates that anesthetics may work by temporarily, and reversibly, disrupting bimolecular lipoprotein cell membranes. Several recent experiments support this view, but it remains unclear whether anesthesia is produced by membrane disruption only, or as a result of yet undiscovered intracellular processes, or by a combination of mechanisms. Other theories of narcosis have been advanced, but the one described appears the best model, based on current evidence.

Proteins and Nucleic Acids. Proteins and nucleic acids are the next important groups of substrates. Both are important for forming protoplasm, building new body tissues, and repairing damaged tissues. Protein buffer systems act to maintain normal pH in cells, body fluids, and lymph. They also help maintain water balance between those tissues. Proteins provide amino acids for synthesis of new nitrogen-containing compounds and can furnish energy stores when both carbohydrate and lipid mechanisms are depleted or fail to function. They also supply ingredients for building enzymes, hormones, and oxygen-carrying hemoglobin.

Proteins are large molecules built by polymerization of various combinations of the 21 known amino acids. Generally, they contain carbon, hydrogen, oxygen, nitrogen, and sulfur. In amino acids, the amino group (NH_2) is attached to the carbon atom of the first CH_2 group, which in turn is attached to the —COOH group. Those amino acids the body can synthesize only to a slight extent or not at all are referred to as essential amino acids. The remainder are termed nonessential. The simplest amino acid is glycine:

$$
\begin{array}{c}
H \\
| \\
H-C-COOH \\
| \\
NH_2
\end{array}
$$

Nonessential amino acids include alanine, asparagine, aspartic acid, cysteine, cystine, glutamic acid, glutamine, glycine, proline, serine, and tyrosine. The essential amino acids include arginine, histidine, isoleucine, leucine, lysine, methionine, phenylalanine, threonine, tryptophan, and valine. Like all simplest sugars, all amino acids except glycine contain an asymmetric carbon and thus polarize light so that isomers could exist; however, all naturally occurring ones have the same L-configuration, comparable with D-glyceraldehyde. Serine has been shown to be convertible to L-glyceraldehyde; therefore, other amino acids are referenced to serine, for example, L(−)-leucine. A plus or minus sign is used to indicate the plane in which the light is polarized.

Conjugated proteins consist of both protein and nonprotein substructures. The latter are termed *nucleic acids*. Nucleic acids are polymers of *nucleotides*, low-molecular-weight molecules that participate in a number of biochemical reactions. Nucleotides are composed of a nucleoside and a phosphate (H_3PO_4). *Nucleosides* are made up of a pentose sugar (either ribose or deoxyribose) and a purine or pyrimidine ring. Cytosine, uracil, and thymine are the main pyrimidine rings used; adenine and guanine are the usually encountered purine rings. Nucleotides serve as precursors for ribonucleic acid (RNA) and deoxyribonucleic acid (DNA). In addition, purine ribonucleotides participate in high-energy and messenger mechanisms in the body. ATP is an example of the former, whereas AMP exemplifies the latter. They are also components of some coenzymes. The pyrimidine nucleotides play a role as high-energy intermediates in carbohydrate metabolism.

Proteins may be classed as simple and conjugated. *Simple proteins* produce only α-amino acids when hydrolyzed. They include albumins, globulins, globins, and albuminoids (scleroproteins). *Conjugated proteins* hydrolyze to other amino acid types and include phosphoproteins, glycoproteins, chromoproteins, and nucleoproteins. Proteins may also be classed according to structure or functionally as structural proteins, enzymes, hormones, antibodies, blood proteins, or contractile proteins. The last group includes actin and myosin, which allow muscles to contract. As proteins are composed of amino acids, it is not surprising that their chemistry is essentially that of amino acids. As pointed out earlier, amino acids contain both an amino group, which is basic, and an acid carboxyl group. They can therefore act as either acids or bases and for this reason are said to have an amphoteric nature. Building of proteins from amino acids involves combining the amino group of one molecule with the carboxyl group of another. When two amino acids are combined in this way, a molecule of water is lost, and the two amino acids become a dipeptide. As additional molecules are added, the structure becomes a tripeptide or polypeptide. The *peptide linkage* (—CO—NH—) is also known as the amide grouping. As each amino acid is added, another peptide bond is formed. If the amino acid contains sulfur, as does cysteine, there may be an oxidation reaction between two cysteine residues, which produces a cystine residue and water. This is known as a *disulfide bond*. Another bond found in amino acid structures is a *salt bridge*. This type occurs when the ionic bond between an acid group and a base, or amino group, forms a salt. *Hydrogen bonds* may form between hydrogen and either carbonyl oxygen or nitrogen atoms within a protein structure. These may occur within the main chain as well as in side chains. Electrostatic bonds are those that form between salt bonds of opposite electrical charge. Peptide bonds are the strongest of all bonds.

From a biochemical viewpoint, proteins may have four structures, referred to as primary, secondary, tertiary, and quaternary. Primary structures show the amino acid/peptide bond chain in ordered sequence with radical groups running to the sides of the chain. Secondary types depend on hydrogen bonding within the molecule and may take one of two forms: a coil-shaped helical arrangement or a pleated sheet in which hydrogen bonds exist between chains. Tertiary structures occur when the protein molecule is folded on itself and held together by various types of bonds. Fibrous collagen tissue is an example. Quaternary structures are formed by bringing the protein's chains together. In hemoglobin, four chains are held together by various bonds, giving the molecule an overall convoluted appearance.

Hemoglobin has two pairs of chains, alpha and beta. The first pair has 141 amino acids per chain, the second pair 146 each. Each chain also contains a heme group. The sequence of the amino acids on each chain is genetically determined. Hemoglobin's function is to transport oxygen necessary for respiration. This is accomplished by hemoglobin altering its structure in such a manner as to envelop the oxygen. When the oxygen is released to the tissues, the hemoglobin returns to its original form. Such conformational alterations of structure are characteristic of proteins.

Proteins are high-molecular-weight compounds, sometimes exceeding a molecular weight of 1,000,000. Most are water soluble, though they tend to form colloidal solutions rather than a true solution. Their size and number enable them to exert considerable osmotic effect; however, they do not traverse membranes well, which accounts for the fact that proteins are not normally recoverable in urine.

Because they can carry electrical charges, proteins readily interact with other charged substances. Although peptide chains bind the greater portion of amino and carboxyl groups, the presence of these groups on side chains means that they will ionize in solution and carry a net charge, which varies with the pH of the solution. At one specific pH point, the *isoelectric point*, all charges are balanced. The protein will not travel to either the cathode or the anode because its electric charge is equal to zero. (See Chapter 7.) To either side of the isoelectric point, the protein will migrate to one or the other pole depending on its electrical charge. This property is useful for separating proteins from one another by electrophoresis, as in the diagnosis of sickle cell disease, where any abnormal hemoglobin will have a different isoelectric point from normal hemoglobin.

Proteins may be broken down or destroyed by a number of processes. Within the body, chemical hydrolysis is facilitated by the presence of enzymes called proteases. The resulting amino acids can be recombined into new proteins. Proteins may also be destroyed by heat and other sterilizing processes. This principle is used in destroying bacterial protein to kill microorganisms and to render items sterile for surgical use. The process is called *denaturation* and consists of physical disruption of the protein's helical structure by disruption of the weak bonds linking various protein chain sections together. This disruption causes the protein to coagulate. Only the weak bonds, not the peptide ones, are broken. Nonetheless, the protein is effectively destroyed. Certain chemicals may also denature proteins. Examples include an alkaloid, tannic acid, which has been used to cauterize bleeding tissues. Other examples are alcohols, used as disinfectants, and heavy metals, which poison by destroying tissue proteins. Strong acids and bases also denature proteins.

The body is incapable of storing proteins and has only a limited capability for building them. Essential amino acids cannot be provided by the body itself and must be provided exogenously by dietary intake. Postsurgery, protein supplements may be useful in hastening tissue healing and recovery. When patients must fast for prolonged periods, supplemental proteins may be given parenterally in solutions that contain amino acids, trace minerals, and other supplements.

Protein metabolism results in salvage of any purine-based structures, which can then be used for rebuilding, but pyrimidine-based structures are degraded to urea and ammonia. Diseases that upset protein metabolism can result in elevated blood urea levels, tissue wasting, and other detrimental changes.

Other Substrates: Enzymes, Vitamins, and Hormones

Enzymes, vitamins, and hormones are three additional substrates necessary for biochemical reactions.

Enzymes. Enzymes function as catalysts for a variety of chemical activities. As catalysts, they reduce the amount of energy required to initiate or sustain a reaction but are themselves not part of it. Enzyme facilitation of reactions is very specific. Proteases act only on proteins, not on carbohydrates or lipids. Each enzyme has two constituents: a protein portion called the *apoenzyme* and a nonprotein portion termed the *coenzyme*. Enzymes fall into six categories. Those that facilitate oxidation–reduction reactions are called oxidoreductases. Transferases move chemical groups between molecules. Hydrolases catalyze reactions between substrates and water. Lyases help form double bonds, and isomerases facilitate production of isomers. Ligases break molecular couplings.

The important coenzymes include adenosine mono-, di-, and triphosphate (AMP, ADP, and ATP), cyclic adenosine monophosphate (3', 5'-cyclic AMP, often abbreviated cAMP), nicotinamide adenine dinucleotide with and without phosphate (NAD^+ and $NADP^+$), flavin adenine dinucleotide (FAD), and coenzyme A (CoA). Coenzymes are all involved in transfer reactions and may be functionally classed into those that transfer hydrogen (NAD^+ and $NADP^+$) and those that transfer other groups (ATP and associated compounds). Most contain an adenine ring coupled to a ribose sugar and phosphate. This gives them a strong resemblance to AMP. They differ only in the attached radical group.

Enzymes are important in electron transport and phosphate bond energy mechanisms. They are named by using the substrate name followed by the type of reaction catalyzed, for example, cytochrome $c:O_2$ oxidoreductase (cytochrome c oxidase). The suffix *-ase* identifies enzymes. Interestingly, enzyme activity is temperature dependent, optimum temperature being that found at cellular level.

Enzyme action may also be altered by changes in pH. Enzyme activity can be diminished or blocked altogether by inhibitors, of which there are two types: competitive and noncompetitive. Competitive inhibitors are so named because they compete with substrates. Generally, they have similar chemical configurations. Noncompetitive inhibitors disable the enzyme by reacting with one or more of its functional groups. For example, cyanide binds iron to render cytochrome c oxidase ineffective. Some enzymes, such as serum glutamic–pyruvic transaminase (SGPT) and serum glutamic–oxaloacetic transaminase (SGOT), can be diagnostic for disease states, often indicating liver or heart muscle damage. A few diseases, phenylketonuria (PKU) for instance, are caused by hereditary enzyme disorders.

Vitamins. Vitamins are important in regulating a number of biochemical reactions. They also serve as essential components of many, though not all, coenzymes. All are classed as either water or fat soluble. Fat-soluble vitamins are associated with lipids found in natural foods and include vitamins A, D, E, and K. Vitamin C and all B-complex members constitute the water-soluble group.

Recognition that particular foods possessed essential nutrients necessary for disease prevention came well before chemical identification of vitamin compounds. For this reason, vitamins have common names based on the alphabet—vitamins A, B, C, D, and so on. Each differs substantially in chemical structure, but all play a role in normal growth and health. Vitamins can be prepared in pure form by pharmaceutical companies, but an average balanced diet generally supplies all recommended daily allowances. Some vitamins have species-specific effects, and lack of even minute amounts of a particular vitamin can sometimes make a life-or-death difference to the organism. Fortunately, severe deficiencies in humans are rare and often easily correctable. When they do occur, they produce symptoms deleterious to optimum health. For example, lack of vitamin C alters formation of collagen-based connective tissues. This results in bleeding gums, loss of teeth, and other pathologic changes. Like essential amino acids, vitamins cannot be synthesized by the body. They must therefore be provided in the diet. Even today, many of their exact functions are not entirely clear. The following briefly summarizes the important points to be noted about each vitamin.

Vitamin A (retinal) is derived from β-carotene, a plant pigment, which serves as a provitamin. The vitamin plays a role in maintaining epithelial tissue. Ocular tissues are especially susceptible to damage if the vitamin is lacking from the diet. This is because light striking the eye causes a splitting of the eye pigment rhodopsin (visual purple) to a protein portion called opsin and the nonprotein retinal. Retinal is also called vitamin A_1 aldehyde or retinene. The light further decomposes the aldehyde to an alcohol, retinol. Then the enzyme, retinene reductase, with NAD acting as coenzyme, causes regeneration of retinal from retinol and, under conditions of darkness, new rhodopsin is formed. Lack of vitamin A retards this regeneration and a prolonged deficiency can result in night blindness or keratinization of the ocular tissues. Keratinization can, over time, result in permanent blindness. Lack of vitamin A also causes a number of other toxic effects, including decreased skeletal and soft tissue growth, damage to the brain and spinal cord, altered collagen formation, decreased mucopolysaccharide production, changes in cell membrane stability, and disturbances of liver cell mitochondria. Excess vitamin A intake can present problems as well. These include periosteal thickening of long bones, loss of hair, and painful joints. Zinc may play a role in maintaining plasma levels of the vitamin. Intestinal diseases such as sprue and dysentery decrease the amount of vitamin A absorbed by the body.

Vitamin D is, in reality, a group of sterol compounds. Some are provitamins. Under the influence of ultraviolet light, they undergo changes that help prevent rickets, a disease characterized by skeletal malformations and decreased bone calcification. The two most important members of the vitamin D group are ergocalciferol (D_2) and activated 7-dehydrocholesterol, also known as cholecalciferol or vitamin D_3. The latter can be synthesized and activated in humans through the action of sunlight. The reaction takes place in the skin. The main functions of vitamin D are to increase absorption of calcium and phosphorus by the intestines and to maintain phosphate regulation in the kidney. Cholecalciferol must first be converted to 1,25-dihydroxycholecalciferol to be metabolically active. This compound enables vitamin D to exert a major impact on calcium mobilization from storage sites in bone. Conversion takes place because of a number of chemical reactions in both the liver and kidneys. Apart from its effects on bone development and calcium absorption and mobilization, vitamin D plays a role in formation of messenger RNA and protein biosynthesis. Excess intake produces hypercalcemia and nephrocalcinosis (renal stone formation).

Vitamin E is derived from tocopherols and tocotrienols in plant oils. The principal ingredient, α-tocopherol, is present in many foods, but its absorption from the intestines is decreased in malabsorption syndromes, especially those involving lipids. Premature infants are susceptible to increased hemolysis, preventable by vitamin E administration. In adults, deficiency often occurs with a concurrent decrease in polyunsaturated fatty acid intake. Macrocytic anemia and decreased survival time of erythrocytes result. Low-birth-weight infants fed vitamin E-deficient formulas develop a syndrome characterized by anemia, thrombosis, edema, and reticulocytosis. Exogenous vitamin E therapy prevents the syndrome. The most important chemical role for vitamin E in the body is as an antioxidant. As polyunsaturated fatty acids easily react with molecular oxygen to form peroxides, it is beneficial that the vitamin prevents their toxic accumulation in tissues. By the same mechanism, it may also prevent lung damage associated with oxidant-containing atmospheres, such as smog. Other antioxidant biologic properties of the vitamin are being discovered. Vitamin E's properties possibly depend on the presence of selenium. Selenium is an essential component of the enzyme glutathione peroxidase, which scavenges hydroperoxides and converts them to primary and secondary alcohols. The vitamin exhibits notable species specificity. Tocopherol deficiency produces infertility in rats, muscular dystrophy in guinea pigs, and vascular degeneration in chickens. No comparable changes have been proven to occur in humans.

Vitamin K's primary physiologic function is to catalyze synthesis of prothrombin by the liver. Its absence causes development of hypoprothrombinemia and prolonged blood-clotting times. For vitamin K to be effective, it is necessary that liver parenchymal tissues be intact and functioning. No effect is produced when the liver has been damaged by cirrhosis or tumor. Its action is also blocked by agents such as dicumarol. (Conversely, bleeding caused by overtreatment with the anticoagulant dicumarol can be treated with vitamin K.) Prothrombin formation and clotting factors VII, IX, and X are all, to some extent, controlled by the presence of the vitamin. One of its two variations, K_1, may play a role in oxidative phosphorylation within mitochondria of tissue cells, though this has not been conclusively proven. Coenzyme Q, important in electron transport and oxidative phosphorylation, is similar in chemical structure to vitamin K and has been observed to exert many of the same effects.

Vitamin K deficiency is very unlikely, given its wide distribution in food and the fact that intestinal microorganisms are capable of producing it. In theory, prolonged fasting combined with administration of agents that destroy intestinal flora could produce a deficiency state. A somewhat analogous situation occurs in newborns where the sterility of the intestines predisposes to hypoprothrombinemia for several days until bacterial flora start producing the vitamin. For this reason, vitamin K may be administered prophylactically at the time of birth to prevent development of hypoprothrombinemia-induced hemorrhage within vital organs. Anesthetists should be aware of this and other aspects of vitamin K therapy. One such aspect is that, like dicumarol, salicylates antagonize the vitamin's effects. Another is that the vitamin is sometimes used in treatment of uncontrolled bleeding at surgery. This may be especially true for surgery of the biliary tract because normal absorption of the vitamin is dependent on bile, and resection of the intestine may alter its bacterial production, even into the postoperative period. In such situations, treatment with water-soluble preparations of the vitamin may be preferred.

Vitamin C, first of the water-soluble vitamins to be discussed, is called ascorbic acid. Its biochemical function is not yet entirely clear. It is known to play a role in maintaining teeth, cartilage, bone, and collagen synthesis. In addition, there are postulated nonspecific roles in oxidation–reduction systems and in metabolism of tyrosine, drugs, and adrenal steroids. It is found in large amounts in the adrenal cortex, where levels are quickly depleted by adrenocorticotropic hormone (ACTH) stimulation. Infectious processes increase the rapidity with which the vitamin is lost. On this basis, it has been suggested that vitamin C may have a role in stress reactions. Ascorbic acid is available in a number of foods, notably citrus fruits, but it is easily destroyed by cooling or oxidation. It is stored throughout the body in amounts corresponding to the metabolic activity of the tissues.

The *B vitamins* include thiamine (B_1), riboflavin (B_2), niacin, pyridoxine (B_6), pantothenic acid, lipoic acid, biotin (also known as vitamin H), inositol, *para*-aminobenzoic acid, cyanocobalamin (B_{12}), and the folic acid group.

Thiamine acts as coenzyme in a number of systems including the oxidative pathway for glucose. Lack of this vitamin impacts on the cardiovascular, gastrointestinal, and peripheral nervous systems. Though it is readily absorbed by the body, it cannot be stored to any appreciable extent. The amount available to the body depends on overall dietary intake of fats, carbohydrates, and proteins. It has been used to treat various neuritic conditions.

Riboflavin occurs naturally as a coenzyme with two flavoproteins: flavin mononucleotide (FMN) and flavin adenine dinucleotide (FAD). Both are involved in hydrogen transport. Riboflavin is combined with phosphate prior to its absorption. This occurs in intestinal mucosa. Phosphate activates the compound to enable it to participate in oxidation–reduction reactions. Deficiencies in humans are rare, and symptoms are similar to those of niacin deficiency.

Niacin helps form nicotinamide nucleotide coenzymes such as NAD^+ or the phosphate form $NADP^+$. Deficiency causes pellagra, whose symptoms include dermatitis, cheilosis (fissuring of the lips), and a dark red tongue. Niacin compounds serve as coenzymes for dehydrogenases and are involved in oxidation–reduction reactions; however, these reactions are not decreased when the vitamin is lacking. Niacin, or nicotinic acid, can be synthesized in small quantities from the amino acid tryptophan.

Pyridoxine is not, of itself, an extremely potent vitamin, but it can be readily converted to two other more active forms: pyridoxal phosphate and pyridoxamine phosphate. All three are generally present in any natural food containing vitamin B_6. Pyridoxal phosphate is involved with enzymes that decarboxylate or dehydrate amino acids and those involved in transamination. It is also involved in some transulfuration reactions. Vitamin B_6 is required for growth and maturation. Deficiency produces a hypochromic, microcytic anemia, which can be reversed with treatment. Infants and pregnant women are most prone to severe deficiency, which may produce a convulsive disorder. This fact, along with other recent evidence, points to a role for pyridoxine in maintaining the integrity of the central nervous system. Demyelination and axonal degeneration of nerves have been demonstrated in animals. Other evidence points to a possible influence on γ-aminobutyric acid (GABA). This substance, found in brain gray matter, seems to exert some control over both central and peripheral neuronal activity.

Pantothenic acid is a constituent of CoA. The A, which stands for acetyl, indicates that the coenzyme is involved in acetylation reactions by contributing the acyl group. These reactions normally involve fatty acid oxidation or synthesis. Deficiency in humans has not been demonstrated, but in animals it produces a number of symptoms including alopecia, gastritis, and skin conditions. Acetyl-CoA is formed from oxidation of pyruvate or fatty acids. A major function of acetyl-CoA is to join with oxaloacetic acid to form citric acid, which initiates the citric acid cycle. Another reaction important to anesthetists is the enzymatic reaction with compounds that are acyl group receptors, such as choline. The two join to form acetylcholine. This reaction also forms CoA-SH, a thio compound capable of providing high-energy bonds much like high-energy phosphate bonds.

Lipoic acid is involved in a number of oxidative decarboxylation reactions, such as for pyruvic acid. In general it functions much like other vitamins involved in the same reactions (e.g., thiamine, riboflavin). Deficiency is unknown and the vitamin plays no outstanding biochemical role.

Biotin functions in carboxylation reactions, attaching and translocating carbon dioxide. It may play a role in purine synthese and may influence other enzymes, especially deaminases.

Folic acid is composed of three parts: glutamic acid, *para*-aminobenzoic acid, and a pteridine nucleus. Variations in the number of glutamic acid structures produces three chemically related substances. All are termed *pteroyl glutamates*. These coenzymes are involved primarily in reactions requiring transfer or utilization of single-carbon groups. Indirectly, they influence synthesis of purines and other compounds and may play a role in cell development. Folic acid deficiency is rare. It seems to induce changes in red cell production and anemia, but these changes are more likely due to concomitant deficiencies of other vitamins. Folic acid can be antagonized by some substances, notably antimetabolites like methotrexate.

Inositol has nine isomers, but only one exerts biologic activity and its importance has not been established.

para-Aminobenzoic acid's prime role is as a member of the folic acid molecule, which has already been discussed.

Vitamin B_{12} has a unique chemical configuration. Consisting of four reduced and substituted pyrrole rings surrounding a cobalt atom, it somewhat resembles the porphyrins. Attached to the cobalt atom is a cyanide group. For this reason, vitamin B_{12} is also known as cyanocobalamin. The cyano- portion may be removed or substituted to form other compounds. Absorption of B_{12} occurs in the ileum, a process that depends on the presence of hydrochloric acid and a substance called intrinsic factor (IF). Prevention of pernicious anemia is dependent on the presence of both IF and B_{12}. The vitamin is sometimes called extrinsic factor. Pernicious anemia is characterized by a macrocytic anemia and neurologic symptoms. Though important for nucleic acid formation, the vitamin's major impact is on the hematopoietic system.

Hormones. Hormones act as chemical messengers for the body and thus augment neuronal pathways in providing integration of bodily functions. They may be produced either by exocrine glands, which secrete into ducts, or by endocrine organs, which secrete the hormone directly into the blood, which then transports it to the target organ. In some respects, hormones resemble both enzymes and vitamins. Like enzymes, they catalyze chemical reactions without participating in them. They are like vitamins in that minute amounts can exert profound effects on the growth, development, and survival of the organism.

Chemically hormones may be proteins, polypeptides, amino acids, or steroids. Protein hormones are associated with the pituitary and parathyroid glands and with the pancreas, whereas thyroid and adrenal gland medullary hormones are mainly amino acids. Hormones associated with the ovaries, testes, and adrenal cortex are steroidal in nature. Hormone secretion is often an autoregulated process involving feedback mechanisms. Some hormones also require conversion to more active forms to exert their effects. The liver and kidneys are the most common sites of degradation. Hormones can change the synthesis rate of enzymes and proteins, alter the catalytic rates of enzymes, and render cell membranes more permeable. They thus influence cellular membrane transport, protein synthesis, and enzyme and coenzyme activity.

Cyclic adenosine 3', 5'-monophosphate (cAMP) is an important mediator of hormonal action. It is sometimes called the second messenger for this reason. cAMP is synthesized from ATP by the action of adenyl cyclase, and it is destroyed by hydrolysis to AMP. The hydrolysis reaction is caused by the action of phosphodiesterase.

Target organs of nonsteroidal hormones usually have receptors on the plasma membrane of their cells. The hormone, also called the first messenger, never enters the cell. Instead, it binds with the receptor to stimulate adenyl cyclase, which is also present in the membrane. The adenyl cyclase activity increases the amount of cAMP within the cell, enabling it to change the rate of one or more reactions within the cell, thus providing the terminal effect of the originally secreted hormone.

Receptor sites are quite specific so that only one hormone is capable of initiating a particular second-messenger effect. Receptors of different target organs can be triggered by the same hormone; however, each organ will respond differently because internal second-messenger effects will vary with the target organ. Phosphodiesterase inhibitors such as caffeine and theophylline can, at least theoretically, act synergistically with those hormones dependent on a second-messenger effect. These include epinephrine, norepinephrine, glucagon, vasopressin, thyroxine, parathyroid hormone, luteinizing hormone, and thyroid- and melanocyte-stimulating hormones. In turn, second-messenger effects produced by cAMP include ketogenesis, gluconeogenesis, glycolysis, lipolysis, insulin release, and renin and gastric hydrochloric acid production. To produce these effects, cAMP must activate protein kinases, which consist of two subunits. One binds with the cAMP, leaving the other free to catalyze reactions within the cell. Prostaglandins may also modulate the effects of hormones, but except for a few instances, their roles have not been clearly defined. Secretion of a number of hormones is dependent on the presence of releasing or inhibiting factors at the secreting gland. Most are associated with the hypothalamus.

Steroidal hormones, such as cortisone, must enter target cells to exert their effect, which tends to be one of gene expression rather than enzymatic alteration. These hormones act at the cell nucleus rather than at its membrane. Steroidal hormones generally take hours to produce their effects, compared with the few minutes required for second-messenger mechanisms. This is because their actions depend on formation of new proteins. As the hormone enters the cell, it binds to a receptor in the cellular cytoplasm. The conjoined hormone and receptor travel to the nucleus to interact with DNA. Messenger RNA may play a role in this interaction, which ends with formation of new proteins. The new protein is, in effect, an induced enzyme. The induced enzyme contributes the terminal action of the hormone. Additional information on hormones is provided elsewhere in this text.

Bioenergetics

The study of energy changes resulting from chemical reactions within living organisms is called bioenergetics. Foods provide basic nutrient substrates for energy. Their assimilation occurs in the alimentary tract, where complex foods are reduced by digestive enzymes, hydrochloric acid, and bile to amino acids, fatty acids, and simple sugars. These are next converted to acetyl groups, phosphoric acid, and other essential compounds necessary for cellular metabolism. Several metabolic pathways use these essential compounds to produce energy. The two main pathways are oxidative phosphorylation and the citric acid cycle. Though proteins and fats can be used for energy, glucose is the foremost energy substrate. (Fructose and galactose are essentially converted to glucose early after ingestion.) The glucose is oxidized to carbon dioxide and water. Metabolic processes concomitantly build ATP, the chemical fuel allowing the body to perform work. Contraction of muscles, nerve conduction, active transport of chemicals, and synthesis of new molecular compounds would not be possible without a continued supply of ATP. Enzymes control the rate of metabolic reactions, but how much energy is produced depends on the amount of available substrate, the amount of free energy involved in each chemical reaction, and a process called electron transport. These last two concepts are discussed next.

Free Energy. Reactions that convert high-binding-energy compounds to ones of a lower energy state must, of necessity, yield their excess energy. This excess is beyond that required to drive the reaction. It may be lost as body heat or coupled to oxidative reactions for transfer and use elsewhere in the body. Because it is freely available to do work elsewhere, it is also called "free" energy. Reactions that generate free energy are called *exergonic*, whereas those that require it for fuel are termed *endergonic*. Excess free heat energy used to be measured in calories or kilocalories. The newer scientific designations are joules and kilojoules per mole.

Exergonic and endergonic reactions can be coupled by various methods. The transfer can be effected by use of a common intermediate capable of interacting in both reactions. This is not a common process in the body, because the intermediate would have to be specific for both reactions. A more efficient method is to synthesize a high-energy compound from the exergonic reaction that can then participate in the endergonic reaction. Given this mechanism, it is possible for the synthesized compound to participate in a number of endergonic reactions. ATP serves as the major, though not exclusive, transfer substance in most biochemical reactions.

The amount of energy freed by a chemical reaction is determined by the laws of thermodynamics. Essentially, the first law is that of conservation of energy. It states that the total energy of a chemical system remains unchanged, energy being neither lost nor gained. The second law states that the extent of molecular disorder or randomness (entropy) in a chemical system must increase if a spontaneous reaction is to occur. This randomness reaches a maximum as the equilibrium point of the reaction is reached. For a reaction occurring under conditions of constant temperature and pressure, the relationship of the change in free energy to the change in randomness is given by the Gibbs equation, which combines both thermodynamic principles. According to the Gibbs equation,

$$\Delta G = \Delta H - T \, \Delta S$$

where G = the free energy change, H = the thermodynamic potential at constant pressure, and S = the change in randomness. If the change in G is equal to zero, the reaction is at equilibrium. When the change in G is negative, a spontaneous reaction can occur and free energy will be available. The reaction will be exergonic. A positive change in G means that additional input of energy will be required as fuel, and the reaction is therefore endergonic.

For laboratory reactions, free energy is standardized at absolute temperature using 1.0 M concentrations of each reactant. This type of free energy is expressed with the designation G^0. Because biochemical reactions occur under conditions found within the body, the standard state of biochemical reactions has been defined by convention to be based on a pH of 7, with a value of 1 being assigned to both the free energy of water and the activity of hydrogen ions. This is called the free energy change at pH 7 and is abbreviated $G^{0'}$. The total free energy available through a series of reactions is equivalent to the algebraic sum of the free energy changes provided by individual steps in the series.

Organophosphate compounds are especially suited for energy transfer. The body possesses two groups of these compounds: a high-energy group and a low-energy group. ATP has a standard free energy at pH 7 ($G^{0'}$) midway between those of the groups. The high-energy group includes (in decreasing order of standard free energy) phosphoenolpyruvate, carbonyl phosphate, 1,3-biphosphoglycerate, creatine phosphate, acetyl phosphate, and arginine phosphate. After ATP, the list continues (low-energy group): glucose 1-phosphate, fructose 6-phosphate, glucose 6-phosphate, and glycerol 3-phosphate. By virtue of its position, ATP is able to donate a high-energy phosphate bond to compounds lower on the list. As ATP breaks down to ADP and a phosphate bond, the ADP can receive a high-energy phosphate bond from compounds in the first part of the list, providing that appropriate enzymes are available to catalyze the process. ATP and ADP can therefore join processes that generate high energy with those requiring energy input.

As was previously discussed, ATP is a nucleotide composed of adenine, a ribose sugar, and three phosphate units. In its active form ATP is part of a complex with magnesium. For energy purposes, the important parts of the molecule are the two phosphoanhydride bonds that make up the last part of the molecule. Hydrolysis releases a large amount of energy as the end bond is split to produce ADP and orthophosphate (P_i). A similar energy release occurs when ADP has its terminal bond split to produce AMP and pyrophosphate (PP_i). Simplified structural formulas for ATP, ADP, and AMP are

High-energy phosphate bonds are sometimes also drawn as

$$\text{(P)} \sim \text{(P)}$$

The amount of energy liberated by these hydrolysis reactions depends to some extent on the concentration of magnesium and the ionic strength of the medium. Other biochemical reactions rely on compounds analogous to ATP. These include guanosine triphosphate (GTP), uridine triphosphate (UTP), and cytidine triphosphate (CTP). Each, in turn, is degraded to a diphosphate—GDP, UDP, and CDP. Enzymes can transfer the phosphoryl group from one nucleotide to another.

Four processes contribute high-energy phosphate bonds to the ATP/ADP cycle. Most come from intracellular mitochondrial reactions involving ATP synthetase and known as oxidative phosphorylation. This process acts to capture energy. Another mechanism involves breakdown of glucose to lactic acid via a glycolytic action known as the Embden–Meyerhof pathway. This pathway is capable of forming a net gain of two high-energy phosphate groups per mole of glucose catabolized. A third mechanism is the citric acid cycle. The last mechanism occurs in muscle and involves both creatine and arginine phosphate.

Electron Transfer and Oxidative Phosphorylation. Oxidation involves loss of electrons, whereas reduction involves electron gain. Activation of one reaction is always matched by an opposing reaction. Hence, the terms *oxidation–reduction* and *redox* are used to describe them. For redox reactions, the amount of free energy available is proportional to the ability of reactants to accept or donate electrons, or their *redox potential*. Biologically, oxygen is the prime electron acceptor, but the process is not a direct one. Instead, electrons are carried (transferred) by pyridine nucleotides or flavins. The reduced forms of these carriers transfer electrons to oxygen by way of an electron transport chain within the inner membrane of mitochondria. It is the flow of electrons down the chain that helps combine ADP and P_i into ATP. This process, known as oxidative phosphorylation, is the major source of ATP for aerobic organisms. The major electron carriers are NADH, NADPH, and $FADH_2$. These were discussed earlier in the sections on enzymes and vitamins, where it was pointed out that the dinucleotide is a carrier of hydrogen ($FADH_2$ carries two). NAD^+ can carry a hydrogen ion and two electrons. This is equivalent to a hydride ion. NADH is the reduced form. NADPH's role is in ATP production. Enzymes control the rate at which ATP-producing reactions occur. Without these catalysts, such reactions would proceed slowly, if at all. Whereas ATP functions as the prime carrier of phosphoryl groups, coenzyme A functions as the main carrier of acyl groups. The acetyl-CoA thus formed is, like ATP, a major essential ingredient in metabolic processes.

Metabolic Pathways of Glucose. Human bodies use three main glycolytic mechanisms: the Embden–Meyerhof pathway, the hexose monophosphate shunt, and the Krebs cycle.

The Embden–Meyerhof pathway (E–M pathway) consists of a series of non-oxygen-dependent reactions. As an anaerobic process, it can provide energy to meet emergency situations where oxygen might be lacking. But under normal

ATP   Adenosine $\underline{\hspace{2cm}}$

(Adenine + ribose)

$$\text{O}-\overset{\overset{\displaystyle O}{\|}}{\underset{\underset{\displaystyle O^-}{|}}{P}}-\text{O}-\overset{\overset{\displaystyle O}{\|}}{\underset{\underset{\displaystyle O^-}{|}}{P}}-\text{O}-\overset{\overset{\displaystyle O}{\|}}{\underset{\underset{\displaystyle O^-}{|}}{P}}-\text{O}^-$$

ADP   Adenosine $\underline{\hspace{2cm}}$

$$\text{O}-\overset{\overset{\displaystyle O}{\|}}{\underset{\underset{\displaystyle O^-}{|}}{P}}-\text{O}-\overset{\overset{\displaystyle O}{\|}}{\underset{\underset{\displaystyle O^-}{|}}{P}}-\text{O}^-$$

AMP   Adenosine $\underline{\hspace{2cm}}$

$$\text{O}-\overset{\overset{\displaystyle O}{\|}}{\underset{\underset{\displaystyle O^-}{|}}{P}}-\text{O}^-$$

conditions, it feeds into the aerobic Krebs cycle, which serves as the final common path for oxidation of ingested nutrients. The E–M pathway is also known as the lactic acid cycle, anaerobic glycolysis, or the Cori cycle. It is but one intermediate path in the metabolism of carbohydrates. Two other intermediate processes, glycogenesis and glycogenolysis, relate to storage of glucose as glycogen and are discussed later. The function of the E–M pathway is to convert glucose to pyruvate or, in the absence of oxygen, to lactic acid. A buildup of lactic acid occurs during periods of strenuous exercise when metabolic processes outstrip available oxygen, causing muscles to become fatigued.

Intermediate substances in the E–M pathway have either three or six carbons; the latter are derived from glucose and fructose, whereas those with three carbons are derived from glyceraldehyde, glycerate, pyruvate, or dihydroxyacetone. As the process converts glucose to pyruvate, a repeated number of phosphorylation reactions occur, which result in phosphoryl groups that have ester or anhydride linkages. Five types of reactions occur:

1. Transfer of phosphoryl groups from ATP.
2. Shifting of phosphoryl groups from one oxygen molecule to another.
3. Interconversion (isomerization) of ketoses and aldoses.
4. Dehydration and removal of a molecule of water.
5. Splitting of aldol linkages.

There are ten steps in the glycolytic pathway. All occur in cell cytosol. The process both consumes and produces energy. Two ATP molecules are lost, one in the conversion of glucose to glucose 6-phosphate (G6P) and one in the conversion of fructose 6-phosphate to fructose 1,6-diphosphate; however, four ATP molecules are produced by the pathway so that there is a net gain of two ATP molecules for the entire process. This gain occurs by conversion of two molecules of 1,3-diphosphoglycerate to two molecules of 3-phosphoglycerate, and by conversion of two molecules of phosphoenolpyruvate to two molecules of pyruvate. Each pathway step involves an enzyme, but the enzyme phosphofructokinase is the major determinant of the rate of gly-

colysis. Steps in the E–M pathway are given in Table 6–2.

Pyruvate formed by the E–M process can be converted to either lactate or acetyl-CoA. When oxygen is limited, pyruvate is reduced by NADH to form lactate, a process catalyzed by lactate dehydrogenase. The reduction reaction causes regeneration of NAD^+ needed to allow the E–M pathway to function past the point at which glyceraldehyde 3-phosphate is formed. Where this is not possible, no ATP would be produced. Pyruvate reduction thereby provides energy for a limited period until oxygen becomes available. Obviously, there is a limit to how long the body can function under anaerobic conditions alone, but the process does provide a safeguard for survival. Once oxygen becomes available, the lactate is reconverted to pyruvate and the acidosis quickly dissipates. Formation of acetyl-CoA occurs when pyruvate combines with NAD^+ and CoA to produce carbon dioxide, NADH, H^+, and acetyl-CoA. The acetyl-CoA then enters the citric acid cycle.

One offshoot of the glycolytic pathway carries additional importance for anesthesia practice. A mutase may convert 1,3-diphosphoglycerate (1,3-DPG) to 2,3-diphosphoglycerate (2,3-DPG). Large amounts of 2,3-DPG are found in hemoglobin of red cells, where it acts to control the transport of oxygen. Changes in hemoglobin oxygen affinity caused by 2,3-DPG can hold important implications for patients.

The *hexose monophosphate shunt* is an aerobic, enzyme-dependent series of reactions that generate ribose and NADPH. Ribose is used for synthesizing nucleic acids and NADPH is important to the formation of fatty acids. Basically, three molecules of glucose 6-phosphate combine with six molecules of NADP to form three molecules of carbon dioxide, two molecules of fructose 6-phosphate, six molecules of NADPH, and one molecule of glyceraldehyde 3-phosphate. Two compounds produced by the series, fructose 6-phosphate and glyceraldehyde 3-phosphate, may be shared with the Embden–Meyerhof pathway. The shunt pathway, sometimes called the direct oxidative pathway, functions mostly in the liver, adrenals, thyroid, erythrocytes, and adipose tissues. It operates only minimally in skeletal muscle. Shunt reactions begin with oxidation but eventually produce a number of sugars, which are enzymatically converted by nonoxidative means. Table 6–3 shows

TABLE 6–2. THE EMBDEN–MEYERHOF PATHWAY

Substrate	Enzyme	Product
*Glucose + ATP	Hexokinase	Glucose 6-phosphate + ADP + H^+
Glucose 6-phosphate	Phosphoglucose isomerase	Fructose 6-phosphate
*Fructose 6-phosphate + ATP	Phosphofructokinase	Fructose 1,6-diphosphate + ADP + H^+
Fructose 1,6-diphosphate	Aldolase	Dihydroxyacetone phosphate + glyceraldehyde 3-phosphate
Dihydroxyacetone phosphate	Triose phosphate isomerase	Glyceraldehyde 3-phosphate
Glyceraldehyde 3-phosphate + P_i + NAD^+	Glyceraldehyde 3-phosphate dehydrogenase	1,3-Diphosphoglycerate + NADH + H^+
1,3-Diphosphoglycerate + ADP	Phosphoglycerate kinase	3-Phosphoglycerate + ATP
3-Phosphoglycerate	Phosphoglyceromutase	2-Phosphoglycerate
2-Phosphoglycerate	Enolase	Phosphoenolpyruvate + H_2O
Phosphoenolpyruvate + ADP + H^{+a}	Pyruvate kinase	Pyruvate + ATP

[a] Nonreversible reactions.

Adapted, with permission, from Stryer L. Biochemistry. *3rd ed. New York: Freeman; 1988:357. Copyright © 1988 by Lubert Stryer. Adapted by permission of W. H. Freeman and Company.*

TABLE 6–3. THE HEXOSE MONOPHOSPHATE SHUNT

	Enzyme	Product
Group I		
Glucose 6-phosphate + NADP$^+$	Glucose 6-phosphate dehydrogenase	6-Phosphogluconolactone + NADPH + H$^+$
6-Phosphogluconolactone + H$_2$O^a	Lactonase	6-Phosphogluconate + H$^+$
6-Phosphogluconate + NADP^{+a}	6-Phosphogluconate dehydrogenase	Ribulose 5-phosphate^b + CO$_2$ + NADPH
Group II		
Ribulose 5-phosphate^b	Phosphopentose isomerase	Ribose 5-phosphate^b
Ribulose 5-phosphate^b	Phosphopentose epimerase	Xylulose 5-phosphate^b
Xylulose 5-phosphate^c + ribose 5-phosphate^b	Transketolase	Sedoheptulose 7-phosphate^c + glyceraldehyde 3-phosphate
Sedoheptulose 7-phosphate^c + glyceraldehyde 3-phosphate	Transaldolase	Fructose 6-phosphate + erythrose 4-phosphate^d
Xylulose 5-phosphate^b + erythrose 4-phosphate^b	Transketolase	Fructose 6-phosphate + glyceraldehyde 3-phosphate

^{a} Nonreversible reactions.
^{b} Five-carbon sugar.
^{c} Seven-carbon sugar.
^{d} Four-carbon sugar.
Adapted, with permission, from Stryer L. Biochemistry. 3rd ed. New York: Freeman; 1988:428. Copyright © 1988 by Lubert Stryer. Adapted by permission of W. H. Freeman and Company.

the steps of both groups of reactions. Sugars produced may contain four, five, or seven carbon atoms. Because two molecules of glyceraldehyde 3-phosphate can regenerate one molecule of glucose 6-phosphate, the shunt pathway can account for complete oxidation of glucose. The oxidative portion of the reactions relies on dehydrogenation, much like the E–M pathway; but NADP, rather than NAD, becomes the hydrogen carrier. Enzymes for shunt reactions are located in cell cytosol. The hexose monophosphate shunt provides metabolic energy through its reducing powers. Unlike the E–M pathway or Krebs cycle, it is not concerned with ATP production.

The body's principal metabolic pathway is the *Krebs cycle*. When combined with Embden–Meyerhof reactions, the complete pathway is termed *aerobic glycolysis*. As with glycolytic and shunt pathways, each step is enzymatically controlled. Enzymes for the Krebs cycle are located within folded areas of mitochondria known as cristae. The cycle also serves to provide intermediate products for building other chemical components for the body (biosynthesis).

Acetyl-CoA formed from pyruvate during the last stages of glycolytic reactions feeds the cycle. The cycle starts with the combining of oxaloacetate, a four-carbon compound, with the two-carbon acetyl group of acetyl-CoA. The combined compound reacts with water to form CoA and citrate under the influence of citrate synthetase. The citrate is then isomerized to isocitrate through a dehydration–hydration reaction that allows for interchange of H$^+$ and OH$^-$ groups. Isocitrate undergoes an oxidative–reduction reaction, which is facilitated by NAD$^+$ and the enzyme isocitrate dehydrogenase. This reaction produces an intermediate, oxalosuccinate. Loss of carbon dioxide from oxalosuccinate leads to formation of α-ketoglutarate. Formation of this compound determines the overall functioning of the cycle. A second oxidative reduction converts α-ketoglutarate to succinyl-CoA. This reaction too results in conversion of the NAD$^+$ to NADH and the release of CO^2, the reaction being much like the one that converted pyruvate to acetyl-CoA

during glycolysis, except that here a three-enzyme complex (α-ketoglutarate dehydrogenase complex) is required to achieve conversion. The succinyl-CoA contains an energy bond similar to ATP. In a dual reaction catalyzed by succinyl-CoA synthetase, the energy bond is released at the same time that GDP is phosphorylated. The reactions end with formation of GTP, succinate, and CoA, but the phosphoryl group of GTP can be transferred to ADP by nucleoside diphosphokinase to form ATP. Formation of the high-energy bond compares with oxidative phosphorylation discussed earlier; however, this energy-bond formation occurs only once in the tricarboxylic cycle. The last step in the cycle involves re-formation of oxaloacetate from succinate. Three substeps are required for this process, two oxidation reactions and one hydration reaction. When oxaloacetate has been re-formed, the cycle may begin again. Steps in the Krebs cycle are outlined in Table 6–4.

In the Krebs cycle, hydrogen is lost through five reactions. The loss is mostly in the form of NADH, which then enters the electron transport chain. In the chain hydrogen is passed between compounds to facilitate oxidation–reduction reactions. A number of these reactions allow energy to be stored as ATP. Finally, the hydrogens combine with oxygen to form water. Three molecules of ATP are formed from each molecule of NADH, but the entire aerobic glycolysis process forms a net 30 molecules of ATP. This can be summarized as follows:

4	from the E–M pathway
6	from the two NADH released in E–M pathway
30*	from the two pyruvic acids in the Krebs cycle
40	
− 2	used in E–M pathway
38	molecules of ATP total

* Each glucose molecule yields two pyruvic acids in the E–M pathway, and each of these produces five NADH molecules, each capable of producing three molecules of ATP: $2 \times 5 \times 3 = 30$.

TABLE 6–4. THE KREBS CYCLE

Substrate	Enzyme[a]	Product
Acetyl-CoA + oxaloacetate + H_2O[b]	Citrate synthetase	Citrate + CoA + H^+
Citrate	Aconitase	cis-Aconitate + H_2O
Isocitrate + NAD^+	Isocitrate dehydrogenase	α-Ketoglutarate + CO_2 + NADH
α-Ketoglutarate + NAD^+ + CoA	α-Ketoglutarate dehydrogenase complex	Succinyl-CoA + CO_2 + NADH
Succinyl-CoA + P_i + GDP	Succinyl-CoA synthetase	Succinate + GTP + CoA
Succinate + FAD[c]	Succinate dehydrogenase	Fumarate + $FADH_2$
Fumarate + H_2O[c]	Fumarase	Maltate
Malate + NAD^+[c]	Malate dehydrogenase	Oxaloacetate + NADH + H^+

[a] Cofactors, as well as enzymes, are required for nearly all of the steps.
[b] Nonreversible reactions.
[c] The last three steps are aimed at reforming oxaloacetate from succinate.

Adapted, with permission, from Stryer L. Biochemistry. 3rd ed. New York: Freeman; 1988:370. Copyright © 1988 by Lubert Stryer. Adapted by permission of W. H. Freeman and Company.

Glycogen is a polymerized, storable form of glucose. Formation of glycogen (*glycogenesis*) from excess glucose ensures that the E–M, hexose monophosphate, and Krebs pathways can continue to function during periods of decreased food intake. Glycogenesis occurs mainly in the liver, with some conversion occurring in muscle. Once stored, glycogen can later be split by hydrolysis to re-form glucose, a process termed *glycogenolysis*.

Glycogenesis involves the following steps:

1. In the presence of magnesium and the enzyme glucokinase, glucose reacts with ATP. The latter is degraded to ADP and the glucose is converted to glucose 6-phosphate (G6P).
2. Phosphomutase converts G6P to glucose 1-phosphate (G1P).
3. G1P reacts with the uracil-containing nucleotide, UTP, under the influence of the enzyme UDPG pyrophosphorylase, forming UDP-glucose.
4. UDP-glucose is polymerized to glycogen under the influence of UDPG-glycogen transglucolase. This reaction releases UDP.
5. UDP reacts with ATP to form ADP and allows regeneration of UTP. (Two molecules of ATP are required for every molecule of glucose stored.)

Glycogenolysis is not merely the reverse process of glycogenesis. It is a much more accelerated process. An (inactive) enzyme, phosphorylase b, is changed to (active) phosphorylase a by a complex interaction termed the *cascade reaction*. Phosphorylase a is then able to split off a G1P from glycogen. The G1P is reconverted to G6P. Glucose 6-phosphatase then removes phosphate from G6P to form glucose. The cascade reaction is generated by a number of hormones including ACTH, glucagon, and epinephrine. Each step of the cascade accelerates the following step by as much as 100 times. Steps in the cascade are as follows:

1. The hormone (e.g., epinephrine) activates adenyl cyclase.
2. Adenyl cyclase converts AMP to cAMP.
3. cAMP activates protein kinase.
4. Protein kinase activates phosphorylase kinase.
5. Phosphorylase kinase converts phosphorylase b to phosphorylase a.
6. Phosphorylase a acts on glycogen to split off G1P.
7. G1P is converted to G6P.
8. G6P is converted to glucose and enters the bloodstream or glycolytic pathways.

The above reaction occurs only in the liver, as muscles lack the enzyme necessary to convert G6P to glucose. Muscle G6P must enter a glycolytic pathway. The bioenergetic and other biochemical reactions discussed in this section impact, in one fashion or another, on every patient who receives an anesthetic. An appreciation by the anesthetist of the often subtle yet complex biochemical balances required to maintain homeostasis contributes substantially to providing patients optimum safe care.

REFERENCES

1. Danielli J, Davson H. In: Lehninger A, ed. *Biochemistry*, 2nd ed. New York: Worth Publishers; 1975; 304. (Note: no later reference for this point could be found.)
2. Singer SJ, Nicolson G. In: Stryer L, ed. *Biochemistry*, 3rd ed. New York: Freeman; 1988; 295.
3. Overton CE, Myer HH. In: Miller RD, ed. *Anesthesia*, 3rd ed. New York: Churchill Livingstone; 1990; 2091.

BIBLIOGRAPHY

Adriani JA. *The chemistry and physics of anesthesia.* Springfield, IL: Charles C Thomas; 1962. (A classic work.)

Darnell J, Lodish H, Baltimore D. *Molecular cell biology.* 2nd ed. New York: WH Freeman (Scientific American Books); 1990.

Furniss BS, Hannaford AJ, Smith PWG, Tatchell AR, eds. *Vogel's Textbook of Practical Organic Chemistry.* 5th ed. New York: Wiley; 1989.

Hill JW, Feigl DM. *Chemistry and life.* 3rd ed. New York: Macmillan; 1987.

Schauf CL, Moffett DF, Moffett SB. *Human physiology: Foundations and frontiers.* St. Louis, MO: Times Mirror/Mosby College Publishing; 1990.

Electronic and Safety Principles Related to Anesthesia

Leo A. Le Bel

Growing use of sophisticated electronic devices in surgery and anesthesia practice makes a basic knowledge of electronic components and circuits virtually mandatory for today's practicing anesthetist. This chapter provides fundamental information about electrical laws and circuits and shows their relevance to anesthesia practice.

ELECTRICAL PRINCIPLES

Electricity is a phenomenon of nature that depends on atomic structure and the difference in force between electrons and protons. Electrons have a negative charge, protons an equal but positive charge. The *charge* each possesses is a function of mass, and it is the gravitational force between their masses that keeps them bound in atomic configuration. Having opposite charges, electrons and protons are mutually attracted to one another. On the other hand, electrons repel other electrons and protons repel other protons. If one thinks of an aggregate of electrons or protons on the surface of two objects, it is easier to envision how electricity flows. If two objects of opposite charge are kept separate, they retain their relative charges. No electricity flows, and the charges are said to be *static*. As the objects are brought close to one another, forces of attraction build between the two into what is termed an *energy field*. At this point, the objects possess potential energy. But once the two are brought close together, the electricity becomes dynamic and electrons from the negatively charged object flow to the positively charged one. This is termed an *electric current*.

Quantity of charge is measured in *coulombs*. The rate at which the charge travels is measured as a function of time. A rate of one coulomb per second is called an *ampere*. While current flows, it also generates a kinetic energy force field, which is termed *magnetism*. The word *electromagnetic* reflects the close association between the two force fields. When electricity flows, the resulting energy can be used to perform work. In most cases, this involves converting the elec-

trical energy to mechanical energy. Electric motors are one example by which the conversion is made.

In addition to *mass*, *force* (charge), and *rate of flow*, a fourth factor, *distance*, determines the sum effect of an electric current. All electrical quantities can be expressed as a function of one or more of these parameters.

When electricity flows, it is the electron that physically moves. Substances that have loosely attached and easily lost electrons in their atomic structure, such as metals, are called *conductors*. Those that have tightly bound electrons, such as glass and plastics, are called *nonconductors* or *insulators*. Positive charges may be thought of as holes in the atom(s) where electrons are missing and whose positions may be constantly changing, much like a ferris wheel with several of its gondolas missing. Substances whose electrical characteristics are determined by the motion of electrons and the position of holes are termed *semiconductors*. These include transistors and integrated circuits, so prevalent in modern solid-state electronic devices.

The *permittivity* of a substance is an indication of how well it conducts an electrical current compared with current flow in a vacuum. Permittivity is also termed the *dielectric constant* of a substance. It gives an indication of the velocity with which current will flow in that material. Dielectric constants are used for making comparisons between substances with respect to their current-carrying ability, for example, copper versus silver. As current flows, magnetic fields that can generate secondary current flows are developed. This process is termed *induction* and occurs when electricity flowing in one wire sets up a current in an adjoining wire. An electric *shield* is anything that prevents development of induced charges.

Devices that store a charge are termed *capacitors* or *condensers*. Devices that oppose current flow are called *resistors*. The term *electromotive force* (emf) describes any source of electrical energy. Electromotive force is measured in *volts*, 1 volt being equal to the potential required to flow a current of 1 ampere through a resistance of 1 ohm (the unit of resistance).

Charges that flow in an electric current have a force of given potential. When that potential is reduced to a zero point level, the charge is said to be *grounded*. Electrical grounds are used to reduce or eliminate unwanted electric charges. This concept has particular applicability to operating room floors, where grounding may be used to rapidly dispel excess charges before they build to levels high enough to cause "static shock." As electricity courses through an electronic circuit, its potential is progressively decreased. This is termed *voltage drop*.

Any combination of electrical source resistors, capacitors, or other components is called an *electrical network* or *circuit*. All electronic equipment is made up of a number of such networks. A circuit may be designed to perform a unique function or to work in tandem with other circuits to effect multiple operations. Anesthesia monitors that simultaneously keep track of temperature, blood pressure, and other parameters require the integration of literally dozens of specific circuits made up of many discrete parts. Whether or not failure of a single component will result in failure of the entire unit depends on the manner in which the unit has been designed. Special diagrams, *schematics*, outline the entire circuitry of an electronic device by means of electronic symbols. A legend that identifies the symbols used is usually provided. By referring to the schematic diagram of an electronic device before using it, the anesthetist can gain some appreciation of how the unit functions. Many manufacturers also supply block diagrams, which provide information about how major circuits within the unit are functionally related.

Alternating Current

Current can be described as one of two types: alternating (AC) or direct (DC). If one imagines looking at a single cross-sectional area of a conductor (wire) and seeing electrons flow first in one direction and then in the other, the impression left by one back-and-forth movement would be that there was no net movement of electrons, merely one cycle of movement by the same electron. The observer would be left to conclude that there was no flow of electricity (net flow of charge). Yet, what has just been described is known commonly as AC. The answer to the illusion lies in the fact that different electrons were seen to be transversing the cross-sectional area. This is because the molecules of metal that make up the wire are constantly exchanging their loose electrons. With DC, movement of electrons would appear unidirectional. AC is more easily carried over large distances, but DC is generally more efficient and is therefore the primary form used in electronic circuits. Charges that occur with alternating current can be visualized by use of a sine wave. With the conventional electricity we use (AC), the direction of travel of electrons is changed 120 times per second, or 60 back-and-forth cycles, hence the term *60-cycle electricity*. Each cycle is identical, and a sine wave pattern describes the algebraic sum of the movement of electrons through one cycle.

Describing electricity as being 60 cycles/second (hertz) says something about its frequency. Certain electronic circuits operate at an optimum frequency, termed *resonance*, where forces that facilitate current flow through the circuit (*conductance*) are balanced by the forces that hamper current flow (*impedance*). Resonant circuits can be easily upset and

flow through the circuit becomes asynchronous, but, if working properly, resonant circuits perform best at their designed frequency. With some circuits, it becomes possible to tune the resonant circuit over a range of frequencies. Radio receivers use this principle, as do certain medical devices, such as ultrasonic equipment and electrocardiographic telemetry units. Antennas also are a form of resonator; that is, the length or physical design of the antenna determines the best frequency range of operation.

Radiations that possess both electrical and magnetic properties are said to lie in the *electromagnetic spectrum*. These range from electrical waves that are very long in wavelength, relatively slow moving, and relatively low energy to very short, high-energy, rapidly moving cosmic rays. In between, the spectrum includes broadcast and short radio waves, very-high- and ultrahigh-frequency (VHF/UHF) radio waves, infrared, visible, and ultraviolet light spectra, x-rays, and gamma radiation.

If current is flowing through a conductor (wire) and that conductor is formed into a coil, the electromagnetic field generated by each turn of the coil works in concert with those generated by all other turns. When an identical but nonconducting circuit is brought into close proximity, an induced current will begin to flow in the second circuit. This is the basis on which *transformers* work; that is, energy from one part of the circuit is transformed to energy within the second part of the circuit. Yet there is no direct linkage between the two. This transfer of energy represents work done by the electromotive source providing current to the first (primary) circuit. Energy lost by the first circuit can be measured as a voltage drop. Certain forces facilitate or inhibit the energy transfer. For example, placing an iron magnetic rod within the first coil makes it an electromagnet, making energy transfer easier. On the other hand, air between the turns of the first coil provides capacitance, thus restricting the energy transfer, air being a poor conductor of electricity. If, however, the current generated through the coil creates enough charge, arcing (voltage breakdown) will occur between coil elements. The example just presented represents mutual inductance between circuits, but it is also possible for a single circuit to be self-inducting.

Electronic Circuits

Mechanical devices and electronic circuits are often conceptually similar. The former's efficiency is determined by the interaction of components that store energy, those that dissipate it (i.e., cause resistance), those that are capable of storing and using kinetic energy, and those that transform the system's energy in some way (e.g., gears). Electronic circuits have resistors that use up energy, capacitors that store it, inductors that can both store and use energy, and transformers that regulate voltage and current carried by the circuit.

The rate at which both systems perform work is termed *power*. In electrical terms, power (P) is measured as watts and is equal to the electromotive force (E) in volts multiplied by the current (I) in amperes ($P = EI$). One watt is equal to 1 volt multiplied by 1 ampere. The same amount of power can therefore be obtained by using high voltage at low current or low voltage at high current.

The efficiency of an electronic circuit can be measured by dividing its power output by its power input. A circuit that outputs 50 watts for every 100 watts input is operating at 50 percent efficiency. The rest of the power is dissipated in performing work within the circuit or as heat loss. Because any electronic circuit consists of imperfect components, there will always be some resistance to electrical flow. Indeed, just as pressure differences occur within anesthesia breathing circuits so, too, are there numerous factors within an electronic circuit that hamper electrical flow. The simplest conceivable electric circuit would consist of a battery (electromotive force source) and a resistor in a closed circuit. Placing a switch in the circuit breaks the current flow and the circuit is said to be open, or broken.

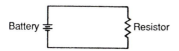

This simple circuit can illustrate basic interactions between voltage (E), current (I), and resistance (R). The relationships are expressed as Ohm's law, which states that current flowing in a circuit is directly proportional to applied electromotive force and inversely proportional to resistance:

$$I \text{ (amperes)} = \frac{E \text{ (volts)}}{R \text{ (ohms)}}$$

The formula can be transposed to solve for any needed value, given that two of the values are known:

$$E = IR \quad \text{and} \quad R = \frac{E}{I}$$

Ohm's law applies to all parts of a circuit as well as to the circuit as a whole. If more than one resistance is present, total resistance will depend on whether the resistances are in series or parallel. For resistances in series, total resistance equals the sum of all resistors, $R = R_1 + R_2 + R_3 + \cdots$. With serial resistances, current remains the same throughout the circuit. With parallel resistances, however, the current becomes divided between the various parallel resistors. This causes total resistance for the circuit to be less than that of the lowest resistance value present. The formula for calculating parallel resistances is

$$R = \frac{1}{1/R_1 + 1/R_2 + 1/R_3 + \cdots}$$

In calculating Ohm's law equations, one must remember to convert known figures to the measurements required by the law. For instance, milliamperes or millivolts must first be converted to their ampere or voltage equivalents by moving the decimal point appropriately. Obtaining values for voltage, current, and resistance normally involves direct measurement by means of voltmeters, ammeters, and ohmeters. The importance of Ohm's law lies in the fact that it is equally applicable to other electronic components within the circuit. For example, capacitors in a circuit can be thought of as resistors and their effect on current and volt-age can be calculated in the same manner. This also applies for series and parallel inductances.

Though electricity has been known since the dawn of humanity through the phenomenon of lightning, only in the past few hundred years have we come to understand its powers and how to control it. By 1900, electricity had some practical applications (e.g., telegraphy), but equipment had to be tied by direct connections. Even early radio frequency transmitters capable of sending signals over distances relied on broad emissions scattered over vast frequency ranges. They required high-energy inputs and were terribly inefficient.

The modern electrical era began with the invention of the vacuum tube. Vacuum tubes allowed the electricity flowing through a circuit to be carefully controlled and directed toward performing specific tasks. A tube contains active elements enclosed in a glass envelope from which air has been evacuated to provide an internal vacuum. Because electrons flow more freely in a vacuum, electrical flow is more efficient. The two primary active elements of a tube are the *cathode* (negative pole from which electrons flow) and the *anode* or plate (positive pole to which electrons flow). A wire filament provides a resistive pathway within the tube, which, by building up heat, enhances electron flow. Interspersed between cathode and anode may be one to several grids, which serve to control electron flux across the tube circuit. Tubes are named for the number of active elements present, excluding filament. A triode has a cathode, anode, and one grid, whereas a pentode has three grids. Connection of tube circuitry to the rest of the electronic circuit is by means of pins located in the base of the tube.

The advent of vacuum tubes meant that, for the first time, sophisticated circuits could be designed for controlling and using electricity. But a few short decades later, tubes gave way to *semiconductors*, electronic components that are part conductor and part insulator, hence their name. In this category are diodes and transistors. Diodes have only two active elements, cathode and anode, and are often named for the substance from which they are made (selenium, silicon, etc.). More sophisticated, transistor semiconductors contain multiple active elements. The basic elements of transistors are the emitter, base, and collector.

Semiconductors perform essentially the same functions as tubes, but their mode of operation is different. In vacuum tubes, electrons function as discrete charged solid particles. Semiconductors rely on the various energy states or levels of the atoms that compose them. When orbital energy levels are such that energy flows, the device conducts. When energy levels prevent energy flow, the device acts as an insulator. The energy levels for both states are partly determined by the amount of electrical energy coming into the device. By the selection of appropriate construction materials and control of their physical assembly, semiconductors can be developed that have relatively positive or relatively negative "poles." These are not specific poles in the usual sense; rather, they represent areas of preponderant negative or positive charges. These preponderant charges relate to the energy levels created within the various sections of the semiconductor, a factor of their design and construction materials. The "positive" charge carriers are the "holes" referred to earlier. The two sections of material within the semiconductor are called P type, for positive, and N type, for negative. When a P type is joined to an N-type material, a one-way current flow occurs. This PN junction is found in all semiconductor devices. A variation, the PNP (positive–negative–positive) transistor, uses a common emitter. Bipolar transistors combine two PN junctions and provide some power amplification for the circuit. A field effect transistor (FET) is another modification that can also amplify. In many respects, FETs resemble pentode vacuum tubes but require much less voltage. Because semiconductors are composed of solid materials, circuits in which they are used are called *solid-state circuits*. *Integrated circuits* (ICs) are, as the name implies, devices that incorporate several interconnected components designed for a particular application. Through the process of microminiaturization it is possible to build complex ICs of very small size, much the way the size of photographs is reduced. Nearly invisible silicon chips now contain all the circuitry that formerly took multiple vacuum tubes, wiring, and other items to accomplish. By designing chips that function when electricity is "on" and do not function when electricity is "off," it is possible to develop what are termed digital–logical ICs. They are termed *digital* because they deal with discrete events and *logical* because they operate in accordance with mathematical principles. Digital–logical ICs form the heart of the modern microcomputer.

With development of semiconductors and microcomputers we have entered the neomodern period of electronics. What are the advantages of solid-state devices besides size and production costs? Principal advantages lie in the fact that they use electricity much more efficiently. Substantially less voltage is required to perform work than was necessary with vacuum tubes. Less heat is generated, equipment operates efficiently for longer periods, repair costs are less, and work can be performed more rapidly. Virtually all electronic equipment used today in both surgery and anesthesia is of solid-state design.

A number of circuits are common to most electronic equipment and a brief description of these is presented next. The power supply circuit receives electrical input from the available commercial power source. In most facilities, this is provided through standard two- or three-prong AC outlets that provide 117 volts at 60 hertz (range: 110–125 volts). With three-prong outlets, one conductor serves as the neutral connection, one is grounded, and one provides the AC. Three-conductor power outlets are now fairly standard, but those used in operating rooms reserved for use of explosive anesthetic agents must have interlocking explosion-proof plugs. These are connected to the surgical suite's isolation transformer, a concept discussed later. As electricity enters the electronic device, a transformer is used to convert line voltage to a value suitable for the unit. A rectifier circuit then converts the AC to a pulsating DC. Filtering circuits may be used to decrease DC pulsation. This smooths the pulses into a relatively constant flow. Power supply filtering circuits serve to regulate voltage and eliminate unwanted (ripple) currents by grounding them through a *bleeder* circuit to ground. A bleeder circuit provides a safety measure for dissipating excess current when the device is turned off. The power supply of any unit normally contains a fuse at the site at which AC electricity enters the unit. This protects the unit from electrical overloading.

Frequency filtering circuits are used either to protect the unit from the effects of extraneous interference or to keep the unit from generating a signal at a frequency that could cause interference to other nearby electronic equipment. Such filters are of four basic types: (1) those that cut out all signals below a specified frequency, (2) those that cut signals above a given frequency, (3) those that pass certain frequency bands while filtering others, and (4) those that inhibit passage of a block of frequencies while passing those above and below.

Oscillator circuits generate signals of either single or multiple frequencies. They are sometimes used to provide an internal standard for calibrating an electronic unit. Multiplier circuits multiply a given frequency, usually two, three, or four times. Divider circuits break down a frequency into smaller units. Mixer circuits combine different frequencies.

Driver circuits generate signals that, in turn, feed into another stage of the circuit. Amplifier circuits enhance or increase signal strength. Metering circuits allow measurement of a specific function. For example, temperature-measuring devices used in the operating room read out either on a needle-and-scale device or on digital displays. Digital readout devices use light-emitting diodes (LEDs), which glow when activated by electrical energy within the circuit. Digital displays may use hundreds of transistors. The combination of energy flow through these determines what numbers appear on the display. Digital devices that read out both letters and numbers are termed *alphanumeric*. Audio circuits convert electrical signals into audible tones. Doppler and ultrasound devices often incorporate such circuits to allow the user to hear changes detected by the device. Another type of readout device is the oscilloscope on which electrical changes are seen as movement of a light beam across a television-like screen. For example, electrocardiographic (ECG) monitors used in surgery provide a readout of heart electrical impulses as they are transmitted across the body. The displayed pattern represents the algebraic sum of impulses traveling to and away from the monitoring electrodes. The pattern changes with the combination of electrodes used, that is, whatever ECG lead is being used. Two types of interference commonly may occur to disrupt the ECG pattern. The first is termed 60-cycle interference, which appears as a sine wave of even amplitude superimposed on the normally isoelectric (zero-voltage) baseline of the ECG pattern. It occurs whenever line-voltage AC enters the monitoring circuit, perhaps as the result of malfunctioning of other electronic devices, improper grounding, or because of capacitive current flow. Complete disruption of the pattern with scattering of the oscilloscope electron beam occurs whenever the monitor is subjected to radio frequency interference (RFI). This is usually caused by electrocautery equipment that disperses energy throughout the operating room environment. This electrical energy enters the monitor to cause disruption of the normal circuitry, which in turn results in disruption of the oscilloscope pattern. Present-day monitoring devices contain circuits designed to dampen electrical interference. Still, high radiant energies may overload these to produce momentary disruptions. A normal pattern is quickly reestablished once the RFI source is eliminated.

Monitoring devices constitute the largest class of electronic devices used by anesthetists. Interestingly, a single circuit forms the basis for most monitors. Known as a *Wheatstone bridge* (Fig. 7–1), it operates by balancing voltages at two different points in such a fashion that a zero potential difference is established between them. Establishing this zero potential difference is termed *balancing, zeroing,* or *nulling the circuit.* Once calibrated in this way, any change in circuit balance can be read as a change in voltage. This voltage change is typically read on a needle-and-scale, oscilloscope, or digital display in terms of the values being monitored, for example, torr pressure and degrees of temperature. The circuit consists of four resistances, of which two are of a fixed, known value (R-1 and R-2 in Fig. 7–1). Once the resistance of standard (R-s) is zeroed, any change it experiences is reflective of the unknown resistance (R-x). To restate this in another fashion, if any three resistances are known, the fourth can be calculated:

$$R\text{-}x = R\text{-}s\,\frac{R\text{-}2}{R\text{-}1}$$

It is important to note that resistance ratios, not actual resistor values, are the basis for the way a Wheatstone bridge functions.

Bridge circuits require a sensing device to provide input capable of changing the reference resistance. The sensing device may be a thermistor probe used for monitoring temperature. Change in heat is carried by cable to the monitor, where it elicits a change in R-s. Another sensing

device is the pressure transducer. A transducer's pressure plate moves in response to mechanical alterations generated by a liquid column attached to an indwelling arterial line catheter. Such a device is often used for continuously measuring blood pressure. Fluctuations at the pressure plate/liquid dome assembly are carried by cable to the monitor to induce changes in R-s. When the monitor has previously been zeroed to air (no mechanical pressure), accurate blood pressure measurements can be made. The monitor may also provide a continuous oscilloscopic pressure wave tracing. Movement of the transducer pressure plate causes nearly imperceptible alterations in cable wire length that act to change its resistance. This variation in electrical resistance is responsible for changing the value of R-s.

The foregoing examples are but two of the more common applications of a Wheatstone bridge circuit. Other circuits (e.g., electromagnetic induction circuits) are also employed in measurement and monitoring devices, but the Wheatstone bridge is the most widely used. Monitors may incorporate amplification and filtering circuits to enhance input to the bridge. They may also be coupled to recording devices to provide permanent recordings of measured changes.

Among the more recent significant advances in monitoring has been the integration of microcomputers, which can take raw measured data, analyze the data, and predict trends. If it appears that the measured parameters (i.e., vital signs) are deteriorating, the monitor can trigger an alarm and thus warn the anesthetist to take corrective action. The more sophisticated computerized monitors identify likely problems, based on probability, and recommend corrective actions to be considered. This can be an invaluable aid clinically, especially if multiple parameters are simultaneously tracked. The fact that the monitor can produce a written record of all measurements will undoubtedly have a future impact on the legal aspects of anesthesia practice.

ELECTRICAL HAZARDS IN THE OPERATING ROOM

Electrical energy, though a common and useful facet of daily life, is not an entirely benign force. In the high-technology environment of the modern operating room, failure to appreciate electricity's potential to maim and kill can lead to disaster for both patients and personnel. Indeed, carelessness has been found to be a major contributing factor to electrically related operating room mishaps.

To appreciate electricity's potential impact on the human body, several concepts should be kept in mind. First, human bodies readily conduct electrical impulses. Second, bodies coming into contact with an electrical circuit become part of that circuit. Third, the extent of physical injury is dependent on the type, amount, and path of electric current. Last, all electrical flow seeks the least resistive path to ground potential.

Major physiologic hazards of electricity include ventricular fibrillation, asphyxia, central nervous system disruption, and burns. Electric shock hazards are divided into two categories based on current density: macroshock and

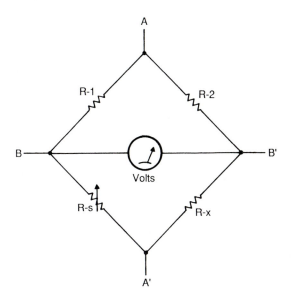

Figure 7–1. Wheatstone bridge circuit. R-1 = R-2; R-1, R-2, and R-x = fixed resistances; R-s = a variable resistance. A and A' are connections to a direct-current power source. B and B' are inputs from a sensing device (transducer).

microshock. Current density refers to the cross-sectional distribution of the electric current. With macroshock, the current is typically distributed throughout the entire body, though not uniformly. Macroshock hazards are typically those to which we are exposed on a daily basis from faulty wiring or improper grounding of electric devices. The mass of the adult human body helps determine the body's resistance to electrical flow. Although various body tissues conduct electricity at different rates, the skin usually takes the brunt of the current, thus providing a protective measure for the body because dangerous currents are shifted away from the heart, the most susceptible organ. However, because currents travel in a conical fashion from the point of entry, some macroshock current can almost always be expected to reach the heart. Happily, the current density or cross-sectional flow of current through the myocardium does not always entirely disrupt its normal electrical conduction system because flow per unit area has been diffused. It is for this reason that not every electric "shock" results in death and that relatively high current flows are required to produce cardiac arrest, compared with current flows associated with microshock. Still, in susceptible patients, currents of even a few hundred milliamperes can cause fibrillation of heart muscle.

Microshock injuries are most often produced by indwelling electrodes of conducting devices, such as cardiac pacemakers. Because the current is applied near or directly on the heart, current densities are high. This means that very little current is required to produce ventricular fibrillation. Thus it is obvious that patients, not operating room personnel, are at greatest risk from microshock. Even just a few dozen microamperes have been known to produce death. Such injuries occur in part because the body's protective mechanisms are bypassed.

How much current flows through a body area determines the type and extent of physiologic injury. Several factors determine the current flow. It has already been mentioned that tissue conductivity plays a role. Dry skin, for example, is highly resistive. But, the presence of sweat can reduce skin resistance by nearly a hundredfold.

The type of current to which the body is exposed is also a determinant of the degree of injury. Although the term *leakage current* is used to describe any unintended current flow, whether through a person or an electrical device, it can make a difference if the current is of the direct or alternating type, and, if the latter, what its frequency is. For example, although both high- and low-frequency ACs are capable of producing heat and burns, only low-frequency currents stimulate nerve and muscles. This can lead to asphyxia secondary to muscle paralysis caused by the electrical stimulus. This is why surgical electrocautery units use high-frequency AC. Almost any device that plugs into 60-hertz electrical outlets can be a source of low-frequency electric current. Unfortunately, 60-hertz current is nearly ideal for producing muscle paralysis.

Cautery units have frequently been implicated as sources of patient injury. The high current densities created by the surgeon's active electrode are supposed to be quickly dissipated through the unit's grounding pad. Safe use requires that the grounding pad be correctly placed, contain a liberal amount of conductive jelly, and be properly con-

nected at all points. Newer electrocautery grounding pads do not require use of conductive jelly but all other precautions still apply. The pad should not be placed over bony prominences or scar areas or near other electrical conducting points such as electrocardiographic electrodes. This is especially to be avoided if the electrodes are of the needle type with small surface areas. All wiring should be intact and connection plugs should be firmly placed in their receptacles. Cautery wiring should not cross or come into contact with wires from other electronic devices.

Electric shock requires two points of contact, the current source and a ground. Because many items within the operating room can serve as a ground, contact with only a current source can cause a person to experience shock. Surfaces wet with blood or irrigating solutions have a lower resistance and facilitate conduction of current, thus adding to the hazard. Virtually any electrical device emits some leakage current, typically below 1000 microamperes. This is below the threshold of perception, the current being quickly carried away by grounding connections. A current of 1 milliampere causes skin tingling. It is considered the lowest level of current that can be perceived. A 16-milliampere current normally causes an individual to let go of the source; however, this current causes paralysis of flexor muscles and a firm grasp of the source may prevent release. Currents of 50 milliamperes cause pain, loss of consciousness, and mechanical injury. A 0.1-ampere (100-milliampere) current is capable of inducing ventricular fibrillation. All of the foregoing (approximate) current values are associated with macroshock injuries from 60-hertz AC. Under microshock conditions, where current is delivered directly to the heart, 20 microamperes can induce ventricular fibrillation. To minimize the potential for electrical injury, all devices used within the operating room should be inspected and labeled by biomedical personnel prior to use. They should also be reexamined on a periodic basis. All items should be operated within the guidelines of manufacturer recommendations. *All suspect equipment should be removed from the operating room environment until repaired and reinspected by biomedical personnel.* Equipment should be inspected carefully before it is used, with particular attention to ensure that ground and other connections are made before the equipment is turned on.

Safety Regulations and Requirements

Although each government municipality is responsible for developing and enforcing its own construction and electrical codes, there exists a high degree of regulatory similarity across the United States. This is because most government agencies look to standards of the National Electrical Code (NEC) and the National Fire Protection Association (NFPA) for guidance in all aspects of electrical and other safety practices. NFPA standards address electrical safety and use of explosive and nonexplosive anesthetic and therapeutic gases and other hazardous substances capable of initiating a fire. Standards are developed by experts who periodically review, update, and publish them in pamphlet form. Though not enforceable as law except where they have been codified by legislative agencies, the standards are still highly regarded by accrediting bodies, which find them useful in making judgments about the quality of care rendered by a health care facility. The governing board of each hospital is responsible for ensuring adherence to legal requirements and for developing internal safety policies and procedures. All anesthetists should be thoroughly familiar with those standards bearing on safe anesthesia practice.

Two primary areas encompassed by safety standards on electrical use by a health facility are testing and grounding. It will be remembered that electrical flow is dependent on a charge difference between two objects. This occurs when a charge-producing substance is brought into contact with a nonconductor. Separation of the two substances leaves each with a charge of "static" electricity. Static electricity has often been implicated as an ignition source in operating room fires and explosions in the past, but the abandonment of explosive anesthetic agents has reduced the hazard. Nevertheless, the principles for dealing with static electricity remain valid for even the most modern operating room because it, like electricity's other forms, can be a source of harm when circumstances allow. For example, a spark could ignite fumes from an open container of volatile cleaning fluid.

A considerable number of electrical items are used in operating rooms. On any given day, most of the following could be employed during just one case: electrocautery, monitors, x-ray equipment, electrical operating room table, microscopes, headlamps, endoscopic equipment, and fluid pumps. The growing use of laser and other high-energy systems will add to the problem. Lasers have already been the source of several operating room fires. Outside the operating room items such as heating lamps and diathermy units can become dangerous sources of electricity. One cannot even consider psychiatric wards safe because electroconvulsive therapy performed in this area has been responsible for patient deaths, probably through cardiac arrhythmias accompanying central nervous system disruption and catecholamine release induced by the therapy. Indeed, no area of a health facility is totally free from the possibility of electrical injury to patients and personnel. For this reason, patient risks for electrical injury have now been classified. Surgical patients represent the highest-risk group because they are exposed to both macro- and microshock hazards. All these considerations underscore the need for careful vigilance and attention to electrical safety requirements.

The most critical factor in operating room safety is electrical grounding. Proper grounding rapidly dissipates static charges and carries away dangerous currents that develop in equipment. As previously mentioned, a power source outlet in the United States consists of three conductors: one is a "live" wire that conducts current; one returns current from equipment back to the power source, at which point it is grounded to earth; and one is locally connected to an earth ground. Conducting wires are normally colored black, white, and green, respectively. The redundant local ground is connected to the equipment chassis by way of the unit's three-conductor power cable. This third conductor serves to remove charges occurring as a result of component malfunction within the unit and as a backup ground should an electrical fault develop to prevent current from being returned via the normal pathway. Providing a redundant

ground for equipment increases safety. Live current flowing through equipment as a result of malfunction presents a macroshock hazard, at least until fuse or circuit-breaker disruption interrupts power to the unit. With an intact redundant ground, current is dissipated quickly, before someone coming into contact with the unit is injured. Extension cords circumvent this safety precaution, and the use of such cords in the operating room is to be condemned.

Both NEC and NFPA standards require patient care areas to use equipotential grounding. This type of grounding joins all equipment, conductive surfaces, and the metal objects in the area in such a way that all are at the same voltage. The point at which these objects are electrically joined is called the *patient reference ground point* because the patient is in contact with many of the conducting surfaces or items. The patient reference ground point is, in turn, connected to the earth ground system of the electrical source. Equipotential environments provide a conductive path for any 60-hertz current accidentally entering a patient-connected system. Proper operation requires that all electrical and ground conductors be well insulated and correctly wired. There may also be specific ground points for special equipment and for a room's conductive metal framework. Potential differences between any two exposed conductive surfaces in an equipotential environment should not exceed 100 to 500 millivolts for frequencies below 1 kilohertz when measured across a 1000-ohm resistance. Specific requirements vary with the degree of patient risk.

Anesthetizing locations require a special type of high-resistance power-delivery circuit using what is called an isolation transformer. Isolated power circuits receive current from the normal electrical service lines by way of the transformer's primary winding. The operating room's electrical outlets are connected to the transformer's secondary winding. Therefore, no direct connection exists between the power source and outlets. Within the transformer, power is transferred from the primary to the secondary by means of magnetic inductance, a concept discussed earlier. Neither of the transformer's output connections is connected to ground. Because energy has been transferred magnetically and not carried as a pure current, the output wires are "isolated." No current will flow through a grounded person coming into contact with either of the wires; hence, the person is not "shocked." Current can, however, flow between the two isolated output conductors. Touching both outputs simultaneously will cause current flow through the individual's arms. Obviously, isolated power circuits increase safety by requiring the individual to make two contacts, rather than one, before receiving a shock. Although they increase safety, isolated power circuits are not perfect. Some capacitive coupling between transformer and person can occur and cause current to be perceived. An additional advantage of isolated power circuits is that a short circuit from either of the lines to a piece of grounded equipment does not disrupt power by activating circuit breakers or fuses. The equipment can be used until the short-circuit defect is repaired. Also, "free-floating" electricity from such a short circuit would not cause sparking that could serve as a fire ignition source.

Because it is possible for an isolated line to become directly shorted to ground and thus present the same hazard as a normal electrical outlet, line isolation monitoring devices are incorporated to warn of the defect. When the monitor detects current flowing to ground, it activates a visual and/or audible alarm. Line monitors are placed in each operating room served by an isolated power system, but they cannot identify a break in equipment grounding systems and should not be relied on to ensure equipment safety.

Explosive anesthetic agents have been abandoned in favor of nonexplosive inhalation agents. When they were in use it was mandatory for hospital facilities to use electrically conductive flooring and equipment. Conductive materials afforded some protection against macroshock injury. Standards required a minimum resistance of 25,000 ohms and a maximum of 1,000,000 ohms. This range best dissipated static charges but created enough resistance to lessen the likelihood of serious macroshock currents from operating room equipment.

Biomedical personnel normally carry out inspection and testing of all operating room equipment. This includes checking wiring, plugs, electrical circuits, and other items. Any equipment needing repair is tagged and removed for servicing. Logs are kept of all test findings and repair work. New equipment should undergo a "shakedown period" before being placed in service within the operating room area.

Special Electrical Hazards

It is a common misconception that battery-operated devices present no hazard. Although battery-operated equipment is typically at low voltage, malfunction under certain conditions can be dangerous. Endoscopic equipment has been responsible for detonating explosions within patient body cavities. Fuel for such explosions can be flammable anesthetics sequestered in the cavity or natural organic by-products. Arcing or heat caused by malfunction of an endoscope bulb can be enough to ignite volatile substances. Use of the electrocautery during laparoscopy is especially dangerous. Laparoscopy involves insufflating a gas into the abdominal cavity to distend it and allow passage of the laparoscope. Carbon dioxide can be the insufflating gas. More often, nitrous oxide is used because patients tolerate it better. Nitrous oxide supports combustion and readily diffuses into the gut to mix with highly explosive methane and hydrogen gas contained there. Heat generated by electrocautery forceps, if they are misapplied to the gut rather than the fallopian tubes, can ignite the gases to cause an explosion.

Another frequently overlooked hazard is that of burns caused by passage of an electric current through an area where electrolyte solution is present. If physiologic saline is pooled under an electrode or on a surface in contact with the patient's skin, passage of the current will ionize the solution to sodium hydroxide and chlorine gas. Contact of these substances with the skin for an extended period results in caustic burns. These are often deep and heal poorly. The anesthetist should always examine the patient's skin for evidence of such burns, particularly under electrode or grounding pads. Even without the presence of an electrolyte solution, leakage current applied to the skin for a long period will produce a thermal injury as current is carried through the patient's body to a grounding site.

Exposure to intense radio frequencies, even when no direct skin contact is made, also results in burns. Recently, questions about the long-term biologic effects of radio frequency exposure have been raised. Research in this area is underway, but no definite information is yet available. Given that nearly every person daily receives radio frequency radiation from the environment, the results of such research could hold important future implications.

In the event that one comes on an electrocution victim, rapid intervention is necessary to prevent death. The following steps should be taken:

1. If possible, shut off the source of electricity.
2. If cutting off power is not possible, separate the victim from the electrical contact using a nonconducting lever (e.g., a piece of wood). *Do not touch* the victim until this is accomplished.
3. Summon aid.
4. Initiate cardiopulmonary resuscitation.
5. Transport the patient to a medical facility.

FIRE AND EXPLOSION HAZARDS

Operating room fires and explosions decreased substantially in the 1970s as anesthesia personnel abandoned the use of flammable anesthetics. Yet, a number of fires are still reported each year, and fire and explosion remain the most frightening and devastating events that can occur in an operating room.

Three factors are necessary for a fire to start: fuel, oxygen, and an ignition source. Any substance capable of chemically combining with oxygen can serve as fuel. This includes most organic compounds, which, because they contain carbon and hydrogen, will lend themselves to burning. A fuel's chemical nature determines the rapidity with which it burns (flammability). For this reason, volatile substances, whether gases, vapors, or liquids, usually burn more easily than solids. Burning involves an oxidative process, but not all oxidative reactions result in fire or explosion. *Combustion* is a term used to indicate those that do. Primary end products of combustion are carbon, carbon dioxide, and water. Oxygen for combustion reactions can be in either pure or combined form. For example, when nitrous oxide is dissociated to its components, nitrogen and oxygen, released oxygen becomes free to enter into oxidative reactions. Therefore, nitrous oxide can support combustion. In relative terms, fire is a slow oxidative process if contrasted with explosions that, on detonation, occur instantly. Burning is an exothermic reaction; that is, heat is produced and liberated. As the reactants of a fire become sufficiently heated, they become luminescent. This glow is seen as the fire flame. Heat in any form can serve as a fire ignition source. This includes open flames, static sparks, electrical arcing, and chemical reactions. Under appropriate conditions, ignition sources need not be intense or applied for a long period.

The oxidative process involves transfer of electrons. As heat from the ignition source accelerates molecular motion within the fuel–oxygen mixture, molecular bonds are bro-

ken and electrons transfer from oxygen to the fuel substance. This results in chemical reduction of the fuel. Heat released with the breaking of the first few bonds activates further molecular activity: more broken bonds bring about greater heat release, which accelerates electron transfer. Certain conditions that facilitate this process include high ambient temperatures, compression of gases, availability of fuel and oxygen, and the extent to which fuel and oxygen are allowed to mix. Conditions that limit either the rate or the extent of burning include low fuel reactivity, a limited supply of either fuel or oxygen, effectiveness of heat dissipation, and presence of quenching agents.

Combustible mixtures are of three types: lean, rich, and stoichiometric. With lean mixtures, oxygen is in greater abundance than fuel. For rich mixtures, the reverse is true, that is, fuel remains after the oxygen has been used up. Stoichiometric mixtures are those in which combustion is complete, where neither fuel nor oxygen remains. The proportions of fuel and oxygen in a mixture determine the flammability range for the mix. Outside the range, oxygen or fuel amounts are insufficient to allow significant combustion. Upper and lower limits of flammability have been determined for all explosive anesthetic agents in combination with oxygen, air, or nitrous oxide. Because explosive agents are not used today, flammability ranges are not covered here. They are available in older standard texts for those desiring more information. Generally, flammable anesthetic concentrations of 1 to 80 percent are sufficiently volatile to cause explosions. With one exception, trichlorethylene, anesthetic concentrations of all explosive agents fall within this range. Mixtures in which oxygen is present at less than 10 percent by volume generally will not self-propagate if ignited. With metabolic oxygen requirements being more than double this amount, it is impossible to entirely eliminate the explosive hazard with flammable anesthetic mixtures.

The fire factor easiest to control is ignition source. A number of sources have already been identified in this chapter. Two ignition source terms that are sometimes confused are flashpoint and ignition temperature. *Flashpoint* is the temperature at which a mixture first burns; however, on removal of the ignition source, the flame goes out. At *ignition temperature*, the mixture continues to burn even after the ignition source has been removed. In most cases of fire and explosion, ignition temperatures are below 500C. Even heat from a small spark is enough to raise the temperature of a portion of flammable mixture above the ignition point. A mixture's *detonation point* is the temperature at which it explodes. Static electricity has been a major ignition source of operating room fires. The use of conductive flooring for removing static charges has been discussed. Another operating room factor serving the same purpose is environmental humidity. At a relative humidity of 55 to 60 percent, air moisture provides enough conductivity on open surfaces to carry away static charges to a ground point. Halogenation of anesthetic compounds has been another approach to reducing operating room flammability hazards.

One ignition source peculiar to anesthesia and inhalation therapy practice is adiabatic compression or expansion. Under most conditions, compression increases and expansion decreases the temperature of a gas. These temperature changes are transferred to the surrounding environment; however, when volume changes occur under conditions that do not allow gain or loss of heat from the environment, they are termed *adiabatic*. Because such volume changes occur very rapidly, high temperatures are generated instantaneously. This is the case within compressed gas cylinders when the tank valve is opened. Gas from the cylinder enters the valve where it is recompressed because of the valve's smaller volume. This creates extremely high temperatures capable of igniting particulate matter lodged in the valve outlet. A flash fire results. Oxygen from the surrounding air or within the gas mixture feeds the fire and adds to the hazard. It is for this reason that cylinder valves should always be kept capped until ready for use. In addition, no oil or other flammable substance should be used as a lubricant around the valve opening. Gas cylinders should be "cracked" (opened slowly to air) prior to attachment of regulating valves. This procedure is not recommended when attaching cylinders to the anesthesia machine. A strainer nipple is present in the machine to filter particulate matter. Adiabatic compression also presents a hazard when cylinders are being filled from bulk supplies. Manufacturers of compressed gas equipment must follow special safety precautions when transfilling cylinders, and anesthesia personnel should never attempt to transfill anesthetic gases themselves.

Another phenomenon seen when releasing gas from a compressed cylinder is the Joule–Thomson effect. As gas leaves the cylinder, its expansion cools the surrounding air, causing condensation of moisture on the tank. The Joule–Thomson effect per se does not represent a fire hazard. But hand contact with the cylinder as cooling takes place can result in a freeze burn to the skin.

The flammability range of explosive mixtures can be narrowed by addition of quenching agents, nonoxidizable inert gases, of which the three most prominent are carbon dioxide, helium, and nitrogen. Quenching agents reduce combustibility because they possess high molal heat capacities or high thermal conductivity. This means they either absorb large amounts of heat readily (thus increasing the amount of heat required for ignition) or rapidly dispel heat, conducting it away before ignition can occur. These agents are often used in safety devices for hazardous locations. Carbon dioxide fire extinguishers are an example.

All anesthetists should be aware of NFPA pamphlets, especially Pamphlets 56A and 56C. These outline proper fire-prevention measures to be used by anesthesia and operating room personnel. Copies of these pamphlets should be available in the surgical suite.

Every operating room should have a fire emergency plan. Prior planning and training can save lives and prevent injury. The following outline reviews the major steps to be taken in the event of an operating room fire or explosion.

Phase I (Notification)

1. The senior operating room charge person initiates the plan at the first hint of a fire.
2. He or she sounds the fire alarm or calls the fire department. Many operating rooms are equipped with automatic alarms to notify firefighters of the emergency. It is possible for such

systems to malfunction. A secondary notification system should also be used. Failure to summon help promptly can be catastrophic.

3. All traffic into the surgical suite is stopped and all personnel alerted to the emergency.
4. Fire doors are closed and emergency exits readied.
5. Personnel are assigned to operate firefighting equipment at all key locations.

Phase II (Preparation)

Within each operating room, personnel should take the following measures:

1. All unnecessary electrical equipment is unplugged.
2. All flammable agents (e.g., alcohols) are removed to a nonpatient area such as a substerile room. Surgical procedures not yet begun should be aborted. Those procedures underway require individual professional judgments as to whether or not to continue.
3. Piped-in anesthesia gases are disconnected, machine reserve cylinders are turned on, and delivered flows reduced if feasible.
4. All unnecessary equipment (e.g., blood warmers, humidifiers) is disconnected.
5. Essential drugs and equipment necessary for patient evacuation are gathered.
6. Plans should be made for maintenance of the patient's vital functions during evacuation.

Phase III (Implementation)

1. Until an all-clear or evacuation signal is given, all personnel should remain at their assigned locations. When notified by the senior person to begin evacuation, personnel should proceed rapidly according to preplanned policies, using designated evacuation routes. How the patient is transported will vary with the circumstances.

It may not be feasible to do more than carry the patient. All equipment may have to be abandoned. Patient vital functions may have to be maintained using cardiopulmonary resuscitation procedures. If the anesthesia machine is abandoned, all gas flows should be shut off.

2. Main electrical and gas lines are disconnected.

Every fire alarm should be treated with the utmost seriousness. Undoubtedly, many alarms will be either false or quickly handled. Callous disregard of an alarm can have dire consequences for both patients and operating room staff.

CONCLUSION

The potential for electrical and fire-related injuries in the modern operating room is virtually unmatched by any other human work environment. Patients trust the nurse anesthetist to ensure their well-being while they are anesthetized. Meeting that responsibility requires an understanding and appreciation of the basic principles underlying operating room hazards. As in all other phases of anesthesia practice, safety resides in constant vigilance.

BIBLIOGRAPHY

Beiser A, Cummings B. *Physics*. 4th ed. Menlo Park, CA: Bubco; 1989.

Blatt FJ. *Principles of physics*. 3rd ed. Boston: Allyn & Bacon; 1989.

Meyer E. *Chemistry of hazardous materials*. 2nd ed. Englewood Cliffs, NJ: Prentice-Hall; 1989.

Neufeld GR. Fires and explosions. In: Orkin FK, Cooperman LH, eds. *Complications in anesthesiology*. Philadelphia: JB Lippincott; 1983.

Scurr C, Feldman S. *Scientific foundations of anesthesia*. 4th ed. Chicago: Year Book Medical; 1990.

The Anesthesia Machine

Linda M. Huffman and
Eddie Bowie

The anesthesia machine is a sophisticated life support system that relies on the principles of mechanics, pneumatics, and electronics to manage pressure, flow, and volume as it delivers anesthetic gases to provide ventilation and oxygenation. Fresh gas sources, the internal machine circuitry, flowmeters, vaporizers, the patient circuit, and the waste gas evacuation systems are major components that require study and understanding because problems can arise at any time. To detect, prevent, or minimize the effects of machine system problems, the anesthetist must be able to verify that all components are functioning properly.

The ability to make an appropriate differential diagnosis of what is happening in the machine system is a learned set of tasks that evolves from a student's work in mastering basic gas flow pathways through the machine. For this reason, the text and figures used in this chapter are generic and may be applied, in principle, to all anesthesia machines manufactured after 1979.

The fundamentals of machine operation are introduced in this chapter to enable students to appreciate and understand the instruction and operations manual, cautions, and warnings that accompany each unique machine and accessory device manufactured for use with an anesthesia delivery system.

The scope of this chapter is limited to the discussion of gas flow, proper function of major system components, and normal machine operations. Recognition of the major parts of the machine and their performance is mandatory preparation for understanding how the system ultimately affects the clinical signs and symptoms exhibited by both the patient and the machine. Without the benefit of understanding these basics, the daily and preuse testing procedures are apt to be inadequate, incomplete, misapplied, and misinterpreted.

Constant vigilance has always been the foundation for accurate and timely assessment of the machine's function and its minimum performance. Vigilance is not adequate, however, unless the user knows how the system is designed to operate and has personally checked and verified its proper working condition. Routine use of appropriate monitoring devices and techniques, an integral part of machine system operation, is also required to ensure that life-sustaining information is accurate, complete, and available.

PRINCIPLES OF GAS DELIVERY

Anesthesia machine systems are basically designed to deliver the right amount of gas, at the right time, and at the right pressure to ensure an appropriate level of surgical anesthesia and to manage ventilation and oxygenation of the patient.

Oxygen and nitrous oxide enter the machine from two sources: the wall supply and the cylinder supply (Fig. 8–1). Oxygen, the dominant gas, flows into the machine through the pipeline inlet check valve (Fig. 8–2) at a pressure of approximately 50 pounds per square inch gauge (psig). Oxygen also provides pressure to the power outlet accessory, where the ventilator may be connected.

At the same time, oxygen travels from the machine inlet to pressurize the oxygen flush valve. As soon as oxygen is connected to the machine, the oxygen flush valve is able to deliver oxygen to the patient circuit. The flow rate delivered by an open flush valve should range from 35 to 75 L/min (Fig. 8–2).[1(p8)]

Aside from pressurizing the power outlet and the flush valve, oxygen flow opens the pressure-sensor shutoff valve (Fig. 8–3), permitting nitrous oxide to be delivered. This sensor is placed in-line, between the nitrous oxide supply and the nitrous oxide flowmeter.

When oxygen supply is adequate and being delivered to the machine at 50 psig, the pressure-sensor shutoff valve opens to direct nitrous oxide to the flowmeter. This valve will remain open as long as the oxygen supply pressure stays above 25 psig. If the oxygen supply pressure falls below this pressure, the shutoff valve closes and stops the flow of nitrous oxide. This mechanical action is responsible for limiting the delivery of nitrous oxide whenever the oxygen pressure is less than appropriate.

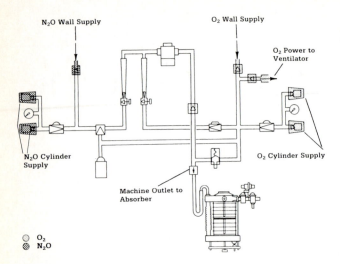

Figure 8–1. Sources of oxygen and nitrous oxide supply within the flow diagram of a basic anesthesia machine. (*Redrawn with permission granted by Ohmeda, a division of BOC Health Care, Inc.*)

The pressure-sensor shutoff valve is essential, but it does not warn the practitioner that it has terminated nitrous oxide flow. The clinician may visually note that the nitrous oxide float is dropping in the flowmeter; however, the oxygen supply failure alarm system is the component that sounds an alarm to provide a warning. This alarm, adjacent to the shutoff valve, contains a reservoir filled with oxygen pressure at 50 psig. When oxygen pressure falls below a predetermined setting of approximately 28 psig, the alarm is activated. It whistles loudly to alert the practitioner that the oxygen pressure in the machine is falling. The alarm begins to sound before the oxygen pressure has fallen to 25 psig, the pressure at which nitrous oxide flow will cease.

Whether the alarm is momentary or prolonged, it indicates that the clinician needs to reestablish an adequate oxygen supply by turning on the reserve oxygen cylinder.

Oxygen pressure is usually, but not always, delivered from the wall supply at 50 psig. Fluctuations do occur, and the pressure may decrease to 40 psig, based on the delivery system and the hospital's demand for oxygen. The second-stage regulator (Fig. 8–4) eliminates the need to continuously adjust the flowmeter based on fluctuations in the wall supply pressure. A constant pressure of approximately 16 psig is maintained by the second-stage regulator at the flow control valve to eliminate changes in oxygen flow resulting from changes in the oxygen supply pressure. This ensures that oxygen is the last gas to cease flowing to the patient if an oxygen supply failure occurs.

Oxygen that is supplied by the cylinders instead of the wall system passes through the hanger yoke check valve(s) and the cylinder pressure regulator before it reaches the second-stage regulator. As the approximate pressure in a full E-size cylinder of oxygen is 2200 psig, it is too high to be easily controlled by the flow control valve. Therefore, it too must be regulated or reduced to 40 to 50 psig. Regardless of the source of oxygen, gas travels the same course within the machine circuitry once it passes through the second-stage regulator.

Oxygen flows upward through the flowmeter once the flow control valve is turned on. It then enters the common manifold, passes through the vaporizer, and proceeds through the machine outlet check valve. This valve, when present, ensures flow in only one direction. The gas mixture continues from the machine outlet through the absorber's inhalation check valve before flowing to the patient (Fig. 8–5). Exhaled gases pass from the patient through the exhalation check valve and enter the rebreathing bag. When the exhaled gases have filled the bag, excess gas will flow through the adjustable pressure-limiting (APL) valve into

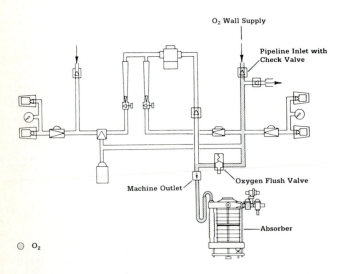

Figure 8–2. Flow pathway of oxygen from the wall supply to the patient circuit. Note that the oxygen flush valve is immediately usable once the hose has been connected. (*Redrawn with permission granted by Ohmeda, a division of BOC Health Care, Inc.*)

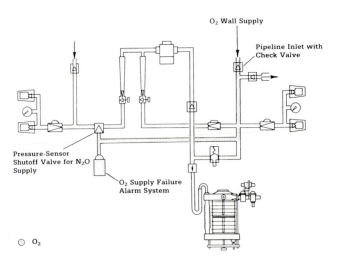

Figure 8–3. Oxygen flow from the wall supply to the pressure-sensor shutoff valve and the oxygen supply failure alarm system. (*Redrawn with permission granted by Ohmeda, a division of BOC Health Care, Inc.*)

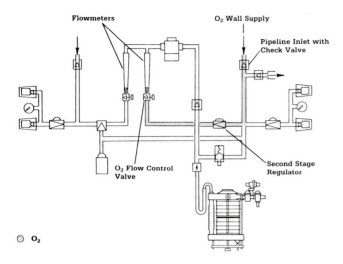

Figure 8–4. Oxygen flows from the wall supply through the second-stage regulator before flowing to the base of the flowmeter. (*Redrawn with permission granted by Ohmeda, a division of BOC Health Care, Inc.*)

the scavenging system that removes waste gases. On the next inspiration, gas remaining in the rebreathing bag passes through the absorber canister(s) where carbon dioxide is removed, before joining the fresh gas flowing into the inspiratory limb of the breathing circuit.

This pattern of gas flow is typically described as a semiclosed breathing system or a circle-with-absorber system. Closed breathing systems have the same flow pattern, but the APL valve is not opened nor regularly adjusted as with semiclosed breathing circuits. Nonrebreathing systems do not use an absorber and employ a specific nonrebreathing

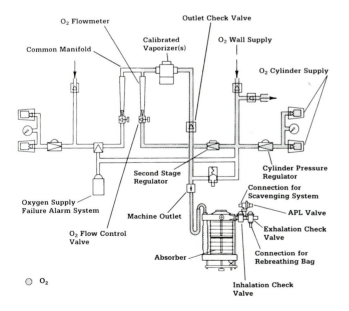

Figure 8–5. Oxygen flow from the wall supply or the cylinder supply through the second-stage regulator, flowmeter, and "in-line" vaporizer to the absorber. (*Redrawn with permission granted by Ohmeda, a division of BOC Health Care, Inc.*)

valve and appropriate delivery hose attached to the common gas outlet.

Closed, semiclosed, and nonrebreathing or partial rebreathing breathing systems may be used with all anesthesia machine systems that meet or exceed the minimum standard for safety and performance, as published by the American Society of Testing and Materials (ASTM).[2] This set of standard specifications, published in 1988, replaced the previous anesthesia machine standard document known as the American National Standards Institute (ANSI) Z.79.8: *Standard for Safety and Performance of Anesthesia Machines for Human Use*. The ANSI Z.79.8 document was the first full consensus standard that defined minimum performance and safety specifications developed by representatives from all sectors of anesthesia practice and interests: CRNAs; physicians; professional engineers; and representatives of manufacturing, government, academic, and consumer groups. Full consensus standards are comprehensively sound and credible because all participants must concur on every aspect of the standard, including words, phrases, terminology, performance specifications, and testing protocols. The standard is also submitted for ballot and vote prior to approval and publication.

The currently applicable ASTM standard document is designated as F1161-88 and is officially titled *Standard Specification for Minimum Performance and Safety Requirements for Components and Systems of Anesthesia Machines*. This standard is under the jurisdiction of the ASTM Committee on Anesthetic and Respiratory Equipment and is the direct responsibility of Subcommittee F29.01.01 on Continuous Flow Anesthesia Gas Machines. ASTM F1161-88, like its predecessor, is a full consensus standard, and is the foundation for ongoing standards writing activity aimed at ensuring that anesthesia machines purchased in the future will meet the minimum expectations for safety.

Manufacturing of anesthesia machines requires compliance with this standard and numerous other standards' specifications relating to circuits, accessories, ventilators, regulators, compressed gases, monitors, and alarms. Each standard is a set of rules established by authority, expertise, custom, and general consensus as a model to be followed. Standards also serve as the basic elements by which quality is defined as part of the overall commitment to public safety. Therefore, it is inappropriate for a clinician or hospital to modify, alter, refine, redesign, or manufacture anesthesia equipment components. Changes and alteration in select equipment configuration are acceptable providing the original product manufacturer describes the intended alteration in the appropriate operations and maintenance manual(s) required for the specific model of machine, component, or accessory used in the anesthesia system.

MACHINE COMPONENTS THAT MANAGE OXYGEN

All anesthesia machines come from the manufacturer with a pipeline inlet consisting of one of two general types of fittings and an enclosed check valve. These fittings are either the diameter-indexed safety system (DISS) type or the "quick-connect" type. Both fittings are indexed to a specific gas and are noninterchangeable between specific gases (Fig.

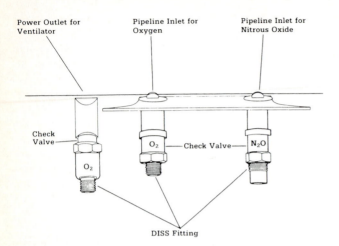

Figure 8–6. Gas supply inlets equipped with noninterchangeable diameter-indexed fittings on the back of the anesthesia machine. (*Redrawn with permission granted by Ohmeda, a division of BOC Health Care, Inc.*)

8–6) so that the appropriate gas flows through the correct inlet. Oxygen and nitrous oxide gas inlet check valves permit gas to flow only into the machine. The check valve in the power outlet permits gas to flow from the machine to a gas-powered accessory such as a ventilator. If the ventilator hose is not attached, the outlet check valve will close to prevent oxygen from flowing into the atmosphere. The mechanical force of attaching the ventilator hose opens the power outlet.

In contrast, pneumatic pressure from the wall supply opens the check valve in the pipeline inlets. The inlet check valve stays in the open position as long as adequate gas pressure is exerted from the wall supply. Gravity and any existing pressure within the gas machine, or the pneumatic pressure from the reserve cylinder supply, close the check valve.[3(p39)]

If the pipeline inlet check valve were not present, gas from a reserve cylinder could escape through the machine and rapidly empty into the piping system in the wall. This would occur any time the pressure in the hospital pipeline was interrupted or dropped below the pressure being supplied to the machine from the reserve cylinder pressure regulator.

Some clinicians feel that when this check valve is present, it is good practice to turn on one cylinder and leave it on as an automatic backup to the wall supply system.[3(p41)] Considering the fact that wall supply pressure changes from time to time, this practice is not acceptable. If a cylinder of oxygen is turned on at the same time that the oxygen pipeline supply is in use, the cylinder could be depleted without warning. The machine will always use oxygen from the source that has the higher pressure. Most cylinder regulators are set lower than the typical wall supply pressure, but the wall pressure can fall even lower than the cylinder regulator's set point during times of peak oxygen demand. In this situation, the higher reserve cylinder pressure closes the inlet check valve, stopping the wall supply and consuming the gas in the reserve cylinder. As there is no loss of

oxygen pressure to trigger the alarm, the reserve supply is depleted without warning. If both reserve cylinders are in use at the same time, the cylinder with the higher pressure will supply the gas machine system until its pressure drops to that of its companion cylinder. At this time, both cylinders will begin to supply the system, ultimately causing both reserve cylinders to empty at the same time. For this reason, it is not appropriate to have both reserve cylinders turned on at the same time.

The reserve cylinders are connected to the gas machine by means of pin-indexed hanger yokes. The pin-indexed configuration for oxygen is readily visible, permitting the pins on the yoke to be inserted into the matching holes located on the cylinder valve (Fig. 8–7). The location of the pins in the hanger yoke is designed to ensure that only cylinders filled with oxygen can be seated on the oxygen yoke (Fig. 8–8). Although the pin system is quite durable, it can be altered or damaged. Therefore, it is important to state that if the cylinder does not attach easily, do not force it. Also, never use more than one cylinder valve gasket on the yoke mechanism. The use of a second gasket may defeat the pin index and permit the wrong gas to be mounted in the yoke.[3(pp37,47),4(p293)]

Once the cylinder is turned on, oxygen enters the yoke and passes through a strainer nipple, a filter that removes dust particles that may be present on the cylinder valve or the contact surface of the yoke (Fig. 8–8). Oxygen flow pushes the check valve off its seat, while the pressure of the gas holds the valve against its retainer and keeps it open. Gas flows around the check valve and retainer into the machine.

When the first cylinder in a double-yoke, two-cylinder assembly is turned on, the flow of gas that enters the machine from the cylinder in one hanger, yoke A, opens the check valve, and its pressure is indicated by the cylinder

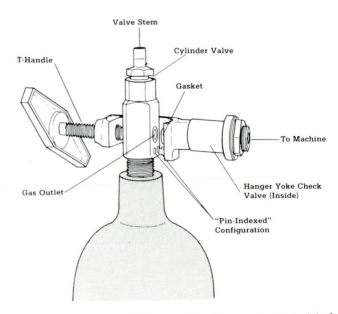

Figure 8–7. Oxygen cylinder positioned in a cutaway model of the hanger yoke. Note the location of the gas outlet and the single gasket. (*Redrawn with permission granted by Ohmeda, a division of BOC Health Care, Inc.*)

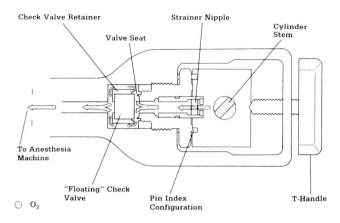

Figure 8–8. Oxygen hanger yoke, cut away to demonstrate the location of the pin-indexed safety system in relation to its placement on the yoke and the flow of oxygen through it. (*Redrawn with permission granted by Ohmeda, a division of BOC Health Care, Inc.*)

pressure gauge (Fig. 8–9). Pressure is exerted on the check valve in yoke B, forcing it onto its seat and closing it. With the valve in hanger yoke B closed, the possibility of gas leaving cylinder A and filling cylinder B is minimized. These hanger yoke valves are intended to reduce cross-filling, the condition in which gas from one cylinder fills the other. Note, however, that the hanger yoke check valve is designed to limit flow, but it is not a leak-free seal. This is another reason why only one cylinder should be opened at a time. Likewise, when only one cylinder is connected to a double-yoke system, the vacant yoke should be sealed with a standard yoke plug and gasket. Without the yoke plug in

place, gas from the cylinder in yoke A could slowly leak from yoke B into the ambient air.[3(pp37,53),5(p129)]

The oxygen flush valve receives its gas supply at approximately 50 psig from the wall or the cylinder and is ready to be used whenever oxygen is present in the machine's system (Fig. 8–10). The flush valve stays in the closed position until the operator opens the valve by pressing the button. Manual depression of this valve moves the pin, which forces the valve off of its seat and creates a path for immediate flow to the machine outlet. The ball valve retaining spring is the opposing force that moves the ball back onto its seat once manual pressure is removed. This spring automatically closes the valve.

The flush valve is used any time more oxygen needs to be added to the rebreathing bag. Flushing the system to add volume results in dilution of the mixture contained in the rebreathing bag and can prolong inhalation inductions. When a poor mask fit is the cause of decreasing volume in the rebreathing bag, using the flush valve is not the preferred method to supplement the loss. Higher flows to the patient circuit can easily be provided by temporarily increasing the liter flow at the flowmeter(s). This will not dilute the agent concentration being delivered when using an integrated calibrated vaporizer.

Indiscriminate, repeated use of the flush valve at the start of the case is generally disruptive to the smooth course of anesthesia. Furthermore, holding the valve in the open position can deliver an unnecessarily high flow, up to 75 L/min,[4(p66)] of positive-pressure gas to the patient circuit. This maneuver may overinflate the patient's lungs and lead to increased intrathoracic pressure and potential barotrauma.[4(pp304,305)]

The pressure-sensor shutoff valve also receives its oxygen supply at approximately 50 psig, and it operates by

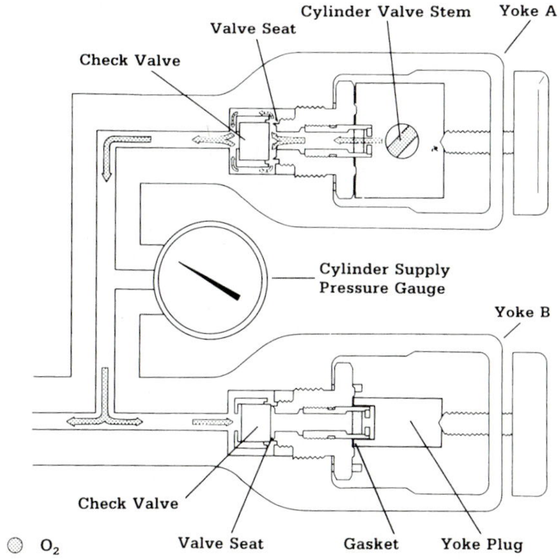

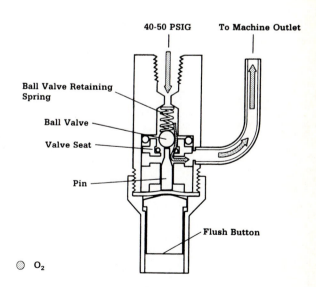

Figure 8–10. Oxygen flow through the activated flush valve. (*Redrawn with permission granted by Ohmeda, a division of BOC Health Care, Inc.*)

Figure 8–9. Oxygen flow through a double yoke when one cylinder is turned on and a yoke plug is present. (*Redrawn with permission granted by Ohmeda, a division of BOC Health Care, Inc.*)

using the lack of adequate oxygen pressure to shut off the nitrous oxide. Oxygen delivered to the machine exerts its pressure on the diaphragm and moves the piston, pin, and valve off the valve seat. This force holds the valve open. As long as at least 25 psig of oxygen pressure is exerted on the diaphragm, the valve will remain open and allow the flow of nitrous oxide from its supply source to the flow control valve (Fig. 8–11). The purpose of this valve is to shut off nitrous oxide or any other gas, for example, medical air, helium, or carbon dioxide, whenever the oxygen pressure drops below 25 psig, as when the wall or cylinder supply fails. Historically, this valve was called a "fail-safe" valve by clinicians who relied on cylinder supply oxygen as the primary source of gas. Before central gas supply systems were common, losing oxygen pressure was a constant aggravation. As a result, this component was a welcome machine monitor and typically the assumption was made that a machine so equipped was "fail-safe" and could not be used to administer a hypoxic mixture. This is a myth and continues to be misleading.

The so-called "fail-safe" valve is a pressure-sensor valve only. It cannot determine flow, volume, ventilation, or fractional inspired oxygen concentration. It is designed to sense the pressure of oxygen in the machine, and it must be checked daily to ensure its proper operation. To test the pressure-sensor shutoff valve, select a midrange flow for oxygen and nitrous oxide. Verify that flow by looking at the position of the floats in the flow tubes. Then disconnect the oxygen wall supply hose and turn the oxygen cylinder supply off. As the oxygen supply is depleted, the nitrous oxide float should fall to the bottom of the flow tube before the oxygen float descends.[3(p69)]

The alarm assembly (Fig. 8–12) warns when a condition of low oxygen pressure develops. It is aptly called the oxygen supply failure alarm system. Oxygen enters this assembly from the wall or cylinder supply through its inlet check valve and flows into the reservoir at approximately 50 psig.

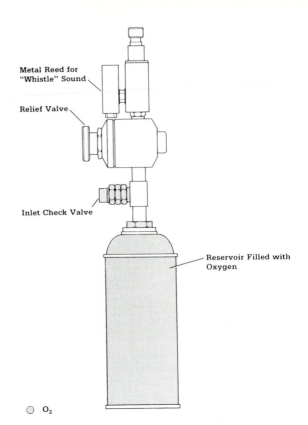

Figure 8–12. Oxygen supply failure alarm system warns when oxygen pressure falls. (*Redrawn with permission granted by Ohmeda, a division of BOC Health Care, Inc.*)

This creates a balance between the pressure inside the reservoir and the supply pressure. When oxygen supply pressure fails and the pressure in the reservoir is slowly depleted to its preset level, oxygen rushes out of the reservoir, passes through the relief valve, vibrates a metal reed, and makes the alarm sound. This event is occurring at the same time as, or slightly before, the pressure-sensor shutoff valve is terminating the flow of nitrous oxide. The alarm sound will continue until the reservoir is depleted, or for a minimum period of approximately 7 seconds. This time interval may vary with different models, but the presence of the alarm condition means the same thing. Oxygen pressure must be reestablished and verified. Unlike smart monitors that cease sounding when the alarm condition is corrected or passed, the ending of the warning tone does not necessarily mean the low-pressure condition has ended. Whenever this alarm is activated, simply turn on the reserve oxygen cylinder before beginning to analyze the cause of the problem.

The second-stage regulator receives a pressure of approximately 50 psig from the wall or reserve cylinder, reduces it to 16 psig, and delivers this constant pressure to the flow control valve. This regulator serves to isolate any pressure changes in either the pipeline or cylinder supply from the flow control valve and ensures that the oxygen supply failure alarm is activated before the falling oxygen pressure affects the oxygen flowmeter.

Although many components that manage oxygen pressure are not visible, the oxygen flowmeter is immediately

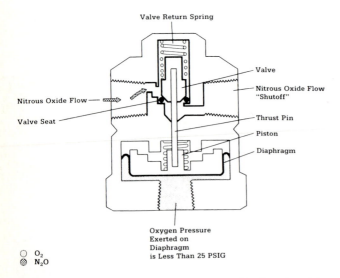

Figure 8–11. Oxygen pressure-sensor shutoff valve closed to prevent nitrous oxide from flowing. (*Redrawn with permission granted by Ohmeda, a division of BOC Health Care, Inc.*)

recognized for its role in the delivery of oxygen flow through the machine to the patient circuit (Fig. 8–13). Turning the knob counterclockwise moves the needle back and away from its seat, allowing oxygen to flow into the tube. Turning the knob clockwise closes the space between the needle and its seat, reducing oxygen flow. In addition to operating the on and off functions, this control is used to adjust the flow delivered to the patient circuit. Each turn makes a precise adjustment in the opening that carefully measures and meters the oxygen flow.

The control knob is designed to be readily identified as the oxygen flowmeter on both touch and sight. The knob is fluted, larger in diameter than other gas knobs, and both color coded and symbol coded for oxygen.[4(p54)] The valve stops on the knob indicate when the valve is closed and oxygen flow has ceased. The stop position feels like an abrupt resistance and is designed to remind the user not to rotate this valve any further.[3(p71)]

Two float stops are present in the flow tube itself. The one at the top of the tube prevents the float from colliding with the surface of the gas outlet, where it could potentially lodge and obstruct gas flow to the common manifold.[6] The stop at the bottom of the tube provides the float with a place to rest in the center of the flow tube, when the oxygen flow is turned off. When the flow control valve is opened, this style of float is centered by the flow of the gas and is read at the point where the top of the float corresponds to the scale.

The flowmeter is a hand-calibrated system that includes a tapered glass tube, a float, and a scale. No two flow tubes are exactly alike. To compensate for differences, the flowmeter scales are individually calibrated to provide a high degree of accuracy over the full range of the scale.[7] The float is inserted into the tube, and the scale is engraved to correspond with each measured flow of the specific gas that passes through that particular tube. After this, the scale becomes specific for that tube and its float, and all parts are regarded as an inseparable unit.[3(p72)] As a result, whenever any flow tube, float, or scale for any gas needs replacement, the complete set must be replaced.

The oxygen flowmeter is always positioned closest to the manifold outlet and to the right of all other flow tubes, as one faces the machine.[3(p73),4(p58),5(p46)] This is a requirement for all American and Canadian machines. With oxygen on the right, it is always downstream of all other gases that flow into the common manifold. Should a crack or leak develop in a nitrous oxide or a third gas flowmeter, oxygen would be the last gas to escape to the atmosphere.

Some older machines and models that do not meet current ASTM standards may have oxygen flowmeters positioned to the left or in the center of a group of flow tubes.[4(p58),5(p46),8] This configuration may be present from time to time when a substitute machine is brought out of storage and placed into service temporarily. Therefore, it is important to examine every machine closely and be aware of this possibility to prevent the unfortunate experience of reaching for the oxygen flow control valve on the right and later discovering that the adjustment made was in the flow of nitrous oxide.[4(p402)]

MACHINE COMPONENTS THAT MANAGE NITROUS OXIDE

Nitrous oxide delivery is less involved in the overall function of the anesthesia machine. Nitrous oxide enters the machine from the wall supply through the nitrous oxide inlet and its check valve at the nominal pressure of 50 psig. It flows freely through the pressure-sensor shutoff valve, providing the machine system is pressurized with more than 25 psig of oxygen. From this point, nitrous oxide travels directly to its flow control valve (Fig. 8–14). When the supply hose for nitrous oxide is connected between the wall source and the machine inlet and the machine system has been pressurized with oxygen, nitrous oxide can be turned on at the flowmeter, even though the oxygen flowmeter remains off. Oxygen pressure needs only to be present to keep the pressure-sensor shutoff valve open; oxygen does not have to be flowing.

Although nitrous oxide is not a gas that is in high demand in other hospital departments, its supply pressure can also fluctuate above or below the usual 50-psig level.[3(p75)] This is caused by the peculiarities of the hospital's central system and the current demand on all of the supply outlets in the surgery suite, as well as any other anesthetizing areas connected to the same supply source.

Unlike cylinder oxygen, which is a compressed gas at room temperature, nitrous oxide is contained in a full cylinder primarily as a liquid and exerts a gas pressure of about 745 psig (Fig. 8–15). As nitrous oxide is withdrawn from the cylinder, some of the remaining liquid vaporizes to a gas and replaces the withdrawn gas. The pressure is maintained

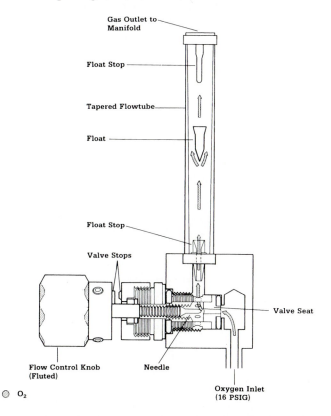

Figure 8–13. Oxygen flowmeter, cut away to illustrate the needle valve in relation to its valve seat. Note the valve and float stops within the component. (*Redrawn with permission granted by Ohmeda, a division of BOC Health Care, Inc.*)

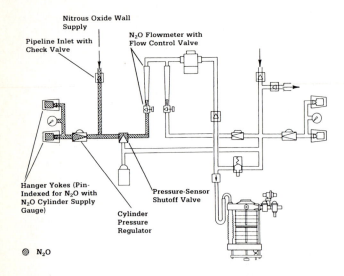

Figure 8–14. Nitrous oxide flows from the wall or cylinder supplies through the cylinder pressure regulator and the pressure-sensor shutoff valve to the base of the flowmeter. (*Redrawn with permission granted by Ohmeda, a division of BOC Health Care, Inc.*)

until all of the liquid has vaporized. As a result, the nitrous oxide pressure gauge will read 745 psig, even though the weight and volume of the contents are both decreasing. For this reason, an additional full cylinder of nitrous oxide should always be available when using nitrous oxide. Once all of the liquid has been evaporated, the cylinder gauge will then reflect actual pressure changes of the remaining gas. A nitrous oxide cylinder can be considered empty when the pressure gauge reads significantly lower than 745 psig. When the cylinder is in use and the pointer on the

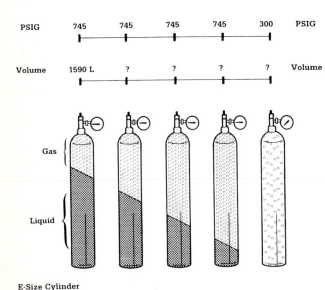

Figure 8–15. Nitrous oxide is stored as a liquid and its pressure gauge does not reflect the volume in the cylinder until all the liquid has been used. (*Redrawn with permission granted by Ohmeda, a division of BOC Health Care, Inc.*)

nitrous oxide pressure gauge is falling, be prepared to replace the cylinder immediately.

Nitrous oxide cylinder yoke assemblies also have check valves to minimize cross-filling, but they too are not designed to be leaktight seals. Nitrous oxide may still escape to the atmosphere and expose health care workers to excess trace gas,[5(pp105–107)] unless a standard yoke plug and its gasket are installed in the empty yoke whenever a single cylinder is mounted on the two-yoke assembly.[3(p81)]

Nitrous oxide reserve cylinders must be managed in the same way as oxygen reserve cylinders. They should be turned on during the machine checking procedure or when the wall supply gas is unavailable. They should not be left on at the same time the wall supply is in use. Although it may be reassuring to have them on and ready to switch over automatically if the wall supply fails, the fact remains that the reserve supply is silently depleted when the wall pressure falls below the pressure delivered by the nitrous oxide pressure regulator.

A nitrous oxide cylinder has its own dedicated regulator, which reduces the pressure to about 50 psig. The regulator is simply an automatic balancing device that balances all gas pressures—those coming in and those going out—against a spring load. The pressure-relief valve will vent to atmosphere when an excessive level of pressure (above 75 psig) develops on the low-pressure side of the regulator.[3(p83)]

The nitrous oxide flowmeter (and flow control valve) is similar to the oxygen flowmeter in its functional role—measuring the flow of gas delivered to the patient circuit. This knob feels different from the oxygen knob and can also be distinguished by sight. Unlike the oxygen control knob, the nitrous oxide knob has a knurled surface and is smaller in diameter.

COMMON AND ISOLATED MANIFOLDS

Oxygen and nitrous oxide leave their respective flowmeters and enter the space just above the flow tubes called the *common manifold* (Fig. 8–16). Here gases mix together as they travel to the vaporizer, where they become the carrier of a volatile anesthetic agent. Gases may also flow through an isolated manifold, one that directs gas around the vaporizer so none of the gas passes over the vaporizing chamber. There are several kinds of manifolds and a vaporizer can be mounted within them in a variety of ways. To understand how the particular manifold on each machine is connected to the flowmeters and vaporizer(s) and what characteristics each configuration presents, the operations manual must be reviewed for each model of anesthesia machine.

CALIBRATED VAPORIZERS

An agent-specific calibrated vaporizer is a device that controls the concentration of a volatile anesthetic agent delivered through the common gas outlet. It is dedicated to one agent only, precisely calibrated, and automatically compensated to perform over the usual range of temperatures and variations in gas flow. For example, if one sets the concentration control knob to deliver 1 percent of anesthetic agent, the vaporizer will make adjustments for temperature and

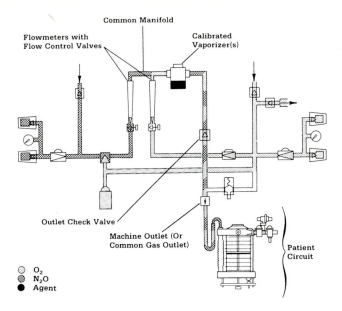

Figure 8–16. Oxygen and nitrous oxide enter the manifold, pass through a vaporizer that is turned off, and flow to the absorber. (*Redrawn with permission granted by Ohmeda, a division of BOC Health Care, Inc.*)

flow to keep its output at 1 percent, plus or minus the small variation (tolerance) specified by the manufacturer. This holds true as the liquid agent warms and cools, if the room is hot or cold, and if the total flow rate is high or low.

In the Ohio calibrated vaporizer (Fig. 8–17), gas flows from the flowmeters through the common manifold to the vaporizer inlet, passes through a filter, and moves on toward the relief valve. Under normal conditions, this relief valve remains closed. It opens only when the rate of gas flow is greater than that which will deliver the concentration set on the concentration control valve. In this situation, the relief valve opens to shunt this gas over to the vaporizer outlet instead of permitting it to flow into the vaporizing chamber.[3(p93)]

A portion of the gas moves up and around the temperature-compensating bypass valve and out through the check valve (Fig. 8–17). Not all of the gas travels to the depths of the vaporizer. The proportion of the gas that goes through the channel at the bypass valve is adjusted according to the temperature. Changes in ambient temperature and cooling caused by vaporization are continuous. The temperature-compensating bypass valve is connected to the temperature-sensing bellows, next to the vaporizing chamber. When energy is lost in the form of heat during vaporization, this sensor responds. It increases in height when the vapor is warm and pushes on the stem, which elevates the bypass valve to increase the size of its opening. As this space enlarges, a greater proportion of the incoming gas can flow to the outlet, reducing the total amount of gas available to the other routes. When the vapor cools, the bellows contracts and the stem and the funnel-shaped bypass valve move down and partially close the channel around the bypass valve. This causes more gas to flow through the pathways of the concentration control valve, where the flow is divided between the mixing chamber and the vaporizing

chamber. In this manner, the vaporizer continually compensates for temperature to maintain the desired concentration.

The desired percentage of agent is obtained by turning the concentration control valve. This valve alters the ratio of flow through the calibrated pathways (orifice) and splits the stream of gas between the two chambers. When a higher concentration is selected, more gas flows into the vaporizing chamber and less gas flows into the mixing chamber.

Once in the vaporizing chamber, gas passes over a series of wicks saturated with liquid anesthetic agent and becomes saturated with anesthetic vapor. High concentration settings require more flow to pass over the agent. Low concentrations require less gas flow through the chamber. The saturated gas leaves the vaporizing chamber and joins the unsaturated gas in the mixing chamber. From here it moves up to the top of the vaporizer, where it meets the gas that was diverted through the temperature-compensating bypass valve. The gas mixture carrying the desired concentration of vaporized anesthetic agent passes through the check valve and flows through the vaporizer outlet to the machine outlet.

The vaporizer outlet is equipped with a check valve to prevent reverse flow into the vaporizer. This minimizes the effects of downstream pressure fluctuations on anesthetic agent concentration. The reason for concern about pressure fluctuations and backflow into the vaporizer is simple. This could cause the patient to receive the desired percentage of agent plus additional agent picked up by the gas that went back into the vaporizer. Thus, the outlet check valve on this type of vaporizer protects the patient from receiving a

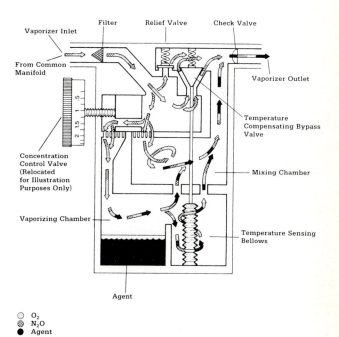

Figure 8–17. Nitrous oxide and oxygen flow through the Ohio calibrated vaporizer. Note the control knob has been graphically moved to the left to better illustrate the gas pathway. (*Redrawn with permission granted by Ohmeda, a division of BOC Health Care, Inc.*)

higher percentage of agent than dialed on the concentration control valve. It must be noted, however, that all vaporizers do not necessarily require a check valve.

In general, a vaporizer should never be tilted beyond 45 degrees when it contains liquid agent because a dangerously high output of agent may result.[4(pp309–310),6] Should this happen, the vaporizer must not be used until it has been drained and dried to purge it. Liquid agent may have spilled into the area above the vaporizing chamber, and when fresh gas flows through it, the agent will vaporize without compensation for temperature and flow. A vaporizer that is calibrated and labeled as agent specific is not designed to be used with any other agent, regardless of molecular similarity.[5(p49)] Never introduce any agent other than the designated agent into any vaporizer. If a vaporizer is inadvertently filled (or charged) with the wrong agent, draining the liquid will not eliminate the agent as some of the agent will have been absorbed by the wick. As a result, the vaporizer must be removed from service and purged of agent by flushing it with 100 percent oxygen or medical air, while the concentration control valve is turned to its maximum setting. This drying procedure must continue until the odor of the agent can no longer be detected at the vaporizer outlet. It should be noted that drying procedures will not remove thymol, the preservative present in halothane, once it is introduced into a nonhalothane vaporizer. In this situation, the vaporizer should be completely serviced in accordance with the manufacturer's recommendation.

When filling a vaporizer, carefully examine the labels on the bottle and the vaporizer. Cap, adapter, and bottle labels are usually color coded to help prevent mixing of agents when the liquid is poured into the vaporizer. Vaporizers may have a funnel-filling system or a keyed-filling receptacle located on the front. Unlike the funnel-fill type, the keyed filler helps prevent the wrong agent from being used in the vaporizer. The TEC 4 vaporizer (Fig. 8–18) is an example of a current design that meets the appropriate ASTM standard, published in 1988.[1(pp9–11)] It is temperature and flow compensated and has a special manifold that completely isolates the vaporizer from the flow of gases to the patient when the vaporizer is in the off position. Unlike the Ohio calibrated vaporizers (Fig. 8–17), the manifold is not "common" to oxygen, nitrous oxide, and anesthetic vapor. Gas supply to the TEC 4 is directed around the device when the vaporizer is turned off.

When the TEC 4 vaporizer is turned on, the port valves are pushed open to permit gas flow to enter the vaporizer (Fig. 8–19). The port valves serve a dual role by allowing gas to flow into the vaporizer and by preventing gas from reaching the vaporizer. Once the gas enters the vaporizer, it is divided into two streams. In the first one, gas passes through the temperature-sensitive valve (also called temperature-compensating valve) and on to the vaporizer outlet, bypassing the vaporizing chamber without being exposed to the anesthetic agent. In the second stream, gas flow is diverted downward through the wick portion of the vaporizing chamber where it becomes saturated with anesthetic agent. The vapor-carrying gas moves up and through the rotary valve to join with the unsaturated gas that was diverted through the bypass stream when it first came into the vaporizer.

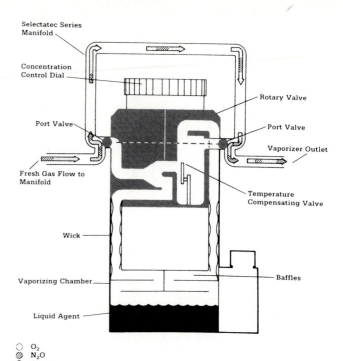

Figure 8–18. Flow of gases through an isolated manifold routes oxygen and nitrous oxide around the vaporizer when it is turned off. Note the location of the port valves in this TEC 4 vaporizer. (*Redrawn with permission granted by Ohmeda, a division of BOC Health Care, Inc.*)

Flow through the vaporizing chamber determines the concentration of anesthetic agent delivered to the vaporizer outlet. The greater the flow, the larger the amount of vapor produced. Flow is regulated by turning the dial, which positions the rotary valve and increases or decreases resistance in the stream. Contraction and expansion of the temperature-sensitive valve also increase or decrease the flow of unsaturated gas within the vaporizer.

This vaporizer and its manifold have a safety interlock system that prevents the turning on of more than one vaporizer at any given time. Another advantage of this design is a release mechanism located adjacent to the control dial that ensures the vaporizer cannot be turned on unless it is correctly mounted.

A system of baffles (Fig. 8–19) inside the vaporizer helps minimize the risk of liquid agent spilling into the rotary valve mechanism when the vaporizer is unintentionally tilted. However, should such tilting occur, it is still necessary to check the vaporizer output with an agent analyzer prior to returning the vaporizer to use. Although baffles minimize the chance of an overdose, they do not prevent liquid agent from flowing out of the vaporizing chamber.

Liquid anesthetic agent corresponding to the label on the vaporizer is poured directly from the bottle into a funnel-fill receptacle, or it is poured into the vaporizer through a keyed-filler adapter. This adapter has an agent-specific configuration that must match on both ends. On one end the adapter must correspond to the keyed collar on

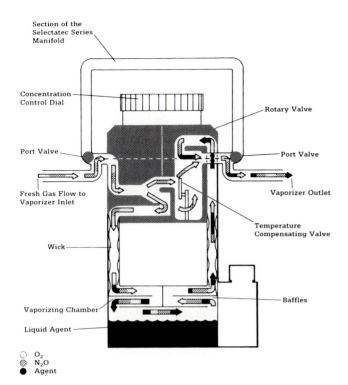

Section of the
Selectatec Series
Manifold

Concentration
Control Dial

Rotary Valve

Port Valve

Port Valve

Vaporizer Outlet

Fresh Gas Flow to
Vaporizer Inlet

Temperature
Compensating Valve

Wick

Baffles

Vaporizing Chamber

Liquid Agent

○ O₂
⊗ N₂O
● Agent

Figure 8–19. Fresh gas flow through the TEC 4 vaporizer and into the vaporizing chamber. (*Redrawn with permission granted by Ohmeda, a division of BOC Health Care, Inc.*)

the bottle of the agent. The other end must correspond to the keyed-filler receptacle on the vaporizer. The keyed-filler system assists in preventing the error of pouring an agent into the wrong vaporizer; however, it is imperative that one always check that the label on the bottle of liquid agent corresponds to the label on the vaporizer. It is equally important to note that any filling system can be defeated if one drains unused agent from the vaporizer back into a bottle. If an agent is drained into the wrong bottle, the risk of pouring unknown agent into a subsequent vaporizer exists.[3(p102),5(p49)]

GAS FLOW THROUGH THE PATIENT CIRCUIT AND ABSORBER

Oxygen, nitrous oxide, and anesthetic agent flow into the absorber from the common gas outlet. The absorber eliminates carbon dioxide from the exhaled gases selectively without affecting the composition of other gases or used agents in the mixture.

If the absorbent granules have been exhausted, the absorber cannot effectively remove carbon dioxide. Therefore, the condition of the granules must be checked at the *end* of each case. Absorbent granules change color at rest and may return to their original color, even though a substantial portion of their absorption capacity is exhausted. Absorbers are most commonly manufactured with two canisters that hold the granules. The top canister is the first one to be exhausted because it is exposed first to the exhaled gases. The absorbent should be discarded when the granules in the top of the lower canister have started to change

color. The upper canister may be removed, refilled with fresh carbon dioxide absorbent, and placed in the lower position, moving the lower canister to the top position.

The patient circuit must be checked for leaks after the canister is refilled. Even though a machine was leaktight before the absorbent was changed, failure to realign the canisters properly can produce a leak. If the system is not checked for leaks before starting a case, the leak produced may become apparent just as the patient requires positive-pressure ventilatory support.

It is important to reemphasize that the entire machine must be inspected and tested daily and the patient circuit must be tested before every case. Guidelines for preuse testing and checking procedures are listed in Chapter 9; however, guidelines do not substitute for the specific machine system checking procedure published in the operator's manual. This document must also be read and applied to ensure the checking procedures are effective for each model of machine to be used.

Gases from the flowmeters and anesthetic agent from the vaporizer leave the machine outlet, enter the fresh gas inlet on the absorber, and flow through the inhalation check valve into the breathing circuit and on through the inspiratory limb of the breathing circuit. When the patient inhales, gas is supplied from the fresh gas flow and from the rebreathing bag via the inspiratory limb of the breathing circuit.

When inhalation is manually assisted, the flow pattern is the same. As the rebreathing bag is squeezed, positive pressure is exerted within the circuit and the flow of gases opens the inhalation check valve. Gas from the rebreathing bag moves down through the absorber canisters and the absorbent granules and then flows up the return tube, where it joins the fresh gas going to the patient.[3(p113)] The exhalation check valve is closed and the weight of the disc keeps it closed.

When the patient exhales (Fig. 8–20), gases enter the breathing circuit, open the exhalation check valve, and fill the rebreathing bag. Excess gas goes out the APL valve. Fresh gas continues to flow from the common gas outlet into the absorber throughout inspiration and expiration. This characteristic makes the anesthesia machine a continuous-flow gas delivery system.

Once the oxygen flush valve is manually opened, a high flow of oxygen (35–75 L/min)[1(p8)] immediately enters the absorber (Fig. 8–21). Most of this supplemental flow takes the path of least resistance and flows through the top of the absorber and inhalation check valve, on to the patient, and back to the rebreathing bag until the pressure rises sufficiently to cause the APL valve to vent the excess. The rest of the flush flow goes down the return tube, up through the absorber, and into the rebreathing bag.[3(pp117,129)]

The inhalation check valve permits flow of gases to the patient during inspiration (Fig. 8–22). When the patient inhales, the valve disc is lifted off its seat. While the inhalation check valve is open, the exhalation check valve is closed. The barrier ring prevents the valve disc from being dislodged and potentially creating an obstruction to inhaled or exhaled gases (Fig. 8–23).

Exhaled gases flow first to the rebreathing bag. The remaining or excess gas goes out the APL valve. Exhaled gases flow from the bag to the absorber during the next

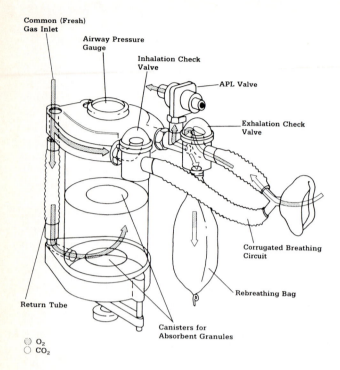

Figure 8–20 labels: Common (Fresh) Gas Inlet, Airway Pressure Gauge, Inhalation Check Valve, APL Valve, Exhalation Check Valve, Corrugated Breathing Circuit, Rebreathing Bag, Return Tube, Canisters for Absorbent Granules

○ O₂
○ CO₂

Figure 8–20. Gas flow during exhalation in a continuous-flow circle system. As the patient exhales, gas flows into the rebreathing bag until it fills; excess gas escapes through the adjustable pressure-limiting (APL) valve. Fresh gas continues to flow into the circle. (*Redrawn with permission granted by Ohmeda, a division of BOC Health Care, Inc.*)

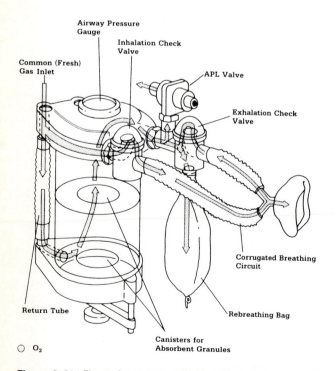

Figure 8–21 labels: Airway Pressure Gauge, Inhalation Check Valve, Common (Fresh) Gas Inlet, APL Valve, Exhalation Check Valve, Corrugated Breathing Circuit, Rebreathing Bag, Return Tube, Canisters for Absorbent Granules

○ O₂

Figure 8–21. Flow of gas during oxygen flush. (*Redrawn with permission granted by Ohmeda, a division of BOC Health Care, Inc.*)

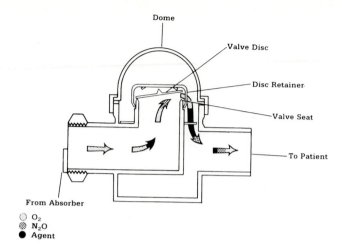

Figure 8–22 labels: Dome, Valve Disc, Disc Retainer, Valve Seat, To Patient, From Absorber

○ O₂
⊗ N₂O
● Agent

Figure 8–22. Gas flow through the inhalation check valve during inspiration. Note the location of the valve disc and the disc retainer, which maintains alignment with the valve seat. (*Redrawn with permission granted by Ohmeda, a division of BOC Health Care, Inc.*)

inspiration. While exhaled gases are opening the valve on the exhalation side of the breathing circuit, the inhalation check valve rests on its seat. This check valve prevents exhaled gas from flowing in a reverse pattern and entering the absorber from the inhalation side; however, fresh gas from the common gas outlet continues to flow into the system.

Also located on the absorber is the APL valve located in the expiratory side of the absorber (Fig. 8–24). The APL valve is adjusted so that the right amount of pressure is applied to assist ventilation. Gas in excess of that needed to achieve the required airway pressure is discharged into the waste gas scavenging system. The APL valve has been commonly called the "pop-off" valve, but this is a misnomer. The term *pop-off* implies a pressure relief function only, as in basic relief valves found in the ventilator and the waste gas scavenger system. The APL valve adjusts the limit of positive pressure attained within the rebreathing bag and vents excess gas once the preset pressure is reached. The knob controls the adjustment by loading the spring with tension. The tension translates into force exerted against the diaphragm. Each turn of the knob alters the force applied against the diaphragm. The circuit pressure gauge reflects this force as pressure delivered to the patient's airway, not the specific pressure within the patient's thorax.

The function of the APL valve is checked daily to be sure that it opens and closes smoothly. In this absorber, the APL valve is attached to the exhalation check valve. The APL valve should be precisely adjusted so that volume intended for the patient is not exhausted into the scavenging system.

An integrated absorber has all the necessary valves and mechanisms built into it, rather than added onto it (Fig. 8–25). Included in its housing are the bag-to-ventilator switch, the APL valve, the oxygen monitor sensor, the circuit pressure-sensing port, a breathing circuit pressure-sensing gauge, and a drain valve to remove water. When

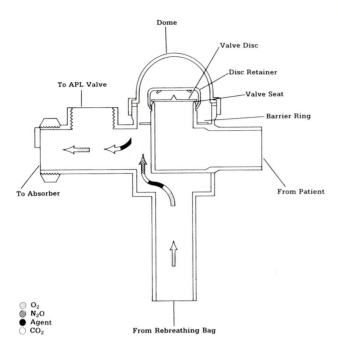

O₂
N₂O
Agent
CO₂

Figure 8–23. Gas flow through the exhalation check valve during inspiration. The barrier ring is designed to reduce the risk of the valve disc becoming lodged in the flow pathway. (*Redrawn with permission granted by Ohmeda, a division of BOC Health Care, Inc.*)

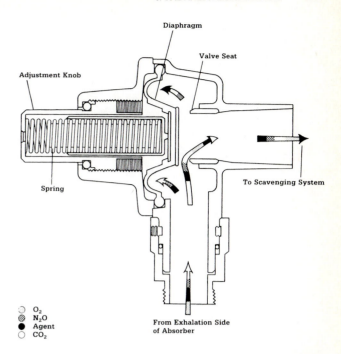

O₂
N₂O
Agent
CO₂

Figure 8–24. Flow of gases through the adjustable pressure-limiting (APL) valve. (*Redrawn with permission granted by Ohmeda, a division of BOC Health Care, Inc.*)

the bag-to-ventilation selector switch is present, the APL valve is usually out of circuit and is not closed. With all other absorbers, the APL valve must be closed during mechanical ventilation.

An oxygen sensor is found in the inhalation chamber of this absorber. If a nonintegrated absorber is used, a T-piece adapter is usually employed to attach a fractional inspired oxygen sensor between the inhalation check valve and the inspiratory limb of the circuit.

WASTE GAS MANAGEMENT

A waste gas scavenging system includes the interface manifold valves (Fig. 8–26) and the hospital's central evacuation system, which receives waste gases from the anesthesia machine and vents them outside the operating room. The interface valve is essentially a manifold with four ports and two relief valves. As gas is pulled into the hospital vacuum system, it flows through the manifold past the two relief valves. One relief valve is for positive pressure, and one is for negative pressure. A 3-L reservoir bag is attached. When more flow is passing into the valve than the vacuum can remove, the gas is temporarily stored in the bag. When a waste gas scavenging system is attached to a vacuum source, it is called an active scavenging system.

The rate of flow through the manifold is controlled by adjusting the needle valve so that the reservoir bag is not allowed to become filled. In the ideal situation, the rate of flow is maintained so the volume in the reservoir is between empty and half-filled.[3(p137),9] Adjusting the needle valve alters the flow of waste gases into the vacuum source. This

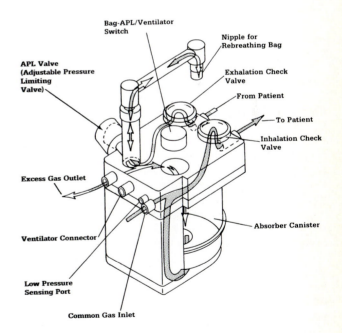

O₂
CO₂

Figure 8–25. Flow of gases through an integrated absorber assembly: the Ohmeda GMS absorber. To illustrate gas flow through this component, the oxygen-sensor socket, the locking lever on the canisters, and the mechanism that attaches it to the machine are not shown. (*Redrawn with permission granted by Ohmeda, a division of BOC Health Care, Inc.*)

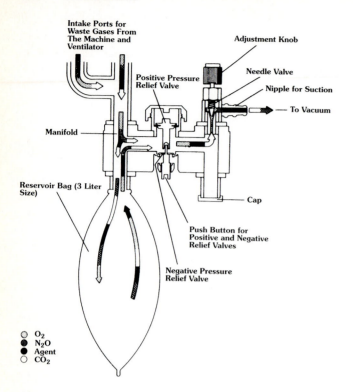

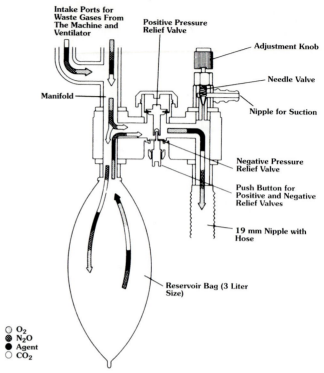

Figure 8–26. Flow of waste gases from the breathing circuit (machine) and the ventilator. The waste gases enter the intake ports of the interface valve, go to the reservoir, and exit through the vacuum in an active scavenging system. (*Redrawn with permission granted by Ohmeda, a division of BOC Health Care, Inc.*)

Figure 8–27. Flow of waste gases through the manifold in a passive scavenging system. Note that the cap has been replaced by a 19-mm hose and the adjustment knob for the vacuum is closed. (*Redrawn with permission granted by Ohmeda, a division of BOC Health Care, Inc.*)

adjustment does not regulate the vacuum or suction level.

If the vacuum flow is insufficient and the reservoir bag is allowed to distend, the positive-pressure relief valve on the interface manifold opens and vents exhaled gases into the room. Exposure to trace gas is minimized by adjusting the needle valve to increase the flow of waste gas to the vacuum. If the flow is too high and the bag collapses, the negative relief valve opens and pulls in room air to satisfy the needs of the vacuum. These valves are installed to protect the patient circuit from extremes in pressure. The positive-pressure relief valve will not be activated if the flow is properly adjusted. In active scavenger systems, any unused nipple must be capped or the vacuum will draw room air instead of waste gases into the central system.

A passive waste gas system (Fig. 8–27) uses the hospital ventilation ducts to exhaust the gas through the air circulation system. Waste gases enter the manifold in the same way and the flow is similarly controlled by the relief valves; however, the needle valve is closed and a 19-mm corrugated hose is connected between the interface valve and the exhaust grille of the air conditioning system.

A waste gas scavenging interface valve is required on every anesthesia machine.[10] The clinician is responsible for verifying that it is properly adjusted to protect operating room personnel from exposure to waste gases. As the anesthesia machine continually receives a supply of fresh gas and the flow is usually more than the patient uses, an efficient means of disposal must be provided. To under-

stand fully how each waste gas system functions and how to adjust it properly, consult the specific manufacturer's operation manual.

CLINICAL CONSIDERATIONS

Problems with oxygen supply have historically been the cause of anesthetic morbidity and mortality, and these problems remain today. The most common problem associated with external pipeline systems is insufficient oxygen pressure.[6] As a result, pipeline pressure gauges are positioned on the front of each machine that meets the current ASTM machine safety and performance standard.[10] Nurse anesthetists should regularly monitor the pipeline gauges to verify adequate pressure before and during the anesthetic course.

If a pipeline source is used, at least one reserve cylinder must be present on the machine. Cylinder contents should be checked to ensure adequate gas supply and then closed so the reserve oxygen is not depleted. If a central pipeline gas source is not available, a machine with a double-yoke assembly for oxygen and nitrous oxide permits the use of one cylinder and the readiness of a reserve cylinder at all times. The pin-indexed safety system (PISS) and the diameter-indexed safety system (DISS) are designed to minimize the risk of making an incorrect connection to a cylinder or pipeline source. Specifically, the gas-specific pin configuration serves to prevent placement of the wrong

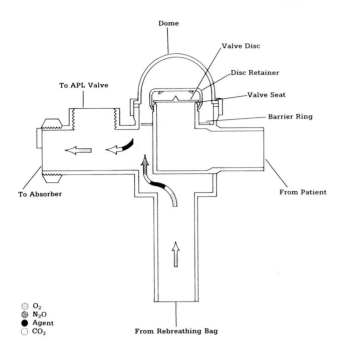

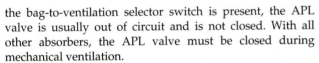

Figure 8–23. Gas flow through the exhalation check valve during inspiration. The barrier ring is designed to reduce the risk of the valve disc becoming lodged in the flow pathway. (*Redrawn with permission granted by Ohmeda, a division of BOC Health Care, Inc.*)

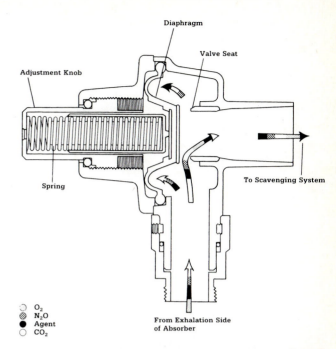

Figure 8–24. Flow of gases through the adjustable pressure-limiting (APL) valve. (*Redrawn with permission granted by Ohmeda, a division of BOC Health Care, Inc.*)

the bag-to-ventilation selector switch is present, the APL valve is usually out of circuit and is not closed. With all other absorbers, the APL valve must be closed during mechanical ventilation.

An oxygen sensor is found in the inhalation chamber of this absorber. If a nonintegrated absorber is used, a T-piece adapter is usually employed to attach a fractional inspired oxygen sensor between the inhalation check valve and the inspiratory limb of the circuit.

WASTE GAS MANAGEMENT

A waste gas scavenging system includes the interface manifold valves (Fig. 8–26) and the hospital's central evacuation system, which receives waste gases from the anesthesia machine and vents them outside the operating room. The interface valve is essentially a manifold with four ports and two relief valves. As gas is pulled into the hospital vacuum system, it flows through the manifold past the two relief valves. One relief valve is for positive pressure, and one is for negative pressure. A 3-L reservoir bag is attached. When more flow is passing into the valve than the vacuum can remove, the gas is temporarily stored in the bag. When a waste gas scavenging system is attached to a vacuum source, it is called an active scavenging system.

The rate of flow through the manifold is controlled by adjusting the needle valve so that the reservoir bag is not allowed to become filled. In the ideal situation, the rate of flow is maintained so the volume in the reservoir is between empty and half-filled.[3(p137),9] Adjusting the needle valve alters the flow of waste gases into the vacuum source. This

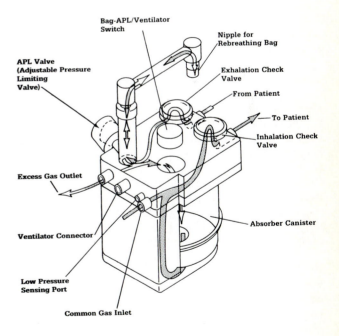

Figure 8–25. Flow of gases through an integrated absorber assembly: the Ohmeda GMS absorber. To illustrate gas flow through this component, the oxygen-sensor socket, the locking lever on the canisters, and the mechanism that attaches it to the machine are not shown. (*Redrawn with permission granted by Ohmeda, a division of BOC Health Care, Inc.*)

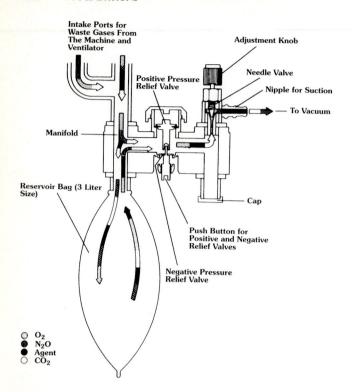

Figure 8–26. Flow of waste gases from the breathing circuit (machine) and the ventilator. The waste gases enter the intake ports of the interface valve, go to the reservoir, and exit through the vacuum in an active scavenging system. (*Redrawn with permission granted by Ohmeda, a division of BOC Health Care, Inc.*)

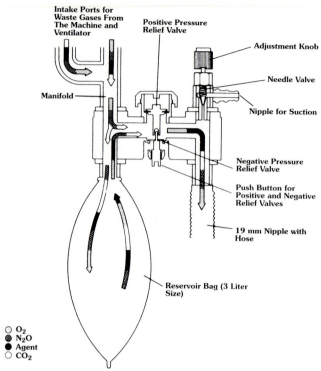

Figure 8–27. Flow of waste gases through the manifold in a passive scavenging system. Note that the cap has been replaced by a 19-mm hose and the adjustment knob for the vacuum is closed. (*Redrawn with permission granted by Ohmeda, a division of BOC Health Care, Inc.*)

adjustment does not regulate the vacuum or suction level.

If the vacuum flow is insufficient and the reservoir bag is allowed to distend, the positive-pressure relief valve on the interface manifold opens and vents exhaled gases into the room. Exposure to trace gas is minimized by adjusting the needle valve to increase the flow of waste gas to the vacuum. If the flow is too high and the bag collapses, the negative relief valve opens and pulls in room air to satisfy the needs of the vacuum. These valves are installed to protect the patient circuit from extremes in pressure. The positive-pressure relief valve will not be activated if the flow is properly adjusted. In active scavenger systems, any unused nipple must be capped or the vacuum will draw room air instead of waste gases into the central system.

A passive waste gas system (Fig. 8–27) uses the hospital ventilation ducts to exhaust the gas through the air circulation system. Waste gases enter the manifold in the same way and the flow is similarly controlled by the relief valves; however, the needle valve is closed and a 19-mm corrugated hose is connected between the interface valve and the exhaust grille of the air conditioning system.

A waste gas scavenging interface valve is required on every anesthesia machine.[10] The clinician is responsible for verifying that it is properly adjusted to protect operating room personnel from exposure to waste gases. As the anesthesia machine continually receives a supply of fresh gas and the flow is usually more than the patient uses, an efficient means of disposal must be provided. To under-

stand fully how each waste gas system functions and how to adjust it properly, consult the specific manufacturer's operation manual.

CLINICAL CONSIDERATIONS

Problems with oxygen supply have historically been the cause of anesthetic morbidity and mortality, and these problems remain today. The most common problem associated with external pipeline systems is insufficient oxygen pressure.[6] As a result, pipeline pressure gauges are positioned on the front of each machine that meets the current ASTM machine safety and performance standard.[10] Nurse anesthetists should regularly monitor the pipeline gauges to verify adequate pressure before and during the anesthetic course.

If a pipeline source is used, at least one reserve cylinder must be present on the machine. Cylinder contents should be checked to ensure adequate gas supply and then closed so the reserve oxygen is not depleted. If a central pipeline gas source is not available, a machine with a double-yoke assembly for oxygen and nitrous oxide permits the use of one cylinder and the readiness of a reserve cylinder at all times. The pin-indexed safety system (PISS) and the diameter-indexed safety system (DISS) are designed to minimize the risk of making an incorrect connection to a cylinder or pipeline source. Specifically, the gas-specific pin configuration serves to prevent placement of the wrong cylinder into a yoke. The diameter-specific fittings help prevent placement of the wrong gas supply hose into a machine inlet or a wall supply outlet.

The oxygen supply failure alarm system is a pressure-related audible alarm component that warns when oxygen pressure is decreasing or has fallen below the machine's predetermined nominal requirement. This alarm always implies that the reserve cylinder should be immediately turned on before the cause of the problem is evaluated and corrected. When the oxygen supply failure alarm is sounding, the pressure-sensor shutoff valve is activated to stop the flow of nitrous oxide or any other gas. This component senses pressure and does not deal with oxygen flow or oxygen concentration.

The airway pressure alarm should also be checked prior to the start of the workday. Numerous models of airway pressure monitors exist and the routine preuse inspection and testing should be conducted according to the manufacturer's instructions. This simple device is able to warn of disconnection in the patient circuit, often before other clinical evidence of change is apparent.

The precision flowmeter requires careful handling and should receive respectful attention during the preuse checking procedure. Forceful closure of this valve should be avoided to prevent wear and tear on the valve seat, which may lead to inaccurate flow readings. The float should be visually inspected to be certain it moves freely within the flow tube. Halting, irregular, or erratic movement of the float may signal the possibility of inaccurate readings. In addition, care should be exercised when turning the flowmeter on to avoid propelling the float to the top of the flow tube where it may lodge, obstructing the flow of gas into the manifold.[4(p54)]

Always verify that the oxygen flush valve is operational to ensure that a supplement of 100 percent oxygen can be delivered to the patient circuit without delay. Monitor the effects of the flush maneuver on the airway pressure manometer or monitor located within the circuit. Indiscriminate use of the flush valve is not appropriate as it can significantly increase the patient's airway pressure. Unintentional opening of the flush valve is also a concern, now minimized by a recessed casing in machines that meet current ASTM standards[4(p66)] for machine safety and performance.

Calibrated vaporizers play an important role in the integrity of gas flow through the machine. Machine function should be tested with the vaporizers closed and opened to ensure their proper alignment within the manifold and to detect potential leaks. Anesthetic agent should be carefully poured into the vaporizer, following the manufacturer's recommendation for funnel-fill and key-filling procedures. Liquid agent drained from a vaporizer should never be poured back into a bottle, and the liquid agent should be disposed of in an appropriate manner to minimize the exposure of trace gas to health care workers.

Vaporizers should be mounted upstream from the common gas outlet and properly placed within their integrated, isolated manifold. It is unacceptable to install a vaporizer downstream of the common gas outlet. Not only is this practice out of date and unnecessary, it fails to meet the minimum ASTM standard of safety and performance

for vaporizers.[1(pp9-11)] Downstream vaporizers are prone to be tilted and may be readily misconnected to the fresh gas flow. Both of these conditions lead to overdose. Use of the flush valve is also problematic with a downstream vaporizer because oxygen flow, up to 75 L/min, may be flushed through the head of the vaporizer without the safeguard of appropriate flow compensation to minimize the risk of uncontrolled vaporization and patient overdose.

Vaporizers are instruments that need periodic maintenance, regardless of the stability of their performance and the apparent clinical verification of their output. The goal of every equipment maintenance program is to minimize the possibility that a device or component will fail or malfunction. These efforts are undertaken with all medical equipment to detect evidence of wear or deterioration long before it causes a patient a problem or results in financial loss. For this reason, the basic foundations of preventive maintenance and equipment safety apply to mechanical vaporizers in the same way as they do to all other mechanical or pneumatic components of the anesthesia system.

Depending on the specific model of vaporizer, manufacturers recommend service on a regular basis, for example, every 1 to 2 years, so that all parts can be inspected, new parts can be installed where there is any doubt about wear, and calibration can be verified with a precision refractometer. This procedure is not to be confused with the practice of spotchecking a vaporizer's output, a routine that is only one phase of a regular maintenance program. Using a portable gas indicator, an agent analyzer, or an agent monitor to follow trends in vaporizer output is not a sufficient reason to justify operating vaporizers that are clearly performing outside the limits of their specifications.[11] A calibration spotcheck can detect a malfunction but it cannot predict one. In addition, a spotcheck can determine the concentration of an agent, but it cannot verify that the temperature-compensating system is operating at its mechanical best.

When a temperature-compensating mechanism fails, the resultant increase in vaporizer output does not cause a gradually changing reading. Instead, the change is usually sudden and develops without subtle indicators. The agent monitor can demonstrate the sudden overdose and sound an alarm, but it cannot protect the patient from exposure to this problem.

Vaporizers may not perform as intended when they suffer from abuse, misuse, or improper maintenance. Currently, all calibrated models are mechanical and prone to the same risks of wear and tear as any other component of the anesthesia machine system. When funnel-filled vaporizers are used instead of key-filled vaporizers, the risks of contamination by dust and particulate matter increase. Dust, when introduced into the vaporizer, contributes to wear on its moving parts. Thymol, normally present in halothane vaporizers, is another example of particulate matter that also adds to the problem of mechanical deterioration. Filling errors continue to be a problem, as the halothane preservative thymol continues to be discovered inside enflurane and isoflurane vaporizers.[4(p312)]

The patient circuit includes all components located between the common gas outlet and the patient's airway, and every component must be checked daily in accordance with the manufacturer's recommendations. Testing for unacceptable leaks in the patient circuit is only one of the concerns that need clinical attention. The gas delivery tube should be inspected to be sure it is not kinked and is, in fact, a high-pressure medical gas delivery hose. Hospital-grade rubber tubing and plastic tubes should not be used as gas delivery hoses when administering anesthesia. The inhalation and exhalation check valves should also be inspected to be certain that the dome is intact, the disc is present, and the guard and the barrier ring are properly positioned.

The patency of the breathing circuit and rebreathing bag should be inspected and functionally tested (along with the entire patient circuit) prior to each case. The absorber must be filled with soda lime or an equivalent absorbent, firmly packed in canisters, and mounted in the absorber with correct alignment. Failure to check absorber alignment and canister placement may result in an undetected leak within the patient circuit.

The color indicator in the absorbent granules signifies when a fresh supply is needed. When the granules in the top canister change color in a two-chamber absorber, place the bottom canister in the upper position and add fresh granules to the bottom canister. This must be done at the end of a case, as the granules can return to their original color between cases.

Test the APL (pop-off) valve daily to be sure it can be fully opened and fully closed and that the airway pressure gauge corresponds to these adjustments. Correct function of this valve is necessary for appropriate management of pressure within the patient circuit and for control of gas flow to the waste gas scavenging system.

The needle valve on the waste gas manifold must be adjusted when excess flow from the patient circuit increases or decreases. The needle valve on this component does not regulate the vacuum (suction) level, but alters the amount of flow allowed to leave the manifold and enter the evacuation system. The vacuum level remains "constant" except for fluctuations that occur when heavy demand decreases the level of vacuum available to the wall outlet or when lower demand increases the vacuum.

The reservoir bag on the waste gas scavenger serves as a temporary storage site so that one does not need to adjust the waste gas flow, minute-to-minute. Changes in total flow of fresh gas do occur, however, and the waste gas needle valve setting must be appropriately adjusted to prevent overinflation or underinflation of the reservoir bag. Visual monitoring of the contour of this bag offers a valuable reminder to the clinician when flow needs to be altered.

Should a higher level of vacuum exist than is needed, the negative-pressure relief valve on the manifold will open to allow room air to enter the evacuation system. If an inadequate vacuum supply occurs, the positive-pressure relief valve will open and exhaust the excess gas into the room. This prevents an accumulation of undesirable high pressure within the manifold that could be referred to the patient circuit.

Although ventilator function is beyond the scope of this chapter (see Chapter 16) it is important to note that most ventilators are accessories to the patient circuit and must be checked prior to use, according to the manufactur-er's recommendations. Ventilator and machine hoses and tubing must be visually examined to verify appropriate connections. If a selector valve is present, its function must be tested in both bag and ventilator modes. Ventilator function should be tested using the breathing system and a test lung at the patient end of the breathing circuit.[6]

After setting an appropriate flow on the anesthesia machine, close the APL (pop-off) valve and turn the ventilator and any accompanying monitors on. This will simulate the patient's breathing, permitting tidal volume and respiratory rates to be set, and will allow for assessment of the system for pressure and leaks. Check the volume delivered by the ventilator with a mechanical or electronic volume monitor located in the exhalation limb of the circuit. The difference between the volume set on the ventilator and the volume measured at the expiratory limb is the result of compliance and resistance in the patient circuit. Tidal volume settings marked on any ventilator bellows, its housing, or any accessory scale are estimates of volume and are not patient measurements.

Anesthesia ventilators are equipped with a bellows that communicates directly with the breathing circuit and moves gases via pressure fluctuations in the housing surrounding it. Two types of bellows exist in anesthesia ventilators: (1) the type that rises during inspiration and falls with gravity during exhalation, and (2) the type in which the bellows falls or descends during inspiration and ascends during exhalation. Both types of bellows fill during exhalation.

A ventilator that ascends during inspiration and falls during exhalation is called a "hanging bellows" and will continue to cycle even in the presence of a disconnection in the patient circuit. A "sitting bellows" ventilator will not appear to be operating normally in the event of a disconnection because exhaled gases from the patient as well as fresh gas flow are required to fill the bellows. Failure to cycle or an interrupted cycle is a visual image that helps warn the anesthetist of a disconnection; however, the bellows configuration does not appropriately substitute for the use of ventilator low-pressure sensors, a volume monitor, an airway pressure monitor,[12] and all analysis monitors for oxygen and carbon dioxide. Regardless of the type of ventilator used, the nurse anesthetist must understand the expected operation and performance of each model of ventilator and routinely use all appropriate monitors to verify the adequacy of both mechanical and manual ventilation.

REFERENCES

1. *Standard specification for minimum performance and safety requirements for components and systems of anesthesia gas machines: F1161-88*. Philadelphia: ASTM; 1988.
2. *Standard specification for minimum performance and safety requirements for anesthesia breathing circuits: F20.01.02*. Philadelphia: ASTM; 1990:2–8.
3. Bowie E, Huffman LM. *The anesthesia machine: Essentials for understanding*. Madison, WI: BOC Group; 1985.
4. Dorsch JA, Dorsch SE. *Understanding anesthesia equipment: Construction, care and complications*. 2nd ed. Baltimore, MD: Williams & Wilkins; 1984.
5. Petty C. *The anesthesia machine*. New York: Churchill Livingstone; 1987.

6. Waugaman WR, Bradshaw H. Monitoring in anesthesia: clinical application of monitoring gas and vapor delivery. *AANAJ.* 1985:5;53:446–452.

7. *Modulus II anesthesia system: Operation and maintenance manual.* Madison, WI: BOC Group; 1985:8.

8. Ward CS. *Anaesthetic equipment: Physical principles and maintenance.* 2nd ed. London: Bailliere Tindall; 1985:48.

9. *Modulus anesthesia system: Operation and maintenance manual.* Madison, WI: BOC Group; 1990:19.

10. Huffman LM. Common problems in waste gas management. *AANA J.* 1991;59:109.

11. Huffman LM. Calibrated vaporizers: Maintaining clinical performance. *AANA J.* 1990;58:119–120.

12. Roth S, Tweedie E, Sommer RM. Excessive airway pressure due to a malfunctioning anesthesia ventilator. *Anesthesia.* 1986;65:532–534.

The Care of Anesthesia Equipment

Leslie Rendell-Baker

The practice of anesthesia, once the simple dripping of ether on a mask while keeping a finger on the pulse, now depends on a wide range of mechanical, electronic, and plastic equipment. All of this equipment is exposed daily to potential contamination with the patient's blood and secretions and with microorganisms carried on the users' hands.

Many anesthesia machines in spite of routine superficial cleaning have been cultured positively for contaminants. Machine design has changed little over the years to reduce dirt-collecting surfaces. The hygienic model of an anesthesia machine by Dupaco eliminated many dirt traps and held the cylinders in a rear enclosure. Although the apparatus introduced after the publication in 1979 of the ANSI Z79.8* Standard on the Safety and Performance of Anesthesia Apparatus were much improved in safety, they were still as difficult to clean as many of the older models.

STERILIZATION, DISINFECTION, AND ANTISEPSIS

The wide range of apparatus we use and their varying tolerance to cleaning and sterilizing procedures require that we have suitable alternatives available. Sterilization is any process that completely destroys all living organisms in or on an object. Disinfection is a process in which an agent is used to kill pathogenic microorganisms, usually on inanimate objects. Antisepsis is any process that prevents or combats infection by killing or inhibiting microorganisms usually on human tissue. Decontamination is the process that frees a person or object from soiling with an infectious material.

The type of sterilization or disinfection is selected contingent on the material of the item to be decontaminated,

---

* The American National Standards Institute Committee Z79, which formerly worked on standards for anesthesia and ventilatory equipment was, in 1983, replaced by the American Society for Testing and Materials Committee F29, which has the same functions.

the microorganism to be destroyed, and the degree of decontamination to be attained. Items that penetrate the skin barrier or come in contact with mucous membranes must be sterilized, whereas equipment in a contaminated room can be properly decontaminated by washing with a germicidal detergent solution.

Cleaning is the first step in any decontamination method. Dirt, body secretions, and other extraneous material inhibit the action of the disinfectant by a mechanical blocking or neutralizing effect. The efficiency of any disinfectant is dependent on time and concentration and especially on the acidity or alkalinity (pH) of the environment. Some disinfectants are more efficacious under neutral conditions. This is important to remember when using alkaline soaps and detergents for preliminary cleaning. If these alkaline solutions are not completely rinsed from the surface to be disinfected, they may neutralize or decrease the effectiveness of a disinfectant requiring an acid environment. Temperature is a determinant of the efficiency of disinfectants. As a general rule, the higher the temperature, the faster acting will be the disinfectant.

Recommended Methods

I. *Sterilization*
   A. Steam autoclaving
      1. This is always the first choice.
      2. Items must tolerate the heat and steam.
   B. Ethylene oxide gas autoclaving
      1. Large enough stock of items must be available to permit proper duration of aeration to eliminate residues of the gas.
      2. Never gas autoclave any item that can be steam autoclaved.
II. *Disinfection*
   A. Alkaline glutaraldehyde (e.g., Cidex)
      1. Mix solution as instructed.
      2. Use solution no longer than 28 days.
      3. Rinse disinfected items properly to remove residues.
      4. Avoid contact with skin.

5. Use in well-ventilated area.
6. Flush splashes to eyes with water and report to employee health service for immediate care.

B. Phenolic solution (e.g., Wexcide)
1. This solution is the hospital germicidal disinfectant of choice and should be supplied from the pharmacy diluted and ready for use.
2. Follow manufacturer's instructions when diluting concentrated product for use.
3. Avoid contact with skin by wearing gloves.
4. Solution is caustic; if splashed in eyes, flood with water and contact employee health service.

C. Sodium hypochloride (chlorine bleach 1 : 5 to 1 : 10 dilution)
1. This is the first-choice disinfectant for destroying hepatitis virus.
2. Bleach solution will decolorize fabric.

III. *Antisepsis*
A. Iodophor (e.g., Betadine)
1. The povidone–iodine surgical scrub, which incorporates liquid soap, is also recommended for hand washing.
2. The povidone–iodine solution is used in surgical preparation and wound cleaning.

B. Chlorhexidine gluconate (e.g., Hibiclens)
This is recommended for hand washing. Rinse hands thoroughly with water.

C. Hexachlorophene
Hexachlorophene is recommended for hand washing for persons who are allergic to iodophor and chlorhexidine gluconate.

D. Alcohol, 70 percent
Keep bottle tightly closed; alcohol is volatile.

E. Unsatisfactory agent: Benzalkonium chloride is not listed as a disinfectant or antiseptic because it is not effective against all gram-negative organisms, some of which can multiply in it. It may be used as a sanitizer only.

Infection Control Guidelines for Anesthesia Equipment

I. *Anesthesia machines and ventilators*
A. Clean all surfaces, including flow control knobs, daily with a phenolic solution.
B. Cover machine counter with clean towel for each patient.
C. After use with an infectious patient, such as one with a lung abscess or open pulmonary tuberculosis, clean all surfaces immediately with a phenolic solution.

II. *Disposable equipment to be discarded after each use*
A. Syringes and needles—into a "sharps" container
B. Breathing systems including breathing bags
C. Tracheal tubes, polyvinyl chloride (PVC) plastic wire-reinforced tubes, plastic endobronchial tubes.
D. Esophageal stethoscopes[†]
E. Face masks

III. *Equipment to be sterilized or pasteurized*
Whenever possible, use steam sterilization. It is simpler, safer, and quicker than ethylene oxide gas sterilization. Pasteurization can be used when clean rather than sterile equipment is acceptable.
A. Rubber breathing systems[*,†]
B. Rubber endobronchial tubes[†]
C. Nondisposable face masks[*,†]
D. Oral airways[*]
E. Temperature probes[*,†]
F. Laryngoscope blades[*,‡]
G. Wash and gas sterilize ventilator bellows on a rotation basis and after use with a contaminated patient.
H. Autoclave the carbon dioxide absorber assembly whenever possible after anesthetizing patients with pulmonary tuberculosis and other pulmonary infections.

Methods of Disinfection and Sterilization

Moist Heat. Moist heat is much more effective in causing coagulation of cellular proteins and death of organisms at lower temperatures than is dry heat, which is of little use for sterilization of anesthesia equipment.

Pasteurization. Louis Pasteur (1822–1895), the French chemist, discovered the bacteria that are responsible for fermentation and disease and developed the process of pasteurization to protect wine and milk against spoilage. Milk is heated to 62C, held there for 30 minutes, and then rapidly cooled. Although pasteurization does not destroy spores, it kills *Mycobacterium tuberculosis*, salmonellae, brucellae, and streptococci, which were the cause of serious milkborne diseases.

Pasteurization is now widely used to disinfect biologicals and plastic and rubber anesthesia equipment. It is most important that blood secretions and other soil be removed first by a thorough washing process. The equipment to be disinfected is then exposed to hot water at 170F (77C) for 30 minutes. This method does not produce sterility, because the outside of the equipment must be handled twice as it is transferred from the washer to the drier and again when it is removed from the drier to be packed into plastic bags; however, anesthesia breathing systems properly processed in this way are as clean as disposable breathing systems. Use of a mechanical rotary washer and pasteurizing equipment, such as the Olympic Pasteurmatic (Fig. 9–1) has proved to be an efficient and economic method of providing clean equipment in some busy anesthesia services. The Cidematic was a similar system that used glutaraldehyde instead of heat to kill the bacteria. Glutaraldehyde is effective against *M. tuberculosis* and vegetative forms of bacteria, even in the presence of blood and mucus. It is an irritant to the skin, so rubber gloves should be worn. The equipment must be rinsed thoroughly to remove the residues and odor. Glutaraldehyde solution has a limited stability and should be discarded after 2 weeks. Most clean equipment can be sealed in plastic bags for storage (Fig. 9–2).

---

[*] May be pasteurized
[†] May be washed, packaged, and gas sterilized
[‡] May be autoclaved

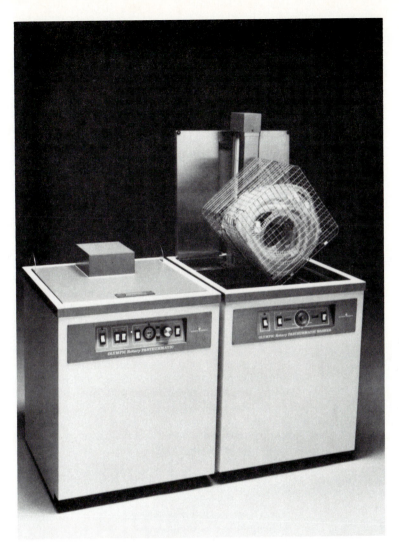

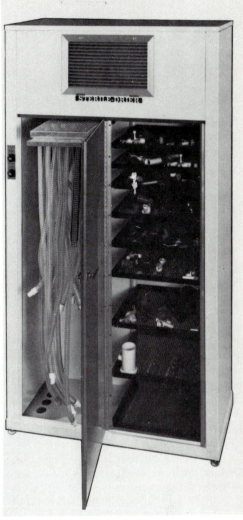

A   **B**

Figure 9–1. The Olympic Rotary Pasteurmatic system. **A.** Rotary washer (30-minute cycle) (right). Up to 20 anesthesia breathing system components are loaded into the stainless-steel baskets, which are lowered into the washer. The baskets rotate as jets of hot water at 60C (140F) spray onto the contents. As the chamber fills, the equipment is repeatedly plunged into the hot detergent solution to dislodge the contaminating soil. At the end of the wash cycle the equipment is rinsed in hot water and allowed to drain. Rotary Pasteurmatic (30-minute cycle) (left). The same baskets are transferred to the pasteurizer, which contains hotter water (77C [170F]), and submerged for 30 minutes after a preliminary period of rotation to release trapped air. **B.** Drying cabinet. Bacteria-free HEPA-filtered air at 57C (135F) is blown over and through the equipment to speed up the drying process. On removal from the drier, the equipment is sealed in plastic bags (see Fig. 9–4) to prevent contamination before its next use.

Boiling. Boiling was once a widely used method of sterilization. Boiling occurs at 100C at sea level (760 mm Hg) and at lower temperatures at higher altitudes, for example, at 94.4C in Denver, Colorado, at 5550 ft, and at 86.6C in LaPaz, Bolivia, at 13,600 ft. There is a drop of about 1C in the temperature at which water boils for each 1000-ft rise in altitude. Boiling at 100C for 30 minutes is lethal to all vegetative forms of bacteria, most spores, and most viruses. It is recommended that the boiling time be extended 5 minutes for each 1000-ft rise in altitude above sea level. These facts are of importance where high-pressure steam sterilization is not available.

Steam Autoclave. At sea level, water in a pan boils at 100C; however, if the water is heated in a pressure cooker, as the pressure rises so will the temperature at which the water boils. The change from liquid to vapor requires a considerable amount of heat (i.e., 580 calories for each milliliter of water). It is the availability of this latent heat in the steam that is given up when the steam condenses on the cool load in the sterilizer that so shortens the time required by steam to produce sterility, compared with hot air at the same temperature. The higher the pressure, the higher will be the steam's temperature and with it the shorter the time

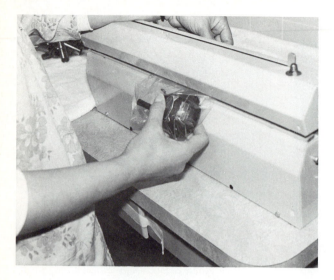

Figure 9–2. Anesthesia technician sealing clean equipment in plastic bag for storage. (© *1987 L. Rendell-Baker.*)

required to heat everything within the sterilizer to the temperature required for sterility.

Before commencing the sterilizing cycle it is important to remove the air from the chamber by vacuum; otherwise the air will reduce the amount of steam entering and, thus, the temperature achieved at any given pressure. Sterilization starts when steam flows into the chamber, penetrating the load and giving up its latent heat as it condenses on the cooler items. Once the desired temperature is achieved, the required duration for sterilization is set. At the end of this period, to avoid residual condensation on the load when the cool air is admitted, the steam is exhausted from the chamber by vacuum.

Most modern autoclaves have automatic controls to ensure that the correct sequence is followed. Commonly used combinations are 15 minutes at 121C and 15 psi and 5 to 10 minutes at 132C and 30 psi.

Steam autoclaving is by far the quickest and most effective method of sterilization, provided the materials to be sterilized can tolerate steam and the temperature. Items that must be sterile for use should be packed in nylon bags or specially made packets that are easily permeable to steam.

Ethylene Oxide Gas Sterilization. Ethylene oxide was first used as a fumigant in 1928 and has been extensively used as a sterilizing agent since the technique for its use, introduced by Phillips and Kaye in 1949,[1] was perfected by McDonald in 1962.[2] It is particularly useful for sterilizing plastic and other equipment that would be damaged by the higher temperatures achieved in the steam autoclave. It was the availability of this convenient, low-temperature method of sterilization that made possible the provision of the sterile disposable equipment now so widely used in our hospitals.

The method was first used to sterilize anesthesia equipment by the anesthesia department of Buffalo General Hospital in 1960 and by Dr. John Snow of Boston in 1962.[3] Very little information was available on the rate of elimina-

tion of the gas from sterilized plastic items, and no one knew how much ethylene oxide human tissues could tolerate. By 1968, reports of skin and tracheal burns and hemolysis of blood began to appear, which led the American National Standards Institute (ANSI) Z79 Anesthesia Standards Committee to form a subcommittee to study this problem. This group has continued its work, now under the aegis of the Association for Advancement of Medical Instrumentation, from whom up-to-date advice on the safe use of ethylene oxide may be obtained (Appendix I).

It became apparent that ethylene oxide, which would not be effective if it were not poisonous, is a much more serious danger to the operator's health than is nitrous oxide pollution in the operating room. As a result, the Occupational Safety and Health Administration (OSHA) set a maximum exposure level of 1 ppm. To maintain this low level and protect employees' health, ethylene oxide sterilizers and aerators should not be placed in a work area, but rather should be kept in a separate well-ventilated area, preferably equipped with a dedicated air extraction system to remove the gas residues to the outside air. In response to concern about the health hazard of the ethylene oxide sterilization process then used in hospitals, the Environmental Protection Agency (EPA) in 1984 set forth its recommendation for modifications in workplace design and practice in hospitals to help reduce the exposure of hospital workers to 1 ppm of ethylene oxide.[4]

Nonrecirculating or dedicated ventilation systems be provided to remove ethylene oxide:
1. from "capture boxes" installed to enclose the floor drain into which the mixture of gas and water discharges at the end of the sterilization cycle.
2. from the aerator unit.
3. from a hood installed over the sterilizer door to capture gas escaping when the door is opened.
4. from a similar arrangement to remove the gas escaping when ethylene oxide cylinders are changed.

As ethylene oxide is highly explosive, large sterilizers have in the past used a mixture of 12 percent ethylene oxide and 88 percent Freon 12, a fluorocarbon gaseous quenching agent, or 10 percent ethylene oxide and 90 percent carbon dioxide, which has the same effect. Since Freon 12 has been implicated in the depletion of the earth's ozone layer, Pennsylvania Engineering has introduced a new environmentally acceptable substitute fluorocarbon, Penngas 2, which in a mixture of 90 percent with 10 percent ethylene oxide functions as well in existing sterilizers as the original mixture.[5] Small sterilizers often use cartridges of 100 percent ethylene oxide.

Among the factors of importance in the use of ethylene oxide sterilization are the following:

1. Unlike steam sterilization, the ethylene oxide process has two phases: one during which the gas is forced into the load, the other during which it slowly escapes from the load. Unfortunately, the second phase is much longer than the first. It may last from 8 hours to 7 days depending on the temperature and airflow. An aerator cabinet providing a flow of warm bacterially filtered air at 140F pro-

duces satisfactory aeration in 8 hours. Contrast this with packets of polyvinyl chloride items left on a shelf at 70F, which will take 7 days to eliminate the large quantity of gas absorbed by the plastic.

2. Before sterilization, clean and remove all gross water droplets; however, equipment must not be heat-dried, for ethylene oxide requires the presence of greater than 45 percent relative humidity for efficient penetration and sterilization of the load.

3. Pack the equipment in 3-mil-thick polyethylene bags or in specifically designed gas sterilization packages. Nylon is impermeable to ethylene oxide and polyvinyl chloride retains the gas, hindering aeration, so neither material should be used with ethylene oxide sterilization. Place the items in the sterilizer and start the sterilization cycle (Fig. 9–3).

4. A vacuum of 29 in. Hg is required to remove the air from the chamber and the load.

5. Apply steam to humidify the load; this is necessary for the gas to penetrate and kill the bacteria.

6. Exposure to ethylene oxide for 4 to 5 hours at a pressure of 8 psi with fluorocarbon mixtures or 25 psig with carbon dioxide mixtures and a temperature of 130° F is necessary. The fluorocarbon facilitates penetration of the gas through the packaging and into the depths of the plastic or rubber items being sterilized.

7. Many modern ethylene sterilizers incorporate a "purge cycle" to remove most of the gas remaining within the sterilizer at the end of the cycle. In sterilizers lacking a purge cycle, a cloud of 2000 to 5000 ppm ethylene oxide is released when the sterilizer door is first opened. (It is for this reason that a gas extraction hood surrounding the sterilizer door and containing a dedicated exhaust system is recommended by the EPA). Therefore, in sterilizers without a purge cycle, open the sterilizer door 6 in. and leave the area for 15 minutes; then open the door fully and leave for another 15 minutes before removing the load. In sterilizers with a purge cycle, remove the load immediately; the purge cycle is completed, thus not allowing time for further ethylene oxide to "degas" from the sterilized items.

8. Transfer the load to an aerator through which a steam of bacterially filtered air at 120F to 140F is drawn. The standard aeration phase usually takes 8 to 12 hours to remove the gas from such items as polyvinyl chloride plastic tubes, which retain the gas much longer than do any other materials.

If an aeration time less than the 8 to 12 hours recommended by the manufacturer is used there is a risk of skin burns or mucosal irritation caused by gas residues retained in the equipment. Therefore, when equipment can withstand high temperatures, steam sterilization is preferred; it is quicker, simpler, and safer for both patient and technician.

SPECIAL PROBLEMS

Precautions Against Infection With Hepatitis B and Human Immunodeficiency Viruses

Anesthesia requires that the practitioner have frequent contact with the patient's mucous membranes and saliva, and this poses the risk of transmission of hepatitis B virus (HBV) and, to a lesser extent, human immunodeficiency virus (HIV). Contact with the patient's blood when starting an infusion, drawing a blood sample, or injecting drugs into an intravenous line is a more evident risk. To put these hazards into perspective it has been reported that 8 to 20 percent of health care workers exposed by needle stick to HBV-infected blood become infected with HBV,[6,7] and that acute and chronic sequelae of hepatitis B are responsible for about 300 deaths per year in health care workers.[7,8] On the

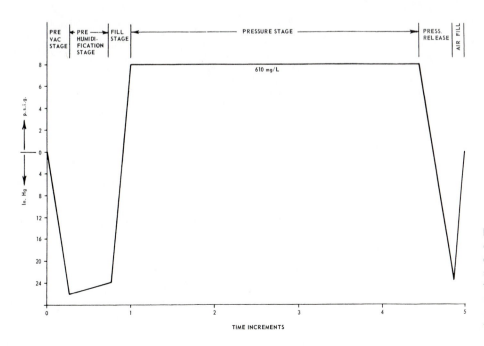

Figure 9–3. McDonald ethylene oxide gaseous sterilization process. The graph shows the pressure changes during the sequential events of the cycle. Note the high degree of vacuum produced at the beginning and at the end of the sequence.

other hand, the Centers for Disease Control (CDC) reported that only 0.47 percent of workers exposed to HIV-infected blood by needle stick became infected.[8,9] Surveys have shown that in an anesthesia staff tested for the presence of hepatitis B surface antibody and antigen, an indicator of prior exposure to the virus, 20 percent in the American studies[6,7] and 31 percent in a German study tested positive. Fortunately, hepatitis B vaccine is now available to provide protection.

Immunization should be encouraged for all high-risk staff, such as surgical, anesthesia, laboratory, and hemodialysis personnel. The hepatitis B surface antigen can survive several days on stainless-steel surfaces, needles, and gloves so that many of the items of equipment used in anesthesia are potential routes of transmission. The virus is resistant to phenol- and chlorine-containing disinfectants so that steam sterilization or disposable equipment should be used.

CDC Universal Precaution Recommendations. As it is not possible to determine which patients are HBV or HIV positive, it is essential to guard one's health by preventing skin or mucous membrane exposure to blood or other body fluids by wearing gloves, goggles, gown, and mask throughout all procedures (CDC Universal Precautions[10]). Provision of these protective items and their use by the staff are now mandated by OSHA 1991 regulations.[11,12]

Hands and other skin surfaces should be washed immediately and thoroughly if contaminated with blood or other body fluids. Hands should be washed after gloves are removed as intact skin may transmit HIV infection. Studies suggest that the Langerhans cells in the skin and mucous membranes are the primary target cells and vehicle for HIV infection. "The assumption that HIV infection occurs exclusively by entry of the virus through wounds in the skin and mucous membranes into the blood can no longer be considered valid."[13-15] Caution should be exercised in the disposal of used needles and other sharp items in the "sharps" container. If unprotected needles are used the CDC's Recommendation, incorporated into the OSHA regulation, is that they not be recapped or removed from disposable syringes.

Minimizing the Impact of HIV Positive Status on the Staff. Though the chance of anesthetists becoming infected with HIV or HBV when using correct CDC precautions is quite low, the impact of the infection on the individual is so severe that leading centers now provide disability insurance coverage for all their house staff. No doubt this insurance will be extended to cover the anesthesia staff.[16,17]

Eliminate the Use of Needles. As most cases of HIV infection in hospital workers have been related to accidental needle sticks it would seem logical to eliminate the use of unprotected needles as far as possible. Fortunately, equipment manufacturers have responded to this need.

1. An intravenous needle cannula placement set has been developed that encloses the needle as the cannula is inserted (Fig. 9–4).
2. If an intravenous extension set such as that shown in Figure 9–5 is used, intravenous doses of drugs may be given from syringes through the one-way valves without the use of needles.

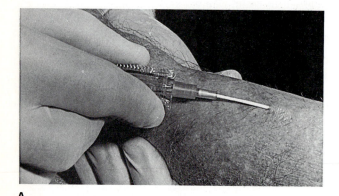

A

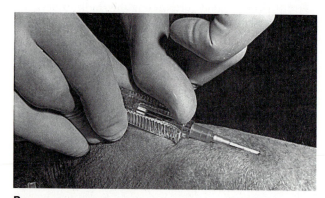

B

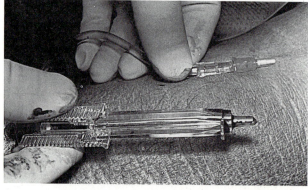

C

Figure 9–4. Steps in insertion of a Critikon Protectiv IV catheter. **A.** Inserting the needle and catheter into the vein. **B.** As the catheter is advanced into the vein the needle is drawn back into and securely locked into its protective sheath. **C.** The sheath with the needle locked inside. (© *1990 L. Rendell-Baker.*)

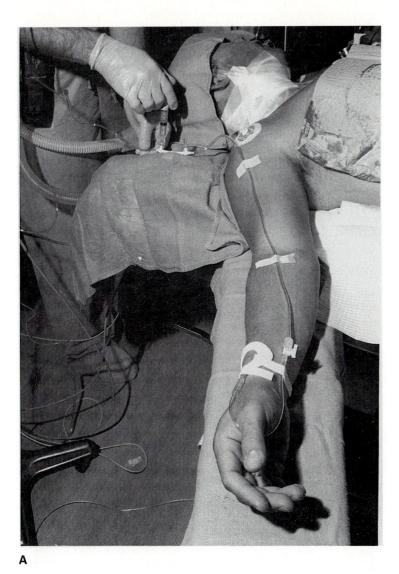

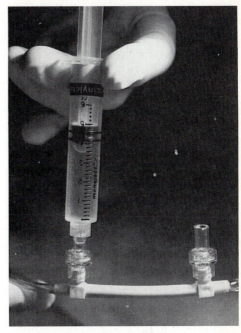

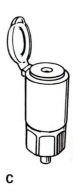

A

B

C

Figure 9–5. **A.** The 36-in.-long Burron AET-36 Anesthesia Extension Set provides two-way valved injection ports close to the anesthetist, which permits injections without the use of needles. **B.** Closeup of the two-way valved injection sites. Note the need to replace the separate caps for good hygiene. **C.** Wallace one-way valved syringe injection site with attached cap, an excellent hygienic feature. (© *1990 L. Rendell-Baker.*)

3. The syringes may be filled with drugs from vials using a minispike inserted into each vial (Fig. 9–6).
4. If, however, the extension set similar to that shown in Figure 9–5 and minispikes are not available, use of shrouded needles (Fig. 9–7) to make injections into the injection ports of a standard intravenous set will greatly reduce the hazard resulting from needle sticks.

Contamination of Apparatus with Mycobacteria

There have been no documented cases of transmission of tubercle bacilli via anesthesia equipment. Of all bacteria, however, the acid-fast bacilli are the most adaptable and are particularly resistant to desiccation. The rising incidence of active pulmonary tuberculosis in HIV-infected patients represents reactivation of old lesions as their immune systems become impaired. Reportedly, this is most commonly seen in intra-

venous drug abusers, Haitian-Americans, and other non-white population.[18,19] As *mycobacterium tuberculosis* is more virulent than other latent intracellular pathogens, tuberculosis tends to occur early in the course of the HIV infection, preceding the diagnosis of AIDS in more than half the cases.[20] In addition, in AIDS patients the lesions seen on chest radiography in tuberculosis may be indistinguishable from those of *Pneumocystis carinii*.[21] The report of pulmonary tuberculosis infection in respiratory therapists treating patients with *P. carinii* infection with pentamidine inhalations stresses the need for a greater degree of vigilance by anesthesia staff when dealing with patients who have pulmonary disease that could be caused by acid-fast organisms.[22,23] This vigilance should include the following precautions:

1. Nondisposable equipment must be subjected to initial sterilization or disinfection with appropriate chemicals (e.g., glutaraldehyde) after use. Subse-

quently, equipment must be washed thoroughly. Finally, wrapping, labeling, and terminal sterilization (preferably with steam) should follow.

2. Use of a disposable circle system and absorber may be helpful.

3. All operating room staff should be aware that the patient is infectious.

4. When possible, the patient should wear a mask.

5. All gowns, gloves, shoe covers, and masks should be discarded in the approved manner on leaving the operating room.

6. Traffic and equipment within the operating room should be kept to a minimum.

7. The anesthesia staff should keep intraoral manipulations to a minimum.

Nontuberculous Mycobacterial Infections. DuMoulin and Stottmeir reported that in Massachusetts there had been a fivefold increase in the incidence of nontuberculous mycobacterial infections, which are difficult to treat with antimycobacterial drugs and are particularly likely to infect patients with HIV and other immunodeficient conditions.[24] Since 1972, a fourfold increase in pulmonary infections in adults and of lymphadenitis in children caused by *Mycobacterium avium-intracellulare* bacilli has been reported in Massachusetts.[25] Transmission of these organisms is by

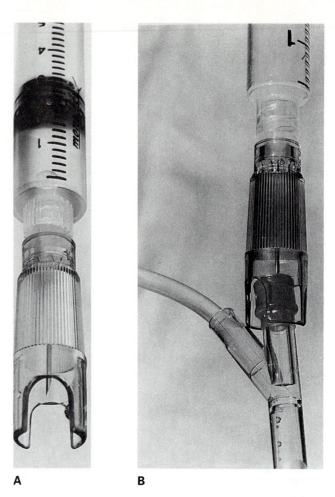

A   **B**

Figure 9–7. A. The IMS 4009 Stick-Gard shrouded needle prevents accidental needle punctures while permitting injections into IV injection sites. **B.** Shrouded needle used to make injection into IV injection site. A Burron Mini Spike (see Fig. 9–6) or similar device must be used to aspirate medications safely

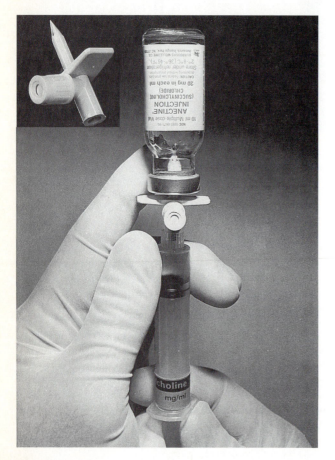

Figure 9–6. Filling the syringe with succinylcholine without using a needle. Instead, a Burron DP 1000 Mini Spike is inserted into the vial. (© *1990 L. Rendell-Baker.*)

environmental contact rather than person to person, with hospital tap water implicated as the primary vehicle of infection. *M. avium* was isolated from water at 41 percent of sites within one hospital. Hot water at 52C to 57C in 11 of 14 sites tested was positive for *M. avium* compared with 3 of 18 cold water sites. The organism was recovered from 5 of 12 hospitals surveyed in Boston as well as one in Chicago. It is resistant to chlorine in the amounts commonly used in drinking.

As a result of these studies, it has been recommended that (1) the hot water temperature be raised to 77C and patients cautioned to avoid the hot water aerosols produced by showers by bathing instead, and (2) novel filtration, disinfection, or decontamination methods be used to reduce the likelihood of transmission. *M. avium* is one of the opportunistic pathogens in patients with AIDS and is frequently isolated from clinical specimens. Patients with chronic obstructive pulmonary disease or with healed tuberculosis may also be at risk of acquiring this pulmonary infection from water.[26]

Hand Washing. To an interested observer, the contrast between the careful hand scrubbing of surgeons and the often total absence of hand washing by anesthesia personnel is marked. We expect dental surgeons to wash their hands before working in our mouths. Should not our patients expect the same standard from us? Scrub sinks for anesthesia personnel should be provided in anesthesia induction areas, particularly in view of the importance of prompt removal of any of the patient's blood from the hands. Anesthetists should wash hands following these patient contacts and between cases.

Use of Disposable Equipment

When the first disposable plastic blood and intravenous administration sets were introduced in 1947, they were such a major improvement over the reusable red rubber sets that they were rapidly accepted in the United States and, later, in other countries. In 1947, up-to-date hospitals employed syringe services to clean and sterilize the syringes and needles used throughout the hospital. Needles were checked and sharpened before each sterilization, although the standard of sharpness achieved would hardly be acceptable today. This service required considerable hand labor, so the introduction in 1957 of disposable plastic syringes and very sharp needles was generally welcomed. These were followed in 1959 by disposable trays for minor procedures, such as catheterization. Since then, the quality and variety of available disposable equipment have expanded so much that it is doubtful whether reusable products of equivalent performance could be produced at a reasonable price, if at all.

Anesthesiology and respiratory therapy came to this field rather late. It was not until 1969 that the first disposable breathing systems and humidifiers were introduced. R. Bryan Roberts, MD, who played a leading role in their development, recounted that

> their introduction is in great part, due to the foresight of a New Jersey businessman, Thomas J. Mahon, who in 1958, having just sold his pharmaceutical business, looked around for new medical problems to tackle. Concerned about the reported incidence of patients, both in hospital and at home, using ventilatory therapy equipment, who were crossinfecting each other and reinfecting themselves, he, with an engineering friend, Samual Cherba, set about designing a low-cost disposable oxygen nebulizer and humidifier.

> It soon became apparent that a length of disposable corrugated hose would be necessary to bridge the gap between nebulizer and patient. However, no company in the United States at that time had the technology to produce corrugated polyethylene hose of 22 mm standard diameter. Further search disclosed that a machine capable of this spiral blow-molding technique had been developed in West Germany, and one of these was imported into the United States. After considerable trial and error a hose of acceptable diameter, weight, flexibility, and distensibility was first made in 1967.[27]

The contribution of Bryan Roberts to the use of disposables in anesthesia practice is exemplified by his design (with Mahon) of a lightweight anesthesia breathing system with a plastic swivel mask and tube adapter, which was first shown at the ASA Convention in Washington, DC, in October 1968 (Fig. 9–8). Since that time, disposable breath-

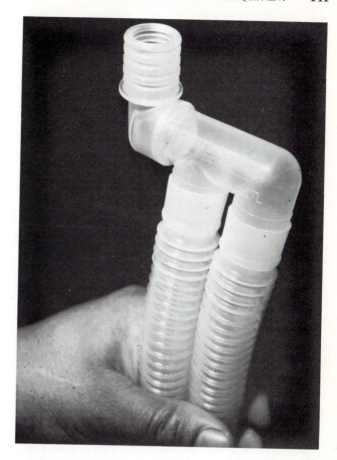

Figure 9–8. U-Mid disposable anesthesia system and swivel Y designed by Bryan Roberts and Thomas J. Mahon in 1968. (© 1987 L. Rendell-Baker.)

ing systems in anesthesia and respiratory care have been adopted almost universally. In addition to the savings in labor costs, part of the attraction of disposable items for hospitals has been that they constitute an easily identifiable cost item for reimbursement purposes; the cost for each use of reusable items is more difficult to calculate.

Problems with Disposable Breathing Systems. Standard 15- and 22-mm fittings were introduced by the ANSI's Z79 Anesthesia Standards Committee between 1960 and 1965.[28,29] Standard "plug-and-ring" gauges were also designed to facilitate checking whether fittings were made to the correct dimensions. Before that time each manufacturer had its own unique size of fittings on the absorber, bag mount, Y-piece, and mask; the user thus had to buy bags, masks, and breathing tubes of that size from the original manufacturer.[29] Adoption of standard fittings by all manufacturers meant that the user had to stock only one supply of expendable rubber components and these could be obtained from a number of suppliers.

Accidental Disconnection. Adoption of standard-sized fittings encouraged plastic molding firms to make tracheal tube connectors, Y-pieces, mask adaptors, and complete breathing systems from plastic. In metal the gradual 1-in-40 taper (1-unit increase in diameter for each 40 units of length) used for conical fittings worked well, but for molded plastic fittings a much steeper taper of about 1-in-20 was better. It is much simpler to achieve the required accuracy in metal than in plastic, which tends to shrink after it leaves the mold. The characteristics of plastic also vary. Polycarbonate is rigid and can be given a highly polished surface that grips securely when the components are wrung together; at the other extreme is polyethylene, which is quite flexible and can have a slippery, waxy surface, which is the reason it is used in artificial hip joints. In addition, female fittings made from softer plastics tend to stretch, and the male fittings "creep" when they are wrung tightly together. Clearly, an anesthetist's confidence in the ability of a breathing system to remain securely connected under the drapes depends on the suitability of the plastic used and the accuracy achieved in the final product.

Unfortunately, manufacturers of plastic components were often unaware of the existence of the standard dimensions and the gauges that should be used to determine the accuracy of their fittings. As a result, they made their components to fit as many other makers' plastic items as possible, which were often incorrectly sized in the first place, so that the value of having all components of standard size and readily interchangeable was lost.

Accidental disconnection was the most frequent anesthesia problem reported to Cooper et al in their Boston "critical incident" surveys in 1978–1984.[30–32] The poor retention of some plastic fittings received most of the blame. The problem of accidental disconnection became so widespread and troublesome that the Food and Drug Administration (FDA) funded a study to determine the cause and, if possible, a cure. According to the January 1986 final report,

1. Disconnection commonly occurred in anesthesia and critical care and resulted in preventable serious injuries and deaths.
2. Most disconnections occurred between the tracheal tube connector and the breathing system for several reasons, among them the need of the user to make and undo the connection easily and repeatedly. This prevents maximum force from being used to make the engagement for fear of then being unable to disengage the components. Also, if the connection is made too securely, extubation might occur.
3. Standards limited to dimensions are obsolete because of the variable properties of the materials.
4. A better connector design and a performance standard were required.
5. Users needed to appreciate the importance of the rotary movement while forcing the components together.[33]

New standard gauges and test methods specially designed to allow for the variable characteristics of plastics have been published[34] by the ASTM F29 Anesthesia Standards Committee (Appendix II), so in the future plastic components should be correctly sized and provide better security from accidental disengagement. An antidisconnect fitting designed to prevent disconnection of the 15-mm male tube connector fitting from the grooved 22-mm male Y-piece fitting has been introduced (Fig. 9–9) that will work

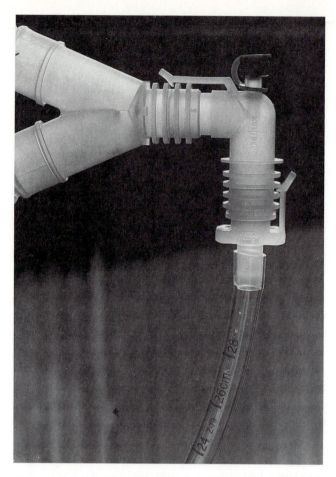

Figure 9–9. In this Kendal Safetrak 11 breathing system, the security clips on the tracheal tube connector and the mask adapter lock onto the rings on the 22-mm male fittings to prevent accidental disconnection. (© *1990 L. Rendell-Baker.*)

satisfactorily with breathing systems which have grooved 22-mm male fittings.

The security with which plastic components grip each other can be assessed by forcing them together while rotating them 45 degrees. Unsatisfactory components cannot be made to grip and will continue to rotate no matter how much force is applied. If the components make a cracking sound as they are fit together and grip so firmly that they cannot be rotated further, it is unlikely they will come apart in use. In everyday use it is essential when fitting plastic or metal components together to rotate them to obtain a secure fit.

Though the poor retention of some plastic fittings received most of the blame for the harm suffered by patients as a result of accidental disconnections, changes in anesthesia practice also played a part. When most patients breathed spontaneously or were manually ventilated, any accidental disconnection was quickly noted; but with the increasing use of volume ventilators, most of which earlier had weighted *dependent* bellows, disconnection was less easily detected. The bellows of such ventilators would rise and fall in a normal manner whether attached to the patient or not. If the ventilator's bellows are designed to ascend only when filled with expired gas, the bellows will collapse and remain motionless if disconnection occurs, thus promptly alerting the anesthetist to the problem. For this reason, the designs of ventilators were changed to incorporate ascending bellows and only these designs should be chosen for use in the future.

Can We Reuse Disposable Equipment? Much disposable equipment can be reused if it is carefully handled, cleaned, tested, repackaged, and resterilized, usually with ethylene oxide. It is likely that most hospitals in the United States are reusing selected, disposable items, such as hemodialyzers,[35] cardiovascular catheters, and respiratory therapy breathing circuits.[36] If a hospital has the necessary staff and wants to reprocess disposables, it should follow the FDA guidelines and be able to demonstrate (1) that the device can be adequately cleaned and sterilized; (2) that the physical characteristics or quality of the device will not be adversely affected; (3) that the device remains safe and effective for its intended use; and (4) they must accept full responsibility for the device's safety and effectiveness (FDA).[37]

When a hospital reprocesses and reuses disposable equipment, the hospital, not the manufacturer, is responsible for its safety and effectiveness. Hedley Whyte reports that "the reuse of disposable anesthesia devices presents a greater medicolegal hazard than other types of equipment, commensurate with the relative size of malpractice awards in anesthesiology. Consequently, anesthesia devices intended for single use are not reused in Harvard Medical School's teaching hospitals."[38]

Disposables or Reusables: Which to Use? The objective of either system is to provide each patient with (1) a sterile tracheal tube; (2) a clean breathing system (face mask, mask adapter, Y-piece, two breathing tubes, and breathing bag)*; (3) a clean oral airway*; (4) a clean esophageal stethoscope*; and (5) a clean telethermometer probe.* Note that hand washing of reusable equipment cannot satisfy these requirements.

Factors to Be Considered. The projected annual number of operations, the number of anesthetists, the number of anesthesia technicians, and the space available in or near the operating room suite are all factors that must be considered.

Reusables. In the past, reusable items were hand-washed, but technicians' hands cannot tolerate the high temperatures necessary, and the equipment is not exposed long enough to hot water at 170F, which is necessary to effect pasteurization. If reusable equipment is selected, a Pasteurmatic or similar system is required.

The Pasteurmatic system (see Fig. 9–1) takes 20 anesthesia breathing systems per load, and a technician can process 5 loads in an 8-hour shift, that is, a total of 100 breathing systems per shift. This type of system produces a clean rather than a sterile final product. The process proceeds in four phases: washing, pasteurization, drying, and bagging. The most time-consuming part of the process is

bagging the clean equipment. This system could handle the equipment for 20 to 25 operating rooms, or more if an evening technician is employed.

Disposables. The small hospital with few operations per day and no anesthesia technicians to clean the equipment between patients can achieve the same hygienic standards by providing a clean, disposable system for each patient. Most hospitals now use disposable tracheal tubes, including disposable double-lumen endobronchial tubes.

Space in or near the operating room is essential for storing the bulky disposable breathing systems and other items. A local equipment dealer may agree to store major portions of a hospital's disposables if awarded the annual supply contract. The quantity required can be delivered once or twice a month to suit the hospital's storage capacity; however, remember that deliveries can be halted by strikes, bad weather, or other factors, so a 2-week supply should be kept in the hospital.

The features of the disposable items chosen should be at least as good as those of the reusable items. The plastic breathing systems are always lighter, and the clear ones permit easy monitoring of the amount of condensation in the system. A clear plastic system should always be chosen when a heated humidifier is to be used to help maintain the patient's body temperature.

If in doubt about whether to choose reusables or disposables, remember that the manufacturers of the Pasteurmatic equipment will produce a cost analysis comparing the cost to your hospital of using their equipment and reusable items with the cost of using disposable items.

Cross-Infection from Anesthesia Equipment: Is It a Real Problem?

Interest in possible cross-infection from anesthesia equipment was stimulated by a dramatic increase in nosocomial infections, particularly those caused by gram-negative bacilli. Studies clearly showed a link between the use of respiratory therapy equipment, particularly nebulizers, and the incidence of necrotizing pneumonia. Because of this correlation, the occurrence of postoperative chest infections was presumed by many clinicians to result from the less-than-ideal standards of hygiene found in many anesthesia departments. Although no good clinical studies demonstrated that anesthesia equipment was the cause of the infections, disposable breathing systems with bacterial filters were strongly advocated as the answer to the problem.

DuMoulin and Saubermann showed that the anesthesia machine and breathing system were not likely to be sources of bacterial contamination, because the breathing system is an inhospitable environment for bacteria.[39] They found that after 75 minutes of anesthesia administration to a patient colonized with *Pseudomonas aeruginosa*, although the expiratory tube nearest the patient was contaminated, neither in this or any of their other patients was contamination of the expiratory valve on the carbon dioxide absorber observed. When the expiratory valve was deliberately inoculated with a bacterial culture and 3 L of nitrous oxide–oxygen flowed through the system for 3 hours, there was a progressive decrease in the bacteria present at the valve, and the organisms failed to propagate to other parts of the system. Feeley

---

* It may be desirable to provide these items in sterile packets for immunosuppressed patients.

et al[40] showed that the use of sterile breathing systems had no effect on the incidence of postoperative pulmonary infection, and Pace et al[41] and Garibaldi et al[42] reported that bacterial filters failed to reduce the incidence of pneumonia after inhalation anesthesia. Commenting on these studies, Mazze[43] stated that bacterial filters in breathing systems probably add $20 to $30 million to the annual health care budget without any apparent influence on patients' outcome. He believed that we should stop using bacterial filters for breathing circuits until better-designed and executed experiments cause us to question the validity of the studies reviewed here.

The incidence of postoperative atelectasis and pneumonia is more directly influenced by the patient's preoperative pulmonary condition, the location and duration of surgery, the amount of postoperative pain and narcotics given, and the efficiency of the "stir up" regimen than by the presence of a small number of skin or surface contaminants in the breathing tubes.

Bacterial Filters

The work by duMoulin and Saubermann, Feeley et al, and Garibaldi et al convinced the Z79 standards committee that bacterial filters were not necessary in anesthesia breathing systems and should not be included in their standard on the safety and performance of these breathing systems. A concern about bacterial filters is that there is no single, universally accepted performance standard against which the efficiency of a filter can be measured. There is the dioctyl phthalate test, in which a fine dust of known particle size is blown through the filter to determine the proportion entrapped. Another test is the bacterial aerosol challenge test, in which a microbial aerosol is directed through the filter and bacteria in the effluent flow are collected on agar plates in an Anderson sampler. Although both tests appear efficient, they often give contradictory results, and filters that satisfy one test may not do well in the other. This situation hardly inspires confidence.

An additional problem with filters is that they add another source of leakage and increase the resistance to breathing. If a heated humidifier is used to help maintain the patient's body temperature during prolonged surgery, condensation within the filter may greatly increase its resistance. There is a tendency, because filters are expensive, to use them for more than one patient, thus increasing the chance that bacteria may accumulate in condensation within the filter. The filter may therefore become a bacterial accumulator rather than a bacterial eliminator.

DESIRABLE FEATURES OF ANESTHESIA APPARATUS*

Preventive Maintenance

Anesthesia apparatus are potentially dangerous, and their internal mechanisms are becoming increasingly complicated. The anesthesia department or the hospital should

* The State of New Jersey has mandated that anesthesia apparatus in that state meet the safety and performance requirements enumerated here. No doubt other states will follow this example.

contract for preventive maintenance for all anesthesia, ventilatory, and monitoring equipment at the recommended three-monthly or six-monthly intervals. The quality of maintenance available locally should always be considered first in selecting anesthesia apparatus. Other features to be considered follow.

Hygiene

The apparatus should be easy to clean. The absorber assembly and absorbent containers should be easily removable for cleaning and should be steam autoclavable (Fig. 9–10). The ventilator's patient breathing system should be easily removable for cleaning and should withstand steam autoclaving or, if not that, ethylene oxide sterilization. If disposable breathing systems are not to be used, the breathing system tubing, Y-piece, mask adapter, and mask should be able to withstand steam sterilization or pasteurization. Because the cylinders are for emergency use only and are changed infrequently, they can be enclosed, as they were on the Dupaco Hygienic model.

Gas Supply

Now that most apparatus are operated entirely from pipeline supplies of gases supplied through standard

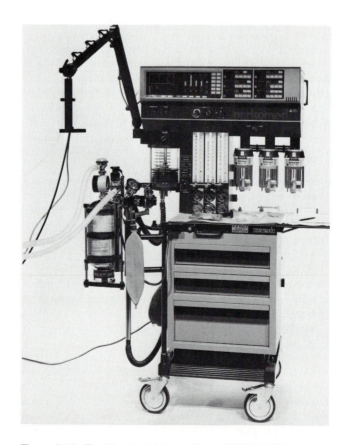

Figure 9–10. The North American Drager Narkomed 3 apparatus showing the autoclavable carbon dioxide absorber, the automatically switched-on oxygen analyzer and other monitors, and the integrated alarms system. (© 1987 L. Rendell-Baker.)

diameter-indexed safety system (DISS) (Appendix III) pipeline inlet fittings on the machine, it is essential to have at least one and preferably two cylinder yokes for oxygen on the machine in case of interruption of pipeline supplies.

All apparatus have oxygen supply failure systems (so-called fail-safe) that shut off the other gases if the oxygen pressure within the machine falls to less than 50 percent normal. (*Note*: this does not prevent the administration of a hypoxic mixture.) A further safety feature should be included in any apparatus chosen: automatic reduction of the flow of the other gases as the oxygen flow is reduced manually, to prevent the accidental administration of less than 25 percent oxygen.

Power Supply

As present traditional "gas machines" give way in the future to all-electronic anesthesia "workstations"[44] a trickle charger-supported battery backup electronic power supply will become essential. Electronic flowmeters and injector-driven vaporizers already exist.[45,46] They have the advantage that their output can be displayed on a panel facing the anesthetist while he or she observes the patient.

Common Gas Outlet

The Z79.8 standard specified a 15-mm female/22-mm male coaxial fitting for the common gas outlet. The 15-mm male fitting has been reported to accidentally detach from the 15-mm female fitting within the common gas outlet, resulting in hypoxia. Some earlier 15-mm female common gas outlet fittings incorporated a rubber O-ring that ensured secure retention of the male fitting. All new apparatus are now fitted with a positive retention mechanism to prevent accidental disconnection at this position. Older apparatus may lack this valuable safety feature.

Flowmeters

The flow controls for oxygen and nitrous oxide should be linked mechanically, pneumatically, or electronically to prevent the accidental administration of a hypoxic mixture. There should be only one flow control knob per gas to prevent the accidental use of milliliters of oxygen when liters were intended, as has happened in the past when two separate flowmeters with separate flow controls were fitted. If two flowmeters, one for milliliters and the other for liters, are desired, they can be placed in series and can be operated by a single control knob. The flowmeter calibration should be etched onto the tube or the tube and its scale should be linked, to prevent accidental incorrect reassembly after cleaning.

A flowmeter for air should be provided for use in anesthetizing neonates, to avoid too high an oxygen tension and with it the danger of retrolental fibroplasia; in surgery for bowel obstruction to avoid the diffusion of nitrous oxide into and consequent distension of the bowel; in laryngeal laser surgery to minimize the danger of fire, ever present when nitrous oxide–oxygen gas mixtures are used; and for use with desflurane to reduce the percentage of oxygen in the gas mixture, as nitrous oxide will no longer be necessary.

Vaporizers

Vaporizers should be permanently mounted between the flowmeters and the machine's fresh gas outlet. Mounting an extra vaporizer between the fresh gas outlet and the absorber or breathing system is a dangerous practice and should be avoided. Dangers include a wrong-way-around gas connection leading to a higher-than-intended vapor concentration[47]; tilting of a filled vaporizer, leading to excessive vapor delivery[48]; and disconnection of the gas flow to a vaporizer incorporating a check valve going undetected and resulting in hypoxia.[49]

The vaporizers can be fitted with an agent-specific filling mechanism, to prevent errors in filling the vaporizer with the wrong agent and to reduce the chance of spillage.

Interlock or other mechanisms should be used to prevent gas from passing through the vaporizing chamber of one vaporizer and then through another, thus contaminating the downstream vaporizer with the agent from the upstream one.

Ventilators

The ventilator controls can be conveniently built into the anesthesia machine. The controls should be arranged to directly determine the parameters of importance in controlling the patient's respiration. Some ventilators require the user to adjust inspiratory flow rate, expiratory flow rate, expiratory pause, and tidal volume before counting the respiratory rate and measuring the minute volume to see if the result is satisfactory. The clinician needs to control (1) the minute volume ventilation, which controls carbon dioxide elimination; (2) the frequency of respiration, which with minute volume ventilation will determine a reasonable tidal volume; and (3) the inspiratory:expiratory time ratio, to provide adequate expiratory time for the circulation to compensate for the abnormal rise in intrathoracic pressure during inspiration produced by the ventilator. On some simpler ventilators, this is fixed at 1 : 2, which is usually satisfactory.

The ventilator's patient breathing system should be easy to disassemble for cleaning and disinfection. For safety, the patient bellows must be designed to ascend as it fills with the patient's expired gas. The bellows will collapse should leakage or breathing system disconnection occur.

Ventilator Alarm

The ventilator should have an alarm that sounds (1) if a subatmospheric pressure is detected or the normal pressure wave is not detected in the patient breathing system within 12 seconds, or (2) if an excessively high or sustained peak pressure is detected. It would be an advantage if the mechanism could also release the pressure in the breathing system promptly until the user can attend to the problem.[50] The North American Drager MDM S monitor is an example of a device that satisfies all these requirements except for the pressure-release mechanism.

Scavenging System

The adjustable pressure-limited valve (APL) or "pop-off" valve of the anesthesia breathing system and the ventilator gas overflow valve are designed to capture surplus anesthetic gases and convey them to the scavenger interface system. This interface system usually incorporates a reservoir bag to hold excess flows of gas, a needle valve to control the suction and with it the rate of gas outflow, and two valves to limit the pressure within the system to a negative pressure of -0.5 cm H_2O and a positive pressure of $+5$ cm H_2O. The interface is an essential safety feature, for it guards against either (1) excessive suction drawing all the gases from the breathing system or (2) a high degree of positive end-expiratory pressure (PEEP) if the scavenger system becomes blocked. The conical fittings in the scavenging system of 19-mm diameter are smaller than the breathing system's 22-mm-diameter fittings. This limits the chance that the breathing tubing will be incorrectly connected to the breathing system scavenging valve.

It may be more convenient to dispose of the surplus anesthetic gases through the air-conditioning system, provided (1) the operating rooms have efficient (20 air changes/hour) nonrecirculating air conditioning and (2) the air-conditioning exhaust grilles are conveniently close to the anesthesia apparatus. In this case wide-bore tubing should be used between the interface and the air exhaust grill to reduce the resistance to gas flow.

No matter how good the scavenging system is, contamination of the operating room atmosphere will occur from time to time, for example, during suction of the patient's airway or during inhalation inductions, so efficient air conditioning is essential to remove these gases.

Suction

An efficient suction system conveniently sited on the anesthesia apparatus is an essential safety feature. This should provide a reservoir container and an on/off control that also permits the degree of suction to be adjusted.

Heated Humidifiers

High laminar-air flow rates of 20 to 25 changes per hour and prolonged surgery with wide exposure of abdominal viscera have combined to make inadvertent hypothermia a serious problem in many modern operating rooms. Heat is lost by evaporation of moisture from the exposed bowel and by evaporation of moisture from the bronchial tree as a result of the dry anesthetic gas mixture.

In addition to a warming blanket under the patient, placement of a heated humidifier in the patient's breathing system has proved invaluable. The humidifier should be controlled by a temperature sensor placed close to the patient's airway, with a servomechanism controlling the heater within the humidifier so that the patient receives gas 80 to 100 percent saturated with water vapor at body temperature. The problem of condensation caused by the temperature drop along the inspiratory tubing can be avoided if the servomechanism also controls a wire heating element within the inspiratory tubing to maintain the desired temperature of 37C within the tubing. The Fisher Paykel is an example of a servomechanism-controlled, heated humidifier that has been found satisfactory (Fig. 9–11). Maintaining the normal humidity within the bronchial tree helps maintain normal mucociliary activity. The dry gases normally pres-

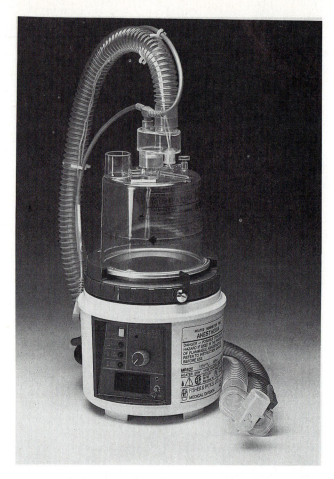

Figure 9–11. The Fisher-Paykel servo-controlled humidifier has a heating element in the main chamber with another flexible element in the delivery tubing to maintain the desired temperature and prevent "rainout."

ent in breathing systems, except during use of low-flow methods, have been shown to damage the cilia and superficial cells of the bronchial tree.[51] This impedes the clearance of secretions postoperatively and increases the incidence of atelectasis and pulmonary complications.

Heat and Moisture Exchangers

For shorter operations without extensive exposure of the viscera a heat and moisture exchanger will be adequate to prevent a fall in temperature and drying of the bronchial mucosa (Fig. 9–12).

A large-capacity warm-air blower (Fig. 9–13) has been found invaluable in rewarming hypothermic patients in the recovery room at Loma Linda University Medical Center (Loma Linda, California). A similar device has been used to maintain the patient's temperature in the operating room during surgery (Fig. 9–14).

CHECKING THE ANESTHESIA APPARATUS PRIOR TO USE

Before commencing each flight, the pilot of a commercial airplane goes through a series of checks to ensure that all systems are functioning correctly. The FDA published such

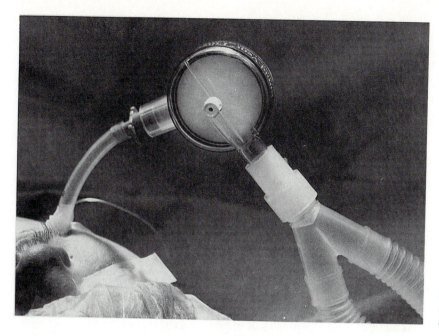

Figure 9–12. This Gibeck Humid Vent heat and moisture exchanger also functions as an efficient bacterial and viral filter.

a recommended checklist for anesthesia apparatus, which was subsequently endorsed by the American Association of Nurse Anesthetists (AANA)[52] (Table 9–1). It is intended that each hospital's staff will evolve their own checklist tailored to the equipment they use.

STANDARDS FOR PATIENT MONITORING DURING ANESTHESIA

The Department of Anesthesia of Harvard Medical School (Boston), as part of a patient safety risk management effort, devised detailed mandatory standards for minimal patient monitoring during anesthesia at its nine component teaching hospitals.[53] These standards were endorsed by the AANA in 1986[54] (Table 9–2). Both the ASA and the AANA have since

updated their standards. Those of the ASA can be found in Table 9–3. It should be noted that in addition to time-honored clinical monitoring, such as frequent checks of the blood pressure, continuous auscultation of the heart rate and breath sounds, and observation of the electrocardiogram (ECG) and movement of the reservoir bag, the standard strongly recommends the following continuous monitoring:

- For ventilation, an end-tidal carbon dioxide monitor is strongly preferred.
- For circulation, pulse oximetry is preferred.
- For breathing systems, an oxygen analyzer with a low-concentration alarm is preferred. A disconnection monitor is to be used when ventilation is controlled by a ventilator.

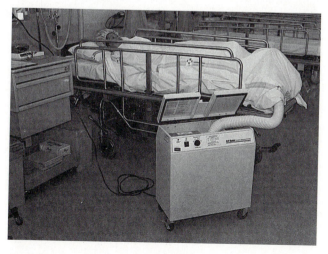

Figure 9–13. An Augustine Medical "Bair Hugger" warm-air unit is used in the recovery room, Loma Linda University Medical Center (Loma Linda, California), to rewarm a patient who was hypothermic after surgery. (© *1990 L. Rendell-Baker.*)

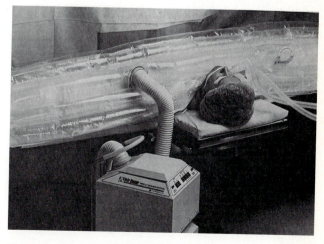

Figure 9–14. This Augustine Medical "Bair Hugger" convective warming unit is designed to maintain normal body temperature during surgery. (*Courtesy Augustine Medical, Inc.*)

TABLE 9–1. ANESTHESIA APPARATUS CHECKOUT RECOMMENDATIONS, 1992[a]

Emergency Ventilation Equipment

1. Verify backup ventilation equipment is available and functioning.

High-Pressure System

2. Check oxygen cylinder supply.
   a. Open O_2 cylinder and verify at least half full (about 1000 psi).
   b. Close cylinder.

3. Check central pipeline supplies.
   a. Check that hoses are connected and pipeline gauges read 45–55 psi.

Low-Pressure System

4. Check initial status of low-pressure system.
   a. Close flow control valves and turn vaporizers off.
   b. Check fill level and tighten vaporizers' filler caps.
   c. Remove O_2 monitor sensor from circuit.

5. Perform leak check of machine low-pressure system.
   a. Verify that the machine master switch and flow control valves are OFF.
   b. Attach "suction bulb" to common (fresh) gas outlet.
   c. Squeeze bulb repeatedly until fully collapsed.
   d. Verify bulb stays *fully* collapsed for at least 10 s.
   e. Open one vaporizer at a time and repeat steps c and d as above.
   f. Remove suction bulb, and reconnect fresh gas hose.

6. Turn on machine master switch
   and all other necessary electrical equipment.

7. Test flowmeters.
   a. Adjust flow of all gases through their full range, checking for smooth operation of floats and undamaged flow tubes.
   b. Attempt to create a hypoxic O_2/N_2O mixture and verify correct changes in flow and/or alarm.

Breathing System

8. Calibrate O_2 monitor.
   a. Calibrate to read 21% in room air.
   b. Reinstall sensor in circuit and flush breathing system with O_2.
   c. Verify that monitor now reads greater than 90%.

> *If an anesthetist uses the same machine in successive cases, the left side of the checklist need not be repeated or may be abbreviated after the initial checkout.*

9. Check initial status of breathing system.
   a. Set selector switch in "bag" mode.
   b. Check that breathing circuit is complete, undamaged and unobstructed.
   c. Verify that CO_2 absorbent is adequate.

10. Install breathing circuit accessory equipment
   to be used during the case.

11. Perform leak check of the breathing system.
   a. Set all gas flows to zero (or minimum).
   b. Close APL valve and occlude Y-piece.
   c. Pressurize breathing system to 30 cm H_2O with O_2 flush.
   d. Ensure that pressure remains at 30 cm H_2O for at least 10 s.

Scavenging System

12. Check APL valve and scavenging system.
   a. Pressurize breathing system to 50 cm H_2O and ensure its integrity.
   b. Open APL valve and ensure that pressure decreases.
   c. Ensure proper scavenging connections and waste gas vacuum.
   d. Fully open APL valve and occlude Y-piece.
   e. Ensure absorber pressure gauge reads zero when:
      • minimum O_2 is flowing.
      • O_2 flush is activated.

Ventilator

13. Test ventilator and unidirectional valves.
   a. Place breathing bag on Y-piece.
   b. Set appropriate ventilator parameters for next patient.
   c. Set O_2 flow to 250 mL/min, other gas flows to zero.
   d. Turn ventilator ON and fill bellows with O_2 flush.
   e. Verify cycling of ventilator and free movement of bellows.
   f. *Check for proper action of unidirectional valves.*
   g. Exercise breathing circuit accessories to ensure proper function.
   h. Turn ventilator OFF, and return breathing bag to bag mount.

Monitors

14. Check, calibrate, and/or set alarm limits of all monitors.

Capnometer	Pulse oximeter
Oxygen analyzer	Respiratory volume monitor (spirometer)

Pressure Monitor with high- and low-airway pressure alarms

Final Position

15. Check final status of machine.

a. Vaporizers off.	d. All flowmeters to zero (or minimum).
b. APL valve open.	
c. Selector switch to "Bag."	e. Patient suction level adequate.
	f. Breathing system ready to use.

---

[a] This checkout, or a reasonable equivalent, should be conducted before administration of anesthesia. These recommendations are only valid for an anesthesia system that conforms to current and relevant standards and includes an ascending bellows ventilator and at least the following monitors: capnograph, pulse oximeter, oxygen analyzer, respiratory volume monitor (spirometer) and breathing system pressure monitor with high and low pressure alarms. This is a guideline which users are encouraged to modify to accommodate differences in equipment design and variations in local clinical practice. Such local modifications should have appropriate peer review. Users should refer to the operators manual for specific procedures and precautions.

FDA DRAFT ver2.7, 2/28/92 HIGH-LOW.CHP, WORKING.wp5.
FDA Revised Draft. February 28, 1992. (Subject to revision after public comment.)

TABLE 9–2. HARVARD MEDICAL SCHOOL STANDARDS FOR MINIMAL PATIENT MONITORING DURING ANESTHESIA

These standards apply for any administration of anesthesia involving department of anesthesia personnel and are specifically referable to preplanned anesthetics administered in designated anesthetizing locations (specific exclusion: administration of epidural analgesia for labor or pain management). In emergency circumstances in any location, immediate life support measures of whatever appropriate nature come first, with attention turning to the measures described in these standards as soon as possible and practical. These are minimal standards that may be exceeded at any time based on the judgment of the involved anesthesia personnel. These standards encourage high-quality patient care, but observing them cannot guarantee any specific patient outcome. These standards are subject to revision from time to time, as warranted by the evolution of technology and practice.

Anesthesiologist's or Nurse Anesthetist's Presence in Operating Room

For all residents initiated by or involving a member of the department of anesthesia, an attending or resident anesthesiologist or nurse anesthetist shall be present in the room throughout the conduct of all general anesthetics, regional anesthetics, and monitored intravenous anesthetics. An exception is made when there is a direct known hazard, e.g., radiation, to the anesthesiologist or nurse anesthetist, in which case some provision for monitoring the patient must be made.

Blood Pressure and Heart Rate

Every patient receiving general anesthesia, regional anesthesia, or managed intravenous anesthesia shall have arterial blood pressure and heart rate measured at least every five minutes, where not clinically impractical.[a]

Electrocardiogram

Every patient shall have the electrocardiogram continuously displayed from the induction or institution of anesthesia until preparing to leave the anesthetizing location, where not clinically impractical.[a]

Continuous Monitoring

During every administration of general anesthesia, the anesthetist shall employ methods of continuously monitoring the patient's ventilation and circulation. The methods shall include, for ventilation and circulation each, at least one of the following or the equivalent.[b]

For Ventilation. Palpation or observation of the reservoir breathing bag, auscultation of breath sounds, monitoring of respiratory gases such as end-tidal carbon dioxide, or monitoring of expiratory gas flow. Monitoring end-tidal carbon dioxide is an emerging standard and is strongly preferred.

For Circulation. Palpation of a pulse, auscultation of heart sounds, monitoring of a tracing of intraarterial pressure, pulse plethysmography/oximetry, or ultrasound peripheral pulse monitoring. It is recognized that brief interruptions of the continuous monitoring may be unavoidable.

Breathing System Disconnection Monitoring

When ventilation is controlled by an automatic mechanical ventilator, there shall be in continuous use a device that is capable of detecting disconnection of any component of the breathing system. The device must give an audible signal when its alarm threshold is exceeded. (It is recognized that there are certain rare or unusual circumstances in which such a device may fail to detect a disconnection.)

Oxygen Analyzer

During every administration of general anesthesia using an anesthesia machine, the concentration of oxygen in the patient breathing system will be measured by a functioning oxygen analyzer with a low-concentration-limit alarm in use. This device must conform to the American National Standards Institute Z79.10 standard.[a]

Ability to Measure Temperature

During every administration of general anesthesia, there shall be readily available a means to measure the patient's temperature.

Rationale. A means of temperature measurement must be available as a potential aid in the diagnosis and treatment of suspected or actual intraoperative hypothermia and malignant hyperthermia. The measurement/monitoring of temperature during *every* general anesthetic is not specifically mandated because of the potential risks of such monitoring and because of the likelihood of other physical signs giving earlier indication of the development of malignant hyperthermia.

[a] Under extenuating conditions, the attending anesthesiologist may waive this requirement after so stating (including the reasons) in a note in the patient's chart.

[b] Equivalence is to be defined by the chief of the individual hospital department after submission to and review by the department heads. Department of Anesthesia, Harvard Medical School, Boston.

Reprinted, with permission, from Eichhorn et al.[53] Copyright 1986, American Medical Association.

Monitors

Though in the past emphasis has been placed on monitoring the circulation, that is, blood pressure, pulse, and ECG, analysis of anesthetic accidents by Katz showed that most accidents stem from problems with the airway and unrecognized hypoxia.[55] To minimize this risk the following monitors are of prime importance:

1. The oxygen analyzer is most important, as it is the only instrument that can give prompt indication that the gas supplied by the oxygen flowmeter is not oxygen. It will also provide the earliest warning of any accidental reduction of oxygen percentage in the gas mixture. The oxygen analyzer should be so designed that it is switched on automatically as the machine's gases are turned on. This is essential to avoid those hypoxic accidents that have occurred when the analyzer is switched on only when hypoxia is suspected.
2. The capnograph or mass spectrometer, by displaying the patient's end-tidal carbon dioxide, indicates correct or incorrect placement of the tracheal tube and adequacy of the minute ventilation.
3. The pulse oximeter indicates the adequacy of peripheral oxygen saturation and the circulation.

TABLE 9–3. ASA STANDARDS FOR BASIC INTRAOPERATIVE MONITORING (1986, AMENDED 1990)

STANDARD I

Qualified anesthesia personnel shall be present in the room throughout the conduct of all general anesthetics, regional anesthetics, and monitored anesthesia care.

Objective

Because of the rapid changes in patient status during anesthesia, qualified anesthesia personnel shall be continuously present to monitor the patient and provide anesthesia care. In the event there is a direct known hazard, e.g., radiation, to the anesthesia personnel that might require intermittent remote observation of the patient, some provision for monitoring the patient must be made. In the event that an emergency requires the temporary absence of the person primarily responsible for the anesthetic, the best judgment of the anesthesiologist will be exercised in comparing the emergency with the anesthetized patient's condition and in the selection of the person left responsible for the anesthetic during the temporary absence.

STANDARD II

During all anesthetics, the patient's oxygenation, ventilation, circulation, and temperature shall be continually evaluated.

Oxygenation

Objective

To ensure adequate oxygen concentration in the inspired gas and the blood during all anesthetics.

Methods

1. Inspired gas: During every administration of general anesthesia using an anesthesia machine, the concentration of oxygen in the patient breathing system shall be measured by an oxygen analyzer with a low oxygen concentration limit alarm in use.

2. Blood oxygenation: During all anesthetics, a quantitative method of assessing oxygenation such as a pulse oximetry shall be employed. Adequate illumination and exposure of the patient are necessary to assess color.

Ventilation

Objective

To ensure adequate ventilation of the patient during all anesthetics.

Methods

1. Every patient receiving general anesthesia shall have the adequacy of ventilation continually evaluated. While quali-

tative clinical signs such as chest excursion, observation of the reservoir breathing bag, and auscultation of breath sounds may be adequate, quantitative monitoring of the CO_2 content and/or volume of expired gas is encouraged.

2. When an endotracheal tube is inserted, its correct positioning in the trachea must be verified by clinical assessment and by identification of carbon dioxide in the expired gas. End-tidal CO_2 analysis, in use from the time of endotracheal tube placement, is encouraged.

3. When ventilation is controlled by a mechanical ventilator, there shall be in continuous use a device that is capable of detecting disconnection of components of the breathing system. The device must give an audible signal when its alarm threshold is exceeded.

4. During regional anesthesia and monitored anesthesia care, the adequacy of ventilation shall be evaluated, at least, by continual observation of qualitative clinical signs.

Circulation

Objective

To ensure the adequacy of the patient's circulatory function during all anesthetics.

Methods

1. Every patient receiving anesthesia shall have the electrocardiogram continuously displayed from the beginning of anesthesia until preparing to leave the anesthetizing location.

2. Every patient receiving anesthesia shall have arterial blood pressure and heart rate determined and evaluated at least every five minutes.

3. Every patient receiving general anesthesia shall have, in addition to the above, circulatory function continually evaluated by at least one of the following: palpation of a pulse, auscultation of heart sounds, monitoring of a tracing of intraarterial pressure, ultrasound peripheral pulse monitoring, or pulse plethysmography or oximetry.

Body Temperature

Objective

To aid in the maintenance of appropriate body temperature during all anesthetics.

Methods

There shall be readily available a means to continuously measure the patient's temperature. When changes in body temperature are intended, anticipated, or suspected, the temperature shall be measured.

Reprinted, with permission, from American Society of Anesthesiologists, 515 Busse Highway, Park Ridge, IL 60068–3189; approved by the October 1990 House of Delegates; implemented 1991.

4. A breathing system pressure monitor should be activated when a ventilator is in use. This monitor should detect failure of the ventilator to achieve either the preset minimum pressure or the minimum tidal exchange. It should also detect either an excessively high or a sustained peak pressure.

In addition there should be (1) an automatic blood pressure apparatus, which, if combined with an automatic chart recorder, indicates what happens during induction and at other times when the user is too busy to record these signs manually; (2) a cathode-ray tube with channels for the display of ECG and arterial and venous pressures and the numerical displays of pulse rate and temperature; (3) a telethermometer, if it is not included in the ECG; (4) a breathing spirometer and a pressure gauge, which are very useful as a cross-check on the influence of the breathing system's compliance on the minute volume delivered to the patient. The ultimate monitor is the anesthetist, who remains in close contact with the patient via a precordial or esophageal stethoscope and whose trained ear will pick up instantly any significant change in heartbeat or respiration.

Monitor Confusion

As the design of anesthesia apparatus has progressed, especially since 1980, more and more monitors have been added, each with its own audible and visual alarms (Fig. 9–15). There is a dangerous tendency to silence these alarms to avoid disturbing surgical composure. A better solution is for the manufacturer to combine all the alarms so that the tone of the single audible alarm indicates its urgency, and the visual display shows which function requires attention (Fig. 9–16).

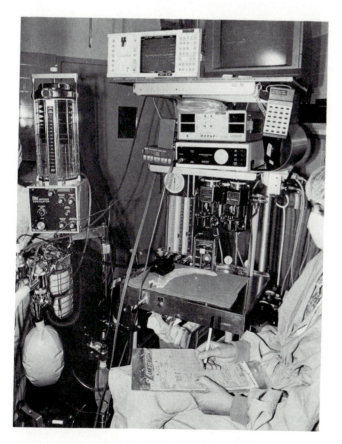

Figure 9–15. Monitor confusion. With each technical advance, more and more monitors have been added. The anesthetist closely monitoring the patient may easily miss changes on the mass spectrometer screen placed well above the line of sight. Good human engineering requires that all important items to be checked frequently occupy the space now taken by the anesthesia ventilator. (© *1987 L. Rendell-Baker.*)

Visibility of Controls

The controls, gauges, and monitors on the apparatus should be arranged so that they can be seen with only minimal movement of the head while the anesthetist is looking at the patient. In other words, they should face the user (Fig. 9–17) as do the airplane pilot's instruments.

Though an apparatus built to achieve this objective was exhibited widely in the 1970s (Fig. 9–18), manufacturers have made little progress in incorporating good human engineering principles and making their apparatus easier and safer to use. Maybe these manufacturers cannot be blamed, as they see users position their present apparatus behind their backs, where the controls are least easily visible (Fig. 9–19).

Standardized Equipment Layout

A policy to standardize widely used equipment in all hospital areas helps to eliminate mishaps, for example, in an emergency, when staff encounter equipment with which they are unfamiliar, or when intravenous sets or arterial line transducers are incompatible and have to be changed. Often, an arterial line with its transducer may be set up in the coronary care unit and then, should the patient require cardiac surgery, the set and transducer are changed and the first ones are discarded. After surgery, if the patient is sent to the surgical intensive care unit, another change is made. Thus, a total of three transducers and arterial sets are expended for one course of treatment. Clearly, adoption of one standard set of equipment would save time and money and would eliminate the inevitable hazards involved in these changes.

Standard Color Code for Sizes of Cannulas

In the past considerable confusion has accompanied the attempt to determine the size of an intravenous cannula inserted elsewhere, for each manufacturer had its own color code. Fortunately, under pressure from the European Community to achieve uniform standards by 1992, manufacturers are now making progress toward an international standard with a uniform color code to identify the sizes of cannulas (Table 9–4). ASTM standard D4775 for labels on prefilled syringes for emergency use greatly simplifies the identification of these syringes, which in the past were difficult to distinguish because of their poor labels (Fig. 9–20).

Servicing of Equipment

The lives of our patients often depend on the correct functioning of our equipment, and to ensure this, gas machines, ventilators, and other devices should be serviced at regular intervals. In addition, it is essential for medicolegal reasons to be able to prove that such maintenance has been carried out. Most authorities advise that apparatus be serviced quarterly. Manufacturers of most equipment offer service contracts; in addition, there are biomedical servicing companies that service a wide range of hospital equipment. It may be advantageous to hire such a company, which can service most makes of equipment at a single visit, rather

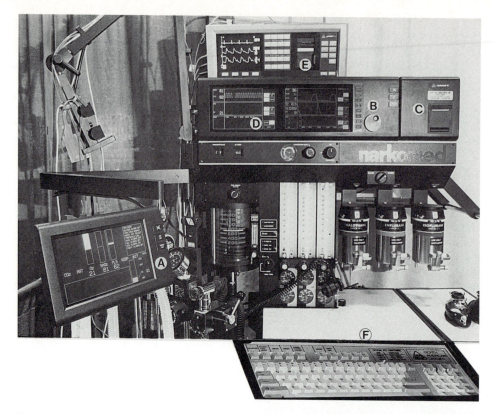

Figure 9–16. NA Drager Narkomed 4 monitor displays. The NA Drager Narkomed 4 apparatus incorporates two 32-bit 25-MHz computers using two central processing units working in parallel in an integrated data management system. **A.** On the mobile remote screen, designed to be placed close to the patient, are displayed as bar graphs and numerically the end-tidal CO_2, the inspired anesthetic agent concentration, the inspired O_2, the tissue O_2 saturation, the pulse rate, and the systolic blood pressure together with a centralized alarm display. **B.** The rotary selection dial facilitates rapid single-finger adjustment of the system parameters and configurations displayed and a review of earlier data. **C.** The strip chart printer provides an immediate hard copy of all numeric and graphic data generated by the unit. **D.** The tiltable touch panel screens respond to the gloved finger to change the monitored data displayed. Monitored are inspired O_2, Nellcor tissue O_2 saturation, minute and tidal volumes, respiratory rate, airway pressure, end-tidal CO_2, inspired N_2O and anesthetic agent, and systolic, diastolic, and mean blood pressures. **E.** The Drager Vitalert 2000 displays the ECG, two invasive pressures, and body temperature in addition to providing a strip chart printer. **F.** The OR Data Manager is controlled by a keyboard which slides out of a compartment under the table top. It captures all operative data and stores it on a floppy disk. These data are displayed on a mobile screen during anesthesia (not shown), and at the end of surgery the data are printed out to provide a detailed anesthetic record. (© 1991 L. Rendell-Baker.)

than the manufacturer's servicing agent, who handles only one make of equipment. Before signing a contract, seek bids from all companies offering this service in the area and check with other hospitals to discuss their experience with the service provided.

Large medical centers with an efficient biomedical engineering department may wish to consider having the servicing of the equipment carried out by the center's own staff. In this way, the staff can become familiar with a wide range of equipment and can advise on the choice of apparatus and inspect it before purchase. Their opinion will be unbiased, unlike that of the local equipment supplier. A biomedical engineering department can help to unify the choice of equipment throughout the hospital, thus avoiding the purchase of incompatible pieces of equipment, all requiring their own specific attachments.

Final Preuse Check

Although some servicing companies check the apparatus after servicing and warrant it to be in good working order, some manufacturers give the user the responsibility for the final check by attaching a prominent label to the apparatus warning that it should be checked before use.

ORGANIZATION OF DEPARTMENTAL ANCILLARY SERVICES

In a large hospital with many operating rooms, it can be difficult to keep apprised of how the operations are progressing, where help may be needed, and which operating rooms are vacant. One method used successfully in a hospital with 22 operating rooms on three contiguous floors was to install

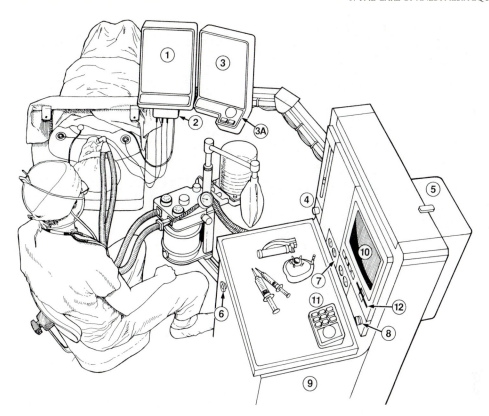

Figure 9–17. Future anesthesia workstation. Good human factors engineering has been used in this design of a future computer-operated servo-controlled anesthesia workstation. It incorporates presently available components arranged so that the patient monitor (1) and the apparatus monitors and controls (2) are close to the patient and face the user when observing the patient.

Featured are: Patient monitor (1) with analog and digital displays of the end tidal CO_2, ECG, pulse rate, noninvasive blood pressure, intraarterial blood pressure and another pressure, pulse oximeter and body temperature, inspired O_2 and anesthetic agent, minute and tidal volumes, respiratory frequency and airway pressure. The connections from the patient are attached to the monitor at (2). Panel (3) contains the monitors and contols for the workstation's functions such as the flow rates of the anesthetic gases and vapors and the ventilation provided. The anesthetist uses the track ball controller (3A) to pull down the desired menu on the screen to set the apparatus parameters. Once these have been set, the computer monitors the function of the apparatus and corrects for any deviation, alerting the user to any problems needing attention. (4) Total gas flow monitor and emergency O_2 flow control in the event of loss of all electrical power supplies. (5) Scavenged cabinet for the bottles of volatile anesthetic agents which are connected to the vaporizer's pump. (6) Emergency O_2 flush. (7) Pipeline gas supply pressure gauges. Emergency cylinder gas pressure gauges. (8) Main ON/OFF control for gases and electrical power. (9) Cabinet containing the electronic gas flow meters, micropump operated vaporizer, and back-up battery power with trickle charger. (10) Display of intraoperative monitored data, which is recorded on floppy disk for later production of the anesthesia record printed out in the recovery room. (11) Track ball controller to permit data to be added to anesthesia record. (12) Floppy disk records data for printout in recovery room. (© *1991 L. Rendell-Baker.*)

a TV surveillance camera in each operating room. It was arranged so that the anesthetist and the anesthesia apparatus appeared on the screen in the foreground, and because the cameras had wide-angle lenses, the picture included the entire operating room. Small TV monitoring screens for each operating room were mounted at the operating room control desk, where they could be seen by the operating room and anesthesia supervisors (Fig. 9–21). A two-way speaker and microphone permitted instant communication with any operating room. The cost of this installation was

modest, as the cameras and monitors were the type used for security monitoring in shops and other commercial establishments. The ease of control provided was invaluable.

Operating Room Intercom System

Communication between the operating rooms and 30 locations, including the equipment rooms, blood banks, laboratories, and operating room supervisor's office, is greatly simplified by the use of a two-way speaker and microphone

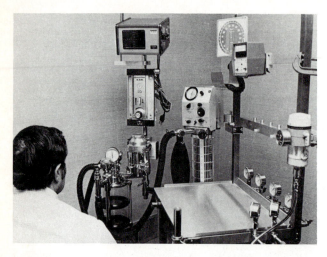

Figure 9–18. Harris-Lake "Line of Sight" anesthesia apparatus, designed by Chalmers Goodyear and Leslie Rendell-Baker, MD, and built for the Department of Anesthesiology, Mt. Sinai Medical Center, New York, in 1976. The engineer is seated to show how the machine's controls face the anesthetist seated at the head of the operating room table and looking at the patient. (© *1987 L. Rendell-Baker.*)

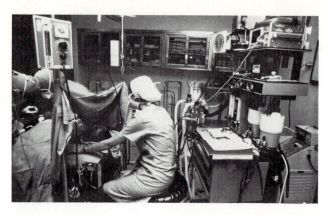

Figure 9–19. How not to arrange your apparatus for greatest safety. Would you fly with an airline that required the pilot to look over his or her shoulder to check the instruments while landing? Should not we also have our instruments in front of us like the pilot? (© *L. Rendell-Baker.*)

on the operating room wall behind the anesthetist (Fig. 9–22).

Anesthesia Technician Call System

A call button for the anesthesia technicians is placed beside the operating room door, where it can be activated as the anesthetist and surgeon move the patient from the operating room to the recovery room (Fig. 9–23). This button sounds a chime and illuminates a number on a call panel in the anesthesia equipment room (Fig. 9–24) to notify the technicians that the operating room is clear and ready for

removal of used equipment and restocking of drugs and apparatus. This system reduces cleanup time between cases and makes the maximum use of the technician's time.

Organization of Anesthesia Supplies

The myriad items needed for the everyday practice of anesthesia no longer fit into the drawers in the anesthesia apparatus. A drug and equipment cart is essential (Fig. 9–25). Many anesthesia departments in the past used the tool cabinets sold by commercial firms. These cabinets, made from painted steel, are much less expensive; however, they are prone to rust if washed down with disinfectant solutions and are not easy to clean. The contrast between a large department without a well-organized disposal and cleaning system (Fig. 9–26) and one with an efficient system (Fig. 9–27) is immediately apparent. Providing one recepta-

TABLE 9–4. COLORS USED ON CATHETERS IN THE UNITED STATES AND THOSE PROPOSED FOR AN INTERNATIONAL STANDARD

	Present U.S. Catheter Colors				
	14 Gauge	*16 Gauge*	*18 Gauge*	*20 Gauge*	*22 Gauge*
Abbocath (Abbot)	Gold/tan	Gray	Green	Pink	Dark blue
Medicut (Argyle)	Orange/tan	Gray	Green	Dark pink	Blue
IV Cath (B-D)	Light gray	Lavender	Light pink	Light yellow	Dark gray
Longdwell (D-B)	Olive	Purple	Pink	Yellow	Black
Angiocath (Deseret)	Pink	Yellow	Tan	Light green	Light blue
Cathlon (Jelco)	Orange	Gray	Dark green	Pink	Dark blue
Quick Cath (Vicra)	Orange	Gray	Light green	Light pink	Light blue
Equivalent metric size	2.0 mm	1.6 mm	1.2 mm	0.9 mm	0.7 mm
ISO/TC84 Proposed International Standard Colors*					
	Orange	Gray	Green	Pink	Blue

* Based on the existing French national standard; note several manufacturers already comply with this.

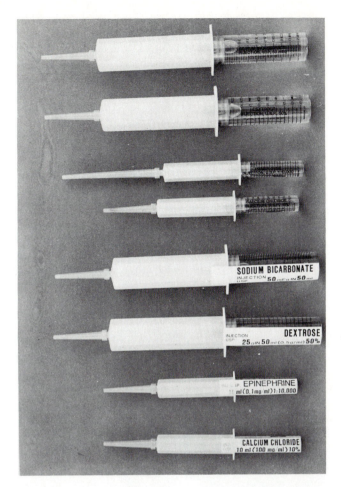

Figure 9–20. New, clearly legible labels for prefilled syringes are shown here on the lower four syringes. The ASTM standard D4775 (see Appendix II.A3) requires that they be legible, through the barrel, at 5 ft, that is, across the patient's bed or litter. They form a vivid contrast with the old, difficult-to-read labels seen on the upper four syringes. (© *1987 L. Rendell-Baker.*)

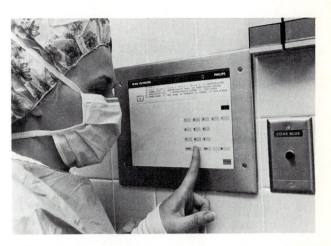

Figure 9–22. Anesthetist using a two-way intercom in the operating room. This provides direct contact with 30 locations, including the anesthesia equipment room, blood bank, blood gas laboratory, pathology frozen-section laboratory, recovery room, and operating room switchboard. (© *1987 L. Rendell-Baker.*)

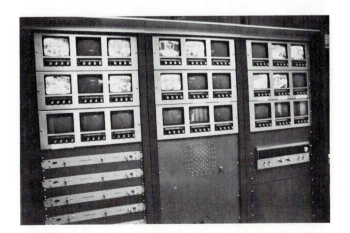

Figure 9–21. TV monitors provide at a glance the information needed from 22 operating rooms on three floors. (© *1987 L. Rendell-Baker.*)

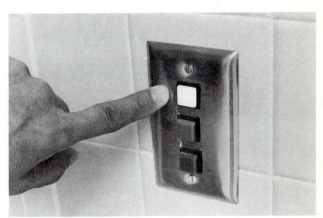

Figure 9–23. Operating room call system. By pressing the yellow top button the anesthetist tells the anesthesia technician and the operating room supervisor that the procedure is completed and that the operating room is ready to receive the next patient; the lowest green button is then pressed. The center red button is pressed when the next patient enters the operating room. This tells the operating room supervisor and the anesthesia staff that the room is occupied. (© *1987 L. Rendell-Baker.*)

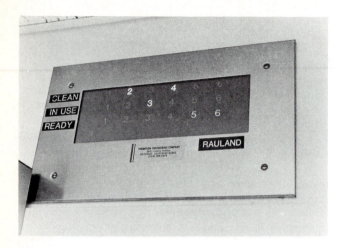

Figure 9–24. Operating room status monitor in anesthesia work room and operating room supervisor's office. The **2** and **4** in the top row indicate that those operating rooms are ready to be cleaned. The **3** in the center row indicates that the room is in use, and the **5** and **6** in the bottom row show that those operating rooms are ready for their next patients. (© *1987 L. Rendell-Baker.*)

cle for contaminated equipment that is to be cleaned and another for trash greatly simplifies the work of the technicians, and the apparatus is quickly readied for the next operation (Fig. 9–28). There have become available modular plastic carts and cabinets (Fig. 9–29) that are more easily cleaned and do not rust or corrode. They can be assembled from interchangeable components to accommodate the specific equipment needed; however, one must check that their drawers slide easily.

Accidental Injection of the Wrong Drug

Because many drugs are drawn up into syringes before the commencement of anesthesia, it is important to ensure that the syringes are clearly labeled. Unfortunately, confusion can easily arise when syringe labels of similar colors are used for drugs as different as succinylcholine and Sublimaze (fentanyl). The inadvertent injection of 5 mL of succinylcholine before the thiopental when fentanyl was intended is an error that neither patient nor anesthetist is likely to forget. The syringe label colors used in each hospital may vary, and anesthetists working in several hospitals can easily be misled. To bring order to this situation ASTM Standards Subcommittee D10.34, comprising anesthetists and other users, drug firms, and label manufacturers, devel-

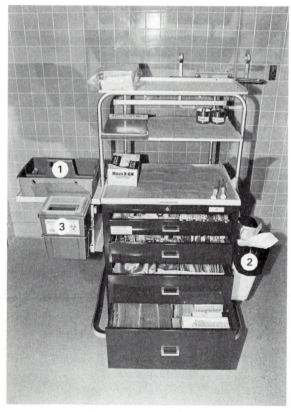

A

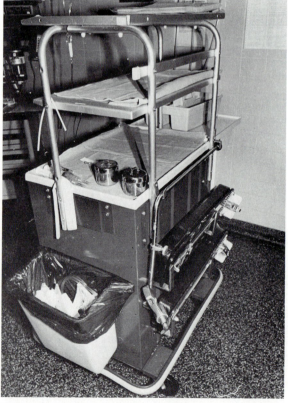

B

Figure 9–25.   A. The anesthesia drug and equipment cart (Blue Bell Biomedical, Blue Bell, Pennsylvania) enables one to separate reusables (laryngoscopes, face masks, etc.), which are placed in the plastic basket **(1)** for cleaning, from disposables, which are placed in the plastic trash bag in the basket **(2).** Syringes, needles, and ampules are placed in the plastic sharps collection system box **(3)** (Devon Industries Inc., 9530 DeSoto Avenue, Chatsworth California). **B.** The back of the cart has hooks for patient screen and arm boards. (© *1987 L. Rendell-Baker.*)

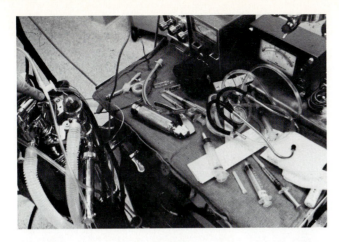

Figure 9–26. An anesthesia department with no cleanup system. This is the way many gas machines looked at the end of an operation before a proper system for the disposal of used equipment was introduced. Note the heavy contamination from used tracheal tub, suction catheter, and laryngoscope lying on the machine. (© 1987 L. Rendell-Baker.)

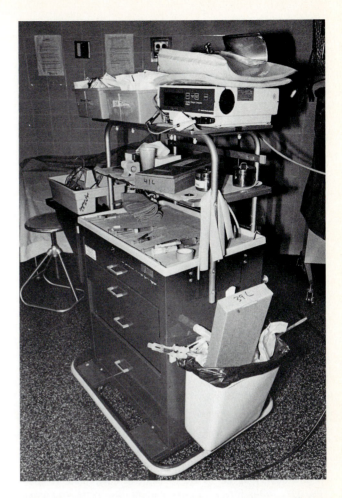

Figure 9–27. An anesthesia department with an efficient cleanup system. Anesthesia drug and equipment cart at the end of a thoracic operation. The reusable equipment to be cleaned has been placed in the plastic caddy on the far end of the cart; the disposables and trash are overflowing the trash basket, indicating that a larger one is needed. (© 1987 L. Rendell-Baker.)

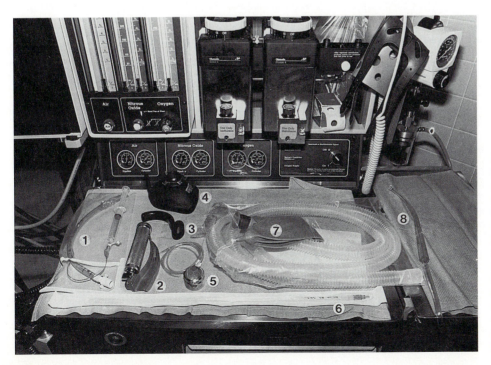

Figure 9–28. Anesthesia apparatus ready for use with clean towel on table top and **(1)** tracheal tube* with attached 10-mL syringe, **(2)** laryngoscope with Macintosh blade,* **(3)** Guedel oral airway,* **(4)** face mask,* **(5)** Wenger precordial stethoscope, **(6)** esophageal stethoscope,* **(7)** disposable breathing system and bag,* and **(8)** Yankauer suction handle.* (Items followed by an asterisk were unpacked for this photograph, but are normally supplied packaged clean or sterile.)

157

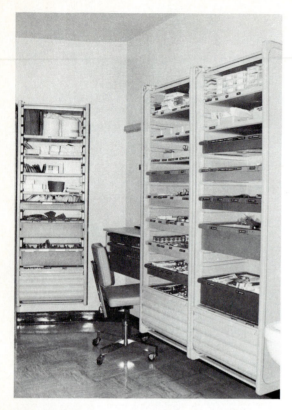

Figure 9–29. Modular plastic anesthesia equipment lockers with roll-up tambour doors are hung from the wall. The depth of the trays may be varied to suit the equipment. A charting desk with drawers forms part of the same equipment installation (Herman Miller Inc., Zeeland, Michigan). (© *1987 L. Rendell-Baker.*)

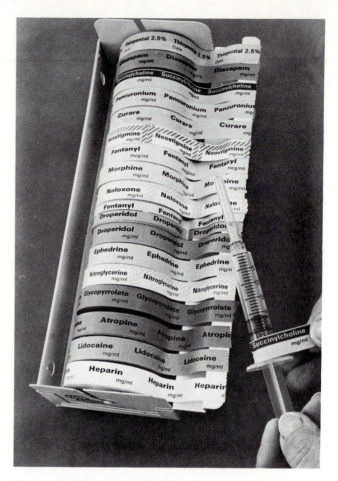

Figure 9–30. Standard syringe labels developed by the American Society for Testing and Materials Subcommittee D10.34 (see Appendix II). Standard colors, defined by the Pantone Matching System for printers' inks, are used to indicate the group to which a drug belongs. Examples: induction agents, Pantone yellow; tranquilizers, PMS 151 orange; muscle relaxants, PMS 811 fluorescent red; narcotics, PMS 297 blue; vasopressors, PMS 256 violet; local anesthetics, PMS 401 gray; anticholinergics, PMS 367 green. The antagonists are distinguished by diagonal stripes of the agonist color alternating with white stripes. (© *1987 L. Rendell-Baker.*)

oped a range of standard colors for syringe labels published as ASTM Standard D4774 (Fig. 9–30). These labels are available from most label firms by quoting ASTM Standard No. D4774 (see also Appendix III footnote).

Dangerous Concentrated Solutions of Drugs

Drugs that must be diluted before use, such as potassium chloride, 1-in-1000 epinephrine, dopamine, and 10 or 20 percent lidocaine, are at present available in ampules, vials, and syringes. This makes a bolus overdose of the concentrated solution fatally easy to administer. Deaths caused by mistakenly injecting potassium chloride when sodium chloride is intended occur with frightening regularity, reported in Britain by the Medical Defence Union in London[56] and in the United States by the U.S. Pharmacopoeial Convention, Inc.[57] Accidental injections of concentrated 23.4 percent sodium chloride have been reported by the FDA.[58] To address this problem ASTM Subcommittee D10.34 evolved Standard D5022-88 to identify vials and ampules of concentrated solutions of drugs that required dilution before use. For identification these vials are fitted with black caps and metal closures, both marked with "Dilute Before Use" or a similar warning. Ampules are identified by a black band(s) above the constriction.*

Until these changes are reflected in the marketplace, these solutions, because they are rarely needed at a

moment's notice, should be kept in the pharmacy where suitable dilutions can be prepared on request. In hospitals without 24-hour pharmacy service concentrated solutions should be kept under lock and key away from the other drug supplies.

Anesthesia Equipment Room

Good storage facilities will greatly simplify the tasks of technicians and anesthetists. Small plastic bins of various sizes can be used for curved tracheal tube connectors and other small parts, and tracheal tubes can be stored in larger bins (Fig. 9–31). These bins hang on racks attached to the wall. Modular plastic lockers with roll-up doors that also hang

---

* These requirements have now been adopted by the U.S. Pharmacopoeia in its requirements for concentrated potassium chloride solutions, and will become effective January 15, 1993.

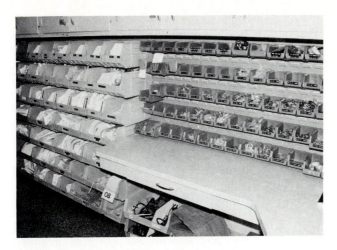

Figure 9–31. Plastic storage bins for tracheal tube connectors and tracheal tubes facilitate the orderly storage of these small parts in the anesthesia equipment room. (© *1987 L. Rendell-Baker.*)

from the wall (see Fig. 9–29) provide excellent flexibility in arranging an equipment room. The depth of the shelves or drawers can be chosen to suit the size and type of equipment to be stored. When the requirements change, the lockers can be rearranged or relocated readily. Manufacturers of modular hospital furniture are always ready to help solve a storage problem or help plan a new facility.

REFERENCES

1. Phillips CR. The sterilization action of gaseous ethylene oxide. II Sterilization of contaminated objects and related compounds. Time, concentration and temperature relationships. *Am J Hyg.* 1947;50:280.
2. McDonald RL. Methods of sterilizing. U.S. Patent No. 3.068.064:1962.
3. Snow JC, Mangiaracine AB, Anderson ML. Sterilization of anesthesia equipment with ethylene oxide. *N Engl J Med.* 1962;266:443.
4. *Federal Register.* June 22, 1984; 49(122):25,801–25,802.
5. Pennsylvania Engineering Co., Recipient of EPA Stratospheric Ozone Protection Award, December 1991. 1107-21 North Howard Street; Philadelphia, PA 10123.
6. Berry AJ, Isaacsen IJ, Hunt D, et al. The prevalence of hepatitis B viral markers in anesthesia personnel. *Anesthesiology.* 1984,60:6.
7. Berry AJ, Isaacsen IJ, Kane MA, et al. A multicenter study of the prevalence of hepatitis B viral serology-markers in anesthesia personnel. *Anesth Analg.* 1984;63:738.
8. Centers for Disease Control. Update: Acquired immunodeficiency syndrome and human immunodeficiency virus infection among health care workers. *MMWR.* 1988;37:229.
9. Centers for Disease Control. Guidelines for prevention of transmission of HIV and hepatitis B to health care and public safety workers. *MMWR.* 1989;38:S6.
10. Centers for Disease Control Update. Universal precautions for prevention of transmission of HIV, HbV and other blood-borne pathogens in health care settings. *MMWR.* 1988;37:24.
11. Occupational exposure to bloodborne pathogens: Final rules. Federal Register Part 2 Department of Labor OSHA. December 6, 1991; 29CFR Part 1910-1030.
12. OSHA Instruction CPL2-2.44B, Feb. 27, 1990. Enforcement procedure for occupational exposure to hepatitis B virus (HBV) and human immunodeficiency virus (HIV).
13. Braathen LR, Ramirez G, Kunze ROF, et al. Langerhans cells as primary target cells for HIV infection. *Lancet.* 1987;2:1094.
14. Niedecken H, Lutz G, Bauer R, et al. Langerhans cells and primary target and vehicle for transmission of HIV. *Lancet.* 1987;2:519.
15. Kay LA. Immunology of human skin and susceptibility to HIV infection. *Lancet.* 1987;2:166.
16. Dunne DW, Keggi JM, Korneck JJ, et al. Physicians in training and HIV. *N Engl J Med.* 1990;322:1392–1393.
17. York E. When a house office gets AIDS. *N Engl J Med.* 1990;322:1155. Letter.
18. Selwyn PA, Hartel D, Lewis VA, et al. A prospective study of the risk of tuberculosis among I/V drug users with human immunodeficiency virus infection. *N Engl J Med.* 1989;320:545.
19. Pitchenick AE, Cole C, Russell BW, et al. Tuberculosis, atypical mycobacteriosis and acquired immunodeficiency syndrome among Haitian and non-Haitian patients in South Florida. *Ann Intern Med.* 1984;101:641.
20. Chaisson RE, Schechter GF, Theurer CP, et al. Tuberculosis in patients with acquired immunodeficiency syndrome, clinical features, response to therapy. *Am Rev Respir Dis.* 1987;136:570.
21. Pitchenick AE, Rubinson HA. The radiographic appearance of tuberculosis in patients with acquired immunodeficiency syndrome (AIDS) and pre-AIDS. *Am Rev Respir Dis.* 1985;131:393.
22. Montgomery AB, Corkery KJ, Baunette ER. Occupational exposure to aerosolized pentamidine. *Chest.* 1990;98:386–388.
23. Centers for Disease Control. Tuberculosis and acquired immunodeficiency syndrome, New York City. *MMWR.* 1987;36:785–795.
24. duMoulin, GC, Stottmeir KD. Water-borne mycobacteria: An increasing threat to health. *ASM News.* 1986;53:525–529.
25. duMoulin GC, Hedley-Whyte J. Bacterial interactions between anesthesiologists, their patients and equipment. *Anesthesiology.* 1982;57:37–44.
26. duMoulin GC, Stottmeir KD, Pelletier PA, et al. Concentrations of *Mycobacterium avium* by hospital hot water systems. *JAMA.* 1988;260:1599–1601.
27. Roberts RB. Infections and sterilization problems. *Int Anesthesiol Clin.* 1972;10:1–177.
28. Rendell-Baker L. Standards of anesthetic and ventilatory equipment. *Int Anesthesiol Clin.* 1982;20:171.
29. Rendell-Baker L. *Standards for anesthesia.* In: Brown BR, ed. *The issues in future anesthesia delivery systems.* Philadelphia: Davis; 1982:59–78.
30. Cooper JB, Newbower RS, et al. Preventable anesthesia mishaps: A study of human factors. *Anesthesiology.* 1978;49:399–406.
31. Cooper JB, Long CD, et al. Multi-hospital study of preventable anesthesia mishaps. *Anesthesiology.* 1979;51:S348. Abstract.
32. Cooper JB, Newbower RS, et al. An analysis of major errors and equipment failures in anesthesia: Considerations for prevention and detection. *Anesthesiology.* 1984;60:34–42.
33. FDA Contract 223-82-5070, Report 86-4205: Accidental breathing system disconnections.
34. ASTM Standard F1054-87; Standard specification for conical fittings of 15 mm and 22 mm sizes.
35. *AAMI recommended practice on reuse of hemodialyzers 1990.* Available from AAMI, 3330 Washington Blvd, Suite 400, Arlington, VA 22201-4598.
36. Greene VW. Reuse of disposable medical devices: Historical and current aspects. *Infect Contr.* 1986;7(10):508–513.
37. *FDA Compliance Policy Guide 7124-16: Reuse of medical devices.* Washington, DC: U.S. Govt. Printing Office; Sept. 24, 1987.
38. Hedley Whyte J. Medicolegal and infection risks of reuse of single use supplies and equipment in anesthesiology. In: *Reuse of disposable medical devices in the 1980's. Proceedings of an International Conference, March 29–30, 1984.* Washington, DC: Institute for Health Policy Analysis, Georgetown Medical Center; 1984;149–155.

39. duMoulin GC, Saubermann AJ. The anesthesia machine and circle system are not likely to be sources of bacterial contamination. *Anesthesiology.* 1977;47:353–358.
40. Feeley WT, Hamilton WK, et al. Sterile anesthesia breathing circuits do not prevent postoperative pulmonary infection. *Anesthesiology.* 1981;54:369.
41. Pace NL, Webster C, et al. Failure of anesthetic circuit bacterial filters to reduce postoperative pulmonary infections. *Anesthesiology.* 1979;51(3):S362.
42. Garibaldi RA, Britt MR, et al. Failure of bacterial filters to reduce the incidence of pneumonia after inhalation anesthesia. *Anesthesiology.* 1981;54:364.
43. Mazze RI. Bacterial air filters. *Anesthesiology.* 1981;54:359. Editorial.
44. Loeb RQ, Brunner JX, Westenskow DR. The Utah anesthesia workstation. *Anesthesiology.* 1989;70:999–1007.
45. Cooper JB, Newbower RS, Moore JW, et al. A new anesthesia delivery system. *Anesthesiology.* 1978;49:310–318.
46. Norlander OP, Krill P, Lassborn O, et al. A new integrated system for anesthesia. Abstract 99. Presented at the 7th European Congress on Anaesthesia, Vienna, 1986.
47. Marks WE, Bullard JR. Another hazard of free-standing vaporizers: Increased anesthetic concentrations with reversed flow of vaporizing gas. *Anesthesiology.* 1976;45:445.
48. Munson WM. Cardiac arrest: Hazard of tipping a vaporizer. *Anesthesiology.* 1965;26:235.
49. Capan L, Ramanathan S, et al. A possible hazard with the use of the Ohio Ethrane vaporizer. *Anesth Analg.* 1980;59:65.
50. Rendell-Baker L, Meyer JA. Accidental disconnection and pulmonary barotrauma. *Anesthesiology.* 1983;58:286.
51. Chalon J, Mahgul A, et al. *Humidification of Anesthetic Gases.* Springfield, IL: Charles C Thomas; 1981.
52. American Association of Nurse Anesthetists. AANA endorses apparatus checklist. *JAANA* 1986;54:494.
53. Eichhorn JH, et al. Standards for patient-monitoring during anesthesia at Harvard Medical School. *JAMA.* 1986;256:1017–1020.
54. AANA endorses Harvard monitoring standards. *AANA J.* 1986.
55. Katz R. Lessons learned from malpractice review. ASA Refresher Course Lecture 134A, 1986.
56. Rendell-Baker L. Paraplegia from accidental injection of potassium chloride. *Anaesthesia.* 1985;40:912–913.
57. U.S.P. Proposal to revise monograph on potassium chloride injections (July–August 1989) PF 15(4), p. 5342.
58. FDA Notice, June 1990.

APPENDIXES: INFORMATION RESOURCES FOR EQUIPMENT STANDARDS AND PROCEDURES

Appendix I

The following documents on steam and ethylene oxide sterilization and performance of medical equipment may be obtained from

Dawn Helsing
Association for Advancement of Medical Instrumentation
3330 Washington Blvd, Suite 400
Arlington, VA 22201–4598
(703) 525–4890

A. *Good Hospital Practices*
1. Steam sterilization and sterility assurance
2. Steam sterilization using the unwrapped method (Flash sterilization)
3. Handling and biological decontamination of reusable medical devices
4. Ethylene oxide gas-ventilation recommendations and safe use
5. Performance evaluation of ethylene oxide sterilizers—EO test packs
6. Ethylene oxide sterilization and sterility assurance

B. *Standards and Recommended Practices*
1. Hospital steam sterilizers
2. Automatic, general-purpose ethylene oxide sterilizers and sterilant sources intended for use in health care facilities
3. Determining residual ethylene oxide, ethylene chlorhydrin, and ethylene glycol in medical devices
4. Chemical sterilants and sterilization methods—A guide to selection and use
5. Selection and use of chemical indicators for steam sterilization monitoring in health care facilities
6. Autologous transfusion devices
7. Infant incubators
8. Infusion devices
9. Sphygmomanometers, electronic or automated
10. Human engineering guidelines and preferred practice for design of medical devices

Appendix II

The following standards applicable to anesthesia practice may be obtained from

American Society for Testing and Materials
1916 Race Street
Philadelphia, PA 19103

A. *Contact Margie Lawlor at (215) 299-5518 for these D10.34 documents:*
1. D4627-89: Standard specifications for the legibility of labels for small-volume (less than 100 mL) parenteral drug containers
2. D4774-88: Standard practice for user-applied drug labels in anesthesiology*
3. D4775-88: Standard specifications for identification and configuration of prefilled syringes and delivery systems for drugs—excluding pharmacy bulk packages

* Syringe labels complying with this standard may be obtained from label manufacturers including the following: United Ad Label, Inc., P.O. Box 2165, 1035 S. Greenleaf Ave., Whittier, CA 90610; TimeMed Labelling Systems Inc., 144 Tower Drive, Hinsdale, IL 60521; Shamrock Scientific Systems, Inc., 34 Davis Drive, Bellwood, IL 60104.

4. D5022-89: Standard specification for identification of vials and ampules containing concentrated solutions of drugs to be diluted before use.

B. *Contact Beth Moran at (215) 299-5517 for these F29 documents:*

1. F920-85: Minimum performance and safety requirements for resuscitation intended for use with humans
2. F927-86: Pediatric tracheostomy tubes
3. F960-86: Medical and surgical suction and drainage systems
4. F965-85: Rigid laryngoscopes for tracheal intubation—hook-on fittings for laryngoscope handles and blades with lamps
5. F984-86: Cutaneous gas monitoring devices for oxygen and carbon dioxide
6. F1161-88: Minimum performance and safety requirements for components and systems of anesthesia gas machines
7. F1208-89: Minimum performance and safety requirements for anesthesia breathing systems
8. F1054-87: Standard practice for conical fittings of 15-mm and 22-mm sizes
9. F1242-89: Cuffed tracheostomy tubes
10. F1205-88: Standard specification for breathing tubes
11. F1243-89: Standard specification for tracheal tube connectors
12. F1100-90: Standard specification for ventilators intended for use in critical care
13. F1101-90: Standard specification for ventilators intended for use during anesthesia
14. In preparation: Standard specifications for blood gas analyzers
15. In preparation: Standard specification for humidifiers for medical use
16. In preparation: Standard specification for oxygen analyzers for monitoring patient breathing mixtures
17. In preparation: Standard specification for home-care ventilators
18. In preparation: Oxygen concentrators for medical use

Appendix III

The following pamphlet can be obtained from:

Don Slee
Compressed Gas Association
1235 Jefferson Davis Highway
Arlington, VA 22202

Pamphlet V5, Diameter
Index Safety System

10

Environmental Safety

M. Regina B. Puno and
Benjamin M. Rigor

Approximately one-quarter million health care professionals and employees and two million surgical patients in the United States are exposed to operating room hazards every year. These hazards or potentially dangerous conditions include the risk of infection with various microorganisms; stress and pressure from hectic work schedules, from interaction with other members of the surgical and operating room teams, from the constant vigilance required, and from other extraneous factors such as noise and hypothermia; risk of addiction from substance use and abuse; such physical agents as radiation, fire and explosion, and electric shock or electrocution; and, finally, medical gases and chemicals, such as ambient and trace levels of anesthetic gases, ethylene oxide fumes, and vapors of methylmethacrylate. This chapter focuses on environmental safety by identifying and discussing proven or suspect hazards in the operating room and the suggested/recommended guidelines or precautions to take.

THE RISK OF INFECTION

The problems of infection and contamination of equipment have been discussed in Chapter 9. This section addresses the risk of infection for patients and hospital personnel.

Nosocomial infections are those infections originating in the hospital that may be transmitted from patient to hospital personnel, or vice versa, and from patient to patient. Anesthesia personnel may also play an important role in the spread of nosocomial infections because of their contact with nasopharyngeal secretions, considered to be a microbiological hazard. The risk of spread of these types of infection confirms the need for the use of gloves in manipulations involving the oropharynx. Occupationally acquired bacterial infection in healthy individuals is not common unless the immune system is already compromised; however, the surgical patient is vulnerable to bacterial infection. Understandably, this risk is minimized by aseptic surgical technique. Additional measures can be used to reduce bacteria in the conventional operating room environment:

1. Decreasing the number of personnel in the room.
2. Keeping doors closed.
3. Using disposable gowns, gloves, and drapes.
4. Using ultraviolet radiation over an open incision or wound.
5. Using occlusive, nonwoven gowns.
6. Regularly washing trolleys or stretchers used to transfer patients into the operating room, particularly around the wheels.

Some type of laminar-airflow system or some other method of environmental control has been suggested as being the most important factor in reducing bacterial contamination in the operating room.

Presently, health care workers in many settings are concerned with being exposed to hepatitis B and acquired immunodeficiency syndrome (AIDS). In the anesthesia practice setting, hepatitis B and herpetic whitlow have been documented as being work-related hazards; AIDS has not been reported.

With our increased knowledge of the mechanics for transmission of infection, we now have specific recommendations and strategies for infection control. In general, these include the use of physical barriers (gloves, masks, eyeglasses, and gowns) and immunologic protection with active or passive immunization. Regular educational programs are essential for all employees involved in the contact of patients, laboratory specimens, or contaminated instruments and supplies. An efficient system for maintaining immunization records, reporting, and follow-up of accidental exposure results in decreased morbidity and absenteeism from infections acquired from the workplace.

Respiratory Viruses

Influenza A and B viruses, parainfluenza, rhinovirus, adenovirus, and respiratory syncytial virus (RSV) are respiratory viruses. Small-particle aerosols or large droplets containing these viruses may be produced by coughing, sneezing, or talking. Transmission may occur by small-particle aerosols propelled over a large distance, as with influenza, or by close person-to-person contact where large nasopharyngeal droplets contaminate hands or inanimate surfaces, as with RSV and rhinovirus, thus transferring the virus to the susceptible individual, usually by self-inoculation from the hand.

Recommendations to prevent the spread of diseases caused by the respiratory viruses include the following:

1. Respiratory isolation precautions for the duration of the clinical illness.
2. Annual immunization of hospital staff against influenza.
3. Use and disposal of gowns, gloves, and masks in an approved manner.
4. Careful, thorough handwashing between patient contacts.
5. Limiting elective hospital admissions and surgery during community epidemics.

Herpesviruses

The herpetoviridines include varicella zoster virus (VZV), herpes simplex virus types I and II, cytomegalovirus (CMV), and Epstein-Barr virus (EBV). VZV is spread by direct contact or by small-particle aerosols, but the remaining herpesviruses are transmitted by close contact. After primary infection with the herpes viruses, the organism becomes latent and may reactivate at a later time.

Nosocomial infection is not common except among pediatric and immunosuppressed patients, because by middle age most individuals have been infected by all the different herpetoviridines and have, as a result, acquired immunity. Herpetic whitlow, or herpetic infection of the finger, however, is a well-recognized occupational hazard for anesthesia personnel. A finger in which skin integrity has been broken may be inoculated by direct contact with oral secretions of infected but asymptomatic patients. A diagnosis of herpes simplex can be made from smears from the vesicle fluid showing giant epithelial cells or nuclear inclusion bodies. Treatment is conservative and surgical drainage is not necessary.

The guidelines recommended for preventing transmission of herpetoviridines are as follows:

1. Performing serologic testing to determine immunity in health care workers without a history of the clinical illness.
2. Administering immune globulin to susceptible personnel who have been exposed.
3. Considering dressings from infected patients as infectious because of the large number of viruses contained in the vesicles.
4. Advising women who are or who may become pregnant not to care for patients carrying CMV because it has the potential to cause congenital malformations.

Rubella

Twenty percent of women of childbearing age are susceptible to rubella infection. In the first trimester of pregnancy,

rubella is associated with congenital malformations or fetal death. Hospital outbreaks of rubella also carry significant loss in cost and in employee morbidity and absenteeism. Serologic documentation of immunity is advised for hospital employees. Vaccination of susceptible women of childbearing age and personnel who might transfer rubella to pregnant patients is recommended.

Viral Hepatitis

Hepatitis A. Infectious hepatitis, or hepatitis A virus (HAV), is spread by the fecal–oral route. This type of hepatitis is responsible for about one fifth of the cases of viral hepatitis in adults in the United States. Because hepatitis A virus usually causes a self-limited illness that does not require hospitalization, hospital employees are not at increased risk for this infection. Yet hospital outbreaks have occurred in which patients in the prodromal stage of infection were admitted. The diagnosis is made from the presence of serum anti-HAV IgM found 4 to 6 weeks after infection. Jaundiced hospitalized patients should be placed on enteric precautions until this etiology has been ruled out. Exposed individuals should be given immune serum globulin to diminish the chances of infection.

Hepatitis B. Serum hepatitis, or hepatitis B virus (HBV), is transmitted by contact with blood, blood products, or body fluids from individuals carrying the virus. Ninety percent of acute hepatitis B infections resolve without significant hepatic damage. The other 10 percent of infected patients become chronic HBV carriers, half of whom are likely to develop chronic active hepatitis if their infection persists for more than 2 years.

Hepatitis B virus is a hardy virus that may remain infectious for a week or longer in dried blood on environmental surfaces. Anesthesia personnel are at risk for accidental infection with HBV. This risk appears to begin when patient contact is initiated during training and continues throughout one's practice years. Surveys conducted both in the United States and in other countries have shown significantly higher prevalence for seropositivity to hepatitis B in anesthesia personnel.[1-11] The range of seropositivity (13 to 49 percent in surveys in the United States) probably reflects the prevalence of hepatitis B carriers in the local population. The prevalence in the general population in the United States is 3 to 5 percent on the basis of serologic screening of volunteers donating blood.[12]

Diagnosis of HBV is based on serologic testing. Within 3 to 4 weeks of infection, while the patient is still asymptomatic but already infectious, hepatitis B surface antigen (HBsAg) can be detected in the serum. Within 8 to 12 weeks of infection, symptoms of hepatitis, jaundice, and elevated liver enzymes occur. When the acute infection resolves, HBsAg disappears from the serum. Antibody to the surface antigen (anti-HBs) that confers lasting immunity from further HBV infections then is detectable.

There is a period or "window" between the decline of HBsAg and the detectability of anti-HBs when antibody to the core antigen (anti-HBc) is measurable. The presence of anti-HBc indicates a past infection with HBV. Anti-HBc and anti-HBs may both be detectable after the hepatitis B infection has resolved, but after many years, only one of them may still be measurable. HBsAg and anti-HBc are both likely to be present in chronic (and infective) HBV carriers.

Groups at very high risk for being HBV carriers have been identified. They include patients on hemodialysis, parenteral illicit drug users, homosexual males, and immigrants from endemic areas. Most of these groups are also at high risk for AIDS. Still, there are many unrecognized HBV carriers who are hospitalized, and routine clinical history and preoperative laboratory tests are rarely helpful in identifying them. Because of this, it is recommended that susceptible health care personnel working in high-risk specialties be given the hepatitis B vaccine.

The first hepatitis B vaccine developed was prepared from the plasma of chronic HBV carriers. Extensive evaluation showed no evidence that AIDS was transmitted by this plasma-derived vehicle.[13] The idea that AIDS could theoretically be transmitted through a vaccine made from the plasma of HBV carriers led to the development of a second hepatitis B vaccine composed of HBsAg made from bread yeast by recombinant technology.[14] This vaccine appears to be safe and effective,[15] but it is less effective in producing antibodies to HBV than vaccine prepared from plasma.[16]

Needle sticks from contaminated needles are very common. To avoid accidental skin puncture, injection of drugs through a stopcock is recommended over recapping of needles. In instances of actual exposure to contaminated needles or to blood from an HBsAg-positive patient, susceptible employees should receive prophylactic treatment as soon as possible with hepatitis B immune globulin (HBIG) and should be given the hepatitis B vaccine simultaneously. The dose of HBIG is repeated after 1 month.

The Centers for Disease Control (CDC) have formulated guidelines for correct handling and disposal of blood, body fluid, and objects soiled with these contaminated fluids.[17,18] These are the same guidelines for preventing transmission of human immunodeficiency virus (HIV), the etiological agent for AIDS; however, the guidelines were based on the epidemiology of hepatitis B as a worst-case model for transmission of bloodborne infections. These guidelines have been particularly successful in dialysis units and are summarized below.

1. All needles, blades, and sharp instruments should be carefully handled to prevent accidental injuries, and all should be considered potentially infected. Disposable sharp items should be placed in puncture-resistant containers located as close as is practical to the area in which they are used. Needles should not be recapped, bent, broken, or removed from disposable syringes by hand prior to their placement in appropriate disposable receptacles.

2. Gloves should be worn when touching mucous membranes or open skin of all patients. When the possibility exists of exposure to blood, body fluids, or items soiled with these, gloves should be used. With some procedures, such as endoscopy, when aerosolization or splashes of blood or secretions are likely to occur, masks, eye coverings, and gowns are indicated. Gloves and body coverings should be removed and disposed of properly after patient contact.

3. Strict attention should be given to handwashing, especially between patient contacts, after gloves are removed, even if there has been no direct contact with blood or fluid. If hands are accidentally contaminated with blood or other body fluids, they should be washed as soon as possible.

4. Resuscitation equipment that prevents the need for emergency mouth-to-mouth contact should be available.

5. Although the pregnant health care worker is not known to have an increased risk of contracting infection, the infant is at risk of infection from perinatal transmission. Pregnant women should be counseled on the precautions for preventing transmission in the health care setting.

6. Health facility workers who have exudative lesions or weeping dermatitis should not participate in direct patient care activities, which include performing or assisting with invasive procedures and handling contaminated equipment.

7. Workers in health care facilities with evidence of any illness that compromises their ability to safely perform invasive procedures should be evaluated to determine whether they are both physically and mentally competent to perform these procedures.

8. Routine serologic testing of health care personnel for infection is not recommended.

9. Disinfection procedures are currently recommended for use in health care institutions. Contaminated instruments should undergo routine sterilization or disinfection, and surfaces exposed to blood and body fluids should be cleaned with an appropriate germicide.

10. Potentially infective wastes should be transported in clearly identified plastic bags. If the outside of a bag is contaminated, a second outer bag should be used.

11. All specimens sent to laboratories should be handled as if infected.

If an exposure incident occurs follow the OSHA standard (see Appendix).

Hepatitis C. Hepatitis C virus (HCV), identified by Choo et al. in 1989,[19] is known to be the major causative agent of parenteral non-A, non-B hepatitis (NANBH). Viral hepatitis in the absence of serologic markers of known hepatotrophic agents, such as HAV, HBV, CMV, and EBV, is termed *NANBH*. NANBH includes two epidemiologically distinct types of hepatitis: parenterally transmitted and enterically transmitted.

Parenterally transmitted NANBH accounts for 20 to 40 percent of acute viral hepatitis in the United States and has epidemiologic characteristics similar to those of HBV.[20] About 90 percent of hepatitis that follows blood transfusion is parenteral NANBH.[21-23] NANBH may cause serious illnesses, including fulminant hepatitis and cirrhosis, and may result in the development of chronic hepatitis in an average of 50 percent of patients.[24] The role of person-to-person contact in disease transmission and the risk and consequences of perinatal transmission have not, however, been well defined and multiple episodes of NANBH observed among the same individuals may be caused by bloodborne agents other than HBC.

In May of 1990, the Food and Drug Administration approved the use of an enzyme immunoassay kit to detect HCV infection. Blood centers and blood banks in the United States now routinely test blood donors for the presence of the antibody to HCV, or anti-HCV. Blood components derived from donors found to be repeatedly positive for anti-HCV are discarded and the donors' names are placed on a deferral registry. Epidemiologic studies suggest that because HCV is the predominant agent of transfusion-associated NANBH, screening of blood donors for anti-HCV should prevent many cases of this disease.[25–27]

Precautions against HCV and parenteral NANBH are similar to those for hepatitis B. It is a reasonable practice to give immune globulin to individuals as soon as possible after percutaneous exposure to blood from patients with NANBH. Additionally, anti-HCV-positive patients should be evaluated for clinical and laboratory evidence of hepatitis. Until confirmatory tests to distinguish infectious from noninfectious anti-HCV-positive blood are developed, all anti-HCV-positive blood and individuals should be presumed infected and capable of transmitting HCV.

Although currently there is no available specific antiviral therapy for HCV, initial reports suggest that α-interferon may moderate HCV-related NANBH.[28,29] Patients with clinical hepatitis should be followed so that they may have access to specific therapy should it become available.

Acquired Immunodeficiency Syndrome

The human immunodeficiency virus (HIV), a retrovirus, is now known to be the agent responsible for AIDS, although not all individuals infected with HIV will develop AIDS or the AIDS-related complex.

Infection is spread by intimate sexual contact, by infected blood and blood products through transfusion or shared needles, perinatally from mother to child, and possibly through infected body secretions. The majority of those individuals with HIV have an antibody detectable through the use of an enzyme-linked immunosorbent assay (ELISA) test, on which a diagnosis is made. This antibody, however, neither results in the eradication of nor confers immunity to the virus.

An individual is considered to be both infected with HIV and infective if the ELISA and a supplemental, more sensitive test (either the Western blot or indirect fluorescent antibody) are repeatedly positive. Results of these tests become positive within weeks of inoculation, but the first opportunistic disease may not appear for 7 years or more.

Studies have shown that health care workers are at very low risk of contracting HIV infection even after parenteral exposure,[30–32] although infection has been documented in individuals who provided care to AIDS patients.[33] In a study of 1201 health care workers exposed to infected blood or body fluid, 95 percent with parenteral exposure, only 0.5 percent developed antibodies to HIV, with seroconversion usually occurring within 3 months of exposure.[34] Of the 1167 health care workers reported by the CDC in Atlanta to have been exposed to HIV-positive blood between 1983 and March 1990, none of the 74 workers with mucous membrane exposure or the 88 with nonintact skin exposure have tested positive.[35]

The minimal dose of contaminated blood needed to infect humans is unknown, but the likelihood of developing antibodies to HIV is probably volume related. The HIV is relatively fragile and several hours of drying will inactivate 90 to 99 percent of viable virus. The amount of HIV usually found on contaminated surgical instruments and equipment can be killed with careful cleaning and disinfection with a 1 : 10 to 1 : 100 dilution of sodium hypochlorite or household bleach.

Because there may be many undiagnosed patients carrying HIV, particularly victims of trauma, the same infection control recommendations as summarized under Hepatitis B should be used during all patient contact. Some centers now advise zidovudine (formerly called azidothymidine or AZT) prophylaxis for health care workers after occupational exposure to HIV-positive blood. The CDC reports increased acceptance of the prophylactic 42-day course of AZT from 1989 to 1990.[35]

Tuberculosis

The incidence of tuberculosis (TB) in the United States is now much lower since the discovery of streptomycin in 1947 and of isoniazid in 1952 and the improvement in the standard of living; however, hospital personnel are at risk from undiagnosed patients who may be hospitalized for initial workup. Routine periodic screening of employees for TB should be an employee health policy of hospitals and ambulatory care facilities, particularly in areas that report a significant number of new cases. Skin testing should be performed on personnel who might have been infected by patients who were later discovered to be contagious with tuberculosis. Those with previously negative skin tests that convert to a positive one should be advised to undergo isoniazid therapy. Active TB patients must be kept in respiratory isolation.

STRESS

Any job that involves accountability for the life or well-being of an individual inevitably carries the element of stress with it. Stress is a recognized potential health hazard of the operating room environment. A hectic or excessive work schedule, the process of making difficult decisions, the constant vigilance required in the operating room, night duty, fatigue, increasing reliance on technology, and interpersonal tensions cause stress for anesthesia and surgery personnel alike. Areas of stress that are very specific to the practice of anesthesia are (1) the induction of anesthesia, (2) overlapping realms of responsibility with the surgeon, and (3) dealing with uncertainty, the critically ill, and the dying patient. This discussion focuses on those sources and variables of stress that are subject to some degree of control.

Maintaining Vigilance

Vigilance is the most critical function performed by the anesthesia practitioner, and although necessary, it is not in itself sufficient for avoiding anesthetic mishaps. A vigilance task is defined as one requiring the detection of changes in stimulus during long monitoring periods when the subject has little or no prior knowledge of the sequence of the changes. Most vigilance tasks are accomplished at a 90 percent level of accuracy.[36] In the field of anesthesia, however, this performance level is still unacceptable because the consequences of an inappropriate response may be catastrophic.

The objective demands of this potentially difficult job can be a source of stress to the anesthesia practitioner, and attempts to improve proficiency in vigilance require the analysis of its components and the identification of factors that can improve or hinder performance.

There are several components to the vigilance task. First, it is a repetitious and monotonous function; however, the unpredictable nature and timing of changes in the parameters being monitored distinguish this task from other monotonous and repetitive tasks. Thus, the individual cannot pace himself or herself but must respond to the monitors' cues. The task is complex, needing manual dexterity, visual attention, and mental alertness; yet, it neither fully occupies mental activity nor leaves one free to perform other mental functions.[12]

As the ability to perform a vigilance task varies inversely with its complexity,[37] the factors that diminish the ability to sustain concentration are important considerations. Poor design in monitor displays, inappropriate equipment positioning in both the vertical and horizontal planes, and alarm artifacts are examples of factors that contribute to distraction from the primary vigilance task[38] and to fatigue from excessive and unnecessary energy expenditure. Even the perpetual use of one color in the operating suite has been suggested as a cause of fluctuation and lapses in concentration.[39]

The consideration of human factors in equipment design is the area of ergonomics, long recognized by industry as important. Work toward modernizing anesthetic equipment and the operating room environment to ergonometric standards has begun.[40–42] Computer technology for data integration to provide trending information and "intelligent" warnings of potential difficulties[43] as well as automation in anesthetic delivery[44–48] is a promising area of current research and development. (See also Standardized Equipment Layout under Standards for Patient Monitoring During Anesthesia in Chapter 9.)

The possibility of adverse influence on vigilance of noise, irregular hours, and exposure to trace anesthetic gases is discussed at length in other sections of this chapter.

Noise

The effects of noise depend on its intensity and duration. Intensity is logarithmically determined in decibels (dB), and an increase of 10 dB means that the intensity has increased 10-fold. The Occupational Safety and Health Administration (OSHA), the federal agency responsible for enacting, investigating, and enforcing health standards, has established levels for safe noise exposure. The maximum safe exposure is 90 dB for 8 hours.[49] Each increase of 5 dB halves the permissible exposure time so that 100 dB is allowed for only 2 hours a day. The maximum permissible exposure in an industrial setting is 115 dB. Ultimately, hearing loss results from excessive exposure to noise pollution.

Noise is an important factor in decreasing work productivity, in disrupting communication, in hindering concentration, and in contributing to physiologic stress.[50] Because the walls of the operating room provide sound-reflecting surfaces, noise levels can approach that which constitutes a health hazard.[51] Conversing in the operating room produces noise levels between 66 and 72 dB. The noise generated by operating power drills, opening packages of gloves, or having various objects strike the floor is even greater than that of normal conversation. Noise not only may affect operating room personnel but may disturb the patient.[52] Unnecessary sources of auditory distractions in the operating room and other acute care areas should therefore be kept to a minimum.

Irregular Work Hours

The body depends on environmental cues such as light and temperature to regulate physiologic functions, such as hormone release, sleep, and alertness. Periods of vulnerability to sleep in humans have been identified, with a major peak between 2 A.M. and 7 A.M. and a smaller peak in the midafternoon. Variable work schedules interfere with this circadian rhythm. In industry, the detrimental effect of sleep deprivation or disruption on work efficiency is well documented.[36,53,54] The finding that the majority of single-occupant motor vehicle and several catastrophic industrial accidents involving shift workers result from human error during these time periods seems to further support this concept.[55]

Fatigue from continuous wakefulness because of irregular work hours produces a measurable deterioration in psychomotor performance[56,57] and in the ability to concentrate on a task that requires sustained attention.[58–60] In surveys of anesthesia-related mishaps, fatigue has been the most frequently reported associated factor.[61,62] As a result, legislation that would limit work shifts has actually been instituted in some states or is being planned in others and is based on the concept that performance returns to normal levels after 24 hours of rest and recovery.

CHEMICAL DEPENDENCE

Questionnaires and treatment centers have been the primary sources of information for estimating the prevalence of the problem of chemical dependency among anesthesia personnel. Although bias may play a role in these types of reporting techniques,[63] the data suggest that a disproportionately high incidence of addictive disease exists in the specialty of anesthesia when compared with any other medical specialty.[64] In fact, some nurses and physicians have reported that they entered the anesthesia specialty because they believed it to be a relatively safe source of drugs.

To understand this serious potential occupational hazard, it is important to define terms relating to the subject.[65] *Addiction* is the compulsive continued use of a substance despite the adverse consequences. *Substance abuse* is the detrimental use of drugs but not to the point of addiction. *Chemical dependence* is a physical *or* psychologic dependence on a drug and implies lack of control over drug usage.

Impairment for physicians and nurses is the inability to perform as a professional person and as a practitioner of the healing arts because of alcoholism, drug abuse, mental illness, senility, or disabling disease.[66] *Recovery* is the process of conquering the disease.

Drug or substance addiction is best understood as a disease with both environmental and genetic factors involved in its etiology. The disease results from a vulnerable host and a favorable environment. Familial transmission of drug addiction has been documented.[67] Children of alcoholics are four times more likely to develop alcoholism.[68] Easily identifiable biologic markers of alcoholism are being looked into.[69,70] In the anesthesia environment, job stress, availability of addicting drugs, and lack of external recognition and respect may be contributing factors.

An individual's response to stress depends on the nature of the stress, modified by the person's level of vocational training, degree of experience,[71,72] age, and personality traits. Personality traits dictate which defense or coping mechanisms will be employed. Traits that have been identified to predispose the individual toward maladaptive behavior include the obsessive–compulsive/dependent character structure. These people typically manifest pessimism, passivity, self-doubt, and feelings of insecurity and respond to stress by internalizing anger and becoming hypochondrial and depressed.[73] A history of maladaptive behavior has been linked to the subsequent development of substance abuse.[74]

The addictive potential of the substance being abused is also a factor in the development of chemical dependence. The risk of addiction from casual abuse of alcohol and even morphine, meperidine, and codeine does not compare with the overwhelming addictive potential of fentanyl, sufentanil, and other potent opioids.[75,76]

Management of the chemically dependent colleague involves identification, intervention, referral for treatment, and help with reentry. Identification is difficult because the disease becomes apparent only in the late phase. Increasing withdrawal and isolation from outside interests occur first, followed by isolation from developing turmoil in the home. Unexpected illnesses, personality changes, frequent job changes, and moves between cities may follow. Job performance is usually the last to be affected because work is the source of the abused drug.

Intervention is the process of demonstrating to a chemically dependent person that he or she is ill and needs treatment. Intervention should never be attempted by just one person. The goal of treatment, which may consist of several months of inpatient therapy followed by several years of outpatient care, is to provide the recovering individual with the ability to remain sober with support from peer groups. Gradual return to work with continuing peer support is important to prevent the likelihood of relapse. Adequate narcotic control mechanisms should be implemented in the workplace to deter drug diversion.

Those individuals that have been previously dependent are referred to as recovering rather than cured, implying that chemical dependency is an incurable disease that can only be controlled. If left untreated, chemical dependency is a fatal illness. Most recovering individuals are able to return to a productive professional life.[77,78] We do not know how successful anesthesia personnel are at recovery as the successful outcomes are not indexed by medical specialty.

PHYSICAL AGENTS

Anesthetic Gases

When the possible biologic effects (Table 10–1) of occupational exposure to trace anesthetic gases were realized in the 1960s, investigators began to make decisions about ways to monitor the concentrations of these gases and to remove the excess or waste gases from the operating room atmosphere. Monitoring techniques were developed so that leaks in the breathing circuit and in anesthesia machines and their connections to the wall and to the breathing system could be detected. With the recognition and prevention of leaks, scavenging systems were developed to collect excess anesthetic gases and dispose of them outside of the building. Hospital equipment workshops were organized with facilities for pressure testing the components of anesthesia machines, and maintenance personnel and anesthesia technicians are made aware of the importance of this work through antipollution programs.

Reports on the effects of chronic environmental exposure to anesthetics have included epidemiologic surveys, in vitro studies, cellular research, and studies in laboratory animals and humans. In 1967, Vaisman,[79] in a survey of 303 Russian anesthetists, found that a wide variety of complaints were common, with headache, irritability, and fatigue being the most frequently reported. Of 31 pregnancies among operating room personnel, 18 ended in spontaneous abortions. Ether and nitrous oxide without scavenging were the most commonly used anesthetics in this survey. Although this study was very small and did not include a control group, Vaisman concluded that these complaints were due to factors in the working environment.

TABLE 10–1. ANESTHESIA POLLUTION: POSSIBLE ADVERSE BIOLOGIC EFFECTS

Behavioral and other constitutional effects
  Learning deficits
  Perceptual, cognitive, and motor skills
  Russian anesthesia study
    Increased irritability (84.4%)
    Recurrent headaches (78.5%)
    Increased fatigability (75.5%)
Ultrastructural abnormalities
  Liver, kidney, and nerve tissues
  Decreased myelin synthesis and brain maturation
Reproductive organs
  Spontaneous abortions
  Premature delivery
  Teratogenesis and congenital malformations
  Infertility and genital prematurity
Hematopoietic organs and systems
  Bone marrow depression and granulocytopenia
  Suppression of immune process
  Neoplasm of the RES
Carcinogenesis

Many other retrospective reports followed, addressing other issues such as increased incidence of congenital anomalies in offspring of anesthesiologists compared with those of other physicians and increased incidence of liver disease among anesthesia personnel. Three large studies conducted with questionnaires in the United States[80] and the United Kingdom[81] all concluded that there was an increased prevalence of spontaneous abortion in women working in the operating room.

A number of review articles[82–86] that critiqued the original data were then published. These articles pointed out the inconsistencies, the lack of control of confounding variables (Table 10–2), and the presence of flaws and biases that are inherent in information obtained by surveys and retrospective studies (Table 10–3). Interest in the adverse effects of waste anesthetic gases waned in intensity after nearly all the data appeared inconclusive. There is a need for well planned long-term prospective studies to assess the possible hazards of exposure to trace anesthetic gases. Such a study involving 11,000 women in Great Britain is currently under way.[87]

Many of the other reported in vitro, cellular research, and laboratory animal studies that attempted to determine the effects of anesthetic exposure were likewise equivocal, with no definite proof of a relationship to irreversible cellular ultrastructural changes and functional abnormalities. The majority of animal studies fail to demonstrate alterations in fertility and reproduction, and the validity of applying data from these studies to humans was also questionable.

The effect of trace anesthetic gases on psychomotor skills has also been addressed. Concentrations of trace gases are usually reported on a volume-per-volume unit in parts per million (ppm) so that 10,000 ppm of halothane equals 1 percent. In 1969, Linde and Bruce[88] sampled air at various distances from the pop-off valve of an anesthesia machine and found average concentrations of 10 ppm halothane and 130 ppm nitrous oxide. They also noted 0 to 10 ppm halothane in the end-tidal air samples of anesthesiologists after work.

TABLE 10–2. OTHER PHYSIOLOGIC OR ADVERSE CONDITIONS MIMICKING BIOLOGIC EFFECTS OF ANESTHESIA POLLUTION

Diet
    Modification and carcinogenesis
    Malnutrition
Stress and anxiety
    Reproductive problems
    Alterations in working schedule
    Fatigue
Effects of hypoxia
    Congenital malformation
    Liver enzymes
    Teratogenic effect
Atmospheric contaminants and pollutants
    Smoking
    Ionizing radiation
Infections

TABLE 10–3. ANESTHESIA POLLUTION: POSSIBLE FLAWS IN REPORTS AND EXPERIMENTAL DESIGNS

Sampling bias and errors
Vague definition of control
Lack of quantification of exposure to anesthetic gases
Losses to follow-up
Inappropriate comparison groups
Lack of independent verification of the reported data
Unreliable retrospective studies
No good prospective and epidemiologic studies

In 1976, Bruce and Bach[89] demonstrated that nitrous oxide as low as 50 ppm, either alone or in combination with 1 ppm halothane, was associated with decreased behavioral performance, but 25 ppm of nitrous oxide with 0.5 ppm of halothane had no effect.

The National Institute for Occupational Safety and Health (NIOSH)[90] created their recommendations (Table 10–4) based on the findings of Bruce and Bach. It should be noted, however, that three investigators were subsequently unable to confirm these findings, so no convincing evidence exists to support the theory that levels of waste gases in unscavenged areas affect the higher mental functions of healthy subjects.

In practice, NIOSH recommendations are nearly impossible to achieve. But the reduction in trace anesthetic gas exposure is remarkable (90 percent) when an active scavenging system is used with an effective air-conditioning system, and it will result in time-weighted averages for nitrous oxide under the 25-ppm limit suggested by NIOSH.

The maximal concentration of halothane recommended by NIOSH is severalfold lower than the lowest concentration that humans can recognize. The threshold of perception ranges from less than 3 ppm to more than 100 ppm. Thus, when one is able to smell the halothane, the level far exceeds the maximum recommended level.

Although there is no firm evidence to support or oppose the concept that trace anesthetic gases are a health hazard, it would be prudent to direct attention toward scavenging waste gases to keep the operating environment levels to a minimum and prevent the spillage of volatile agents.

In addition to monitoring, preventive maintenance, adequate air-conditioning, and scavenging, it is very important that the anesthetist pay attention to the following details:

TABLE 10–4. NATIONAL INSTITUTE FOR OCCUPATIONAL SAFETY AND HEALTH (NIOSH) STANDARDS

Anesthetic Gas	Criterion
Nitrous oxide	Not more than 25 ppm
Halogenated anesthetics + nitrous oxide	Not more than 0.5 ppm
Halogenated anesthetics	Not more than 2.0 ppm

Note. 100% of a gas = 1,000,000 ppm; 1% of a gas = 10,000 ppm; 0.00001% of a gas = 1 ppm.

TABLE 10–5. POSSIBLE SOLUTIONS TO ANESTHESIA POLLUTION

Use of regional or conduction anesthesia
Use of low-flow and closed systems
Engineering control procedures
　Air conditioning
　Scavenging or evacuation
Modification of work practices
Leak testing and equipment maintenance
Air monitoring and personnel surveillance

TABLE 10–7. MEDICAL SURVEILLANCE PROCEDURES

Comprehensive medical and occupational histories
Placement and annual physical examination
Employee awareness and education
Reporting of abnormal outcome of pregnancies
Record keeping and filing

1. Ensure that gas disposal lines are connected.
2. Avoid turning on the nitrous oxide flowmeter or the vaporizers before the patient is connected to the circuit. Turn them off when they are not in use.
3. Select the optimal-size endotracheal tube for the patient and ensure that the cuff is adequately inflated.
4. Disconnect the patient from the circuit as infrequently as possible. Brief periods of discontinuity in a breathing circuit result in marked rises in anesthetic spillage.
5. Empty the breathing bag into the scavenging system rather than into the room.
6. At the end of the surgical procedure, continue to administer oxygen as long as possible, using high fresh gas flow rates to wash the anesthetic gases out of the circuit and the patient. Leave the patient attached to the circle as long as it is convenient, allowing the anesthetic to be collected by the scavenging system. Also, it is good patient care to give oxygen on recovery.
7. Use low-flow anesthesia systems. It is possible to close an anesthetic circle by reducing fresh gas flows. In a circle system wherein oxygen is the only carrier gas, any fresh gas inflow greater than the patient's metabolic oxygen requirement is popped off as waste. A 70-kg man may require about 240 mL/min oxygen. For a fresh gas flow of 1 L/min, 760 mL is unused. If the system has been carefully assessed as leak free, the adequacy of low fresh gas flow rates can be determined by monitoring distension of the breathing bag. Without oxygen monitoring equipment, however, relatively high fresh gas flow rates are necessary to ensure an inspired oxygen concentration of 50 percent when nitrous oxide is being used.
8. Use a mask that fits the contour of the face properly.

9. Perform the following high-pressure tests on the anesthesia equipment.

- Test 1: Turn on the nitrous oxide cylinders with the flowmeters off. Then turn the cylinder off and observe the time taken for the pressure gauges to fall. A good machine will hold its pressure for several hours; less than 1 hour is unacceptable.
- Test 2: Connect the outlet of the machine to a manometer. A rate greater than 100 mL/min to maintain a pressure of 30 mm Hg is unacceptable.

Repeat the second test, this time using the manometer connected to the Y-piece of the circle absorber. This will tell you if there is any leakage in the machine itself or leakage in the breathing circuit.

Possible solutions to anesthesia pollution are listed in Table 10–5. Table 10–6 gives work practice recommendations, and Table 10–7, medical surveillance procedures.

Radiation

Ionizing Radiation. X-rays and occasional encounters with radioactive isotopes are sources of ionizing radiation in the operating room environment. By driving electrons out of their stable orbitals, ionizing radiation creates free radicals and ionized molecules in tissue. Depending on the severity of the exposure, enzymes, structural proteins, genetic material, or any other cell part may be altered (as in malignant degeneration) or completely destroyed. Exposure is commonly reported in rem, an abbreviation for *roentgen equivalent man*. The rem is a measure of the biologic damage from radiation adjusted to apply to all tissues.[91]

Exposure from natural sources comes primarily from cosmic rays and radioactive compounds found in soil, brick, and concrete, and averages about 80 to 200 millirem (mrem) per year. The maximum yearly occupational exposure is mandated to be no more than 5 rem. During pregnancy, personnel are advised to limit exposure to a maximum of 500 mrem.

Although there has been an upsurge in the use of x-rays, fluoroscopy, and image intensifiers in the operating room for the care of the surgical patient (particularly in the specialties of orthopedics, neurosurgery, and urology), radiology personnel rarely absorb more than 10 percent of the maximum exposure advised. One study showed that anesthesiologists received an average of 13 milliroentgens per week.[88]

TABLE 10–6. WORK PRACTICE RECOMMENDATIONS

Functional waste gas disposal systems
Use of tight-fitting masks
Tests for low- and high-pressure leaks
Filling of vaporizers
No premature gas flow starts
Awareness of disconnection
Emptying of bags into scavenging system

One chest film results in about 25 mrem of exposure to the patient. The amount of radiation generated during fluoroscopy depends on the length of time the fluoroscopic beam is on. Intraoperative radiation measurements have shown that exposure is inversely related to the experience of the surgeon and that the amount of radiation received by the anesthetist during orthopedic procedures is not measurable.[92]

X-rays reflected from surfaces account for most occupational exposure. Physical separation is the best protection, as the intensity of scattered radiation is inversely proportional to the square of the distance from the source. A distance of at least 3 ft from the patient is recommended. Six feet of air provides protection equivalent to 9 in. of concrete or 2.5 mm of lead.[93] Aprons containing 0.25 to 0.5 mm of lead are effective in blocking most of the scattered radiation; however, uncovered areas, such as the human eye lens, still bear risk of injury. The implementation of radiation protection policies that include education and monitoring programs (with film badges or dosimeters) can reduce maximum exposure to the limit.

Nonionizing Radiation. Exposure to nonionizing radiation occurs with the use of lasers. This kind of radiation may excite electrons to move from ground state to higher orbitals, but the electrons stay within the molecule. The damage to tissues results from the heat produced by the absorbed radiation.

The word *laser* is an acronym for *light amplification by stimulated emission of radiation*. Lasers produce infrared, visible, or ultraviolet light depending on the laser medium (carbon dioxide, argon, or neodymium:yttrium aluminum garnet [Nd:YAG]). The patient's greatest risk from laser surgery is from laser burns or inadvertent laser fires.[94] Eye injuries from direct or reflected radiation are the greatest risk to personnel working near lasers. The intensity of reflected radiation is not diminished significantly by the distances traveled in the operating suite, so protective eyewear is recommended for all personnel.

Aside from the heat that lasers give off, matter is released from cells during treatment. The commonly malodorous *plume*, the vapor and cellular debris produced by lasers, contains particles whose median size is too small to be trapped by most surgical masks. Intact DNA from human papillomavirus has been detected in the vapor from laser-treated plantar warts. Whether this could be infectious or harmful to operating room personnel is unknown, but care should be taken to scavenge vaporized debris.

Chemicals

Hundreds of different chemicals are used throughout the hospital from the clinical laboratory to the housekeeping and maintenance areas. Knowledge of the appropriate use, risks, and precautions associated with these chemicals is important. For example, ethylene oxide, used in gas sterilization, is an occupational health hazard, as exposure can result in cancer, reproductive abnormalities including genetic damage, and neurologic disease.[95] For every 8-hour shift, a concentration ceiling of only 1 ppm is allowed. Glutaraldehyde and formaldehyde are two chemicals commonly used for disinfection and sterilization. The recommended ceiling threshold limit value for glutaraldehyde is only 0.2 ppm; that for formaldehyde is 1 ppm.

The mixing of chemicals, whether inadvertent or intentional, can present additional hazards. Even common cleaning agents can present problems if mixed. Formaldehyde mixed with hydrochloric acid in sufficient quantities can produce bis(chloromethyl) ether (BCME), a potent carcinogen. Formation of toxic chlorine fumes from mixing bleach and ammonia or bleach and toilet bowl cleaners has been reported.[96]

Occupational exposure to methylmethacrylate, or bone cement, has been associated with respiratory, cutaneous, gastrointestinal, and genitourinary problems. OSHA has established an 8-hour, time-weighted average allowable exposure of 100 ppm, yet factory workers exposed to levels below this have experienced problems.[97] Allergic reactions manifesting as occupational asthma have been reported after exposure to methylmethacrylate.

Some general guidelines that should be followed to minimize effects from chemicals follow:

1. Ensure adequate ventilation in areas where chemicals are used. Scavenging devices should be available for areas where concentrations of these vapors exceed recommended levels.
2. Wear appropriate protective clothing.
3. Read and follow all labels and signs concerning proper use, storage, and first-aid.
4. Do not mix chemicals unless you know the end products and are aware of any necessary precautions.
5. Know the location of the nearest wash area.
6. Have chemicals periodically reviewed to determine if a less hazardous chemical could be used.

OTHER POTENTIAL HAZARDS IN THE SURGICAL ENVIRONMENT

Concerns about safety in the operating room and other acute care areas of the hospital should take into consideration both the patient and the health care provider. The major issues have been discussed. Others, such as electrical safety, are covered in other chapters. Hazards associated with controlling patient temperature and with patient transport/transfer activities have been identified and guidelines for recommended practices have been issued by the Association of Operating Room Nurses.[98]

It is important to recognize that the identification of potential safety hazards in the workplace is an ongoing process. Policies and procedures related to the establishment of safe practice should be developed as new concerns arise within the practice setting and should comply with applicable local, state, and federal regulations.

REFERENCES

1. Berry AJ, Isaacson IJ, Hunt D, et al. The prevalence of hepatitis B viral markers in anesthesia personnel. *Anesthesiology.* 1984;60:6.

2. Denes AE, Smith JL, Maynard JE, et al. Hepatitis B infection in physicians. Results of a nationwide seroepidemiologic survey. *JAMA*. 1978;239:210.

3. Berry AJ, Isaacson IJ, Kane MA, et al. A multicenter study of the prevalence of hepatitis B viral serologic markers in anesthesia personnel. *Anesth Analg*. 1984;63:738.

4. Berry AJ, Isaacson IJ, Kane MA, et al. A multicenter study of the epidemiology of hepatitis B in anesthesia residents. *Anesth Analg*. 1985;64:672.

5. Fyman PN, Hartung J, Weinberg S, et al. Prevalence of hepatitis B markers in the anesthesia staff in a large inner-city hospital. *Anesth Analg*. 1984;63:433.

6. Malm DN, Mathias RG, Turnbull KW, et al. Prevalence of hepatitis B in anaesthesia personnel. *Can Anaesth Soc J*. 1986;33:167.

7. Chernesky MA, Browne RA, Rondi P. Hepatitis B virus antibody prevalence in anaesthetists. *Can Anaesth Soc J*. 1984;31:239.

8. Siebke JC, Degre M. Prevalence of viral hepatitis in the staff in Norwegian anaesthesiology units. *Acta Anaesthesiol Scand*. 1984;28:549.

9. Carstens J, Macnab GM, Kew MC. Hepatitis B virus infection in anaesthetists. *Br J Anaesth*. 1977;49:887.

10. Sinclair ME, Ashby MW, Kurtz JB. The prevalence of serological markers for hepatitis B virus infection amongst anaesthetists in the Oxford region. *Anaesthesia*. 1987;42:30.

11. Janzen J, Tripatzis I, Wagner U, et al. Epidemiology of hepatitis B surface antigen (HBsAg) and antibody to HBsAg in hospital personnel. *J Infect Dis*. 1978;137:261.

12. Berry AJ, Katz JD. Hazards of working in the operating room. In: Barash PG, Cullen BF, Stoelting RK, eds. *Clinical anesthesia*. Philadelphia: JB Lippincott; 1989:chap 4.

13. Francis DP, Feorino PM, McDougal S, et al. The safety of the hepatitis B vaccine. Inactivation of the AIDS virus during routine vaccine manufacture. *JAMA*. 1986;256:869.

14. Scolnick Em, McLean AA, West DJ, et al. Clinical evaluation in healthy adults of a hepatitis B vaccine made by recombinant DNA. *JAMA*. 1984;251:2812.

15. Brown SE, Stanley C, Howard CR, et al. Antibody responses to recombinant and plasma derived hepatitis B vaccines. *Br J Med*. 1986;292:159.

16. Okada N, Eldred L, Cohen S, et al: Comparative immunogenicity of plasma and recombinant hepatitis B virus vaccines in homosexual men. *JAMA*. 1988;260:3635.

17. Centers for Disease Control. Recommendations for prevention of HIV transmission in health-care settings. *MMWR*. 1987;36(suppl 2S):3S–18S.

18. Centers for Disease Control. Recommendations for preventing transmission of infection with human T-lymphotropic virus type III/lymphadenopathy-associated virus in the workplace. *MMWR*. 1985;34:681, 691.

19. Choo QL, Kuo G, Weiner AJ, et al. Isolation of a cDNA clone derived from bloodborne non-A, non-B hepatitis genome. *Science*. 1989;244:359.

20. Alter HJ, Hadler SC, Francis DP, et al. The epidemiology of non-A, non-B hepatitis in the United States. In: Dodd RY, Barker LF, eds. *Infection, immunity and blood transfusion*. New York: Alan R. Liss, 1985:71.

21. Stevens CE, Aach RD, Hollinger FB, et al. Hepatitis B virus antibody in donors and the occurrence of non-A, non-B hepatitis in transfusion recipients. *Ann Intern Med*. 1984;101:733.

22. Koziol DE, Holland PV, Alling DW, et al. Antibody to hepatitis core antigen as a paradoxical marker for non-A, non-B hepatitis agents in donated blood. *Ann Intern Med*. 1986;104:488.

23. Alter HJ, Holland PV. Indirect tests to detect the non-A, non-B hepatitis carrier state. *Ann Intern Med*. 1984;101:859.

24. Dienstag JL, Alter HJ. Non-A, non-B hepatitis: Evolving epidemiologic and clinical perspectives. *Semin Liver Dis*. 1986;6:67.

25. Alter HJ, Purcell RH, Shih JW, et al. Detection of antibody to hepatitis C virus in prospectively followed transfusion recipients with acute and chronic non-A, non-B hepatitis. *N Engl J Med*. 1989;321:1494.

26. Stevens CE, Taylor PE, Pindyck J, et al. Epidemiology of hepatitis C virus: A preliminary study in volunteer blood donors. *JAMA*. 1990;263:49.

27. Mosley JW, Aach RD, Hollinger FB, et al. Non-A, non-B hepatitis and antibody to hepatitis C virus. *JAMA*. 1990;263:77.

28. DiBisceglie AM, Martin P, Kassianides C, et al. Recombinant interferon alpha therapy for chronic hepatitis C: A randomized, double-blind, placebo-controlled trial. *N Engl J Med*. 1989;321:1506.

29. Davis GL, Balart LA, Schiff ER, et al. Treatment of chronic hepatitis C with recombinant interferon alfa: A multicenter randomized, controlled trial. *N Engl J Med*. 1989;321:1501.

30. Kelen GD, Fritz S, Qaqish B, et al. Unrecognized human immunodeficiency virus infection in emergency department patients. *N Engl J Med*. 1988;318:1645.

31. Weiss SH, Saxinger WC, Rechtman D, et al. HTLV-III infection among health-care workers: Association with needle-stick injuries. *JAMA*. 1985;254:2089.

32. The Cooperative Needlestick Surveillance Group. Occupational risk of the acquired immunodeficiency syndrome among health care workers. *N Engl J Med*. 1986;314:1127.

33. Centers for Disease Control. Update: Human immunodeficiency virus infections in health-care workers exposed to blood of infected patients. *MMWR*. 1987;36:285.

34. Marcus R. Surveillance of health care workers exposed to blood from patients infected with the human immunodeficiency virus. *N Engl J Med*. 1988;219:1118.

35. Slim J. AIDS update. Reports about the epidemiology, diagnosis and treatment of acquired immunodeficiency syndrome. *Hosp Phys*. 1991;27:17.

36. Morgan BB, Brown BR, Alluisi EA. Effects on sustained performance of 48 hours of continuous work and sleep loss. *Hum Factors*. 1974;16:406.

37. Baker RA, Ware JR. The relationship between vigilance and monotonous work. *Ergonomics*. 1966;9:109.

38. Drui AB, Behm RJ, Martin WE. Predesign investigation of the anesthesia operational environment. *Anesth Analg*. 1973;52:584.

39. Belkin NL. Is your OR giving you the blues? It could be color. *AORN J*. 1986;43:792.

40. Boquet G, Bushman JA, Davenport HT. The anaesthetic machine—A study of function and design. *Br J Anaesth*. 1980;52:61.

41. Cooper JB, Newbower RS, Moore JW, et al. A new anesthesia delivery system. *Anesthesiology*. 1978;49:310.

42. Waterson CK. The anesthesia machine: Current design and alternatives. *Med Instrum*. 1983;17:379.

43. Arnell WJ, Schultz DG. Computers in anesthesiology—A new look ahead. *Med Instrum*. 1983;17:393.

44. Smith NT, Quinn ML, Flick J. Automatic control in anesthesia: A comparison in performance between the anesthetist and the machine. *Anesth Analg*. 1984;63:715.

45. Kraft HH, Lees DE. Closing the loop: How near is automated anesthesia? *South Med J*. 1984;77:7.

46. Sykes MK, Sugg BR, Hahn CE, et al. A new microprocessor-controlled anesthetic machine. *Br J Anaesth*. 1989;62:445.

47. Wallroth CF. Technical conception for an anesthesia system with electronic metering of gases and vapors. *Acta Anaesthesiol Belg*. 1984;35:279.

48. Gaba DM, DeAnda A. A comprehensive anesthesia simulation environment: Recreating the operating room for research and training. *Anesthesiology*. 1988;69:387.

49. NIOSH recommendations for occupational safety and health standards. *MMWR*. 1986;35:33S.

50. Kryter KD. *The Effects of Noise on Man*. 2nd ed. New York: Academic Press; 1985.

51. Shapiro RA, Berland T. Noise in the operating room. *N Engl J Med*. 1972;287:1236.

52. Falk SA, Woods NF. Hospital noise-levels and potential health hazards. *N Engl J Med.* 1973;289:774.

53. Gordon NP, Cleary PD, Parker CE, Czeisler CA. The prevalence and health impact of shiftwork. *Am J Public Health.* 1986;76:1225.

54. Friedmann J, Globus G, Huntley A, et al. Performance and mood during and after gradual sleep reduction. *Psychophysiology.* 1977;14:245.

55. Arnold WP. Environmental safety including chemical dependency. In: Miller RD, ed. *Anesthesia.* 3rd ed. New York: Churchill Livingstone; 1990:chap 80.

56. Denisco RA, Drummond JN, Gravenstein JS. Effect of fatigue on performance of a simulated anesthetic task. *Anesthesiology.* 1984;61:A467.

57. Narang V, Laycock JRD. Psychomotor testing of on-call residents. *Anaesthesia.* 1986;41:868.

58. Friedman RL, Bigger JT, Kornfield DS. The intern and sleep loss. *N Engl J Med.* 1971;285:201.

59. Jerison HJ, Pickett RM. Vigilance: A review and reevaluation. *Hum Factors.* 1963;5:221.

60. Wallace-Barnhill GL, Florex G, Turndoff H, et al. The effect of 24 hour duty on the performance of anesthesiology residents on vigilance, mood, and memory tasks. *Anesthesiology.* 1983;59:A460.

61. McDonald JS, Peterson S. Lethal errors in anesthesiology. *Anesthesiology.* 1985;63:A497.

62. Cooper JB, Newbower RS, Long CD, et al. Preventable anesthesia mishaps: A study of human factors. *Anesthesiology.* 1987;49:399.

63. Jones RE. Do psychiatrists cover up addiction of physicians? *Psychiatr Opinion.* 1975;12:31.

64. Talbott DG, Gallegos KV, Wilson PO, et al. The Medical Association of Georgia's impaired physicians program. *JAMA.* 1987;257:2927.

65. Rinaldi RC, Steindler EM, Wilford BB, Goodwin D. Clarification and standardization of substance abuse terminology. *JAMA.* 1988;259:555.

66. Canavan DJ. The impaired physicians program: The subject of impairment. *Med Soc NJ.* 1983;80:47.

67. Cadoret R, Troughton E, O'Gorman TW, Heywood E. An adoption study of genetic and environmental factors in drug abuse. *Arch Gen Psychiatry.* 1986;43:1131.

68. Cloninger CR. Neurogenetic adaptive mechanisms in alcoholism. *Science.* 1987;236:410.

69. Reich T. Biologic-marker studies in alcoholism. *N Engl J Med.* 1988;318:180.

70. Mueller GC, Fleming MF, LeMahieu MA, et al. Synthesis of phosphatidylethanol—A potential marker for adult males at risk for alcoholism. *Proc Natl Acad Sci USA.* 1988;85:9778.

71. Azar I, Sophie S, Lear E. The cardiovascular response of anesthesiologists during induction of anesthesia. *Anesthesiology.* 1985;63:A76.

72. Pinnock CA, Elling AE, Eastley RJ, et al. Anxiety levels in junior anaesthetists during early training. *Anaesthesia.* 1986;41:258.

73. Vaillant GE, Brighton JR, McArthur C. Physician's use of mood-altering drugs. *N Engl J Med.* 1970;282:365.

74. Vaillant GE, Sobowale NC, McArthur C. Some psychological vulnerabilities of physicians. *N Engl J Med.* 1972;287:372.

75. McAuliffe WE, Rohman M, Santangello S, et al. Psychoactive drug use among practicing physicians and medical students. *N Engl J Med.* 1986;315:805.

76. Gallegos KV, Browne CH, Veit FW, et al. Addiction in anesthesiologists: Drug access and patterns of substance abuse. *QRB.* 1988;14:116.

77. Shore JH. The Oregon experience with impaired physicians on probation: An eight-year follow-up. *JAMA.* 1987;257:2931.

78. Morse RM, Martin MA, Swenson WM, Niven RG. Prognosis of physicians treated for alcoholism and drug dependence. *JAMA.* 1984;251:743.

79. Vaisman AL. Working conditions in surgery and their effect on the health of anesthesiologists. *Eksp Khir Anesteziol.* 1967;3:44.

80. American Society of Anesthesiologists Ad Hoc Committee on the Effect of Trace Anesthetics on the Health of Operating Room Personnel. Occupational disease among operating room personnel: A national study. *Anesthesiology.* 1974;41:321.

81. Spence AA, Cohen EN, Brown BW Jr, et al. Occupational hazards for operating room-based physicians: Analysis of data from the United States and the United Kingdom. *JAMA.* 1977;238:955.

82. Ferstandig LL: Trace concentrations of anesthetic gases: A critical review of their disease potential. *Anesth Analg.* 1978;57:328.

83. Lecky JH. Problems of trace anesthetic levels. In: Orkin FK, Cooperman LH, eds. *Complications in anesthesiology.* Philadelphia: JB Lippincott; 1983:715.

84. Buring JE, Hennekens CH, Mayrent SL, et al. Health experiences of operating room personnel. *Anesthesiology.* 1985;62:325.

85. Vessey MP. Epidemiological studies of the occupational hazards of anaesthesia—A review. *Anaesthesia.* 1978;33:430.

86. Spence AA, Knill-Jones RP. Is there a health hazard in anaesthetic practice? *Br J Anaesth.* 1978;50:713.

87. Spence AA. Environmental pollution by inhalation anaesthetics. *Br J Anaesth.* 1987;59:96.

88. Linde HW, Bruce DL. Occupational exposure of anesthetists to halothane, nitrous oxide and radiation. *Anesthesiology.* 1969;30:363.

89. Bruce DL, Bach MJ. Effects of trace anaesthetic gases on behavioral performance of volunteers. *Br J Anaesth.* 1976;48:871.

90. National Institute for Occupational Safety and Health. *Criteria for a recommended standard: Occupational exposure to waste anesthetic gases and vapors.* DHEW (NIOSH) Publication No. 77-140. Washington, DC: U.S. Govt. Printing Office; 1977.

91. Voelz GL. Ionizing radiation. In: Zenz C, ed. *Occupational Medicine: Principles and practical applications.* 2nd ed. Chicago: Year Book Medical; 1988:426.

92. Kiviniitty K, Lahti Lahde S, Torniainen P. Radiation doses from x-ray units used outside radiology departments. *Health Phys.* 1980;38:419.

93. Barker D. Protection and safety in the x-ray department. *Radiography.* 1978;44:45.

94. Hayes DM, Gaba DM, Goode RL. Incendiary characteristics of a new laser-resistant endotracheal tube. *Otolaryngol Head Neck Surg.* 1986;95:37.

95. Haney PE, Raymond BA, Lewis LC. Ethylene oxide. An occupational health hazard in the surgical environment. *AORN J.* 1989;50:396.

96. Chemical hazards in the hospital. *Health Devices.* 1980;9:320.

97. Cromer J, Kronoveter K. *A study of methylmethacrylate exposure and employee health.* DHEW Publication No. 77-119 (NIOSH). Washington, DC: U.S. Govt. Printing Office; 1976.

98. Proposed recommended practices. Safe care through identification of potential hazards in the surgical environment. *AORN J.* 1989;50:396.

APPENDIX

Brochures addressing *Bloodborne Pathogens and Acute Care Facilities* (OSHA 3128) and *Occupational Exposure to Bloodborne Pathogens* (OSHA 3127) may be obtained from:

> OSHA Publications Office
> 200 Constitution Avenue, N.W., Room N3101
> Washington, D.C. 20210
> (202) 523-9667

Please send a self-addressed label with the request for a single copy

A. What to Do if an Exposure Incident Occurs?*

The standard requires that the postexposure medical evaluation and followup be made available immediately for employees who have had an exposure incident. At a minimum, the evaluation and followup must, at least, include the following elements:

- Document the routes of exposure and how exposure occurred.
- Identify and document the source individual, unless the employer can establish that identification is infeasible or prohibited by state or local law.
- Obtain consent (If consent is not obtained, the employer must show that legally required consent could not be obtained. Where consent is not required by law, the source individual's blood, if available, should be tested and the results documented.) and test source individual's blood as soon as possible to determine HIV and HBV infectivity and document the source's blood test results.
- If the source individual is known to be infected with either HIV or HBV, testing need not be repeated to determine the known infectivity.
- Provide the exposed employee with the source individual's test results and information about applicable disclosure laws and regulations concerning the source identity and infectious status.
- After obtaining consent, collect exposed employee's blood as soon as feasible after the exposure incident and test blood for HBV and HIV serological status.
- If the employee does not give consent for HIV serological testing during the collection of blood for baseline testing, preserve the baseline blood sample for at least 90 days. (If, during this time, the exposed employee elects to have the baseline sample tested, testing shall be done as soon as feasible.)
- Provide HBV and HIB serological testing, counseling, and safe and effective postexposure prophylaxis following the current recommendations of the U.S. Public Health Service.

The employer must give the health care professional responsible for the employee's hepatitis B vaccination and postexposure evaluation and followup a copy of the OSHA standard. The employer also must provide to the health care professional evaluating the employee after an exposure incident a description of the employee's job duties relevant to the exposure incident, documentation of the route(s) of exposure, circumstances of exposure, and results of the source individual's blood tests, if available, and all relevant employee medical records, including vaccination status.

Within 15 days after evaluation of the exposed employee, the employer must provide the employee with a copy of the health care professional's written opinion. The written opinion is limited to whether the vaccine is indicated and if it has been received. The written opinion for postexposure evaluation must document that the employee has been informed of the results of the medical evaluation and of any medical conditions resulting from the exposure incident that may require further evaluation or treatment. All other diagnoses must remain confidential and not be included in the written report.

B. Recordkeeping of Exposure

Employers also must preserve and maintain for each employee an accurate record of occupational exposure according to OSHA's rule governing access to employee exposure and medical records, *Title 29 Code of Federal Regulations*, Part 1910.20

Under the bloodborne pathogens standard, however, medical records also must include the following information:

- Employee's name and social security number;
- Employee's hepatitis B vaccination status including vaccination dates and any medical records related to the employee's ability to receive vaccinations;
- Results of examinations, medical testing, and postexposure evaluation and followup procedures;
- Health care professional's written opinion;
- A copy of the information provided to the health care professional.

Medical records must be kept confidential and maintained for at least the duration of employment plus 30 years.

The bloodborne pathogens standard also requires employers to maintain and to keep accurate training records for 3 years and to include the following: training dates, content or a summary of the training, names and qualifications of trainer(s), and names and job titles of trainees. Upon request, both medical and training records must be made available to the Director of the National Institute for Occupational Safety and Health (NIOSH) and to the Assistant Secretary of Labor for Occupational Safety and Health. Training records must be available to employees or employee representatives upon request. An employee's medical records can be obtained by that employee or anyone having that employee's written consent. Also, if the employer ceases to do business, medical and training records must be transferred to the successor employer. If there is no successor employer, the employer must notify the Director, NIOSH, U.S. Department of Health and Human Services, for specific directions regarding disposition of the records at least 3 months prior to intended disposal.

In addition to other requirements of the standard, employers in research laboratories and production facilities engaged in the culture, production, concentration, experimentation, and manipulation of HIB and HBV (not clinical or diagnostic laboratories) must comply with other standards which are included in the OSHA 3127 publication.

* Reprinted, with permission, from *Occupational Exposure to Bloodborne Pathogens.* Washington, DC: U.S. Department of Labor, Occupational Safety and Health Administration publication OSHA 3127, 1992.

Perioperative Considerations

Perioperative Considerations

Preoperative Assessment and Evaluation

Christine S. Zambricki

Preanesthetic evaluations afford the CRNA a unique opportunity to make a significant impact on a patient's response to surgery and anesthesia. The perception of what constitutes an adequate preanesthetic screening has undergone developmental changes in recent years primarily because of identification of physiologic factors that directly affect a positive anesthetic outcome. Too, the spiraling costs of health care have necessitated a closer look at routine laboratory testing relative to its effectiveness and necessity in preoperative assessment and outcome prediction. Historically, the majority of presurgical evaluation and preparation of patients occurred several days prior to surgery. Ideally, such evaluations should occur at least 48 hours prior to surgery if possible, especially in elderly patients or those with multisystem disease processes. This period is often required to secure necessary specialty consults and to return patients to an optimal state of health; however, because many patients undergo surgery on an outpatient or same-day admissions basis, alternatives such as phone screening and advanced testing without hospital admission are being evaluated.

Within the conceptual framework of holistic approaches to patient care, preoperative assessment is as important to patient outcome as intraoperative or postanesthetic management, regardless of the setting in which the evaluation takes place. Although students in the field of anesthesiology acknowledge the value of the preanesthetic visit, a surprising number of graduates enter the work force ill prepared to comprehensively evaluate their own patients. This has resulted largely from the need to accommodate the surgical outpatient schedule, where time constraints prevent students and practitioners from doing their own evaluations on every patient they anesthetize. It is expected that the reader will be convinced of the importance of a goal-directed preanesthetic assessment and insist on carrying out that responsibility with the same precision required in other phases of anesthetic care. It should also be noted that current standards of care require that all patients shall have received a thorough workup and that the anesthetist be apprised of such information, with adequate time to assimilate information and plan the anesthetic course.

Many institutions use the team approach to anesthesia care. Teams usually consist of an anesthesiologist, certified registered nurse anesthetist, and a student or resident. Every member of the team must become knowledgeable about the patient before surgery, through communication with the patient and each other. One team member may be designated to do a thorough preanesthetic evaluation and complete a written summary, which is placed on the chart; however, all team members remain responsible for reviewing data preoperatively and for introducing themselves to the patient as part of the anesthetic care team. All patients have the right to know and accept their anesthesia providers. In addition, the patient will not be surprised or frightened to find a "team" in attendance rather than one individual practitioner.

The anesthetist can most effectively direct the course of the preoperative visit by being cognizant of the goals to be achieved:

1. Procurement of information
2. Reduction of patient anxiety
3. Education of the patient
4. Securing informed consent
5. Evaluation and documentation of anesthetic risk
6. Optimization of preoperative status; reduction of perioperative morbidity
7. Selection of premedication
8. Formulation of anesthetic care plan

PROCUREMENT OF INFORMATION

The most obvious goal of the preoperative visit is the acquisition of factual information about the patient. This information can come from several sources including a chart review, a personal patient interview to discuss a detailed health history, and a thorough physical and psychologic assessment of the patient. This information provides a baseline of data for planning anesthesia management, comparing intraoperative and postoperative physiologic events, and planning timely and rational anesthetic interventions. A chart review alone is rarely considered adequate for a proper and comprehensive anesthetic assessment.

Chart Review

There are several reasons why the preanesthetic assessment begins with careful scrutiny of the patient's chart. The name and identification number found on the chart should be matched with information from the operating room schedule, and the anesthetist should note the surgeon's name and planned procedure to be sure that the visit is being made to the correct patient. Patients find it disquieting to be asked several times when and what type of surgery is to be performed and this can be avoided if a careful chart review is conducted. Consent forms should be checked for completeness, and any question regarding the legality of signatures should be determined at this time. In general, primary documents for review should include diagnostic reports and admitting progress notes including the history and physical obtained by the surgeon. Every attempt should be made to review primary data, not information that is copied from primary sources. If time permits, a comparison can be made between primary and secondary sources to detect additions, deletions, or contradictions. The surgical procedure listed on the consent form should be compared with the operating schedule. Any questions in this regard should be clarified before the patient's arrival in the operating suite. Preliminary chart review provides the anesthetist with a basis for the patient interview and eliminates the need to return to question the patient again after identifying a contradiction or potential area of concern.

A preanesthetic assessment questionnaire may be part of the patient's chart. The questionnaire is given to the patient to complete as soon as surgery is scheduled so that it can be reviewed in a timely manner. Correctly completed, this document helps the anesthetist focus attention on the patient at risk and allows for efficient use of time available for the preoperative visit. The preanesthetic assessment questionnaire cannot, however, substitute for a careful health history and physical assessment of the patient. Drawbacks to the use of such a form include misinterpretation by the infirm or elderly patient which may result in omissions or incorrect information. Logistic difficulties of getting the form distributed, completed, and returned to the chart before the anesthetist's visit can also be anticipated on occasion.

Valuable information about the course of the patient's illness can be obtained from the progress notes. The admitting history and physical should be reviewed for any points that might indicate the need for special attention during patient assessment; for example, a diagnosis of thyroid disease may be cause for a detailed inquiry about endocrine disease and related sequelae during the preoperative interview. The progress notes describe the primary diagnosis as well as the patient's other coexisting disease states.

Nursing notes provide information related to a particular patient's disabilities that might affect the approach to the patient interview. Is the patient's hearing impaired? If so, a standard printed questionnaire can be supplemented with handwritten questions, and a translator for signing may be of help. Recent federal legislation prevents health care institutions from discriminating against patients with disabilities; therefore, the standard of care for completeness of the pretreatment evaluation must be equal to that offered to the nondisabled patient. The nursing portion of the patient record may include nursing diagnoses and descriptions of the patient's current condition, progress, complaints, and ability to cope with the diagnosed condition. Planned nursing interventions may also provide the anesthetist with clues to how best to obtain pertinent information. The graphic sheet is a source of information about daily temperature, weight, pulse, blood pressure, respiration, and possible intake and output. These background data can be logged on the preanesthetic evaluation sheet before the patient is seen. The anesthetist is responsible for providing care consistent with the nursing care plan, within the limitations of the operating room environment. In some cases, it may be useful to speak with the patient's primary care nurse prior to interviewing the patient.

The preoperative chart review includes attention to pharmacologic agents the patient currently receives or has taken in the past. These drugs should be considered in the development of the anesthetic care plans, with a focus on potential drug interactions. For example, succinylcholine is potentiated by a wide range of drugs, including some antibiotics, lithium, quinidine, echothiophate iodide, cyclophosphamide, and other antineoplastic drugs. Augmentation of nondepolarizing neuromuscular blockade has been reported in patients receiving local anesthetics, antibiotics, or antiarrhythmics, such as digitalis or quinidine, propranolol, and phenytoin. The drug history will help determine the focus of the interview. For example, the patient taking beta blockers should be questioned regarding the reason for the drug, relief of symptoms by the drug, and the person's cardiovascular history. A decision as to the continuance of drug therapy on the day of surgery must be made. Recent literature indicates that antihypertensives, antiseizure medications, and some cardiac drugs should be administered on the day of surgery to provide optimal physiologic support. Attention to the patient's pharmacologic regimen may alert the anesthetist to request further diagnostic tests to complete the patient assessment.

Diagnostic Tests

The results of preoperative laboratory tests and diagnostic studies should be reviewed before the patient is seen. Although "normal values" vary from institution to institution, many departments have codified the "action limits" of abnormality as those that require some alteration in management (Table 11–1). The selection of preoperative screening tests has been the subject of recent controversy.[1–5] At the heart of the debate rests the issue of routine batteries of screening tests versus minimum testing based on patient condition and protocol. Health care providers have been scrutinized both by the federal government and by private insurers for cost efficiency, and as a result, the list of "routine" preoperative tests has dwindled. One surprising

TABLE 11–1. RANGES OF LABORATORY TEST VALUES WITH ACTION LIMITS

Test	Adult Reference Range	Action Limits
Complete blood cell count		
Hemoglobin level (g/dL)	M 13.5–17.5	10.0–18.0
	F 12.0–16.0	
White blood cell count (1000/cu mm)	3.1–11.0	3.0–15.0
Sodium (mEq/L)	136–144	130–150
Potassium (mEq/L)	3.5–5.3	3.2–5.8
Creatinine (mg/dL)	0.5–1.2	≤1.5
Glucose level (mg/dL)	65–110	50–180
Platelet count (1000/cu mm)	140–450	115–800
Prothrombin time (s)	10.5–12.5	10.0–13.0
Partial thromboplastin time (s)	24.0–38.0	22.0–40.0

advantage to ordering fewer tests is the resultant improvement of patient care through risk reduction. Routine testing rarely yields unanticipated diagnoses and may give false-positive results or clinically insignificant borderline positive results. In these cases, more testing may be done and necessary surgery delayed. Frequently, reports of unexpected abnormalities are not on the chart prior to surgery, placing the anesthetist in an indefensible position when the results become known.

Beyond those tests or studies required by local departmental policy, several criteria must be met if a preoperative study is considered essential for assessment of the healthy patient: (1) The condition tested for must manifest symptoms and/or represent a significant deviation from previous health and physical examination histories. (2) The condition would likely increase surgical morbidity or mortality or represent significant risk to those associated with the patient's care. (3) Preoperative diagnosis established by such testing must be more beneficial in terms of patient outcome than diagnosis established postoperatively by the same testing. (4) The abnormality would influence anesthetic or surgical approaches. (5) The available tests must be specific and sensitive enough to allow for accurate detection of the condition. (6) A test should not be used if there exists an alternative that compares in sensitivity at less cost (e.g., serum potassium only versus 12-factor automated multiple analysis of electrolytes). Suggested indications for common preoperative diagnostic studies as well as guidelines for their clinical interpretation are found in Tables 11–2 and 11–3.

Few tests are of value as routine indicators or predictors of positive anesthetic outcomes in apparently healthy people. Only the complete blood count seems indicated for every patient based on cost/benefit analysis. A pregnancy test should be done if pregnancy is possible. Pulmonary function studies may provide valuable information in patients at high risk for postoperative pulmonary sequelae. This population often includes patients with preexisting pulmonary disease presenting for upper abdominal or tho-

racic operations, those with a protracted and heavy smoking histories in which pulmonary compromise is apparent, patients with morbid obesity or other etiologies of severe restrictive disease, and unstable asthmatics (Table 11–4).[6–8]

Many authors have questioned the value of routine preoperative chest x-ray and electrocardiogram (ECG).[9] Routine use of the preoperative chest x-ray is expensive and patients may bear the risk of unnecessary irradiation. In addition, interpretation of chest x-ray is often not available until after surgery, and the results may make no difference in anesthetic management in the asymptomatic patient. Specific indications for preoperative chest x-ray include demonstrated lung disease, cardiovascular disease, malignant disease, major surgical emergencies, current smoking history in patients 50 and older and those on immunosuppression drugs where various pneumonias may be identified. Similarly, the ECG has not proven itself to be a cost-effective component of routine preanesthetic screening for the apparently healthy patient. Both the chest x-ray and ECG may, however, be indicated on the basis of clinical examination, health history, and the proposed surgery. Should the anesthetist choose to obtain an ECG or chest x-ray, the abnormalities listed in Table 11–5 may serve as criteria for evaluation.

One practical approach to decreasing indiscriminate preoperative testing, is the use of previous test results.[10] Some practitioners feel that diagnostic studies completed in the year prior to elective surgery can be safely substituted for preoperative screening tests, if the previous tests are normal and no clinical indication for retesting exists. Other hospitals require that all requisite lab work be obtained within the last 1 to 3 months and chest x-rays, within the preceding 6 months. Until more definitive information is available on the cost/benefit ratios of these common testing modalities, every anesthetist should be aware of existing departmental/hospital policy regarding requisite preoperative laboratory testing for both the inpatient and outpatient. It is against these local standards that a CRNA's performance will be measured, especially by a court of law, quality assurance committees, or various licensing agencies.

The Health History

Personal interview of the patient to obtain an accurate and complete health history is an extremely important component of the preanesthetic process. Through this process, the anesthetist is able to gather an organized, comprehensive set of data from which to formulate the anesthetic care plan. This interview also helps to establish a trusting relationship between the anesthetist and patient and to inspire patient confidence in the CRNA. The anesthetist and patient can then proceed to define the therapeutic goals of the anesthetic plan of care.

The anesthetist should set the stage for a positive interaction by deliberate manipulation of the environment. If the preanesthetic interview is conducted by phone, the anesthetist should make sure that the time and location are convenient and private for the patient. If the interview is conducted in person, the location of the interview should be quiet, private, and free from interruption. If the patient is eating or receiving therapy, a return visit should be made.

TABLE 11–2. SUGGESTED INDICATIONS FOR COMMON PREOPERATIVE DIAGNOSTIC STUDIES

Test	Indications
Chest x-ray	Any lung disease, any cardiovascular disease, known malignant disease, major surgical emergencies, current smoking history in patients more than 50 years old, immunodepression (malnutrition, steroid therapy, chemotherapy)
Electrocardiogram	Age 60 or over; history of or symptoms related to cardiac disease, cardiac medications (such as beta blockers, calcium channel blockers, digitalis preparations, antidysrhythmics), hypertension or diabetes mellitus long-standing or with poor control
Glucose level	Diabetes mellitus, hypoglycemia, corticosteroid therapy, pancreatic disease, pituitary disease, hypothalamic disease, adrenal disease
Hemoglobin	Potentially bloody operation (determined by need for preoperative crossmatch), chronic renal failure, known anemia, bleeding disorder, hemorrhage, hematologic malignancy, radiation/chemotherapy, other potentially relevant diseases (e.g., some infections, liver disease, malnutrition)
Platelet count	Known platelet abnormality, hemorrhage, purpura, hypersplenism, hematologic malignancy (e.g., leukemia), radiation/chemotherapy, thrombosis, some anemias (e.g., aplastic), other potentially relevant diseases (e.g., systemic lupus erythematosus, von Willebrand's disease, paroxysmal nocturnal hemoglobinuria, renal transplant rejection)
Prothrombin time/partial thromboplastin time	Known coagulation disorder, anticoagulant therapy, hemorrhage, anemia, liver disease, malabsorption, malnutrition, other potentially relevant diseases (e.g., systemic lupus erythematosus)
Sodium, potassium, chloride, CO_2 content, BUN,[a] creatinine	Age 60 or over, diuretic or digitalis usage, renal disease, other fluid/electrolyte abnormalities (e.g., diarrhea, syndrome of inappropriate secretion of antidiuretic hormone, diabetes insipidus, severe liver disease), other potentially relevant abnormalities (e.g., convulsions)
Triiodothyronine thyroxine	Treatment with levothyroxine sodium (Synthroid), hyperthyroidism or hypothyroidism, not necessary for nontoxic modular goiter
White blood cell count and differential cell count	Infection, diseases of white blood cells including leukemia, radiation/chemotherapy, immunosuppressive therapy, hypersplenism, aplastic anemia, other potentially relevant abnormalities (e.g., rheumatoid arthritis)

Note. Blood levels of certain pharmacologic agents, such as phenytoin (Dilantin) and digitalis preparations, may be indicated.
[a] Blood urea nitrogen.

Visitors can be asked to step out while the interview takes place unless the visitor functions as a history provider for pediatric or unreliable patients. For patient comfort, the interview should be conducted at eye level, several feet distant from the patient. Lighting should also be adequate for proper visual inspection and the anesthetist should have a properly functioning stethoscope. The patient must be alert and not under the influence of narcotics or tranquilizers.

Care taken with the initial approach can do much to create a good first impression. The anesthetist should appear tactful and unhurried, and clothing should be clean, neat, and professional. In no circumstances should the preoperative visit be made in a bloodstained scrub suit or with a dirty tourniquet wrapped around the stethoscope. It has been demonstrated that the proper use of names is a critical determinant of the patient's attitude, and the patient who is treated with respect is more likely to be satisfied and comply with instructions. The patient should be greeted using proper names, that is, Mrs. Katz, rather than impersonal nicknames. Pediatric patients may be addressed by first name.

The anesthesia practitioner should always indicate what his or her title and role are in the anesthetic care of the patient. The patient has the right to know if the preoperative visitor is a student, certified registered nurse anesthetist, or anesthesiologist. Furthermore, the patient needs to know if there is a chance that the person making the preoperative assessment will not be the same person administering the anesthetic.

Because a significant amount of information is needed from the health history, it is useful to follow an organized interview schedule. Use of silence, posture, and actions and projection of an accepting attitude encourage the patient's response. Direct questions should proceed from the general to the specific, avoiding leading questions. A graded response is preferable to a yes or no answer, for example, How many pillows do you sleep with at night? rather than Do you sleep with your head up? It is less confusing to the patient if the interviewer poses one question at a time, rather than ask a list of questions such as Have you ever had heart disease, lung disease, or liver disease? Language must be clearly understood and appropriate to the patient. Current medical jargon should be avoided and the anesthetist must also take pains to avoid any attitude of condescension or arrogance.

The health history can be organized in many ways.

TABLE 11–3. GUIDELINES FOR INTERPRETATION OF CLINICAL LABORATORY SERUM VALUES

Diagnostic Test	Interpretation
Hemoglobin/hematocrit	Concentrations vary depending on age and sex. High values (hemoconcentration) indicate polycythemia or dehydration. Low concentrations indicate anemia, hemorrhage, or fluid overload resulting in hemodilution.
Potassium	High concentrations may result from excessive exogenous intake such as oral supplements, succinylcholine, chemotherapy, familial periodic paralysis, renal disease, acidosis, or infusion of old blood. Common in trauma and burn victims are hypokalemia caused by GI losses, decreased oral intake, diuretic therapy, and respiratory and metabolic alkalosis.
Sodium	Disorders are associated with loss or gain of free water or sodium ion. Hypernatremia can result from inadequate fluid intake, impaired renal function, severe vomiting, or diarrhea. Hyponatremia results from excessive gastrointestinal suction, use of diuretics, sweating, renal insufficiency, or burns.
Chloride	Hyperchloremia results from aldosteronism, hyperventilation, severe dehydration, or renal failure. Hypochloremia results from gastric suctioning, renal failure, prolonged vomiting, gut fistulas, or any state causing excess extracellular fluid (edema).
Bicarbonate	Derangements indicate acid–base imbalances caused by changes in pulmonary or renal function.
Calcium	Hypercalcemia (excess) is associated with hyperparathyroidism and neoplastic disorders, multiple fractures, prolonged immobilization, and adrenal insufficiency. Hypocalcemia (deficiency) is associated with Cushing's syndrome, renal failure, pancreatitis, hypoparathyroidism, and malabsorption syndromes.
Magnesium	Disorders result from renal failure, Addison's disease, or drug therapy. Hypomagnesemia is associated with chronic alcoholism, malabsorption, diarrhea, burns, hyperparathyroidism, and prolonged gastric aspiration.
Blood urea nitrogen (BUN)	Elevated levels indicate possible renal failure, dehydration, urinary obstruction, burns, or other etiologies of protein catabolism. Low levels are present during malnutrition states or hepatic failure. BUN must be evaluated in relation to other renal function studies.
Creatinine	Elevation above 1.5 mg/dL indicates serious loss of nephron function. High levels are also associated with gigantism and acromegaly.
Aspartate transaminase (AST)	AST corresponds linearly with disease processes signifying extent of cellular necrosis. Low values (2–5 times normal) indicate metastatic tumors, pulmonary emboli, hemolytic anemia, biliary duct obstruction, and acute pancreatitis. Moderate levels (5–15 times normal) are present in chronic hepatitis, Duchenne muscular dystrophy, and resolving stages of a disease process. High values (20 times normal) may indicate acute viral hepatitis, severe skeletal muscle trauma, myocardial infarction (MI), cirrhosis, or hepatic congestion.
Alanine transaminase	Slight elevations are associated with acute MI or hepatic congestion. Moderate elevations indicate hepatic dysfunction. High levels (50 times normal) indicate drug-induced or viral hepatitis.
Lactic acid dehydrogenase (LDH)	LDH is elevated in many disease processes and indicates tissue necrosis. It is often used in diagnosis of acute MI after electrophoresis when LDH_1 is greater than LDH_2.
Creatine phosphokinase (CPK)	CPK may be elevated in severe hypokalemia, CO poisoning, MH, pulmonary or cerebral infarction, malignant tumor, or shock. It is indicative of myocardial cellular necrosis and attendant to skeletal muscle injury.
Alkaline phosphatase	Alkaline phosphatase may be indicative of skeletal disease, biliary obstruction, cirrhosis, viral hepatitis, malignant disease, or hyperparathyroidism.
Total proteins	Increased levels are associated with leukemia, myeloma, vomiting/diarrhea, dehydration, arthritis, and infection. Decreased levels are associated with congestive heart failure, hemorrhage, hepatic dysfunction, gastrointestinal disease, severe burns, surgical trauma, toxemia, malnutrition and diabetes mellitus and hyperthyroidism and renal disease.
Albumin	Increased levels are associated with multiple myeloma. Decreased levels are associated with hyperthyroidism, carcinoma, malnutrition, peptic ulcers, systemic lupus erythematosus, renal impairment, arthritis, and plasma loss resulting from burns.
Bleeding time	Prolongation in view of normal platelet count indicates platelet dysfunction, associated with leukemias, disseminated intravascular coagulation (DIC), severe hepatic disease, or deficiency of factors I, II, V, VII, VIII, IX, and XI.
Platelet count	Thrombocytosis is associated with infection, malignancies, anemias, pregnancy, and splenectomy. Thrombocytopenia is associated with carcinoma, leukemias, B_{12} deficiency, DIC, sequestration of platelets in the spleen, or mechanical breakdown.
Prothrombin time	Prolonged values are associated with deficiencies in fibrinogen, prothrombin, factors V, VII, or X, anticoagulant therapy (coumadin), hepatic diseases, or vitamin K deficiency.
Activated partial thromboplastin time	Prolonged times indicate deficiency in all procoagulants except VII and XIII or the presence of heparin.
Fibrinogen	Decreased levels may indicate DIC, fibrinolysis, malignancies, severe hepatic disease, or trauma. Elevated levels are associated with malignant states or inflammatory disorders.

TABLE 11–4. LABORATORY ABNORMALITIES THAT CORRELATE WITH HIGH RISK CAUSED BY PULMONARY DYSFUNCTION

Function	Value
Maximum voluntary ventilation (MVV)	50% predicted or 50 L/min
$Paco_2$	>45 torr
Forced expiratory volume (FEV_1)	<0.5 L
Forced expiratory flow (FEF)	25–75% 0.6 L
Forced vital capacity (FVC)	<1 L
Electrocardiogram (ECG)	Abnormal
Pao_2	<55
Maximum expiratory flow rate (MEFR)	100 L/min

Table 11–6 shows a suggested method of organizing the data. It should be kept in mind that the sequencing of information is not as important as thoroughness. The topics listed should be rephrased in layperson's terms. For the beginning anesthetist, the formulation of proper questions to elicit required data can be problemmatic, especially when trying to use language that the patient can comprehend. In Table 11–7 are some examples of questions that seek to explore particular organ systems on what would be considered a healthy patient (American Society of Anesthesiologists [ASA] classes I and II). On the basis of positive answers to these questions, the anesthetist can pose more explicit questions to pinpoint specific problems, therapies, and so on. For most healthy adults undergoing routine surgery, the preoperative examination and interview should take about 15 to 20 minutes. Above all, the oral history should be taken in an organized fashion usually by organ system, once preliminary data have been obtained relative to past surgical history, anticipated surgery, anesthetic-related problems in self or family, drug history, current medications, allergies, potential pregnancy, and other items.

TABLE 11–5. ECG AND CHEST X-RAY ABNORMALITIES

ECG Abnormalities	Chest X-ray Abnormalities
Atrial fibrillation or flutter	Pneumonia and atelectasis
Atrial or ventricular prematurities	Tracheal deviation
Ventricular hypertrophy	Pulmonary edema/effusions
ST segment changes	Mediastinal/pulmonary masses
Peaked T-waves/prolonged QT	Bony fractures
Previous/evolving myocardial infarction	Cardiomegaly/aneurysms
Atrioventricular block	Foreign body

THE PHYSICAL ASSESSMENT

In practice, the physical assessment and health history can be obtained simultaneously. Organization and thoroughness are the hallmarks of a good preanesthetic physical assessment. In some institutions, the complete physical assessment may be done by the surgeon or clinical nurse specialist. The CRNA then reviews the findings and focuses his or her physical assessment on areas most pertinent to anesthesia. This, however, does not obviate the anesthetist from the responsibility of meeting with the patient, even if before the surgery in the operating holding area, and confirming pertinent anesthetic-related data.

In the event that the CRNA conducts the entire physical assessment, a relaxed, unhurried, professional approach is imperative for the patient's comfort and confidence. The patient's privacy and freedom from interruption are of primary importance. Ideally the patient should sit on the edge of the bed for most of the examination, allowing examination of the front and back of the chest. As the physical assessment is carried out, the anesthetist explains the procedures to be done, gives appropriate instructions, and warns the patient of any maneuver that may produce discomfort. The examination is conducted systematically, from head to foot. The following equipment may be used: flashlight, tongue depressor, stethoscope with diaphragm and bell, and blood pressure cuff.[11]

General Impression

The physical examination begins with inspection of the patient's general appearance, including general observations such as the patient's chronologic age to age of appearance, race, extent and appropriateness of physical development, skin color and turgor, height, weight and proportion, gait, and posture. Personality characteristics and emotional status can also be observed. Abnormalities in any of these areas deserve further exploration during the physical assessment.

Head and Neck

It is paramount that the physical examination of the patient always include a thorough examination of the head and neck, primarily to assess potential problems with intubation and general airway management. The head is inspected to evaluate general size, shape, and proportion; to note symmetry and normalcy of ears; and to identify the presence of maldistribution of hair. The eyes are examined for redness or drainage, and the pupils inspected with a flashlight for reaction to light and accommodation. Inspection of the nasal cavity through the anterior naris reveals the degree of nasal symmetry, septal position, patency of nares, and condition of the turbinates. This information is essential if nasoendotracheal intubation is planned. The patient is asked to breathe through each nostril independently to compare patency. Dark red nasal mucosa indicates inflammation, rhinitis, or hemorrhage.

The mouth and pharynx are inspected using a tongue depressor and flashlight. The tongue is evaluated for size, deviation, and the presence of lesions. The size of the

TABLE 11–6. THE PREANESTHETIC HEALTH HISTORY

General Health History	*Cardiovascular History*
General state of health	Hypertension
Age, height, weight	Myocardial infarction
Activities of daily living/work	Heart failure
Previous hospitalization/surgery/anesthesia	Anemia
Medications/dosage/efficiency	Angina
Allergies	Exercise tolerance
Alcohol intake/drug use	Paroxysmal nocturnal dyspnea
Nutrition	Coagulopathy
Personal or Family History of Surgical or	*Neuromuscular History*
Anesthetic Complications	Headaches
Postoperative bleeding	Seizures
Perioperative cardiac arrest	Transient ischemic attacks
Cancellation of surgery	Paralysis/paresis
Postoperative jaundice	Muscular disorders
Prolonged apnea	Back pain
Malignant hyperthermia	Syncope/paresis
''Allergies'' to anesthesia	*Gastrointestinal Tract*
Respiratory History	Most recent intake
Dyspnea/orthopnea	Hiatal hernia
Exercise tolerance	Ulcers
Asthma/bronchitis	*Endocrine History*
Tuberculosis	Diabetes
Pneumothorax	Liver disease/jaundice
Smoking history	Thyroid disease
Cough/wheezing	*Renal History*
Colds	Kidney disease
Epistaxis	Genitourinary disease
Hoarseness	*Gynecologic History*
	Vaginal bleeding
	Pregnancy

tongue is an important consideration when use of a mask is planned. A large tongue is seen with such conditions as acromegaly, cretinism, and mongolism. Beyond the tongue and above it is an arch formed by the anterior and posterior pillars, soft palate, and uvula. A long, narrow oral cavity has minimal space within the dental arch, making intubation difficult, as the laryngoscope blocks the anesthetist's view of the larynx. Absence of a clear view of the uvula on oral examination may indicate a difficult, anterior intubation. A narrow, V-shaped arch can compromise placement of the laryngoscope as well, because the blade catches on the maxillary teeth. The normal soft palate is pink, moist, and smooth without inflammation or masses. There are usually 32 teeth in the adult mouth. Dental abnormalities, such as missing, chipped, or diseased teeth and gums, are identified. Incisors that are widely spread apart or protruding may present a problem with instrumentation, and dental malocclusion can lead to difficulties with airway management.

The mouth is examined for the presence of loose teeth. Newly erupted deciduous teeth appear at approximately 6 months of age. At this time, the roots are only partially formed. Permanent teeth begin to erupt at 6 years of age; therefore, loose deciduous teeth can be expected between the ages of 6 and 12. The location of loose teeth is noted on the chart and the parents warned of possible damage. It is recommended that the patient or parent (in the case of minors) sign a sheet describing the condition of the teeth.

Besides damage to the teeth, the possibility of a dislodged tooth migrating to the pharynx, larynx, or trachea is also a danger. The existence and position of dental crowns and bridges are noted on the preoperative evaluation to minimize the possibility of damage. The patient is advised to remove any dentures preoperatively. The patient's teeth should also be assessed for evidence of an overriding maxilla or receding jaw which portends difficulty in intubation.

Some congenital anomalies result in unusual problems in airway management, which can be anticipated. Pierre Robin syndrome is characterized by a small mandible, micrognathia, and downward displacement or retraction of the tongue; Treacher Collins syndrome presents with a receding chin; and hemifacial microsomia is a deformity consisting of hypoplasia of the mandible and soft-tissue structures of the face and cranium.

Joint function is an additional anatomic factor that is important when considering airway management. Two distinct motions are involved in the joint function of the mouth. The hingelike action of the condyle allows the mouth to open partially, whereas the wider opening of the mouth results from a motion of anterior displacement and forward gliding. Ankylosis of the temporomandibular joint or progressive arthritic changes may limit mandibular opening. Mobility of the temporomandibular joint is assessed by asking the patient to open his or her mouth as wide as possible. The patient is then asked to touch chin to chest, to extend the head posteriorly as far as possible, and

TABLE 11–7. EXAMPLES OF QUESTIONS THAT MAY BE USED TO OBTAIN THE HEALTH HISTORY

To Assess the Cardiovascular System
1. Have you ever had a heart attack or stroke? If so, when, and how would you describe your recovery?
2. Do you ever have chest pain or heart palpitations?
3. Do you have high blood pressure?
4. Have you ever had rheumatic fever or been told you had a heart murmur?
5. What is the most physically strenuous activity you have done in the last 2 weeks?
6. How many pillows do you sleep on at night?

To Assess the Respiratory System
1. Do you normally have shortness of breath conducting everyday activities such as vacuuming, gardening, carrying groceries, or walking up a single flight of stairs?
2. Do you ever wake up at night short of breath?
3. Do you smoke? If so, how much?
4. Do you have a history of any type of lung disease, especially pneumonia, asthma, and chronic bronchitis?
5. Do you currently have any symptoms of a cold, sore throat, or flu?
6. Do you cough frequently on awakening in the mornings?

To Assess the Renal System
1. Have you ever had a kidney disease?
2. Do you eat a normal diet or on any type of oral fluid restriction?
3. Have you ever taken medications for anemia?

To Assess the Gastrointestinal System
1. Do you have problems with abdominal pain or bloating?
2. Do you have heartburn, especially after eating?
3. Do you have problems with intermittent nausea and vomiting, excessive thirst, or diarrhea?

To Assess the Hepatic System
1. Have you ever had hepatitis, yellow jaundice, or malaria?
2. Have you recently been exposed to anyone with those conditions?
3. Do you drink wine, beer, or hard liquor? If so, how much and how frequently?
4. Do you have exposure to abused drugs? If so, when did you last use them?
5. Do you bleed easily, for example, when you brush your teeth?

To Assess the Nervous System
1. Have you ever had a seizure, convulsion, or fit?
2. Have you ever had an arm or leg go numb or been paralyzed?
3. Do you have problems with headache or double vision?

---

to turn the head to the right and to the left to assess range of motion. Normally the chin can be touched to the chest and the head can be bent through at least 45 degrees and rotate 90 degrees to either side, parallel with the shoulder axis. The neck is examined for physical characteristics, keeping in mind that airway management is more difficult when the patient has a short, muscular neck. The neck is inspected for symmetry and abnormal swelling or masses and the trachea palpated. The presence of nodules or swelling of the thyroid gland is noted.

The mobility of the cervical vertebrae is dependent on 23 joints extending from the occiput to the thoracic verte-brae. The joint movement consists of sliding, rotation, flexion, and extension. The normal flexion and extension of the head vary from 165 to 190 degrees, with a 20 percent decrease in range of motion expected after the age of 75. Impaired cervical mobility may not be apparent on casual observation, and the patient may be unaware of the disability because limited extension at the lower cervical vertebrae is possible. An anterior intubation may be anticipated when the distance between the superior ridge of the cricoid cartilage is less than three fingerbreadths from the tip of the mandible.

The vasculature of the neck is also inspected at this time. The jugular veins are the most visible veins proximal to the mediastinal and cardiac structures. The jugular veins are observed for venous congestion and for suitability for cannulation. The internal jugular veins and carotid artery cross superior to the neck just lateral to and slightly behind the trachea. Atherosclerosis frequently affects the carotid arteries, producing audible bruits that may be auscultated with a stethoscope. Carotid pulsations are palpated for quality and symmetry.

Lungs and Thorax

Examination of the lungs and thorax is accomplished by inspection, palpation, percussion, and auscultation. The posterior thorax is inspected while the patient is in the sitting position, with arms folded across the chest. Anterior thorax and lungs can be examined with the patient in Fowler's position. The midsternal, midclavicular, and anterior axillary line provide imaginary vertical reference points for localization of pertinent anatomic landmarks (Fig. 11–1). Ribs can be numbered by using the sternal angle to locate the adjacent second rib. The external measurement along the body surface from the upper border of the cricoid cartilage to the tip of the xiphoid process corresponds to the internal distance from the upper teeth to the carina. Knowing that the trachea bifurcates at the level of the second interspace is helpful when judging endotracheal tube length.

Assessment of the chest begins with observation of the rate, rhythm, and effort of respiration. The ratio of inspiration to expiration (normal approximately 1:2) is noted and the depth of respiration estimated. The slope of the ribs and shape of the chest are assessed. Abnormal retractions or a widened costal angle indicate the presence of obstructive disease. Palpation is used to assess respiratory excursion and to evaluate tactile fremitus. The anesthetist places his or her hands parallel to the tenth rib posteriorly and the costal margin anteriorly (Fig. 11–2). The range and symmetry of respiratory movement are observed as the patient inhales deeply and exhales. The patient is then asked to repeat the word *ninety-nine*. Simultaneously the anesthetist uses the lateral aspect of his or her hand to palpate the vibration transmitted through the bronchopulmonary system to the chest wall (Fig. 11–3). Fremitus is decreased when a bronchus is obstructed or the pleural space is filled with fluid or air. Lung consolidation is manifested by increased fremitus. Percussion causes vibration of the chest wall and underlying tissue, which produces audible sounds. Per-

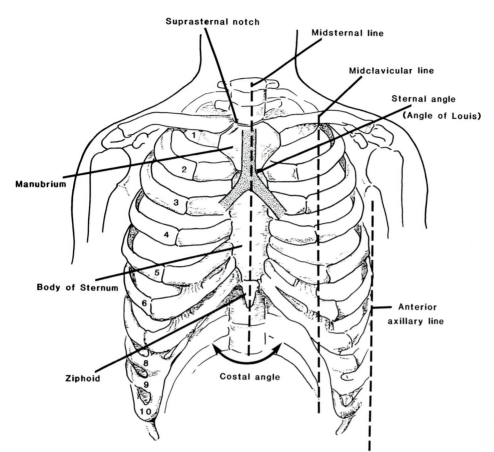

Suprasternal notch

Midsternal line

Midclavicular line

Sternal angle
(Angle of Louis)

Manubrium

Body of Sternum

Ziphoid

Costal angle

Anterior
axillary line

Figure 11-1. Anatomic relationships of surface and internal structures.

cussion can be done either directly or indirectly. Direct percussion is accomplished by striking the body surface with the tips of all four fingers held together; however, the indirect method is most commonly used (Fig. 11–4). The examiner hyperextends the middle finger of the left hand, firmly pressing the distal phalanx on the body surface to be

percussed. This stationary finger is referred to as the pleximeter. The middle finger of the other hand (plexor) is used to strike the base of the distal phalanx of the left middle finger. The sounds produced by percussion are described in Table 11–8.

Auscultation of the chest with the diaphragm of a

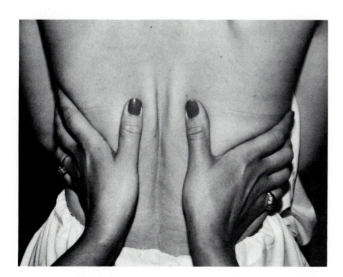

Figure 11-2. Palpation technique for respiratory excursion.

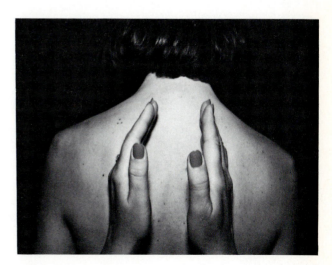

Figure 11-3. Palpation technique for transmission of bronchopulmonary vibrations.

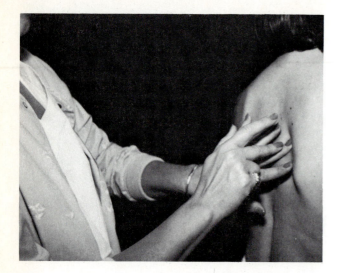

Figure 11–4. Indirect method of palpation.

stethoscope yields information about the quality of breath sounds and the presence of any abnormal sounds. The pitch, intensity, and duration of respirations are noted in all lung fields. Adventitious sounds are superimposed on breath sounds and are not normally heard. Rales are discrete, crackling sounds heard most often on inspiration. They are caused by the bubbling of air through a fluid medium. Rales often disappear with deep breathing or coughing. Rhonchi and wheezes are more prominent during expiration and are caused by air passing through a partially obstructed airway. Pleural friction rubs are rough, multiphasic, rubbing sounds that are present when the pleura is inflamed. Adventitious sounds should be identified by type, timing in the respiratory cycle, and location.

Semiquantitative screening tests of pulmonary function may be employed when bedside spirometry is not available. The anesthetist may accompany the patient walking down the hall or climbing one flight of stairs to quantify "breathlessness." Another semiquantitative test of pulmonary function is carried out with the anesthetist applying a stethoscope to the interscapular region and asking the patient to breathe in as much air as possible. The anesthetist times the expiratory effort until expirations are inaudible. The patient with obstructive lung disease will take considerable time to exhale, and expiratory sounds will be heard longer than 3 seconds. Vital capacity can be measured with a spirometer. A simple test to evaluate the presence of retained secretions

is to ask the patient to take a deep breath and forcibly exhale a few times. In the patient with chronic bronchitis, this maneuver will usually produce an attack of paroxysmal coughing with rhonchi and wheezing.

Cardiovascular System

Physical examination of the heart requires that the patient be supine or with the upper body slightly elevated. The anterior chest is inspected for abnormal pulses, which can sometimes be felt as "thrills." The point of maximum impulse is identified relative to superficial landmarks. A stethoscope is used to auscultate the first and second heart sounds (S_1 and S_2). S_2 is normally louder than S_1 at the aortic (second right interspace close to the sternum) and pulmonic (second left interspace close to the sternum) areas. Extrasystolic or diastolic sounds are identified and noted for location, timing, intensity, pitch, and effects of respirations on the sounds. The heart rate is counted for a minute and the heart rhythm evaluated. The patient should have the blood pressure and pulse rate taken in both the sitting and supine positions to demonstrate presence of orthostatic hypotension. Blood pressure readings should be taken in both upper extremities when occlusive disease is expected. The carotid arteries should be palpated and pulsations of the jugular vein examined. Evidence of jugular engorgement should be noted as should any evidence of associated heptomegaly or splenomegaly. Such evidence may indicate congestive heart failure and symptoms may be associated with peripheral edema.

The tricuspid (lower left sternal border) and mitral (fifth interspace medial to the midclavicular line) areas are auscultated for abnormal sounds. The patient is positioned with the left side down for accentuation of mitral murmurs and presence of S_3 or S_4. S_4 is common in the presence of coronary heart disease. The clinical features of peripheral vascular disease of the lower extremities include diminution or absence of pulses, systolic bruits, ischemic skin changes, and muscle wasting. The anesthetist palpates peripheral pulses bilaterally and compares one side against the other. An Allen test is done if arterial catheterization is planned. The blood pressure is measured with a sphygmomanometer in both arms. Average mean arterial pressure is calculated based on readings for a 24-hour period.

Vertebral Column and Back

The back should be inspected for symmetry, presence of lesions, rash, scar tissue indicating previous surgery, and

TABLE 11–8. QUALITIES OF PERCUSSION SOUNDS

Quality	Intensity	Pitch	Duration	Normal Location	Pathology
Resonant	Loud	Low	Long	Lung	
Hyperresonant	Very loud	Lower	Longer		Emphysema
Flat	Soft	High	Short	Thigh	Pleural effusion
Dull	Medium	Medium	Medium	Liver, diaphragm	Pneumonia, fluid in pleural space
Tympany	Loud	High	Long	Stomach, intestine	

curvature of the vertebral column. If regional anesthesia is planned, the patient's ability to flex the back should be evaluated and the appropriate intervertebral spaces palpated.

REDUCTION OF PATIENT ANXIETY

The short-term effects of patient psychologic preparation and teaching before surgery cannot be overemphasized relative to their importance to postoperative outcome. Research has shown that effective preoperative preparation reduces the need for pain medication in the postoperative period. This advantage could conceivably translate into a shorter hospital stay, making the time spent in psychologic preparation of the patient well worth the effort. The quality of the CRNA–patient interaction is more critical than the timing of this interaction. Reduction of anxiety can effectively occur by telephone conversation, by preoperative visit, or in the preoperative holding area.

Despite the safeguards of modern medicine, many patients experience intense fear in anticipation of the anesthetic and subsequent surgical procedure. Common preoperative concerns include fear of not awakening, experiencing pain, being paralyzed, awakening during the operation, being temporarily out of control of physiologic functions, and disclosing personal matters while under the influence of drugs.[12] Because this anxiety continues through the operation and beyond, it is imperative to decrease anxiety preoperatively. When properly done, the preoperative visit compares favorably with a purely pharmacologic approach. By demonstrating concern, the anesthetist can employ strategies aimed at reducing the patient's anxiety and educating the patient in ways that will strengthen his or her coping mechanisms.

Patients scheduled for surgery are likely to be experiencing many types of stresses, induced either at home or experienced in the hospital. The patient may be experiencing personal injury or illness that requires radical changes in personal habits and life-style, even if on a temporary basis. Normal routines of sleeping, eating, recreating, and spiritual activities are disrupted. Socially, the patient may undergo changes in marital relations or work setting, and his or her financial picture may be altered. The anesthetist must be sensitive to these possible stressors during the preanesthetic interview.

There is evidence that a striking relationship exists between preoperative fear and postoperative behavior.[13] Three distinct coping patterns have been noted in patients facing surgery:

1. *High anticipatory fear.* Patients in this category manifest a heightened level of anxiety and fear of pain, mutilation, and death. After surgery the patient continues to be extremely anxious.
2. *Moderate anticipatory fear.* Patients in this category worry occasionally and are anxious about specific details of the operation. After the operation they are cooperative and participate in their postoperative care.
3. *Low anticipatory fear.* Patients in this category exhibit an absence of anxiety coupled with an unrealistic, optimistic outlook. After surgery, they often demon-

strate difficult, obstinate, or recalcitrant behaviors such as refusing postoperative treatments or drugs or self-care routines.

During the preoperative visit, the anesthetist must give special attention to the patient's perception of anticipated effects or results of surgery and of recovery. It may be helpful to elicit details of the surgical and anesthetic experiences of relatives and friends as perceived by the patient to help him or her clarify expectations and quell undue fear or trepidation. Special attention should be given to the patient's past surgical history, especially if previous surgical experiences were unpleasant and can be avoided in the future.

The duration of the preoperative visit and characteristic interview techniques have been compared relative to their effectiveness in patients who demonstrate failed coping patterns. A cursory preoperative interview, one with minimal information and the absence of rapport, results in increased anxiety levels and increased thiopental sodium requirements in patients with low anticipatory fear. This same interview technique results in decreased anxiety and lower thiopental dosage in patients with high anticipatory fear. A supportive interview, of reasonable duration, including establishment of rapport and provision of information, has little effect on the patient with initial low anxiety levels. In the extremely anxious patient, this supportive interview also reduces the anxiety level. Clearly, the highly anxious patient needs a preoperative visit to reduce anxiety, regardless of the characteristics of that visit. It appears that maximum benefit in the patient's psychologic preparations will occur if the anesthetist supplies reassuring information about the events that will occur and identifies coping mechanisms that the patient can use to handle stress and pain.

EDUCATION OF THE PATIENT

Significant evidence exists to demonstrate that preoperative instruction has a positive and beneficial effect on postoperative outcomes. The development of the educational component of the preanesthetic interview must include characteristics of high-quality patient teaching. This includes (1) active participation by the patient focusing on the patient's learning needs; (2) content stressing what the patient should *do*, not just what the patient should *know*; and (3) use of a combination of written, visual, and personalized approaches to patient instruction.

The anesthetist first needs to evaluate the level of the patient's desire for information.[14] Care must be taken to avoid overbriefing. Some patients want only a minimal-to-moderate amount of simple, factual information; some want no information at all. A simple explanation of the preoperative holding room, intravenous lines, and anesthesia induction will usually suffice. The patient may then lead the interviewer to answer specific questions. If questions are asked about diagnosis and surgical treatment, the anesthetist must be careful that answers do not conflict with those provided by others. Patient-focused education in anesthesia practice is based on knowledge of common causes of anxiety in presurgical patients as well as procedure-specific facts.[15,16] For example, surveys have demonstrated that the majority of patients prefer general anesthesia induced by intravenous injection. With this preference in mind, sufficient time should be spent explaining planned regional techniques and answering questions regarding these techniques. It is never a good idea to instill fear in patients as a strategy for convincing them to accept a nondesired technique.

Preoperative information allows the patient to mentally "rehearse," to develop realistic expectations and plans for coping with the perioperative experience. As well as providing information, the anesthetist can counsel the patient about coping mechanisms. The anesthetist can provide active emotional support by fostering the patient's sense of control over density, for example, by teaching the technique of coughing and deep breathing, with a return demonstration by the patient, and at the same time explaining how this technique helps prevent atelectasis and maintain optimum lung function. In addition, reassurance can be given that postoperative analgesics will be available. The patient can also be shown how to splint the incision to reduce pain during coughing and deep breathing. Options for post operative pain control, such as use of an indwelling epidural catheter or patient-controlled anesthesia (PCA) pump, can be discussed. The anesthetist can also review the techniques for deep breathing and relaxation as a method for coping with stress and postoperative pain.

SECURING INFORMED CONSENT

Securing informed consent for anesthesia services is a primary duty of the anesthetist making the preoperative visit. This responsibility can be difficult if the anesthesia care provider is unclear as to the patient's ability or desire to assimilate this new and sometimes threatening information. Most hospitals require patients to sign a dual-purpose consent form that covers both surgery and administration of anesthesia. Some departments of anesthesiology have developed a separate form that specifically describes the type of anesthesia proposed and risk assessment. Should such a form exist, the anesthetist should not assume that the surgical permit alone will suffice for permission if a separate anesthesia form exists. If both types of permission forms exist, both must be signed.

Regardless of the type of form used, the quality and comprehensiveness of the anestheisa provider's explanation of the anesthetic course to the patient and the patient's understanding of this information are required for a bona fide informed consent. Courts generally agree that a proper informed consent must include three components: (1) the nature of the treatments proposed; (2) risks, complications, and expected benefits; and (3) alternative forms or modalities of treatment. Consent forms usually also contain verification that the provider has provided an accurate explanation of alternative anesthesia techniques available and a chronology of events that will occur in the operating room. The anesthetist must also identify the other anesthesia care providers who will be involved in the anesthetic care. Any particular concerns of the patient should be documented in the chart.

Special problems with informed consent arise in patients with limited intelligence, depressed levels of consciousness, or language barriers or in those who on reli-

gious grounds refuse a certain type of treatment or blood products. The anesthetist must assess the degree of limitation imposed before giving explanations or asking for written consent. If a language barrier exists, a neutral, objective translator must be located. The translator should be instructed to interpret and summarize information carefully. In the case of refusal of certain treatment modalities, a notation should be made on the chart including the potential risks of refusal. This addendum is most often included in the progress notes and bears the patient's signature designating approval. When the level of consciousness or intelligence is impaired, the anesthetist should retain permission from a family member or court-appointed guardian. Even after informed consent is obtained, the anesthetist should offer to answer any questions about the planned anesthetic agent or technique. Legally the patient is free to withdraw consent at any time even when on the operating room table, without future prejudice to care and treatment. To not comply with such wishes could leave the CRNA liable to charges of assault and battery.

EVALUATION AND DOCUMENTATION OF ANESTHETIC RISK

One of the goals of the preoperative visit is to evaluate the physical status or condition of the patient and, subsequently, the relative risk of anesthesia.[17] Identification of accurate estimates and predictors of risk remains elusive as many variables play a role in comprehensive assessment. Traditionally, practitioners have used subjective criteria based on factors such as the anesthetist's previous experience with similar patients and operations, clinical history, physical examination, laboratory results, the skill of the surgeon, and the characteristics of the institution or operating room environment. Classification systems have been devel-

TABLE 11–9. AMERICAN SOCIETY OF ANESTHESIOLOGISTS CLASSIFICATION OF PHYSICAL STATUS

Class I	The patient has no organic, physiologic, biochemical, or psychiatric disturbance. The pathologic process is localized and does not entail a systemic disturbance.
Class II	The patient has a mild to moderate systemic disturbance caused by either the conditions to be treated surgically or other pathophysiologic process. (Example: controlled hypertension.)
Class III	The patient has severe systemic disturbances that impact on activities of daily living. (Example: brittle diabetic.)
Class IV	The patient has severe systemic disorders that are life-threatening and not necessarily correctable by surgical means. (Example: widespread vascular disease and kidney failure.)
Class V	The patient is moribund and is not expected to survive 24 hours. (Example: head injury with stroke.)
Emergency	The patient is in one of the classes listed above and is having surgery on an emergency basis.

Reprinted, with permission, from Dripps et al.[18]

TABLE 11–10. MODIFIED CHILD'S INDEX FOR GRADING SEVERITY OF LIVER DISEASE

Clinical or Laboratory Feature	Points Scored for Increasing Abnormality*		
	1	**2**	**3**
Encephalopathy	None	Mild–moderate	Severe
Ascites	None	Slight	Moderate
Bilirubin	34.2 µmol/L (<2 mg/dL)	34.2–51.3 µmol/L (2–3 mg/dL)	>51.3 µmol/L (>3 mg/dL)
Albumin	35 g/L	28–34 g/L	<28 g/L
Prothrombin time (prolonged)	4 s	4–6 s	>6 s

* Patients with 5 to 6 points are considered good operative risks; those with 7 to 9 points, moderate risks; and those with 10 to 15 points, poor risks.
Adapted, with permission, from Pugh et al.[19]

oped to more accurately and objectively quantify the physical condition of patients. Often, practitioners consider these classification systems synonymous with risks of anesthesia. This practice, however, is not entirely reliable as research has failed to produce clear evidence that patient classification systems are, in fact, predictive of patient outcome. The reason for this is that most of the common systems, such as the ASA Classification of Physical Status, speak only to pathophysiologic characteristics of patients and do not include other factors such as human error or equipment failure which still account for a large segment of adverse patient outcomes. There is general agreement that the ASA Classification of Physical Status should not be construed as a risk classification.

TABLE 11–11. GOLDMAN CARDIAC OPERATIVE RISK INDEX SCORING SYSTEM (CRIS)[a]

Factors	Points
1. History	
Age > 70	5
Myocardial infarction within previous 6 months	10
Aortic stenosis	3
2. Physical examination	
Early diastolic gallop	11
Jugular venous distension or congestive heart failure	
3. ECG	
Nonsinus rhythm	7
>5 premature ventricular contractions per minute	7
4. General information	
Pao_2 < 60 mm Hg	3
$Paco_2$ > 50 mm Hg	3
Potassium 3 mEq/L	3
BUN > 50 mg/dL	3
Creatinine > 3 mg/dL	3
Bedridden	3
5. Operating	
Emergency	4
Intrathoracic	
Intraabdominal	3
Aortic surgery	3
Total	72

[a] Class I: 0–5 points, Class II: 6–12 points, Class III: 13–25 points, Class IV: 26 points or more.
Reprinted, with permission, from Goldman and Caldera.[20]

The ASA Classification of Physical Status, developed by Dripps et al.,[18] is one of the most commonly used systems to classify a patient's physical condition. On the basis of preoperative assessment, the patient is assigned to a particular classification. The categories of physical status (known as ASA Classes I–V, E or PS Classes I–V, E) are listed in Table 11–9.

Various other indexes for patient physical classification have been developed in addition to the Dripps system and some of these may be considered more akin to a traditional risk classification. A liver disease scoring system exists to predict patient outcome based on the presence of encephalopathy, ascites, bilirubinemia, increased prothrombin time, and decreased blood albumin (Table 11–10).[19] The Goldman Cardiac Operative Risk Index Scoring System (CRIS) is a multifactor index that has been used extensively for patients with cardiac disease to determine the risk and advisability of surgery (Table 11–11).[20] The authors recommend that elective surgery not be performed on patients with total CRIS scores over 26 points, which is considered a Class IV risk. The preoperative interview should include identification of factors contributing to cardiac risk. Coronary artery disease should be suspected if predisposing factors are noted. The risk of developing coronary artery disease is doubled by smoking, increased four times by the combination of smoking and hypertension, and increased eight times in the presence of smoking, hypertension, and elevated serum cholesterol. Additional danger signals include obesity, glucose intolerance, occlusive vascular events, and a family history of heart disease.

Despite the many objective scoring systems devised to estimate patient risk, the Dripps system has prevailed as the standard in anesthesia practice. Other systems, such as CRIS, may be employed in special situations. The ASA classification is entered on the patient's record before anesthesia, thereby providing a baseline for anesthesia planning and management decisions and as a later reference in guiding postoperative care.

OPTIMIZATION OF PREOPERATIVE STATUS: REDUCTION OF PERIOPERATIVE MORBIDITY

One of the primary goals of the preoperative visit is to use the data obtained to plan and implement strategies that will optimize the patient's preoperative status. The preanesthetic evaluation that is done in sufficient time to allow fur-

TABLE 11–12. PREEXISTING DISEASE, RISK, AND OPTIMIZATION OF PATIENT STATUS

Preexisting Disease	Risk	Management
Cardiac		
Coronary artery disease	Postop MI[a] with peak incidence on third postop day MI in past 3 months, 30% risk of reinfarction MI in past 3–6 months, 10% risk of reinfarction MI in past 6 months, 5% risk of reinfarction; rate remains constant	ECG within a day of surgery and on third and fifth postop day in high-risk patients Delay nonemergent surgery until 6 months post-MI Exercise tolerance test for major vascular procedures and in patients with unstable angina or new ECG findings Delay elective surgery to 30 days post-coronary artery bypass graft
Congestive heart failure	Postoperative pulmonary edema occurs in 2% of patients with no history of CHF, in 6% of patients with history of CHF and no current symptoms, and in 30% of patients with jugular venous distension or S_2 gallop Peak occurrence is immediate postop or 24–48 h later	Hemodynamic monitoring Preoperative diuretics, digitalization
Valvular heart disease	Aortic stenosis poses the greatest operative risk	Preoperative echocardiography Hemodynamic monitoring Endocarditis antibiotic prophylaxis if substantial valvular heart disease or undergoing contaminated procedures
Hypertension (diastolic > 110 mm Hg)	Postop hypertension occurs in 30% of patients > 60 with history of hypertension	Continue medication through morning of surgery Parenteral regime if patient incapable of oral intake postop
Pulmonary		
COPD is primary risk Asthma has significant reversible component	Increased risk of postoperative pulmonary complications include smoking history, obesity, age > 60, duration of anesthesia > 3 h, upper abdominal or thoracic operations Low risk: FEV > 2000 Medium risk: FEV 1000–2000 High risk: FEV < 1000 FEV_1 75% of predicted: high risk FEV_1 declines by 60% following thoracic and upper abdominal procedures MMV < 50%	Especially FEV_1 and % of predicted pulmonary function tests in patients with pulmonary symptoms such as dyspnea or chronic cough, and those undergoing upper abdominal procedures Arterial blood gases for baseline Cessation of smoking at least a week prior to surgery Theophylline or aerosolized bronchodilators Antibiotics for purulent cough Teach incentive spirometry in preparation for postop care Chest physiotherapy
Hematologic		
Anemia	Unknown	Transfuse to HCT 30% Transfuse to HCT 20% in cases of sickle cell anemia or chronic renal disease Transfuse 24 h prior to OR to allow regeneration of 2,3-DPG and reequilibration of blood volume Treat cause of anemia
Leukocytes	Wound healing unimpaired until granulocyte count of 500	
Platelets	Unknown	Platelet transfusion to 100,000 for major procedures, 30,000 for minor procedures Each unit of transfused platelets raises platelet count by 10,000 Posttransfusion platelet count Discontinue aspirin 5–7 days prior to surgery Stop nonsteroidal anti-inflammatory drugs 1–2 days prior to surgery
Clotting factor deficiency	Unknown	PT, PTT Increased PT usually due to warfarin therapy; stop warfarin 3–4 days preoperatively; 10 mg vitamin K may be given initially and repeated 12 h later; FFP therapy (20 mL/kg) is a more rapid means of reversing warfarin

TABLE 11–12. PREEXISTING DISEASE, RISK, AND OPTIMIZATION OF PATIENT STATUS (*continued*)

Preexisting Disease	Risk	Management
Hematologic (continued)		
Clotting factor deficiency (*continued*)		Administer FFP to patients with liver failure Increased PTT usually due to heparin Stop heparin 6 h prior to surgery May reverse heparin with protamine-specific factor replacement for hemophiliacs Low-dose heparin (5000 units SC, bid to tid) is standard regimen for prophylaxis of thromboembolism; indications include age > 40, cancer, obesity, immobilization, hypercoagulable states, and venous stasis
Endocrinologic		
Insulin-dependent diabetes mellitus	Unknown	Fasting blood sugar One-half insulin dose of intermediate-acting before surgery with glucose containing intravenous infusion Some advocate "no glucose–no insulin" for minor procedures
Non-insulin-dependent diabetes mellitus	Unknown	Stop long-acting sulfonylureas, such as chlorpropamide, 3 days prior to surgery to avoid hypoglycemia Discontinue short-acting agents the day before surgery
Obesity	By itself, unknown risk	Preoperative weight loss, cessation of smoking, optimization of pulmonary and cardiac function, and prophylactic heparinization
Steroid therapy	Adrenal suppression in patient who has been on steroids for a week or more in the preceding 12 months	Corticosteroid supplements
Hepatic		
Chronic liver dysfunction	Chronic liver dysfunction increases likelihood of postoperative pulmonary, renal, bleeding, and healing abnormalities	Monitor volume status Laboratory workup including Hgb, PT, creatinine, lytes, and liver function tests Correct clotting and electrolyte abnormalities, reduce ascites, alleviate encephalopathy, and improve nutritional status
Acute hepatitis	Relative contraindication to surgery	Avoid elective surgery until a month after liver function tests have returned to normal
Renal	If renal insufficiency is glomerular, intestinal, or obstructive, risk increased by decline in creatinine clearance If nephrotic syndrome is present, amount of azotemia determines operative risk	Management of total body sodium, serum potassium, and acid–base status Fluid restriction and avoidance of hypotonic IV solution if Na^{2+} less than 125 mm/L Antihypertensive or loop diuretics Dialysis or ultrafiltration Patients on maintenance dialysis must be dialyzed within 24 h of surgery. Avoid dialysis in the 4 h preceding surgery Preoperative infusion of cryoprecipitate, deamino-8-D-arginine vasopression, or conjugated estrogens may reduce bleeding in uremic patients

[a] MI, myocardial infarction; CHF, congestive heart failure; COPD, chronic obstructive pulmonary disease; HCT, hematocrit; PT, prothrombin time; PTT, partial thromboplastin time; FFP, fresh-frozen plasma; Hgb, hemoglobin.

ther diagnostic tests and preparation of the patient may significantly reduce perioperative morbidity or mortality. Frequently facts come to light in the preoperative assessment that call for review of previous charts. Any suggestion that a personal or family history of anesthetic complications exists should be examined in greater detail. If the patient has had previous surgery at the same institution, old anesthesia records should be retrieved and studied. Old patient records can provide valuable insights into future care. For instance, if the patient describes a history of prolonged apnea after a previous anesthetic, a thorough probe of possible causes is carried out; this may include securing a

TABLE 11–13. DRUG MANAGEMENT AND PREOPERATIVE PREPARATION

Drug	Preoperative Preparation	Potential Intraoperative Problems
Antianginal medications	Sublingual tablets can be continued until induction with IV nitroglycerin or paste administered intraoperatively. Met-hemoglobin levels of heavy nitrate users should be monitored.	Potentiate hypotensive effects of some anesthetic agents, particularly in hypovolemic patients.
Antiarrhythmics	Continue to day of surgery.	Potentiate neuromuscular blockers.
Antibiotics	Avoid aminoglycosides (i.e., neomycin).	Aminoglycosides potentiate neuromuscular blockers and anesthetics that provide muscular relaxation.
Anticoagulants	Replace oral anticoagulants with subcutaneous heparin to ensure prompt reversal, if necessary, with IV protamine sulfate.	Oral anticoagulants are not reversed by protamine sulfate and it takes 24–48 h for IV vitamin K_1 (phytonadione [AquaMEPHYTON]) to return prothrombin time to normal.
Antidiabetics	Measure preoperative blood sugar. Discontinue chlorpropamide 3 days before surgery and continue all other oral hypoglycemics until the evening before surgery. Begin glucose/insulin infusion before surgery if indicated.	Intraoperative fluctuations in blood sugar.
Antihypertensives	Continue methyldopa, reserpine, and guanethidine to day of surgery. Continue clonidine parenterally to avoid severe rebound hypertension.	Unstable blood pressure with wide fluctuations.
Antiparkinson medications	Continue levodopa until night before surgery. If antiemetic is needed, antihistamine type (diphenhydramine) is preferred over phenothiazine.	Phenothiazines nullify antiparkinson effects of levodopa. Aminoglycosides may interact to cause neuromuscular blockade.
Antiseizure medications	Phenytoin augments nondepolarizing neuromuscular blockade.	Continue phenytoin and phenobarbital to day of surgery.
Beta blockers	Continue to day of surgery. May be given IV if oral route is contraindicated.	Potentiate cardiac depressant effects of some anesthetics.
Cardiac glycosides	Continue to day of surgery. Assess patient for signs of digitalis toxicity or potassium depletion and correct if present.	Potentiate nondepolarizing muscle relaxants.
Corticosteroids	Continue to day of surgery. Administer 100 mg hydrocortisone 1 h before surgery.	Patients who are on corticosteroid therapy (7.5 mg daily prednisone or equivalent) for at least 2 months preceding surgery require intraoperative and postoperative supplementation.
Psychotropes	MAO[a] inhibitors should be discontinued 2 weeks before surgery.	MAO inhibitors interact with narcotic analgesics (i.e., meperdine [Demerol]), local anesthetic/epinephrine combinations, and other vasopressors.
	Continue tricyclic antidepressants, lithium, and phenothiazine antipsychotics to day of surgery.	Lithium prolongs the effect of depolarizing muscle relaxants.

[a] MAO, monoamine oxidase.

dibucaine number and a pseudocholinesterase level. Similarly, a patient who describes an episode that sounds like malignant hyperthermia can be further assessed with creatine phosphokinase levels or muscle biopsy with in vitro testing. Should the preoperative diagnosis of malignant hyperthermia be substantiated, strategies can be undertaken to minimize the patient's risk, including administration of preoperative dantrolene sodium and heavy sedation on the morning of surgery.

The nutritional status of the patient can be cause for preoperative intervention. Preoperative parenteral nutrition has been shown to decrease wound infections significantly in patients with low serum albumin. Preoperative measures can be instituted to minimize risk in the patient with pulmonary disease if the patient is taught the use of incentive spirometry and the importance of coughing and deep breathing. At this time the anesthetist explains the adverse effects of anesthesia, postoperative medication, dressings, and immobilization in the supine position on respiratory function. If postoperative ventilation is probable, the patient is so informed. The patient is encouraged to quit smoking, recognizing that although carboxyhemoglobin levels will

decrease immediately on cessation of smoking; improvement in pulmonary function requires several weeks. Administration of antibiotics, bronchodilators, steroids, or sympathomimetics may reverse bronchospasm. Mobilization of secretions should be attempted by hydration, aerosol therapy, expectorants, and chest physiotherapy.

General guidelines have been developed for the scheduling of anesthesia and surgery on the patient with pulmonary disease. Surgery is scheduled late in the day if the patient has chronic bronchitis, to allow for morning mobilization of sputum. A 2-week interval between the occurrence of upper respiratory tract infection and elective surgery is advisable to minimize the chance of pulmonary complications. Hyperirritability of the airways is present for several weeks after acute asthma attacks; therefore, it is recommended that the disease symptoms be pharmacologically controlled before surgery and anesthesia.

The various body systems must be considered in relation to optimization of physical status. Patient factors that increase the risk of surgery and recommendations on how to minimize surgical risk are listed in Table 11–12. With the recent advances in pharmacology, it is common to find patients taking a number of prescription and over-the-counter drugs. This is especially true in patients over 55 years of age. Preoperative management of pharmacotherapeutic agents is specific to the individual drugs (Table 11–13).

SELECTION OF PREMEDICATION AND MANAGEMENT PLANS

After preoperative assessment, a choice of preoperative medication is made. The primary factor in this decision is the individual patient's psychologic need for pharmacologic intervention to relieve anxiety or control pain. The patient's physical status and the planned surgery are also considerations. For some patients, such as the patient in shock, no preoperative medication may be required. In contrast, the patient presenting for cerebral aneurysm clipping will require significant premedication. A multitude of drugs are used for premedication purposes (Table 11–14). It is preferred that the drugs chosen have a synergistic effect with the planned anesthetic. A narcotic–tranquilizer combination may be an excellent preanesthetic medication when a balanced anesthetic technique is planned. Anticholinergics are avoided when regional anesthesia is used. Preoperative medications are discussed more extensively in Chapter 14. A preoperative holding area is the ideal setting for administration of preanesthetic medication for most patients. In this setting the anesthetist can safely administer intravenous medications, thus sparing the patient an additional intramuscular injection. Administration of intravenous premedications by the CRNA and subsequent observation allow for a more accurate estimation of patient response to the planned intravenous anesthetic agents. Close nursing supervision of the patient is available in the preoperative holding area, allowing for optimum titration of the drugs.

The primary purpose of preoperative evaluation and preparation of the surgical patient is to allow for the generation of an anesthetic care plan that will provide maximum

TABLE 11–14. PREANESTHESIA MEDICATION

Classification	Drug	Adult Dosage (mg)
Narcotics	Butorphanol tartrate	2.0
	Fentanyl	0.05–0.015
	Meperidine	50.0–100.0
	Morphine	5.0–15.0
	Sufentanil	0.005–0.010
Anticholinergics	Atropine	0.4–0.6
	Glycopyrrolate	0.2–0.3
	Scopolamine	0.3–0.5
Tranquilizers/sedatives	Diazepam	5.0–10.0
	Droperidol	2.5–5.0
	Hydroxyzine	50.0–150.0
	Lorazepam	1.0–4.0
	Midazolam	1.0–4.0
	Promethazine	25.0–50.0

safety for the patient. The choice of anesthetic technique and agent is based on many factors, including patient condition and preference, type and duration of surgery, skill and preference of the anesthetist, and characteristics of the surgeon and institution. The foundation of the anesthetic care plan lies in the analysis of information gleaned during the preoperative evaluation process. Synthesis of patient-specific information with learned physiologic, pharmacologic, anesthesia, and nursing principles results in generation of an optimum plan of care.

In the educational setting, completion of a verbal or written anesthetic care plan is integral to the process of learning. Planning should be characterized by a series of decisions that are based solidly on a competent theoretical base, accurate patient data, and compliance with accepted standards of care. Rarely are specific drugs or techniques strictly contraindicated, allowing significant flexibility in decision making and planning; however, it is incumbent on the CRNA to be able to justify decisions, provide alternative care plans, incorporate patient data germane to the surgical procedure, and anticipate potential postanesthetic problems. The CRNA should plan for all phases of patient care—pre, intra, and post—during the perioperative course. Perhaps it is this single characteristic of practice that has earned CRNAs the deserved reputation as providers of comprehensive and systematic care. The surgeon depends significantly on the CRNA to keep him or her informed of the patient's condition at all times. This trust must become the hallmark of clinical practice for all CRNAs.

REFERENCES

1. Cebul R, Beck J. Applications in ambulatory screening and preadmission testing of adults. *Ann Intern Med.* 1987; 106:403–413.
2. Kaplan E, Sheirer L, Boeckmann A, et al. The usefulness of preoperative laboratory screening. *JAMA.* 1985;253(24):3576–3581.
3. Roizen MF. The compelling rationale for less preoperative testing. *Can J Anaesth.* 1988;35:214–215. Editorial.
4. Corman LC, Bolt RJ, eds. Symposium on medical evaluation of the prospective patient. *Med Clin North Am.* 1979;63:1129–1390.

5. Elliot D, Linz DH, Kane JA. Medical evaluation before operation. *West J Med.* 1982;137:351–358.

6. Luce JM. Preoperative evaluation and perioperative management of patients with pulmonary disease. *Postgrad Med.* 1980;67:201–207.

7. Hodgkin JE, Dines DE, Didier EP. Preoperative evaluation of the patient with pulmonary disease. *Mayo Clin Proc.* 1973;48;114–118.

8. Mohr D, Jett J. Preoperative evaluation of pulmonary risk factors. *J Gen Intern Med.* 1988;3:277–287.

9. Charpak Y, Blery C, Chastang C, et al. Prospective assessment of a protocol for selective ordering of preoperative chest x-rays. *Can J Anaesth.* 1988;35(3):259–264.

10. Macpherson D, Snow R, Lofgren R. Preoperative screening—value of previous tests. *Ann Intern Med.* 1990;113(12):969–973.

11. Bates B. *A guide to physical examination.* 34th ed. Philadelphia: JB Lippincott; 1983.

12. Sheude K, Panagopoulos G. A survey of 800 patients' knowledge, attitudes, and concerns regarding anesthesia. *Anesth Analg.* 1991;73(2):190–198.

13. Williams J, Jones JR, Workhover MN. The psychological control of preoperative anxiety. *Psychophysiology.* 1975;12:50–54.

14. Elsass P, Eikard B, Junge J, et al. Psychological effect of detailed preanesthetic information. *Acta Anesthesiol Scand.* 1987;31:579–583.

15. Twerksy R, Frank D, Lebovits A. Evaluation for surgical outpatients—Does it matter? *Anesthesiology.* 1990;73:3A.

16. Bartlett E. How can patient education contribute to improved health care under prospective pricing? *Health Policy.* 1986;6:290–298.

17. Kroehke K. Preoperative evaluation: The assessment and management of surgical risk. *J Gen Intern Med.* 1987;2:257–269.

18. Dripps RD, Lamont A, Eckenhoff JE. The role of anesthesia in surgical mortality. *JAMA.* 1961;178:261–266.

19. Pugh RNH, Murray-Lyon IM, Dawson JL, et al. Preoperative management of patients with liver disease. *Surg Clin North Am.* 1968;48:907–930.

20. Goldman L. Caldera DL. Multifactorial index of cardiac risk in non-cardiac surgical procedures. *N Engl J Med.* 1977;297:845–850.

Perioperative Monitoring

Scot D. Foster
and J. L. Reeves-Viets

The primary role of the nurse anesthetist is to provide a safe anesthetic with optimal patient outcomes, according to the needs of the patient and the requirements of the surgeon. A safe anesthetic may be defined to include several discrete functions.

1. Obtain and collate data sufficient for preoperative evaluation and perioperative planning.
2. Administer a physiologically sound anesthetic according to the patient's condition and the type of surgery anticipated.
3. Collect appropriate perioperative data to evaluate the patient's course and extrapolate pertinent information which allows timely and efficacious interventions, if required.
4. Competently evaluate all instituted therapies.
5. Document in writing all events of the perioperative course on the medical record.
6. Conduct all decision making and clinical judgments within the framework of accepted clinical and academic practice/theory, as well as accepted standards of patient care.

The clinical practice of anesthesia and monitoring specifically has changed rapidly with the advent of new technologies. It is incumbent on the practicing nurse anesthetist to make himself/herself aware of the changes and to incorporate them into practice. This chapter deals with the basics of intraoperative monitoring and interpretation of data obtained to benefit clinical decision making.

ISSUES OF PATIENT SAFETY AND ANESTHESIA RISK

Perhaps the greatest influence on the quality of anesthesia care, within the last decade, has been the attention given to patient safety. These concerns have been manifest in a variety of ways; predominant among them was the development of quality assurance and risk management programming and written standards for clinical monitoring of patients undergoing anesthesia. Most practitioners agree that the introduction of capnometry and pulse oximetry has been largely responsible for the recent declines in patient morbidity and mortality. Prior to 1984, it was estimated that the risk of anesthesia-related deaths was 1 in 10,000. Barely a decade later, those risks have fallen to at least 1 in 30,000.[1] It should be noted that these statistics apply across all patient populations and risk categories. For the healthy patient undergoing an elective procedure, the incidence may be as low as 1 : 50,000 to 1 : 100,000.[1] Aukberg et al found that the greatest improvement in mortality statistics was in the area of preventable respiratory incidents, from 0.84 : 10,000 to 0.15 : 10,000, in a retrospective comparative study involving anesthesia-related cardiac arrests during our two most recent decades.[2] In addition to improved patient outcomes, the recent decline in payout for anesthesia malpractice claims has resulted in a reduction of malpractice premiums providers must pay annually. In some cases, malpractice rates are being reduced by up to 25 percent, further reflecting the increased safety of anesthesia administration.

It is generally believed that 70 to 80 percent of major anesthesia mishaps are related directly to human error and most annual deaths could at least, in part, be preventable. Pierce and Cooper contend that most anesthetic mishaps, malpractice claims, or deaths strongly implicate failure in vigilance as a primary cause of injury.[3] Some of these human errors occur with relative frequency in routine practice including, among others, breathing circuit disconnect or leak, syringe or ampule swap, drug overdose, loss of oxygen supply or inadvertent changes in gas flow, esophageal intubation or unintentional extubation, hypotension, and wrong blood transfused.[4] Other behavioral or psychologic variables that may influence the incidence of anesthesia mishaps are carelessness, fatigue, lack of adequate supervision or assistance, lack of familiarity with equipment, and failure to perform proper machine and equipment checks prior to induction of anesthesia. With the development of monitoring standards, there has been some argument that the proliferation of monitoring equipment is not only costly, but distracts the practitioner from focusing on the patient. Undoubtedly, the combination of sophisticated physiologic monitoring equipment in conjunction with practitioner vigilance is the most effective method of secure patient safety. It should be noted that relative to the factor of cost in the provision of comprehensive monitoring, the actual cost of providing malpractice insurance for each surgical patient is about 10 times greater than the cost of providing an electrocardiogram (ECG), oxygen monitor, disconnect alarm, blood pressure cuff, and precordial stethoscope. Duberman and Bendixen found that monitoring equipment costs about $7 per patient over the lifetime of the equipment.[5]

Definitions and Purposes of Monitoring

The ultimate goal of monitoring is to enhance patient safety. Physiologic monitoring of patients involves the systematic collection of data that reflect the patient's homeostatic state, the timely recognition of aberrant clinical parameters, the estimation of the efficacy of therapy instituted, and the documentation of proper machine and equipment function. Monitoring data are required for every patient, regardless of procedure, type of anesthetic technique, or patient physical state, when there is an anesthesia provider in attendance. Monitoring data also provide documentation that the CRNA provided proper and timely care throughout the perioperative course. In addition, it is the right of every patient to have a complete and comprehensive record of his or her medical care from which evaluations of past care can be determined or future therapies can be based.

The process of monitoring includes several discrete sets of technical and cognitive skills with which the CRNA should be fluent. First, effective monitoring requires that equipment be operational and applied correctly. Second, data acquired are valuable only to the extent they are capably and accurately interpreted, in context to the particular patient and surgical circumstance. Finally, the selection of monitors should be individualized to each patient according to his or her physical condition, type of surgical procedure undertaken, and inherent risk of application, especially when invasive monitors are contemplated. In addition, monitors must be sufficiently accurate, sensitive, and reliable to detect changes in the patient's condition.

Routine monitors are those considered applicable to every patient. These are noninvasive and consist of equipment to measure blood pressure, a precordial or esophageal stethoscope, continuous ECG, and pulse oximetry to determine the extent of oxygen saturation. Relative to the anesthesia machine, it is required that the breathing circuit be equipped with a disconnect alarm, an oxygen analyzer with a low-concentration-limit alarm, as well as a fail-safe system to warn of low oxygen pressures to the anesthesia machine. In addition to these minimums, it is a standard of care to routinely employ the use of capnometry or mass spectrometry to determine expired concentrations of CO_2

and, in the case of the latter, to determine exhaled concentrations of life gases as well as the common inhalation anesthetic agents. A peripheral nerve stimulator should be used when muscle relaxants are employed both to quantify the extent of muscle relaxation and to effectively document extubation criteria. When appropriate, urine output should be recorded to document adequate renal function.

For patients whose surgical procedure requires more sophisticated monitoring, other devices can be used including intraarterial blood pressure, central venous pressure, and/or Swan-Ganz pulmonary artery catheters. For selected cases, evoked potentials may be used to assess spinal cord patency and general neurologic function.

Clinical Anesthesia Monitoring Standards

The most widely accepted written standards for monitoring of patients undergoing anesthesia were first introduced in 1986 by the anesthesiology staff of the Harvard Medical School. The American Association of Nurse Anesthetists (AANA) adopted their own standards of patient monitoring which were part of the standards of practice adopted in 1974. These have since been revised, most recently in 1992, to reflect current trends in monitoring technology.[6] It is the assumption of the legal community that these standards have been adopted by the professional organization and anesthesia community at large and, as such, represent the standard of care to which any CRNA should adhere. Although most malpractice litigation involving questions of monitoring are determined according to local community standards, the AANA Monitoring Standards are sufficiently broad to incorporate a variety of practice settings and circumstances, yet maintain basic principles of patient safety (Appendix 1). Standards of monitoring should be used in conjunction with the AANA Clinical Practice Standards, which provide the context for application of the monitoring standards (Appendix 2).[7] The AANA Monitoring Standards apply to patients undergoing general, regional, or monitored anesthesia care for diagnostic or therapeutic procedures. They call for the CRNA to use clinical judgment in prioritizing and implementing these standards. The standards do not normally apply to epidural analgesia for labor or pain management therapy; however, it should be noted that most prudent anesthetists will, in fact, employ part of these standards in specialized care settings. Should the anesthetist not follow the standards as written, especially for obstetric patients, it is suggested that documentation appear on the chart citing substitute modalities afforded the patient. Standards may be exceeded in any or all respects at any time at the discretion of the anesthetist, as required by individual patient needs. It should also be emphasized that unless the patient's anesthetic record documents the use of data for each monitoring modality, peer review officials or those reviewing the chart as expert witnesses may consider no equipment was used that was not charted, regardless of practitioner claims to the contrary. The balance of this chapter discusses the range of monitoring equipment commonly used in anesthesia practice, stressing the interpretation of data obtained.

ASSESSING ANESTHETIC DEPTH

Since Guedel's introduction of the classic signs and stages of ether anesthesia during World War I, practitioners have explored ways of determining the anesthetic depth of patients at any moment in the course of anesthesia. Although newer agents have rendered this evaluation tool less applicable, some autonomic signs remain useful in assessing the various stages and planes of anesthesia (Fig. 12–1). Too, it provides convenient nomenclature to describe relative depth. Eger has provided us with another measurement tool for assessment of anesthetic depth. Minimum alveolar concentration defines an anesthetic state in which there is an absence of movement in 50% of patients when a surgical incision is made, depending on other variables of temperature, age, and use of adjunct agents such as nitrous oxide or narcotics.[8] This measure also has its vagaries as the clinician must assume that delivery of gas from the machine is absolutely accurate and the patient presents with few or no impediments to uptake and distribution. As clinicians and researchers have yet to delineate a functional measurement tool to accurately assess anesthetic depth, we continue to rely on acute patient observations to surgical response.

Autonomic Responses

Monitoring signs of respiration, muscle tone, pupil size, and eye movement is basic to Guedel's scheme. If an inhalation anesthetic has been administered without muscle relaxants, rate and depth of respiration are excellent indicators of depth of anesthesia. An increase in rate or depth, or an irregular rhythm, may signal inadequate anesthesia. The use of muscle relaxation, hyperventilation, or mechanical ventilation eliminates the possibility of using changes in respiration as accurate indicators of depth of anesthesia. Similarly, the value of observing muscle tone has been lost because of the routine use of muscle relaxants.

General anesthesia affects pupil size and eye movement. A concentrically fixed, nonreactive pupil that is relatively "tight" is thought to be an accurate index of satisfactory anesthesia. If balanced anesthesia techniques are employed, the predictability of this index is decreased. For example, miosis associated with narcotic administration is well appreciated; however, this phenomenon has been shown to vary significantly with age.[9] Thiopental dilates the pupil inconsistently.[10] Halothane and isoflurane tend to constrict the pupil. The combination of enflurane, nitrous oxide/oxygen, and succinylcholine produced miosis in virtually all patients studied by Larsen.[9] Therefore, pupil size appears to be a variable indicator of the response of the central nervous system to anesthesia.

Heart rate and blood pressure are probably the most frequently used indicators of the activity of the adrenergic nervous system. With the inhalation agents, deeper levels of anesthesia generally correlate with lowered blood pressure. Yet, there are a number of potentially confounding vari-

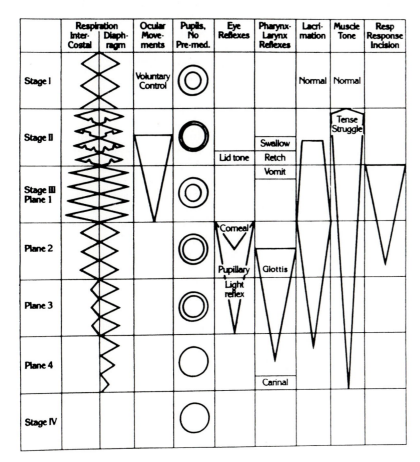

Figure 12–1. Signs and reflex actions of the stages of anesthesia. The converging lines indicate progressive loss of reflex activity as anesthesia deepens. (*Reprinted, with permission, from Gillespie NA. Anesth Analg. 1943;22:275.*)

ables including preexisting physiologic conditions, surgical stimulation, volume status, and preoperative use of medications. In general, hypertension and tachycardia are signs of inadequate depth of anesthesia; however, some patients under balanced anesthesia have no major changes in blood pressure or heart rate, yet experience awareness during surgery.[11,12] So, heart rate and blood pressure, although useful indicators of anesthetic depth, must be used with regard for mitigating factors and in concert with other signs.

Electrophysiologic Assessment

The usefulness of the electroencephalogram (EEG) in clinical practice is limited by the idiosyncratic effect of individual agents at various doses, the complexity and nonspecific nature of the EEG information, the difficulty in assessing trends in conventionally displayed EEG tracings, the emphasis on complex analysis of frequency, cost, and space requirements, and the need for a well-trained interpreter. The EEG consists of highly complex waveforms that are not as morphologically well defined as those of the ECG. The EEG waveform is the end product of many electrical impulses that are filtered through the skull from different locations in the cerebral cortex. Although the cerebral function monitor and the cerebral function analyzer monitor facilitate the clinical integration of the EEG, they still appear deficient in monitoring subtle changes in depth of anesthesia. The strength of these two devices lies in their ability to sense ischemic changes during certain cerebrovascular manipulations such as carotid endarterectomy and bypass procedures.

Somatosensory evoked potential (SEP) is basically an electrophysiologic response to sensory or motor stimulation. By evaluating the SEP, one can assess the transmission of information from a receptor to the central nervous system. The SEP may be a potentially useful neurophysiologic index of the depth of anesthesia. Recent evidence indicates that induction of anesthesia is associated with a reduction in SEP amplitude and an increase in latency, whereas recovery from anesthesia is associated with an increase in amplitude to preinduction values. Relatively consistent changes occur in SEP amplitude with narcotic and volatile anesthetics.[13] Surgical stimulation correlates with activation of the evoked response in the form of an observed increase in amplitude. Clearly, anesthetics depress cortical evoked responses. Whether or not this response is an effect of anesthetic depth or is due merely to a poorly elucidated drug effect awaits further research and better correlation with autonomic indices of depth of anesthesia. In the future, SEP appears to be a promising guide to the neurophysiologic effect of anesthetic agents. For now, its major function is to assess the integrity of neural pathways, the monitoring of which is especially beneficial in patients who have sustained spinal cord damage or require corrective surgery of the spine, cranial tumor resection, or major vascular procedures.

Monitoring the smooth muscle of the lower portion of the esophagus may indicate depth of anesthesia, as this musculature is unaffected by muscle relaxants. Nonperistaltic esophageal contractions are affected by various levels of anesthesia.[14] The usefulness of this relatively simple monitoring strategy may be hampered by any condition affecting lower esophageal contractility such as disease of the esophagus, various systemic disorders, and drugs. This modality is still undergoing investigations regarding its actual clinical applicability.

MONITORING THE CARDIOVASCULAR SYSTEM

No other area of anesthesia practice has undergone such rapid development over the past 20 years as has cardiovascular monitoring. During that time, monitoring has progressed from blood pressure cuffs using a mercury manometer and palpation of a peripheral pulse, to the availability of oximetry, multiple venous and arterial pressure monitors, and calculations of cardiac output. In terms of definition, all modalities of monitoring the cardiovascular system are used as indices of the adequacy of blood flow and oxygenation to critical organs. A variety of devices are employed for specific assessment of cardiac output, perfusion pressure, and other parameters of organ perfusion and oxygenation. This section presents an overview of the variety of hemodynamic monitoring devices available, in a framework that describes their use and interpretation of data.

Hemodynamic monitoring usually assesses four critical parameters: the electrical mechanism of myocardial contraction, intravascular or intracavitary pressures, net forward flow, and adequacy of organ perfusion. For those purposes, the usual clinical monitors include continuous ECG; measurement of arterial, venous, or chamber pressures with invasive or noninvasive techniques; calculation of cardiac output with a thermodilution technique via Swan-Ganz catheter; and assessment of perfusion with mixed venous and/or peripheral arterial pulse oximetry.

The ECG remains the most uniformly applied monitor in anesthesia. Continuous monitoring of the ECG permits the practitioner to assess the electrical mechanism and rate and demonstrates dysfunctional rhythms that would have a deleterious effect on cardiac output. ECG monitors employed in anesthesia are generally either three- or five-lead systems. Both rely on measurement of electrical impulses using silver–silver chloride gel electrodes which may be placed either on the limbs or over the precordium for assessment of selected regions of the heart. Impulses are measured from a negative ground electrode to a second, distant positive reference electrode. The resulting electrical impulse is then transmitted to the monitor for display. The relationship between the electrical impulse generated and cardiac activity in the atria and ventricles is demonstrated in Figure 12–2.

The standard, color-coded electrode assignment is as follows: white to right upper limb, black to left upper limb, green to right lower limb, red to left lower limb, and brown to the precordial lead. In the three-lead system, only the right upper limb and left upper and lower limb electrodes are used, which provides assessment of limb leads I, II, and III (Fig. 12–3). Summation of the limb leads as a ground with a unipolar limb electrode for reference permits assessment of leads R, L, and F (Fig. 12–4). The use of a precordial reference electrode permits assessment of electrical activity over selected regions of the ventricles and across the septum (Fig. 12–5).

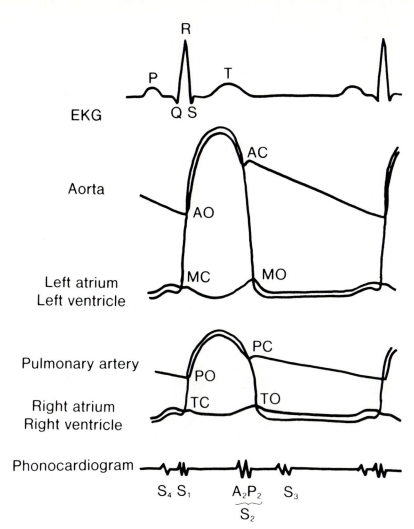

EKG

Aorta

Left atrium
Left ventricle

Pulmonary artery

Right atrium
Right ventricle

Phonocardiogram

Figure 12–2. Correlation of the electrical and mechanical activities of the heart. AO, aortic opening; AC, aortic closure; MC, mitral closure; MO, mitral opening; PO, pulmonic opening; PC, pulmonic closure; TC, tricuspid closure; TO, tricuspid opening. A vertical line at any point gives the simultaneous events occurring at that time. (*Reprinted, with permission, from Burnside.*[23(p154)])

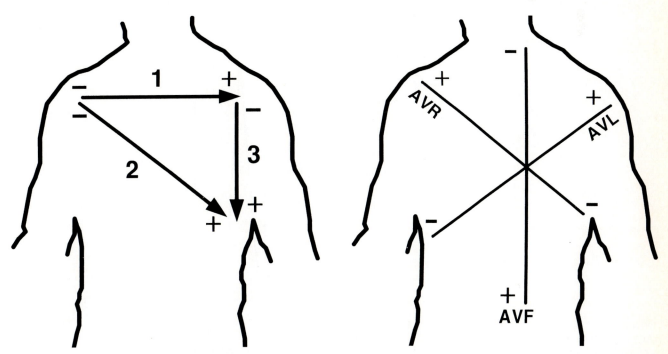

Figure 12–3. Electrode placement for ECG limb leads 1, 2, and 3. The – refers to negative electrode; + to positive electrode.

Figure 12–4. Axes defined by ECG leads AVR, AVL, and AVF. The – is negative; +, positive.

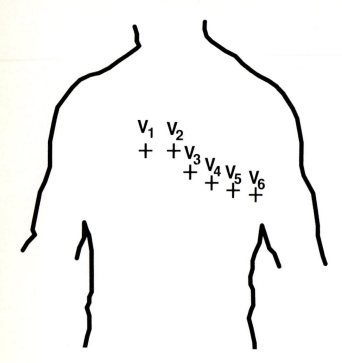

Figure 12–5. Electrode placement for ECG chest leads V1 through V6. The + is placement of positive electrode.

The normal range of time intervals for each phase of the ECG complex is demonstrated in Figure 12–6. The normal electrical mechanism begins at the level of the sinoatrial (SA) node, located at the juncture of the superior vena cava and the right atrium. Impulses are transmitted from the SA node through the atria by way of Bachman's bundles, and traverse the atria to the atrioventricular (AV) node located in the septum. Propagation of the impulse across the AV node permits depolarization of the ventricles by way of a single right and dual left anterior and posterior bundle branches, and the Purkinje system.

The elements of the cardiac cycle may be demonstrated with varying ease depending on the lead chosen. Limb lead II is most commonly used for identification of the p-wave; the precordial leads may be used for identification of ischemic changes. With a three-lead system, relocating limb electrodes permits approximation of precordial leads. Placing the left upper limb electrode in the V-5 position and monitoring the AVL lead will approximate a V-5 precordial lead. The modified chest lead I (MCL-I) permits approximation of any of the selected precordial leads by placing the left upper limb electrode near the shoulder or under the clavicle and the left lower limb electrode in the selected precordial lead position, and monitoring on lead III. Placing the negative electrode on the right scapula and the positive electrode in the V-5 position creates a lead CB5, which provides a prominent p-wave and permits detection of anterolateral ischemia (Fig. 12–7). When choosing leads for continuous monitoring, it is useful to remember that leads III and AVF display greater variation in amplitude with the respiratory cycle than other leads.[15] Assessment of the informa-

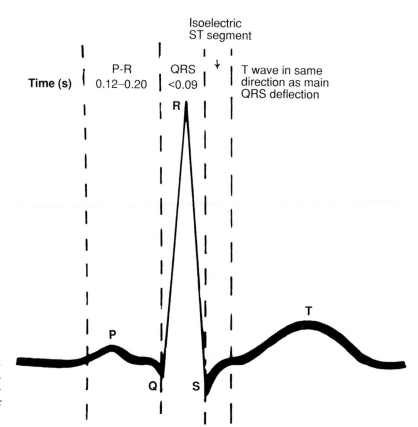

Figure 12–6. Normal ECG time intervals. (*Reprinted, with permission, from Wylie WD, Churchill-Davidson HC. A practice of anesthesia. 5th ed. Chicago: Year Book Medical; 1984:419.*)

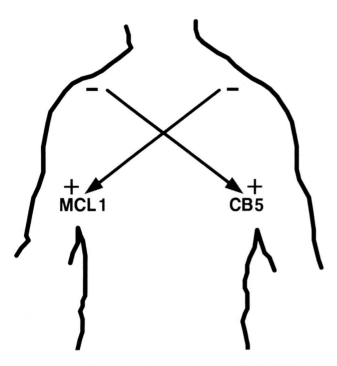

Figure 12–7. Electrode placement for modified ECG leads MCL-1 and CB-5. The – is negative electrode; +, positive electrode.

tion provided by ECG analysis provides a variety of parameters. Heart rate is directly measured. Disturbances in the electrical mechanism, including abnormal origin of rhythm, disturbances in synchronicity, and appearance of ectopic beats, are demonstrable. Evidence of myocardial ischemia or infarction may be demonstrable. Finally, analysis of the ECG may provide clues to electrolyte abnormalities or toxic responses to various anesthetic agents. Guidelines for rapid analysis of ECG activity are valuable to the practitioner. Although complete and detailed analysis is difficult in clinical practice, a simplified diagnostic scheme follows (Table 12–1).

The normal sinus mechanism produces synchronous depolarization of the atria, followed by the ventricles. Although the rhythm is generally regular, it is normal to note a pattern of variation in the beat-to-beat interval that corresponds with the respiratory cycle. That variation may be accentuated in the healthy young patient, and should not be mistaken for the irregularly irregular rhythm of atrial fibrillation. The normal rate of depolarization in the SA node produces a resting heart rate of about 70 beats per minute in the typical adult, which masks the intrinsic rates of 40 to 60 for the AV node or 30 to 40 for intrinsic ventricular depolarization.

Atrial dysrhythmias may present as prematurities, tachycardias, flutter, or fibrillation. Premature atrial contractions generally present with anomalous p-wave morphology and a shortened P-P interval, and may have a shortened P-R interval. Atrial tachycardias present with a 1:1 ratio between the p-wave and QRS complex, although the p-wave may be superimposed on the T-wave when the heart rate is rapid, making identification difficult. The P-R

interval may be decreased with rapid ventricular responses. Although the QRS complex is generally normal in appearance, aberrant ventricular conduction or the presence of a rate-dependent bundle branch block may mimic the appearance of ventricular tachycardia, unless p-waves are identified. Atrial flutter generally presents with a regular rhythm and conduction of only a fraction of the atrial rate of 300 beats per minute. The degree of block may vary according to the responsiveness of the AV node. With a 2:1 AV block, atrial flutter may mimic sinus tachycardia as the nonconducted p-wave is hidden in the preceding T-wave. Atrial fibrillation presents with the appearance of the classic jagged baseline representing "f-waves" which are irregular in both form and frequency. As conduction across the AV node is inconsistent, the rhythm is irregularly irregular.

AV conduction abnormalities may appear either as dissociation or as junctional or nodal dysrhythmias. The latter may appear as premature complexes or as escape beats in the presence of severe sinus bradycardia. The p-wave may not be present or may follow the QRS complexes. Shortened P-R intervals which may appear with an aberrant atrial focus should not be confused with an actual nodal rhythm. The former represents an atrial focus near the AV node; the latter represents a failure to maintain normal sinus or atrial mechanisms entirely. Premature complexes usually occur at an accelerated rate with a shortened R-R interval. Junctional escape beats usually occur with sinus bradycardia when the sinus mechanism fails to maintain a resting rate above the normal AV nodal rate of 40 to 60 beats per minute. Several

TABLE 12–1. CLINICALLY RELEVANT CLUES FROM ELECTROCARDIOGRAPHIC ANALYSIS

Possible Condition	Indication on ECG
Hyperkalemia	Appearance of tall "tented" T-wave
	Appearance of wide, bizarre QRS complex merging with T-wave
	Disappearance of p-wave
	Ventricular extrasystoles, fibrillation, or asystole
Hypokalemia	Flattening or inversion of T-wave
	Increase in P-R interval
	Depression of ST segment
	Appearance of U wave
	Apparent prolongation of Q-T interval (a normal Q-U interval)
	Atrial, ventricular extrasystoles, ventricular tachycardia
Hypercalcemia	Reduction in $Q\text{-}T_c$* interval
	Blending of T with QRS
Hypocalcemia	Prolongation of $Q\text{-}T_c$* interval
Hypomagnesemia	Prolongation of $Q\text{-}T_c$* interval
Venous air embolism	Rightsided heart "strain" pattern
	Atrial and ventricular extrasystoles

* The Q-T interval varies with heart rate and, when corrected for a heart rate of 60 beats per minute, is signified "$Q\text{-}T_c$" ($Q\text{-}T_{corrected}$). (Kessin M, Schwartzchild M, Bakst H. A nomogram for rate correction of the QT interval in the electrocardiogram. Am Heart J 1948;35:990–992.)
Reprinted, with permission, from Gray TC, Nunn JF, Utting JE, eds. General anaesthesia. 4th ed. Boston: Butterworths; 1980;1:613 and 651, p 2:1002.

AV conduction abnormalities may present. Each represents a block at one or another level in the conduction system. A first-degree block, with an extended P-R interval, represents a delay in conduction of the impulse generated in the SA node across the atria to the AV node, and is generally not clinically significant in early stages. A second-degree block may present in two forms. Type I (Winkebach) represents progressive failure of the AV node to transmit an impulse, and shows a progressive lengthening of the P-R interval with eventual failure to conduct an atrial impulse. Rhythm is regularly irregular. Type II block generally occurs in the ventricular conductive pathway as spontaneous failure to propagate an impulse. Therefore, it occurs without a progressive lengthening of the P-R interval. When the conduction block occurs in the bundle branches, the QRS may be widened. A third-degree block presents a complete dissociation of the atrial and ventricular mechanisms, in which each chamber beats at its own intrinsic rhythm without any coordination. QRS complexes and p-waves are often normal but unrelated. Ventricular response rates depend on the site or origin of the ventricular mechanism.

Ventricular dysrhythmias occur in four primary forms. Premature ventricular complexes (PVCs) are defined as ventricular contractions appearing prior to the next normally conducted beat. The QRS complex is generally broad and abnormal in conformation. It is generally reversed in polarity to the normal QRS complex. As it is associated with a refractory pause in the AV node, there is a compensatory pause following a PVC. Fixed, unifocal PVCs are more frequently benign. Multiform PVCs, multiple PVCs in sequence and those occurring near the preceding T-wave, predispose to ventricular tachycardia and are thus of greater concern. Ventricular tachycardia is defined as more than three ventricular prematurities in sequence with a rate greater than 100 beats per minute. Arterial pressure may or may not be transmitted, depending on the rate of ventricular filling. Morphology of the QRS complex is broad, generally inverted, and similar to that of PVCs. Ventricular fibrillation presents as a highly irregular rhythm with no discernible pattern. There is no effective forward arterial flow with ventricular fibrillation. Finally, bundle branch blocks may occur in conduction of the impulse to the ventricles. These represent failure to conduct the wave of depolarization in the normal antegrade fashion, with conduction in a retrograde manner from a point distal to the block. Hence, the QRS complex is broad and atypical. A single bundle branch block is generally benign, and the pattern may appear in patients with ventricular hypertrophy or discrete conduction abnormalities. Bundle branch blocks involving the right bundle and left anterior branch are generally benign, with only 10% progressing to complete AV block. Right bundle branch block and left posterior hemiblock carry a 90% incidence of progression to complete AV block and are consequently more grave. Analysis of the ECG complex provides evidence of a variety of pathologies. Ischemic changes present in the form of ST segment depression, with depression greater than 2 mm considered critical. Myocardial injury may be demonstrated by the presence of ST segment elevation in the early phase or the presence of Q-waves associated with old infarction.

PRESSURE MONITORING

Monitoring pressure provides the most common mechanism for assessing volume status and circulatory adequacy. A variety of methods of measurement are employed, which can be broken down into noninvasive and invasive systems. In general, the clinical practice is to employ noninvasive measurements of arterial pressure for intraoperative monitoring of healthy patients having routine procedures, and invasive techniques for measurement of arterial, venous, or chamber pressures in patients with selected disease states and for selected surgical procedures requiring additional information for clinical management.

Noninvasive Monitoring

The accepted standard for monitoring arterial blood pressure during routine cases on healthy patients is the noninvasive technique. Two general methods may be employed: (1) manual techniques using either sphygmomanometer or mercury column with auscultation; (2) automated systems which operate on an ultrasonic technique. Each of these has applications and selected drawbacks, and both are well described (Table 12–2).

Auscultatory methods generally employ the upper extremities as the site for measurement, largely for sake of convenience. Lower-extremity cuffs may also be employed, although the inability to readily auscultate Korotkoff sounds limits their application. The auscultatory technique requires turbulent flow in the artery to produce the Korotkoff sounds which form the basis for determining systolic and diastolic pressures. The first sound heard represents the systolic pressure, and the point at which sounds

TABLE 12–2. FACTORS AFFECTING THE ACCURACY OF INDIRECT BLOOD PRESSURE MEASUREMENTS

Factor	Consequence
Hearing ability	Variable sensitivity to Korotkoff sounds
Stethoscope	Design and positioning determines intensity of sounds
Touch	Variable sensitivity to pulse palpation
Cuff size	Falsely high BP[a]—too small or loose-fitting cuff Falsely low BP—too large a cuff
Aneroid manometer	Inaccurate BP with improper calibration
Deflation of sphygmomanometer	Falsely low BP—too rapid deflation
Oscillometry	Imprecise detection of first and last oscillations, indicating systolic and diastolic pressures, respectively

[a] BP, blood pressure.
Reprinted, with permission, from Hug CC Jr. Monitoring. In: Miller RD, ed. Anesthesia. 2nd ed. Edited by Miller RD. New York: Churchill Livingstone; 1986;1:411–463.

are lost represents the diastolic pressure. In those instances where auscultatory sounds are continued to zero, the point at which a distinct diminution in auscultated sounds is noted is taken as the actual diastolic pressure.

Physiologic changes that alter the distensibility of the arterial wall may alter the readings obtained from auscultatory or oscillometric techniques. Thus, extremes of body temperature with consequent vasoconstriction or vasodilation may reduce the accuracy of measurement, as may the use of vasoconstrictors or dilators. This is particularly true with the use of auscultatory methods, and less prominent with the use of ultrasonic systems such as the Dinamap or Doppler detected pulses. Likewise, stiffening of the arterial walls with progressive atherosclerosis may reduce the ability to auscultate pressure.

A final drawback to the use of noninvasive techniques for measurement of arterial pressure is their relatively cumbersome and time-inefficient operation. Noninvasive techniques provide only intermittent measurements of arterial pressure, and require varying time intervals to obtain measurement. In comparison, invasive techniques provide immediate, beat-to-beat analysis. Hence, in complex cases or cases that include significant disturbances in normal pulsatile flow, noninvasive techniques prove unsuitable for monitoring.

Invasive Monitoring

Vascular cannulation provides the practitioner with the ability to directly measure pressures in the peripheral arterial or venous system, as well as chamber and central venous or pulmonary artery pressures. The availability of vascular and chamber pressure measures increases precision in assessment of hemodynamic and volume status. The techniques for transducing vascular pressures remains constant regardless of the vessel or chamber, although interpretation of the information gained from cannulation is dependent on the particular monitoring modality selected for evaluation.

Mechanisms of Transducing

Mechanically, the system for transduction of pressures should be the same whether transducing high-pressure arterial or lower-pressure venous sites. The system should include a stiff, low-compliance pressure tubing connecting the vascular cannula to a pressure-sensing diaphragm. Transduction of the physical pressure wave to that diaphragm produces bending of the diaphragm, resulting in a small volume change in response to the applied change in pressure.[16] The arterial compliance measurement should be 0.01 cu mm per 100 mm Hg pressure; that for venous compliance should be 0.1 cu mm per 100 mm Hg pressure. Three forms of transducers are generally employed in translating the pressure waveform into an electrical waveform: electromagnetic, capacitive, and strain gauge transducers.[17]

In electromagnetic transducers, the diaphragm moves a soft iron core between the primary and secondary coils of a transformer. An alternative current passing through the primary coil sets up an alternative magnetic field, which in turn induces a current in the secondary coil that is modified in

amplitude by the extent to which the iron core concentrates the magnetic field through the coils. In capacitative transducers, the diaphragm forms one plate of a capacitor. As the capacitor is incapable of transmitting a unidirectional current, an alternative current is used to energize it. The impedance of the transducer changes with displacement of the two plates of the capacitor, creating the changes in current that are later interpreted as the waveform in display.

In strain gauge transducers, the sensing elements are composed of electrically conductive elastic materials that respond reversibly to pressure deformation with a change in electrical resistance. That resistance is converted into a voltage signal by connecting the elements in the form of a Wheatstone bridge circuit. The elements are assembled in the transducer so that two elements are stretched and two compressed by the physical pressure applied to the diaphragm, with each pair being incorporated into the opposite sides of the bridge. A stable, unidirectional voltage is then applied across the bridge. The output voltage is proportional to the physical pressure applied and to the excitation voltage. It is characteristic of strain gauge transducers that they tend to drift electrically when first connected to a voltage supply, because the current produces a heating effect on the strain gauge elements themselves. This drift usually settles within 15 minutes as temperature stabilizes in the elements of the strain gauge, after which pressure measurements remain reliable.

Frequency responses in transducer systems should be at least 1.5 times the fastest component being measured. The frequency response of the arterial trace is normally 20 to 30 Hz, whereas that of the transducer is normally 150 to 1000 Hz.[18] The presence of air in the tubing or stopcocks and increases in the length of the tubing between the vessel and the transducer itself lower the frequency response. These may approach the frequencies encountered in the vascular waveform, and are particularly demonstrated in the systolic upstroke. The resulting distortion, commonly referred to as ringing, may produce an overshoot in measurement of systolic pressure.

An alternative was employed prior to the current, reliable, and easily managed monitoring systems that still provides an effective means of monitoring systemic pressure when the clinician is unable to readily access a monitoring screen, as during transport, or in selected sites external to the operating theater. By connecting the arterial line through an extension to a stopcock, and a second extension to an aneroid manometer, one can identify the mean arterial pressure, which provides important clinical information regarding perfusion pressure. This system, however, does not provide immediate waveform analysis or information regarding the true systolic or diastolic pressures.

The Arterial Waveform

Physically, the conduction of an arterial waveform is not exclusively related to the flow of blood within the vessel.[19] The waveform demonstrated on the monitor represents a summation of the force of blood flow through the vessel and the propagation of the elastic forces in the wall of the vessels themselves. The left ventricular pulse wave travels at a speed of 10 m/s, in contrast to the aortic elastic recoil wave, which travels at 0.5 m/s.[20]

In arterial waveforms, the initial upstroke is considered to be a reflection of the inotropic component of ventricular contraction. The contour of the rounded, sustained portion of the curve, referred to as the dicrotic notch, is composed of three elements: the ventricular stroke volume, the distension of the ascending aorta and aortic arch, and runoff into the various major branches of the aorta. A second, smaller peak in pressure that may be seen in some waveforms is felt to represent the reflection of waves from the head, neck, and upper extremities (Fig. 12–8).

In general, as the pressure wave is measured progressively further from the heart in the normal vascular tree, there is a delay in the transmission of the waveform, a steeper inotropic upstroke, and loss of the dicrotic notch. This results in a steeper, more peaked systolic upstroke. This altered waveform results in part from the fact that peripheral arteries include proportionately less elastic fiber in the arterial wall, making them stiffer and less compliant. Further, tapering of the vessel diameter as the artery proceeds peripherally serves to amplify the arterial waveform, in a fashion similar to the manner in which the ear trumpet amplifies sound waves[21,22] (Fig. 12–9).

The presence of atherosclerotic arterial occlusive disease may reduce all these components, resulting in a reduction in the measured pressure distal to the site of occlusion. The presence of aneurysmal dilation of the major vessels may blunt the systolic upstroke in the peripheral arteries, as well as form a "buffer zone" in the vascular tree which reduces the transmitted pressure in the peripheral artery.

Interpretation of Arterial Monitoring

In clinical practice, the only information obtainable from arterial monitoring is the systemic blood pressure. As previously indicated, when no physical cause is demonstrable for damping or ringing which would alter the measured pressure, the pressures measured by arterial cannulation are presumed more reliable than noninvasive means of monitoring. In those states that are nonphysiologic, such as induced hypotension, extremes of temperature, or nonpulsatile flow such as seen in conjunction with cardiopulmonary bypass, measurement of intraarterial pressures may be the only reliable means of measuring systemic pressure.

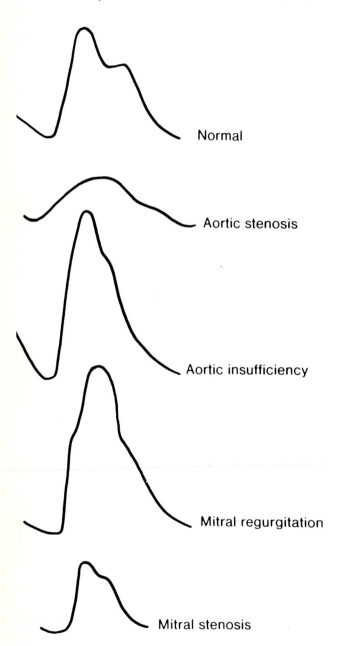

Figure 12–8. Arterial waveforms: normal and with valvular disease. (*Reprinted, with permission, from Burnside.*[23(p149)])

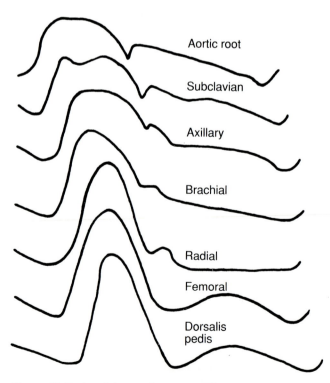

Figure 12–9. Arterial waveforms at different anatomic locations. (*Reprinted, with permission, from Blitt CD. Monitoring in anesthesia and critical care medicine. New York: Churchill Livingstone; 1985:50.*)

Despite the fact that there is no absolute correlation between arterial pressure or waveform and cardiac output or other indices of perfusion, a variety of information can be gained by observation and analysis of the arterial waveform. Although these indirect indices are not absolute, they provide valuable clues in the management of patients with arterial monitoring. When assuming that there is no mechanical cause for damping or ringing, the upstroke provides an index of the contractile mechanism, or inotropic state of the left ventricle. Stroke volume may also be estimated by the area under the waveform, although not in a quantifiable fashion. Comparison of the arterial waveform with the respiratory cycle may demonstrate fluctuations in arterial pressure in conjunction with respiration. Fluctuations in excess of 10 mm Hg are considered abnormal, and may represent vascular hypovolemia.[23] Further, the dicrotic notch may be seen to fall with the development of hypovolemia. Caution should be employed in making absolute guides of changes in arterial waveforms, as the physiologic impact of anesthetic agents on hemodynamics includes the reduction of inotropic state, peripheral arterial dilation, and shunting of flow. Therefore, changes should be compared between two similar intervals. Waveforms observed prior to induction and volume shift should not be relied on solely as evidence of the development of hypovolemia following stabilization postinduction. It should also be noted that aortic valvular lesions may also produce typical abnormalities in the conformation of the arterial waveform, making interruption, without a baseline prior to induction of anesthesia or any physiologic change during the course of anesthesia, unreliable.

Cannulating the Artery

When cannulating vessels, it is important to consider the physical nature and structure of both the catheter and the monitoring system. In general, the smaller the catheter used in proportion to the lumen of the vessel, the lower the incidence of vascular thrombosis. The material composition of the catheter determines other physical characteristics. Being stiffer, polypropylene proves more resistant to kinking. In contrast, Teflon is less stiff and more prone to kinking, but is more widely used because it proves least thrombogenic.[24] It should be noted that as many as 20 percent of 20-gauge Teflon arterial catheters kink within 24 hours of placement.[25] Finally, the size of the catheter used determines the likelihood or degree of ringing that occurs. Smaller-gauge catheters demonstrate less ringing in transmission of the waveform as a result of dampening of the underdampened catheter extension tubing system.

The site, technique, and route employed for cannulation also determine the incidence of complications. Localized infection rates of 4 to 6.5 percent are reported, with *Staphylococcus epidermidis* being the most common agent.[26,27] In catheters inserted via cutdown, the rate increases to 30 to 39 percent for catheters in place for more than 4 days.[28] Local antibiotic treatment is effective in reducing the infection rate. Catheters treated at the puncture site with iodophor demonstrated a 2.2 percent incidence of infection, compared with 3.6 percent for triple-antibiotic preparation and 6.5 percent for controls.[28] There are commercial systems available that purport to act as bio-

logic filters, usually impregnated with antibiotic material, which may be placed about the catheter or over the catheter for insertion under the skin surface. Data on the efficacy of these systems have not yet been conclusive for prevention of sepsis, particularly in short-term cannulations.

In sharp contrast to many other studies, one group demonstrated that the use of 18- to 20-gauge propylene catheters for periods not to exceed 48 hours in patients with no history of peripheral small-vessel disease such as Raynaud's had no associated, significant complications.[29] Further, there was no predictive value in the Allen test, based on a total of 16 patients with an abnormal Allen test on examination prior to cannulation. Nevertheless, it is generally recommended that an Allen test be performed prior to cannulation of a radial artery, and an alternate site be chosen, if possible, when filling from the ulnar artery takes more than 5 seconds.

Interpretation of Central Venous Monitoring

The interpretation of data from central venous monitoring is dependent on an appreciation of the physiologic basis for that particular monitor. In general, central venous pressure (CVP) is measured as an assessment of volume status. The purpose in monitoring volume status is to establish the patient's relative position on the typical volume/pressure curve or volume/cardiac output curve, which is the clinical correlate to the Frank–Starling curve. The normal patient demonstrates a roughly linear relationship between vascular volume and CVP within a limited physiologic range, as described in Chapter 20.

As CVP measurements in the normal population cover a broad range, absolute values are not reliable guides to volume status. Each patient operates within an individualized, normal range. CVP measurements outside that range may represent extremes of volume for the single patient while still being within normal range for a larger population, or vice versa. Hence, the use of CVP in conjunction with additional nonhemodynamic parameters such as maintenance of satisfactory urinary output supports an assessment of normovolemia. Measurements taken within that range may be presumed to be rough indices of volume status and, therefore, cardiac output, when no interventions have been undertaken that would impair ventricular function or alter the normal relationship.

Additional valuable information can be gained from analysis of the venous waveform. The normal CVP waveform, with its component elements, is demonstrated in Figure 12–10. The a-wave represents the wave of atrial contraction. In the normal patient, it remains a comparatively low-amplitude wave. In the case of ventricular nondistensibility, however, this atrial contraction occurs against an incompletely relaxed ventricle. The additional pressure generated by contraction against a stiff, unyielding ventricle presents as an exaggerated a-wave, which may be the first clue to ventricular diastolic dysfunction. Further, a-wave amplitude is exaggerated with the development of a nodal mechanism. In the presence of atrial fibrillation, the a-wave is lost in the CVP waveform. Late in the cardiac cycle, the v-wave appears as a reflection of the force generated during ventricular contraction. The amplitude of the v-wave may

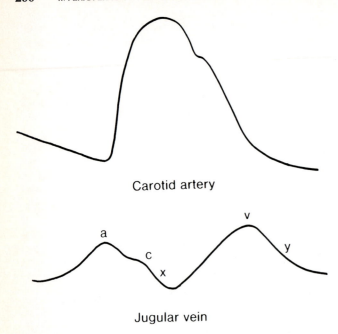

Figure 12–10. Typical central venous pressure waveform in the jugular vein. a, atrial contraction; c, tricuspid valve closure (may be seen only in right atrial pressure tracings); x, atrial relaxation and filling; v, ventricular contraction; y, tricuspid valve opening and ventricular filling. (*Reprinted, with permission, from Burnside.*[23])

be grossly exaggerated in the presence of tricuspid regurgitation. Changes in the amplitude of the v-wave may serve as a rough index of the degree of regurgitation, and it should return to normal when the cause for regurgitation is corrected.

Interpretation of Pulmonary Artery Monitoring

Pulmonary artery monitoring is achieved with the use of the Swan-Ganz catheter. This long, flexible balloon-tipped catheter is designed to drift with blood flow from the point of insertion into the central circulation. It has a distal port at the tip of the catheter, which is protected when the balloon is inflated with the recommended 1.5 cc of air. A proximal port, located 30 cm from the tip of the catheter, provides a site for measurement of central venous pressure when inserted into the normal-sized adult. A thermistor probe is located in the tip of the catheter for cannulation of cardiac output by means of thermodilution techniques. In more recent developments, continuous measurement of mixed venous oxygen saturation is available via this catheter. The final common pathway is through the right atrium and ventricle into the pulmonary artery, where pressure and other measurements are made. Typical waveforms for central venous pressure, right atrial and ventricular pressures, and pulmonary artery and capillary wedge pressures are found in Figure 12–11.

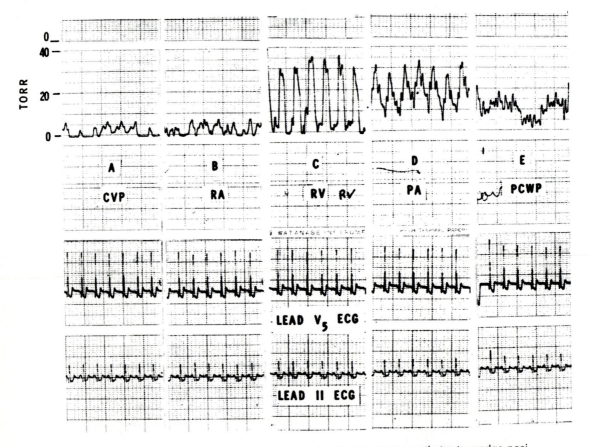

Figure 12–11. Typical tracing with advancement of pulmonary artery catheter to wedge position. RA, right atrium; RV, right ventricle; PA, pulmonary artery; PCW, pulmonary capillary wedge. (*Reprinted, with permission, from Dizon CT, PG Barash. The value of monitoring pulmonary artery pressure in clinical practice. Conn Med. 1977;41:622.*)

A variety of information is available from a Swan-Ganz catheter. These measurements may be direct measurements, calculated parameters made using only the Swan-Ganz, or integrated parameters calculated using information derived from alternate invasive modalities. For this reason, sophistication in the management and interpretation of data derived from the Swan-Ganz catheter is critical for management of complex cases. A table of normal Swan-Ganz values can be found in Table 12–3.

Directly Measured Parameters

Parameters directly measured with the Swan-Ganz catheter typically include central venous pressure, pulmonary artery pressure, wedge pressure, and injectate and patient core temperatures. In sequence, these offer indices of right ventricular preload, integration of cardiac output and pulmonary vascular resistance, and index of left ventricular preload. Recent developments add the potential for measurement of mixed venous oxygen saturation. Interpretation of data derived by monitoring with a Swan-Ganz should be tempered with consideration of the individual patient's hemodynamic and cardiac status. Factors that alter the interpretation of pressure data derived from the Swan-Ganz include valvular dysfunction, vascular and chamber compliance, ventricular function, and alterations in the normal electrical conduction pattern.

Clinical Interpretation of Data

Valvular dysfunction may make pressure data derived from the Swan-Ganz less reliable as a measure of ventricular pre-

load. Regurgitant valvular lesions produce a retrograde "v-wave" which artificially elevates the upstream vascular pressure measurement (Fig. 12–12). Hence, actual ventricular preload may be substantially lower than the measured pressures indicate. Stenotic valvular lesions reduce the orifice across which blood flows during the diastolic filling interval, requiring higher atrial pressures to generate sufficient flow across the valve to maintain ventricular filling volume. As a result, increased CVP or wedge pressures may follow the degree of stenosis and may not reflect actual ventricular preload directly.

Vascular and chamber compliances may also affect the interpretation of pressure data derived from central venous and pulmonary artery monitoring. Vasodilators such as nitroglycerine may produce increases in venous or pulmonary artery compliance, resulting in lowered pressures, without reducing the actual vascular volume or flow. Conversely, vasoconstrictors and physiologic derangements such as hypoxemia and hypercarbia may produce increases in measured pressures without actually altering the vascular volume or flow. Similarly, changes in chamber compliance may alter the normal volume–pressure relationship. Hypertrophy, ischemia, use of inotropic agents, and increases in afterload may all reduce ventricular compliance and make pressure data less reliable as guides to ventricular filling volume.

Although alterations in valvular and vascular status disrupt the typical pressure–volume relationship, each patient follows an individualized clinical Starling curve. Therefore, certain guidelines may be developed to support clinical decisions based on expected pressure alterations with selected lesions. Patients with long-standing systemic hypertension or outflow obstruction generally require higher filling pressures to maintain preload in a less compliant ventricle. Aortic insufficiency results in dilation and hypertrophy of the left ventricle. Higher diastolic pressures reflect the degree of regurgitant flow, as insufficiency exposes the left ventricle to aortic root pressures. Hence, patients with long-standing hypertension or aortic valvular dysfunction may require a wedge pressure as great as 16 to 18 torr to maintain adequate left ventricular filling volume for a suitable cardiac output. Patients with mitral stenosis may require higher-than-normal atrial pressures to generate sufficient flow across a constricted valve area for adequate left ventricular filling. Thus, a wedge pressure of 18 to 22 torr may be required to maintain a suitable cardiac output. Patients with mitral insufficiency frequently demonstrate a regurgitant v-wave in the pulmonary artery tracing, making it impossible to obtain a wedge tracing. Estimation of reductions in the magnitude of the v-wave may provide a crude guide to improvement of forward low, provided that the cardiac output remains constant. Because the Swan-Ganz follows the venous circulation into the pulmonary circulation, its use is not generally recommended in patients with stenotic valvular lesions involving the right side of the heart. In patients with right-sided valvular insufficiency, it may prove difficult to pass the Swan-Ganz. Data derived from the wedge will still be accurate, although data gathered on right-sided filling pressures will be subject to the same errors described for the left ventricular and pulmonary artery or wedge pressures.

As would be expected, patients with a history of ven-

TABLE 12–3. NORMAL RESTING HEMODYNAMIC VALUES

	Systolic	Diastolic	Mean
Pressure (mm Hg)			
Right atrium	—	—	–2 to +6
Right ventricle	15–30	0–8	5–15
Pulmonary artery			0–12
Left atrium			0–12
Left ventricle	100–140	60–90	70–105
Volume			
Left ventricle			
End-diastolic	70–95 mL m^{-2}		
End-systolic	24–36 mL m^{-2}		
Performance			
Cardiac index	2.5–4.2 L min^{-1} m^{-2}		
Stroke volume index	50–70 mL/m^{-2}		
Ejection fraction	0.67 ± 0.08 (SD)		
Resistance			
Pulmonary vascular	20–120 dyn·s cm^{-5}		
Systemic vascular	770–1500 dyn·s cm^{-5}		
Oxygen measurements			
Oxygen consumption	110–150 mL min^{-1} m^{-2}		
Arteriovenous oxygen difference	3–5 mL dL^{-1} blood		
Valve measurements			
Aortic valve area	2.6–3.5 cm^2		
Mitral valve area	4.0–6.0 cm^2		

Reprinted, with permission, from Nunn JF, Utting JE, Brown BR. General anaesthesia. 5th ed. Boston: Butterworths; 1980:474.

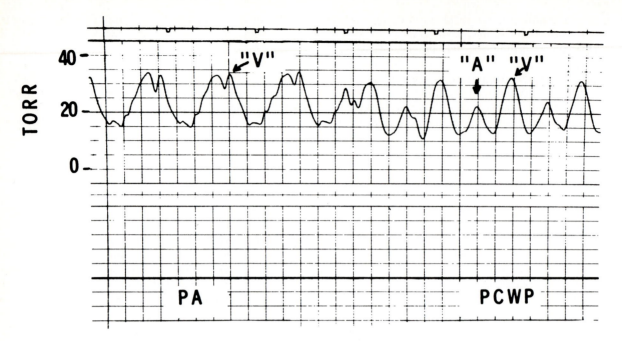

Figure 12–12. v-wave morphology in pulmonary artery wedge tracing. PA, pulmonary artery; PCWP, pulmonary capillary wedge pressure; "V," v-wave; "A," a-wave. (*Reprinted, with permission, from Miller.*[15(p451)])

tricular dysfunction also frequently have a dilated and less compliant ventricle, requiring higher-than-normal filling pressures. As a result, it is typical to find that patients with chronic left ventricular dysfunction require a wedge pressure as great as 18 torr to maintain adequate filling pressures for a suitable cardiac output. Similarly, patients with chronic right ventricular dysfunction or pulmonary hypertension may require elevated filling pressures as evidenced by CVP measurements that may exceed 20 torr; however, those filling pressures may be limited to the right side, and left ventricular filling pressures may remain relatively normal. As the prognosis for patients with chronic pulmonary hypertension is ominous, it becomes critical to monitor right-sided filling pressures, and assessment of right ventricular function may prove the most critical determinant of successful management.

Finally, conduction defects may alter the normal volume–pressure relationship. In general, it may be deduced that abnormalities in conduction, particularly those that disturb the normal pattern of atrioventricular synchronicity, result in the need for increased filling pressures. Patients with mitral stenosis frequently maintain a rhythm of atrial fibrillation, in which no atrial kick is present to augment left ventricular filling. That atrial kick is also lost in patients with a nodal rhythm or those with a paced ventricular mechanism. As a compensatory measure, elevated atrial pressures may be reflected as an increased CVP or wedge pressure, and patients may require higher venous or atrial pressures to maintain normal ventricular filling volumes. Patients with paced or nodal mechanisms generally maintain suitable cardiac output with a wedge pressure of about 16 torr, whereas patients with atrial fibrillation

may require a wedge pressure of 18 to 22 torr. The amplitude of the normal a-wave of atrial contraction is increased in patients with nodal mechanisms, as the atria contract against a closed atrioventricular valve. Patients with acutely induced nondistensibility, as occurs in the presence of myocardial ischemia, may also demonstrate an exaggerated a-wave amplitude.

Oximetric Measurements

The development of the oximetric Swan-Ganz has offered an additional benefit in invasive monitoring. The measurement of mixed venous oxygen saturation provides additional information on the global adequacy of circulatory function. The normal patient extracts approximately 25 percent of available oxygen in the awake, resting state. This corresponds to a mixed venous oxygen saturation of approximately 75 percent, or a mixed venous PO_2 of about 40 torr. Reductions in mixed venous oxygen saturation provide a relatively sensitive index of global oxygen balance. Disturbances that decrease mixed venous oxygen saturation may result from decreased oxygen-carrying capacity through reductions in cardiac output with ventricular dysfunction, reductions in circulating hemoglobin levels as seen with acute bleeding, or increases in systemic oxygen utilization as seen in the toxic or septic patient.

Anesthesia accommodating the use of muscle relaxants produces a shunting of blood from the muscle bed and eliminates the work of breathing, which reduces oxygen utilization and increases the mixed venous oxygen saturation. A typical mixed venous oxygen saturation for the anesthetized, mechanically ventilated patient is 85 to 90 percent.

Progressive decreases in body temperature, whether from deliberate induction of hypothermia or passive dissipation of heat into a cold operating room, account for progressive reductions in oxygen utilization and increases in mixed venous saturation, when cardiac output and hemoglobin concentrations remain constant. Thus, by incorporating factors of cardiac output, hemoglobin concentration, and oxygen-carrying capacity, the clinician can approximate the appropriate mixed venous oxygen saturation for the anesthetized patient.

Calculated Parameters

In addition to those pressure parameters measured directly, the use of a Swan-Ganz permits the calculation of a variety of derived parameters. The most commonly employed calculation is the cardiac output. Cardiac output is most often calculated by a variety of available self-contained units, using an algorithm that employs the measured difference in temperature across time; hence the term *thermodilution cardiac output*. Alternative methods of measuring cardiac output, such as dye dilution, are relatively more cumbersome and less adaptable to the clinical setting. Calculations of cardiac output using the classic Fick method require assumptions about the utilization of oxygen that are not valid in the anesthetized, mechanically ventilated, and frequently hypothermic patient. For those reasons, current standards in clinical practice support the use of the thermodilution cardiac output technique derived from a Swan-Ganz catheter.

Measurement of cardiac output with a Swan-Ganz thermodilution catheter necessitates a variety of assumptions, and these incorporate the opportunity for error in measure. These include the speed of the injection, error in volume of injectate, discrepancies in the temperature gradient between the patient and the injectate, and internal error of measure. Slow injection of excessive volumes may produce erroneously low output readings, as may reductions in the difference between the temperature of the patient and the injectate, or the use of warmer injectate than incorporated in the coefficients dialed into the output computer. In contrast, too rapid injection, use of volumes less than indicated, extreme differences in temperature, and use of colder-than-indicated injectate tend to magnify the cardiac output calculation. Finally, the error of measure makes absolute interpretation of cardiac output measurements unreliable. Within the normal range of cardiac output, the error of measure may be accepted as approximately 10 percent. As cardiac output deviates more than a standard deviation from the mean, the error in measure increases. At measurements greater than two standard deviations from the mean, the error of measure may approach 50 percent. In general, error of measure increases more rapidly in measurements below the mean, making low cardiac output measurements less reliable than correspondingly high measurements. For those reasons, most experienced clinicians rely heavily on trends in cardiac output rather than absolute calculations, and use collateral data such as arterial blood gases, acid–base balance, and mixed venous oxygen saturation in making judgments of the adequacy of systemic circulation and oxygenation.

Finally, it must be remembered that the thermodilution

cardiac output technique actually measures right ventricular cardiac output. Thus, the clinician assumes that right and left ventricular outputs are consistently and directly related. In the normal state, that assumption remains accurate. In patients with ventricular failure, however, that rule is violated. Acute left ventricular failure does not result in an immediate decrease in right ventricular output, and other indices of left ventricular function, such as changes in wedge pressure or waveform analysis, may prove necessary to obtain a more complete analysis.

Integrated Calculations

A variety of integrated calculations can be made when the cardiac output is estimated using the thermodilution technique. Both systemic and pulmonary vascular resistances may be calculated, using the formula in Table 12–4, which also lists normal values. These determinations may support the decision to employ vasodilators or vasoconstrictors. They may also indicate the requirement for therapy in the patient with left ventricular failure, or direct the management of patients requiring higher-than-normal systemic vascular resistance to maintain coronary perfusion, as patients with ventricular hypertrophy. The development of a variety of drugs that are effective pulmonary dilators has made it possible to manage the patient with pulmonary hypertension with greater sophistication than previously possible, by using integrated parameters.

In addition to vascular resistances, it is possible to gather an estimate of the ventricular stroke work from calculations provided by the Swan-Ganz catheter. The stroke work indices outlined in Table 12–4 permit the clinician to

TABLE 12–4. PARAMETERS DERIVED FROM INVASIVE MONITORING

Formula	Normal Value
$SV = \dfrac{CO}{HR} \times 1000$	60–90 mL beat^{-1}
$SI = \dfrac{SV}{BSA}$	40–60 mL beat^{-1} m^{-2}
$LVSWI = 1.36 \times \dfrac{(\overline{MAP} - \overline{PCWP}) \times SI}{100}$	45–60 g·m m^{-2} beat^{-1}
$RVSWI = 1.36 \times \dfrac{(\overline{PAP} - \overline{CVP}) \times SI}{100}$	5–10 g·m m^{-2} beat^{-1}
$SVR = \dfrac{(\overline{MAP} - \overline{CVP}) \times 80}{CO}$	900–1500 dyn·cm^{-5}
$PVR = \dfrac{(\overline{PAP} - \overline{PCWP}) \times 80}{CO}$	50–150 dyn·s cm^{-5}

Abbreviations used. SV, stroke volume; CO, cardiac output; HR, heart rate; BSA, body surface area; LVSWI, left ventricular stroke work index; $\overline{MAP}$, mean arterial pressure; $\overline{PCWP}$, mean pulmonary capillary wedge pressure; RVSWI, right ventricular stroke work index; $\overline{PAP}$, mean pulmonary artery pressure; $\overline{CVP}$, mean central venous pressure; SVR, systemic vascular resistance; PVR, pulmonary vascular resistance; SI, stroke index.
Note. All of these parameters are rapidly derived in both the operating room and intensive care unit using programmable portable calculators available at the present time.
Reprinted, with permission, from Hug CC. Monitoring. In: Miller RD, ed. Anesthesia. 2nd ed. New York: Churchill Livingstone; 1986:453.

estimate the workload against which either ventricle is operating by incorporating indices of preload, afterload, and stroke index. For these calculations, it is necessary to convert absolute stroke volume to stroke index, which is done by dividing the stroke volume by the patient's body surface area (BSA) in square meters. That area can be approximated from a variety of nomograms that use the patient's height and weight, such as that shown in Figure 12–13. The use of BSA-adjusted figures permits adjustment for the individual patient's relative size, which is not otherwise addressed in calculation. As it is inherently obvious that a 90-kg patient requires greater cardiac output and correspondingly higher indices than a 60-kg patient, or that a tall muscular 70-kg patient requires a greater cardiac output than a short obese 70-kg patient, the conversion of absolute

calculations to indices provides a more precise and meaningful estimate of cardiovascular function.

The single drawback to these increasingly complex integrated calculations is the accumulation of error of measure with each successive calculation. It must be remembered that cardiac output itself is a calculated parameter subject to inherent assumptions. Violation of these assumptions renders the calculated result less reliable. In similar fashion, each of the successive derivations of additional integrated indices are dependent on assumptions for greater accuracy. With each additional calculation, these indices are rendered less reliable as absolute measurements. That progressive accumulation of error in measure may render values that are far outside the norm less reliable as absolute indicators; however, trends and the use of collateral supportive data and measurements supplement their use in clinical practice and form the basis for decisions in clinical management.

MONITORING THE RESPIRATORY SYSTEM

Anesthetic management imposes many physiologic, mechanical, and biochemical changes on respiration. Administration of potent inhalation agents, endotracheal intubation and control of the mechanics of respiration, and use of positive-pressure ventilation all affect the respiratory system. These manipulations require careful monitoring to assess physiologic hemostasis and to prevent an adverse outcome from the administration of anesthetics. Cooper et al, in an analysis of major equipment failure, found that breathing circuit failures accounted for 23 percent of all equipment failures.[30] The percentage of failures with ventilators, anesthesia machines, and airway devices is also high. Thus, monitoring of the respiratory system and its components is paramount in the delivery of a safe anesthetic.

It should be noted before proceeding that no amount of respiratory monitoring equipment will automatically impart to patients an implied or explicit level of safety. That task falls largely on the vigilance of the anesthesia provider in conjunction with today's highly sophisticated monitoring equipment. There is no substitute for the character of vigilance, which includes consistent observation of the patient, surgeon, and conduct of the surgical procedure; anticipation of future events; procedures for periodic machine and equipment checks intraoperatively; and, above all, concentration and attention to detail and trend. In addition, the nurse anesthetist should consistently employ all skills of chest inspection, palpation, and auscultation, which include assessment of color, chest movement, and breath sounds. There is no doubt that equipment such as the pulse oximeter and capnometer has extended our ability to recognize early signs of impending problems; however, the equipment does not substitute in any way for the use of our senses of touch, sight, and sound as the mainstay of competent patient monitoring.

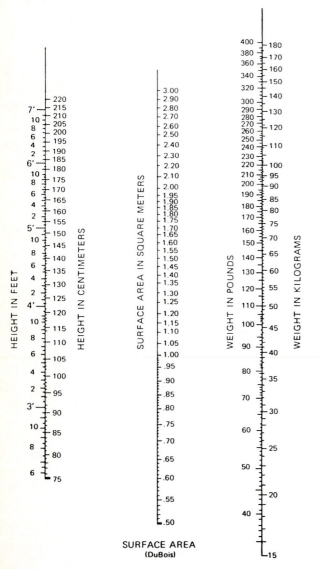

Figure 12–13. Body surface area nomogram. (*Reprinted, with permission, from DuBois D, Dubois EF. Clinical calorimetry. A formula to estimate the approximate surface area if height and weight are known.* Arch Intern Med. *1916;17:863.*)

Precordial/Esophageal Stethoscope

The precordial or esophageal stethoscope is a basic and inexpensive mode of monitoring that can be used with every patient. Changes in breath or heart sounds can be detected easily and early with this instrument. An esophageal or precordial stethoscope is particularly valuable in patients in whom the airway cannot be easily reached or observed, as in those procedures involving the head or neck or in patients in a prone position.

The precordial stethoscope should be bell-shaped, with or without a diaphragm, and made of material of adequate weight to provide an airtight seal. Proper placement in an adult is usually at the supraclavicular notch or at the apex of the left lung. Placement over the right side of the chest may fail to detect an endobronchial intubation in the adult patient, as it is much easier to inadvertently intubate the right lung preferentially because of the configuration of the mainstem bronchi. By maintaining a left-sided position, the anesthetist can determine a right mainstem intubation by the lack of breath sounds on the left, in addition to hearing heart sounds more clearly. The esophageal stethoscope is a balloon-tipped tube used when endotracheal anesthesia is employed. Both devices can be reused after proper cleaning. Causes for failure of the devices include improper placement, kinking or obstruction of the tubing, tubing long enough to attenuate sound, and improper fit of the earpiece. These devices are especially effective in identifying changes in heart rate or rhythm and changes in breath sounds, which may indicate endotracheal tube movement, breathing circuit disconnect, need for suctioning, or regurgitation.

Minimal Respiratory Monitoring Standards

Minimum respiratory monitoring equipment and techniques as recommended by the Harvard Standards and adopted by the AANA consist of the following: ventilatory assessment by continuous auscultation of breath sounds and observation of chest excursion, an oxygen analyzer, and a circuit disconnect alarm. The use of pulse oximetry is required on all cases and monitoring of the end-tidal concentrations of gases is employed by most astute clinicians. The most basic aspect of respiratory monitoring again involves observing the rate and quality of breathing. The combination of this practice and observation of skin color provides a simple yet valuable assessment of respiratory function.

Pulse Oximetry and Capnography

Pulse oximetry and capnography (infrared determination of CO_2 in expired gases) provide a more comprehensive analysis of ventilation and oxygenation. The use of these two monitoring techniques is now considered to be the standard of care. Continuous assessment of arterial oxygenation is important in the management of both sedated and anesthetized patients, especially when access to patients is limited by surgical requirements. Arterial oxygenation can be determined noninvasively and continuously by spectophotoelectric oximetric techniques. This technology is the basis for the pulse oximeter, which became commercially available in 1981. A sensor that emits two wavelengths of light is placed on a pulsatile arterial bed such as fingers, toes, ear lobe, or bridge of the nose. The sensor detects an arterial pulse and counts the pulse rate. A graphic representation of the pulse wave and a numerical indication of the oxygen

saturation of hemoglobin (SpO_2) are produced. Some models also provide a signal strength indicator that confirms adequate perfusion and the accuracy of SpO_2 determinations. The circuit control, calculation of saturation, and display are controlled by microprocessor and do not require calibration by the user.

Evaluating its accuracy in healthy volunteers, Yelderman and New found pulse oximetry to be accurate and precise over the range 70 to 100 percent saturation.[31] Pulse oximetry also accurately reflects SpO_2 values for infants with high levels of fetal hemoglobin.[32] A variety of physiologic and environmental factors can, however, affect the accuracy of pulse oximetry: high-intensity light, patient movement, electrocautery, peripheral vasoconstriction, cardiopulmonary bypass, dyshemoglobinemias, and hypothermia. In addition, intravenously administered dyes can cause spurious decreases in saturation, the largest decreases from baseline saturation occurring with methylene blue.[33,34] Dyshemoglobinemias, most notably, elevated carboxyhemoglobin levels, can cause the pulse oximeter to overestimate arterial hemoglobin saturation.[35]

Clinical use of pulse oximetry requires a familiarity with the relationship between saturation and PO_2 as demonstrated by the oxyhemoglobin dissociation curve (Fig. 12–14). Decreases in oxygen saturation of hemoglobin promote precipitous drops in PO_2 in accordance with the sigmoid shape of the curve. For example, an SaO_2 of 90% is equivalent to a PO_2 of 58 mm Hg. The clinician can therefore estimate PO_2 when given an SaO_2 value from the pulse oximeter. Assessments of SaO_2 provide trend information in the awake patient before administration of anesthetic agents. The display of these trends allows evaluation of arterial saturation and minute-to-minute corrective action. It should be noted, however, that the pulse oximeter provides only the oxygen saturation. Therefore, when PaO_2 remains above 100 torr, the SpO_2 remains 100%. Monitoring with pulse oximetry does not guarantee against the risk of inadvertent endobronchial intubation, when the shunt created does not produce a decrease in PaO_2 below that level. The use of pulse oximetry does not replace the necessity to monitor ventilatory adequacy by other means such as precordial or esophageal stethoscopy. Similarly, when deliberate endobronchial intubation is employed for intrathoracic cases, the pulse oximeter serves more effectively as an alarm for unacceptable declines in oxygen tension than as a means of continuous monitoring of oxygen transfer at the alveolocapillary level. The development of continuous intraarterial pH, PaO_2, and $PaCO_2$ monitoring remains in the developmental stage at present.

Pulse oximetry has found wide acceptance in a variety of clinical circumstances. It is a useful tool in detecting hypoxemia before development of cyanosis, a late indicator of hypoxia. Values of SpO_2 of 70 percent (PO_2 = 35 mm Hg) have been observed in children without noticeable cyanosis.[36] Because general anesthesia is associated with decreases in functional residual capacity and increases in alveolar–arterial oxygen tension gradients, the use of pulse oximetry during patient transport and recovery room care facilitates postoperative care. Tyler et al found a high incidence of hypoxemia (SpO_2 90 percent = PaO_2 58 mm Hg) in healthy adult ASA physical status I and II patients after

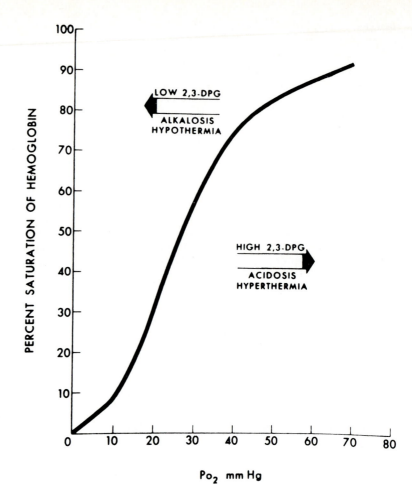

Figure 12–14. Low levels of 2,3-DPG, alkalosis and hypothermia shift the dissociation curve to the left resulting in an increased affinity for oxygen to remain tightly bound to hemoglobin. A shift of the curve to the right enhances release of oxygen to the cells. (*Reprinted, with permission, from Miller RD. The oxygen dissociation curve and multiple transfusions of ACO blood. In: Howland WS, Schweizer O, eds.* Management of patients for radical cancer surgery. Clinical Anesthesia Series, *vol. 9. Philadelphia: FA Davis; 1972:43–52.*)

anesthesia.[37] Pulse oximetry is particularly helpful when access to the airway is limited. The anesthetist can titrate sedative medication more safely when monitoring the competency of ventilatory efforts by means of oximetry.

Capnography: General Principles

The definitive indicator of ventilatory function is the measurement of arterial CO_2 by blood gas analysis. In some clinical situations, however, determination of arterial blood gases cannot be justified because of cost, invasiveness, or need for diagnostic criteria. In such instances, capnography provides a valuable assessment of the quality of ventilation and the patency of the airway and circuit. Capnographic techniques measure exhaled CO_2 at the airway by digital and graphic display. The reported value for the end-tidal concentration of CO_2 is expressed in percentage or millimeters of mercury.

Capnography uses two types of gas sampling, aspiration and in-line sampling. The most common, aspirating capnographs, take in respiratory gas through a small-bore tube from a lightweight adapter at the Y-piece. A disadvantage of the aspirating capnographer is that this tubing can become clogged with water and airway mucus, thereby obstructing the flow of gas to the sensing device and producing a falsely high CO_2 value. The aspiration and analysis of gas produce a lag time in reporting the true end-tidal concentration of CO_2. Aspirating capnographs do not require intubation of the trachea.

In-line sampling is accomplished by placing a heated sensor in connection with the endotracheal tube. The respiratory gas sample is analyzed by this sensor, and information is relayed by cable to the machine. The sensor adds bulk and dead space to the airway; however, the in-line sampling capnographer is not prone to obstruction because there is no transport of the sample. Also there is no fresh gas mixing and no significant lag time in reporting end-tidal CO_2. In-line sampling requires endotracheal intubation.

Figure 12–15 shows the normal expiratory CO_2 curve. The curve should be examined for height, shape, baseline positioning, and frequency. The normal end-tidal CO_2 waveform has a baseline of zero, unless the patient is inspiring CO_2. The waveform rises sharply from the baseline, the first portion of exhaled air (P-Q) having a low concentration of CO_2. The curve continues to rise as alveolar air displaces the initially exhaled air (Q-R) and reaches a peak (R). The peak of the curve is the end-tidal concentration of CO_2. The concentration of CO_2 decreases rapidly (R-S) with the beginning of inspiration, eventually reaching the baseline of zero.

Carbon dioxide is a product of metabolism produced by tissue and is transported via the circulation to the lungs for elimination. Therefore, changes in CO_2 levels reflect the general efficiency of circulation, respiration, and metabolism. Although end-tidal CO_2 and arterial CO_2 are not iden-

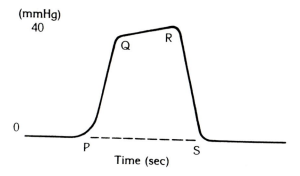

(mmHg)
40

0

Time (sec)

Figure 12–15. A normal expiratory CO_2 waveform. Exhalation begins at **P**. The slope between **Q** and **R** reflects the alveolar concentration, and **R** is the peak expired concentration of CO_2. (*Reprinted, with permission, from Jordan J, Huffman LM. Monitoring in anesthesia: Clinical application of monitoring oxygenation and ventilation. AANA J. 1985;53:521.*)

tical, measurement of end-tidal CO_2 provides a continuous and accurate record of respiratory function and is a reliable index of arterial CO_2 in a resting state. As with other monitors of respiratory function, such as the oximeter, the relationship between end-tidal CO_2 and $PaCO_2$ is not a static one. Changes in cardiac output, or one-lung ventilation (deliberate or inadvertent), alter the normal ventilation–perfusion relationship, making it necessary to evaluate ventilatory function with blood gases when indicated for management of complex cases and cases involving intrathoracic procedures. Swedlow described capnography as an "anesthesia disaster early warning system."[38] Equipment failures such as malfunctioning of the ventilator, disconnection of the breathing circuit, and changes in the position of airway devices are preventable intraoperative mishaps.[39] Figure 12–16 provides common expiratory CO_2 waveforms that the clinician might encounter during equipment failure or other catastrophic physiologic events.

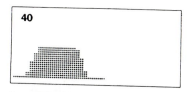

Low etCO₂ with normal rate

· Minute volume of ventilator may be too high.

· Shock

· Low body temperature

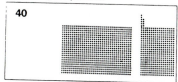

Disconnect and Reestablishment

· Sudden drop to zero at point of disconnect

· Slight increase in etCO₂ for short while following reestablishment of airway

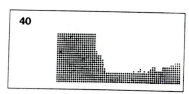

Air Embolism

· Sudden fall in exhaled CO_2.

· Could also be a kinked endotracheal tube.

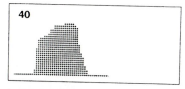

Leak in Respiratory System

· Dilution during exhalation

· Slope flattens

· Size and shape of irregularity depends on location and severity of leak.

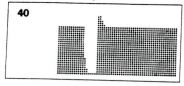

Circulatory arrest

· Patient developed ventricular fibrillation.

· etCO₂ level dropped as blood flow slowed and ceased.

· Following defibrillation, etCO₂ rose to above normal levels for a few breaths.

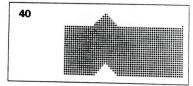

Rebreathing

· Baseline representing inspired CO_2 fails to return to zero.

· Both baseline and peak rise.

· Following elimination of rebreathing, back to normal.

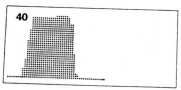

High etCO₂ with normal rate

· Minute volume of ventilator may be too low.

· May indicate onset of malignant hyperthermia.

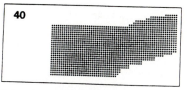

Saturation of CO₂ absorbent.

· Both baseline and etCO₂ levels rise.

· Would not be readily detected by etCO₂ monitor, which automatically readjusts to zero with each inspiration.

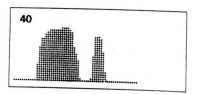

Patient fighting the ventilator

· Normal capnogram when ventilator institutes a normal breath

· Secondary capnogram when patient attempts to breathe spontaneously

Figure 12–16. These are common anesthesia-related incidents which will change the configuration of the normal capnograph. (*Reprinted, with permission, from Jordan F, Huffman LM. Monitoring in anesthesia: Clinical application of monitoring oxygenation and ventilation. AANA J. 1985;53:522–523.*)

The end-tidal level of CO_2 is perhaps the best indicator of successful endotracheal intubation, providing a waveform confirmation of entry into the trachea. Entry into the esophagus produces either no waveform or a waveform dampened in quality as compared with the control. There are a variety of conditions affecting the end-tidal concentrations of carbon dioxide (Table 12–5). Table 12–6 lists relative response times of the pulse oximeter and the capnometer in various clinical conditions, during simultaneous use of both monitors.

Mass Spectrometry: General Principles

Currently, the mass spectrometer (MS) is the only commercially available device that analyzes respiratory gases including carbon dioxide, oxygen, nitrogen, and the anesthetic gases halothane, enflurane, and isoflurane. The MS provides both numerical displays as percentages and millimeters of mercury and graphic displays of inspired and expired concentrations of these respiratory gases. Approximately 30 percent of the operating rooms in this country use a mass spectrometer, the principles of which have been reviewed elsewhere.[38,40]

The mass spectrometer is normally used in several operating rooms simultaneously. These areas are usually within 150 ft of the central unit. Each area has a gas sampling outlet and a computer terminal that receives information from the MS. The anesthetist installs an elbow connector at the Y-piece with an attached sampling tube, which transports the gas to the central unit. Sampling of respiratory gas depends on a number of factors: distance from the MS, the number of rooms being sampled, and the room priority. Because of the lag time between aspiration of the sample and display of the recorded value, breath-to-breath analysis of respiratory gases is not possible. Research is ongoing to eventually produce an MS that displays breath-to-breath analysis of end-tidal CO_2 that continues in the event of a malfunction with the central unit. A centrally located printer provides a hardcopy record of the data for inclusion in the anesthesia record. Also available are single, self-contained units which are free standing and provide sampling of a range of physiologic and anesthetic gases for a single operating room.

TABLE 12–6. RELATIVE RESPONSE (TIME) SEQUENCE OF ETco2 VERSUS Sao2[a] MONITORS

Clinical Conditions:	ETco2	Sao2
Low Flo2	↓	↓↓
Hypoventilation	↑↑	—
Hyperventilation	↓↓	—
Shunt	↑	↓↓
Esophageal intubation	↓↓	↓
Endobronchial intubation	↑	↓↓
Apnea or disconnect	↓↓	↓
Exhausted absorber/rebreathing	↑↑	↓
Embolism	↓↓	—
Low O_2 flow	↓	↓↓
Circulatory arrest	↓↓	↓
Malignant hyperthermia	↑↑	↓

[a] ETco2, end-tidal CO_2; Sao2, saturation with oxygen, arterial blood. *Reprinted, with permission, from Jordan J, Huffman LM. Monitoring in anesthesia: Clinical application of monitoring oxygenation and ventilation. AANA J. 1985;53:521–524.*

The MS alerts the clinician to acute or potentially dangerous anesthetic conditions, such as equipment failure, initial stages of malignant hyperthermia, and disconnection of the ventilator. Equipment failures identifiable by MS include malfunctioning valves in circle absorber systems, exhausted soda lime, malfunctioning pop-off valves, and errors in polarographic oxygen sensors. The MS can also be used clinically to diagnose hyperventilation, hypoventilation, and residual muscle relaxation. The information supplied by the MS regarding the inspired and expired concentrations of volatile anesthetic helps the clinician assess uptake and distribution of these agents and promotes a more timely recovery from anesthesia. Additionally, by measurement of inspired concentration, the MS can reveal when a vaporizer is malfunctioning or when it does not contain the correct agent. Because presence of an end-tidal concentration of nitrogen is a sensitive indicator of the presence of air in the pulmonary or cardiovascular system, detection of air embolus by this method is 30 to 90 seconds faster than detection by changes in precordial Doppler sounds.[41]

The greatest potential for the MS is the integration of all monitoring functions into a centralized alarm system that directs the anesthetist to the source of the problem. Cooper found that equipment failures accounted for 5 percent of adverse anesthetic outcomes, and approximately half of these incidents would have been detected by mass spectrometry.[30] The functions of the individual monitoring devices discussed earlier can all be performed by the MS. It provides a reliable backup system to the individual monitors employed; however, because of the reporting time lag in gas analysis, additional monitoring devices such as the oxygen analyzer, disconnect alarms, and low-flow alarms are still critical for early detection of problems.

MONITORING BODY TEMPERATURE

The measurement of body temperature is considered a standard of anesthesia care in contemporary operating rooms, especially for the pediatric patient. Current standards

TABLE 12–5. CLINICAL CONDITIONS AFFECTING THE END-TIDAL CONCENTRATION OF CARBON DIOXIDE

Decreased CO_2	Increased CO_2
Hyperventilation	Hypoventilation
Hypothermia	Hyperthermia
Impaired pulmonary circulation	Increased transport to lungs
Shock	IV sodium bicarbonate
Air embolism	Rebreathing air (e.g., exhausted CO_2 absorbent, faulty breathing circuit)
Contamination	Intraabdominal CO_2 (laparoscopy)

Reprinted, with permission, from McLaughlin G. Respiratory gas monitoring. Curr Rev Nurse Anesthetists. 1985;8:9.

require that unless otherwise indicated by the type and extent of surgery, a way of continuously measuring a patient's temperature must be available. Inherent in anesthesia is some loss of body heat and a lowering of core temperature generally 0.5C to 1C per hour, usually no more than 2C to 3C. Temperatures below 34C, however, may lead to significant morbidity. The degree of loss depends on many factors including ambient room temperature, scope and length of surgery, degree of depression of hypothalamic control, surgical prevention, intraoperative fluid replacement, and the vigilance of the anesthetist in preserving and maintaining core temperature.

Recent advances in thermotechnology have produced more sophisticated methods of measuring core body temperature. Such methods use liquid crystals, miniaturized electronic devices, computer enhancements, and nuclear magnetic resonance.[42] For the anesthetist, the goal of measuring body temperature remains the same, to keep core temperature within the normal range of $37 \pm 0.5C$, to ensure that homeostatic functions of the body are maintained. Theoretically, core temperature varies minimally, with surrounding peripheral tissue interacting with the environment through temperature gradients. True core temperature is thought to be the temperature of the hypothalamus, which acts as the control center for regulation of temperature. To estimate core temperature accurately, using measurements of surface body temperature, one would need 4 to 10 measurements at each of a variety of peripheral sites.

In the two most common methods of monitoring temperature during anesthesia, a variety of probes are used to determine core temperature and liquid crystal material is applied to the surface of the body to assess temperature in regional sections of the body. Some anesthetists believe that the concurrent use of both techniques provides a more accurate reflection of temperature trend. This reduces the possibility of overshoot or "drift" where temperatures continue to drop 2C to 3C even after cooling measures have been stopped, such as during intentional hypothermia.

Liquid-Crystal Thermometers

Liquid-crystal thermometry uses Mylar strips impregnated with microencapsulated cholesteric liquid crystals. Variations in skin temperature change the molecular arrangement of the crystals. These strips are most often applied to the forehead and show only regional temperatures. They are easily applied to the awake patient for regional anesthesia or monitored anesthesia care, where further invasiveness or discomfort is not warranted. Although this technique produces values that correlate in a linear fashion with esophageal measurements, temperature at the two sites differ consistently by several degrees. This type of measurement technique is relatively inexpensive, easy to apply, noninvasive, and safe.

Probes

Temperature probes are of two types, the thermocouple and the thermistor. The thermocouple circuit consists of two dissimilar metals between which an electromotive force is generated. The voltage or electromagnetic frequency is proportional to the difference between the temperatures of the two metals. Thermistors are semiconducting elements that are thermally sensitive resistors having a high temperature coefficient. Because of their sensitivity and ease of application, thermistor probes are among the most common types of measurement devices now being used in anesthesia.

Probes can be placed in the nasopharynx, rectum, esophagus, tympanic membrane, axilla, and bladder. Because all those sites have specific advantages and disadvantages (Table 12–7) final selection usually depends on the degree of invasiveness (and hence, risk), the application, the precision of the temperature measurement site, and the type of anesthetic technique employed. Temperatures produced by esophageal and tympanic membrane devices correlate highly with cerebral and thoracic temperatures.

Tympanic membrane temperature is considered the most accurate estimate of core temperature because the probe is placed close to the tympanic blood supply from the posterior auricular and internal maxillary arteries, branches of the external carotid artery. The correlation between tympanic membrane temperature and esophageal temperatures seems to be good as long as the probe has been placed properly and exposure of the probe to ambient

TABLE 12–7. SITES FOR MONITORING BODY TEMPERATURE

Site	Characteristics, Advantages, and Disadvantages
Skin	Varies with subcutaneous blood flow, sweating, radiation, and conduction of heat to or from extracorporeal objects
Axilla	Varies with blood flow
Tympanic membrane	Closely approximates temperature of blood perfusing the brain when probe is against tympanic membrane; discrepancies arise when probe is located away from membrane or impacted in cerumen, which acts as an insulator; risks of membrane perforation and hemorrhage
Nasopharynx	Reflects temperature of blood going to brain; nasal probes can cause epistaxis
Oropharynx and upper esophagus	Reflects temperature of respiratory gases
Lower esophagus (20 cm below pharyngoesophageal junction)	Closely approximates temperature of aortic blood (core temperature)
Rectum	Varies with blood flow; fecal mass acts as an insulator
Urinary bladder	Catheter with thermistor can be used to measure core temperature
Pulmonary artery (Swan-Ganz thermodilution catheter)	Measures the temperature of blood in the body core, except with pericardial irrigation during cardiac operations
Muscle	Requires special probe; varies with blood flow

Reprinted, with permission, from Hug CC Jr. Monitoring. In: Miller RD, ed. Anesthesia. 2nd ed. New York: Churchill Livingstone; 1986:411–463.

temperature is minimized. To avoid damage to the tympanic membrane and to ensure that measurements are accurate, the probe should be placed only while the patient is awake. Caution in placement is mandatory because the incidence of bleeding into the external auditory canal as a result of rupture of the membrane is 2 to 3 percent.[43]

Some investigators believe that measurements in the lower esophagus correlate well with cerebral temperature in non-open-chest procedures. These probes must be placed in the lower one third or one quarter of the esophagus, or about 45 cm from the nostril. In children, placement can be guided by the following formula, which gives the number of centimeters below the corniculate cartilages at which the probe should be placed[44]:

$$10 = \frac{(2 \times \text{age in years})}{3}$$

Probe Sites: Advantages, Disadvantages, and Risks

The monitoring of intraoperative temperature for all patients undergoing general anesthesia constitutes rational patient care. For selected patients for whom traditional probe placement may be difficult, such as burn victims, intermittent use of rectal or axillary probes allows the anesthetist to follow temperature trends. For most routine cases, the esophageal probe is most desirable because of its linear correlation with core temperature, ease of application, and lower rate of complications. For open chest procedures, concurrent use of esophageal and rectal probes is advisable, with periodic temperature readings from the pulmonary artery catheter. When deliberate hypothermia is used, several sources of temperature measurement are warranted because there may be significant regional variations in body temperature during rewarming.

Following are some disadvantages and risks associated with various temperature probe placements. Although a thermistor-tipped pulmonary artery catheter may provide the most accurate estimate of core temperature, it is not applicable for most anesthetic procedures. Tympanic, nasopharyngeal, needle, and rectal probes present some element of clinical risk and inconvenience that has limited their widespread acceptance for intraoperative monitoring. Rectal temperature may be unreliable because of contact with bowel content. Nasopharyngeal readings can be dampened by excessive contact with ambient temperature in the airway. Bladder probes cause discomfort and may lead to urinary tract infection. Despite the close correlation between tympanic membrane and cerebral temperature, potential damage to the membrane and spurious readings after inadequate placement of the probe have placed pragmatic limits on the clinical effectiveness of measuring tympanic membrane temperature.

SUMMARY

It is incumbent on all anesthetists to become quite familiar with the written standards of care expected of every provider. Should logistic barriers arise that do not allow use of these standards (even if only on a temporary basis), notation of such should be made on the patient's record with a thorough, written justification. In no circumstance should an elective case proceed without full monitoring equipment available, functional, and used. Periodic checks and maintenance records of equipment and the machine should also be documented in departmental files. In the opinion of the authors, after having reviewed substantial numbers of case records involved in litigation, lack of monitoring use, documentation, or inability to interpret competently the data obtained still constitute a major basis for determinations of negligence.

The technology of monitoring has increased substantially over the past decade, as concerns for patient safety under anesthesia have justifiably increased. Still, vigilance remains our strongest defense in protecting patients from deleterious outcomes.

The authors recognize Mr. John Aker CRNA, MSNA, Research Medical Center; Dr. Chuck Biddle, CRNA, University of Kansas Medical Center; and Dr. D. E. Supkis, Baylor College of Medicine, for their valued work and contributions to this chapter.

REFERENCES

1. Stein RH. Reporters ask safety questions during ASA media tour. *Anesth Patient Saf Found Newslett.* Winter 1990–1991:41.
2. Aukburg SJ, Gilbert H, Owens W, Polk S, Vender J, Pertlin G. Decreasing anesthesia cardiac arrests. In: *Abstracts, 1990 ASA Annual Meeting.*
3. Pierce EC, Cooper JB Jr, eds. *Analysis of anesthetic mishaps.* Boston: Little, Brown; 1984;22:2.
4. Cooper JB. Toward Prevention of Anesthetic Mishaps. In: Pierce EC Jr, Cooper JB, eds. *Analysis of anesthetic mishaps. International anesthesia clinics.* Boston: Little, Brown; 1984.
5. Duberman SM, Bendixen HH. Concepts of fail-safe anesthesia practice. In: Pierce EC Jr, Cooper JB, eds. *Analysis of anesthetic mishaps. International anesthesia clinics.* Boston: Little, Brown; 1984:149–165.
6. American Association of Nurse Anesthetists. Patient monitoring standards. In: *Professional practice manual for the CRNA: Standards for nurse anesthesia practice.* 1989:5–6.
7. American Association of Nurse Anesthetists. Standards for nurse anesthesia practice. In: *Professional practice manual for the CRNA: Standards for nurse anesthesia practice.* 1989:3–4.
8. Eger E. The concept of MAC. In: *Uptake and distribution of anesthetic agents.* Baltimore: Williams & Wilkins; 1974.
9. Larsen MD. Pupillary effects of general anesthesia. *Anesthesiol Rev.* 1986;13:25–31.
10. Larsen MD. Dilation of the pupil in human subjects after intravenous thiopental. *Anesthesiology.* 1981;54:246.
11. Wong KC. Narcotics are not expected to produce unconsciousness and amnesia. *Anesth Analg.* 1985;62:625–626. Editorial.
12. Russell IF. Balanced anesthesia: Does it anesthetize? *Anesth Analg.* 1985;64:941–944. Letter to the Editor.
13. Sebel PS, Heneghan CP, Ingram DA. Evoked responses—A neurophysiological indication of depth of anesthesia? *Br J Anesth.* 1985;57:841–842. Letter to the Editor.

14. Evans JM, Davis WL. Monitoring anesthesia. *Clin Anesthesiol.* 1984;2:249.

15. Miller RD, ed. *Anesthesia.* 2nd ed. Edinburgh: Churchill Livingstone; 1986:467.

16. Lee AP. Biotechnological principles of monitoring. *Int Anesthesiol Clin.* 1981;19:204.

17. Mishin WW, Jones PL, eds. *Physics for the anaesthetist.* 4th ed. Blackwell Scientific; 1986:489–499.

18. Hunter FP, Eastwood DW. Manometry. In: *Instrumentation and anesthesia.* Philadelphia: FA Davis; 1986, 2964.

19. Brunner JMR. *Handbook of blood pressure monitoring.* Littleton, MA: PSG; 1978.

20. Remington JW. Contour changes of the aortic pulse during propagation. *Am J Physiol.* 1960;199:331.

21. Brunner JMR, Krenis LJ, Kunsman JM, et al. Comparison of direct and indirect methods of measuring arterial blood pressure. Part 1. *Med Instrum.* 1981;15:11.

22. O'Rourke MF, Taylor MG. Vascular impedance of the femoral bed. *Circ Res.* 1966;18:126.

23. Burnside JW. *Physical diagnosis.* 16th ed. Baltimore: Williams & Wilkins; 1981:49.

24. Brown AE, Sweeney DB, Lumley J. Percutaneous radial artery cannulation. *Anaesthesia.* 1969;24:532.

25. Bedford FR. Radial arterial function following percutaneous cannulation with 18 and 20 gauge catheters. *Anesthesiology.* 1977;47:37.

26. Bedford FR. Long-term radial artery cannulation: Effects on subsequent vessel function. *Crit Care Med.* 1978;6:64.

27. Pinella JC, Ross DF, Martin T, et al. Study of the incidence of intravascular catheter infection and associated septicemia in critically ill patients. *Crit Care Med.* 1983;11:21.

28. Hayes MF, Morello DC, Rosenbaum, et al. Radial artery catheterization by cutdown technique. *Crit Care Med.* 1973; 1:151.

29. Slogoff S, Keats AS, Arlund C. On the safety of radial artery cannulation. *Anesthesiology.* 1983;59:42.

30. Cooper JB, Newhower RS, Kitz RJ. An analysis of major errors and equipment failures in anesthesia management: Consideration for prevention and detection. *Anesthesiology.* 1984;60:34–42.

31. Yelderman M, New W Jr. Evaluation of pulse oximetry. *Anesthesiology.* 1983;59:349–352.

32. Deckardt R, Steward DJ. Non-invasive arterial hemoglobin oxygen saturation versus transcutaneous oxygen tension monitoring in the preterm infant. *Crit Care Med.* 1984;12:935–939.

33. Scheller MS, Unger RJ, Kilner MJ. Effects of intravenously administered dyes on pulse oximetry readings. *Anesthesiology.* 1986;65:550–552.

34. Kessler MR, Eide T, Humayun B, Poppers PH. Spurious pulse oximeter denaturation with methylene blue injection. *Anesthesiology.* 1986;65:435–436.

35. Barber SJ, Tremper KR. The effect of carbon monoxide inhalation on pulse oximetry and transcutaneous P_{O_2}. *Anesthesiology.* 1987;66:677–679.

36. Motoyama EK, Glazener CH. Hypoxemia after general anesthesia in children. *Anesth Analg.* 1986;65:267–272.

37. Tyler IL, Tantisira B, Winter PM. Continuous monitoring of arterial oxygen saturation with pulse oximetry during transfer to the recovery room. *Anesth Analg.* 1985;64:1108–1112.

38. Swedlow DB. Capnometry and capnography: The anesthesia disaster early warning system. *Semin Anesth.* 1986;5:194–205.

39. Cooper JB. Preventable mishaps in anesthesia practice. *ASA Refresher Course Lectures.* 1984:217.

40. Jameson LC. Application of mass spectrometry in clinical anesthesia. *ASA Refresher Course Lectures.* 1986:226.

41. Matasko J, Petrozza P, MacKenzie CF. Sensitivity of endotidal nitrogen in venous air embolism detection in dogs. *Anesthesiology.* 1985;63:418–423.

42. Maziarski FT. Clinical monitoring in anesthesia: Applied technology in monitoring temperature. *AANA J.* 1985;53:272–285.

43. Whitby JD, Dunkin LJ. Cerebral, oesophageal and nasopharyngeal temperatures. *Br J Anaesth.* 1971;43:673–676.

44. Gravenstein JS, Paulus DA. *Monitoring practice in clinical anesthesia.* Philadelphia: JB Lippincott; 1982:170–172.

APPENDIX 1: PATIENT MONITORING STANDARDS*

Basic to safe anesthesia care is the application of qualitative and quantitative monitoring which enables the anesthetist to administer anesthesia and evaluate its effect in a manner that optimizes desired responses while minimizing the risks of anesthesia. Fundamental to this endeavor is the use of multiple monitoring modalities which play vital roles in assisting anesthetists to provide conscientious care to patients receiving anesthesia.

These patient monitoring standards are intended to assist the CRNA practitioner in providing consistent, safe anesthesia care.

These standards apply to patients undergoing general, regional, or monitored anesthesia care for diagnostic or therapeutic procedures in designated anesthetizing locations. In extenuating circumstances, the CRNA must use clinical judgment in prioritizing and implementing these standards. All of these standards do not normally apply to epidural analgesia for labor or pain management therapy. The standards may be exceeded in any or all respects at any time at the discretion of the anesthetist, as required by individual patient needs.

While the standards are intended to encourage high-quality patient care, they cannot insure specific patient outcomes. It is recognized that appropriately used monitoring modalities may fail to detect untoward clinical developments. Further, it is recognized by the AANA that under some circumstances certain monitoring standards may not be applicable. While this is a fact of practice, the omission of one or more monitoring standards should be documented and the reason stated on the patient's anesthesia record. Interruptions in monitoring may be unavoidable. Occasionally, the anesthetist must work at some distance from the patient because of an environmental hazard such as, but not limited to, radiation. Under such circumstances, provisions for monitoring the patient must be made and documented on the patient's anesthesia record.

Adequate facilities must exist to enable remote patient monitoring.

The standards are subject to review and revision from time to time, as indicated by technology and practice.

Anesthesia Providers

Continuous clinical observation and anesthetist vigilance are the bases of safe anesthesia care. The anes-

* Reproduced, with permission, from American Association of Nurse Anesthetists.[6]

thetist, or nurse anesthesia student, shall be in constant attendance of the patient until the responsibility for care has been accepted by another qualified health care provider.

Patient Monitors

Ventilation

Purpose. To assess adequate ventilation of the patient.

Standard. Intubation of the trachea shall be verified by auscultation, chest excursion and confirmation of carbon dioxide in the expired gas. Controlled or assisted ventilation during the anesthetic shall be monitored continuously with an end-tidal CO_2 monitor. Additionally, spirometry and ventilatory pressure monitors may also be used.

Breathing system disconnect monitor: When the patient is ventilated by an automatic mechanical ventilator, the integrity of the breathing system must be monitored by a device that is capable of detecting the disconnection of any component of the breathing system. Such a device shall be equipped with an audible alarm which is activated when its limits are exceeded.

Oxygenation

Purpose. To assess adequate oxygenation of the patient.

Standard. Adequacy of patient oxygenation shall be monitored continuously with pulse oximetry. In addition to pulse oximetry, oxygenation shall also be monitored by observations of skin color, the color of the blood in the surgical field, and arterial blood gas analysis when indicated.

During general anesthesia, the oxygen concentration delivered by the anesthesia machine shall be monitored continuously with an oxygen analyzer with a low-oxygen-concentration limit alarm. An oxygen supply failure alarm system shall be operational to warn of low oxygen pressure to the anesthesia machine.

Circulation

Purpose. To assess adequacy of the cardiovascular system.

Standard. Blood pressure and heart rate shall be determined and recorded at least every 5 minutes.

The patient's electrocardiogram shall be monitored continuously during the course of the anesthetic.

Circulation also shall be assessed by at least one of the following measures: digital palpation of pulse, auscultation of heart sounds, continuous intraarterial pressure monitoring, electronic pulse monitoring, or pulse oximetry.

Body Temperature

Purpose. To assess changes in body temperature.

Standard. Body temperature shall be intermittently or continuously monitored and recorded on all patients receiving general anesthesia; the means to monitor temperature shall be immediately available for use on all patients receiving local or regional anesthesia and used when indicated.

Neuromuscular Function

Purpose. To assess neuromuscular function.

Standard. The means to evaluate the patient's neuromuscular function by the use of a nerve stimulator shall be available immediately when neuromuscular blocking agents have been used.

Anesthesia Equipment

A complete equipment safety check shall be performed daily and an abbreviated check of all equipment shall be performed before each anesthetic is administered.

All anesthesia machines and monitoring equipment shall conform to the appropriate national and state standards. An ongoing preventive maintenance program shall be established and enforced.

APPENDIX 2: STANDARDS FOR NURSE ANESTHESIA PRACTICE*

Introduction

A characteristic of any profession is its responsibility to the public for promulgating standards by which the quality of practice rendered by its members can be assessed. Standards, based upon sound philosophy, theory, science, and principles, serve to upgrade clinical practice.

As the representative of the profession, the Board of Directors of the American Association of Nurse Anesthetists adopts and promulgates standards of practice with input from the members of the Association. The primary responsibility for implementing these standards rests with the practitioners, Certified Registered Nurse Anesthetists (CRNAs). As an organization composed of health care providers, the American Association of Nurse Anesthetists recognizes that the principles of anesthesia practice should be clearly described as professional standards which guide the practitioner in maintaining and improving the delivery of quality anesthesia care.

Purpose of Standards

These standards are intended to assist the CRNA practitioner in providing consistent, safe anesthesia care. The standards are descriptive, providing a basis for evaluation of the practice and reflecting the rights of those receiving anesthesia care. The AANA recognizes it may not be possible for the CRNA to comply with each of

---

* Reprinted, with permission, from American Association of Nurse Anesthetists.[7]

these standards in certain extraordinary or emergency situations. It is expected that the CRNA should assess each patient situation and utilize professional judgment in selecting a course of action, and that in each case, the CRNA can demonstrate that the decisions made were in the best interest of the patient. In addition, while the standards are intended to encourage high-quality patient care, they cannot insure specific patient outcomes.

Their intent is to

1. assist the profession in evaluating the quality of care provided by its practitioners,
2. provide a common base for practitioners to use to coordinate care and unify their efforts in the development of a quality practice,
3. assist the public in understanding what to expect from the practitioner,
4. support and preserve the basic rights of the patient.

Standard I. A thorough and complete preanesthetic assessment shall be performed.

Interpretation. The responsibility of a CRNA begins before the actual administration of the anesthesia. Except under unusual or emergency situations, the CRNA has an obligation to determine that relevant tests have been completed and thorough assessment of the patient has been made.

Standard II. Informed consent for the planned anesthetic intervention shall be obtained from the patient or legal guardian.

Interpretation. The CRNA shall obtain or verify that an informed consent has been obtained by another qualified provider. Anesthetic options and risks should be discussed with the patient and/or legal guardian in language the patient and/or legal guardian can understand. The patient's medical record should reflect that informed consent was obtained.

Standard III. A patient-specific plan for anesthesia care shall be formulated.

Interpretation. The plan of care is developed by the CRNA in coordination with appropriate health care providers in a systematic manner based upon assessment, analysis, anticipated procedure, patient preference, and current anesthesia principles. It must be coordinated with appropriate health care providers.

Standard IV. The anesthesia care plan shall be skillfully implemented and the plan of care adjusted as needed to adapt to the patient's response to the anesthetic. Vigilance shall be maintained for untoward identifiable reactions and corrective actions initiated as required.

Interpretation: The CRNA shall induce and maintain anesthesia at required levels. The CRNA shall continuously assess the patient's response to the anesthetic and/or surgical intervention and intervene as required to maintain the patient in a homeostatic, physiologic condition.

Standard V. The patient's physiologic condition shall be monitored consistent with both the type of anesthesia care and specific patient needs.

Interpretation: Monitoring modalities shall be instituted in accordance with AANA *Patient Monitoring Standards.* [*See Appendix 1.*]

Standard VI. There shall be prompt, complete, and accurate documentation of pertinent information on the patient's record.

Interpretation: Documentation should be criteria-based, reflecting the standards of anesthesia practice. Documentation should include all anesthetic interventions and patient responses.

Accurate recording facilitates comprehensive patient care, provides information for retrospective review and research data, and establishes a medical-legal record. The CRNA is responsible for assuring that the care provided by the CRNA is properly documented.

Standard VII. The responsibility for the care of the patient shall be transferred to other qualified providers in a manner which assures continuity of care and patient safety.

Interpretation: The CRNA shall assess the patient's status and determine when it is safe to transfer responsibility for care to other qualified personnel. The CRNA shall accurately report the patient's condition and all essential information to the personnel assuming responsibility for the care of the patient.

Standard VIII. Appropriate safety precautions shall be taken to minimize the risks of fire, explosion, electrical shock, and equipment malfunction.

Interpretation: Safety precautions and controls, as established within the institution, shall be strictly adhered to, so as to minimize the hazards of electricity, fire, and explosion in areas where anesthesia care is provided. The anesthetic machine shall be inspected by the CRNA according to guidelines before use. The CRNA shall check the readiness, availability, cleanliness, and working condition of all equipment to be utilized in the administration of the anesthesia care. Documentation shall be made of the patient's medical record that the anesthesia machine and equipment were checked. Policies for routine safety and maintenance checks of anesthesia equipment and monitors shall be developed and adhered to by the appropriate individuals and departments within the institution.

Standard IX. Appropriate safety precautions shall be taken to minimize the risk of infection for the patient, CRNA, and other staff.

Interpretation: Written policies on infection control shall be developed and followed in order to minimize the risks of infectious disease.

Standard X. **Anesthesia care shall be assessed to assure its quality.**

Interpretation: The CRNA shall participate in the ongoing review and evaluation of the quality and appropriateness of anesthesia care that he or she provides. Evaluation shall be performed based upon appropriate outcome criteria and reviewed on an ongoing basis.

Standard XI. **The CRNA shall participate in a continual process of self-evaluation and strive for excellence in anesthesia practice.**

Interpretation: Self-evaluation is accomplished in several ways, including quality assurance, peer review, annual performance appraisal, review of clinical privileges, and ongoing assessment of clinical practice. The CRNA shall incorporate into practice new techniques and knowledge which have been acquired through formal, self-directed study.

Standard XII. **The CRNA shall respect and maintain the basic rights of patients, demonstrating concern for personal dignity and human relationships.**

Interpretation: The CRNA shall support and preserve the basic rights of patients to privacy, independence of expression, decision, and action.

Positioning for Anesthesia and Surgery

*Everard R. Hicks and
Kathleen C. Koerbacher*

Alterations in body physiology caused by positioning for surgical procedures are well documented but often ignored until a catastrophe occurs. Perhaps the earliest recorded death under anesthesia caused by posture change occurred on January 19, 1849. The patient was John Griffith, age 31, a seaman in the U.S. Navy. He received chloroform by open mask in the sitting position and, as soon as he was anesthetized, he was placed in the lateral position for the removal of some hemorrhoids. History records that as soon as the posture change occurred, he ceased to breathe and was found to be pulseless. All efforts to restore the deceased failed.[1]

Obviously there is little comparison between anesthesia in the 1840s and anesthesia in the 1990s. Nevertheless, body physiology has changed little. Despite our advanced knowledge, profound changes in the circulatory and respiratory systems do occur as a result of posture changes. Nerve injuries associated with malpositioning of the patient on the operating table are not infrequent occurrences.

The purpose of this chapter is to present an overview of the alteration in the body physiology caused by posture changes, with special emphasis being placed on the circulatory and respiratory systems, and of common nerve injuries associated with the commonly used surgical positions.

POSITIONING

Not only do we have a moral obligation to care properly for those we anesthetize, but we also have a legal one. The court has made a clear statement in this regard: "During general anesthesia, the patient is unconscious. The protective reflexes have now been attenuated and the patient is no longer able to protect himself against injury. The patient cannot cry out in pain. Responsibility for the patient then falls solely upon the anesthesia care provider." One is also reminded of the motto of the Canadian Anesthetists Society: "We watch closely those who sleep."

The type of surgery and the anatomic location of the surgery dictate the posture of the patient for that particular surgical intervention. Some of these positions do indeed "defy the muscular and skeletal mechanics possible to the human body."[1]

It may be worthwhile for all anesthetists to be placed in each of the common postures to allow them to experience the discomfort associated with various surgical positions.

For example, in tests done on awake patients subjected to many of the modifications of the prone position, it was found that no subject could be made to feel comfortable, and these subjects complained of severe pain and numbness in various parts of their bodies within 5 to 10 minutes.[2]

Because the role of anesthesia is to relieve the pain of surgery, the pain of positioning is also relieved. Often the patient has been heard to remark that he or she is not concerned with the surgical position because "I will be asleep and I will not feel any pain." These same patients in the conscious state, however, could not and would not tolerate this discomfort.

Circulation

The role of the pressoreceptors in the regulation of systemic blood pressure should be well known to all students of physiology.

These receptors—located in the carotid sinuses, aortic arch, pulmonary arteries, and other arteries—respond to pressure changes. An increase in blood pressure causes impulses to inhibit the medullary vasoconstrictor center and excite the vagus nerve. Once the vagus is stimulated, the heart rate slows, the peripheral vessels dilate, and the myocardial contractility is decreased, resulting in a compensatory fall in blood pressure.

A sudden fall in arterial blood pressure has somewhat the opposite effect. There is now a sympathetic effect that increases the heart rate, causes a constriction of peripheral vessels, and increases myocardial contraction.

The Bainbridge reflex, located in the right atrium, also responds to returning blood flow and pressure and adjusts the heart rate to allow for more effective filling.

All these compensatory reflexes attempt to regulate blood flow to the vital organs of the body, especially the brain, heart, and kidney, as well as other vessel-rich organs.

In the normal, healthy, awake person, these reflexes rapidly regulate blood pressure and tissue perfusion. The vigor of these protective mechanisms is impaired by disease, injury, and anesthesia. Postural changes that normally cause little or no change in blood pressure and tissue perfusion will cause a significant fall in both blood pressure and perfusion in the anesthetized patient.[3]

Any drug producing a sympatholytic effect will seem to accentuate these changes to varying degrees. The effects of these depressant drugs usually can be considered dose related, so it becomes important to avoid deep or even moderate levels of anesthesia prior to position changes. Agents known for their circulation-depressing effects should be avoided until the posture change has been completed.

Most authorities agree that the safest anesthesia prior to position change would be a thiopental, nitrous oxide, oxygen, muscle relaxant technique. Use of the fluorinated agents prior to a posture change will almost always result in blood pressure drops caused by their sympatholytic action.

Caution should also be taken with postural changes at the termination of surgery. Blood pooling in body areas below heart level will reenter the general circulation; however, those areas above the heart level will rapidly receive a large volume of blood when lowered to heart level. Many times one will see a precipitous fall in blood pressure unless the rate of posture change is slow. Even rapid, rough movement from the operating room table to the stretcher can adversely influence circulatory homeostasis.

Alterations in position from the horizontal to the upright or tilted to head down cause little or no alteration in blood pressure in the conscious person. The head-down tilt is extremely uncomfortable in conscious subjects because of increased pressure in the cranial veins, capillary distention with possible edema, and petechial hemorrhage.

In the 1950s, the importance of blood pressure and blood flow to the brain during anesthesia and surgery when the patient is tilted away from the horizontal position was noted. When blood pressure is taken in the arm, the blood pressure may stay the same after tilt, because the limb remains at the approximate level of the heart. If blood pressure were taken in both the elevated and lowered portions of the body, a dramatic difference in pressure would be seen.

Wylie and Churchill-Davidson[4] suggested that "As a general rule the difference in pressure in a particular area may be calculated on the basis of allowing plus or minus 2 mm Hg for each one inch (2.5 cm) of tilt below or above the level of the heart."

Nerve Injuries Associated with Anesthesia

Stretching or direct compression of a nerve is the chief cause of nerve damage from positioning.

Either stretching or compression interferes with the blood supply to the nerve and can result in permanent damage and necrosis.

Blood is supplied to the peripheral nerves via small arterioles that anastomose with each other at regular intervals. Because these vessels are so small, they are easily compressed, resulting in ischemia.

General anesthesia produces two conditions ideal for nerve damage: muscle tone is lost and perceptive power is no longer intact to warn the patient of impending danger.

Space limits broad coverage here of each peripheral nerve subject to damage caused by improper posture. The reader is referred to Britt and Gordon's excellent article on this subject.[5]

Brachial Plexus. The brachial plexus is the group of nerves most vulnerable by far to damage from malpositioning.

Stretching is the chief cause of damage to the brachial plexus. This stretching can be produced by many factors, but one of the most common is abduction and dorsal extension of the arm on an arm board at an angle of more than 60 degrees to the operating table.[6] With the arm extended to a maximum of 90 degrees and the hand forcibly pronated, the brachial plexus is stretched across the humeral–clavicular joint, leading to injury (Figs. 13–1 and 13–2).

Suspension of the arm from the ether screen in the lateral position, or in any position that causes the plexus to stretch, should be avoided (Fig. 13–3).

Ulnar Nerve. The ulnar nerve is especially vulnerable as it passes posteriorly under the medial epicondyle of the elbow. The ulnar nerve and the ulnar collateral artery pass through the cubital tunnel at the elbow as they course from

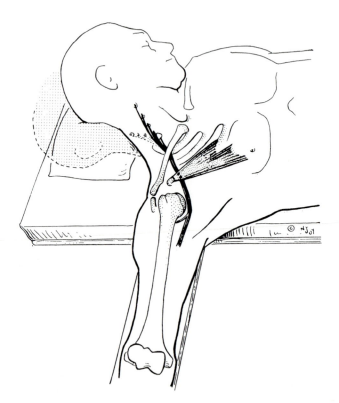

Figure 13–1. Nerve damage occurs when the brachial plexus is stretched when the arm is abducted, extended, and externally rotated, and the head is deviated to the opposite side. (*Courtesy Department of Art as Applied to Medicine, Faculty of Medicine, University of Toronto.*)

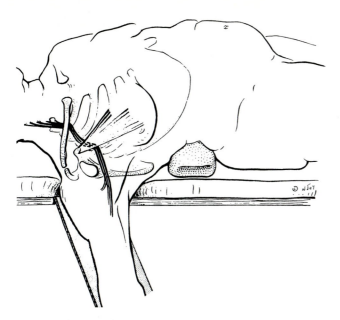

Figure 13–2. Damaging stretching of the brachial plexus around the tendon of pectoralis minor when the shoulder girdle falls back with the arm abducted, extended, and externally rated. (*Courtesy Department of Art as Applied to Medicine, Faculty of Medicine, University of Toronto.*)

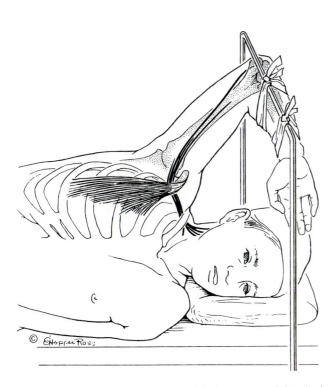

Figure 13–3. Stretching of the brachial plexus around the clavicle and tendon of pectoralis minor by fixation of the abducted arm to the frame of an ether screen is to be avoided. (*Courtesy Department of Art as Applied to Medicine, Faculty of Medicine, University of Toronto.*)

the arm to the forearm. External compression on this cubital tunnel can produce the "cubital tunnel external compression syndrome."[7] This syndrome can be the consequence of rest in an armchair, but more often it occurs because of external pressure during anesthesia and operation. Controversy exists as to whether the arm should be placed on the arm board with the hand in the pronated or supinated position.[5,7] With the arm extended and supinated, the cubital tunnel is free from compression, but the brachial plexus is stretched. If the hand is pronated, the cubital tunnel is exposed to compression. This tunnel must be protected with soft pads and judicious positioning to prevent pressure on the ulnar nerve.[6]

Compression of the ulnar nerve may also result when the elbow is allowed to sag slightly over the side of the operating table or when the arms are folded across the abdomen or chest (Fig. 13–4).

A patient with damage to this nerve has clawing of the ring and little finger and sensory deficit in the ulnar nerve distribution.

Radial Nerve. When the arm is compressed between the body and ether screen there is danger of damage to the radial nerve if the nerve is pinched between the screen and spiral groove of the humerus (Fig. 13–5).

Clinically, with radial nerve injury there is wrist drop and inability to extend the metacarpophalangeal joints because of paralysis of the extensor muscles in the forearm.

Peroneal and Saphenous Nerves. The most frequently damaged nerves of the lower extremities are the common peroneal and the saphenous.[8]

The common peroneal nerve is injured in the lithotomy position when the nerve is allowed to be compressed between the lithotomy stirrup and the neck of the fibula. This occurs when the legs are inside the stirrups in the lithotomy position. Soft padding should be used between the leg and the stirrup (Fig. 13–6).

The saphenous nerve is damaged in the lithotomy position when the legs are suspended lateral to the vertical

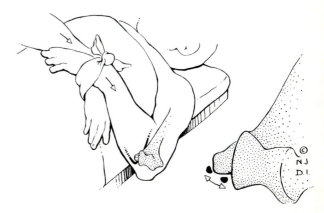

Figure 13–4. Ulnar nerve injury is caused by compression between the medial epicondyle of the humerus and the edge of the operating table. Inset: Anomalous position of ulnar nerve. (*Courtesy Department of Art as Applied to Medicine, Faculty of Medicine, University of Toronto.*)

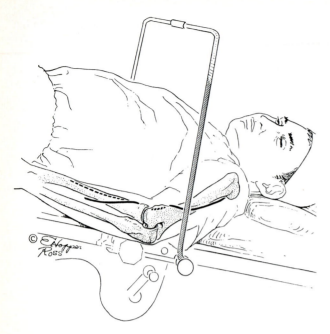

Figure 13–5. Damaging compression of the radial nerve between the humerus and an ether screen. (*Courtesy Department of Art as Applied to Medicine, Faculty of Medicine, University of Toronto.*)

braces or stirrups. This nerve can be compressed between the stirrup and tibia (Fig. 13–7). Soft padding between leg and stirrups can help prevent this nerve injury.

Malpositioning compression damage has also been reported on a host of other nerves, including the pudendal, femoral, and obturator. Other nerves have been injured by injections and slippage of anesthesia airway equipment. These include the phrenic nerve, stellate ganglion, lumbar spinal, optic and supraorbital, facial, abducens, and trigeminal nerves.[5]

Respiration

Mechanical interference with chest movement, which limits expansion of the lung, is perhaps the single most important effect of posture on respiration.

In normal respiration the lung expands in an inferior–superior direction with movement of the diaphragm. The thorax expands in all directions, except posteriorly because it is prevented by the spine.

Because the diaphragm is responsible for movement of about 60 percent or more of intrathoracic volume, any limitation on this muscle's movement can become "the most significant postural influence on respiration [, one that] contributes most to the deleterious effects of posture."[9]

It is well documented that in the conscious subject any variation from the sitting position will produce decreases in vital capacity. These decreases are brought about by a variety of causes, but all surgical positions mechanically restrict air flow into the lungs.

Little[1] described four effects of posture on respiration: (1) changes in pulmonary blood flow, (2) changes in lung compliance, (3) changes in intrapulmonary distribution of inspired air, and (4) most important, limitation of expansion of the lungs from simple mechanical interference with normal movements.

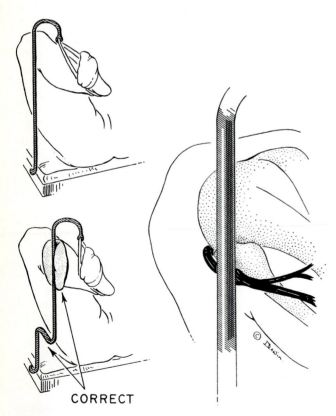

CORRECT

Figure 13–6. Common peroneal nerve compression between lithotomy stirrup and neck of fibula. This may be avoided by padding (see inset). (*Courtesy Department of Art as Applied to Medicine, Faculty of Medicine, University of Toronto.*)

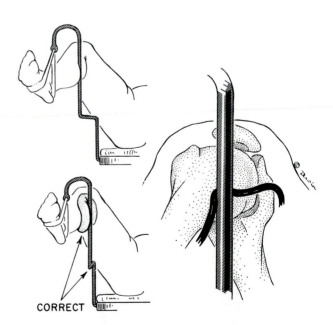

CORRECT

Figure 13–7. Saphenous nerve compressed between lithotomy stirrup and tibia. (*Courtesy Department of Art as Applied to Medicine, Faculty of Medicine, University of Toronto.*)

In his studies, Little compared the decrease in vital capacity from the sitting position with that in all of the common surgical positions. It is to be noted that all positions did restrict diaphragmatic movement and all positions, with the exception of supine and reverse Trendelenburg, restricted movements in the lateral as well as anterior–posterior expansion of the chest.

The following respiratory effects of surgical postures are all extracted from Little's chart.[1] These figures show the decrease in vital capacity from the sitting position to common surgical positions in the normal, awake subject. These figures may be decreased further in the anesthetized patient.

Supine	9.5%
Reverse Trendelenburg	9.0%
Prone	10.0%
Lateral	10.0%
Jacknife	12.5%
Gallbladder	13.5%
Kidney	14.5%
Trendelenburg	14.5%
Lithotomy	18.0%

Because gravity influences the blood flow as well as the gas volume in the lungs, it is well to think of the lungs as two distinct areas functionally. There will always be a lower, or dependent, portion and an upper, or independent portion.

In the lateral position, because of the weight of the viscera and increased hydrostatic pressure, the down or dependent side will afford the diaphragm on that side a markedly increased excursion. Radiologic evidence indicates that ventilation is always greater in the dependent portion of the lungs no matter what the surgical posture is.[10]

With spontaneous breathing, both ventilation and perfusion are increased when the patient is in the lateral position. If the patient is paralyzed and artificially ventilated, the upper or independent lung now becomes preferentially ventilated; its compliance is greater because of less pressure from abdominal contents and partly because of less perfusion.[4] Anesthesia has a marked effect on pulmonary compliance by decreasing it.

Men have a greater compliance than women in the awake state but also have a greater reduction in compliance in the anesthetized state. Men also have a greater incidence of postoperative pulmonary complications.

One should be constantly reminded that the most deadly and persistent enemy of the anesthetist is hypoxia. The clinical manifestations of hypoxia and hypercarbia are not always immediately recognized because of "masking" of signs and symptoms by the anesthetic drugs. Be assured that hypoventilation will eventually take its toll and will produce problems over a period of time. Any decrease in tidal volume should be avoided by assisted or controlled breathing.

Obesity

Obesity constitutes one of the gravest hazards in anesthesia today. Excess weight markedly restricts the diaphragm, with a reduction of tidal exchange and functional residual capacity.[11] "Extreme obesity, therefore, exaggerates all of the deleterious effects of surgical posture and accelerates the clinical manifestations of respiratory insufficiency."[9]

A study by Jenkins[10] of 1000 obese surgical patients disclosed a precipitous drop in vital capacity, expiratory reserve volume, and maximum inspiratory and expiratory reserves in the postoperative period. It took these obese patients 5 days to return even to sublevels of their preoperative values.

Judicious use of endotracheal tubes with assisted positive pressure is recommended for the postoperative period if obesity presents a ventilation problem. One patient in Jenkins' series was improved significantly by sitting up, which removed the weight that was restricting movement of the diaphragm.

Along with assisted or controlled respiration, it is recommended that arterial blood gases be monitored postoperatively as well as during surgery.

Intragastric Pressure

A potential complication associated with posture changes under anesthesia is the change in intragastric pressure.

If the patient is in a steep foot-down position during induction there is a lowering of intragastric pressure, helping to prevent regurgitation. If, however, gastric contents enter the oropharynx, the chance of aspiration is enhanced. Use of a steep head-down position causes an increase in intragastric pressure, which encourages the flow of gastric contents into the oropharynx but makes aspiration into the trachea improbable. To some degree the supine horizontal position combines the disadvantages of the two positions described. The writer recommends a head-up position with cricoid pressure until the patient is intubated with a cuffed tube.

Muscular System

General anesthesia with the use of muscle relaxants produces complete muscle relaxation, as does spinal anesthesia. This profound muscle relaxation causes the legs to lie flat on the operating table and unduly stretches ligaments and muscles of the lower spine. This stretch is responsible for most cases of backache in the postoperative period. Soft padding should be placed under the legs and back to prevent this discomfort.

Use of the lithotomy position has been shown to cause backache in 37 percent of patients, whereas the lateral position caused backache in only 12 percent when compared with reported incidence of backache following surgery performed in the supine position.

The other important factor affecting the likelihood of backache was the duration of surgery. In cases lasting 1 to 60 minutes, 18 percent of the patients developed postoperative backache, whereas in those procedures lasting 181 to 240 minutes, 34 percent developed backache.

SUPINE

Supine is perhaps the position given least thought in anesthesia and surgery. The patient is moved onto the flat, minimally padded, cold operating table, adjusted so that she feels like she is in the middle of the table, and extensions placed to support heels and occiput as necessary. As she lies flat on the table, the patient's weight is distributed to occiput, shoulder, spine, hips, and heels, which are bone prominences. The skin on these areas receives minimal protection and maximum pressure, ideal conditions for rapid development of ischemia. In the harsh environment of the operating theater this ischemia can be more pronounced and occurs even more rapidly than otherwise.

Martin advocates a "lawn chair" position that is more physiologic than the anatomic supine (Fig. 13–8).[12] It incorporates hip and knee flexion, with slight head elevation on a small pillow. This position not only redistributes the weight, but also brings the hips and knee joints into a more neutral position, thereby decreasing pull or tension on muscles and nerves. This position will alleviate some of the postoperative complaints of leg and back muscle pain often voiced by patients. If the procedure is long or drapes unduly heavy, the feet require support to prevent foot drop.

The leg strap should be applied across midthigh on top of a smooth sheet and around the table for maximum patient protection and safety. The arm, when positioned by

the side, must fit on the mattress and not hang off. Touching the metal table causes pressure on the ulnar nerve at the elbow, and it is a possible site for unintentional cautery grounding. The arms, when positioned at the side, should not be tucked under the buttocks but should be placed under the lift sheet. This sheet should extend above the elbow to midupper arm for support and be tucked under the mattress. Anything placed beneath the patient should be smooth and wrinkle-free because wrinkles or any distortion will increase pressure areas (Fig. 13–9).

The arm when placed on an arm board must be in a neutral position to protect neural and vascular structures, as discussed earlier. During prolonged mask cases, damage can occur to the optic nerve from direct mask pressure or mask strap tension. The facial nerve as it passes around the mandibular rami is at risk from a tight mask strap or the hand supporting the upper airway and mask (Fig. 13–10).

PRONE

The prone position is most awkward for patients of all ages and sizes. Irrespective of size, the patient's abdominal wall must not touch or dig into the mattress. Support on two "shoulder rolls" that extend from the shoulder to the iliac crest frees not only the abdominal wall but the anterior thoracic wall as well. This markedly improves circulation and respiration. There are numerous variations of this position: Georgia position, Smith's modification of the Georgia position, Overholt position, and Sellor-Brown position, to mention a few. In addition, several tables that carry the inventor's name for the prone position have been developed. All of these modifications provide for free space between table and mattress and anterior abdominal wall to prevent resis-

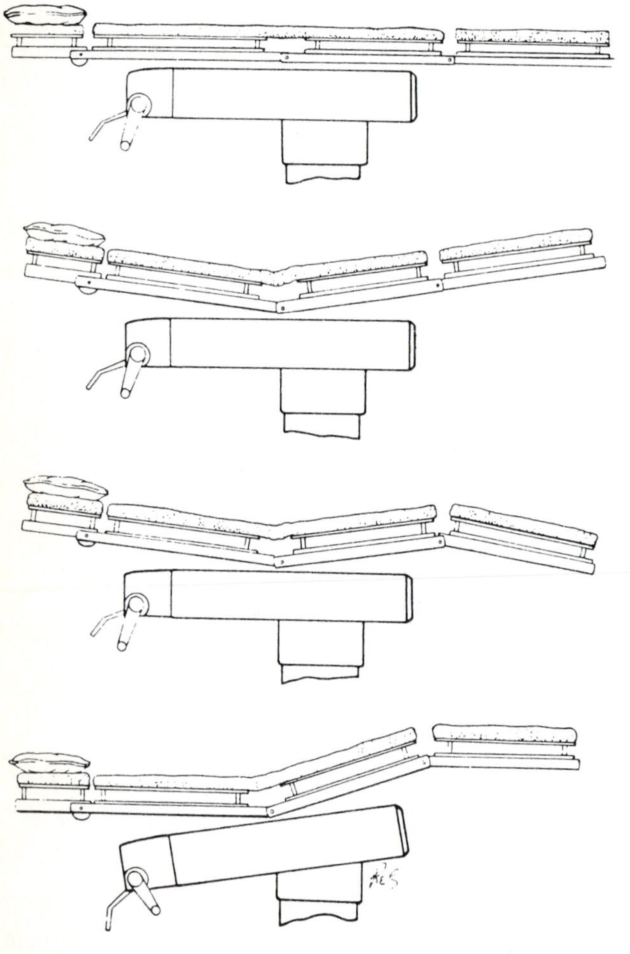

Figure 13–8. Supine position: Establishing the "lawn chair" position with hip and knee flexion and a pillow for the head. (*Reprinted, with permission, from Martin.*[12])

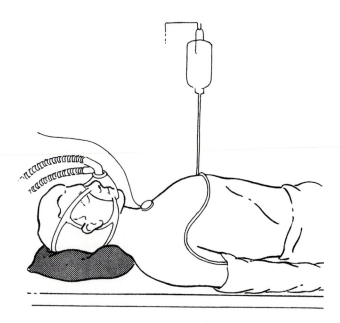

Figure 13–9. Supine position: head on small pillow, arm by side, well on mattress, with lift sheet extending above the elbow to provide support. (*Courtesy Department of Art as Applied to Medicine, Faculty of Medicine, University of Toronto.*)

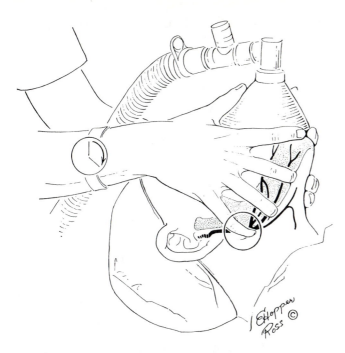

Figure 13–10. Motor root of facial nerve injured by traction on the angle of the mandible. (*Courtesy Department of Art as Applied to Medicine, Faculty of Medicine, University of Toronto.*)

tance to respiration, compression of vena cava and lymphatic system, and stability so that the patient does not give or slip during surgical procedures. The male genitalia must also be protected by ensuring that the patient is not lying on them, that they are not caught between patient and table, and that the electrosurgical ground pad is well away from the area. The female breasts can pose problems, especially large pendulous breasts and the high, firm breasts of the young. Large breasts, because of their elasticity, can be swept away from the midline so that the shoulder-to-hip roll can be placed between them. The arms of the patient must then be placed above her head. The arms must be rotated through the natural arch when positioning them overhead. The upper arm biceps–triceps area must be supported to the same elevation as the thorax to prevent pull and stretch on brachial plexus. If arms must be by the side, often the breasts are swept inward and the shoulder rolls placed distal to them. In this way the arms can easily be accommodated at the side. The buxom nullipara often presents more of a challenge as these breasts are firm and immobile, offering little or no opportunity for movement. Though some of the mass may be shifted, it is often impossible to reduce the pressure on them significantly.

Obviously the dorsum of the foot is at grave risk and must be supported and protected by rolls or pillows or both. Injury to the eyes, ears, and nose can easily occur from protracted pressure from the weight of the head against the table or mattress. The possibility of spinal cord and bony spine injury during the act of turning the patient exists because of the lack of muscular support. Consequently the head, neck, shoulders, hip, and thigh must be kept in alignment and the patient turned as a unit, logrolling. A mini-

mum of three people are required to turn patients from the supine position: one to turn the head and neck, coordinate the team, and maintain the airway, one to turn shoulders and thorax, and one to turn the hips and legs (Fig. 13–11). Many methods are used to achieve the prone position; two are more desirable than the others. The first one is to anesthetize the patient on the stretcher and then logroll him or her onto the operating room table. The advantage is that shoulder rolls, head support, foot rolls, and arm board can be prepositioned, and the patient can be rolled into the arms of the team, lifted, and placed on the supports. Naturally some adjustments will be required. In those instances when the patient must be anesthetized on the operating room table, the second method is used. Again with the turning team of three, after the patient is anesthetized, he or she is turned to lateral and then to prone. Supports are placed one at a time—shoulder roll, head support, arm boards, foot rolls, and so on. Final adjustments are made when all supports have been placed. This ensures that the extremities are in alignment and position of function, with no pressure areas, capillary refill is good, and distal pulse is present and easily palpable. A check is made to ensure that the eyes are closed, ears are flat, anterior abdominal and thoracic walls are free, and no instruments, tubes, or other objects are under the patient to cause pressure. The catheter drainage tubing, if a Foley is in place, can be run down between the legs and off the caudal end of the table or passed under the muscular anterior thigh and over the side of the table.

Because many anesthetic agents cause depression of the cardiovascular system, including diminished pressure response, the likelihood of acute protracted hypotension exists whenever an anesthetized patient's position is altered.

LITHOTOMY

Since ancient times the lithotomy position has been used by both obstetrician and urologist; it is only within the last century that this position has been used by gynecologists. To prevent injury it is imperative that the equipment fit the patient. Both legs must be flexed and extended simultaneously to prevent joint and spinal injury, including hip disarticulation (Fig. 13–12). Whichever type of stirrups is chosen, the right and left devices must be a pair. The leg support with an adjustable foot plate is preferable because it evenly distributes the weight; however, it is time consuming to adjust the angles of both the hip and knee joint and shorten or lengthen the foot plate. Consequently this stirrup is often abandoned in favor of the ankle strap or, more unfortunately, the leg support is misused. With the ankle strap, the upright rods are at right angles to the table and the leg is flexed inside the uprights. When more exposure is necessary the legs are placed outside the uprights which is one of the modified positions for radical peroneal surgery. When the ankle straps are used, the legs must not rest against the upright. The common peroneal nerve, running lateral and very superficial to the fibular head, is at risk from pressure of the upright support (Fig. 13–6). The superficial peroneal nerve, as the name implies, runs between the subcutaneous fat and muscles of the lateral calf. The surgical assistant will often push the calf against the rod to obtain a keener view

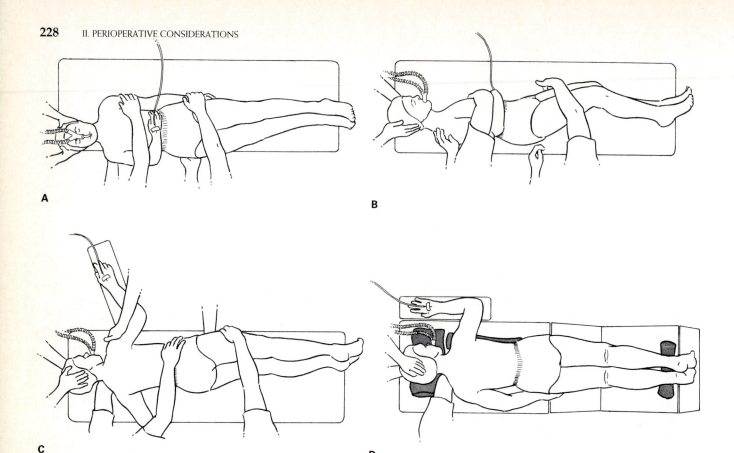

A

B

C

D

Figure 13–11. A, B, C. Three people—one for head and coordinator, one for shoulder thorax, and one for hips and legs—turn patient as a unit. **D.** Placement of supports. (*Reprinted, with permission, from Martin.*[12])

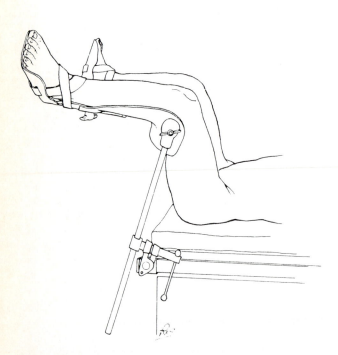

Figure 13–12. Lithotomy position. Note placement of legs into stirrups and buttocks on table. (*Reprinted, with permission, from Martin.*[12])

of the surgical field, compressing the superficial peroneal nerve between the tibia and upright. With the legs on the outside of the upright, undue stretch is often placed on the muscle, tendons, and joints by the surgical assistants who crowd in for a better view of the operative field. The saphenous nerve is at risk from assistants who stand outside and lean against the leg in an effort to obtain a better view of the surgical field from "above."

The obturator, saphenous, and femoral nerves are all at risk when the leg support stirrup is used because of the compression of the legs in the supports and accompanying straps. It goes without saying that venous pooling is a problem with this position, its severity depending on patient condition, anesthetic management, position, and length of time requiring this surgical position. When the legs are returned to the supine position they should be lowered simultaneously and slowly in stages, to prevent hypotension secondary to filling of the dilated peripheral vascular bed.

The arms may be positioned in several ways: both on arm boards, one on an arm board and one on the chest, or both on the chest; however, the precautions discussed regarding the supine position must be adhered to if either or both arms are extended on arm boards. When positioning the arm or arms on the chest, care must be taken that the elbow does not rest on the table. This causes pressure on the ulnar nerve and is an unintentional cautery ground site.

The arm should not be acutely flexed across the chest. An angle of more than 100 degrees at the elbow can compromise the arterial supply to the lower arm and hand. Placement of the arm by the side is not recommended because the fingers can extend beyond the table break, becoming entrapped between the two table sections and, as the lower piece is raised after completion of the surgical procedure, resulting in damage to or even amputation of one or more fingers.

LATERAL

This position bears a number of labels, depending on the purpose for which it is used: thoracotomy, kidney, lateral, and decubitus. The position has been used by thoracic surgeons for a multitude of surgical procedures. The flexed lateral is used most frequently by urologists and nephrologists for access to the kidney via various types of incisions.

Essentially, the patient is turned 90 degrees to the horizontal surface of the table and stabilized. Flexion or extension of the extremities modifies this perpendicular position. Flexion of the lower leg causes the patient to roll backward to achieve a greater-than-90-degree angle, useful for the anterior thoracic incision. The upper arm then must be supported in an elevated position on an accessory or double-deck arm board or on a Mayo stand, or hung from the ether screen (Fig. 13–13). The precautions that must be observed are the same as those previously discussed. The upper arm must be positioned to protect its arterial and nerve supply and must be in good body alignment; the nail beds should be checked for capillary refill; the radial pulse should be readily palpable before securing the patient. Care must be taken when using either an accessory arm board or Mayo stand that the edge does not press into the tissue, causing pressure on the brachial artery or median or ulnar nerves. A tunnel must be created for the lower arm to prevent compression of the dependent brachial artery and overstretching of the brachial plexus. A small rolled towel, a covered sandbag, or a covered intravenous (IV) fluid bag placed under the upper chest, not in the axilla, all work nicely.

Flexion of the upper leg causes the patient to roll forward to achieve a less-than-90-degree angle. The upper arm can be supported on a small pillow in either an extended or a flexed position. Again, the radial pulse should be checked along with capillary refill before securing the patient.

The flexed position used for approaches to the kidney is a modification of any of the three above-mentioned positions. The "kidney rest," or break in the table between upper and lower sections, must be at the level of the iliac crest (Fig. 13–14). The table sections are lower, causing the muscle to be stretched. The table can be placed in reverse Trendelenburg, making the operative sets parallel to the floor. The lower leg is usually slightly flexed, the upper remaining extended. The legs must not overhang or touch the metal table and must be separated by a pillow. This removes the weight of the upper leg and promotes venous drainage. The upper arm is extended on a support (double arm board, Mayo, etc.). The head and neck are supported on folded sheets or pillows in line with the thoracic spine (Fig. 13–15).

Broad straps or strips of nonelastic adhesive tape, placed across the hips just below the iliac crest and across the shoulder, are secured to the undersides of the table to ensure stability.

Again, as in prone positioning, the patient must be turned as a whole or unit, ensuring that body alignment is maintained at all times. A minimum of three people are required: one, a coordinator, to turn the head and maintain the airway; one, to turn shoulders and thorax; and one to turn the hips and legs. It is highly desirable to have additional personnel to place the required folded sheets and pillows and support patients while straps are being secured.

OTHER POSITIONS

The sitting or "park bench" position is used for posterior fossa craniotomies and some posterior cervical surgical procedures. The use of the skeletal positioning device has improved the stability and decreased complications of this position.[13] The older horseshoe face masks and opposing pads offered little stability, and ocular damage resulted from intraoperative movement. Skull-pin head-holder assemblies are available from a number of surgical instrument manufacturers (Fig. 13–16). All contain the same essentials, including a bar or rod for table attachment, a connecting rod from the upright to the head-holding unit,

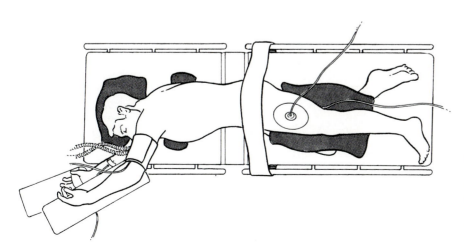

Figure 13–13. Lateral position. Note placement of support, flexion of lower leg, extension of upper leg, separation by pillow, placement of IV catheter, grounding pad, blood pressure cuff, and strap across iliac crest. (*Reprinted, with permission, from Martin.*[12])

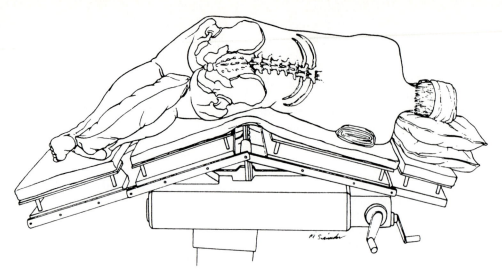

Figure 13–14. Kidney position. Note support of head, neck, and upper thorax, separation of legs by pillow and elevation of foot of upper leg, position of dependent flexed leg with foot on mattress, and position of nonelastic adhesive tape across iliac crest and under table to provide stable positioning. (*Reprinted, with permission, from Martin.*[12])

the head-holding units, and three pins. The head-holding unit is a C-shaped clamp with two pins on one arm of the C and one pin on the opposite side. When placed, however, *no* two pins should be opposite each other; rather, the two closer pins should be equidistant from a point directly opposite the third pin in the same plane. These pins should pierce the outer table of the skull for maximum stability.

Naturally, for individuals with thin skulls, hydrocephalic infants, and others, the possibility of penetrating both tables of the skull contraindicates use of this device. It is also useful for positioning patients for surgical procedures requiring access to more than a single surgical plane, for example, frontal and temporal, both temporal areas, when prone position with marked neck flexion is necessary.

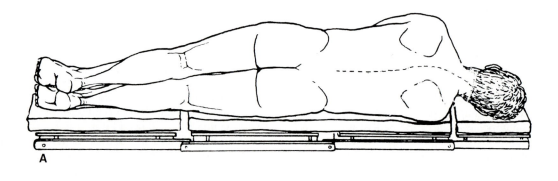

A

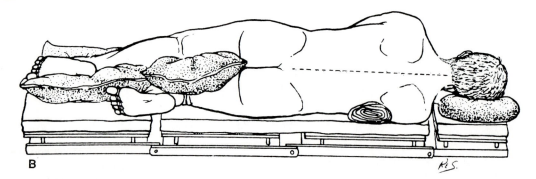

B

Figure 13–15. Spinal alignment in the lateral position. **A.** Note lack of support for head, upper thorax, and poor spinal alignment. **B.** Proper support of head and upper thorax. (*Reprinted, with permission, from Martin.*[12])

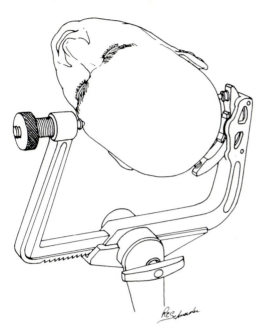

Figure 13–16. Head holder. Typical of the variety commercially available. Note pin placement. Two pins equidistant from midpoint of opposing third pin also piercing the outer but not the inner table of skull. (*Reprinted, with permission, from Martin.*[12])

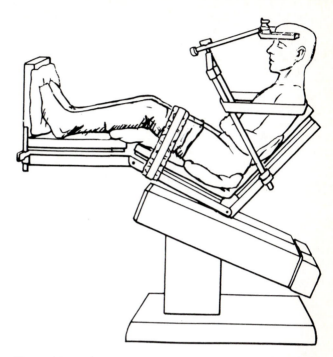

Figure 13–17. Park bench position. Head in skeletal holder, legs flexed and at heart level, with support hose to thigh level. Access to anterior thoracic wall. (*Adapted, with permission, from GE Morgan, MS Mikhail. Clinical Anesthesiology. Norwalk, CT: Appleton & Lange, 1992.*)

When the sitting position is used, the legs should be wrapped in woven elastic bandages or elastic stockings applied as far as the groin. Some institutions use "antigravity" units or military antishock trousers (MAST) to improve venous return. The legs are flexed at both hips and knees, with the lower legs and feet at the level of the heart (Fig. 13–17). The arms are crossed in the patient's lap. This provides access to peripheral lines, both arterial and venous. Care should be taken to see that the elbows are not touching the metal table. Access to the anterior thoracic wall is also provided, allowing access to the heart should percutaneous removal of air from the right ventricle become necessary. Because the head is securely supported by the skull pins and assembly, it can be flexed to accommodate surgical requirements.

The use of various "frames," "traction," or "fracture" tables to provide access to the operative sites pose potential problems and complications too numerous for the scope of this chapter; however, the basic principles of positioning apply, irrespective of the specific device required: stability; protection of bony prominences, superficial nerves, extremities including ears and nose, and external male genitalia; and maintenance of homeostasis.

SUMMARY

All surgical postures have been shown to be potentially harmful because they interfere with circulation, respiration, and the musculoskeletal system and may cause injury to peripheral nerves.

Postural interference with the circulatory system during anesthesia includes vasodilation, peripheral pooling of blood, obstruction to blood flow, and obtundation of compensatory cardiovascular reflexes. These deleterious effects are increased by an increase in depth of anesthesia.

The effects of posture on respiration include changes in lung compliance, vital capacity, blood flow, and distribution of inspired air, as well as mechanical interference with movements of the diaphragm. These changes lead to respiratory fatigue, hypercapnea, and hypoxia secondary to hypoventilation.

The harmful effects of posture on the skeletal system, muscular system, and peripheral nerves are due to compression and stretch while the patient is relaxed and pain free. All of these potentially harmful effects can be avoided or lessened by the judicious (1) use of soft pads to prevent compression of peripheral nerves, (2) use of assisted or controlled breathing to ensure adequate ventilation, (3) avoidance of deep anesthesia prior to postural changes to prevent cardiovascular collapse, and (4) modification of extreme positions whenever possible to prevent stretch of muscles, ligaments, and nerves.

REFERENCES

1. Little DM. Posture and anesthesia. *Can Anesth Soc J.* 1960;7:2–15.
2. Smith RH, Grambling ZW, et al. Problems related to the prone position for surgical operations. *Anesthesiology.* 1961;22:189.
3. Biddle C, Caunady M. Surgical positions, their effect on cardiovascular, respiratory systems. *AORN J.* 1990;52(2):350–359.

4. Wylie WD, Churchill-Davidson HC. *A practice of anesthesia.* 5th ed. Chicago: Year Book Medical; 1984.

5. Britt BA, Gordon RA. Peripheral nerve injuries associated with anesthesia. *Can Anaesth Soc J.* 1964;11:514.

6. Proposed recommended practices. Positioning the surgical patient. *AORN J.* 1990;51(1):216–218, 220–224.

7. Wadsworth TG. The cubital tunnel and the external compression syndrome. *Anesth Analg.* 1974;53:303.

8. Schindler H. *Operating room techniques: Patient positioning.* New York: Thieme Medical; 1988.

9. Courington FW, Little DM Jr. The role of posture in anesthesia. *Clin Anesth.* 1968;3:24.

10. Jenkins LC. The interaction of drugs with particular reference for anesthetic practice. *Can Anaesth Soc J.* 1968;15:111–117.

11. Castenacchi AJ, Anderson JD, Boersma D. Anesthetic hazards of obesity. *JAMA.* 1961;175:657.

12. Martin JT. *Positioning in anesthesia and surgery.* 2nd ed. Philadelphia: WB Saunders; 1987.

13. Miller RA. Neurosurgical anesthesia in the sitting position. *Br J Anaesth.* 1972;44:495.

Preoperative Medications and Techniques of Induction and Maintenance

Ceil E. Vercellino

The rationale for anesthetic premedication is to achieve certain specific and desirable objectives prior to the induction of anesthesia. There are no specific premedication regimens; rather, the choice of premedication techniques is often based on the practitioner's experience and institutional traditions. As there is no defined standard regarding the exact premedications to be administered, the anesthesia practitioner must consider the goals of premedicant therapy for each individual patient.

The goals of anesthetic premedicant therapy include anxiolysis, analgesia, control of sympathetic response to induction and intubation, reduction in the maintenance doses of anesthesia, antiemesis, and vagolysis (Table 14–1). The goals of premedicant therapy also include maintenance of therapeutic regimens to provide an optimal preanesthetic condition, such as optimization of antiepileptic and bronchodilator therapies, elevation of gastric pH and an increase in gastrointestinal motility in the event of obesity or an incompetent esophageal sphincter, control of hemodynamic instability, and the use of premedication as adjunctive agents to regional anesthesia.

PREOPERATIVE EVALUATION

A variety of medications can be used to achieve any one or a combination of these objectives, but before the anesthesia practitioner can decide what goals will best satisfy the patient's needs, a thorough preanesthetic interview and evaluation must be conducted. The evaluation serves to identify individual patient requirements and specific factors to be considered when determining the type of premedication necessary. The patient variables to be taken into account when administering premedications include age, physical status, preexisting medical and surgical conditions, preoperative level of anxiety, allergies, inpatient versus outpatient status, type of surgery to be performed, elective versus emergent procedures, coexisting pain and debilitations,

potential drug interactions with the patient's current medical therapy, and potential routes of administration of the premedication.

In the evaluation of the need for and quantity of premedication necessary to provide anxiolysis, the preanesthetic interview and visit also permit the development of a relationship between the anesthetic provider and the patient in order to establish trust, to communicate individual idiosyncracies, and to retrieve a past medical and anesthetic history, all of which function to allay anxiety in the presurgical patient. The well-known study by Egbert et al[1] demonstrated that a preoperative visit by the anesthesia provider was more effective than a barbiturate in decreasing preoperative anxiety. A clinical report by Lichtor et al[2] demonstrated that patient anxiety in the preoperative waiting area correlated significantly to the level of anxiety identified the afternoon before surgery.

The preoperative evaluation of the patient's preexisting anxiety level can then be used as a guide for predetermining the degree of expected immediate presurgical anxiety, and an appropriate premedication can be administered. One may conclude that patients experience less anxiety when given complete and detailed explanations of what to expect from their anesthetic experience. It is for these reasons that the preanesthetic interview itself is a highly valued premedication for the relief of anxiety.

PREMEDICANT DRUGS

Anxiolysis can be achieved pharmacologically through the administration of sedative hypnotics such as benzodiazepines, phenothiazines, butyrophenones, diphenhydramine, and barbiturates. The benzodiazepine agents are the most frequently employed premedications. The most commonly used benzodiazepines are midazolam (Versed), diazepam (Valium), and lorazepam (Ativan).

Benzodiazepines

Benzodiazepines produce sedation, anxiolysis and amnesia (Table 14–2). Benzodiazepines also produce muscle relax-

233

TABLE 14-1. GOALS OF PREMEDICANT THERAPY

Anxiolysis

Analgesia

Sedation

Vagolysis

Sympatholysis

Antiemesis

Elevation of gastric pH

Antisialogogy

ation and anticonvulsant activity. The mechanisms of action by which these effects are mediated are receptor-specific facilitation of the inhibitory actions of γ-aminobutyric acid (GABA) and mimicking of the inhibitory actions of glycine in the central nervous system. It is possible, however, in certain patient populations, such as in the elderly and parturient groups, that agitation, restlessness, and delirium can potentially result from a reaction to benzodiazepines. This reaction is unpredictable and can be recognized only after the drug has been given.

Benzodiazepines are indicated in patients experiencing alcohol withdrawal syndrome for the treatment and prevention of delirium tremens. They should be included as part of the premedication routine in any patient with a history of alcohol abuse to prevent the onset of withdrawal throughout any portion of the perioperative period.[3]

Benzodiazepines are often combined with narcotics to provide amnesia and sedation, as narcotics are primarily analgesics and lack specific amnestic and hypnotic properties. The additive side effects of these two categories of agents may be synergistic, as in an augmentation of narcotic-produced respiratory depression, cardiovascular depression, and sedation.[4] When used in combination these agents may be highly effective in producing a calm, pain-free patient. Careful consideration should be given to the dosages employed. The dose of each agent should be modified from that which would be given if administered individually. Often it is prudent to administer the narcotic as an intramuscular injection 1 hour prior to the surgical time, and then administer the benzodiazepine intravenously in a titrated fashion in the preoperative holding area.

Benzodiazepines are considered to be of benefit in the reduction of the dysphoric reactions associated with ketamine administration. Patients have reported hallucinations, dysphoria, and disturbing dreams after the administration of ketamine anesthesia.[5] These responses correlate with age (the elderly), sex (females greater than males), prior psycho-

logic history, and use of other premedications, such as the combination of droperidol and ketamine which seems to worsen the dysphoria. It has been noted that use of any of the benzodiazepines reduces the likelihood and severity of these side effects, although it does not guarantee protection against their occurrence.[6]

Midazolam. Midazolam is a water-soluble benzodiazepine that is supplied in either 1 or 5 mg/mL preparations. As midazolam is water soluble, it has an extremely low incidence of venous irritation and therefore a high acceptance from patients for both intramuscular and intravenous administration because of the lack of pain on injection. It is a rapid-acting agent, with onset times between 60 and 90 seconds when given intravenously and approximately 15 minutes when given intramuscularly. The duration of action is 6 to 15 minutes intravenously and 60 to 90 minutes intramuscularly.[7]

The pharmacokinetics of midazolam make it an excellent choice for outpatients, as the alpha half-life is short and the elimination half-life is approximately 2 hours. It can be given intramuscularly at doses in the range 0.07 to 0.1 mg/kg, 1 hour prior to surgery,[8] and additional doses of the drug can be titrated intravenously in the preoperative holding area to achieve a somnolent and calm but arousable patient. When titrating midazolam intravenously, it is recommended to start with 0.5 to 1 mg IV, followed every 2 to 5 minutes with additional doses up to 0.03 to 0.1 mg/kg, until the desired level of sedation is achieved.[9] The optimal level of sedation is reached in a patient who appears calm and relaxed yet is still cooperative.

Recently, midazolam has become increasingly used for premedication in pediatric patients. Intramuscular injections for pediatric patients are restricted to only the most necessary cases, to reduce the traumatic and painful experience of an injection. The benefit of midazolam is its potential for oral administration. Midazolam is diluted to a dose of 0.5 to 0.7 mg/kg (taken from the intravenous dose vial as this is the only preparation of midazolam presently available in the United States) in 3 to 10 mL of clear liquid solution such as apple or grape juice.[10,11] To ameliorate the slightly bitter taste, a sugar substitute may be added to the preparation. Because the child has been NPO (nothing by mouth) for several hours prior to arrival in the preoperative holding area, he or she generally welcomes "a little something to drink." The presence of the child's parents in the preoperative holding area and the administration of fluid perceived by the patient as a feeding may lessen his or her anxiety. Routinely, 10 to 20 minutes is required to achieve sedation in this manner. It is also recommended that this be done in the presence of anesthesia personnel who are quickly able to manage a sedated child properly; this technique is not recommended for use with an unattended child on the hospital ward. The duration of action of midazolam given orally is approximately 50 to 60 minutes.

Diazepam. Diazepam has largely been replaced by midazolam as a premedicant in anesthesia. There are several reasons for this change, the most clinically significant of which is that propylene glycol is the vehicle used to make diazepam solution for injection, and this substance produces significant pain and venous irritation on injection. To

TABLE 14-2. BENZODIAZEPINES AND COMMON PREMEDICANT DOSES

Drug	Average Dose
Midazolam (Versed)	0.07–0.1 mg/kg IM
	0.03–0.1 mg/kg IV
	0.50–0.7 mg/kg PO
Diazepam (Valium)	5–10 mg PO
	0.05–0.15 mg/kg IV
Lorazepam (Ativan)	1–4 mg PO or IV

avoid this irritation, it may be useful to inject 1 to 2 mL of 1 percent xylocaine intravenously prior to injection of diazepam. Diazepam also has a significantly longer half-life than midazolam, and some reports indicate an elimination half-life as long as 32.9 ± 8.8 hours.[12] This makes it less desirable for a quick emergence from anesthesia, especially in the outpatient population.

Diazepam still has a place in the premedication arena. It is especially useful when given as an oral medication, generally 5 to 10 mg, 1 hour prior to surgery with a sip of water. It is an excellent anxiolytic administered orally on the morning of surgery for an afternoon operation. In this way the patient remains calm and relaxed until the additional premedications are given, especially if that is to be done in the preoperative holding area. Diazepam can be given intravenously in the preoperative holding area in doses of approximately 0.05 to 0.15 mg/kg. This dose should be titrated at 1.25- to 2.5-mg intervals at least 3 minutes apart.[13] Caution should be exercised in patients concomitantly receiving cimetidine, as diazepam clearance has been shown to be delayed in patients receiving cimetidine therapy.[14]

Lorazepam. Lorazepam is a long-acting benzodiazepine, with a mean half-life of 14 to 15 hours. It is an excellent amnestic agent and is four times as potent as diazepam, with a longer onset time and duration of action.[15] It can be given parenterally but is generally administered orally the night before surgery for inpatients in doses of 1 to 4 mg. The beneficial effects of anxiolysis and amnesia should still be present well into the next surgical day. Because of lorazepam's long duration of action, it is probably not an appropriate choice for outpatient anesthesia.

Phenothiazines

The phenothiazines are antipsychotics and major tranquilizers. The phenothiazines most often used as premedications are promethazine (Phenergan) and chlorpromazine (Thorazine). These medications are useful for their sedative, antihistaminic, anticholinergic, and antiemetic effects. Chlorpromazine is rarely used as an anesthetic premedication; however, promethazine is still employed in combination with a narcotic to enhance sedation and prevent nausea. Generally it is given as a 12.5- to 25-mg intramuscular injection with the narcotic.[16] It is associated with prolonged recovery from anesthesia[17] and is therefore given to patients who require somnolent premedication or who are expected to have a lengthy operation, such as patients for cardiac surgery, aortic aneurysm repair, or major oncologic resections.

The phenothiazines may cause hypotension as a result of central depression of the vasoactive centers, direct vasodilation, and peripheral adrenergic blockade. They may also exacerbate extrapyramidal symptoms and therefore should be used judiciously, especially in patients receiving antiparkinsonism medications.

Butyrophenones; Droperidol

Droperidol (Inapsine) is the most widely used agent in this category, employed primarily for its antiemetic properties.

It also produces a state in which the patient appears somnolent, indifferent to the surroundings, and has reduced motor activity. In doses ranging from 0.25 to 1.25 mg IV, it provides additional ataraxia as well as prevention and treatment of postoperative nausea and vomiting. Droperidol also is an alpha-adrenergic antagonist, usually in doses of 2.5 mg and higher, and therefore may cause hypotension. When droperidol is administered as a sole premedicant, the incidence of dysphoria is high. It is recommended that it be given in combination with benzodiazepines. Patients have been known to refuse surgery after receiving droperidol.[18] Droperidol can cause extrapyramidal reactions in a small percentage of patients because of its dopaminergic antagonism.[19] This can be treated effectively with diphenhydramine.

Droperidol, when used in combination with fentanyl, is known as Innovar and is used to produce a neuroleptic anesthetic. In this case, each milliliter of Innovar contains 2.5 mg of droperidol and 50 µg of fentanyl. A dose of 2 to 4 mL of this mixture in a young, healthy adult is an effective premedication for use in semiawake intubations, minor surgical procedures such as bronchoscopy or endoscopy, and dressing changes for burn patients.

Antihistamines

Hydroxyzine. Hydroxyzine (Vistaril) is an antihistamine that is not related to the phenothiazines. It is most commonly used to enhance the analgesic properties of narcotics. It has minor physiologic effects including bronchodilation, antisialagogy, antiemesis, antiarrhythmic properties, and ataraxis, adding to the premedication. It is normally administered intramuscularly in doses ranging from 50 to 150 mg. Hydroxyzine has not been demonstrated to prolong the recovery from anesthesia.[20]

Diphenhydramine. Diphenhydramine (Benadryl) is an antihistamine that can serve several purposes. It produces sedation and drowsiness without respiratory or cardiac depression. This makes it useful for debilitated or geriatric patients. It can also be given to ameliorate pruritus or allergic reactions in a patient who is known to be sensitive to certain drugs.[21] Diphenhydramine may be given orally or parenterally, in 25- to 50-mg doses to produce sedation, 30 to 60 minutes prior to induction of anesthesia. Diphenhydramine can also be used as a sleep medication the night before surgery at the same doses.

Barbiturates

Barbiturates have largely been replaced by newer agents that have much shorter half-lives and therefore are less likely to interfere with the intraoperative anesthetic and recovery from anesthesia. They are employed for their sedative-hypnotic properties and do not cause cardiac or respiratory depression in normal premedication doses. Barbiturates should not be used in patients with a history of porphyria. The most frequently administered barbiturate premedications are secobarbital (Seconal) and pentobarbital (Nembutal).

Secobarbital is given in doses ranging from 50 to 200 mg intramuscularly for adult patients. Its sedative effects can last 4 hours or longer. Neurologic impairment secondary to the administration of barbiturates has been reported to persist 10 to 22 hours.[22] Pentobarbital is usually administered in doses of 50 to 150 mg orally, and it can also be given parenterally. Its biotransformation half-life is about 50 hours,[23] and this makes it undesirable for short procedures and outpatient anesthesia.

Analgesics

Analgesics are administered to relieve pain prior to the induction of anesthesia. They are most useful in patients already experiencing discomfort from a preexisting condition. Narcotics are the most frequently used analgesics for a variety of reasons, mainly because they offer superior pain relief. Narcotic premedications can be used to establish a baseline level of narcosis prior to induction when a nitrous oxide–narcotic general anesthetic technique is planned. They decrease sympathetic response to intubation and induction.[24] Opioids also decrease the minimum alveolar concentration of inhalational agents and therefore less inhalational agent is required to produce sufficient anesthesia to blunt the physiologic effect of surgical stimulation.[25,26] Preoperative administration of intramuscular narcotics may provide pain relief postoperatively in relatively short surgical cases, and may reduce postoperative narcotic analgesic requirements. Side effects include drowsiness, mood alteration, and occasionally euphoria. They do not have hypnotic or amnestic properties, and should not be employed as a sole anesthetic agent.[27]

All the narcotics have certain side effects that are dose dependent (refer to Chapter 26). Briefly, respiratory depression via direct centrally acting mechanisms is the most severe and life-threatening side effect. The opioids do not, with the exception of meperidine, cause direct myocardial depression and therefore can be used in anesthetic doses with remarkable cardiac stability (refer to Chapters 26 and 41 for a full discussion of the cardiovascular effects of opioids). Histamine release is associated with morphine and meperidine. Nausea and vomiting are common complications of narcotic administration. Narcotics may also induce spasm of the sphincter of Oddi which may result in biliary colic; therefore they should not be administered to patients prior to a cholecystectomy or a biliary tract exploration procedure. Narcotics should be used judiciously, and possibly not at all, in a patient with increased intracranial pressure because of the possibility of elevating the intracranial pressure secondary to enhanced cerebral blood flow via hypoventilation-induced hypercarbia.

It is important to premedicate patients with a narcotic addiction with an appropriately long-acting narcotic, such as methadone, to prevent the sudden onset of withdrawal syndrome during the perioperative period. It is appropriate to use narcotics when indicated in these patients, realizing, however, that their tolerance to usual doses of narcotics may be overwhelmingly high.[28(p318)] Additionally, the anesthetist must ascertain via direct questioning the extent of the addiction, the type of narcotic, the last known use of that drug, and the quantity ingested. If the ingestion of the substance was recent, the patient may require less than the usual amount of narcotic, inhalational anesthesia, or both.

Morphine and meperidine (Demerol) are the most commonly used preoperative narcotic agents, but hydromorphone (Dilaudid) may also be used for intramuscular premedication (Table 14–3). Fentanyl is not recommended for intramuscular injection, as the pharmacokinetics of fentanyl preclude its effectiveness when given intramuscularly. The magnitude of fentanyl's clinical effects depends on the rapidity with which it crosses the blood–brain barrier; therefore it is usually given via intravenous bolus or infusion.

Morphine. Morphine is widely used in all patient populations. It is normally given in a dose of 0.1 mg/kg intramuscularly approximately 1 hour prior to surgery. In the immediate preoperative period, it can be titrated intravenously in 1- to 2-mg increments for a total dose of 0.1 to 0.25 mg/kg or until the desired effect of narcosis is achieved. When given intravenously, the onset of action of morphine is about 3 to 5 minutes and the peak effect occurs at about 10 minutes. The duration of action of morphine is 4 to 5 hours.[29]

Morphine, via histamine release and its sympathologic properties, may act as a peripheral vasodilator. Care should be exercised in those patients who are hypovolemic or who otherwise exhibit a condition where the risk of hypotension is significant.

Meperidine. Meperidine (Demerol) is largely used as an intramuscular premedication agent at doses of 1 mg/kg. The onset of action of meperidine is faster than that of morphine, and the duration of effect is approximately 2 to 3 hours[30] when used in analgesic doses. It is effective for pain relief and has a narrow therapeutic index. In the doses recommended for premedication and pain relief, the risk of tachycardia is relatively low.

Fentanyl. Fentanyl (Sublimaze) is a short-acting narcotic used primarily in the intravenous form. It is commonly administered in the immediate preoperative/preinduction period. Dosages of fentanyl depend on the desired sympatholytic effect, age, and condition of the patient. Generally, doses of 1 to 2 µg/kg prior to induction of anesthesia contribute to the blunting of the sympathetic response to intubation.[28(p314)] Doses up to 5 to 7 µg/kg will not only blunt the response to intubation but will also decrease the dosage of other induction agents (e.g., thiopental).[31,32] The onset of action of fentanyl is 1 to 2 minutes, and it has a duration of action of 10 to 30 minutes. The elimination half-life is 2 to 4 hours. Because of its rapid onset of action, it is imperative that the anesthetist have resuscitation equipment and drugs readily available when fentanyl

TABLE 14–3. COMMONLY USED NARCOTIC ANALGESIC PREMEDICATIONS

Drug	Average Dose
Morphine	0.1–0.25 mg/kg IM
	0.05–0.25 mg/kg IV
Meperidine	1 mg/kg IM

is administered. Rapid administration of the short-acting (fentanyl) and ultrashort-acting (sufentanil and alfentanil) narcotics may result in chest wall rigidity that is manageable only with administration of an intravenous muscle relaxant and subsequent intubation. For these reasons, these agents should not be used for premedication on the ward, but may be given in the preoperative holding area, where the patient can be closely observed.

Anticholinergics

The anticholinergic agents used routinely in anesthesia include glycopyrrolate, atropine, and scopolamine. Anticholinergics were once almost routinely administered preoperatively to prevent excessive salivation, to prevent bradycardia (especially in pediatric patients when succinylcholine was employed), and to promote sedation (especially with scopolamine). These agents competitively inhibit the muscarinic actions of acetylcholine. Presently, anticholinergics are used when necessary for a specific indication. Potential indications for preoperative administration of anticholinergics for their antisialogogue properties may include the use of a fiberoptic laryngoscope, in situations when it is desirable to prevent secretions from interfering with visualization, or for surgery in the oral cavity or tracheobronchial area. Indications for use as vagolytic agents include situations of extreme bradycardia resulting from fentanyl, sufentanil, or alfentanil administration, acute treatment of the oculocardiac reflex, or a vagally mediated bradycardia during intraperitoneal surgery.

Glycopyrrolate is generally given in 0.2-mg doses intravenously or intramuscularly. It produces less tachycardia, sedation, and blurred vision than either atropine or scopolamine.[33] Glycopyrrolate is a quaternary ammonium compound that is unable to cross the blood–brain barrier and elicit central nervous system effects. Its effects are mediated at the peripheral cholinergic receptors. At equipotent doses, glycopyrrolate, atropine, and scopolamine produce the same degree of antisialogogy.[34]

Atropine is the most potent vagolytic agent of the three.[35] Atropine and scopolamine are both tertiary amines and therefore can cross the blood–brain barrier and produce the central nervous system side effects of delirium, restlessness, flushing, pyrexia, and confusion. Atropine exhibits fewer central nervous system effects than scopolamine. Atropine produces dryness of the mouth and blurred vision within 10 to 15 minutes of intramuscular injection of 0.4 to 0.6 mg. Vagolytic effects occur at doses closer to 1 mg.[33]

Scopolamine is 8 to 10 times more potent as an amnestic agent than atropine.[36] This property is used most effectively when combined with morphine.[37] The combination provides a potent sedative premedication and can be given as an intramuscular injection to premedicate cardiac surgery patients. Scopolamine is generally given in 0.3- to 0.6-mg doses, either intramuscularly or intravenously.

Anticholinergics have been implicated as agents that reduce lower esophageal sphincter tone.[38] Although this has never been documented in a clinical setting, theoretically the use of an anticholinergic agent could increase the risk of esophageal reflux through a reduction in this pressure gradient.

Premedications to Decrease Sympathetic Nervous System Response

Premedications are often effective in attenuating the sympathetic response to induction and intubation. These responses include hypertension, hypotension, tachycardia, and bradycardia. Selective premedication can aid in controlling the extremes of the sympathetic responses and thereby provide for a more stable and predictable anesthetic course.

Generally, all patients arrive at the preoperative holding area with some degree of anxiety. This manifests itself as a sympathetic response mediated through the release of catecholamines. The degree to which the patient exhibits this response is highly individual. Many patients present to the operating room with a high degree of preexisting sympathetic tone. Often, the administration of small doses of benzodiazepines, narcotics, or droperidol will reduce the blood pressure and heart rate simply because of the sedative effects of those agents. When the patient is in a relaxed state, catecholamine levels are reduced.

Narcotic premedication assists in diminishing the sympathetic response to intubation and surgical incision. Narcotics act by decreasing the central sympathetic outflow and by increasing the parasympathetic outflow at the level of the medullary neurons.[39-41] The narcotic used should be titrated to achieve the desired effects, which are a stable heart rate and blood pressure, without depressing the respiratory status.

An agent that has recently been reported to be effective in blunting the sympathetic response to intubation without depressing respiratory status is clonidine (Catapres). Clonidine is a centrally acting alpha-2 agonist whose effects result in a decrease in the release of norepinephrine. The dosages described for effective control of blood pressure and heart rate range from 0.1 to 0.3 mg (or about 5 µg/kg) given orally 1 hour prior to surgery.[42] Clonidine has been shown to reduce the minimum alveolar concentration of inhalational maintenance anesthesia and narcotic requirements during nitrous oxide–narcotic maintenance technique.[43,44] It has been suggested that clonidine itself contains analgesic and sedative properties.[45]

Premedications to Decrease Maintenance Doses of Anesthesia

Generally, all premedication will decrease the maintenance dose of anesthesia, but the extent of this effect is dependent on the amount and type of premedication, the patient's response to the premedication, and, of course, the type of operation and degree of surgical stimulation. It is generally desirable that the patient enter the operating suite with a lowered level of circulating catecholamines to attenuate the magnitude of the stress responses. The maintenance doses of anesthesia are then prescribed according to patient need and tolerance, response to surgical stimulation, and, of course, any other existing medical condition. Caution should be exercised in depressing catecholamine levels in patients with serious cardiovascular disease, as some of these patients may depend on sympathetic drive for maintenance of their hemodynamic stability.

Premedications to Provide Postoperative Antiemesis

Nausea and vomiting are probably the most frequent postanesthetic complaints. There is a correlation between type of surgery, sex, inpatient versus outpatient status, and the likelihood of the development of nausea with or without vomiting. Nausea occurs frequently in patients undergoing therapeutic abortions, middle ear surgery, and laparoscopies. Females have almost twice the incidence of nausea than males.[46] Outpatients also have a higher incidence of nausea and vomiting than inpatients.

The antiemetics most frequently employed as premedications include promethazine, droperidol, and transdermal scopolamine. As mentioned earlier, promethazine is given intramuscularly at least 1 hour prior to surgery in doses of 12.5 to 25 mg. Droperidol employed for antiemesis can be given intramuscularly or intravenously, with the intramuscular dose being 2.5 to 5 mg given 1 hour prior to induction of anesthesia. The intravenous dose is 0.25 to 1.25 mg and this can be administered in the preoperative holding area or throughout the course of the anesthetic period. Wetchler et al[47] gave droperidol in doses as low as 0.25 mg intravenously to outpatients undergoing laparoscopic surgery immediately postintubation and found it to be effective as an antiemetic. Transdermal scopolamine is given as a patch, placed behind the ear, which maintains low circulating levels of scopolamine up to 72 hours.[48] Its effects are comparable to those of droperidol.[49] The patch may be applied the night before surgery and remain on postoperatively. One study using the technique of the transdermal scopolamine patch has shown the incidence of nausea to be 45 percent less than in patients given a placebo when undergoing minor gynecologic surgery.[50]

Premedications to Reduce Risk of Gastric Acid Aspiration

Gastric acid aspiration is a potential complication in all surgical patients. Some patients are predisposed to increased incidence of aspiration. Patients who are at increased risk include those who are obese (20 percent above ideal body weight), those who have a hiatal hernia or otherwise incompetent gastroesophageal sphincter, parturients in their second or third trimester, outpatients, those with peptic ulcer disease, patients exhibiting extreme anxiety, patients with diabetes mellitus, and the elderly. Esophageal regurgitation may be promoted by fasciculations from succinylcholine, use of the Trendelenburg position or the prone position, palpation of the abdomen, and increased intragastric pressure secondary to positive-pressure mask ventilation. The risk of aspiration pneumonitis following aspiration of gastric contents has been correlated with a gastric volume greater than 25 mL and a pH less than 2.5.[51]

The goals of premedication are to reduce gastric volume and to raise gastric pH above 2.5. The medication that is most widely used in anesthesia to reduce gastric volume is metoclopramide (Reglan). Metoclopramide is a dopamine antagonist that promotes gastric emptying by stimulating gastric motility, increasing lower esophageal sphincter tone, and is thought by some to act as an antiemetic.[52] Metoclopramide can be given in doses of 10 mg orally, 1 to 2 hours prior to induction of anesthesia, or 10 mg intravenously, 30 to 90 minutes prior to induction of anesthesia,[53] with a resultant decrease in gastric volume. As metoclopramide is a dopamine antagonist, it may produce the undesirable side effect of extrapyramidal symptoms. Caution should be exercised when administering metoclopromide to patients on antiparkinsonian agents.

There are basically two methods of increasing the gastric pH. One method is via H_2 receptor antagonists, which include cimetidine and ranitidine; the other method is through the use of oral antacids. The oral antacids should be of the clear liquid type, rather than suspension antacids, as the suspension antacids contain particulate matter which can be dangerous if aspirated. Cimetidine and ranitidine are histamine H_2 receptor antagonists that prevent histamine from inducing gastric acid secretion with a high hydrogen ion content (low pH). They can prevent the secretion of gastric acid but have no effect on the pH of preexisting gastric contents. They are both competitive and selective H_2 receptor antagonists.

Cimetidine given in a dose of 300 mg orally at least 1 hour prior to surgery increases the pH of the gastric contents to greater than 2.5 in at least 80 percent of the patients who receive it.[54] Cimetidine does not affect gastric volume.[55 (p378)] Cimetidine can also be administered parenterally to those in whom oral administration may be impossible. The effects of cimetidine on gastric contents last 3 to 4 hours, and the elimination half-life is 1.5 to 2 hours.[55 (pp387–389)]

The side effects of cimetidine administration include central nervous system dysfunction because of its ability to cross the blood–brain barrier. These effects may manifest as confusion, agitation, hallucinations, and seizures, especially in the geriatric age group.[56] Rapid administration of cimetidine (intravenously in less than 2 minutes) results in a direct peripheral vasodilation and hypotension in critically ill patients.[57] In healthy volunteers, however, there were no changes noted in blood pressure or ejection fraction with rapid injection of cimetidine.[58] Lastly, cimetidine has been implicated in retarding the metabolism of drugs that normally undergo high hepatic extraction, such as lidocaine, propranolol, and diazepam.[59,60] The mechanism is thought to be inhibition of the cytochrome P450 enzyme system in the liver which results in a reduction of the metabolization of such drugs.[61] Caution should be exercised when administering cimetidine to patients with these concurrent therapies.

Ranitidine is also an H_2 selective and competitive antagonist. It has an imidazole structure and is five to eight times as potent as cimetidine.[55 (p381)] It is absorbed from the gastrointestinal tract within 30 to 60 minutes. Recommended doses are 50 mg intravenously and 150 mg orally. Its elimination half-life is 2 to 3 hours, but its effect on inhibition of gastric acid secretion lasts 8 to 12 hours.[62] As the structure of ranitidine differs from that of cimetidine, it does not produce the same side effects as cimetidine. It has limited ability to cross the blood–brain barrier, infrequent cardiac effects, and less inhibition of hepatic microsomal enzyme systems.

The use of H_2 antagonists in the asthmatic population may be problematic as it has the potential for inducing unopposed H_1 receptor responses which may cause bronchoconstriction. Although the H_2 antagonists have been safely administered to patients with bronchospastic disease, the anesthetist should be aware of this potential side effect.

The oral antacid in clear suspension most frequently used in anesthesia is Bicitra, which is a commercial preparation of sodium citrate and citric acid. The use of oral antacids clearly represents an effective means of raising the pH of gastric contents, but does nothing to promote gastric emptying or change lower esophageal sphincter pressure. In fact, the use of oral antacids is associated with an increase in gastric volume, especially when compared with the use of an H_2 blocker and metoclopramide.[53] The oral antacids are effective only in alkalinizing the existing acid present in the stomach, and are not effective in preventing further secretion of acid from the parietal cells. Oral antacids are generally given in doses of 15 to 30 mL, at least 15 minutes before the induction of anesthesia. They are commonly given to parturients, as there is no placental transfer and hence no adverse effects on the fetus.

Premedication for Common Medical Problems

Frequently encountered medical problems that require special attention to premedicant therapy include epilepsy, bronchospastic disorders, alterations in cardiovascular stability, diabetes mellitus, and steroid dependency. The general goal of premedicant therapy in these instances is to optimize and maximize the patient's current medical therapy to prevent exacerbation of the underlying condition in the perioperative period. Generally, preexisting medical therapies are maintained throughout the perioperative period.

Seizure Disorders. It is important to identify the etiology of the seizure activity to evaluate the indications for current therapy. Differentiation must be made between seizures secondary to increased intracranial pressure (e.g., mass lesions) and those resulting from specific epileptic foci. Seizure activity should ideally be reduced as much as possible prior to the induction of anesthesia. Commonly used anticonvulsants include phenytoin, phenobarbital, carbamazepine, and valproic acid. A serum level of the anticonvulsant medication should be obtained prior to surgery to determine the extent to which the patient has a therapeutic level and the effectiveness of that level of medication. All anticonvulsant medications should be continued until the time of surgery.[64] They either can be given parenterally when indicated or can be taken orally with a sip of water on the morning of surgery.

Asthma. Antiasthmatic medications include inhalation therapies (such as pocket inhalers of beta agonists or steroids) and oral agents. Commonly used oral agents include xanthines, antihistamines, corticosteroids, anticholinergics, and beta-adrenergic stimulants. Again, serum levels should be obtained for therapeutic index levels in those patients on oral bronchodilators (xanthines and beta-adrenergic stimulators), especially in those patients who are symptomatic in the perioperative period. Agents that are available in oral and parenteral preparations can be given either parenterally or orally with a sip of water on the morning of surgery. The inhalational agents can be used as indicated until the time of surgery, and additionally 2 to 4 puffs of the hand-held nebulizer can be given just prior to the induction of anesthesia (or even in the preoperative holding area). During anesthesia, up to 10 puffs of a beta agonist can be administered through the endotracheal tube to provide further bronchodilation if necessary.[65] In the case of a severe asthmatic, evaluation of pulmonary function testing may be necessary to determine the severity of the patient's preoperative bronchoconstriction and response to bronchodilators. If the patient is actively wheezing prior to surgery, it is may be necessary to cancel any surgery except that required to treat a life-threatening condition. Consultation with the medical team may be necessary to reevaluate the patient and treat the active bronchospasm most effectively.

Alterations in Cardiac Stability. Complicating factors in the maintenance of cardiac stability include dysrhythmias, hypertension, coronary artery disease, and congestive heart failure. Again, it is generally advised to continue the patient's preoperative medical regimen before and during the anesthetic course, as well as to ensure therapeutic serum levels of currently used agents, especially in patients who are symptomatic preoperatively. The premedication regimen should include the patient's current cardiac medications as well as a sedative, opiate, or both to attenuate the patient's response to intubation and incision.

Antiarrhythmic therapy may include digitalis preparations, beta-adrenergic blockers, calcium channel blockers, local anesthetics (lidocaine, procainamide), quinidine, and antiadrenergic drugs (disopyramide, amiodarone). If the patient requires any of these medications prior to surgery, they should be continued throughout the perioperative period. The anesthetist should also investigate any drug interactions that occur in response to the use of anesthetic agents with these cardiac medications and be prepared to direct the patient's anesthetic management accordingly.

Antihypertensive regimens include alpha-adrenergic blockade, beta-adrenergic blockade, inhibition of angiotensin-converting enzymes, diuretic therapy, and calcium channel blockers. The most frequent complications of hypertension affecting the management of anesthesia include an increased systemic vascular resistance and a decreased intravascular volume. These two factors may cause wide variation in blood pressure, an exaggerated vasopressor response, and edema.[66] These complications are also associated with an increased incidence of ischemia, myocardial infarction, dysrhythmias, and stroke. Stone et al noted that even a single dose of a beta blocker 90 minutes prior to induction significantly reduced the occurrence of these problems.[67] Clonidine, if discontinued prior to surgery, may result in a "rebound" hypertensive episode and hypertensive crisis; therefore this medication must be continued until and during surgery.[68]

Controversy exists as to whether or not to continue preexisting diuretic therapy into the preoperative period. The most common complications of diuretic therapy are hypovolemia and hypokalemia. Most frequently, patients on diuretic therapy either are hypertensive or have congestive heart failure. They may be diuretic dependent for maintenance of hemodynamic stability and also have some degree of renal insufficiency. Premedications including diuretic therapy are individualized to the patient's needs, and no set standard exists. Consideration of the patient's medical condition and type and length of surgery should be taken into account when determining whether to administer diuretics as a premedication. In the patient with coronary artery disease, a full preoperative evaluation must be performed and the patient's usual medical regimen is continued until the time of surgery.

Diabetes Mellitus. Premedication regimens for diabetics who are insulin dependent can be managed by one of two methods. If the patient is scheduled for surgery early in the day, the patient is made NPO after midnight and instructed not to take a morning insulin dose. On arrival at the hospital (same day surgery) or preoperative holding area, serum glucose is measured. The anesthetist can either administer regular insulin or start an intravenous infusion of a 5 percent glucose solution, or both. Walts et al found better control over blood glucose levels when no insulin was given the morning of surgery and the intravenous glucose and insulin were titrated according to the frequent blood glucose analysis (every hour).[69] The 5 percent glucose solution should be given at the rate of 2 mL/h/kg body weight.[70] Blood glucose analysis is conducted at 1- to 2-hour intervals throughout surgery and insulin and glucose are titrated to obtain the patient's optimal blood glucose level. Alternatively, the patient can be instructed to take (or be given) half of their normal morning or daily insulin dose (if the patient takes insulin only once per day), followed by an intravenous solution of 5 percent glucose at 2 mL/h/kg body weight. A preoperative blood glucose level is obtained, and insulin and glucose levels are titrated in the same fashion as above.[70] The reader is referred to the aforementioned reference for a complete and excellent review of the management of the diabetic surgical patient.

Patients receiving oral hypoglycemics are usually instructed not to take their hypoglycemic agent the day of surgery. Blood glucose analysis proceeds as described above. It may be necessary to administer parenteral regular insulin should these patients experience hyperglycemia. All diabetic patients should carry with them, or have immediately available in the hospital, a means of ingesting glucose orally if they begin to experience a hypoglycemic episode. Orange juice and candy are commonly used for self-treatment of a hypoglycemic episode.

Steroid Dependency. A daily regimen of steroids (greater than 7.5 mg prednisone) will suppress endogenous cortisol production and lead to atrophy of the adrenal gland. General guidelines for the premedication of patients who have received these doses of steroids within the past 6 months prior to surgery include consideration of a preoperative steroid bolus. The maximum recommended steroid bolus is 300 mg of hydrocortisone, given in three 100-mg doses. The first dose is given either orally or parenterally the night before surgery, the second dose is given the morn-

ing of surgery, and the last dose is given in the preinduction/induction period. The least amount of exogenous cortisol to be administered should be 100 mg. Consideration must be given to the patient's past use of steroids (quantity, frequency, last dose) and the type of surgery (minor versus major). In determination of the amount of a steroid bolus, minor surgeries do not necessarily induce the maximal stress response and therefore smaller doses of hydrocortisone may be administered.[71]

Premedications as Adjuncts to Regional Anesthesia

Premedications are used as adjuncts to regional anesthesia to provide sedation and comfort by relieving residual pain and anxiety. A combination of an opiate and a benzodiazepine is generally effective in accomplishing this goal. The premedication is helpful in assisting the patient through the discomfort of positioning and the initial placement of the regional anesthetic. The patient should not be so sedated that she or he becomes unresponsive or uncooperative.

Consideration of Patient Variables

The specific and general goals of premedications have been discussed, as have the psychologic and pharmacologic methods of accomplishing them. The anesthetist must consider factors including the patient's age, physical status, preexisting medical and surgical conditions, preoperative level of anxiety, allergies, inpatient versus outpatient status, type of surgical procedure, elective versus emergency surgery, coexisting pain, potential routes of administration, and potential drug interactions when determining the appropriate premedication (Table 14–4). The premedication regimen selected must meet the patient's needs and satisfy the anesthetist's objectives.

Age is an important factor in prescribing premedications. Significant caution and judgment are to be exercised when approaching extremes of age. The elderly have a decreased volume of distribution and decreased levels of total protein; are often hypovolemic, malnourished, or both; and have a decreased rate of metabolism of drugs. Young healthy patients are generally very anxious and have a high level of circulating catecholamines, making premedication

TABLE 14–4. PATIENT VARIABLES TO CONSIDER IN PREMEDICANT THERAPY

Age

Sex

Physical status

Preexisting medical/surgical conditions

Allergies

Outpatient status

Type of surgery

Emergency surgery

Current medical therapy

Potential routes of drug administration

very desirable and generally requiring higher doses. Pediatric patients offer many challenges in consideration of proper premedication.

Pediatric patients should be as well prepared psychologically as possible to prevent a traumatic surgical experience by lessening the fear and pain associated with illness and an operation. Some centers do not premedicate pediatric patients, especially with intramuscular injections, to decrease the severity of the trauma of the hospital experience. In this circumstance, "preinduction" medications are administered in the preoperative holding area. This may be accomplished by administration of rectal methohexital, oral midazolam, or intranasal sufentanil. Allowing parents to accompany the pediatric patient to the preoperative holding area is usually effective in reducing the stress of surgery. Parents can also assist in administering the nonparenteral medication to help allay the child's anxiety.

The patient's preexisting medical and surgical conditions must be examined carefully before selecting appropriate premedication. Some of those conditions were mentioned in the preceding section. All disease states must be addressed and the patient's condition optimized by the appropriate medical regimens, prior to surgery. Discretion must be exercised when premedicating debilitated patients, patients less than 1 year of age, the very aged, and those with altered levels of consciousness, increased intracranial pressure, hypovolemia/shock, and severe pulmonary disease. The addition of a sedative or analgesic premedication has the potential to worsen or generate respiratory and cardiac depression or to make patients obtunded so that they lose their protective airway reflexes and suffer from pulmonary aspiration or cardiopulmonary arrest.

Choice of outpatient premedication should recognize several differences between inpatients and outpatients. Outpatients need to be recovered and fully awake soon after surgery, making long-acting premedications inappropriate. Outpatients tend to have a higher gastric volume and lower gastric pH than inpatients so they are theoretically at greater risk for gastric acid aspiration.[72] Control of nausea and vomiting is of prime importance, as the patient will not receive intravenous fluids postoperatively and must be able to maintain oral intake. Lastly, any coexisting disease process should be well controlled (i.e., diabetes mellitus, hypertension) as the patient will return to an unsupervised area following discharge.

Elective surgeries allow time for proper planning, institution of premedicant therapy, and optimization of the patient's physical status. Consideration must be given to the type of surgery to be performed, owing to the fact that major procedures are more threatening and anxiety producing than minor procedures. For example, a patient scheduled for cardiac surgery or a major oncologic resection will have more apprehension and fear than a patient scheduled for an inguinal hernia repair. Hence, the premedication for each patient in those categories must be adjusted accordingly.

Emergency surgery, in contrast to elective surgery, allows little time for premedication and evaluation. All emergency surgical patients should be carefully examined and evaluated to determine what, if any, premedication is necessary. All emergency surgical patients are generally considered to have a full stomach and are at maximum risk for vomiting and aspiration of gastric contents. These patients should have some form of protection from gastric acid aspiration. A rapid sequence induction should be performed if a general anesthetic is planned. Patients having surgery for multiple trauma are typically hypovolemic and clinically in shock. These patients are dependent on their high level of sympathetic tone and circulating catecholamines to maintain hemodynamic stability. Premedications should be given judiciously, if at all, to prevent worsening of an already compromised hemodynamic status. Patients with head injuries are at risk for increased intracranial pressure and may have mass effects from cerebral swelling and hemorrhage. They are at significant risk of respiratory depression and worsening of the increased intracranial pressure, with increased cerebral blood flow secondary to hypoventilation-induced hypercarbia as a side effect of a narcotic premedication. Premedications that place the patient in jeopardy of respiratory depression or loss of consciousness should not be given. Patients who present in the emergency room with a compromised airway should not be sedated or premedicated because of the risk of possibly losing what little remains of an intact airway. Emergent procedures always require careful planning and prioritization to keep the patient as safe as possible and maintain or control homeostatic mechanisms.

Finally, the anesthetist must consider the patient's condition and tolerance level for potential routes of administration of the premedication. Patients who are extremely fearful of injections should not be forced to receive one. Patients who cannot ingest oral medications because of a medical problem or severe nausea and vomiting should receive parenteral premedications. Timing of the premedications is also important. Most premedications require time for absorption and onset of action (except those premedications given intravenously in the preoperative holding area or the immediate preinduction period). It is not helpful to give a high-dose intramuscular injection immediately prior to the patient's arrival in the operating room. It will not have time to take effect, and the patient will arrive in the operating room without sedation, only to have the medication take effect sometime during the induction or postinduction period. The anesthetist must therefore consider the route and timing of the premedications to be given, to achieve its maximal effect.

TECHNIQUES OF INDUCTION AND MAINTENANCE OF ANESTHESIA

Techniques of induction are generally categorized as intravenous, inhalational/mask, rapid sequence, mask induction with cricoid pressure, and intramuscular ketamine methods (Table 14–5). The selection of the technique for induction is based on the same patient variables discussed for premedications. The goals of induction and maintenance of anesthesia include providing optimal conditions for laryngoscopy and intubation, establishing a sufficient depth of anesthesia to attenuate the sympathetic and stress responses to incision and surgery, maintaining a stable hemodynamic profile throughout induction and maintenance of anesthesia, producing a hypnotic state for lack of recall of surgi-

TABLE 14–5. TECHNIQUES OF INDUCTION OF ANESTHESIA

Technique	Average Dose
Intravenous induction	
Barbiturates	
Sodium pentothal	3–5 mg/kg IV
Methohexital	1–2 mg/kg IV
Thiamylol	3–4 mg/kg IV
Etomidate	0.2–0.3 mg/kg IV
Ketamine	1–2 mg/kg IV
Narcotics	
Fentanyl	5–7 µg/kg IV
Sufentanil	0.5–1.5 µg/kg IV
Alfentanil	10–50 µg/kg IV
Benzodiazepines	
Midazolam	0.2–0.35 mg/kg IV
Propofol	1–2.5 mg/kg IV
Mask/inhalation induction	Titration
Rapid sequence induction	Maximum ranges of IV doses
Intramuscular ketamine induction	5–10 mg/kg

cal events, keeping the patient immobile throughout surgery, and achieving a rapid time to awakening.

The induction technique should correlate to the maintenance technique. Maintenance techniques use inhalation agents, narcotics combined with nitrous oxide, propofol, benzodiazepines, and muscle relaxants. For example, if a narcotic induction is performed, a narcotic–nitrous oxide anesthetic may be the most appropriate maintenance technique. The maintenance anesthetic can be an extension of the induction technique (as just described) or a combination of techniques, such as use of a barbiturate induction followed by an inhalational agent combined with small doses of a narcotic for maintenance. Full discussions regarding the pharmacokinetics and pharmacodynamics of the intravenous anesthetic agents and inhalational agents can be found in Chapters 25, 26, and 28. The reader is referred to these chapters for a complete review of these agents.

Preinduction Technique

Obviously the anesthetist must have secured an intravenous line to perform an intravenous induction. Sometimes, especially in pediatric or uncooperative patients, this is not easily accomplished. It is often necessary to use an adjunct preinduction anesthetic agent to establish the conditions necessary to place an intravenous line. In children less than 5 years old, rectal methohexital in doses of 20 to 30 mg/kg of a 10 percent solution can be given in the preoperative holding area to sedate the child. Other techniques include oral midazolam (described earlier) or intramuscular ketamine in doses of 2 to 4 mg/kg before entry into the operating room. Intramuscular ketamine can also be used in adults who are mentally disabled and do not have the capacity to cooperate (as in organic brain syndrome or severe mental retardation). Once the patient is in the operating room, an intravenous line can be placed and an intravenous induction can take place. The intravenous induction

dosage is generally reduced if a preinduction medication has been given.

Intravenous Induction

Use of the intravenous induction agents can result in either a rapid or slow onset of anesthesia, depending on the dose, speed, and rapidity of titration of the intravenous agent employed. The major benefit of intravenous agents is that they can induce anesthesia in a matter of seconds when the situation is required. The basic procedure for an intravenous induction is first to preoxygenate/denitrogenate the lungs by allowing the patient to spontaneously breathe 100 percent oxygen for 5 minutes. The intravenous induction agent is then administered. Once the patient has lost the eyelid reflex and has become apneic, a breath is given by mask to ensure the capability of artificial ventilation through a competent airway. Once the airway is established, the muscle relaxant of choice is given and, at the appropriate time, the patient can be intubated. If the patient is not going to be intubated but rather ventilated by mask, no muscle relaxant is given and the maintenance agent, such as an inhalational agent or an intravenous anesthetic infusion, is initiated.

Intravenous induction techniques include the use of barbiturates, etomidate, ketamine, narcotics, midazolam, and propofol. The barbiturates are the most frequently used induction agents. The barbiturate induction agents currently in use are sodium thiopental, thiamylol, and methohexital. Thiopental is given in doses of 3 to 5 mg/kg, thiamylol is given in doses of 2 to 4 mg/kg, and methohexital is administered as a 1 to 2 mg/kg bolus. These agents have a rapid onset time, from 30 to 60 seconds or one arm–brain circulation time, when given intravenously. They rapidly produce stage 3, plane 3 levels of surgical anesthesia for approximately 3 to 7 minutes (which typically produces apnea). This is necessary to effectively attenuate the stress of laryngoscopy and intubation. During that induction time a muscle relaxant can be given and the patient can be intubated. If the patient is to be maintained on a mask technique, no muscle relaxant is given, but the airway is established and the maintenance anesthetic begun.

Etomidate is a short-acting intravenous induction anesthetic. It contains an imidazole nucleus and is structurally unrelated to any other anesthetic. It lacks analgesic properties, and therefore narcotic premedication may be beneficial for the patient for whom an etomidate induction is planned. Etomidate is administered in doses of 0.2 to 0.4 mg/kg. It does not depress cardiovascular function and prevents hypertension and tachycardia during laryngoscopy.[73,74] It is painful on injection and has been associated with suppression of adrenocortical function.[75]

Ketamine is a phencyclidine derivative that has a rapid intravenous onset and a relatively rapid (5 to 10 minutes) intramuscular onset. It provides analgesia, anesthesia, and a state of catatonia. This has been referred to as dissociative anesthesia. Intravenous dosage for induction is 1 to 2 mg/kg. It is most useful in providing support to the cardiovascular and respiratory systems, as it does not cause hypotension and usually does not depress ventilation, except in higher doses. It is a very useful agent for the induction of patients in shock. It is not recommended for patients with hypertension, increased intracranial pressure, or prior cerebrovascular accident. It is associated with hallucinations, restlessness, and disorientation. Some of these side effects can be prevented with the use of a benzodiazepine premedication. Ketamine can be used as the sole maintenance anesthetic if administered as an infusion. The infusion rate for maintenance of anesthesia is 50 µg/kg/min.

Narcotics are often used as induction agents. The most popular opiate induction agents include fentanyl, sufentanil, alfentanil, and, to a lesser extent, morphine. Morphine has largely been supplanted by the short- and ultrashort-acting narcotics because of its potential for the release of histamine and lengthier duration of action. It is possible to use hydromorphone and meperidine, but because of extended durations of actions and a large number of side effects, they are used rather infrequently. The goal behind a narcotic induction is to "front-load" the narcotic, that is, administer doses that render the patient with a respiratory rate from 6 to 10 up to the maximum recommended dosage and then administer either intermittent bolus injections or an infusion for maintenance of anesthesia. Narcotics may not provide amnesia or hypnosis and, therefore, should be combined with either nitrous oxide, benzodiazepines, or a low-dose inhalational agent to provide hypnosis and prevent recall. The benefits of narcotic inductions include excellent control of hemodynamics during the induction and maintenance of anesthesia as well as reliable analgesia. Disadvantages of a narcotic induction and maintenance technique include a high incidence of nausea and vomiting, prolonged respiratory depression, somnolence, a prolonged time to awakening, and the possibility of postoperative renarcotization.

The benzodiazepines may be employed as induction agents. Before midazolam was available, diazepam was used. At the present time, when a benzodiazepine induction is chosen, midazolam is the agent of choice. Midazolam can induce anesthesia in doses of 0.2 to 0.35 mg/kg.[76] Midazolam is a slower induction agent when compared with the barbiturates. It has a prolonged amnestic effect postoperatively for 1 to 2 hours. It does not have adverse effects on cardiovascular stability when used alone.

Propofol is an induction agent recently made available in the United States. It is an alkyl phenol and is structurally unrelated to the other anesthetics. It is insoluble in water and is prepared in an opaque oil-in-water emulsion. It is painful on injection to the small veins of the hand, and is best given through the larger vein in the forearm and antecubital area. It is an extremely rapid-acting agent with a half-life of only 2 to 3 minutes. This property makes it a useful agent for outpatient surgery. The induction dose of propofol is 2.5 mg/kg, and the induction dose should be decreased to half of the recommended dose in the elderly and debilitated. Propofol is also associated with significantly less nausea and vomiting than are other anesthetics. Patients can be managed on a propofol infusion for maintenance of anesthesia, and awaken in approximately 13.9 ± 2.6 minutes.[77] Propofol does not have analgesic properties and is recommended for use in combination with a narcotic for pain relief. It has been shown to cause cardiac depression in

the elderly and debilitated, but not the young and healthy. It is not yet approved for use in pediatric patients.

With the exception of the benzodiazepines and etomidate, all of the above intravenous anesthetics used for induction are commonly used in either infusion or intermittent bolus forms to maintain anesthesia. The agents are titrated to the desired effect for control of hemodynamic responses to the stress of the surgical procedure. The infusions or boluses are stopped when nearing the end of the procedure. The anesthetist must also study the pharmacokinetic profiles of each agent to determine predicted serum levels and use that information to calculate the appropriate time for cessation of the medication. This will aid in a smooth and timely patient awakening.

Mask/Inhalation Induction

Preoperative medication is useful in the course of a mask induction because it facilitates a smoother induction and less tracheobronchial irritation from the inhalational agent. Benzodiazepines in clinical doses do not cause respiratory depression, whereas a high dose of narcotic premedication might. It is often helpful for the patient to be breathing spontaneously on induction. This may avoid the need to provide positive-pressure mask ventilation and risk gastric distension. Mask inductions are commonly used in pediatric patients to achieve a baseline anesthetic level to allow placement of the intravenous line. The patient is generally allowed to breathe spontaneously a mixture of 70 percent nitrous oxide and 30 percent oxygen. After the patient experiences a period of nystagmus and excitation, the inhalational agent of choice is titrated up in incremental doses to the desired alveolar concentration of the agent. This procedure is followed to reduce the irritating effects of the inhalational agent in the tracheobronchial tree. For example, halothane is increased in 0.2 percent increments every three to five breaths until the patient has achieved the surgical plane of anesthesia. The inhalation agent of choice can then be continued as the maintenance agent throughout the remainder of the procedure.

Rapid Sequence Induction

The rapid sequence induction technique is used for patients with a full stomach (those who have eaten or taken liquid within 8 hours of induction), hiatal hernia, esophageal reflux, or diabetic gastroparesis or parturients in the second and third trimesters. In addition, any patient undergoing emergency surgery is usually considered to have a full stomach. The goal of the rapid sequence induction is to avoid gastric distension during positive-pressure mask ventilation during the induction period (to prevent vomiting and aspiration). The Sellick maneuver is an attempt to close off the esophagus through the application of cricoid pressure in the event of reflux. The patient is allowed to breathe spontaneously 100 percent oxygen by mask to denitrogenate the lungs and ensure adequate preoxygenation. The induction agent and either succinylcholine or a high-dose nondepolarizing muscle relaxant are administered in rapid sequence, without ventilation of the patient between administration of the induction agents and muscle relaxants, while simultaneously holding pressure on the cricoid cartilage. The patient is then rapidly intubated, the cuff is inflated, breath sounds are identified, and confirmation of correct endotracheal tube placement should be ensured by positive end-tidal carbon dioxide measurements. Only when endotracheal tube placement is confirmed is the cricoid pressure released in the event of misplacement of the endotracheal tube. This procedure is not necessarily 100 percent effective in preventing vomiting or reflux. If the patient does begin to vomit, cricoid pressure must be released; otherwise the potential exists for esophageal rupture from the force of vomiting and rapid increase in pressure in the esophagus. The patient should be suctioned immediately with the head turned to the side. Controversy exists as to whether the patient should be placed in the head-up or head-down position to prevent aspiration.

An alternative to the rapid sequence induction is to hold cricoid pressure during the routine intravenous induction. The rapid sequence induction can be very stressful to the hemodynamics of the patient and those with unstable cardiovascular hemodynamics may not be able to tolerate such an insult. Mask induction with cricoid pressure allows for a slower induction with some protection against pulmonary aspiration of gastric contents.

Intramuscular Ketamine Induction

Full induction with ketamine is sometimes used in specific circumstances. One example is pediatric radiology procedures. In this case the pediatric patient may need a short burst of radiation therapy and must remain completely still, and alone, in the radiation room. In this case ketamine can be given intramuscularly in 5 to 10 mg/kg doses and will provide for the induction and maintenance of anesthesia for about 10 to 15 minutes. The respiratory drive is not depressed, pharyngeal and laryngeal reflexes are potentially slightly depressed, and the cardiovascular system remains intact.

Rectal barbiturate (methohexital) anesthesia can be used for induction, but it is usually reserved for sedation for mask compliance or to start an intravenous line. The usual dose is 20 to 30 mg/kg of the viscous form of the preparation.

SUMMARY

The reader must understand that very rarely are these induction techniques used in a pure form. In other words, it is rare to use one method exclusive of the other concepts and methods involved in the other techniques. Generally, a combination of the above techniques is used to tailor the induction to the individual needs of the patient. Those individual needs take into consideration all the variables in the patient's medical status and the best anesthetic agents to effectively manage the patient's condition. An intravenous narcotic induction, for example, may be followed by an inhalational maintenance technique. Or both narcotics and barbiturates may be used to induce the patient, and a combination of inhalational agent and small titrated doses of the same narcotic used for maintenance of anesthesia. The choice of premedication, induction, and maintenance techniques is ultimately based on the specific goals of the anesthetist regarding the management of the patient's medical and surgical needs.

REFERENCES

1. Egbert LD, Battit GE, Turndorf H, Beecher HK. The value of the preoperative visit by an anesthetist. *JAMA.* 1963;185:553.
2. Lichtor JL, Johanson CE, Mhoon D, Faure EAM, Hassan SZ, Roizen MF. Preoperative anxiety: Does anxiety level the afternoon before surgery predict anxiety level just before surgery? *Anesthesiology.* 1987;67:4:595–599.
3. Roizen MF. Anesthetic implications of concurrent diseases. In: Miller RD, ed. *Anesthesia.* 3rd ed. New York: Churchill Livingstone; 1990:847.
4. Tomicheck RC, Rosow CE, Philbin DM, Moss J, Teplick RS, Schnieder RC. Diazepam–fentanyl interaction—Hemodynamic and hormonal effects in coronary artery surgery. *Anesth Analg.* 1983;62:881–4.
5. Fine J, Finestone SC. Sensory disturbances following ketamine anesthesia: Recurrent hallucinations. *Anesth Analg.* 1973;52:429–430.
6. Ramasubramanian R, Rawle PR, Verma R. Attenuation of psychological effects of ketamine anesthesia by midazolam: A dose response study. *Anesth Analg.* 1988;67:S182.
7. Fragen RJ, Funk DI, Avram MJ, et al. Midazolam versus hydroxyzine as an intramuscular premedicant. *Can Anesth Soc J.* 1983;30:136.
8. Vinik HR, Reves JG, Wright D. Premedication with intramuscular midazolam—A prospective double-blind controlled study. *Anesth Analg.* 1982;61:933.
9. White PF, Vasconez LO, Mathes SA, Way WL, Wender LA. Comparison of midazolam and diazepam for sedation during plastic surgery. *Plas Reconstr Surg.* 1988;81:703–710.
10. Weldon BC, Watcha M, White PF. Oral midazolam premedication: Optimal timing and effect of atropine. *Anesthesiology.* 73:No. 3A, A1243, 1990;73(3A):A1243.
11. O'Boyle CA, Harris D, Barry H, et al. Comparison of midazolam by mouth and diazepam intravenously in outpatient oral surgery. *Br J Anaesth.* 1987;59:746.
12. Klotz U, Antonin K-H, Bieck PR. Pharmacokinetics and plasma binding of diazepam in man, dog, rabbit, guinea pig and rat. *J Pharmacol Exp Ther.* 1976;67:199.
13. Wetchler BV, ed. *Anesthesia for ambulatory surgery.* 2nd ed. Philadelphia: JB Lippincott; 1990:203.
14. Greenblatt DJ, Abernathy DR, Morse DS, Harmatz JS, Shader RI. Clinical importance of the interaction of diazepam and cimetidine. *N Engl J Med.* 1984;310:1639.
15. Dundee JW, McGowan WAW, Lilburn JK, et al. Comparison of the actions of diazepam and lorazepam. *Br J Anaesth.* 1979;51:439.
16. Baldessarini RJ. Drugs and the treatment of psychiatric disorders. In: Goodman AG, Gilman LS, eds. *The pharmacological basis of therapeutics.* 7th ed. New York: Macmillan; 1985:412.
17. Howatt DDC. Antiemetic drugs in anaesthesia. *Anaesthesia.* 1960;15:289–297.
18. Lee CM, Yeakel AE. Patients refusal of surgery following Innovar premedication. *Anesth Analg.* 1975;54:224–226.
19. Rivera VM, Keichian AH, Oliver RE. Persistent parkinsonism following neurolept anesthesia. *Anesthesia.* 1975;42:635–637.
20. Wallace G, Mindlin LJ. A controlled double blind comparison of intramuscular lorazepam and hydroxyzine as surgical premedicants. *Anesth Analg.* 1984;63:571–576.
21. Stoelting R. *Pharmacology and physiology in anesthetic practice.* Philadelphia: JB Lippincott; 1987:376–378.

22. Koch-Weser J, Greenblatt DJ. The archaic barbiturate hypnotics. *N Engl J Med.* 1974;291:790.

23. Moyers JR. Preoperative medication in clinical anesthesia. In: Barash PG, Cullen BF, Stoelting RK, eds. *Clinical Anesthesia.* Philadelphia: JB Lippincott; 1989:490.

24. Black TE, Kay B, Healy TW. Reducing the hemodynamic responses to laryngoscopy and intubation. A comparison of alfentanil and fentanyl. *Anaesthesia.* 1984;39:883–887.

25. Murphy MR, Hug CC. The enflurane sparing effect of morphine, butorphanol and nalbuphine. *Anesthesia.* 1982;57:489.

26. Lake CL, DiFazio CA, Moscicki JC, Engle JS. Reduction in halothane MAC: Comparison of morphine and alfentanil. *Anesth Analg.* 1985;64:807.

27. Wong KC. Narcotics are not expected to produce unconsciousness and amnesia. *Anesth Analg.* 1983;66:625. Editorial.

28. Bailey PL, Stanley TH. Narcotic intravenous anesthetics. In: Miller RK, ed. *Anesthesia.* 3rd ed. New York: Churchill Livingstone; 1990.

29. DeCastro J, Van de Water A, Wouters L, Xhonneux R, et al. Comparative study of cardiovascular, neurological, and metabolic side effects of eight narcotics in dogs. *Acta Anaesth Belg.* 1979;30:6–96.

30. Murphy MR. Opioids. In: Barash PG, Cullen BF, Stoelting RK, eds. *Clinical Anesthesia.* Philadelphia: JB Lippincott; 1989:265.

31. Katz RI, Alexander G. Hemodynamic stability and thiopental, ketamine, thiopental/fentanyl and ketamine/fentanyl anesthetic induction. *Anesthesia.* 1990;73(3A):A324.

32. Flacke JW, Bloor BC, Kripke BJ, et al. Comparison of morphine, meperidine, fentanyl and sufentanil in balanced anesthesia. A double-blind study. *Anesth Analg.* 1985;64:897–910.

33. Smith TC, Wollman H. History and principles of anesthesiology. In: Goodman AG, Gilman LS, eds. *The pharmacological basis of therapeutics.* 7th ed. New York: Macmillan; 1985:272.

34. Sengupta A, Gupta PK, Pandey K. Investigation of glycopyrrolate as a premedicant drug. *Br J Anaesth.* 1980;52:513.

35. Weiner N. Atropine, scopolamine and related antimuscarinic drugs. In: Goodman AG, Gilman LS, eds. *The pharmacological basis of therapeutics.* 7th ed. New York: Macmillan; 1985:133.

36. Ketchum JS, Sidell FR, Crowell EB, et al. Atropine, scopolamine and ditran: Comparative pharmacology and antagonists in man. *Psychopharmacologia.* 1973;28:121–125.

37. Conner JT, Bellvill JW, Wender R, et al. Morphine, scopolamine and atropine as intravenous surgical premedicants. *Anesth Analg.* 1977;56:606.

38. Brock-Utne JG, Rubin J, Welman S, et al. The effect of glycopyrrolate (Robinul) on the lower esophageal sphincter. *Can Anaesth Soc J.* 1978;25:144.

39. Laubie M, Schmitt H, Canellas J, Roquebert J, Demichel P. Centrally mediated bradycardia and hypotension induced by narcotic analgesics: Dextromoramide and fentanyl. *Eur J Pharmacol.* 1974;28:66–75.

40. Laubie M, Schmitt H, Drouillat M. Central sites and mechanisms of the hypotensive and bradycardic effects of the narcotic analgesic agent fentanyl. *Naunyn Schmiedeberg's Arch Pharmacol.* 1977;296:255–261.

41. Laubie M, Schmitt H. Action of the morphinomitic agent, fentanyl, on the nucleus tractus solitarii and the nucleus ambiguous cardiovascular neurons. *Eur J Pharmacol.* 1980;67:403–412.

42. Ghignone M, Quinton L, Duke PC, et al. Effects of clonidine on narcotic requirements and hemodynamic response during induction of fentanyl anesthesia and endotracheal intubation. *Anesthesia.* 1986;64:36–42.

43. Maze M, Tranquilli W. Alpha 2 adrenoreceptor agonists: Defining the role in clinical anesthesia. *Anesthesia.* 1991;74:593.

44. Bloor BC, Flacke WE. Reduction in halothane anesthetic requirement by clonidine, an alpha adrenergic agonist. *Anesth Analg.* 1982;61:741–745.

45. Northfield KM, Stead SW. Effects of clonidine premedication for monitored anesthesia. *Anesthesia.* 1990;73(3A):A24.

46. Burtles R, Peckett BW. Postoperative vomiting. Some factors affecting its incidence. *Br J Anaesth.* 1957;29:114.

47. Wetchler BV, Collins IS, Jacob L. Antiemetic effects of droperidol on the ambulatory surgical patient. *Anesth Rev.* 1982;9:23.

48. Lichtor JL. Psychological preparation on preoperative medication. In: Miller RD, ed. *Anesthesia,* 3rd ed. New York: Churchill Livingstone; 1990:920.

49. Tigerstedt I, Salmela L, Aromaa U. Double blind comparison of transdermal scopolamine, droperidol and placebo against postoperative nausea and vomiting. *Acta Anaesthesiol Scand.* 1988;32:454.

50. Tolksdorf W, Meisel R, Miller P, Bender HJ. Transdermales Scopolamin (TTS-Scopolamin) zur Prophylaxe Postoperativer Ubelkeit und Erbrechen. *Anaesthesist.* 1985;34:656.

51. Mendelson CL. Aspiration of stomach contents into lungs during obstetric anesthesia. *Am J Obstet Gynecol.* 1946;53:196–205.

52. Dundee JW, Clark RSJ. The premedicant and antiemetic action of metoclopramide. *Post Grad Med J.* 1973;48:34–37.

53. Manchikanti L, Blane Grow J, Colliver J, et al. Bicitra (sodium citrate) and metoclopramide in outpatient anesthesia for prophylaxis against aspiration pneumonitis. *Anesthesiology.* 1985;63:378–384.

54. Pandit SK, Kothary SP, Pandit UA, Mirakhur RK. Premedication with cimetidine and metoclopramide. *Anaesthesia.* 1986;41:486–492.

55. Stoelting RK. *Pharmacology and physiology in anesthetic practice.* Philadelphia: JB Lippincott; 1987.

56. Schentag JJ, Cerra FB, Calleri G, DeGlopper E, Ross JQ, Bernhard H. Pharmacokinetic and clinical studies in patients with cimetidine associated mental confusion. *Lancet.* 1979;1:177–181.

57. Iberti TJ, Paluch TA, Helmer L, Murgolo VA, Benjamin E. The hemodynamic effects of intravenous cimetidine in intensive care patients: A double-blind, prospective study. *Anesthesiology.* 1986;64:87–89.

58. Mangiameli A, Condorelli G, Data A, Monaco S. Cardiovascular response to the acute intravenous administration of the H_2 receptor antagonists ranitidine and cimetidine. *Curr Ther Res.* 1984;36:13–17.

59. Donovan M, Hagerty A, Pael L, Castleden M, Pohl JEF. Cimetidine and bioavailability of propranolol. *Lancet.* 1981;1:164.

60. Klotz U, Reimann I. Delayed clearance of diazepam due to cimetidine. *N Engl J Med.* 1980;302:1012–1014.

61. Puurumen J, Pelkonen O. Cimetidine inhibits microsomal drug metabolism in the rat. *Eur J Pharmacol.* 1979;55:335–336.

62. Konturek SJ, Obtulowicz W, Kwiecian N, Kopp B, Oleksy J. Kinetics and duration of action of ranitidine on gastric secretion and its effect on pancreatic secretion in duodenal ulcer patients. *Scand J Gastroenterol.* 1981;69:91–99.

64. Dierdorf SF. Rare and co-existing diseases. In: Barash PG, Cullen BF, Stoelting RK, eds. *Clinical Anesthesia.* Philadelphia: JB Lippincott; 1989:445.

65. Bishop M. Bronchospasm: Managing and avoiding a potential anesthetic disaster. ASA Annual Refresher Courses. American Society of Anesthesiologists Publications; 1990:A272.

66. Barash PG: Anesthesia for the patient with cardiac disease undergoing non-cardiac surgery. ASA Refresher Course Lectures. American Society of Anesthesiologists Publications; 1990:A111.

67. Stone JG, Foex P, Sear JW, et al. Myocardial ischemia in untreated hypertensive patients: Effect of a single small dose of beta-adrenergic blocking agent. *Anesthesiology.* 1988;68:495–500.

68. Hansson L. Clinical aspects of blood pressure crisis due to withdrawal of centrally acting antihypertensive drugs. *Br J Clin Pharmacol.* 1983;15(suppl 4):485S–489S.

69. Walts LF, Miller J, Davidson MB, Brown J. Perioperative management of diabetes mellitus. *Anesthesia.* 1981;55:104–109.

70. Hirsh IB, McGill JB, Cryer PE, White PF. Perioperative management of surgical patients with diabetes mellitus. *Anesthesia.* 1991;74:346–359.

71. Apfelbaum JL, Kallar SK, Wetchler BV. Adult and geriatric patients. In: Wetchler BV, ed. *Anesthesia for ambulatory surgery.* Philadelphia: JB Lippincott Co.; 1990:272.

72. Ong BY, Palahniuk RJ, Comming M. Gastric volume in outpatients. *Can Anaesth Soc J.* 1978;25:36.

73. Tempelhoff R, Modica PA, Jellish WS, Spitznagel EL. Etomidate-induced EEG burst suppression maintains hemodynamic stability during induction and tracheal intubation. *Anesth Analg.* 1990;70:S406.

74. Ebert TJ, Kanitz DD, Berens RJ, Kampine JP. Etomidate induction maintains sympathetic outflow in humans: Direct observations from sympathetic recordings. *Anesthesia.* 1990;73(3A): A342.

75. Wagner RL, White PF. Etomidate inhibits adrenocortical function in surgical patients. *Anesthesia.* 1984;61:647.

76. White PF. Comparative evaluation of intravenous agents for rapid sequence induction—Thiopental, ketamine and midazolam. *Anesthesia.* 1982;57:279.

77. Kortilla K, Nuotto E, Lichtor JL, Ostman P, Apfelbaum J, Rupani G. Recovery and psychomotor effects after brief anesthesia with propofol and thiopental. *Anesth Analg.* 1989;68:S151.

Intubation and Airway Management

Christine S. Zambricki

Airway management, including the placement of various pharyngeal or endotracheal airway devices, is recognized as an area in which the CRNA possesses significant skill and proficiency. In the operating room, the CRNA routinely assesses and manages airway problems ranging from simple to complex with the aid of a variety of equipment, techniques, and pharmacologic agents. The CRNA also functions as a resource person outside of the operating room, providing airway management during cardiopulmonary resuscitation and situations where respiratory failure or insufficiency occurs.

The physical placement of an endotracheal tube is a technical skill that improves with practice and consistent attention to careful technique; however, successful airway management involves more than adept manual skills. It is an art requiring (1) sound clinical judgment based on knowledge of airway anatomy and physiology and a thorough history and physical assessment, (2) familiarity with state-of-the-art equipment and techniques, and (3) an understanding of the risks related to instrumentation and placement of artificial airways.

This chapter provides the reader with a thorough review of the principles of airway management as well as the technical aspects of instrumentation. The discussion covers the anatomy and physiology of the respiratory passages, airway assessment techniques, equipment, techniques, and potential complications in management.

ANATOMY AND PHYSIOLOGY OF THE AIRWAY

The respiratory passages provide a mechanism for the exchange of air between a person and the environment. These passages have been divided into two areas in series, the upper airway and the lower airway (Fig. 15–1). The term *upper airway* designates those portions of the respiratory passages superior to and including the larynx and comprising such structures as the nose, nasopharynx, oral cavity, laryngopharynx, and the larynx.

The nasal cavity is divided into two channels by the nasal septum, which is covered by vascular mucous membranes and supported by both bone and cartilage. Curving bony projections, called turbinates (superior, middle, and inferior), protrude into the nasal cavity from the lateral wall. Turbinates are covered by a mucous membrane well supplied with blood and provide additional surface area for the cleansing, humidification, and warming of inspired air. The rich blood supply of the nasal passages presents a hazard when trauma is incurred during nasal intubation. Pharmacologic agents such as cocaine may be used to constrict the nasal vasculature, thereby expanding the size of the nasal inlet and facilitating passage of a nasopharyngeal airway or nasoendotracheal tube.

The nasopharynx extends from the sphenoid and occipital bones superiorly along the posterior nasopharyngeal wall to the level of the soft palate, where it joins the oropharynx. The nasopharynx is of significance because it houses the lymphoid tissue called the pharyngeal tonsils or adenoids. This tissue may swell and cause nasal obstruction in children, an important consideration when attempting to ventilate a child with a mask. In these cases, the anesthetist must take care to keep the mouth open with an oropharyngeal airway or by maneuvering the mandible to achieve effective ventilation. The nasopharynx is connected to the middle ear by the eustachian tube.

The oropharynx is continuous with the nasopharynx, extending to the epiglottis inferiorly, and can be seen through the oral cavity. The paired palatine tonsils can be seen in the fossae between the anterior and posterior pillars and may impede visualization of the larynx if enlarged. The vallecula is the space lying between the base of the tongue and the epiglottis. As a point of reference for intubation, the tip of a cured laryngoscope blade is placed in the vallecula. The oral cavity is bound by the palate, oropharynx, tongue, and cheeks. Significant anatomic landmarks for the endoscopist include the uvula, soft palate, and posterior wall of the oropharynx. The tongue can be compressed and deflected, thereby enlarging the size of the oral cavity and improving visualization of anatomic structures.

The laryngopharynx extends from the epiglottis superi-

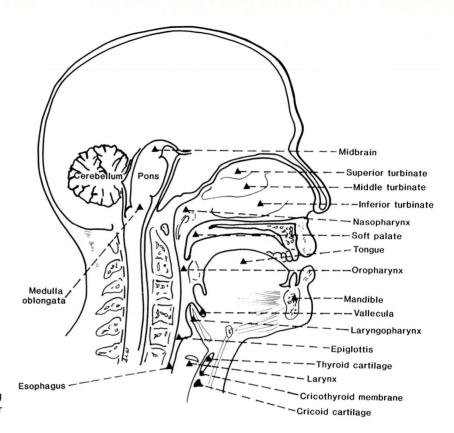

Figure 15–1. Sagittal section illustrating upper airway and superior portion of lower airway.

orly to the esophagus inferiorly. The laryngeal inlet lies anterior to the laryngopharynx at the level of C-4 to C-6. Important landmarks of endotracheal intubation, such as the epiglottis, aryepiglottic folds, and mucous membrane-covered arytenoid cartilages, are located within the laryngopharynx. The primary function of the pharyngeal musculature is to coordinate the act of swallowing with motor innervation via the vagus nerve (cranial nerve X). Sensory supply to the pharynx is provided by the glossopharyngeal nerve (cranial nerve IX).

Transition between the upper and lower airways occurs at the larynx. The opening to the larynx is called the rima glottidis. The predominant single cartilages forming the laryngeal skeleton are the thyroid, cricoid, and epiglottis. The three sets of paired cartilages (arytenoid, corniculate, and cuneiform) articulate to effect vocal cord functioning. The cricoid cartilage, located below the larynx, is the narrowest point in a child's airway, a fact of clinical significance because its size cannot be estimated by direct visualization. The cricoid cartilage is the only complete tracheal ring and as such there is no room to accommodate swelling without increasing airway resistance. Because the cricothyroid membrane is below the level of the vocal cords, it is the site most commonly used for emergency entry into the trachea.

The epiglottis, a flexible cartilage that lies superior to the vocal cords and attaches to the thyroid cartilage, provides an important anatomic landmark for endotracheal intubation. Its function is to occlude the glottic opening during swallowing. The vocal cords are composed of muscle,

ligament, submucosal soft tissue, and laryngeal mucosa. No cilia are present in the larynx. The vocal cords insert into the thyroid cartilage anteriorly and into the arytenoid cartilages posteriorly. Reinke's space, located just beneath the mucous membrane covering the vocal cords, is a space of potentially poor lymphatic drainage where fluid may accumulate and occlude the laryngeal inlet. Even slight swelling in this area will cause a tremendous amount of airway resistance, particularly in children.

The laryngeal ventricles lie above the true vocal cords. The false vocal cords, or vestibular folds, are located immediately superior to them. The false vocal cords function sphincterally to prevent aspiration of foreign material.[1]

The larynx functions primarily as (1) a gas-conducting conduit between the laryngopharynx and the trachea; (2) a sphincter to protect the lower airway from foreign substances; (3) a site of reflex origination, generating the cough reflex as well as cardiovascular and pulmonary changes; and (4) a speech generator, by modifying expired air in voice production. The sensory and motor innervation to structures of the larynx is of clinical significance to the anesthetist. Sensory innervation to the superior surface of the epiglottis is via the glossopharyngeal nerve (IX), whereas the superior laryngeal nerve (a branch of cranial nerve X) is the primary motor supply to all muscles of the larynx except the cricothyroid, which is supplied by an external branch of superior laryngeal nerve. Injury to the recurrent laryngeal nerve will result in vocal cord dysfunction. Recurrent laryngeal nerve function can be checked in the nonparalyzed patient by direct laryngoscopy. (Refer to

Chapter 36 for a more detailed discussion of vocal cord nerve damage and its sequelae.)

THE LOWER AIRWAY

The lower airway extends from the tracheobronchial tree to the lung parenchyma. The function of the tracheobronchial tree is to conduct, humidify, and heat inspired air. Alveolocapillary membrane exchange occurs distal to the terminal bronchioles. The trachea extends from the cricoid cartilage of the larynx to its bifurcation at the level of T-5. The trachea is approximately 14 cm in length and branches into two main bronchi at the carina. External landmarks for the tracheal bifurcation are the sternal angle anteriorly and the fourth thoracic spinous process posteriorly. The walls of the trachea are formed by a series of 16 to 20 C-shaped cartilages, whose open ends face posteriorly. The trachea is separated from the esophagus posteriorly by a muscle layer. A portion of the thyroid gland lies in front of the trachea at the second, third, and fourth tracheal cartilages. The trachea is near several large vessels of the neck, including the anterior and internal jugular veins, the inferior thyroid veins, and the innominate and carotid arteries. The vascular relationships are of obvious significance in the performance of tracheostomy or cricothyrotomy.

The trachea bifurcates into right and left mainstem bronchi with a 25-degree angle on the right and a 50-degree angle on the left. In the infant, both mainstem bronchi form angles of approximately 55 degrees, making it possible for the endotracheal tube to slip into either mainstem bronchus. Because pediatric tubes are cuffless, it is very easy for unintentional endobronchial intubation to occur. The mainstem bronchi are in series with the lobar bronchi, which then divide into segmental and subsegmental bronchi. Cartilage begins to disappear in the bronchioles at the end of the terminal bronchioles, where tissue is composed of simple epithelial cells. Distal to the terminal bronchioles are the alveoli, where the diffusion of gas occurs.

ASSESSMENT OF THE AIRWAY

Evaluation of the patient's airway is of primary concern to the anesthetist during the preoperative visit (see Chapter 11). This assessment begins with a thorough review of the patient's chart with special attention given to any suspicious findings related to potential airway problems such as altered arterial blood gases, abnormal pulmonary function studies, or genetic or anatomic alterations affecting normal head and neck anatomy. A lateral neck film may show a soft-tissue mass impinging on the trachea. Cervical films may demonstrate severe arthritic changes of the cervical spine. Whenever anticipated surgery involves the upper or lower respiratory passages, the patient's old charts should be scrutinized for information about previous diagnostic or surgical procedures. Not only should the anesthetist ascertain what agents and techniques were used, but she or he should also scan narrative comments that may indicate that there were multiple attempts at intubation. This should serve as ample warning for subsequent airway difficulties.

The overwhelming importance of the airway to the anesthetic care of the patient makes a thorough history and physical examination imperative. The patient interview should include questions about the presence of dyspnea, orthopnea, exercise tolerance, previous surgery, or pathology involving the airway, as well as a smoking history. The physical examination should routinely include inspection of the nose, nares, nasal septum, temporomandibular joint, dentition, oropharynx, and structures contained therein. The neck should be observed for symmetry and size, and the thorax should be examined for signs of chronic lung disease. The anterior neck should be palpated for masses and the orientation of the trachea to midline assessed. At the same time, an enlarged thyroid gland can be detected, if present. Maneuvers such as flexion/extension of the head and opening of the mouth should be requested of every patient. Lateral neck x-rays or indirect laryngoscopy with a dental mirror may be useful diagnostic adjuncts. The chest should always be auscultated in all fields.

Of special importance is the quality of the patient's dentition. The eruption of deciduous teeth generally begins by age 6 months and is complete by 2.5 years. Beginning at approximately 5 years and continuing until the 12th year, deciduous teeth are being replaced by permanent ones and are consequently loosely attached. The exposed incisors and canine teeth are most easily dislodged, being secured to the alveolar parts of the maxilla and mandible only by a single root. The adult patient may have loose or diseased teeth, which are susceptible to accidental extraction. Dental abnormalities such as missing teeth, chips, and the presence of crown or bridges should be noted on the anesthesia record or patient's chart preoperatively.

Anatomic characteristics that may make endotracheal intubation difficult under direct visualization include (1) a short muscular neck, (2) protruding maxillary incisors, (3) receding mandible, and (4) poor temporomandibular mobility (less than two fingerbreadths opening in mouth).[2] A simple test for predicting difficulty with endotracheal intubation can be conducted at the bedside. While viewing the base of the tongue, if the facial pillars (palatoglossal and palatopharyngeal arches) and uvula cannot be seen in a sitting patient with tongue protruding, visualization of the glottis is likely to be difficult. Another test to assess relative difficulty of intubation involves placing three fingers between the superior ridge of the thyroid cartilage and the tip of the mandible. If this distance is less than three fingerbreadths (5 to 6 cm), it is likely that the larynx is placed anteriorly and normal lines of vision, via laryngoscopy, may be interrupted.[3]

OBSTRUCTION

Upper airway obstruction is the most common type of obstruction encountered in clinical practice. The causes of upper airway obstruction are varied, and efforts must be made to distinguish the source of the problem so as to be able to relieve the obstruction effectively and quickly.

Soft-tissue obstruction is encountered frequently both in patient units and in the operating room. One common cause of soft-tissue obstruction is the loss of muscle tone, caused either by pathologic conditions of the central nervous system or by the effect of anesthetic agents, resulting in relaxation of the voluntary pharyngeal–laryngeal muscles. In a patient in the supine position, the tongue has a tendency to fall back into the pharynx, obstructing the laryngeal inlet. Soft-tissue obstruction is exaggerated in the edentulous patient, who may have resorption of alveolar bone.

Foreign materials such as food, vomitus, chewing tobacco, gum, and dentures may lead to upper airway obstruction. Retching or vomiting during induction or emergence may result from opioid premedication, suction, airway insertion, movement of the patient, or distension of the abdomen with air. Esophageal reflux may occur secondary to the use of muscle relaxants or in patients with bowel obstruction or ascites or in those who have recently eaten. Excessive manipulation of the airway to gain visual exposure may cause edema, hematoma, or bleeding, precipitating complete obstruction. Occasionally, the cause of upper airway obstruction may be direct injury of the pharynx or larynx. If a patient passes through a protracted excitement phase during induction or emergence, the jaw may clench tightly and the neck flex, resulting in obstruction. Accumulation of secretions during the induction phase of general anesthesia may potentiate upper airway obstruction. This condition is aggravated by repeated injections of succinylcholine, which tend to have a parasympathomimetic effect. Concomitant hypercarbia and hypoxemia potentiate the effect of respiratory distress and lead to additional problems in airway management.

Respiratory obstruction in the anesthetized patient is recognized by the sound of snoring or the feel of vibrations when the mask is being held. The reservoir bag may or may not continue to move, but the characteristics of the movement will be different from those in the unobstructed state. Direct inspection and chest auscultation of the patient to determine the quality of respirations is the best method for detection of airway obstruction. Indications of an obstructed airway are (1) the use of accessory muscles or presence of retractions; (2) jerking, downward movement of the trachea known as "tracheal tug"; or (3) a "rocking boat" respiratory pattern characterized by restricted chest movement resulting in a jerking abdominal motion as the diaphragm descends against the closed or obstructed glottis. These signs indicate the need for immediate clinical intervention.

The cause of upper airway obstruction dictates the strategy to be employed to relieve it. The anesthetist should proceed from simple corrective measures to more complex maneuvers involving actual instrumentation. Initially, an attempt should be made to hyperextend the neck, thereby positioning the tongue and soft tissue away from the posterior pharyngeal wall. A useful technique known as "angling of jaw" or subluxation is employed next. The mandible is displaced forward, with the anesthetist holding the angles of the patient's jaw slightly below and in front of each ear with bent forefingers. The thumbs assist in holding the mouth open. The mandible is pulled forward and maintained in this position. This strategy should be employed for only a short period because it may result in tenderness or swelling. The technique manually moves the tongue upward and may stimulate vigorous respiration. Should mechanical positioning not relieve soft-tissue obstruction,

an oropharyngeal or nasopharyngeal airway may be employed. If the obstruction persists, an endotracheal tube is placed. As a last resort, cricothyrotomy or tracheostomy may be considered.

Treatment of laryngospasm requires strategies different from those used to relieve soft-tissue obstruction. Laryngospasm is marked by a high-pitched crowing sound (partial laryngospasm) or the absence of sound and the inability to ventilate (complete laryngospasm). Dealing with laryngospasm requires distinguishing between partial and complete laryngospasm. Partial laryngospasm often occurs during light planes of anesthesia in response to surgical or pharyngeal stimulation. Attempts should be made to deepen anesthesia without additional airway manipulation. The anesthetist relaxes his or her grip on the mandible and mask and observes the reservoir bag for the quality of excursion, providing gentle positive pressure, if needed. Pharmacologic deepening of anesthesia must take place before further stimulation is continued. Partial laryngospasm can progress to complete laryngospasm with closure of the glottic opening. Sustained, moderate positive airway pressure of approximately 20 cm H_2O applied to the reservoir bag for 10 seconds is the first and primary strategy employed to "break" complete laryngospasm. This maneuver is particularly successful in children. Continual assessment is essential while the patient is in spasm, because no air exchange or ventilation is taking place. Succinylcholine (20 to 40 mg) is commonly used to relieve total laryngospasm in cases that are refractory to positive pressure.

LOWER AIRWAY OBSTRUCTION

Lower airway obstruction may be caused by a foreign body, lesions, excessive secretions, or bronchospasm. Pediatric patients are often found to have lower airway obstructions such as coins, food, and toys when they are brought to the operating room for bronchoscopy and removal of the foreign body. Adult patients may present with a pathologic lesion of the lower airway. This can be bypassed with a flexible wire-reinforced endotracheal tube. Depending on the level of the lesion, tracheostomy or cardiopulmonary bypass may be necessary for resection. Excessive, tenacious secretions may be sufficient to obstruct the bronchial lumen totally; subsequently pulmonary toilet or careful lavage may be required for secretion removal.

Bronchospasm is a form of lower airway obstruction manifested by bronchial smooth muscle contraction. The hallmark of bronchospasm is the patient's unexpected, total inability to ventilate in the absence of upper airway obstruction. Wheezes on both inspiration and expiration may precede bronchospasm; however, bronchospasm does not always follow wheezing. Intraoperatively, bronchospasm is treated by the administration of bronchodilating pharmacologic agents such as halothane, aminophylline, and terbutaline. In addition, endotracheal intubation may be necessary to ensure adequate oxygenation and ventilation. When aminophylline is selected, it can be administered in a loading dose of 5 to 7 mg/kg over 20 minutes, followed by a maintenance drip of 7 µg/kg/h. The patient should be carefully monitored by electrocardiogram for dysrhythmias during this period.

AIRWAY MANAGEMENT: EQUIPMENT, TECHNIQUES, AND COMPLICATIONS

Use of a Face Mask

The anesthetist must rely on the use of a variety of respiratory equipment in the administration of anesthesia or at times when manual techniques fail to relieve airway obstruction. Anesthesia apparatus and airway equipment can be lifesaving in skilled hands but can be the cause of iatrogenic complications when used by the inexperienced clinician.

Masks may be disposable or nondisposable (Fig. 15–2). A clear plastic mask allows detection of cyanosis or vomitus while the patient is wearing it; however, many anesthetists prefer the standard black masks, which conform better to facial structures. These masks are available in several shapes. A rubber mask may be surrounded by a pad that conforms to the shape of the patient's face. Some clear masks have a preinflated cushion designed for a tight seal. The preformed mask has no padding but is contoured to fit the patient's face and has minimal dead space. This is of particular importance in the pediatric patient. A mask should be selected to provide the best fit for a given patient. It should be pliant enough to be adjusted to the shape of a patient's face, but rigid enough not to dent when held tightly. A mask with a metal or plastic ring and hooks for head strap attachment allows easier airway management.

Selection of the proper size mask is of prime importance. After inspection of the patient's facial characteristics, the mask can be molded or manually shaped to approximate the patient's facial contours. A good fit can be obtained by spreading the bottom of the mask and placing it on the patient's chin before positioning the remainder of the mask (Fig. 15–3). The anesthetist holds the mask in place with the left hand, using the thumb to hold the top of the

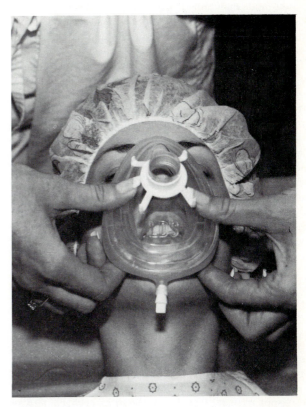

Figure 15–3. A good mask fit can be obtained by spreading the bottom of the mask and placing it on the patient's chin before positioning the remainder of the mask.

mask down and the third, fourth, and fifth fingers to direct the mandible cephalad. If the mask fit is good (Fig. 15–4), the anesthetist will not experience excessive fatigue or hand tremors. In some difficult or prolonged mask cases, the anesthetist may position his or her left elbow on the operating table to provide additional strength; however, with

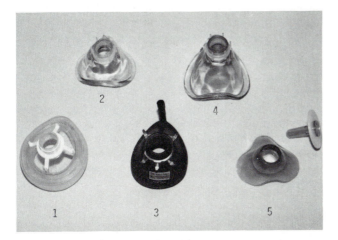

Figure 15–2. 1. Cushion-Flex single-use face mask by Life Design Systems. **2.** Transparent preformed single-use pediatric face mask by Dryden Corporation. **3.** Multiple-use rubber face mask by Ohio Medical Products. **4.** Transparent preformed single-use adult face mask by Dryden Products Corporation. **5.** Pediatric anesthesia mask (PAM), scented with pacifier, by Plasmedics.

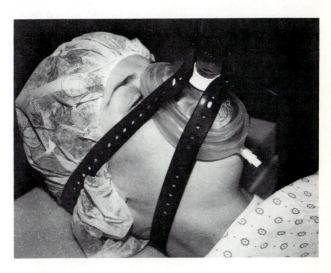

Figure 15–4. Proper mask fit with head strap attached.

experience this is not usually necessary. Anesthesia can be induced and maintained with a mask alone in many patients having minor surgery. Mask management is not appropriate for patients in the prone, sitting, or true lateral position.

Caution must be exercised when applying manual pressure on the mask to achieve a better fit and, consequently, a more patent airway. Excessive pressure will not correct the problem of respiratory obstruction and may damage the facial nerve. Once the mask is properly positioned and the airway secured, head straps may be applied to help stabilize the mask. The patient's ears must not be pinched or bent by the head strap, nor should the head strap apply undue pressure to the sides of the face or the eyes. Eye care is particularly important for the patient having general anesthesia by mask. The mask must not apply pressure to the orbital area. Eyes should be lubricated and taped closed, with eye patches applied if necessary. The danger of inadvertent damage by the anesthetist's fingers on the mask is compounded by the drying effect of gases that may blow on the eyes from small leaks at the superior bridge of the mask.

Use of Pharyngeal Airways

Pharyngeal airways are employed when respiratory obstruction is refractory to manual corrective measures. Two types of pharyngeal airways are in use: oropharyngeal and nasopharyngeal (Fig. 15–5). The oropharyngeal airway is inserted along the tongue and separates the posterior oropharynx and the base of the tongue. There are two basic styles of oropharyngeal airway, the Berman and the Guedel. Oropharyngeal airways are very stimulating to the awake or lightly anesthetized patient and may cause retching, vomiting, or laryngospasm. Care must be taken to select the proper size of oropharyngeal airway. Too large an airway may traumatize the oropharynx and mouth, whereas too

small an airway may push the back of the tongue against the posterior pharyngeal wall, thus potentiating obstruction. In cases where obstruction to lymphatic drainage of the head is expected, one size smaller airway may be selected because macroglossia can occur. Such situations include head and neck surgery or sitting cervical laminectomy.

The oropharyngeal airway should be placed quickly and carefully to avoid injury to the lips, teeth, or gingiva. With the left hand, a tongue blade is placed toward the posterior aspect of the tongue and the tongue drawn forward. The airway is inserted with the right hand. In no circumstances should the airway be twisted into place or forced between the clenched teeth of a lightly anesthetized patient. Occasionally the condition of the tongue or teeth precludes the use of an oral airway. After airway insertion, the teeth and gums should be inspected for pressure or trauma. A suction catheter can be passed along with the oral airway as required.

The nasopharyngeal, or Robertazzi airway, is a soft rubber tube designed to be inserted through the naris, passing along the curvature of the nasopharynx and oropharynx. When positioned correctly, this airway rests between the base of the tongue and the posterior pharyngeal wall. Because insertion of a nasopharyngeal airway is less stimulating than that of an oropharyngeal airway, it can be used in the awake or lightly anesthetized patient who develops airway obstruction and may not tolerate an oropharyngeal airway.

Nasopharyngeal airways come in different sizes ranging from pediatric to adult. To minimize trauma and bleeding, this airway should be coated with a local anesthetic lubricant before insertion. Its use should be avoided in patients with nasal septal deformity, leakage of cerebrospinal fluid from the nose, or coagulopathy. The nasopharyngeal airway should be inserted gently with one hand while the other hand is used to deflect the tip of the nose upward. The airway should be angled toward the occiput, following the natural contours of the nasal cavity, rather than superiorly. If resistance is encountered, the other naris should be tried.

The nasopharyngeal airway is too often an underused piece of anesthesia equipment. It may be inserted easily, requiring little skill, and is useful in patients who are unable or unwilling to open their mouths. A suction catheter can be passed through the middle of the airway if necessary to facilitate suction. Clinicians have reported circumstances in which airway obstruction was unrelieved by oropharyngeal airway insertion but was responsive to nasopharyngeal airway insertion. Regardless of whether an oropharyngeal or nasopharyngeal airway is selected, the anesthetist must develop the skill to insert the airway quickly and atraumatically.

Endotracheal Intubation

Although technology has made tremendous strides in the manufacture of endotracheal tubes, the advantages of endotracheal intubation are the same as they were in the 19th century. First and foremost, the patency of the airway is

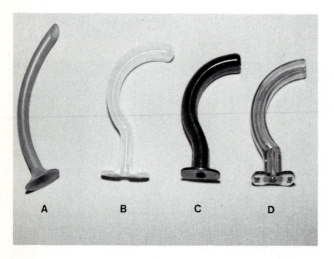

Figure 15–5. Pharyngeal airways: **A.** Robertazzi nasopharyngeal airway. **B.** Berman plastic oropharyngeal airway. **C.** Guedel rubber oropharyngeal airway. **D.** Guedel plastic oropharyngeal airway.

maintained with a high degree of reliability if the endotracheal tube is in position and unobstructed. The endotracheal tube allows positive-pressure ventilation and at the same time minimizes intragastric air. In addition, a cuffed endotracheal tube provides marked protection against aspiration of regurgitant, in contrast to pharyngeal airways, which provide no protection. Respirations can be maintained artificially by the anesthetist despite the position of the patient or the distance from the patient to the anesthetist. The tracheobronchial tree can be suctioned with relative ease. A further benefit is that the endotracheal tube reduces dead space by one half. Thus, it is clear that the placement of an endotracheal tube, when indicated, will allow the CRNA a degree of security not present when oropharyngeal or nasopharyngeal airways are used.

Indications. The numerous indications for endotracheal intubation can be classified in two broad categories: those mandated by patient characteristics and those mandated by the surgical procedure. Airway problems may arise unexpectedly, and the anesthetist must learn to look for them even when they do not fall into one of these categories.

The features that mandate endotracheal intubation can often be assessed during preanesthetic evaluation. The patient may possess anatomic traits that cause difficulty with a mask fit, such as protruding teeth or long-standing lack of teeth with concomitant resorption of alveolar bone, micrognathia or a malformed jaw, or facial features such as a prominent or broad, flat nose. The patient who presents with a short, fat, or thick neck should be elevated carefully. Beards or facial burns can also make mask management difficult.

Certain skeletal malformations such as kyphoscoliosis, cervical arthritis, or severe pectus excavatum predispose the patient to difficulties with ventilation. Traumatic injuries resulting in fractured ribs and an unstable chest wall require immediate intubation. Respiratory failure or insufficiency is also an indication for endotracheal intubation. Any type of severe respiratory dysfunction should be regarded as an indication for immediate intubation; however, the cause of respiratory distress must be determined to anticipate the possibility of prolonged postoperative intubation and ventilation.

The patient's general physical condition may be so poor that endotracheal intubation should be planned, even for the simplest procedure. For example, severe cardiac dysfunction, cachexia, or kidney failure may render the patient a poor risk; thus, the anesthetist should plan to have two hands available for case management. Although the critically ill patient can be managed with mask ventilation, the anesthetist must also plan for the postoperative period when the patient will most likely require mechanical ventilation with an endotracheal tube.

For general anesthesia, intubation is required for any patient with known or suspected gastric contents. This includes the intoxicated patient, the patient with pyloric stenosis, bowel obstruction, or ascites, and the pregnant patient. Although the cuff on the endotracheal tube does not provide a waterproof barrier to aspiration, it is the safest technique of aspiration prevention available for airway management when general anesthesia is necessary.

The position of the patient during surgery can preclude the use of a mask as the primary mechanism for ventilation. Patients assuming the prone or sitting position require endotracheal intubation. The true lateral position is an indication for placement of an endotracheal tube; however, mask management for patients in a modified lateral position has been reported. Although the lithotomy position does not require endotracheal intubation, the exaggerated lithotomy position makes mask management very difficult, especially when coupled with steep Trendelenburg.

Surgical procedures that involve the oral cavity, pharynx, or neck require that the patient be intubated as the surgeon and anesthetist will be sharing the airway. Surgical procedures of the head, such as neurosurgery, tympanomastoidectomy, or cleft palate repair, usually necessitate positioning the anesthetist distant from the patient's airway and from the surgical site. In addition, intracranial pressure increases can be avoided by accurate maintenance of $PaCO_2$ and PaO_2. Intrathoracic surgery clearly indicates endotracheal or endobronchial intubation. The majority of patients undergoing thoracic surgery have lung disease and require careful monitoring of their respiratory status intraoperatively. General anesthesia coupled with thoracic surgery profoundly affects the ventilation : perfusion ratio, thereby exacerbating existing problems. If pneumothorax is induced on incision into the thorax, the patient must receive controlled positive-pressure ventilation via the endotracheal tube to prevent paradoxical respiration and mediastinal shift.

Intubation is required for intraabdominal procedures for several reasons. Surgical retractors in the abdomen push abdominal contents cephalad against the diaphragm, making mask ventilation difficult. Unintentional introduction of air into the stomach with mask ventilation hinders the surgeon's work and prolongs the duration of anesthesia. Patients undergoing abdominal surgery often have delayed gastric emptying times, enhancing the risk of aspiration. Relaxation of the abdominal muscles must be adequate to allow the surgeon to explore the area unhindered. Once paralyzed, the intubated patient can be mechanically ventilated with ease and oxygenation uncompromised, especially when mechanical retraction is used.

Although practice varies, it is generally agreed that any surgical procedure lasting longer than 2 hours justifies endotracheal intubation. Longer procedures frequently require massive fluid and blood replacement, multiple anesthetic agents, and adjunct drugs. Endotracheal intubation allows the anesthetist freedom to respond to the demands of major surgery. If the surgical procedure is long but not major, such as multiple tendon repairs of the hand, the anesthetist may elect to intubate as a matter of convenience when administering a general anesthetic.

In addition to these indications, other circumstances may dictate the choice of endotracheal intubation. Rather than following a memorized list of indications, the anesthetist should apply the principles of sound airway management to the needs of the individual patient in the particular surgical situation. Sound clinical judgment and skilled technique are necessary to prevent mishaps caused by inappropriate airway management.

Equipment. Basic equipment for intubation includes a laryngoscope, endotracheal tube, and assorted connectors, adaptors, forceps, and stylets.

Laryngoscopes may be divided into two broad categories: those with straight blades and those with curved blades (Fig. 15–6). The straight (e.g., Miller) laryngoscope blade is designed to allow the tip of the blade to reach below the epiglottis and lift the epiglottis (Fig. 15–7). Because the underside of the epiglottis is innervated by the vagal nerve (cranial nerve X), some clinicians believe that this approach is more likely to lead to cardiac dysrhythmias. Nevertheless, the glottic structures are visualized in their entirety more frequently with the straight blade because of its direct lifting action. In the event of difficult intubation, a Harlan lock may be fitted between the blade and the laryngoscope handle to alter the laryngoscope configuration and help expose anatomic structures.

The curved blade (e.g., MacIntosh) conforms to the curvature of the tongue, with the tip of the blade being placed at the vallecula (Fig. 15–8). As the laryngoscope is lifted forward and upward, the glottis is pulled anteriorly and the underlying cords are exposed. The blade tip is said to stimulate the glossopharyngeal nerve (cranial nerve IX) with less risk of vagal-induced cardiopulmonary changes. The

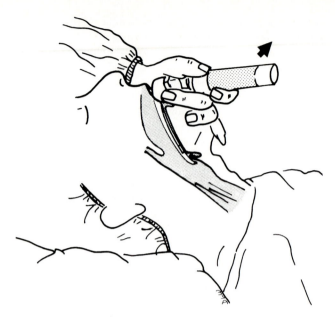

Figure 15–7. Proper placement of the straight blade on the inferior side of the epiglottis.

curved blade allows more room for maneuvering the endotracheal tube in the mouth and for this reason may be more appropriate for use in the obese patient.

Curved and straight-blade laryngoscopes have several features in common. The blades are interchangeable and are connected to the laryngoscope handle by means of a hook-and-bar mechanism. Contact is made between the blade, which contains a bulb, and the battery-containing handle

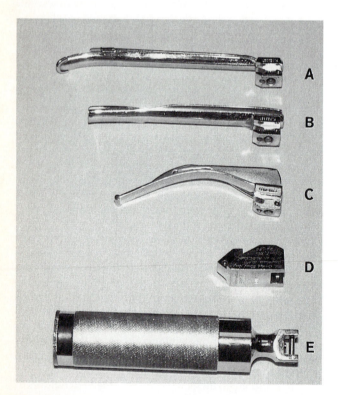

Figure 15–6. Laryngoscopes: **A.** Miller blade (straight). **B.** Wis-Foreggar blade (straight). **C.** MacIntosh blade (curved). **D.** Harlan lock. **E.** Laryngoscopy handle with bar latch; batteries are inside cylinder, which is entered by unscrewing the bottom of the handle.

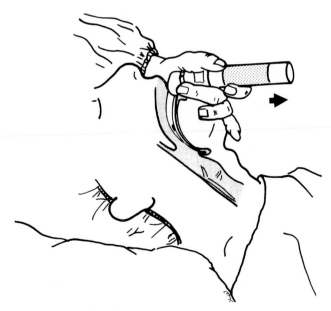

Figure 15–8. Proper placement of the curved blade, with blade tip in the vallecula.

when the laryngoscope is open and ready for use. Batteries can be replaced by unscrewing the base of the handle. Blades are manufactured in sizes ranging from 0 to 4. The handle of the laryngoscope comes in different diameters and may be constructed of aluminum or steel.

Nontraditional laryngoscopes have been developed in recent years for specific functions. Plastic, disposable laryngoscopes, designed for one-time use, are now available. Fiberoptic laryngoscopes have a brighter, whiter light than traditional laryngoscopes, without the electrical problems caused by wires and bulbs in the blade.[4] A plastic laryngoscope costs less than an ordinary laryngoscope, but the plastic can be used only once. A fiberoptic laryngoscope costs about twice as much as a traditional laryngoscope. The fiberoptic Bullard laryngoscope employs a unique blade–handle configuration and is said to facilitate difficult intubations. Teaching scopes and cameras are available for fiberoptic laryngoscopes.

Because the traditional-design laryngoscope has few working parts, troubleshooting in the event of malfunctions is simple. The laryngoscope is checked before use by attaching the handle securely and opening it such that the blade and handle are at 90-degree angles. The hook-and-bar latch must be securely in place or the equipment will not work. If the light does not go on, the bulb is checked to make sure it is screwed in properly. A new bulb may be substituted. The base of the handle can be unscrewed and the batteries checked. Rarely, if the laryngoscope has been damaged, the wire connection between the bulb and the proximal portion of the blade may be broken and the blade will not work. The laryngoscope should always be cleaned after use by disconnecting the blade from the handle, scrubbing the handle and blade, and immersing the blade in a disinfectant solution before the next use.

Most endotracheal tubes in use today are disposable and made of polyvinylchloride (PVC) (Fig. 15–9). The tube wall is generally marked with radiopaque lines for checking tube placement by x-ray. Some hospitals still use tubes of natural or synthetic rubber. Rubber substances have been found to be rigid, difficult to clean, and more irritating to tissue than the plastic substances available. PVC has gained popularity for artificial airways because it usually does not cause tissue reactions and is flexible within the airway. The PVC tube must be watched for kinking, especially when it is long and weighty rubber or metal corrugated tubes are attached to it. Kinking may take place inside the mouth or nose.

Endotracheal tube sizes reflect their internal diameter in millimeters, ranging from 2.0 to 10.0 mm in 0.5-mm increments (Table 15–1). The internal diameter of the tube is the most critical factor in determining airflow resistance. According to the laws of physics, resistance varies inversely with the fourth power of the radius of the tube. Tube selection for oral intubation is generally determined by the age and size of the patient: a size 7.5 for the average woman and a size 8.5 for the average man. A size 8.0 nasal endotracheal tube is the largest size used for female or male patients. Pediatric oral endotracheal tube sizes can be estimated by the following formula, which takes into account conversion from the French number: age + 18 divided by 4 = size of tube. A tube one size larger and a tube one size smaller than the one selected should be immediately available at the intubating location to account for unexpected patient variation. The tube used should be the largest one that can pass without force. The thickness of the tube may vary from 1 to 2 mm; therefore, a thin-walled tube will be easier to pass for a given size.

Tube length ranges from 11 to 28 cm and is designated on the tube, starting at the distal end. Oral endotracheal tubes may require cutting before use if they are not precut by the manufacturer. Proper length required can be estimated by placing the endotracheal tube along the patient's face and measuring from the level of the mouth to the angle of Louis, which is assumed to be the level of the carina. The tube should be of the proper length to position the cuff in the upper portion of the trachea and extend slightly out of the nose or mouth to allow attachment of ventilatory equipment to the endotracheal tube connector.

Manufacturers have designed variations of endotracheal tubes suited for the particular needs of the patient and

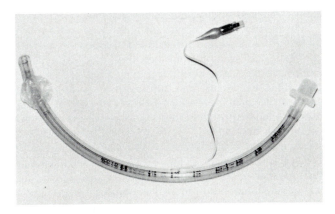

Figure 15–9. Disposable endotracheal tube with cuff and pilot balloon with valve.

TABLE 15–1. ENDOTRACHEAL TUBE SIZES FOR AVERAGE PATIENTS BASED ON AGE AND SEX

Age/Sex	Internal Diameter (mm)
Premature	2.0–2.5
Newborn	2.5
6 months	3.5
1 year	4.5
2 years	5.0
4 years	5.5
6 years	6.0
8 years	6.5
10 years	7.0
12 years	7.5
14 years	8.0
Adult	
Female	8.0–8.5
Male	9.0–9.5

anesthetist (Fig. 15–10). The anode, or armored, tube has a coiled wire within the wall of the tube, which prevents collapse or kinking. Because the wire support is not continuous to the proximal end of the tube, kinking may still take place between the connector and the wire. Noncollapsible tubes are preferred in procedures such as a radical neck surgery, where the surgeon may be manipulating the tube to a sharp angle. The anode tube is also used in instances of tracheal stenosis or when tumor compression of the trachea is present. Some clinicians prefer this type of tube whenever the head will be sharply flexed intraoperatively.

The oral or nasal Rae tubes were developed with a natural curvature in the tube to eliminate the need for additional curved connectors or adaptors during special procedures. The oral Rae tube is useful when the anesthetist will be positioned to the side of the patient, whereas the nasal Rae can be used in oral surgery, when the tube and ventilating hoses must be directed toward the anesthetist at the head of the table.

Double-lumen endobronchial tubes such as the Carlens, White, and Robertshaw have been developed to provide preferential ventilation of one lung during anesthesia (Fig. 15–11). These tubes are also used to isolate one lung in the event of massive hemorrhage or infection and are constructed differently from endotracheal tubes. Within the endobronchial tube, there is a double lumen through the length of the tube with both a tracheal and bronchial cuff to allow for distribution of ventilation.

Federal standards have been developed for artificial airways and influence the endotracheal tube design. The designation *I.T.* stands for "implantation tested," meaning that rabbits have been injected with the material and have not reacted to it. Standards for substance toxicity and tissue irritation are reviewed and revised by the American Society for Testing and Materials (ASTM) Committee F-29.

The tracheal tube cuff is generally built into the distal portion of the adult endotracheal tube and may be either

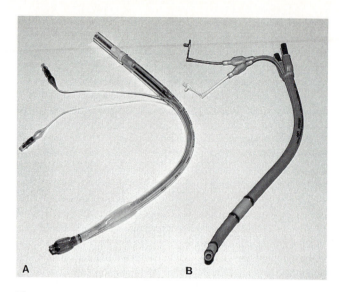

Figure 15–11. Endobronchial tubes. **A.** Robertshaw tube. **B.** Carlens tube.

"high residual volume" (low pressure) or "low residual volume" (high pressure). Pediatric tubes do not have a cuff because of the small diameter of the pediatric airway. The purpose of the cuff is to form a seal against the tracheal wall, thereby facilitating positive-pressure ventilation while at the same time discouraging aspiration of foreign material. Capillary blood flow in the area contacted by the cuff must be maintained and, as such, cuffs must not be overinflated. This is usually ensured if instillation of air into the cuff stops immediately after "leak" obliteration.

The intraarterial pressure of the tracheal wall has been estimated at 30 torr, whereas the venous end of the capillary bed has a pressure of 20 torr. Lymphatic flow in the tracheal area operates at a pressure of 5 torr. Sensitive devices implanted into the anterior tracheal wall have shown that pressures exerted by the cuff during endotracheal intubation may exceed 100 torr. Studies have demonstrated that maintaining intracuff pressure in high-residual-volume, thin-walled cuffs between 17 and 23 torr during spontaneous or controlled ventilation forms an effective seal and allows adequate capillary mucosal blood flow.

In recent years, a significant number of studies have looked at the characteristics of tracheal tube cuffs and the complications resulting from their use.[5–9] Various types of cuffs have been developed, including prestretched cuffs, cuffs filled with foam, and cuffs with pressure-regulated systems. The goal in developing these cuffs was to present the clinician with a high-residual-volume cuff that produced less tracheal wall pressure than the narrow, low-residual-volume cuff. Tracheal wall changes reported with the high-pressure cuff follow a distinct pattern. Mucosal inflammation and ciliary denudation occur under the cuff site within 2 hours. Within 24 hours mucosal edema is evident. Necrotic areas over the cartilaginous rings of the anterior tracheal wall will follow. Secondary infection may set

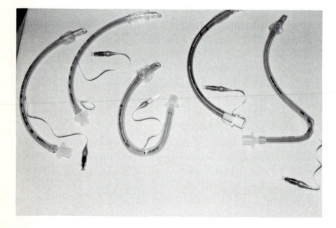

Figure 15–10. Variations of endotracheal tubes: **A.** Traditional endotracheal tube. **B.** Endotrol by National Catheter, with plastic ring for deflecting tip of endotracheal tube. **C.** Rae tube for oral use. **D.** Disposable armored tube. **E.** Rae tube for nasal use.

in, and with continued cuff inflation, tracheal rings may soften. Further pressure can lead to posterior erosion into the esophagus or anterior erosion into the innominate artery. The changes are explained by the physical principles of cuff inflation within a closed space. As air is introduced, elastic forces within the cuff cause expansion until the cuff touches the walls of the trachea. As more air is added to the cuff, the trachea is further compressed. High-residual-volume cuffs have the advantage of conforming to the shape of the trachea with minimal increase in cuff or mucosal pressure. Although data suggest that endotracheal tubes with compliant cuffs should be chosen over those with stiff cuffs, certain precautions still must be observed. The compliant cuffs are easy to overinflate because little resistance is felt. Although inadvertent overinflation of the cuff is less likely to produce damaging pressure on the trachea, the cuffs can occlude the beveled end of the endotracheal tube, obstructing the airway.

Nitrous oxide and other gases diffuse into air-inflated tracheal tube cuffs and increase volume and pressure in all cuffs. Intraluminal pressure may also increase as the air in the cuff is warmed to body temperature. Cuff volume increases will vary with exposure time, cuff thickness, partial pressure of nitrous oxide, and cuff composition. The anesthetist must assume that there is nitrous oxide diffusion into a cuff inflated with air and must deflate the cuff to the minimal occluding volume approximately every 30 minutes. The anesthetist can fill the cuff with the anesthetic gas mixture to prevent diffusion. Cuff pressure can then be adjusted with a syringe to allow sufficient tracheal capillary blood flow. A device that monitors the intraluminal pressure of the cuff is available.

Desirable cuff characteristics include (1) a thin wall, (2) a large diameter and high compliance, (3) a large enough residual volume to allow for positive endotracheal pressure, and (4) tear resistance. Cuff thickness determines the size of folds on channels formed when the cuff is inflated in the trachea. Thin folds decrease the channeling of liquids and offer better protection against aspiration. Although thick cuffs slow the diffusion of nitrous oxide, eventually the same volume of nitrous oxide will diffuse.

The anesthetist's armamentarium for airway management includes other equipment (Fig. 15–12). Endotracheal tubes are supplied with straight 15-mm connectors, but curved connectors of plastic or metal may be substituted for convenience of positioning. Straight or curved adaptors can be used to link the connector with corrugated tubing or other ventilatory equipment. A specialized connector has been developed for use with a fiberoptic bronchoscope, allowing ventilation via the endotracheal tube during the procedure.

A stylet is a malleable probe used to give shape and form to the endotracheal tube. Stylets are constructed of copper or aluminum and may be plastic coated. The stylet is inserted into the endotracheal tube with its tip approximately one-half inch from the beveled end of the tube. The stylet should never extend into or beyond the bevel because tracheal perforation or vocal cord damage may result. The stylet is bent once, away from the operator at the tube connector, to prevent it from inadvertently going too far down

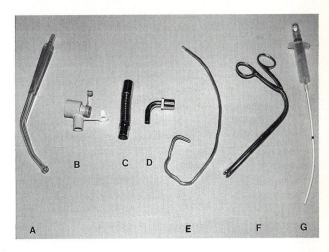

Figure 15–12. Additional airway equipment: **A.** tonsil suction; **B.** connector for use with fiberoptic bronchoscope; **C.** metal flex connector; **D.** metal curved connector; **E.** stylet; **F.** McGill forceps; **G.** laryngeal–tracheal anesthesia kit.

into the tube. Stylets should be avoided in nasal intubation, especially in patients with head trauma.

The lighted stylet is a flexible light source placed in the endotracheal tube prior to attempting intubation. The stylet is flexed to a "hockey stick" configuration. When the room lights are turned off, transillumination during tube advancement results in a diffuse circle of light visualized on the anterior surface of the neck as the lighted stylet approximates the larynx. The endotracheal tube can be advanced over the lighted stylet into the trachea.[10,10a]

McGill forceps are long-necked forceps that are commonly used to direct the tip of the tube anteriorly during nasoendotracheal intubation. These forceps grasp the tube immediately superior to the cuff. They may be helpful in guiding an oral endotracheal tube or nasogastric tube as well. Caution must be used to keep the forceps from inadvertently grabbing mucosal tissue or the uvula with their serrated tips. This complication may result in hemorrhage requiring surgical intervention. A tonsil suction has an advantage over the traditional flexible suction catheter in that it can be manipulated with one hand during laryngoscopy. One disadvantage of the tonsil suction is that it cannot be used through an endotracheal tube.

The laryngeal tracheal anesthesia kit contains local anesthetic for topical application to the lower pharynx, larynx, and trachea. This anesthesia technique requires laryngoscopy and is applied before placement of the endotracheal tube. The usual dose is 100 to 120 mg of Xylocaine absorbed through mucous membranes. Full effect is achieved within a few minutes.

Technique. The trachea can be cannulated using either the oral or nasal route. Many of the principles are the same regardless of the route employed. Before beginning the procedure, the patient must be positioned on a stationary table or bed with the head at the level of the anesthetist's xiphoid process. The anesthetist should be positioned behind the patient's head. A 4-in. pad or pillow should be positioned under the patient's head to provide optimum alignment of the oral, pharyngeal, and laryngeal axes. Good lighting is essential to allow continual assessment of the patient's mucosa and integument for cyanosis. A tonsil suction is set up for use before the actual insertion of the endotracheal tube, and a suction catheter should be available for deep tracheal suctioning afterward.

A resuscitation bag and mask of the appropriate size are necessary, not only for checking placement of the endotracheal tube but for use in the event that the anesthetist is unable to intubate a patient experiencing airway distress. The reservoir bag that is part of the anesthesia circuit may be used for the same purpose. Universal precautions, including the use of gloves, mask, and protective eyewear, must always be employed when conducting airway maneuvers. This technique provides protection against inadvertent exposure to body fluids.

Oral Intubation. All required equipment should be assembled before beginning the procedure. For oral endotracheal intubation, the following equipment is necessary: local anesthetic lubricant, oral airway, tongue blade, laryngoscope, oral endotracheal tube with 15-mm connector, stylet, 10-mL syringe, and suction and positive-pressure ventilation apparatus. Laryngoscope function should be checked and the endotracheal tube cuff assessed for airtightness.

The technique for oral endotracheal intubation is best learned through study of the following sequence and practice. Initial attempts at intubation should concentrate on maintaining good technique rather than on success of the placement. Common errors and difficulties of the novice are (1) insertion of the laryngoscope blade too far, (2) excessive hyperextension of the head, (3) loss of control of the tongue, (4) failure to position the blade midline, and (5) prying on the teeth and bending the wrist.

Immediately before intubation, the patient's head must be properly positioned to maximize visualization. Two head positions are commonly used for endotracheal intuba-

tion (Fig. 15–13). The "sniffing" or "amended" position has been shown to improve alignment of the axis of the oral cavity, pharynx, and trachea (Fig. 15–13A). This position is achieved by placing a 4-in. pad or pillow under the patient's occiput, without elevating the shoulders. Extreme hyperextension of the head is not required; gentle extension of the atlantooccipital junction will facilitate intubation. Although this position improves visualization, it does require the pad or pillow, which may not be readily available in an emergency situation. The sniffing position is contraindicated in patients with known or suspected injury of the cervical spine.

In contrast to the sniffing position, the classic or Jacksonian position is one in which the patient's shoulders and head remain on the bed or table (Fig. 15–13B). The disadvantage of this position is that the lip-to-glottis distance is elongated and the larynx rotated anteriorly. Gentle hyperextension of the head with the right hand at the occiput will stabilize the head during intubation (Fig. 15–14).

Table 15–2 summarizes the oral endotracheal intubation technique. When learning the technique of laryngoscopy, it is helpful to memorize the anatomic landmarks in sequence (Table 15–3). These can be used as checkpoints while performing laryngoscopy to ensure successful visualization.

Nasal Intubation. Certain situations indicate the need for a nasal approach to tracheal cannulation. A nasal tube is necessary for patients who are unable to open the mouth or hyperextend the neck, making laryngoscopy and ventilation impossible. It is desirable for oral surgical cases where the surgeon will be doing extensive work in the mouth or on the jaws. Nasoendotracheal intubation is a good choice for patients who will require long-term ventilation postoperatively because the tube is easier to stabilize and more comfortable for the patient. Patient oral hygiene is more readily maintained without an oral endotracheal tube in the mouth.

Contraindications to the nasal approach do exist.

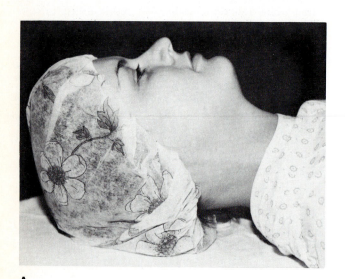

A

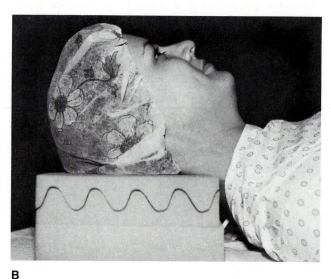

B

Figure 15–13. Positioning the head for endotracheal intubation: **A.** Sniffing or amended position. **B.** Classic or "Jacksonian" position.

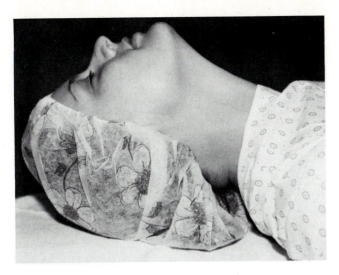

Figure 15–14. Classic Jacksonian position with gentle hyperextension.

Patients with coagulopathies are not good candidates for nasoendotracheal intubation because of the vascularity of the nasal mucosa. This technique should be avoided in patients suffering from a dural tear presenting with cerebrospinal fluid draining from the nose, and in those with a nasal injury, acute sinusitis, or mastoiditis. If the patient has an extremely deviated septum or difficulty breathing through the nose, nasal intubation should be avoided if possible.

All equipment for nasoendotracheal intubation must be assembled before beginning the procedure. Necessary equipment includes vasoconstricting nose drops, laryngoscope, soft nasal airway, local anesthetic lubricant, nasal endotracheal tubes with 15-mm connector, oral tubes, 10-mL syringe, McGill forceps, and suction and positive-pressure ventilation apparatus. A stylet is never used for nasal intubation.

Immediately before intubation, the patient is properly positioned in the sniffing position. If the procedure is to be carried out on an awake patient experiencing respiratory distress, the patient may remain in a semi-Fowler's position. Oral endotracheal tubes are available for use in the event of difficulty with the nasal approach. Before attempting nasal intubation, the anesthetist should identify which naris is more patent by asking the patient which side of the nose he or she can breathe through better. If there is no surgical or patient-based indication to use the left naris, the right naris is preferred for mechanical convenience to the anesthetist. The anesthetist may also measure the length of the nasotracheal tube using anatomic landmarks (Fig. 15–15). The tube should be cut at the level of the naris and the connector reinserted to prevent kinking.

Table 15–4 summarizes the technique for nasal endotracheal intubation in the anesthetized patient.

Intubation via the nasal route has some disadvantages. It is not uncommon for the pressure of the tube to cause necrosis in the area of the ala nasi in patients requiring long-term intubation. Once in place, the nasal tube can totally obstruct sinus drainage, leading to acute sinusitis. It

TABLE 15–2. ORAL ENDOTRACHEAL INTUBATION TECHNIQUE

1. Obtain good lighting. Position the patient on a nonmoving surface in sniffing position, with the head at the level of the anesthetist's xiphoid process.
2. Open the mouth with the right hand by gently depressing the mandible with the thumb. It is not usually necessary to put the fingers in the mouth; on rare occasions, if the anesthetist's fingers are placed in the patient's mouth to facilitate opening, gloves should be worn.
3. Using the left hand, place the laryngoscope blade in the right side of the mouth. Move the laryngoscope to the midline, deflecting the tongue to the left. The blade should be perpendicular to the patient's body.
4. Maintaining a midline orientation, continue to direct the laryngoscope blade down the pharynx. The anatomic landmarks seen will be the uvula, the oropharyngeal wall, and the epiglottis.
5. If a straight laryngoscope blade is used, advance the blade approximately 1 cm beyond the epiglottis. At this point, the blade tip lifts up the epiglottis as the anesthetist lifts the laryngoscope forward and upward, and the glottis is exposed (direct exposure).
6. If a curved laryngoscope blade is used, advance the blade and place the tip in the vallecula. The laryngoscope is lifted upward and forward, thereby exposing the glottis (indirect exposure).
7. Using the right hand, direct the endotracheal tube into the right side of the oral cavity and pharynx and through the vocal cords. If a stylet is used, it is withdrawn as the tube passes through the vocal cords. The anesthetist must watch the cuff pass through the cords.
8. Connect the apparatus for positive-pressure ventilation to the endotracheal tube. Listen to breath sounds bilaterally in all quadrants and auscultate the stomach. Observe chest excursion and note the appearance of humidity in the oral endotracheal tube. Capnography should be checked for the presence of a CO_2 waveform.[11] Inflate the cuff of the endotracheal tube by injecting air into the pilot balloon until there is no leak.
9. Insert an oral airway and secure the tube.

may also block the eustachian tube in the nasopharynx, resulting in otitis media. The nasal tube may kink within the nose, leading to acute airway obstruction. This most commonly occurs as the tube warms to body temperature.

Intubation of the Awake Patient. There are situations in which awake intubation is indicated, either in the operating room before surgery or in the patient's room. The nasal route is preferred for awake intubation unless contraindications to this approach exist. The nasal tube can often be

TABLE 15–3. ANATOMIC LANDMARKS USED IN INTUBATION

Mouth

Uvula

Posterior pharynx

Epiglottis

Glottis

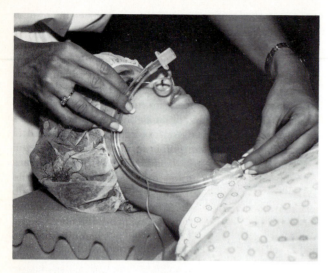

Figure 15–15. Measuring the length of a nasotracheal tube using external landmarks: suprasternal notch, earlobe, and naris.

placed "blindly," that is, without laryngoscopy and visualization of the glottis. There is currently available a nasal tube that has at the proximal end a ring connected via the tube wall to the tip of the tube. Pulling up on the ring curves the tip of the tube upward so that it can pass through the vocal cords more easily. Blind nasal intubation can be facilitated by changing the position of the patient's head

**TABLE 15–4. NASAL ENDOTRACHEAL
INTUBATION TECHNIQUE**

1. Position the patient. Apply vasoconstricting drops to both nares. Anesthetize the patient.

2. Insert a well-lubricated soft nasal airway in the naris to be used for intubation to ascertain nasal patency. Ventilate.

3. Remove the nasopharyngeal airway. Using the left hand to gently push up on tip of the nose, insert the lubricated nasal endotracheal tube, following the contours of the vestibule of the nose, going from the nostril and backward and down into the nasopharynx. With steady pressure, advance the tube until loss of resistance occurs.

4. Using the right hand, open the mouth by depressing the mandible and insert the laryngoscope blade into the right side of the mouth using the left hand.

5. As the laryngoscope is moved midline, the tip of the nasal tube should be seen in the pharynx. If it is not, advance the tube further until the tip is identified.

6. Advance the endotracheal tube and laryngoscope simultaneously. Exposure of the glottis is obtained and the tube inserted. The cuff of the tube should bypass below the vocal cords.

7. Remove the laryngoscope and attach the endotracheal tube connection to the breathing circuit. Apply positive pressure and check tube placement by auscultating the chest bilaterally, followed by ausculation over the stomach. Capnography should be checked for the presence of a CO_2 waveform. The cuff is inflated until no leak is present and the nasal tube is secure.

from side to side or from flexion to extension. The anesthetist listens to breath sounds from the endotracheal tube and advances the tube toward them. Loss of breath sounds is cause to withdraw the tube slightly and redirect it or reposition the patient. When the breath sounds become very audible or the patient coughs, the tube should be firmly advanced. Cessation of breath sounds, lack of humidity appearing on the tube, or regurgitant material in the tube is evidence of failure to pass the tube through the glottis. At times the tube may appear as a bulge on the outside of the neck. It should then be withdrawn slightly and redirected.

It is not possible to intubate every patient using the blind technique. If there have been several attempts, it is best to open the patient's mouth and proceed with direct laryngoscopy. McGill forceps may be necessary to direct the tube into the trachea. The patient in respiratory distress is a poor candidate for multiple intubation attempts; if the tube cannot be passed easily by the blind technique, it is best to move quickly to direct laryngoscopy. Often, lifting the patient's head up slightly at the occiput will facilitate movement of the tube into the larynx in those patients who have anteriorly placed laryngeal anatomy.

Oral endotracheal intubation can also be performed in the awake patient, although it is not usually attempted without using laryngoscopy. Awake oral intubation is chosen for the patient suspected of impending respiratory or cardiac arrest and for patients with nasal injuries requiring general anesthesia if the ability to ventilate the patient is in question. Awake intubation is the safest technique for a patient who has a full stomach and requires general anesthesia.

Awake intubation using either the nasal or oral approach is not without risk. The procedure is extremely stimulating and uncomfortable for the patient. Laryngoscopy can elicit violent cough and gag reflexes in the awake patient. This reaction is of particular danger to the patient with suspected cervical injury, increased intracranial pressure, or increased intraocular pressure. Complications may be induced in the patient with coronary artery disease, hypertension, or asthma. For these patients, awake intubation should be avoided if at all possible.

Before beginning awake intubation, the anesthetist should prepare the patient so as to minimize discomfort and maximize cooperation. The proposed procedure should be explained in simple terms, along with the reason why this approach is desirable. Whenever possible, time should be taken to provide maximum analgesia and amnesia for the procedure via traditional intravenous agents, ever cautious not to overdose and compromise ventilation. The patient can receive titrated doses of sedatives with an amnesic effect such as diazepam and lorazepam. Small doses of short-acting narcotics, such as fentanyl, can be given incrementally to minimize discomfort. The use of a fentanyl citrate and droperidol (Innovar) drip has also been reported for sedation. Again, caution must be taken to avoid respiratory depression lest the patient develop the airway problems that awake intubation is meant to avoid.

If nasal intubation is planned, vasoconstrictive drops should be applied at least 1 minute before beginning. A well-lubricated nasopharyngeal airway should first be passed to provide local anesthesia to the mucosal surface of the nose. Cocaine can be applied to the mucosa with either pledgets or cotton swabs, to minimize bleeding and achieve local anesthesia. If laryngoscopy is necessary, the laryngoscope should be rinsed with warm water and the local anesthetic lubricant applied to the blade. A local anesthetic spray can be applied in stages to the oral cavity and pharynx. Once the tongue is anesthetized, it can be displaced forward with a tongue blade and the lower portion of the pharynx sprayed. The patient, if cooperative, can gargle with viscous lidocaine for additional anesthesia. A recurrent laryngeal or superior laryngeal nerve block may also be performed, mindful that such a maneuver in the compromised or obtunded patient is unwise.

Complications with an Endotracheal Tube in Place. An endotracheal tube in place interferes with the normal functions of the airway, such as coughing, humidification, and speech. Because the patient cannot mobilize secretions with a cough, the anesthetist must suction the tracheobronchial tree via the endotracheal tube. Most patients will require suctioning periodically during lengthy surgery and at the end of the procedure; patients with copious secretions may require suctioning more frequently.

Serious complications may result from improper suctioning. Therefore, it is most important to incorporate sound procedure into the anesthetic care plan. Sterile technique, using a sterile glove for the hand holding the catheter, must be used whenever possible. The suction catheter should never pass from the oropharynx to the endotracheal tube as this may prompt bronchial infections. The suction catheter is inserted without vacuum, and intermittent suction is applied during removal. Suctioning during the surgical procedure is best performed during periods of maximal relaxation. The patient should be well oxygenated before and after tracheal suctioning. The suction catheter should remain in the airway no longer than 15 seconds. Various humidified circuits are now available for use on anesthesia machines. These devices are particularly helpful for patients undergoing prolonged surgery or for pediatric patients receiving anesthesia via a nonrebreathing system. When intubation is expected to continue in the recovery room, the patient should be instructed preoperatively about ways to communicate while the tube is in place. A pencil and pad can be available at the bedside. All attempts at talking with the tube in place should be discouraged, because trauma to the vocal cords can occur. Despite the many advantages of endotracheal intubation, the procedure is not without risk. Intubation may cause chipped or broken teeth and damage to the lips, tongue, or mucous membranes of the oral cavity and pharynx. Epistaxis and hemorrhage are possible.

Airway emergencies can still occur once the endotracheal tube is inserted. Tube obstruction may result from a variety of causes. The cuff can slip or overinflate, occluding the end of the tube. This can be relieved by deflating the cuff. The tube may kink or collapse. This can be corrected by manipulating the tube or the patient's head. Secretions or a foreign body may also occlude the tube. In normal circumstances, suction will remove the obstructing material; however, in certain situations the tube will have to be replaced. The bevel of the tube may lodge against the tra-

cheal wall; this problem can be remedied by tube manipulation.

Cuff leaks are not only bothersome but dangerous, and ventilation must be maintained with increased tidal volumes while the cause of the problem is ascertained. In the case of nasal intubation, cuff leakage is assumed to result from damage to a cuff during insertion. Sudden air leakage and failure to maintain a closed system require performance of a direct laryngoscopy. Often the problem is that the cuff is superior to the cords. Passage of a nasogastric tube into the trachea resulting in a large air leak has been reported. If tube replacement is necessary because of a damaged cuff, the new tube is inserted along the existing tube while the larynx is visualized. The malfunctioning tube is then removed and a new tube inserted under direct visualization.

Malpositioning of the tube is another airway problem that can occur after the anesthetist has completed the intubation procedure. The tube may slip down into the bronchial tree, resulting in unilateral ventilation or ventilation–perfusion inequality. Sometimes it is difficult to hear breath sounds over the lung fields because of abnormal chest configuration. In other instances, auscultation of the chest produces the sound of air although the tube is positioned in the esophagus. When any doubt exists, the anesthetist should quickly auscultate over the stomach. If doubt lingers, laryngoscopy should be performed and the tube position verified visually. Observation of chest excursion and auscultation of breath sounds should always be repeated after the patient's position is changed intraoperatively.

The tube may become dislodged and unintentional extubation occur. This airway emergency can have dire consequences if the patient is in the sitting or prone position. Prevention requires that the tube always be secured properly from the start. Continuous monitoring of lung sounds via a precordial stethoscope allows the anesthetist to detect intraoperative extubation immediately. In the event of accidental extubation, the surgeon should be informed and the patient ventilated with 100 percent oxygen. Reintubation should take place as soon as possible.

Airway emergencies also occur when the tube is patent and properly positioned but there is a break in the ventilating circuit. This circumstance is characterized by complete loss of the patient's breath sounds and chest excursion. Systematic checking of the entire circuit, from patient to gas machine, will usually reveal the cause. If the cause is difficult to diagnose, the patient must be ventilated meanwhile, either by Ambu bag or mouth-to-tube ventilation. Intubation during light planes of anesthesia can result in breath holding, prolonged cough, and spasm of the chest wall or bronchi. Deepening of the anesthetic usually relieves the difficulty. Additional measures, such as the administration of succinylcholine or aminophylline, may be required.

Extubation. At the end of the surgical procedure, the patient is extubated if there are no indications for continued endotracheal intubation. If no muscle relaxant has been used, the patient may be extubated either at a deep plane of anesthesia or when reflexes have returned. Extubation during light planes of anesthesia can result in breath holding and laryngospasm. Deep extubation takes place when spontaneous respirations are present but the patient has not begun to cough on the tube or move. The procedure for carrying out deep extubation is as follows.

When spontaneous respirations are present, the nitrous oxide is turned off and the anesthetic deepened by increasing the concentration of inhalation agent. Spontaneous respiration must be maintained. Gentle suctioning may take place at this time (reflex response to suctioning occurs when the patient is at too light a plane of anesthesia). If the patient is assessed to be in a sufficiently deep plane, the cuff is deflated and the tube removed while positive-pressure ventilation is applied. Extubation on inspiration is less likely to cause laryngospasm. If laryngospasm should occur, the lungs are full of oxygen so that passive diffusion may take place during the temporary lapse in ventilation. Once the tube is removed, 100 percent oxygen is administered via mask and the patient is allowed to awaken. Miscalculation in timing of deep extubation may result in complications such as breath holding or laryngospasm. Deep extubation is indicated when the patient's condition demands the absence of coughing or bucking on the endotracheal tube (e.g., with increased intraocular or intracranial pressure, asthma, or severe cardiovascular disease). Deep extubation is contraindicated in patients with a full stomach or airway difficulties.

Administration of muscle relaxant intraoperatively adds another dimension to the question of when to extubate. In this instance, the anesthetist is not only concerned that the patient be awake and reflexic but that an adequate number of skeletal muscle receptors be unoccupied. There are several methods for assessing adequacy of muscle relaxant reversal. The patient who can demonstrate a "train of four" in response to peripheral nerve stimulation has somewhat less than 75 percent of receptors occupied. This tool is useful for assessment in the operating room but less suitable for the emerging or awake patient because the stimulus is painful. The emerging patient should also be checked per peripheral nerve stimulator (PNS) for presence of sustained tetanus.

Sustained antigravity movement, such as lifting the head on request, is a better alternative. The patient must begin in a supine position and deliberately raise his or her head without the use of handrails. The movement should be purposeful and sustained for 5 seconds. Jerking, coughing movements of the head in response to a tracheal stimulus does not qualify the patient for extubation. Grip strength is an indicator of receptor occupancy. Bilateral grip strength can be compared with preoperative norms. This measure, although difficult to quantify, is useful for patients who were unable to lift their heads preoperatively.

Measurement of the negative inspiratory pressure is a useful indicator of muscle power and the patient's ability to generate an effective cough. The equipment required is relatively inexpensive and simple to use. A manometer is connected via plastic tubing to a three-way adaptor, which is connected to the endotracheal tube. While the anesthetist occludes the port, the patient is instructed to breathe. The pressure measured on the manometer reflects the negative "pulling power" of the lungs and diaphragm. A negative inspiratory pressure (NIP) of -20 cm H_2O correlates with a vital capacity of 15 mL/kg or greater and compares well

with the train of four for assessment of muscle relaxant reversal.

The patient's ability to self-extubate is never considered an appropriate measure of muscle relaxant reversal. The patient is receiving a strong airway stimulus from the indwelling endotracheal tube and possibly an oropharyngeal airway. The patient may muster all possible strength to remove the endotracheal tube, only to lapse into respiratory depression once the tube is out. Self-extubation does not guarantee that the patient has adequate muscle power to generate an effective cough or handle secretions. Damage to the vocal cords can result from self-extubation with the cuff inflated.

Once the decision has been made to extubate, the procedure should be explained to the patient in simple terms if the patient is alert enough to understand. The trachea, pharynx, and oral cavity should be suctioned. Oxygen is delivered after tracheal suctioning, before extubation. The cuff on the endotracheal tube is deflated and the tube removed on inspiration. The awake patient should be instructed to open his or her mouth and take a deep breath to facilitate a quick, safe extubation. Oxygen is administered after extubation and the patient is carefully observed for signs of obstruction or laryngospasm. The period immediately after extubation is a critical one because of the many complications that can follow extubation.

Postextubation Complications. Laryngospasm may occur when the patient is in a light plane of anesthesia and has been extubated. Laryngospasm may be caused by retained secretions that are at the vocal cords postextubation. Treatment of laryngospasm includes the administration of oxygen using positive-pressure apparatus and possibly succinylcholine. Tracheal collapse after extubation has been reported in patients with prolonged intubation, which weakens the cartilaginous rings of the trachea. Thyroid disease or large cervical or mediastinal tumors may also result in tracheal collapse. Immediate reintubation is clearly indicated in this event.

Extubation is contraindicated in any patient suffering from respiratory distress. Poor arterial blood gas values should warn of the danger of proceeding with a planned extubation. In no circumstances should a patient be extubated without the presence of someone who can ventilate the patient and replace the airway if necessary. Many complications of endotracheal intubation manifest themselves only after extubation. Predisposing factors are varied and, in many cases, avoidable. Clinicians report that complications are more frequent in elderly, debilitated patients, with women affected more often than men. Factors that contribute to complications include excessive movement of the tube while in place, use of too large a tube for the patient's larynx,[12] traumatic intubation or multiple attempts at intubation, and poor sterile technique. The most common complaints expressed by patients postextubation are sore throat and laryngitis because during the process of intubation the epithelial layer of the mucous membrane lining the respiratory tract is traumatized. This condition spontaneously clears within 2 to 3 days with adequate hydration.

Glottic and subglottic edema may occur as a result of traumatic intubation by a tight-fitting tube.[13] Rarely, a patient may develop edema in response to the polyvinyl chloride tube. Ventilatory obstruction results from subepithelial edema of the epiglottis, vocal cords, and subglottic area. High-pitched, progressive inspiratory stridor is a key indicator of subglottic or glottic edema. This condition is treated by reassurance, topical decongestant via aerosol, and possibly steroids. The patient must be kept immediately available in case reintubation is necessary. Ulceration of the tracheal mucosa may occur at the cuff site or the anterior wall where the tip of the tube has denuded the epithelium. Infection may occur as a secondary complication.

Vocal cord injury or paralysis after endotracheal intubation has been reported. Ulceration, granuloma, or polyps on the vocal cords are suspected when hoarseness persists several days. The definitive diagnosis is made via laryngoscopy. Trauma, excessive movement, allergic reaction to polyvinyl chloride, and tight-fitting tubes are all possible causes of these complications. Surgery of the head and neck or mediastinum may lead to inadvertent ligation of the recurrent laryngeal nerve, resulting in vocal cord paralysis.

Tracheal stenosis or malacia are complications most often seen in patients undergoing long-term endotracheal intubation and ventilation. The development of tracheal stenosis or tracheal malacia is a result of several factors such as cuff pressure, duration of intubation, mean arterial blood pressure, and sensitivity to endotracheal tube materials.[14] These complications rarely occur in patients undergoing short-term intubation for general anesthesia.

REFERENCES

1. Proctor DF. The upper airway. II. Larynx and trachea. *Am Rev Respir Dis.* 1977;115:315.

2. Burtner D, Goodman M. Anesthetic and operative management of potential upper airway obstruction. *Arch Otolaryngol.* 1978;104:657–661.

3. Mallampati SR, Gatt SP, Guigino LD, et al. A clinical sign to predict difficult tracheal intubation: A prospective study. *Can Anaesth Soc J.* 1985;32:429.

4. Ovassapian A, Dykes MHM. The role of fiberoptic laryngoscopy in anesthesia. *Anesth Analg.* 1974;53:708.

5. Bernhard AN, Cottrell JE, Sivakumaran C. Adjustment of intracuff pressure to prevent aspiration. *Anesthesiology.* 1979;50:363.

6. Bernhard MN, Yost LC, et al. Physical characteristics of the rates of N_2O diffusion into tracheal tube cuffs. *Anesthesiology.* 1978;48:413–417.

7. Cooper JD, Grillo HC. Analysis of problems related to cuffs on endotracheal tubes. *Chest.* 1972;52:2115.

8. Knowlson GTC, Bassett HFM. The pressures exerted on the trachea by endotracheal inflatable cuffs. *J Anesthesiol.* 1970;42:824.

9. Stanley TH. Effects of anesthetic gases on endotracheal tube cuff gas volumes. *Anesth Analg.* 1974;53:480.

10. Ellis DG, Jakymec A, Kaplan RM, et al. Guided orotracheal intubation in the operating room using a lighted stylet: A comparison with direct laryngoscopic technique. *Anesthesiology.* 1986;64:823.

10a. Benumof JL. Management of the difficult adult airway. *Anesthesiology.* 1991;75:1087–1110.

11. Birmingham PY, Cheney FW, Ward FJ. Esophageal intubation: A review of detection techniques. *Anesth Analg.* 1986;65:886.

12. Stout DM, Bishop MJ, Sverstg JF, et al. Correlation of endotracheal tube size with sore throat and hoarseness following general anesthesia. *Anesthesiology.* 1987;67:419.

13. Stauffer JL, Olson DE, et al. Complications and consequences of endotracheal intubation and tracheostomy. *Am J Med.* 1981;70:65–76.

14. Gainer AS, Turndorf H, et al. Surface alterations due to endotracheal intubation. *Am J Med.* 1975;58:674.

Respiratory Therapy and Mechanical Ventilation

Cecil B. Drain

Nurse anesthetists use both respiratory therapy and mechanical ventilation in their particular practice setting. This chapter discusses methods of oxygen therapy and mechanical ventilation including modes of ventilation, indications, and the process of weaning from mechanical ventilation.

RESPIRATORY THERAPY

Oxygen Therapy

There are two types of oxygen therapy systems: high flow and low flow.[1,2] When determining which system is better suited for the patient, the comfort of the patient, humidification, and desired oxygen concentration should be considered.

A low-flow system for the administration of oxygen exists when air entrainment varies to provide the patient's inspiratory flow requirement. A low-flow system for the administration of oxygen supplies less than the total inspired volume of gas needed by the patient. The additional volume of gas required to meet the patient's inspiratory demand is supplied by room air entrained during active inspiration.

The actual concentration of inspired oxygen provided by a low-flow system depends on four factors. A reservoir for the accumulation of oxygen which will increase the inspired oxygen concentration must be available. The larger the reservoir, the greater the resultant increase in inspired oxygen concentration. The nasopharynx and oropharynx act as an anatomic reservoir, with a volume of approximately 50 mL. The oxygen therapy device itself can also serve as a reservoir of varying volume; for example, the area under a face mask or the reservoir bag, which is a part of many oxygen systems, serves as a reservoir. The oxygen flow rate provided also varies with the inspired oxygen concentration. In general, the greater the flow rate of oxygen into the system, the higher the inspired concentration. This effect is limited by the volume of the available oxygen reservoir. Once this reservoir is filled, the excess flow escapes into the atmosphere. In addition, the patient's ventilation pattern affects the inspired oxygen concentration. A more rapid respiratory rate and a greater-than-normal tidal volume reduce the inspired concentration. The degree to which this occurs varies with the degree of change in the patient's ventilatory pattern. Finally, the oxygen therapy device must fit properly to achieve the desired result.

The nasal cannula and catheter are classified as low-flow devices that deliver low to midrange oxygen concentrations. The nasal cannula is comfortable for the patient, but it is easy to dislodge from its desired position. Mouth breathing or any obstruction to the flow of oxygen through the nasal route will reduce the concentration of inspired oxygen (FIO_2). The nasal catheter is not as comfortable for the patient but does offer greater stability. Both the cannula and the catheter, when used at excessive flow rates of oxygen, can cause considerable discomfort, such as drying of secretions, nasal bleeding, and gastric distension. The recommended flow rate for operation of the cannula and catheter is 1 to 6 L/min.[3] Actual inspired oxygen concentrations range from approximately 24 to 44 percent (Table 16–1).[2]

Oxygen masks offer slightly higher oxygen concentrations than nasal devices. With the addition of a reservoir bag, masks of various types can deliver very high concentrations of inspired oxygen. To deliver the highest concentration possible, the mask must fit tightly, which may be uncomfortable for the patient. The oronasal face mask may be hazardous for patients at risk of regurgitation and aspiration. Oxygen masks should be operated at flow rates from 5 to 8 L/min. The inspired oxygen concentration ranges from approximately 40 to 60 percent.[4] A concentration greater than 60 percent is difficult to achieve because of the limited reservoir available. Oxygen masks with an added reservoir bag can deliver very high inspired oxygen concentrations. These devices must be operated at flow rates high enough to prevent the reservoir bag from being emptied during inspiration. If this occurs, the patient will supplement the inspired volume with room air and dilute the oxygen concentration. Masks with a reservoir bag should be operated at a minimum flow rate of 6 L/min, with a maxi-

TABLE 16–1. OXYGEN DELIVERY SYSTEMS (F_{IO_2} ASSUMED ON EUPNEA)

Delivery System	Liter (L/m) Flow	F_{IO_2}	Comments
Low-flow delivery systems			
Nasal cannula	1–6	24–44	F_{IO_2} increases at 4% per L/m increase; Comfortable
Nasal catheter	1–6	24–44	Same as nasal cannula
Simple mask	5–8	40–60	F_{IO_2} increases at 5% per L/m increase; less comfortable
Partial rebreathing mask	6–10	55–70	High F_{IO_2} delivered; same as simple mask; flow should be sufficient to keep reservoir bag from deflating on inspiration
Nonrebreathing mask	6–10	70–100	High F_{IO_2} delivered; same as partial rebreathing mask
High-flow delivery systems			
Venturi mask	Variable	24–50	Exact F_{IO_2} delivered to patient; device of choice for patient with hypoxic drive
Nebulizer with face tent, aerosol mask, or T-piece	6–12	30–100	Used to deliver oxygen and/or aerosol in high concentration; controls temperature of gas

mum flow rate of about 10 L/min.[4] The concentration of inspired oxygen will range from approximately 60 percent to approximately 80 percent, depending on the patient's ventilation pattern.

Tracheostomy masks and T-tubes are similar to other masks in their oxygen delivery capabilities; however, because the upper airway is bypassed in the tracheotomized or intubated patient, the nasopharynx and oropharynx cannot be used as an oxygen reservoir. The loss of this reservoir causes a slight decrease in the inspired oxygen concentration. Loss of the anatomic reservoir can be compensated for, if necessary, by using an oxygen therapy device with a larger reservoir.

The simple, clear plastic face tent is a low-flow oxygen therapy device. It is well tolerated by the patient recovering from anesthesia and supplies extra humidity to the patient. The recommended flow rate for the face tent is 4 to 8 L/min through a bubble-through humidifier. The actual inspired oxygen concentration ranges from approximately 30 to 55 percent.[2]

A high-flow system for the administration of oxygen is one in which the flow rate and reservoir capacity are adequate to provide the total inspired volume to the patient.[1,2] Consequently, the F_{IO_2} is premixed and predictable. An air entrainment principle is used to create this very high flow of gas. This type of system is capable of delivering both low and high concentrations of oxygen. The most common example of a high-flow system is the Venturi-type mask, which uses a Venturi device to produce a specific oxygen concentration. A relatively low flow of 100 percent oxygen is delivered through the Venturi device, creating a high velocity as it escapes. As a result of this high velocity, room air is entrained to mix with the 100 percent oxygen. This mixing, which is designed to occur at a specific ratio, produces a high flow with a relatively specific and consistent oxygen concentration. Depending on the manufacturer, various concentrations are available ranging from a low of 24 percent to a high of 50 percent. Because of the high flow created with this type of system, changes in the patient's ventilatory pattern do not greatly affect the inspired oxygen concentration. To achieve the desired oxygen concentration, the manufacturer's guidelines pertaining to oxygen flow rate to achieve a desired F_{IO_2} should be adhered to.

When a patient's drive to breathe is due mainly to the

hypoxic or secondary drive, oxygen therapy should not be omitted merely because of the fact that the patient will become apneic as a result of cessation of the hypoxic drive from high oxygen concentrations.[4] The patient who is breathing on the hypoxic drive should receive oxygen at a precise F_{IO_2}. In this case, a high-flow oxygen delivery system using the Venturi principle should be used. The minimal oxygen concentration for the patient can be dialed in on the Venturi mask. The patient can be monitored by oxygen saturations or arterial blood gases. For patients whose control of ventilation is through the secondary drive, the PaO_2 should be in the range of 60 to 70 torr and the oxygen saturation should be greater than 96 percent.[4]

Humidity Therapy

Humidity therapy, which is basically the addition of moisture to therapeutic gases, is a major therapeutic intervention used in the practice of anesthesia nursing. Humidification is indicated to enhance bronchial hygiene and when continuous gas therapy is being administered.[1] The intended outcomes of humidity therapy are hydration of inspired secretions, maintenance of the mucus blanket, and reduction of airway inflammation. Humidity therapy can be classified into two major categories based on purpose: (1) to supply enough water vapor to the inspired gas to enhance the patient's comfort and (2) to heat the gas to prevent a reduction in the patient's body temperature by providing a more normal body humidity. The efficiency of humidification devices is increased by enhancing the time of contact between gas and water by increasing the surface area involved in the water–gas interface or heating the water.[2]

Humidification devices are basically of two major types: simple humidifiers and heated humidifiers.[1] Simple humidifiers are nonheating devices. Examples of simple humidifiers are given in Table 16–2. Heated humidifiers, on the other hand, enhance the efficiency of humidification by focusing on the heating properties of humidification. More specifically, bubble diffusion humidifiers or cascade humidifiers are used to replace the heat and moisture normally supplied to the upper airways. In these humidifiers the gas is broken up into small bubbles that pass through heated water, which allows a greater production of small bubbles at higher flow rates than do cold-bubble humidifiers.

TABLE 16–2. AEROSOL AND HUMIDITY THERAPY DELIVERY SYSTEMS

Delivery System	Use	Comments
Aerosol Nebulizers		
Small-reservoir nebulizer: sidestream, mainstream, mininebulizer	Used to deliver aerosolized medications to a patient intermittently; usually 2–5 mL of solution, 1–40 μm particle size	Only precautions are those for the medications; use air for patients on hypoxic drive
Large-reservoir jet nebulizer	Used for continuous oxygen and/or aerosol therapy; 1–40 μm particle size, ½ to 1 mL/min output	Condensation collects in tubing; correct solution level must be maintained
Ultrasonic nebulizer	Used to mobilize thick secretions in lower airways; 90% of the particles are 1–5 μm; usually used only intermittently, but can be used for continuous therapy, output is about 1–6 mL/min	Provides 100% humidity; may precipitate bronchospasm; may cause overhydration
Humidifiers		
Bubble diffuser	Used with all low-flow devices and Venturi masks	Provides only 20 to 40% of body humidity; may be heated to deliver 100% humidity; should not be used for patients with endotracheal tube or tracheostomy
Passover humidifier	Used for either low- or high-flow devices and ventilators	Effective humidity only when heated
Cascade humidifier	Mainstream humidifier for ventilators, for patients with endotracheal tube or tracheostomy	100% humidity at body temperature; correct H_2O level is required

Reprinted, with permission, from Oakes.[3]

Heated humidifiers are preferred for patients receiving mechanical ventilation in the intra- or postoperative period.

Aerosol Therapy

Devices that deliver water vapor along with very fine particles of liquid suspended in a gas are termed *aerosol therapy devices*.[1] These devices are used in patients in which secretions need to be effectively diluted and mucus production enhanced. Aerosol particles are usually spherical and range from 0.2 to 0.7 μm in diameter. Penetration and deposition of an aerosol particle are dependent on the size of the particle, the patient's breathing pattern, and gravity. Particles larger than 30 μm are deposited in the upper airways, 5- to 30-μm particles penetrate the larger airways, and particles smaller than 5 μm enter the small airways.[1] A slow ventilatory frequency with large tidal volumes will enhance aerosol penetration.

The two most common types of nebulizers are the jet nebulizer and the ultrasonic nebulizer. Jet nebulizers can produce particles between 0.5 and 30 μm; ultrasonic nebulizers produce particles of about 5 μm. Intermittent therapy is advised because of the possibility of fluid overload and acute respiratory distress from airway obstruction, as the dried secretions can swell with water over time. Consequently, patients receiving aerosol therapy should never be left unattended.

MECHANICAL VENTILATION

The use of mechanical ventilatory support and the subsequent weaning of the patient from this support have evolved to include numerous methods of ventilation. The various methods used clinically are briefly described in this section.

Modes of Mechanical Ventilation

Spontaneous Ventilation. In certain circumstances when the muscles of ventilation are not capable of supporting the total ventilatory needs of the patient, ventilator assistance is necessary. As it is commonly believed that spontaneous breathing is physiologically more effective in the distribution of ventilation than is positive-pressure ventilation, the patient should be permitted to breathe spontaneously to the clinical extent possible. When the patient has enough muscular power to ventilate adequately but an oxygenation problem exists, a ventilator may not be necessary. Various techniques associated with spontaneous ventilation are available to improve oxygenation without the use of a ventilator. Each technique uses positive end-expiratory pressure (PEEP) to improve the oxygenation level of the patient.[5] It is therefore logical to begin the description of the various techniques with a discussion of PEEP.

PEEP is the application of a pressure greater than atmospheric to the airway at the end of exhalation. This positive pressure is usually created by using some mechanical device that ends the exhalation phase of ventilation early. A certain volume of gas is maintained in the lung over and above the normal volume, to achieve the desired airway pressure level. Basically, PEEP therapy improves oxygenation by expanding the gas-exchanging areas of the lung. Therefore, the clinical goal of PEEP is to raise the functional residual capacity (FRC). By successfully increasing the FRC, oxygenation can be improved without increasing the inspired oxygen concentration, and often the oxygen concentration can be reduced to nontoxic levels while maintaining an adequate PaO_2 and oxygen saturation level.

The therapeutic range of PEEP varies depending on the respiratory pathophysiology being treated. In most clinical situations, the therapeutic range of PEEP is 5 to 30 cm H_2O.

The level of PEEP should be increased or decreased in increments of 2.5 to 5 cm H_2O. An appropriate level of PEEP is achieved when there is adequate arterial oxygenation and cardiac output with an inspired concentration of oxygen of 40 percent or less. Physiologic PEEP is equal to about 5 cm H_2O of positive end-expiratory pressure and is considered to be the same as the resistance normally offered by the intact respiratory system during expiration. "Best" PEEP is the level at which the patient has the best lung compliance.[6] "Optimal" PEEP is the level at which optimal lung function is obtained.[6] It is the level of PEEP that provides a maximum decrease in V_D/V_T and a maximum increase in P_{VO_2}.

Expiratory positive airway pressure (EPAP) is the application of PEEP to the spontaneously breathing patient. Expiratory airway pressures are maintained above atmospheric pressure, whereas inspiratory pressures occur at subatmospheric levels created during normal inspiration. EPAP is indicated in patients who are capable of performing all the work of breathing but require PEEP therapy.

Continuous positive airway pressure (CPAP) is the application of PEEP to the spontaneously breathing patient (EPAP) and the maintenance of inspiratory pressure at a level greater than atmospheric pressure. CPAP is clinically more effective when PEEP therapy is indicated.[7] However, as a result of the CPAP, cardiovascular function may be reduced, and, therefore, EPAP may be more beneficial for the administration of PEEP.

Assisted Ventilation. Assisted ventilation augments the patient's spontaneous breathing efforts. The patient, by initiating a spontaneous inspiration, creates a subatmospheric pressure that is sensed by the ventilator, triggering the inspiratory phase of ventilation. Once the ventilator initiates gas flow in response to the patient's breathing efforts, it takes control of inspiration, overriding the patient's efforts. The assisted mode of ventilation is commonly referred to as intermittent positive-pressure ventilation (IPPV) or positive-pressure ventilation (PPV). This mode of ventilation is used for both long-term ventilatory support and intermittent therapy. When it is used with a volume/time-cycled ventilator, the patient has control over respiratory rate only. During intermittent therapy, a pressure-cycled ventilator is usually used. In this situation, the patient not only controls the respiratory rate but can also influence the delivered tidal volume and inspiratory flow of the assist mode of ventilation, but this has little physiologic advantage over the control mode of ventilation. It does, however, alleviate the need for pharmacologic assistance in controlling the patient's ventilation.

Intermittent Mandatory Ventilation. As with assisted ventilation, intermittent mandatory ventilation (IMV) is a method of augmenting the patient's spontaneous ventilation. IMV differs from assisted ventilation in that the patient's spontaneous breath does not trigger the ventilator into the inspiratory phase. The patient breathes spontaneously from a flow of gas from the ventilator circuit. Intermittently, the ventilator provides a mandatory volume of gas at a predetermined rate. The IMV rate is determined by the patient's ability to assume a portion of the work of breathing. The patient's ventilatory pattern and delivery of the mandatory inspiration are independent of one another.

In an attempt to synchronize the mandatory breath from the ventilator with the patient's ventilatory pattern, various techniques have been developed. Synchronized intermittent mandatory ventilation (SIMV), intermittent assisted ventilation (IAV), and intermittent demand ventilation (IDV) are all systems designed to provide the mandatory breath in response to a spontaneous inspiration at predetermined intervals. This is nothing more than assisted ventilation during the mandatory cycle. The use of IMV, SIMV, IAV, and IDV as methods of weaning has increased significantly in recent years. The patient may assume more of the work of breathing while reducing the mandatory ventilation rate. An advantage to using one of these systems during weaning is that the patient is weaned while remaining attached to the ventilator. The patient thus can be better monitored and receives the same oxygen concentrations and humidification during both spontaneous and mandatory ventilation as during the weaning process.

Controlled Ventilation. Use of intermittent positive-pressure ventilation has decreased significantly in recent years, primarily because of the use of intermittent mandatory ventilation as a method of short- and long-term ventilatory support. The use of controlled ventilation (CV) is, however, still advocated in certain circumstances, such as in patients with central nervous system disorders, anesthetized patients, and critically ill patients whose condition has not been stabilized. The respiratory rate, tidal volume, and inspiratory/expiratory flow rates may all be manipulated during controlled ventilation to obtain the desired physiologic effects. Total control of the patient's ventilatory pattern is the only advantage of IPPV as compared with other modes of ventilation. See Table 16–3 for the initial setup of a ventilator for controlled ventilation.

Inverse Inspiratory : Expiratory Ratio Ventilation. In the early 1970s, it was determined that infants were successfully ventilated using a technique that had an inspiratory phase longer than the expiratory phase, with a pressure hold. This technique has been used on adults in which the inspiratory : expiratory (I : E) ratio reaches 4 : 1 and is combined with low levels of PEEP or CPAP.[2]

Pressure Support Ventilation. In pressure support ventilation (PSV) a gas is applied at a preset level above PEEP. When the patient's spontaneous inspiration is sensed, a demand valve is opened and the ventilator delivers a pressurized breath. Once a particular pressure is reached or flow is decreased, inspiration is ended and exhalation occurs.[2]

Pressure support ventilation is particularly useful for patients requiring weaning from mechanical ventilation who have increased airway resistance. Consequently, PSV offers adjustable breath-to-breath ventilatory assistance and helps to reduce the work of breathing.

High-frequency Ventilation. High-frequency ventilation (HFV) is a method of ventilation that uses rates higher than 60 per minute or greater than four times the standard positive pressure ventilation rate.[2] Although the exact mechanism of action is not clearly defined, it has been established

TABLE 16–3. RECOMMENDED VENTILATOR SETUP PARAMETERS

Parameter	Setting Range	Discussion
Minute ventilation ($\dot{V}_E$)	5–10 L/min	$\dot{V}_E$ determines alveolar ventilation ($\dot{V}_A$) as $\dot{V}_E = 1/Paco_2$, which is usually controlled by V_T and f
Tidal volume (V_T)	10–15 mL/kg	Large V_T is preferred to improve $\dot{V}_A/\dot{Q}_C$, prevent atelectasis, and account dead space lost to tubing
Peak pressure	< 40 cm H_2O	Keep as low as possible to prevent pneumothorax and yet deliver desired V_T
Rate (f)	12–18 breaths/min	Combined with V_T to give desired $\dot{V}_E$ ($Paco_2$). Keep rate (f) low for large V_T
Fio_2	≤40%	Adjust in 5–10% increments to keep the Pao_2 between 60 and 100 torr
Sigh	6–12/h 1½–2 × V_T	Prevent miliary atelectasis, not critical if high V_T values are used
Flow rate ($\dot{V}_I$)	25–60 L/min	Used to provide desired inspiratory pattern
PEEP/CPAP	5–10 cm H_2O	Indicated when Pao_2 < 50 torr on 50% oxygen
Inspiratory time (T_I)	0.5–1.0 s	Normal physiologic time
I:E ratio	1:2 to 1:3	Longer time for obstructive lung disease
Sensitivity	–1–2 cm H_2O	Allows triggering of ventilator in assist mode
Pressure limit	10 cm H_2O above peak pressure	Prevents excess pressure from reaching lungs, warning for increased airway resistance or decreased compliance

that in HFV, carbon dioxide exchange can and does occur even when the tidal volume is less than the patient's dead space.

High-frequency ventilation uses a commercially available ventilator called a high-frequency jet ventilator (HFJV) that delivers a pulse of gas from a high-pressure source between 5 and 50 psi. The pulse of gas is delivered through a small-bore cannula at rates up to 150 per minute. Advantages to the HFJV are few; however, it may have a place in one-lung ventilation, in patients with bronchopleural fistulas, and in anesthetic cases where minimal movement in the surgical field is desirable as in computerized lithotripsy.

Indications for Mechanical Ventilation

Mechanical ventilation is instituted to correct one of three pathophysiologic processes: acute hypoventilation or apnea, high $\dot{V}_A/\dot{Q}_C$, and low $\dot{V}_A/\dot{Q}_C$. Acute hypoventilation may be caused by inadequate skeletal muscle relaxant reversal, prolonged emergence from anesthesia, or overdosage of narcotic agonist. The arterial blood gases of a patient with acute hypoventilation will demonstrate a decreased Pao_2 and an increased $Paco_2$ along with a reduced pH. Apnea, on the other hand, can result from multiple causes. When acute hypoxemia caused by acute hypoventilation or apnea is present, a volume-limited ventilator should be used. In this case, the intervention is intended to restore the patient's normal alveolar ventilation. The initial setup should be in accordance with the parameters described in Table 16–3. Twenty to thirty minutes after the institution of the mechanical ventilation, arterial blood gases should be drawn and evaluated, and the ventilator setting changed accordingly.

High $\dot{V}_A/\dot{Q}_C$ (dead space) occurs when alveolar ventilation exceeds alveolar perfusion. A patient with an acute elevation of the FRC, as occurs during acute respiratory insufficiency caused by chronic obstructive pulmonary disease (COPD), is one example of a high $\dot{V}_A/\dot{Q}_C$. Another example is a pulmonary embolism. The arterial blood gases of a patient with a high $\dot{V}_A/\dot{Q}_C$ will demonstrate acute

hypoxemia and minimal hypercarbia. Another helpful test is to determine the amount of dead-space breathing by using the Bohr equation, commonly referred to as the V_D/V_T[8]:

$$\frac{V_D}{V_T} = \frac{Paco_2 - Peco_2}{Peco_2}$$

Here, $Peco_2$ = mixed expired partial pressure of CO_2 and $Paco_2$ = partial pressure of arterial CO_2. If V_D/V_T is greater than 0.6, mechanical ventilation should be instituted. The same basic considerations in setting up the ventilator (Table 16–3) should be used for the patient with high $\dot{V}_A/\dot{Q}_C$ as for the patient with acute hypoventilation.

Low $\dot{V}_A/\dot{Q}_C$ (shunt) is a pathophysiologic process that can occur intraoperatively and postoperatively. Severe atelectasis is a common cause of low $\dot{V}_A/\dot{Q}_C$. Arterial blood gases in the patient with low $\dot{V}_A/\dot{Q}_C$ usually demonstrate hypoxemia, hypercarbia, and a low pH. Another helpful test to determine the amount of shunt is the $\dot{Q}_S/\dot{Q}_T$. The shunt equation can be used to determine the exact amount of right-to-left shunt; however, if the Fio_2 and the Pao_2 are known, the isoshunt line graph can be used to determine the approximate percentage of shunted blood (Fig. 16–1). If a patient has a shunt ($\dot{Q}_S/\dot{Q}_T$) that is greater than 15 percent, mechanical ventilation should be considered.[8]

FRC is usually low in patients with low $\dot{V}_A/\dot{Q}_C$ because the patient will usually have low lung compliance ($\downarrow C_L$) and high lung recoil ($\uparrow P_{stL}$). Consequently, hyperinflation or PEEP may be required to return the FRC to normal levels. By returning the FRC to normal levels, the V_T will be elevated out of the closing capacity (CC) range, and ultimately alveolar ventilation will improve because there will be better matching of ventilation to perfusion in the lungs.

In patients who have undergone major operations and do not have underlying lung disease, mechanical ventilation may be required until the effects of anesthesia and surgery have dissipated. The patient initially should be provided with 100 mL/kg per minute total ventilation. An IMV rate of 8 to 10 is usually acceptable, and a PEEP of 5 cm H_2O may be added to the ventilator circuit. The use of IMV has

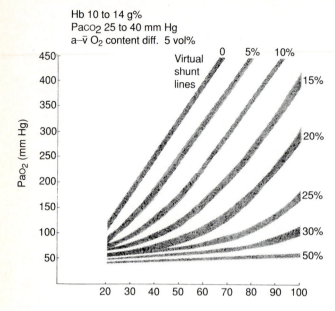

Hb 10 to 14 g%
$Paco_2$ 25 to 40 mm Hg
$a-\bar{v}\ O_2$ content diff. 5 vol%

Figure 16–1. Isoshunt chart indicating the relationship between partial pressure of arterial O_2 (Pao_2) and inspired O_2 concentration (Fio_2) for a range of shunt fractions (0 to 50 percent). (*Reprinted, with permission, from Benatar SR, Hewlett AM, Nunn JF. The use of isoshunt lines for control of oxygen therapy.* Br J Anaesth. *1973;45:713.*)

decreased the period of mechanical ventilatory support slightly and has probably made weaning safer.

Weaning from Mechanical Ventilation

While the patient receives mechanical ventilatory support, cardiovascular stability is of utmost importance. This is particularly true when the patient is being weaned from mechanical ventilation. Special attention should be given to fluids and electrolyte balance. The patient should be afebrile and in a good nutritional state before the weaning process is instituted (Table 16–4).

The patient's respiratory status must be assessed before the weaning process can be started. The assessment parameters are usually grouped into three major categories: ventilation, mechanics, and oxygenation (Table 16–5).[7]

Assessment of ventilation centers around the arterial blood gas analysis. The $Paco_2$ should be within normal limits (35 to 45 torr). VD/VT should be less than 0.6. If PEEP was used, it should be less than 5 cm H_2O at the beginning of the weaning process. Finally, if the minute ventilation

TABLE 16–4. PHYSIOLOGIC PARAMETERS TO BE CORRECTED BEFORE WEANING FROM MECHANICAL VENTILATION

Cardiovascular stability
Improvement in underlying disease
Absence of fever/shivering
Absence of acid–base abnormalities
Absence of electrolyte abnormalities
Adequate nutrition

TABLE 16–5. PHYSIOLOGIC CRITERIA FOR WEANING A PATIENT OFF MECHANICAL VENTILATION

Ventilation
$Paco^2$ = 35–45 torr (CO_2 retains about 55 torr)
VD/VT < 0.6
$\dot{V}E$ < 10 L/min
Mechanics
VC > 10–15 mL/kg
MIF = −20 cm H_2O
MVV = 2 $\dot{V}E$
Oxygenation
Pao_2 > 70 torr (PEEP < 5 cm H_2O and Fio_2 < 0.4)
P(A-a)O_2 at Fio_2 = 1 between 300 and 350 torr
$\dot{Q}s/\dot{Q}T$ at Fio_2 = 1.0 at < 10–20%

($\dot{V}E$) is less than 10 L/min, the weaning process should be allowed to proceed.

As with ventilation, oxygenation is assessed by obtaining arterial blood gases. Before weaning is attempted, the Pao_2 should be greater than 70 torr with a Fio_2 less than 0.4 and less than 5 cm H_2O PEEP. Pao_2 appears to be the best assessment parameter to evaluate adequacy for weaning from mechanical ventilation. The alveolar–arterial oxygen difference or gradient P(A–a)O_2 and the shunt equation ($\dot{Q}s/\dot{Q}T$) add little information compared with the use of Pao_2 alone.

The best tests for assessing mechanical function are vital capacity (VC) and maximal inspiratory force (MIF). Assessment of VC reflects respiratory system compliance and mechanical muscle strength. The VC should be 10 to 15 mL/kg and the MIF should be more negative than 20 cm H_2O. Maximum voluntary ventilation (MVV) can be used as an assessment criterion; however, the VC and MIF are usually adequate to make a decision on weaning from mechanical ventilation.

When the patient fulfills the criteria of the three categories of assessment, the actual process of weaning can begin. It is important to restate that the patient must possess good cardiovascular stability, including adequate nutrition and blood volume. The patient should not receive any drugs that would sedate or depress the respiratory drive. During the weaning process, constant psychologic and physiologic monitoring of the patient is mandatory. Vital signs, arterial blood gases, and mechanics should be recorded on a flowsheet. Once the patient is allowed to breathe spontaneously without the aid of mechanical ventilation, vital signs are recorded every 5 to 10 minutes for about half an hour and then every 30 minutes after that. Arterial blood gases are checked 15 minutes after spontaneous breathing off the ventilator has begun and thereafter on an hourly basis. Mechanical ventilation is resumed if any of the following signs appear: arrhythmia, hypertension or hypotension (change of 15 torr from baseline), tachycardia (> 120 beats per minute), pallor, cyanosis, agitation, increasing $Paco_2$ greater than 1 torr/min, pH less than 7.25, or Pao_2 less than 70 torr.[4]

Most patients who are receiving short-term mechanical ventilation can be weaned in several hours. Mechanical ventilation can be discontinued in two ways: (1) periodic removal from the ventilator using the Briggs' T-piece or (2)

use of IMV. If the first method is used, the Briggs' T-piece ensures that the patient will be adequately oxygenated. The patient who has received long-term ventilator care may tolerate only short periods (< 30 minutes) every 2 to 4 hours of the T-piece weaning process. As tolerated, these patients should spend less time receiving mechanical ventilation and more time using the T-piece. If it is anticipated that the weaning process will be lengthy, the discontinuance from mechanical ventilation should be commenced in the morning when the patient can physiologically tolerate the weaning process.

IMV is an acceptable method of weaning a patient from mechanical ventilation and offers many advantages. IMV increases safety, decreases weaning time, preserves respiratory muscle strength and coordination by allowing ongoing spontaneous breathing efforts, and improves psychologic adjustments to weaning. This method focuses on reducing the number of breaths per minute and allowing the patient to increase control over ventilation. Finally, the patient breathes spontaneously without the aid of mechanical ventilation. The weaning process with IMV is the same as with the T-piece regarding time off the ventilator.

Some patients develop intolerance to the IMV method.

The intolerance may be caused by increased resistance in the IMV circuit (as compared with the T-piece circuit), malfunctions in ventilator setup, or overoxygenation during the weaning period. Patients who are difficult to wean via IMV may respond well to the T-piece method.

REFERENCES

1. McPherson S. *Respiratory therapy equipment.* 4th ed. St. Louis, MO: CV Mosby; 1990.
2. Shapiro B, Cane R. Respiratory care. In: Miller R, ed. *Anesthesia.* 3rd ed. New York: Churchill Livingstone; 1990.
3. Oakes D. *Clinical practitioners pocket guide to respiratory care.* Old Town, ME: Health Educator Publications; 1988.
4. Drain C. *The recovery room: A critical care approach to post anesthesia nursing.* 3rd ed. Philadelphia: WB Saunders; 1992.
5. Nunn J. Positive end-expiratory pressure. *Int Anesthesiol Clin.* 1984;22(4):149.
6. Barash P, Cullen B, Stoelting R. *Clinical anesthesia.* Philadelphia: JB Lippincott; 1989.
7. Kirby R, Smith R, Desautels D. *Mechanical ventilation.* New York: Churchill Livingstone; 1985.
8. Harper R. *A guide to respiratory care.* Philadelphia: JB Lippincott; 1981.

Regional Anesthesia Techniques

Francis R. Gerbasi

Regional anesthesia offers the patient a safe and effective alternative to general anesthesia for certain types of surgical and diagnostic procedures. It provides a relatively pain-free state without necessitating a loss of consciousness.

Analgesia and motor blockade result from the interruption of nerve impulses before they reach and after they leave the spinal cord. This is accomplished by the administration of a local anesthetic solution at a specific site along the pathway of a nerve. Local anesthetic solutions act by inhibiting ion transfer and stop propagation of nerve impulses. Various types of regional anesthetics can be used and are designated according to the specific site of blockade (e.g., field blocks, specific nerve or plexus blocks, and ganglionic blocks).

This chapter discusses four major regional anesthetic techniques: spinal, epidural, brachial plexus, and intravenous regional anesthesia. The primary intent is to emphasize the administration process. The anesthetist sincerely interested in neural blockade must have a thorough understanding of pertinent anatomy, physiology, and pharmacology related to the local anesthetic agents. *It is recommended that additional references be consulted along with supervised clinical experience prior to performing any of the regional anesthetics discussed.*

PREOPERATIVE ASSESSMENT

The patient must be evaluated to determine if a specific regional anesthetic technique is suitable. This assessment should encompass four primary areas:

1. Patients should always willingly give permission for a regional anesthetic to be done. If a block is attempted without authorized permission from the patient or guardian, the anesthetist may be liable for assault and battery charges.
2. Initially the patients' anatomic and pathophysiologic status should be evaluated. Specific anatomic landmarks must be identified for all regional anesthetics. Conditions such as obesity and severe arthritis may hamper the identification of these landmarks and the administration of a specific block. A thorough history and physical examination should be completed including allergies, drug therapy, and evaluation of any pathophysiologic condition. Conditions such as infections, hypovolemia, neurologic disease, and coagulopathies may contraindicate a regional anesthetic.
3. A positive rapport should be established and the patients' psychologic status evaluated. One should explain the regional anesthetic being considered, its benefits/risks, and consent to its use. Usually, increased patient understanding will promote acceptance and facilitate successful anesthetic management. Psychologically the patient must have a positive mental attitude to be cooperative during a regional anesthetic. Conditions such as hysteria and disorientation make administration and management of a regional anesthetic difficult. Often, when there is a language barrier between the patient and provider, administration of blocks is difficult.
4. Finally, the proper anesthetic management is determined. This decision should be based on the findings of the aforementioned evaluation, the specific instructions and contraindications for a given block, the operative procedure, and the needs of the surgeon. No regional anesthetic can be guaranteed effective, and one should always be prepared to administer a general anesthetic.

Preoperative preparation should include nothing by mouth (NPO) for a minimum of 6 to 8 hours before surgery and the possible use of a narcotic and/or sedative as premedication. Although various opinions exist regarding the use of specific premedicants, a sedative (e.g., midazolam) and narcotic (e.g., meperidine, fentanyl) may be given to healthy patients to relieve anxiety and to facilitate anesthetic management. Anticholinergics are not commonly used because of their antisialogue effect; however, they may be indicated for intraoperative treatment of bradycardia. Premedicants should be used with caution in the elderly or poor-risk patient.

SPINAL ANESTHESIA

A spinal anesthetic, or subarachnoid block, consists of the injection of a local anesthetic solution into the subarachnoid space, with resultant blockade of the spinal nerve roots. August Bier is credited with the first planned spinal anesthetic in 1898 but it was not until 1921, when Gaston Labat published an article discussing methods to decrease the dangers of spinal anesthesia, that it became a relatively popular technique.[1]

Advantages and Disadvantages

In selecting a subarachnoid block, as in the process of determining any anesthetic management, the anesthetist must consider the patient's emotional makeup and physical status and the needs of the surgeon.

Usually, spinal anesthesia is administered for surgical procedures performed on the lower abdomen, inguinal region, or lower extremities. It may, however, be used in certain situations for upper abdominal procedures. The degree of muscle relaxation and contraction of bowel obtained with spinal anesthesia is unrivaled by any other anesthetic technique.

A subarachnoid block also presents certain disadvantages. The anesthetist must remember that the duration of anesthesia is limited and that there is a statistical chance of failure associated with administration. The possibility of hypotension, resulting from sympathetic blockade, may present concerns, particularly in the patient who has preoperative cardiovascular disorders. Also, the patient's airway and respiratory systems are not under direct control of the anesthetist as with general anesthesia.

Anatomy

A basic knowledge of the vertebral column, spinal cord, and surrounding structures is of the utmost importance to the anesthetist administering a spinal anesthetic. The following discussion highlights the main areas that directly relate to spinal anesthetic administration.

The vertebral column comprises four curves, the thoracic and sacral being concave anteriorly and the cervical and lumbar being convex anteriorly (Fig. 17–1).[2] Prior to the administration of a spinal anesthetic, the lumbar curve is often modified by having the patient arch his or her back posteriorly. This modification facilitates spinal needle placement by opening the interspinous spaces. Kyphosis, scoliosis, and lordosis can represent variations in the natural curvature of the spine and make the administration of a spinal anesthetic difficult.

The vertebral column is bound together by the ligamentum flavum and supraspinous, interspinous, and longi-

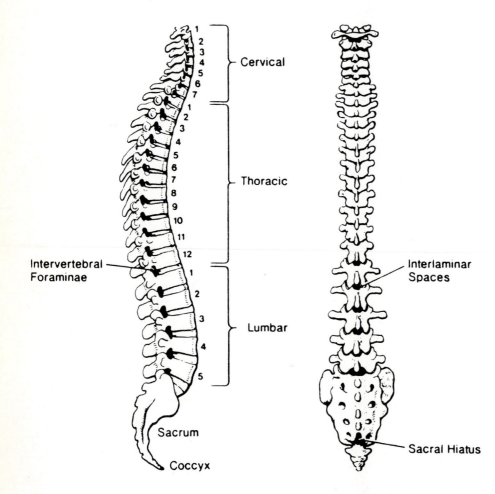

Cervical

Thoracic

Intervertebral Foraminae

Lumbar

Sacrum

Coccyx

Interlaminar Spaces

Sacral Hiatus

Figure 17–1. Illustration of the vertebral column curvatures and interlaminar spaces in the lateral (left) and posterior (right) views. (*Reprinted, with permission, from Cousins and Bredenbaugh.*[2])

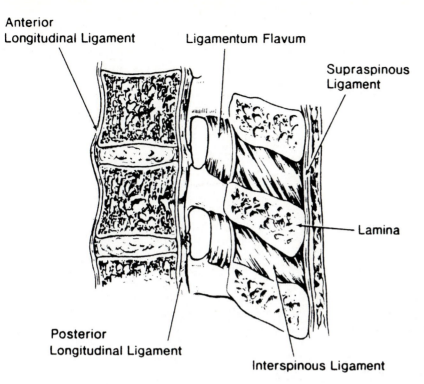

Figure 17–2. Cross section of the vertebral column, showing ligaments. *(Reprinted, with permission, from Cousins and Bredenbaugh.[2])*

tudinal ligaments (Fig. 17–2).[2] The vertebral canal runs vertically in the vertebral column and is bounded anteriorly by the bodies of the vertebrae and the intervertebral discs. The vertebral canal is bounded posteriorly by the arch bearing the spinous process and the interspinous ligaments. The vertebral canal contains the spinal cord, spinal nerve roots, cerebrospinal fluid, and membranes that enclose the spinal cord. The spinal cord is protected by the vertebral column and three tissue membranes. These membranes are the dura mater, arachnoid mater, and pia mater. Although some anatomic variations are seen, the spinal cord usually extends down the spinal canal to the lower border of L-1 (Fig. 17–3).[3] *A spinal needle, therefore, should not be inserted above the second lumbar vertebrae to prevent possible spinal cord damage.*

The initial placement of the spinal needle is determined by the specific relationship between the fourth lumbar vertebra and the top of the iliac crests. Based on the fact that these two structures lie at corresponding levels, each vertebra's location and respective interspaces can be determined. The most commonly used interspace is that between the third and fourth lumbar vertebrae. The interspaces between the second and third lumbar vertebrae may also be used, but only with caution, because occasionally the spinal cord may extend to this level.[4,5]

To place a spinal needle in the subarachnoid space, the correct intervertebral space must be identified and the needle inserted at an appropriate angle. Each of the spinal vertebrae has a spinous process extending posteriorly. The direction in which these spinous processes extend determines, to a large extent, the angle at which the spinal needle must be inserted. The spinous process of the last four lumbar vertebrae, as compared with the other spinous processes, extends in a more horizontal plane. The spinal

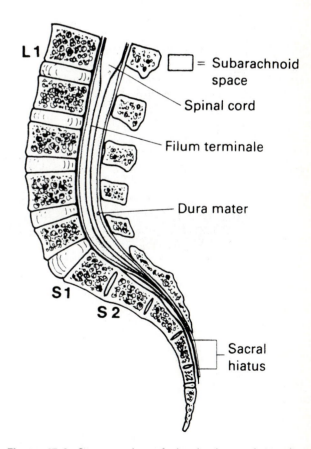

Figure 17–3. Cross section of the lumbosacral vertebrae, showing spinal cord ending at lower border of L-1 with subarachnoid space continuing to S-2. *(Reprinted, with permission, from Miller.[3])*

needle must be introduced parallel to this angle to reach the subarachnoid space (Fig. 17–4).

If a midline approach is used, the spinal needle pierces various ligaments while being introduced into the sub-arachnoid space. These ligaments, in order of their penetration, are the supraspinous ligament, interspinous ligament, and ligamentum flavum. If a paramedian or lateral approach is used only the ligamentum flavum is pierced.

Spinal anesthesia results primarily from blockade of the spinal nerve roots.[6] These spinal nerves originate from the spinal cord as the anterior and posterior roots. The nerve roots unite in the intervertebral foramen to form the spinal nerve, which then extends and divides into anterior and posterior divisions supplying specific areas of the body, termed *dermatomes* (Fig. 17–5).[3]

Sympathetic nerve fibers run with the spinal nerves and supply various organs. Figure 17–6 indicates the sympathetic innervation corresponding to specific levels of the vertebral column. Primarily because of the small size of the sympathetic fiber, it is thought that the sympathetic impulses are blocked above the corresponding sensory block; however, recent investigators have suggested that sympathetic block has less extent and intensity than sensory analgesia.[7] Motor blockade usually occurs approximately two spinal levels below the sensory level.[8] A decrease in blood pressure is often the result of sympathetic blockade and may indicate a relatively high block if it occurs rapidly after spinal administration.

Indications and Contraindications

The indications for and contraindications to a spinal anes-thetic are listed in Table 17–1. Contraindications can be viewed on an absolute or relative basis. A spinal anesthetic should not be administered in the presence of an absolute

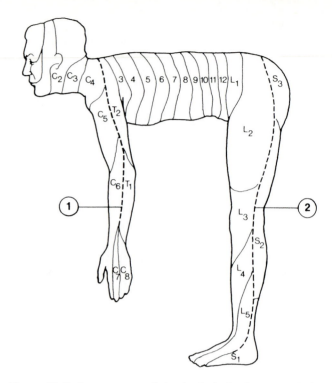

Figure 17–5. Dermatomes of the body indicating an orderly cranial-to-caudad sequence. The numbers **1** and **2** indicate the axial line around which the dermatomes of the upper and lower extremities are distributed. (*Reprinted, with permission, from Foerster I. Brain. 1933; 56:1.*)

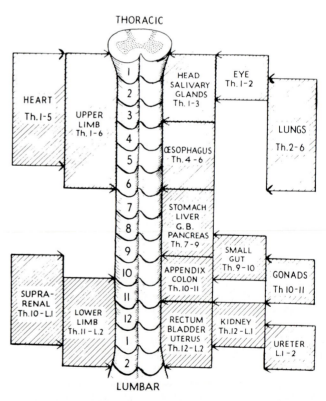

Figure 17–6. Spinal levels of sympathetic innervation. (*Reprinted, with permission, from Last RJ. Anatomy, regional and applied. 6th ed. Edinburgh: Churchill Livingstone, 1978.*)

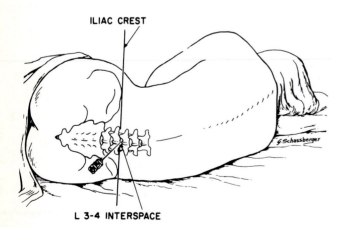

Figure 17–4. Anatomic orientation for spinal needle placement at the L3–4 interspace. Note that the top of the iliac crest corre-sponds to the fourth lumbar vertebra.

TABLE 17–1. INDICATIONS FOR AND CONTRAINDICATIONS TO SPINAL (SUBARACHNOID) ANESTHESIA

Indications
- Procedures involving lower abdomen and extremities
- Obstetric procedures
- Patient preference

Contraindications
- Absolute
  - Anticoagulant therapy or coagulation abnormalities
  - Systemic or localized infection
  - Allergy to anesthetic drug
  - Increased intracranial pressure
  - Presence of acute neurologic disease
  - Patient refusal
- Relative
  - Chronic neurologic disorders
  - Backache
  - Headache
  - Psychologic disorders

contraindication. If a relative contraindication is present, one must weigh the advantages and disadvantages of the technique to arrive at the appropriate anesthetic management decision.

Generally, spinal anesthesia is indicated for lower abdominal procedures, such as transurethral prostatectomy and inguinal herniorrhaphy. It is particularly useful in a patient whose condition may be aggravated by a general anesthetic or in the patient who fears losing consciousness. Spinal anesthesia has been extremely useful in obstetrics for vaginal deliveries or cesarean sections, although epidural anesthesia presently is gaining preference.

Procedure

The following procedure describes the administration of a spinal anesthetic using a 25-gauge standard spinal needle and introducer. Compared with larger-bore needles, the 25-gauge offers the advantage of a decreased incidence of postspinal headache[9]; however, larger-gauge pencil-point needles (e.g., 22-gauge Whitacre) may provide a better "feel" for identifying the various structures and still have a relatively low incidence of spinal headache.

The importance of adequate preparation prior to administration of a spinal anesthetic cannot be overstressed. Table 17–2 indicates some important points with respect to preparation and actual administration of the block. As with any anesthetic technique this procedure should not be performed without the immediate availability of proper resuscitation equipment and medications. The anesthetist must remember that this is a sterile procedure; consequently, sterile technique must be used. Also, in preparation, the healthy patient should receive a preload of fluid (0.5 to 1 L) and have blood pressure, pulse, and respirations measured and recorded.

One of the most important aspects in preparing to administer a spinal anesthetic is patient positioning. Proper positioning of the patient ensures good anatomic orientation and maximum opening of the interspinous spaces. An assistant should be available at all times to help position

and support the patient during the administration of a spinal anesthetic. Opening of the interspinous spaces can best be accomplished in the lateral position by having the patient "curl up" as much as possible and flex his or her back posteriorly. Anatomic orientation is best accomplished by having the patient assume a sitting position. This may be particularly useful in the obese patient. The utilization of a marking pen to indicate anatomic landmarks can also assist in maintaining good anatomic orientation.

There are many variations in skin preparation, each an individual decision by the provider according to institutional policy or accepted practice standards of aseptic technique. Informing the patient of disinfectant solution application and impending needle insertion is particularly important in helping ensure against movement and provides the patient with a more pleasant experience. Several sponges are used to remove the disinfectant solution and the area is draped to maintain sterility.

Presently, a number of spinal trays are commercially available and provide all the necessary syringes, needles, and medications to administer a subarachnoid block. The spinal tray may be prepared between application and removal of the disinfectant solution or prior to application of the solution. It should be prepared so that the medications and needles can be obtained easily. The spinal tray is

TABLE 17–2. IMPORTANT STEPS IN THE ADMINISTRATION OF A SPINAL (SUBARACHNOID) ANESTHETIC

I. Preparation
  A. Prepare equipment.
    1. Arrange resuscitation equipment and medication so that they are immediately available.
    2. Obtain sterile gloves and prep solution.
    3. Verify spinal anesthesia tray sterility and prepare it for easy use.
  B. Prepare patient.
    1. Explain procedure.
    2. Check vital signs.
    3. Position appropriately—sitting or lateral.
      a. Back at edge of table
      b. Proper body alignment with support
      c. Knees and head flexed
      d. Patient relaxed
II. Performance
  A. Identify landmarks.
  B. Raise skin wheal at site.
  C. Insert spinal needle.
    1. Insert 21-gauge introducer to ligamentum flavum.
    2. Introduce 25-gauge spinal needle, bevel parallel to dura fibers.
    3. Advance needle gently.
    4. Frequently check for CSF.[a]
    5. Identify subarachnoid space.
    6. Rotate needle 90 to 180 degrees.
  D. Inject medication.
    1. Attach needle-stabilized syringe.
    2. Aspirate CSF, inject medication.
    3. Aspirate postinjection.
  E. Remove needle and syringe assembly.
  F. Reposition patient.

[a] CSF, cerebrospinal fluid.

then placed on the side of provider dominance, which will facilitate maintaining the needle site with one hand while obtaining equipment with the other.

The medications are prepared using standard techniques to ensure proper identification of medications and sterility. Various agents may be used, including lidocaine, bupivacaine, procaine, and tetracaine. Table 17–3 provides dosages of tetracaine and bupivacaine in relation to specific spinal levels. It should be noted that individual dosages may vary according to patient characteristics and operative requirements. The effect of gravity in relation to patient positioning is a very important factor in determining the spinal level achieved. If a hyperbaric spinal solution is desired, tetracaine should be mixed with 10 percent dextrose in water solution. This may be done by combining equal volumes, on a millimeter basis, although individual variations of this ratio are often seen.

Utilizing the top of the iliac crest as a reference, the fourth lumbar vertebra (L-4) is identified and the appropriate interspace determined. One should not go above the second lumbar vertebra. The step-by-step technique is reviewed in Table 17–2. An introducer is used to facilitate placement of the small-gauge spinal needles and prevent their contact with the skin. The spinal needle is inserted through the introducer with the bevel parallel to the fibers of the dura, which run cephalad to caudad. This decreases the number of transected dura fibers. When initially introduced, the spinal needle should be held securely; then two hands should be used to gently guide the needle inward. The anesthetist must maintain a firm understanding of the anatomic orientation during insertion. It is on this basis that he or she directs the needle into the subarachnoid space (Fig. 17–4).

The needle is advanced until a give or "pop" is elicited. The stylet is removed and a return of cerebrospinal fluid indicates entry into the subarachnoid space. The normal "pop" felt on entering the subarachnoid space is less pronounced when the smaller-gauge needles (e.g., 25- or 26-gauge) are used and the return of cerebrospinal fluid will be relatively slow.

Occasionally, blood is obtained on stylet removal. Usually, this clears after a few drops. If clearing does not occur, the needle may be repositioned until clear cerebrospinal fluid is obtained. *At no time should the agent be injected in the presence of a blood tap or abnormally appearing cerebrospinal fluid.*

Rotating the needle 90 to 180 degrees after obtaining cerebrospinal fluid will help ensure appropriate placement. Then, while the needle is firmly supported, the syringe is attached. One should support the needle with the hand, using the patient's back to assist in stabilizing the spinal needle. This is a very crucial point in the technique. The importance of maintaining needle placement cannot be overstressed. Even a very slight movement may reposition the needle outside the subarachnoid space. Cerebrospinal fluid is then aspirated to confirm needle placement and the local anesthetic is injected. After injection, cerebrospinal fluid is again aspirated as an indication of efficacy and the needle/syringe assembly removed. The patient should then be repositioned according to the level of analgesia desired.

Occasionally, a nerve fiber is touched by the spinal needle, causing a temporary paresthesia which dissipates rapidly. The medication may be injected in this situation but *at no time should the local anesthetic agent be injected in the presence of persistent paresthesia.*

Management

Generally, a spinal anesthetic is administered to obtain a desired level of anesthesia. Specific factors that influence the level obtained are (1) the specific gravity of the agent employed, (2) the volume injected, (3) the speed of injection, and (4) the patient's position immediately after administration.

Of these factors, patient positioning should be instituted immediately after injection. If a hyperbaric solution is used, the effect of gravity will move the medication to the lowest point of the vertebral column. If a unilateral block is desired, the patient should remain on the side to be anesthetized for approximately 5 minutes after administration. If the patient is supine, the table may be placed in a Trendelenberg position to increase the height of the block.

After the patient is repositioned, the vital signs should be assessed and recorded every minute for the first 20 minutes, then monitored every 5 minutes. Oxygen should be administered on a routine basis and significant hypotension should be treated with appropriate fluids and a vasopressor (i.e., ephedrine or mephentermine).

The patient's respirations must be closely monitored. Although an approximate fixing time of 20 minutes is expected with tetracaine, this may vary and the spinal level can rise, causing respiratory embarrassment.

The level of anesthesia can be assessed, after administration, by using a large-gauge needle and touching the skin lightly to determine patient sensitivity (pinprick method). Characteristically, onset of the block proceeds in the following order: sympathetic blockade, superficial pain and temperature, motor, proprioception, and, finally, loss of sensation to touch and deep pressure. Therefore, a patient may feel the touch and pressure associated with disinfectant solution application but be insensitive to pain.

Effective communication is essential at this time to alleviate anxiety and assess the patient's status. Symptoms of a high spinal, such as numbness in the hands or difficulty in breathing can be detected and the appropriate treatment initiated.

Duration of action will vary and depends on the dosage of agent employed, level of anesthesia, type of local anes-

TABLE 17–3. DOSAGES OF 1 PERCENT TETRACAINE AND 0.75 PERCENT BUPIVACAINE (IN 8.5 PERCENT DEXTROSE) NECESSARY TO ACHIEVE AN APPROXIMATE T-10 ANESTHETIC LEVEL IN RELATION TO PATIENT'S HEIGHT[a]

Height (in.)	Tetracaine Dosage (mg)	Bupivacaine Dosage (mg)
60	10	8–10
66	12	10–12
72	14	14–16

[a] Tetracaine dosages assume mixture with an equal volume, on a milliliter basis, of 10 percent dextrose–water. Please refer to text for factors that influence analgesic level achieved.

thetic used, and the patient's age. If epinephrine or phenylephrine has been added, a clinically significant prolongation of regression of analgesia and anesthesia with tetracaine is seen.[10]

Recovery is due primarily to diffusion and vascular absorption of the local anesthetic agent from the subarachnoid space.[11] Characteristically, nerve function recovers in reverse order of onset.

EPIDURAL ANESTHESIA

The injection of a local anesthetic agent into the posterior lumbar epidural space that surrounds the dural sac in the vertebral canal is termed *epidural anesthesia* or *epidural block*. In 1885, Corning produced the first epidural block and since that time various administration techniques have been developed. The following describes the loss of resistance technique and indicates specific points of importance in its administration.

Advantages and Disadvantages

As compared with a subarachnoid block, epidural anesthesia offers distinct advantages. An epidural block has a slower onset of sympathetic blockade, which allows for compensatory vasoconstriction to occur. This may decrease the incidence of hypotension after administration. A larger number of agents are available for an epidural block compared with a subarachnoid block, which allows the anesthetic to be tailored to the specific needs of the procedure. A distinct advantage is the absence of postlumbar puncture headache as long as the dura has not been penetrated.

A disadvantage of the technique is its relative difficulty. *The technique requires careful administration and the importance of proper training and supervised experience cannot be overemphasized.*

Anatomy

An understanding of the anatomic relationships discussed earlier in regard to spinal anesthesia is also important in the administration of an epidural block.

The epidural space, which extends from the foramen magnum to the sacral hiatus, lies between the periosteal and investing layers of the dura. It is approximately 6 mm at its widest point and is bordered posteriorly by the ligamentum flavum.[12] It contains the spinal nerve roots, blood vessels, and fatty areolar tissue.

The anterior and posterior spinal nerve roots pass through the epidural space, surrounded by a dural cuff, and then unite and exit through the intervertebral foramen. These nerves are characteristically less movable in the epidural space and, therefore, are vulnerable to needle trauma. It is postulated that an epidural anesthetic blocks the spinal nerves by a variety of pathways, including diffusion of the local anesthetic through arachnoid villi. The arachnoid villi are located in the dural cuff, which surrounds the nerve roots.

Another important feature of the epidural space is the demonstrable negative pressure that is encountered on initial entry. This is believed to be caused by the transmission of negative thoracic pressure through the intervertebral foramina. The negative pressure may be used to locate and verify the epidural space and can promote the cephalad spread of a local anesthetic agent. An exception is noted in advanced pregnancy, where a positive epidural pressure is present.[13,14]

Indications and Contraindications

Epidural anesthesia may be used for many types of operative and diagnostic procedures. Its popularity has increased in obstetrics because of its ability to provide a relatively pain-free labor and analgesia for either cesarean or vaginal delivery. Contraindications are similar to those associated with a subarachnoid block and are listed in Table 17–4.

Procedure

Initially, the procedure should be discussed with the patient and his or her consent obtained. Prior to administration, an intravenous cannula must be inserted and the appropriate fluid therapy initiated. Vital signs should be measured and recorded and standard resuscitation equipment should be immediately available to treat possible complications.

A standard commercial epidural tray generally contains all the necessary equipment to administer the block, with the possible exception of the local anesthetic agent and the disinfectant solution.

A wide range of local anesthetic agents of various concentrations may be used. The proper selection depends on the characteristics of the block required. Some specific local anesthetic agents are indicated in Table 17–5, along with their respective dosages and approximate durations of action. Currently, the use of narcotics (e.g., fentanyl) in combination with a local anesthetic agent is gaining popularity. Fentanyl 50 to 100 μg can be mixed with bupivacaine 0.125 to 0.25 percent to provide better analgesia without increasing volumes or concentrations of the local anesthetic.

The patient is positioned and disinfectant solution applied using a technique similar to that described for subarachnoid block administration (Table 17–6).

The appropriate interspace is identified according to the desired area being blocked. A skin wheal of local anes-

TABLE 17–4. INDICATIONS FOR AND CONTRAINDICATIONS TO EPIDURAL ANESTHESIA

Indications
    Postoperative pain relief
    Lower abdominal operative procedures
    Normal- and high-risk obstetric procedures
Contraindications
    Absolute
        Anticoagulant therapy
        Hypovolemia
        Systemic or localized infection near needle puncture site
        Increased intracranial pressure
        Patient refusal
    Relative
        Inexperience with the technique
        Active disease of central nervous system
        Previous laminectomy

TABLE 17–5. LOCAL ANESTHETIC AGENTS: CONCENTRATIONS AND APPROXIMATE DURATIONS OF EPIDURAL ANESTHESIA[a]

Agent	Concentration (%)	mg/Segment	Duration (min)
2-Chloroprocaine	3.0	45	60
Lidocaine	2.0	31	46
Mepivacaine	2.0	31	60
Bupivacaine	.5	7	170

[a] These dosages should be decreased in the elderly patient.

thetic is raised, and then a secondary skin puncture is made with a 15-gauge needle. This helps prevent the epidural needle from removing a piece of epidermis, which could lead to cyst formation.

Using a midline approach, the anesthetist inserts an epidural needle in a median plane. The stylet must be firmly held in place during insertion to prevent possible tearing of the epidermis. On entry into the interspinous ligament, which is identified by increased resistance, the stylet is removed.

A well-lubricated air- or normal saline-filled 5-mL glass

TABLE 17–6. IMPORTANT STEPS IN THE ADMINISTRATION OF AN EPIDURAL BLOCK: LOSS OF RESISTANCE TECHNIQUE[a]

I. Preparation
  A. Prepare equipment.
    1. Arrange resuscitation equipment and medication so that they are immediately available.
    2. Obtain sterile gloves and disinfectant solution.
    3. Verify epidural tray sterility and prepare it for easy use.
  B. Prepare patient.
    1. Explain procedure.
    2. Position appropriately
II. Performance
  A. Identify landmark and select site.
  B. Apply disinfectant solution.
  C. Raise skin wheal at site.
  D. Pierce skin with 15-gauge needle.
  E. Insert epidural needle.
    1. Introduce epidural needle.
    2. Attach lubricated 5-mL glass syringe to needle and check resistance.
    3. Advance slowly, checking resistance.
    4. Identify epidural space and check for cerebrospinal fluid or blood.
  F. Inject medication.
    1. Aspirate, introduce test dose, and monitor for symptoms of spinal or toxic reaction.
    2. If negative, administer remaining dosage in incremental doses.
  G. Insert catheter.
    1. After test dose, insert catheter 3 cm beyond needle tip.
    2. Remove needle.
    3. Tape catheter securely and attach syringe assembly.
  H. Reposition patient.

[a] Refer to text for additional information.

syringe is then attached and the feeling of resistance noted in the plunger. The needle is advanced a few millimeters at a time and the plunger retested. If no change in resistance is noted after continued advancement, the needle may be withdrawn and redirected. Penetration into the epidural space is identified when a distinct "pop" through the ligamentum flavum is noted, associated with a loss of resistance to injection. At this point, if no paresthesia is present, the syringe is disconnected and viewed for cerebrospinal fluid or blood. If negative, a test dose of 2 to 3 mL is slowly administered and the patient is observed for signs of spinal anesthesia[15] (e.g., numbness of the extremities); an additional 3 to 5 mL is then administered to test for intravascular injection (e.g., metallic taste, dizziness). If no adverse symptoms are noted, a loading dose is administered in incremental injections, and the needle removed. This is termed the *single administration* technique.

If cerebrospinal fluid is noted after removal of the stylet, one may elect to administer a spinal anesthetic at that time or use an adjacent space. Sixty milliliters of normal saline should then be administered in the epidural space at termination of the technique. If blood is present, the needle should be repositioned to ensure against intravascular injection.

Continuous epidural analgesia is obtained by insertion of a catheter through the epidural needle into the epidural space after administration of a test dose to verify needle position. Once the catheter has passed the tip of the needle, it is advanced approximately 3 cm. The needle is removed over the catheter and the catheter taped securely. *At no time must the catheter be removed from the needle after insertion because of the possibility of catheter shearing.* Prior to local anesthetic injection, catheter position should be verified by administration of a test dose to ensure that the catheter does not communicate with a blood vessel or cerebrospinal fluid. Repeat dosages of the local anesthetic agent may then be administered to maintain continuous analgesia. The repeat dosages should consist of a test dose, with aspiration before and after injection, followed by repeated fractional doses to obtain the refill dose.[16]

Problems may be encountered in association with catheter placement, such as difficulty in advancement and unilateral analgesia. These may be corrected by various catheter and needle maneuvers, but at no time should the catheter be removed from the needle.

Management

After administration the patient should be repositioned according to the procedure to be performed. The parturient may be positioned on her left side, thus providing left lateral displacement during labor. If a lower extremity or abdominal procedure is to be performed, the patient can be placed in a supine position. As with a spinal anesthetic, the patient's vital signs should be measured every minute for the first 20 minutes, and then monitored every 5 minutes.

An appropriate level of analgesia can be expected in approximately 20 minutes, although time varies according to the agent employed. Generally, the shorter-acting local anesthetic agents (e.g., 2-chloroprocaine) have a faster onset than the longer-duration anesthetics (e.g., bupivacaine). The level of analgesia can be determined by using the pinprick technique that was previously discussed in relation to spinal anesthesia assessment. After repositioning and initial assessment, the anesthetist must monitor the patient for possible complications such as hypotension, respiratory insufficiency, and toxic reactions throughout the procedure.

The epidural catheter is removed when analgesia is no longer required. At this time the catheter should be inspected to ensure complete removal and the findings should be documented in the patient's record.

Epidural catheters may remain in place for continuous postoperative pain relief. Continuous infusion of the local anesthetic using an infusion pump is gaining popularity; however, nurses caring for these patients must be able to detect and treat possible complications, such as respiratory depression.

BRACHIAL PLEXUS ANESTHESIA: AXILLARY APPROACH

The technique of blocking nerve impulses to and from the arm by injecting a local anesthetic solution into the group of nerves, or plexus, innervating the extremity is termed *brachial plexus anesthesia.*

Blocking of the brachial plexus can be performed in a variety of ways, for example, the subclavian, interscalene, and axillary techniques. These methods vary with respect to the approach used to reach the plexus and the extent to which the extremity is blocked.[17] Blockade of the brachial plexus by the axillary approach is discussed in this section, with an emphasis on aspects of administration.

Advantages and Disadvantages

Brachial plexus anesthesia by the axillary approach has distinct advantages and disadvantages in comparison to the subclavian and interscalene techniques and to general anesthesia. The axillary approach has the advantage of being less disturbing to general body physiology than general anesthesia, which may be of special importance in the poor-risk patient. Postoperative nausea and vomiting are lessened and other complications of general anesthesia are avoided. As compared with the subclavian and interscalene techniques of blocking the brachial plexus, the axillary approach eliminates the risk of pneumothorax and thus is considered a safer technique. It is also impossible to block the phrenic, vagus, and recurrent laryngeal nerves or the stellate ganglia with the axillary approach.

As with any anesthetic technique, the axillary approach has disadvantages. It has a prolonged onset time and produces less muscle paralysis in comparison to other approaches. Analgesia may be spotty and may be inadequate for surgery beyond the hand into the forearm. Complete anesthesia of the entire upper extremity is not possible, because the injection is made where the nerve fibers begin to leave the axillary sheath.

Anatomy

An understanding of the distribution and anatomic location of the various nerve fibers supplying the arm is useful in administering an axillary block (Table 17–7). On the basis of this knowledge, the anesthetist can relate paresthesias

TABLE 17–7. MAJOR NERVES IN THE ARM AND THEIR DISTRIBUTION

Nerve	Area Supplied
Musculocutaneous	Brachial muscle
Medial	Lateral arm and thumb
Ulnar	Medial arm
Radial	Posterior arm and hand

elicited during needle insertion to the needle's anatomic orientation. This can help to ensure adequate analgesia to a particular area of the extremity.

The brachial plexus is an arrangement of nerve fibers supplying both sensory and motor nerve impulses to and from the arm. The nerve fibers originate from the fifth cervical vertebra (C-5) through the first thoracic vertebra (T-1).[18] The nerves leave their respective vertebral foramina and the nerve roots form three groups, the upper, middle, and lower trunks (Fig. 17–7). An extension of the prevertebral fascia surrounds the nerves as a multicompartmented sheath.[19]

The upper trunk is formed by the fifth and sixth cervical nerves. As the upper trunk progresses, it gives rise to the suprascapular and subclavicular nerves. The upper trunk then forms the lateral cord, which has two primary branches. One branch forms the musculocutaneous nerve and a second branch assists in forming the median nerve.

The lower trunk is formed by the eighth cervical and first thoracic nerves. The lower trunk progresses into the medial cord, which has two primary branches. One branch assists in forming the median nerve; a second branch forms the ulnar nerve.

The middle trunk is formed by the seventh cervical nerve. The middle trunk, along with a branch from the upper and lower trunks, forms the posterior cord. The pos-

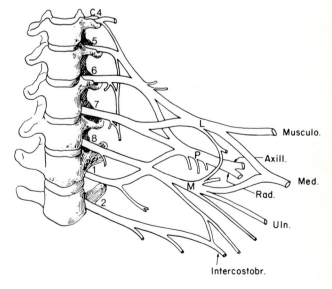

Figure 17–7. The nerve fibers composing the brachial plexus. The lateral, medial, and posterior cords give rise to the musculocutaneous axillary, median, radial, and ulnar nerves.

terior cord branches into the suprascapular, axillary, and radial nerves. The intercostal brachial nerve, originating from the second thoracic vertebra (T-2), is important because it innervates the proximal inner arm.

Indications and Contraindications

Axillary block of the brachial plexus is indicated for surgical procedures involving the arm and hand. It can be used to differentiate central and peripheral pain. The technique is useful for surgical procedures on patients with a full stomach, patients who fear losing consciousness, and patients with complicating conditions.

Axillary block is contraindicated in patients with active infections of the extremity resulting from lymphadenopathy. The block is also contraindicated in patients with coagulation disorders and in patients whose injury would prevent them from abducting the arm. The presence of a nerve injury may also be a contraindication because of legal implications. Difficulty should be anticipated in the markedly obese patient, whose axillary artery may be difficult to palpate.

Procedure

Proper preparation is very important. Table 17–8 offers a step-by-step approach for administration of an axillary block.

One should have all the necessary equipment available for resuscitation before proceeding with the block. If it is performed in the holding area, resuscitation equipment should be readily available. *At no time should this anesthetic technique be performed without equipment on hand for the treatment of complications.*

The specific local anesthetic agent used may vary and there is no one ideal agent. In deciding which agent to use, one must consider the duration of action needed and degree of block required. Also, the agent's potency, duration of action, toxic dosage, effective concentration, and presence of allergies must be considered.

Table 17–9 lists commonly used agents, including their concentrations and approximate duration of action. Use of a sufficient volume (40 to 50 mL) will help ensure adequate spreading of the agent, but the recommended maximum dose should not be exceeded. The use of epinephrine prolongs the action of shorter-acting agents but is of little benefit to agents of longer duration.

The local anesthetic agent is drawn up into two 20-mL syringes in an appropriate dosage, which are then labeled. The extension tubing and syringes are attached to a stopcock and any air is removed. The extension tubing is used to facilitate needle placement and injection.

Before proceeding with the block the patient's full cooperation must be obtained. The importance of this cannot be overstated. If the patient is aware of what is to occur, success is more likely. Prior to administration of the block, an intravenous catheter should be inserted and appropriate fluid therapy initiated. The appropriate monitoring equipment, such as cardioscope, blood pressure cuff, and precordial stethoscope, should be used.

After the appropriate monitoring equipment has been

TABLE 17–8. IMPORTANT STEPS IN THE ADMINISTRATION OF A BRACHIAL PLEXUS BLOCK VIA THE AXILLARY APPROACH*a*

I. Preparation
  A. Prepare equipment.
    1. Arrange resuscitation equipment and medication so that they are immediately available.
    2. Obtain sterile gloves and disinfectant solution.
    3. Obtain two 20-mL syringes, stopcock, extension, and B-beveled needle.
  B. Prepare patient.
    1. Explain procedure.
    2. Position patient supine, with arm abducted 90 degrees and dorsum of hand by head.
    3. Note anatomic landmarks.
    4. Apply disinfectant solution.
II. Performance
  A. Identify landmarks and select site.
  B. Raise skin wheal at site.
  C. Insert needle.
    1. Insert and advance 22-gauge B-beveled needle.
    2. Aspirate continuously while inserting needle.
    3. Allow needle to enter sheath until "pop" is felt.
    4. Redirect needle until paresthesia is elicited.
  D. Inject medication.
    1. Withdraw needle slightly and apply digital pressure distal to injection site.
    2. Inject medication and monitor symptoms of toxicity.
    3. Leave medication in extension tubing for T-2 block.
  E. Withdraw needle to subcutaneous tissue.
  F. Institute blockade of intercostal brachialis (T-2).
    1. Advance needle upward in axilla and inject medication.
    2. Advance needle downward in axilla and inject medication.
  G. Remove needle and abduct arm with gentle massage of axilla.

a Refer to text for additional details on each point.

secured and checked, the patient's arm is abducted 90 degrees and the hand placed under his or her head. The artery is then identified by palpation and appropriate landmarks noted. Removal of axillary hair may be performed at this time. Using sterile technique, the area is prepared with a disinfectant solution. The disinfectant solution is removed with a sterile sponge and the axillary artery is palpated. It is useful at this point to have an assistant manage the syringe and stopcock assembly. The artery is retracted downward

TABLE 17–9. VARIOUS ANESTHETIC AGENTS USED FOR BRACHIAL PLEXUS BLOCK BY THE AXILLARY APPROACH, THEIR CONCENTRATIONS, AND APPROXIMATE DURATIONS OF ACTION

Agent	Concentration (%)	Duration
Bupivacaine	0.5 or 0.25	Long (4–6 h)
Lidocaine	1	Intermediate (2 h)
Mepivacaine	1	Intermediate (2 h)
2-Chloroprocaine	1, 2, 3	Short (1 h)

by the underfinger and the needle is introduced above the artery just under the greater pectoralis muscle. A skin wheal of local anesthetic is then raised and the needle is advanced toward the axillary sheath. An assistant must keep aspirating during needle insertion to detect if a blood vessel is entered.

When the axillary sheath is entered, a distinct "pop" is felt. The needle should then be advanced until a paresthesia is elicited in an area close to the surgical site. The needle is withdrawn slightly, digital pressure is applied distal to the needle site, and the local anesthetic solution is injected slowly. The patient must be carefully monitored for any symptoms of a toxic reaction during injection. The needle is removed to the subcutaneous tissue of the axilla and the remaining solution is injected caudad to and cephalad from the insertion site to block the intercostal brachialis nerve (T-2) supplying the upper axilla. This helps eliminate tourniquet pain.

If during insertion the axillary artery is penetrated, as revealed by aspiration, the needle may be advanced dorsally, through the artery, and one half of the anesthetic agent injected. The needle is then removed until it is located ventral to the artery and the remaining half of the anesthetic agent is injected. A T-2 block is performed as previously described.

After the intercostal brachial nerve has been blocked, the arm should be adducted as soon as possible and the axillary area gently massaged to assist in spreading the anesthetic agent.[20]

Variations

As is true of most anesthetic techniques, individual variations of this technique exist. Generally, variations are adopted as the anesthetist finds his or her success rate increasing with a particular variation.

In one such variation a tourniquet is applied to the upper arm, just below the axilla. This prevents the local anesthetic from spreading distally and encourages its upward movement, although digital pressure may be just as effective.[20] Also, the use of a peripheral nerve stimulator has been advocated.[21] It is set at a low voltage and attached to the needle. This may assist by detecting the location of specific nerves and provides a better perception of needle positioning. This variation can cause discomfort to the patient during testing.[22]

After administration of the block the anesthetist must constantly assess the patient's status. Onset time varies depending on the local anesthetic agent employed, but enough time must be allowed for onset to occur. Informing the surgeon of the time necessary for onset may prevent undue stress. The first sign of onset is characterized by a loss of proprioception in the arm as evidenced by an inability of the patient to touch his or her nose. Then, motor blockade usually develops, followed by sensory blockade, depending on the agent used.[23]

Management

Adequate sedation during the procedure will help ensure effective patient management and aid in making the opera-

tion a pleasant experience. Diazepam and fentanyl are useful agents in increasing patient comfort and allaying anxiety. Diazepam offers the advantage of raising the seizure threshold.

As with any anesthetic technique, the anesthetist must be aware of the possible complications and their treatment. Although this technique is considered to be a very safe means of blocking the brachial plexus, there are still some possible complications that must be considered.

Formation of a hematoma as a result of axillary artery puncture is always possible because the axillary artery lies in the axillary sheath with the plexus. Clinically, it usually has little significance and vigorous massage of the injection site will aid in avoiding its formation. Also, intravenous or interarterial injection must be avoided because of the toxic reactions and arterial damage that may result. Aspiration while advancing and positioning the needle helps avoid this complication.

A spotty block is always a possibility and is due to incomplete blockade of all nerve fibers within the plexus. If this occurs, additional sedation and patient reassurance may be adequate to complete the operative procedure. If not, additional local infiltration or a specific nerve block may be administered to ensure that adequate anesthesia is present.

Whatever the route of administration, the local anesthetic eventually enters the bloodstream, and the possibility of a toxic reaction always exists. Prevention, of course, should be the primary goal. Toxic reactions can be prevented by limiting the dosage of local anesthetic and closely monitoring the patient. Premonitory signs, such as anxiety, muscle twitching, headache, drowsiness, and slurring of speech, may indicate an impending toxic reaction. Should a reaction occur, 100 percent oxygen should be administered with assisted ventilation. Diazepam may help by decreasing limbic system excitability and precluding focal seizure generation. Also, sodium thiopental may be used as an anticonvulsant. The aim in treatment of a toxic reaction is to prevent cerebral hypoxia.

INTRAVENOUS REGIONAL ANESTHESIA

Injection of a local anesthetic agent into a tourniquet-occluded arm is termed intravenous regional anesthesia. It is one of the oldest forms of peripheral nerve blockade and is often used today because of its simplicity and relative safety.

Advantages and Disadvantages

Intravenous regional anesthesia offers distinct advantages. It is relatively easy to perform as long as a step-by-step process is followed. Also, the onset of anesthesia after injection is rapid (5 to 10 minutes) and the recovery time is short after tourniquet deflation.

A major disadvantage of the technique is the limited amount of time the tourniquet can remain inflated without causing tissue damage to the extremity. Generally, the tourniquet should not remain inflated longer than 2 hours, after which time it must be deflated, resulting in a loss of anesthesia.[24,25]

Anatomy

The technique of administering an intravenous regional anesthetic does not require specific anatomic landmarks, as is true of spinal or brachial plexus anesthesia. It is important to note that the local anesthetic, postinjection, is distributed throughout the extremity and is thought to work at three principal sites: (1) the peripheral nerve endings, (2) the neuromuscular junction, and (3) the nerve trunk.[26] The primary site of action is controversial but appears to be on the small peripheral nerve branches.[27,28]

Indications and Contraindications

Indications for and contraindications to intravenous regional anesthesia are listed in Table 17–10. This technique is very useful for soft-tissue operations of the arm or hand (e.g., ganglion removal). The block provides a bloodless field and anesthesia of relatively rapid onset and recovery.

If the surgery is expected to last more than 2 hours, use of this technique is not advised. After 2 hours, the tourniquet must be deflated to prevent tissue damage. It is possible to reinflate the tourniquet and reinject but, in actual practice, this is hard to accomplish.

Procedure

Administering an effective intravenous regional anesthetic requires specific attention to details. Table 17–11 emphasizes some of the important aspects in performing the block on a step-by-step basis.

Various local anesthetic agents have been used, but only lidocaine hydrochloride is presently approved by the U.S. Food and Drug Administration (Fisher LB. 1980. Personal communication: Professional information, Astra Pharmaceutical Products, Worcester, Massachusetts). It is effective at low concentrations (0.5 percent) and relatively safe in large volumes. A dosage of 3 mg/kg lean body weight of a 0.5 percent solution is recommended.

Before proceeding with the block the anesthetist must check all equipment for proper operation. This is true with any anesthetic technique but is particularly important with an intravenous regional anesthetic. Many unsuccessful blocks can be attributed to a leaky cuff or failure of the pressure system supplying the tourniquet. Prior to administration of the block, the anesthetist must pressurize the tourniquet system to ensure that no leaks are present and identify

TABLE 17–10. INDICATIONS FOR AND CONTRAINDICATIONS TO INTRAVENOUS REGIONAL ANESTHESIA

Indications
 Suturing of lacerations
 Reduction and manipulations of fractures
 Amputations
 Minor external operations (e.g., ganglion removal)
Contraindications
 Severe peripheral vascular disease
 Infections of the extremity
 Patient refusal

TABLE 17–11. IMPORTANT STEPS IN THE ADMINISTRATION OF AN INTRAVENOUS REGIONAL BLOCK[a]

I. Preparation
 A. Prepare equipment.
  1. Arrange resuscitation equipment and medications.
  2. Obtain double tourniquet with switch valve and inflationary device.
  3. Obtain Esmarch bandage and roller gauze.
  4. IV catheter (20 gauge), extension tubing, and 50-mL syringe.
 B. Prepare patient.
  1. Perform standard IV insertion.
  2. Explain procedure.
  3. Position patient supine.
  4. Apply cottonwool (Webril) to upper arm.
  5. Apply double tourniquet.
II. Procedure
 A. Insert IV catheter and connect to syringe assembly.
 B. Elevate extremity and wrap tightly with Esmarch bandage.
 C. Inflate proximal cuff.
 D. Remove Esmarch and examine extremity for blanching.
 E. Inject local anesthetic agent and monitor for toxic symptoms.
 F. Remove IV catheter (optional).
 G. Inflate distal cuff and deflate proximal cuff to treat tourniquet pain.

[a] Refer to text for additional information.

that the connections are correct between the double-cuffed tourniquet and the selection switch.

The patient is placed in a supine position and cottonwool (Webril) and a double-cuffed tourniquet are applied to the proximal aspect of the extremity. The cottonwool should be applied wrinkle free and in an adequate amount to prevent skin damage from tourniquet pressure. The double-cuffed tourniquet should then be applied snugly to ensure that cuff pressure is applied to as large a surface area as possible on tourniquet inflation.

An intravenous catheter is inserted into a good-sized vein using an appropriate aseptic technique. Individual opinion varies as to the best site for catheter placement but, generally, the closer the catheter site is to the operative field, the better the anesthesia will be in that specific area.[29] Leaving the catheter in place can facilitate reinjection of the local anesthetic, but it makes placement near the operative site difficult.

One of the most important points in administering an intravenous regional block is to ensure complete exsanguination of the extremity. Early elevation of the limb and wrapping of the extremity distally to proximally tightly with an Esmarch bandage should facilitate adequate exsanguination (Fig. 17–8).

The Esmarch bandage should be wrapped tightly up to the tourniquet and the proximal cuff inflated 100 to 150 mm Hg above the patient's systolic pressure. A maximum pressure of 300 mm Hg for the upper extremity should not be exceeded.[30]

After the Esmarch bandage has been removed, the extremity should have a pale, blanched appearance with an absence of pulses. If this is not the case, it is advisable to ommended local anesthetic dosage should not be exceeded, a reliable tourniquet should be used, and tourniquet release should be delayed 20 to 30 minutes after injection.[32,33]

To terminate the block, the anesthetist should use an inflation–deflation technique, especially if the time from injection is less than 45 minutes. The cycled deflation technique consists of deflating the tourniquet for 5 seconds and then reinflating it for 2 to 3 minutes.[34] This procedure is repeated two to three times. This decreases the local anesthetic bolus effect associated with tourniquet release.

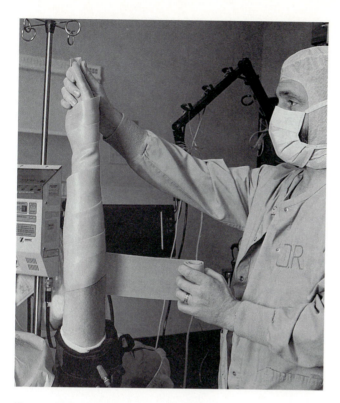

Figure 17–8. Application of double-tourniquet cuff to an extremity wrapped with an Esmarch bandage.

rewrap the extremity to obtain better results. The presence of blood in the extremity will significantly decrease the action of the local anesthetic agent.

After the extremity has been exsanguinated adequately, the anesthetist slowly injects the local anesthetic agent while monitoring for signs of adverse reactions. After injection, the intravenous catheter may be removed and the disinfectant solution applied in preparation for the surgical procedure. The onset of anesthesia should occur within 5 to 10 minutes of injection.

Management

Management of an intravenous block is similar in many respects to management of other regional anesthetic techniques. Adequate sedation and effective communication alleviate patient anxiety and help to ensure a pleasant experience.

Tourniquet pain may occur after prolonged tourniquet occlusion.[31] Often, it can be eliminated by inflating the distal tourniquet and deflating the proximal one. This must be performed with caution. If at any time both cuffs become deflated, the block has been terminated. If this occurs, the anesthetist must monitor for signs of a toxic reaction caused by the bolus effect of local anesthetic agent entering the bloodstream.

A local anesthetic toxic reaction may occur any time but is more likely immediately after tourniquet release. The occurrence of a toxic reaction can be directly related to the duration of ischemia and the dosage and volume of medication administered. To help prevent toxic reactions, the rec-

REFERENCES

1. Lund PC. Reflections upon the historical aspects of spinal anesthesia. *Regional Anaesth.* 1983:8.
2. Cousins MJ, Bredenbaugh PO. *Neural blockade.* 2nd ed. Philadelphia: JB Lippincott; 1982.
3. Miller RD. *Anesthesia.* New York: Churchill Livingstone; 1990.
4. Reimann AF, Anson BJ. The spinal cord and meninges. *Anat Rec.* 1944;88:127.
5. Macintosh R. *Lumbar puncture and spinal analgesia.* Edinburgh: Livingstone; 1957.
6. Greene NM. *Physiology of spinal anesthesia.* 3rd ed. Baltimore: Williams & Wilkins; 1981.
7. Bengtasson M, Lofstrom JB, Malmquist LA. Skin conductance responses during spinal analgesia. *Acta Anesthesiol Scand.* 1985;27:67–71.
8. Freund FG, Bonica JJ, et al. Ventilatory reserve and level of motor block during high spinal and epidural anesthesia. *Anesthesiology.* 1967;28:834.
9. Greene NM. Present concepts of spinal anesthesia. *Refresher Courses Anesthesiol.* 1979;7:131.
10. Armstrong IA, Littlewood DG, Chambers WA. Spinal anesthesia with tetracaine—The effect of added vasoconstrictors. *Anesth Analg.* 1983;62:793–795.
11. Greene NM. Uptake and elimination of local anesthetics during spinal anesthesia. *Anesth Analg.* 1983;62:1013–1024.
12. Ching D. Epidural space. Anatomical and clinical aspects. *Anesth Analg.* 1963;42:398–407.
13. Moya F, Smith B. Spinal anesthesia for cesarean section: Clinical and biochemical studies of effects on maternal physiology. *JAMA.* 1962;179:608.
14. Abouleish E. *Pain control in obstetrics.* Philadelphia: JB Lippincott; 1977.
15. Reisner LS, Hockman BN, Plumer MH. Persistent neurologic deficit and adhesive arachnoiditis following intrathecal 2-chloroprocaine injection. *Anesth Analg.* 1980;59:452–454.
16. Covino BG, Marx GF, et al. Prolonged sensory/motor deficit following inadvertent spinal anesthesia. *Anesth Analg.* 1980;59:399–400.
17. Lanz E, Theiss D, Janicovic D. The extent of blockade following various techniques of brachial plexus block. *Anesth Analg.* 1983;62:55–58.
18. Reese C. Conduction anesthesia of the upper extremity—A literature and technique review. *AANA J.* June 1977:269.
19. Thompson G, Rorie D. Functional anatomy of the brachial plexus sheaths. *Anesthesiology.* 1983;59:117–122.
20. Winnie A, Radenjic R, et al. Factors influencing distribution of local anesthetic injected into the brachial plexus sheath. *Anesth Analg.* 1979;58:225–233.
21. Montgomery SJ. The use of the nerve stimulator with standard unsheathed needles in nerve blockade. *Anesth Analg.* 1973;52:827–831.
22. Smith BL. Efficacy of a nerve stimulator in regional analgesia: Experience in a resident training programme. *Anaesthesia.* 1976;31:778–782.

23. Winnie AP, Tay C, et al. Pharmacokinetics of local anesthetics during plexus blocks. *Anesth Analg.* 1977;56:852–862.

24. Kessler F. The brachial tourniquet and local analgesia in surgery of the upper limb. *J Trauma.* 1966:43–47.

25. Bruner JM. Safety factors in the use of the pneumatic tourniquet for hemostasis in surgery of the hand. *J Bone Joint Surg.* 1951;3A:221–224.

26. Reese C. Intravenous regional conduction anesthesia—A technique and literature review, Part I. *AANA J.* August 1981: 357–373.

27. Holmes CM. *Intravenous regional neural blockade in clinical anesthesia and management of pain.* Philadelphia: JB Lippincott; 1980:343–354.

28. Urban B, McKain C. Onset and progression of intravenous regional anesthesia with dilute lidocaine. *Anesth Analg.* 1982;61: 834–838.

29. Dunbar RW, Mazzee RI. Intravenous regional anesthesia—Experience with 779 cases. *Anesth Analg.* 1967;46:806–813.

30. Thorn-Alquist AM. Intravenous regional anesthesia—A seven year survey. *Acta Anaesthiol Scand.* 1971;15:23–32.

31. Cole F. Tourniquet pain. *Anesth Analg.* 1952;31:63–64.

32. Bier A. Concerning a new method of local anesthesia of the extremities. *Arch Kin Chir.* 1908;86:1007–1016. [English translation by Hellijas CS. *Survey of Anesthesiology, Classical File* 1967;11:294–300.]

33. Morrison JT. Intravenous local anesthesia. *Br J Surg.* 1931;18:642–647.

34. Merrifield AJ, Carter SJ. Intravenous regional anesthesia—Lignocaine blood levels. *Anaesthesia.* 1965;20:287–293.

Fluid and Electrolyte Therapy

Lorraine M. Jordan

The management of fluids and electrolytes is an essential part of the anesthetic care of the surgical patient. The surgical procedures can impose great stress on the fluid and electrolyte status of the patient. A thorough knowledge of the anatomy and physiology of body fluids and electrolytes provides the foundation for perioperative therapy. This chapter outlines fluid derangements and their treatment.

ANATOMY OF BODY FLUIDS

The isotope tracer techniques are perhaps the most accurate means of measuring the different fluid compartments of the body. There is a wide range of normal values based on age, weight, body size, and sex. The compartments remain relatively constant throughout life, once adulthood is reached, as long as the patient remains in a normal steady state. This state is referred to as *dynamic equilibrium*. Dynamic equilibrium attempts to maintain the composition of fluids in balance regardless of the intake and output of fluids.

TOTAL BODY WATER

Total body water (TBW) is the water in the intracellular and extracellular compartments. Water accounts for between 50 and 70 percent of total body weight. If deuterium oxide (D_2O) or titrated water is used for measurement of TBW, the average value for young adult men is 60 percent of body weight, and that for young adult women, 50 percent. The average volume of total body water is 42 L. The amount of total body fluid in adults is based on the percentage of body fat. Fat contains little water, and lean body mass has more body fluid. Obese persons have as much as 25 to 30 percent less TBW than do lean persons of the same height and average weight.

Age has a significant effect on TBW. Moore and Ball[1] have shown that TBW as a percentage of total body weight decreases steadily with age. As age increases, TBW de-

creases to as low as 52 percent for men and 47 percent for women. Just the opposite is true for infants. In premature infants, TBW is approximately 90 percent of the total body weight. The full-term infant has approximately 70 to 80 percent TBW compared with total body weight. As an infant becomes older, there is a gradual reduction of TBW. The 1-year-old has a TBW of approximately 65 percent.[2] The TBW remains relatively constant throughout childhood and puberty. TBW ranges from 500 to 600 mL/kg for an average adult[3] (Table 18–1).

The TBW is divided into two compartments: intracellular fluid (ICF) and extracellular fluid (ECF).

Intracellular Fluid

ICF is the water within the body's different cells. The ICF makes up 30 to 40 percent of the body weight. The largest amount of ICF is in the skeletal muscle mass. ICF contains large amounts of potassium, magnesium, and phosphate ions and small amounts of sodium and chloride. The principal cations of ICF are potassium and magnesium, and the principal anions are proteins and phosphates.

Extracellular Fluid

ECF is the body water outside the cells. The ECF helps to maintain the internal environment of the body. It provides nutrients and removes waste from the cells. The ECF constitutes 20 percent of body weight and 25 percent of TBW. ECF is further categorized into two major types: the intravascular volume (plasma), which totals 5 percent of body weight, and the interstitial volume (fluid between the cells), which totals 15 percent of body weight[3] (Fig. 18–1).

Approximately 80 percent of the ECF is interstitial fluid. Interstitial fluid includes lymph and the extracellular portion of dense connective tissue and the transcellular compartment. Transcellular water includes fluid such as cerebrospinal fluid, intraocular fluid, joint fluid, salivary fluid, and mucous secretions of the respiratory and gastrointestinal tract. This nonfunctional component represents approximately 10 percent of the interstitial fluid volume

TABLE 18–1. APPROXIMATE VALUES OF TOTAL BODY FLUID AS A PERCENTAGE OF BODY WEIGHT IN RELATION TO AGE AND SEX

Age	Total Body Fluid (% body weight)	
Full-term newborn	70–80	
1 year	64	
Puberty to 39 years	Men:	60
	Women:	52
40–60 years	Men:	55
	Women:	47
> 60 years	Men:	52
	Women:	46

Reprinted, with permission, from Metheny.[3]

and should not be confused with "third-space fluid" found in burns and soft-tissue injury. The interstitial fluid also possesses a functional equilibrating component in which dissolved substances move through spaces.

The plasma is approximately 20 percent of the ECF and is the fluid portion of the blood. The plasma interchanges continuously with the interstitial fluid through pores, exchanging oxygen and other metabolic substances as it passes through the capillaries. Colloid osmotic pressure

minimizes the loss of plasma from the circulatory system through the capillary pores.

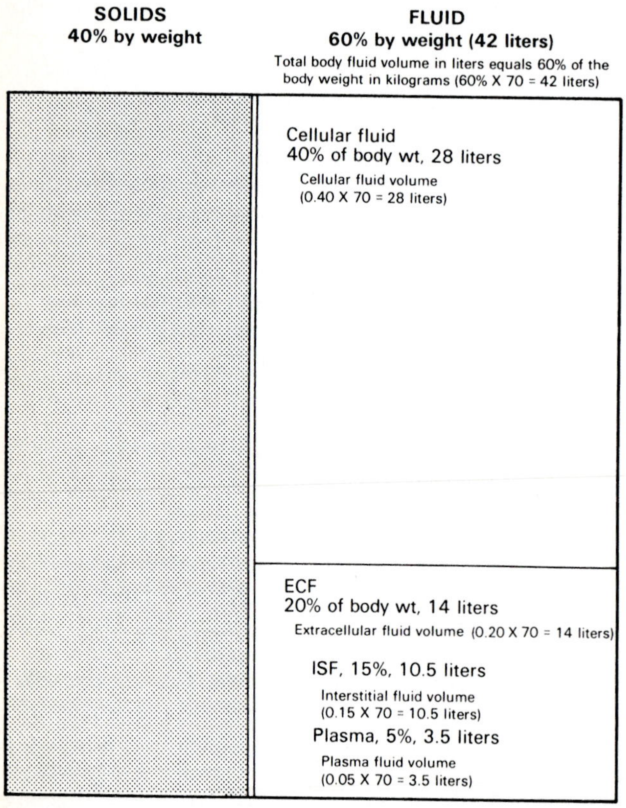

ELECTROLYTES

Continuous interactions occur between the various body fluid compartments. To aid in understanding some of these changes, an explanation of the terminology follows.

Electrolytes are electrically charged particles within the body fluids. These charged particles are ions. The term *ion* describes chemical reactivity. Ions possess negative (anions) and positive (cations) charges. ICF and ECF have different concentrations of ions. The chemical reactivity of ions in each compartment is expressed as milliequivalents per liter (mEq/L) (Fig. 18–2). Molecules of substances found in fluid compartments are expressed in mg/100 mL or in g/1000 mL of fluid. The number of particles per unit volume is expressed in moles (*mol*) or millimoles (*mmol*).[3]

One millimole is 1/1000th of a mole. A mole is the molecular weight of a substance expressed in grams. One mole of $CaCl_2$ is 110 g of $CaCl_2$; to determine the number of grams in $CaCl_2$ the sum of the atomic weights of Ca and Cl is determined. The atomic weight of Ca is 40 and that of Cl is 35. The sum of the atomic weights is known as the *molecular weight*. An example follows for $CaCl_2$.

$$\text{Atomic weight of Ca} = 40$$

$$\text{Atomic weight of Cl} = 35$$

$$\text{Atomic weight} + \text{atomic weight} = \text{molecular weight}$$

$$40 + 35(2) = 110$$

$$110 \text{ g} = 1 \text{ mol of } CaCl_2$$

If 1 mol of a substance is mixed with 1 L of water, the solution would be expressed as 1 mol/L.

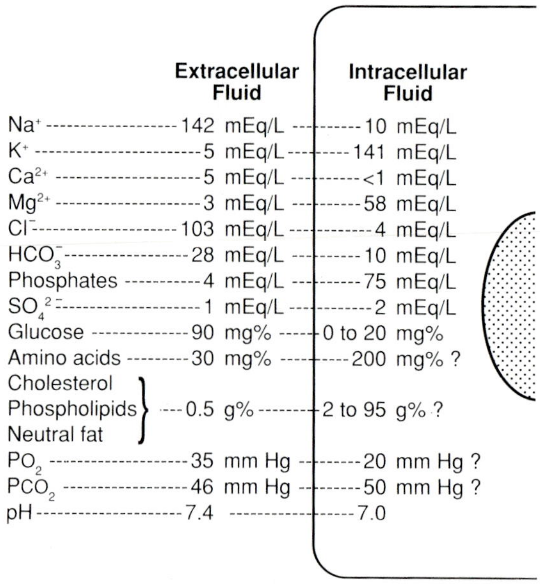

Figure 18–1. Fluid compartments and the amount of fluid in a 70 kg (154 lb) young adult male. (*From Metheny N: Quick Reference to Fluid Balance. Philadelphia, JB Lippincott, 1984*).

Figure 18–2. Chemical compositions of extracellular and intracellular fluids. (*From Guyton A: Textbook of Medical Physiology, 5th ed. Philadelphia, WB Saunders, 1976.*)

OSMOLARITY

Osmolarity is an expression of total solute concentration of body fluids. The solute concentration exerts a pressure that is attributed to the number of osmotically active particles in solution. The osmole (osm) is a unit of measure used to quantify osmolarity. The osmotic pressure of body fluid is often expressed in a smaller unit, the milliosmole (mosm). An example is the dissociation of sodium chloride (NaCl) into Na and Cl, which constitutes 2 mosm.

Calcium (Ca$_2$) and magnesium (Mg$_2$) are divalent ions. Divalent ions carry two charges in the molecule. Therefore, 1 mmol of a divalent cation equals 2 mEq. For elements that are monovalent, such as sodium (Na), 1 mmol of the ion is equivalent to 1 mEq.[4]

There remains an ionic difference between the two compartments (ICF and ECF). The osmotic pressure exerted is dependent on the number of osmotically active particles. The number of substances that fail to pass through the semipermeable membrane contribute to the effective osmotic pressure. Sodium is the principal cation of ECF and is the major contributor of osmotic pressure, whereas the dissolved proteins in the plasma are responsible for the osmotic pressure between the plasma and the interstitial fluid compartment.

The osmotic pressures of the ECF and ICF are essentially equal. The number of osmotically active particles in the ECF and ICF ranges from 290 to 310 mosm. The semipermeable membrane between the ECF and ICF is freely permeable to water and allows the two compartments to maintain essential osmotic equilibrium. The osmotic pressure of compartments can become altered. A change in osmotic pressure of ECF and ICF compartments will lead to changes in fluid volume. For example, a loss of sodium from the ECF would cause an efflux of H$_2$O from the ECF to the ICF.

Osmosis is the net movement of water across a semipermeable membrane, from higher water concentration to lower water concentration, or from an area of lesser concentration of solute to one of greater concentration of solute.[5] The greatest exchange of fluid occurs with the ECF compartment.

BODY FLUID CHANGES

Disorders in fluid balance can be categorized as disturbances in volume, concentration, and composition.

Volume Changes

Volume changes that occur are either a volume deficit or a volume excess.

Volume Deficit. ECF volume deficit is frequently referred to as fluid deficit, hypovolemia, or dehydration. An ECF volume deficit is due to a loss of water and electrolytes, a greater loss of fluid than intake of fluid. The body loses fluid from the kidneys, skin, lungs, and gastrointestinal tract. An adult typically excretes 1 to 2 L of urine per day. The skin loses water through perspiration, which varies widely with the temperature of the environment. Insensible loss of water through the skin occurs by evaporation. The loss of fluid via the lungs occurs at a rate of 300 to 400 mL every day. This loss can increase greatly with an increased respiratory rate and tidal volume. The body loses 100 to 200 mL of fluid daily through the gastrointestinal tract. Therefore, the average adult requires at least 2000 mL of water per day as maintenance.

ECF volume deficit may be caused by vomiting, diarrhea, loss of nasogastric secretions, and fistula drainage. During surgery, the patient loses a great deal of ECF via evaporation, blood loss, and third spacing as a result of surgical trauma. Other causes of ECF loss include burns, peritonitis, intestinal obstruction, and sequestration of fluid from soft-tissue injury.

Two systems primarily affected by volume changes are the cardiovascular and nervous systems. The cardiovascular system displays such signs as a postural decrease in systolic blood pressure in excess of 10 mm Hg, increased heart rate, flat neck veins in supine position, and a decreased central venous pressure. Other signs and symptoms noted when there is an ECF deficit are oliguria (less than 20 to 40 mL/h), nausea, vomiting, weight loss, a depressed anterior fontanel in infants, an increase in specific gravity of the urine, longitudinal wrinkles in the tongue, dry skin, weakness, and apathy.

A severe loss of ECF may lead to shock or cardiovascular collapse, as well as permanent renal damage. The decrease in ECF may lead to hypotension and inadequate perfusion of the kidneys. Inadequate perfusion of the kidneys may cause the nephrons and tubules to deteriorate and to become permanently damaged.

Volume Excess. Excess of ECF volume is often caused by fluid excess, which develops when fluid input exceeds output. The kidneys are unable to rid the body of excess water and electrolytes. Volume excess often develops from overloading the body by oral or parenteral administration of excessive quantities of fluid or as a result of renal failure. Excess ECF indicates an increase in both plasma and interstitial fluid volume.

Some signs generally encountered with volume excess include circulatory overload manifested by pulmonary hypertension, dyspnea, cyanosis, coughing, frothy sputum, elevated pulmonary artery wedge pressure, ascites, effusions into third spaces, peripheral edema, bounding pulse, distended neck veins, moist rales, and increases in central venous pressure and blood pressure. Volume excess in the elderly often presents as congestive heart failure. Patients more susceptible to volume overload are those with chronic heart failure, chronic renal failure, excessive adrenocortical hormones, and excessive administration of intravenous fluids, especially isotonic solutions.

The treatment for volume excess includes fluid restriction, administration of diuretics, restriction of sodium intake, administration of vasodilators, and positive-pressure ventilation. Positive-pressure ventilation increases the intracellular pressure, forcing the fluid out of the alveoli.

Changes in Serum Concentration

Sodium. Sodium (Na) is the most abundant cation of the ECF, and is the most important ion exerting osmotic pressure on the cellular membrane. Concentrations of sodium in the ECF range from 135 to 145 mEq/L. Sodium is a primary determinant of ECF and water distribution. Sodium is regulated in part by the kidneys. It helps to maintain normal composition of ECF, as well as chemical–electrical equilibrium. Sodium also mediates action potentials within the nerves and muscles. The regulation of sodium in the body is controlled by the secretion of antidiuretic hormone (ADH) and aldosterone.

ADH is secreted by the hypothalamic posterior pituitary. The secretion of ADH causes an increase in water reabsorption by the kidneys, decreasing urinary output and increasing urinary concentration. The reabsorption of water in the kidneys occurs at the collecting tubules. The production and release of ADH are influenced by receptors in the hypothalamus known as osmoreceptors. The osmoreceptors are sensitive to osmotic pressure of the plasma. ADH assists in regulation of osmotic pressure. Aldosterone is a hormone secreted by the adrenal cortex. It is a mineralocorticoid that exerts its effect on the kidneys, stimulating reabsorption of sodium and excretion of potassium ions.

Hyponatremia. Hyponatremia is low sodium concentration in the ECF. Hyponatremia may be caused by excessive loss of sodium via vomiting, diarrhea, and diuretics, and by loss through body cavities as in peritonitis, draining ascites, and burns. Sodium deficit may also result in excessive intake of water. The resulting water intoxication dilutes the serum sodium. Examples of serum sodium dilution include excess water intake, depressed renal blood flow, repeated water enemas, congestive heart failure with water retention, and parenteral administration of electrolyte-free solutions.[6] The hyponatremic state lends itself to an osmotic shift out of the ECF compartment and into the ICF compartment. This shift of fluid causes fluid depletion in the ECF compartment and leads to hypovolemia. A severe shift of fluid causes cerebral edema, leading to the development of neurologic symptoms.

The clinical signs associated with hyponatremia resulting from sodium loss are weakness, confusion, nausea, vomiting, neurologic signs, postural hypotension, and lethargy. Some serious neurologic symptoms that may develop are loss of reflexes, the Babinski sign, and seizures. These signs develop when the serum sodium drops below 115 mEq/L. The treatment of sodium deficiency is aimed at restoration of sodium in the ECF compartment. Treatment may entail oral sodium intake and intravenous fluid replacement of sodium with 3 or 5 percent sodium chloride. The treatment may require free-water fluid restriction in an effort to increase the sodium in the ECF compartment.

The disease state frequently associated with hyponatremia is Addison's disease, which results from degeneration of the adrenal cortex and leads to aldosterone deficiency. The decrease in aldosterone secretion is followed by the loss of sodium. Addison's disease may lead to hypovolemia and cerebral edema if left untreated. The treatment of Addison's disease includes corticosteroid supplements and controlled salt intake. Left untreated, Addison's disease will result in death. Another syndrome in which there is inappropriate secretion of ADH is associated with the dilution of sodium and with water gain. The inappropriate

secretion of ADH is often associated with certain tumors frequently found in the bronchus of the lung or in the basal regions of the brain. The effects are a decrease in the sodium concentration in the ECF and a slight increase in ECF volume. The inappropriate secretion of ADH leads to very concentrated urinary output and a loss of sodium. Treatment includes correcting the serum sodium levels and alleviating water retention. Restriction of fluid alone may not provide adequate relief, and a diuretic may be a necessary adjunct. The use of 3 or 5 percent intravenous sodium chloride is suggested for treatment of decreased sodium levels.

The administration of oxytocin may also lead to water intoxication. The hormone oxytocin has an intrinsic antidiuretic effect, leading to an increase in water reabsorption. Therefore, a patient in labor and on a continuous drip of oxytocin needs to be continually assessed for signs of water intoxication. The symptoms of water intoxication must be carefully assessed and must not be mistaken for signs of eclampsia. The best diagnostic aid is a serum sodium determination.

Hypernatremia. Hypernatremia is increased sodium concentration in the ECF. Some causes of hypernatremia include decreased water intake, excessive loss of body fluids particularly via the bronchial tree, increased aldosterone, and excessive administration of sodium-containing fluids. Excessive retention of sodium occurs in the chronically ill patient in whom water is also retained. The retention of sodium by the kidneys is an effort by the body to restore the plasma volume; however, the attempt to restore adequate plasma volume by the renin–angiotensin–aldosterone mechanism results in retention in the interstitial space. Accumulation in the interstitial space leads to edema, ascites, and pleural effusion.

Hypernatremia can be caused by overzealous administration of sodium bicarbonate during resuscitative efforts. Another cause of hypernatremia that the anesthetist may encounter is a hypertonic saline abortion. The hypertonic saline may accidentally enter into the maternal circulation via direct access or by amniotic fluid absorption, possibly elevating the serum sodium. Signs of hypernatremia include furrowed tongue, restlessness, lethargy, increased deep tendon reflexes, sticky mucous membranes, flushed skin, and thirst. The treatment of hypernatremia is to limit sodium intake and administer diuretics and water.

Potassium. Most potassium within the body is found in the intracellular compartment, where it is the major cation. Potassium plays a vital role in the transmission of nerve impulses and the contraction of muscle. Potassium moves freely between the intracellular and extracellular compartments. The sodium–potassium pump controls the movement of potassium between the cells and the ECF. The normal value of serum potassium is 3.5 to 5.5 mEq/L. The normal dietary intake of potassium is 50 to 100 mg daily; however, 80 percent of the potassium is excreted via the renal system and the other 20 percent is lost through the bowel and sweat glands. The normal range of potassium secreted through the kidneys is 40 to 80 mEq/24 h. The kidneys excrete a large amount of potassium daily and do not conserve potassium; therefore, a daily intake of potassium is vital for body functions.

Regulation of potassium is influenced by dietary intake. A high dietary intake of potassium is reflected in an increase in the excretion of potassium. Renal failure inhibits the secretion of potassium and allows the serum levels of potassium to reach potentially fatal levels. A low potassium level may result from diarrhea, surgical stress, or acidosis. Another means of controlling potassium is by the regulation of aldosterone. The release of aldosterone facilitates potassium secretion and sodium reabsorption. Increased potassium intake stimulates the renin–angiotensin–aldosterone mechanism, and the kidneys increase tubular potassium secretion. If the extracellular potassium concentration is low, a decrease in aldosterone production results, conserving potassium at the tubular level. Both excess and deficit alter the resting membrane potential of the cell.

Hypokalemia. Hypokalemia is defined as low serum levels of potassium. Many of the causes of hypokalemia are iatrogenic. Hypokalemia is frequently evidenced in patients on diuretic therapy. Because hypertension is becoming relatively common and one of the modalities of treatment is the use of diuretics, the frequency of hypokalemia in the surgical patient has increased. Other factors leading to hypokalemia are starvation, diarrhea, loss of body fluids particularly gastric secretions, crushing injuries, primary aldosteronism, reduced renal absorption, and stressful situations (fever, sweating, thyroid storm). Prolonged administration of some antibiotics such as sodium carbenicillin and sodium penicillin may also lead to hypokalemia. Hypokalemia also occurs in patients undergoing surgery. In the first 2 postoperative days, the patient may lose 100 mmol of potassium and will continue to lose 25 mmol/d in the immediate postoperative period.

Hypokalemia is frequently associated with metabolic alkalosis. Respiratory and metabolic alkalosis results in increased renal excretion of potassium. Hydrogen and potassium compete for exchange with sodium in the renal tubule. Therefore, potassium is excreted in exchange for sodium. Hypokalemia results in alkalosis because there is an increase in hydrogen ion excretion, compensating for the lower potassium concentration. Movement of hydrogen ions into the cell results in the potassium loss responsible for alkalosis. Chloride depletion often accompanies hypokalemia.

Signs and symptoms of hypokalemia result from an alteration of the body systems. The neuromuscular dysfunctions that are due to hypokalemia are anorexia, weakness, loss of muscle tone, and loss of muscle reflexes. The cardiovascular system displays signs of a weak pulse, arrhythmias, decreased intensity of heart sounds, and a decrease in blood pressure when hypokalemia is evident. The electrocardiogram (ECG) displays a low to flattened T-wave, depressed ST segment, and predominant U-wave (Fig. 18–3). Cardiac arrest may eventually follow. The gastrointestinal tract decreases peristaltic movement, and abdominal distension may result. A pseudodiabetic glycosuria may result because of an inability to move glucose across the cell membrane. Hypokalemia is treated by replacing the potassium and correcting the reason for its loss. If mild hypokalemia is evident, potassium may be replaced by dietary or oral supplements.

Decreased serum potassium levels may threaten the patient's life, and potassium may be given at a rate of 40 mEq/h in intravenous fluid. ECG monitoring should be continuous when administering intravenous potassium. In crisis situations, rapid administration of potassium is potentially dangerous; close and constant monitoring is essential. During rapid potassium replacement, a rapid rise in potassium can predispose the patient to hyperkalemia. In cases of large potassium deficit, replacement and restoration of normal serum values may take days to weeks.

Hyperkalemia. Hyperkalemia is an excess of potassium in the ECF volume. A common cause of hyperkalemia is renal

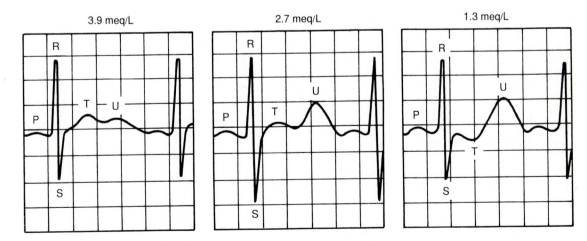

Figure 18–3. Electrocardiographic effects of hypokalemia. Note progressive flattening of the T-wave, an increasingly prominent U-wave, increased amplitude of the P-wave, prolongation of the PR interval, and ST segment depression. (*Reprinted, with permission, from Morgan GE, Mikhail MS.* Clinical Anesthesiology. *Norwalk, Connecticut, Appleton & Lange; 1992:468.*)

failure and an inability of the kidneys to excrete potassium. Life-threatening situations such as crushing injuries, burns, and myocardial damage allow a sudden release of potassium into the ECF. The sudden release of potassium into the ECF compartment can lead to diastolic cardiac arrhythmia, a flaccid myocardium, and cardiac arrest. Other factors associated with hyperkalemia include transfusion of aged blood, adrenocortical insufficiency (Addison's disease), and too rapid or excessive administration of potassium.

Hyperkalemic signs are associated with nerve and muscle function. The muscular system demonstrates signs of weakness and flaccid paralysis. The myocardium becomes flaccid, and arrhythmias and cardiac arrest develop. The conduction system throughout the myocardium is affected, and the ECG demonstrates high, center T-waves. P-waves disappear, the QRS complex widens, and bradycardia develops (Fig. 18–4). Heart block may occur during a severe state of hyperkalemia. The gastrointestinal tract of a patient in a hyperkalemic state demonstrates signs of hyperactivity: nausea, vomiting, intestinal colic, and diarrhea.

The treatment of hyperkalemia entails reduction of serum potassium levels. Restriction of potassium administration and intake is one corrective measure. The use of a cation-exchange resin helps to prevent hyperkalemia in certain patients. The treatment of severe hyperkalemia may include intravenous administration of calcium gluconate, sodium bicarbonate, or regular insulin and hypertonic dextrose. The administration of 5 to 20 mL of 10 percent calcium gluconate or calcium chloride temporarily reverses the chronotropic effects on the myocardium. A continuous ECG will display the altered conduction through the Purkinje fibers, and, should bradycardia develop, the infusion should cease. Sodium bicarbonate raises the pH and drives the potassium into the cell. Administration of sodium bicarbonate should be used carefully in reversing hyperkalemia because of the potential for sodium excess; furthermore, the effect of the drug lasts a few hours. Intravenous administra-

tion of regular insulin, a hypertonic dextrose, stimulates the synthesis of glycogen, resulting in the uptake of potassium. Insulin drives the potassium into the cell but should be limited to 1 unit/5 g of glucose to prevent a rebound of hypoglycemia. For the chronically hyperkalemic patient, other means of potassium excretion are needed. Treatment of these patients may include cation-exchange resins, peritoneal dialysis, and hemodialysis.

Calcium. Calcium is the most abundant cation in the body. It is found in the protoplasm and is present in large proportions in the bone and teeth. Calcium is involved with cellular permeability, neuromuscular activity, and normal blood clotting mechanisms. The normal daily intake of calcium is 1 to 3 g. The body cannot store calcium, and daily consumption of calcium is therefore necessary to sustain adequate calcium levels in the body. Intake of 1 g of calcium is considered adequate for the average adult, but children and pregnant women require larger amounts (1.5 to 2g/d). The normal serum level is 8.6 to 10.5 mg/100 mL. About 50 percent of serum calcium exists in the ionized form, which is responsible for neuromuscular function.

Calcium has a reciprocal relationship with phosphorus. Parathyroid hormone and calcitonin facilitate the transfer of calcium from bone to plasma and therefore raise the plasma level of calcium. The normal urinary calcium content is 100 to 250 mg/24 h. Calcium disturbances are generally not encountered in the postoperative patient, in whom routine calcium supplementation is seldom indicated. Surgical hypoparathyroidism, acute pancreatitis, excessive administration of citrated blood, and maternal diabetes all are circumstances that may require a calcium supplement.

Hypocalcemia. Hypocalcemia is a low serum level of calcium. Common causes of hypocalcemia include hypoparathyroidism, removal of the parathyroid glands, acute pancreatitis, vitamin D deficiency, and chronic administration

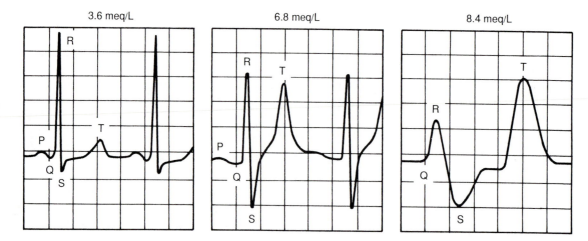

Figure 18–4. Electrocardiographic effect of hyperkalemia. Electrocardiographic changes characteristically progress from symmetrically peaked T-waves, often with a shortened QT interval, to widening of the QRS complex, prolongation of the PR interval, loss of the P-wave, loss of R-wave amplitude, and ST segment depression (occasionally elevation—to an ECG that resembles a sine wave—before final progression into ventricular fibrillation or asystole. (*Reprinted, with permission, from Morgan GE, Mikhail MS.* Clinical Anesthesiology. *Norwalk, Connecticut, Appleton & Lange; 1992:470.*)

of cimetidine. The symptoms of hypocalcemia include tingling and numbness of the fingers, toes, and circumoral region; cramps in the extremities; hyperactivity of deep tendon reflexes; Trousseau's sign; Chvostek's sign; and mental confusion leading to convulsions. The ECG manifests a prolonged QT interval and ST segment (Fig. 18–5).

The sign of hypocalcemia that particularly concerns anesthetists is the spasm of laryngeal muscles leading to airway obstruction. Hypocalcemia can result from accidental damage to the parathyroid glands, potentially occurring in patients undergoing a thyroidectomy or a radical neck dissection. Treatment is aimed at restoration of calcium to normal values. Acute management of hypocalcemia includes intravenous administration of calcium gluconate or calcium chloride. The administration of calcium on a routine basis after massive blood transfusion is controversial. Monitoring calcium levels during massive transfusions is a guide for calcium replacement. The ECG and observation of the QT interval are rough guidelines in assessing serum calcium levels. Mild calcium deficit may be treated with oral supplements and vitamin D. Vitamin D enhances the absorption of calcium by the gastrointestinal tract.

Hypercalcemia. Hypercalcemia may result from hyperparathyroidism, malignant neoplastic disease, overuse of calcium-containing antacids, and prolonged immobilization. Clinical signs of hypercalcemia are vague. Symptoms of hypercalcemia that may be encountered are fatigue, anorexia, nausea, vomiting, urinary calcium stones, somnambulism, stupor, polydypsia, polyuria, and thirst. The two major causes of hypercalcemia are hyperparathyroidism and cancer with bony metastasis. The ECG displays a shortened ST segment and QT interval. Acute hypercalcemia may be treated with 0.45 or 0.9 percent NaCl to dilute the serum calcium and aid in urinary excretion. Other measures of treatment used to lower serum calcium include chelating agents, steroids, and hemodialysis.

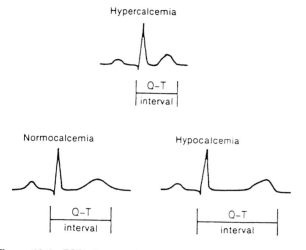

Figure 18–5. ECG changes by serum calcium level variation. (*With permission from Wilson RF (ed): Principles and Techniques of Critical Care, Philadelphia, FA Davis, Co: 1976:26.*)

Magnesium. Magnesium is necessary as a catalyst for intracellular enzymatic reactions. The majority of magnesium is in the intracellular compartment. The extracellular magnesium concentration ranges from 1.5 to 2.5 mEq/L. An increase in the extracellular concentration of magnesium depresses the nervous and skeletal muscular systems. Magnesium imbalance is not a frequent cation imbalance. The normal dietary intake of magnesium is approximately 20 mEq daily. A large amount of magnesium is lost in the urine. The regulation of magnesium is not well understood.

Hypomagnesemia. Magnesium deficiency has been associated with chronic alcohol abuse, gastrointestinal irritability, diuretics, primary aldosteronism, acute pancreatitis, diabetic acidosis, hyperthyroidism, and the use of certain drugs such as gentamicin and cisplatin. Magnesium depletion is characterized by neuromuscular and central nervous system hyperactivity. Coarse tremors, muscle cramps, hyperactive reflexes, tachycardia, paresthesias of the feet and legs, and arrhythmias all are clinical signs of magnesium deficiency. Hypomagnesemia on the ECG demonstrates a prolonged PR interval, wide QRS complex, ST depression, and broadened and flattened (inverted) T-waves.

Hypomagnesemia is treated by restoring the magnesium levels. Oral administration of magnesium salts can be given for mild depletion. Severe depletion may be treated with intravenous magnesium sulfate or magnesium chloride. A dose of 2 mEq/kg body weight in 24 hours is given for severe depletion, providing the renal function is within normal limits. Vital signs should be carefully monitored when administering magnesium supplement. In the event of a rapid rise in plasma magnesium levels, calcium gluconate and calcium chloride should be available to counteract the adverse effects.

Hypermagnesemia. Renal failure is one of the major causes of hypermagnesemia. Other conditions associated with hypermagnesemia are Addison's disease, untreated ketoacidosis, and hypothyroidism. Clinical signs of hypermagnesemia include lethargy, loss of deep tendon reflexes, flushing hypotension, depressed respirations, bradycardia, and ECG changes. The ECG displays an increased PR interval, widened QRS complex, and prolonged QT interval.

In severe hypermagnesemia, treatment is the administration of calcium gluconate or calcium chloride to antagonize the action of magnesium. Correcting acidosis and limiting magnesium intake will aid in lowering the serum level. If conventional means of correcting magnesium are not successful, hemodialysis may be used.

Normal Exchange of Fluid and Electrolytes

The body attempts to maintain a homeostatic environment. The internal and external environments of the body fluids attempt to maintain stable conditions, in which the responses of compensatory mechanisms may be activated. The regulatory system assists in keeping the fluctuations of body fluids and electrolytes at a minimum. The internal environment is maintained by the kidneys, brain, lungs, skin, and gastrointestinal tract. Surgical stress may alter the internal environment.

The body exchanges the fluid and electrolyte requirements on a daily basis. The average needs of a 60- to 80-kg adult man are outlined in Table 18–2.[7] Daily water losses include 250 mL in the stool, 800 to 1500 mL as urine, and approximately 600 to 900 mL as insensible loss. Insensible water losses occur from the lungs by the humidification of inspired air and through the skin by evaporation. The insensible water loss that occurs is approximately 500 mL/m^2 of body surface; however, this insensible loss can become greatly increased under conditions of hypermetabolism, hyperventilation, and fever. This loss through the breathing circuit during anesthesia is a major concern that must be considered particularly during long cases.

The minimal urinary output for a patient who has been totally restricted of fluids is 500 to 800 mL. This is the minimal amount of urinary excretion necessary to rid the body of products of catabolism. There are two variables that help in the regulation of body fluids. The sensation of thirst is the body's sensory drive for fluid replacement. A person experiences thirst by a feeling of deprivation of fluid intake demonstrated by dry mucous membranes and decreased salivary secretions. The second variable associated with thirst is the secretion of ADH. A change in the tonicity of ECF inhibits the release of ADH, and water reabsorption by the renal tubules occurs. The sensation of thirst may be induced by pharmacologic means, such as the administration of atropine, and can also be stimulated by withholding fluids or by hemorrhage. Many factors influence the thirst mechanism.

FLUID AND ELECTROLYTE THERAPY

Parenteral Solution

The selection of parenteral solution should be based on the needs of the individual patient. The type and amount of parenteral solution should be carefully reviewed and estimated according to the physical status, weight, and cardiovascular status of the patient; daily maintenance requirements based on weight or body surface area; and the present fluid status of the patient prior to fluid therapy. Maintenance fluids provide replacement of normal fluid loss, such as loss via the lungs, urine, and skin. Maintenance fluids are isotonic. Replacement fluids are given to correct a loss of isotonic fluid from the body. The loss of isotonic fluid may include ascites and interstitial edema.[8] Table 18–3 can be used as a guide for the most appropriate fluid therapy for maintenance or replacement therapy.

Rate of Fluid Administration

The rate of fluid administration varies considerably, depending on the type of fluid loss, the severity of the fluid loss, and the cardiac and renal status of the patient. Severe fluid loss can be replaced with isotonic solution at a rate of 2000 mL/h or as indicated by the vital signs. Patients who are ill and have compromised body functions will not tolerate rapid fluid loss and replacement as well as patients who are in good physical condition. Therefore, patients who have cardiovascular and renal disease will not tolerate shifts in fluid as well as healthy patients. Fluid administration must be monitored with special care in infants and the elderly.

Preoperative Fluid Therapy

The majority of surgical patients have been fasting 8 to 10 hours prior to surgery. Therefore, patients coming to surgery are depleted of solutes and water as a result of normal body function. In general, adult patients have intravenous fluids started prior to induction of anesthesia to replace these losses and to provide access to the circulatory system.

An adequate assessment of preoperative fluid and electrolyte balance and subsequent correction is necessary for successful surgical intervention. Observation and an accurate history of the patient's fluid intake are means of

TABLE 18–2. WATER EXCHANGE (60- TO 80-KG MAN)

	Average Daily Volume (mL)	Minimal (mL)	Maximal (mL)
H$_2$O gain—routes			
Sensible			
Oral fluids	800–1500	0	1500/h
Solid foods	500–700	0	1500
Insensible			
Water of oxidation	250	125	800
Water of solution	0	0	500
H$_2$O loss—routes			
Sensible			
Urine	800–1500	300	1400/h (diabetes insipidus)
Intestinal	0–250	0	2500/h
Sweat	0	0	4000/h
Insensible			
Lungs and skin	600–900	600–900	1500

Reprinted, with permission, from Sabiston DC. Textbook of surgery: The biological basis of modern surgical practice. 11th ed. Philadelphia: WB Saunders; 1977.

TABLE 18–3. COMMERCIALLY AVAILABLE FLUIDS FOR PARENTERAL USE

Symbol	Type	Dextrose (mg/mL)	Sodium (mEq/L)	Other Cations (mEq/L)	Chloride (mEq/L)	Other Anions (mEq/L)
D_5W^a	Maintenance	50	—	—	—	—
D_4MLR	Maintenance	40	26	K^+, 0.8; Ca^+, 0.5	22	Lactate, 5.5
D_5NaCl 0.45	Maintenance	50	77	—	77	—
LR	Replacement	—	130	K^+, 4; Ca^+, 3	109	Lactate, 28
D_5LR	Replacement	50	130	K^+, 4; Ca^+, 3	109	Lactate, 28
0.9% NaCl	Replacement	—	154	—	154	—
D_5NaCl	Replacement	50	154	—	154	—
Normosol-R	Replacement	—	140	K^+, 5; Mg^+, 3	90	Acetate Gluconate, 50
Plasmalyte	Replacement	—	140	K^+, 5; Mg^+, 3	98	Acetate, 27 Gluconate, 23
5% NaCl	Special purpose	—	855	—	855	—

[a] D5W, 5% dextrose in water USP; D4MLR, 4% dextrose in modified lactated Ringer's solution; D5NaCl 0.45, 5% dextrose in half-strength saline USP; LR, lactated Ringer's solution (also known as Hartman's solution); D5LR, 5% dextrose in lactated Ringer's solution; 0.9% NaCl, 0.9% sodium chloride solution USP (frequently called isotonic saline, "normal saline," or simply "saline" and abbreviated NS); D5NaCl, 5% dextrose in 0.9% sodium chloride solution USP; 5% NaCl, 5% sodium chloride solution (also called hypertonic saline).

Reprinted, with permission, from Miller RD. Anesthesia. 2nd ed. New York: Churchill Livingstone; 1986.

appraising a patient's fluid intake and fluid status. If the patient's fluid status indicates abnormalities in fluid balance, these should be corrected before entering the surgical suite. Abnormalities of fluid balance can easily be categorized into three classes: volume, concentration, and composition.[8] Guidelines for administering fluids on the day of surgery are listed in Table 18–4.

Volume Changes. Disturbances in the ECF compartment are the most common fluid disturbances in the preoperative patient. Withholding fluids prior to surgery causes depletion of ECF because of continuous sensible and insensible losses. This deficit may be strictly volume related, and there may be coderangement of concentration or composition. The diagnosis of severe volume depletion in the ECF compartment is demonstrated clinically by tachycardia and hypotension. In third-space loss, fluid is registered into a nonfunctional space from the extracellular compartment. Third-space loss may occur in patients who have ascites, burns, massive crush injuries, and gastrointestinal inflammation and swelling. A sequestration of fluid into the third space may require replacement treatment to combat the potential for hypotension and tachycardia. The nonfunctional loss of fluids may also occur in patients who have considerable swelling and tissue trauma as a result of surgical manipulation. Third-space sequestration also occurs in patients who have bowel obstructions and injury to the peritoneum.

Estimating fluid deficit is difficult and can best be accomplished by evaluating clinical signs. A mild deficit represents approximately 4 percent, a moderate deficit 6 to 8 percent, and a severe loss 10 percent of the body weight. When a patient has an extracellular volume deficit of 6 to 8 percent, orthostatic hypotension can generally be observed. Signs of ECF loss are manifested by tachycardia, dry mucous membranes, hypotension, furrowed tongue, apa-

thy, oliguria, collapsed veins, poor skin turgor, cool and dry skin, and subnormal temperature.

Restoration of ECF balance is the target of treatment and is directed at achieving stable vital signs and adequate urinary output. Urinary output should be 30 to 50 mL/h or 0.5 to 1 mL/kg/h as a general guideline. The use of a balanced salt solution such as lactated Ringer's is a good choice to replace the pure ECF loss without causing derangements in concentration or composition.

Concentration Changes. The two primary factors involved in concentration changes are the serum sodium concentration and the serum osmolality. The initial and major

TABLE 18–4. GUIDELINES FOR ROUTINE FLUIDS ON THE DAY OF SURGERY

1. Start intravenous line, replace insensible loss with maintenance-type solutions, 2 mL/kg/h, for interval since last oral intake.
2. Change to replacement-type solutions for intraoperative insensible losses. Administer LR, Normosol-R, or, in some cases, NaCl, 2 mg/kg/h.
3. Estimate surgical trauma and add appropriate volume of replacement-type solution to that given in step 2:
   Minimal trauma: add 4 mL/kg/h.
   Moderate trauma: add 6 mL/kg/h.
   Extreme trauma: add 8 mL/kg/h.
4. Give appropriate colloid solution for each volume of blood lost over 20 percent of the patient's estimated blood volume.
5. Monitor vital signs and urine output. Adjust fluids to keep urine output at 1 mL/kg/h.

Reprinted, with permission, from Miller RD. Anesthesia. 2nd ed. New York: Churchill Livingstone; 1986.

concern is the replacement of fluid volume; the concentration abnormality can be corrected at a slower rate.

Serum sodium evaluation is one of the best indicators of concentration in the ECF. A volume deficit is often associated with increased serum sodium. The increased sodium is due to a decrease in extracellular electrolyte-free water and an increase in dissolved substances in plasma. Elevated serum sodium levels can be corrected with hypotonic solutions.

Hyponatremia may be present in increased, decreased, or normal ECF volume. Therefore, the treatment varies according to the condition in which hyponatremia exists. In the hyponatremic patient with a normal ECF volume, the suggested action is observation and detection of the cause of the underlying sodium loss. This type of condition may develop from failure of the kidneys to conserve sodium. The neonate is a sodium loser because the kidneys have an inability to conserve sodium. Inappropriate secretion of ADH and early stages of renal disease may also result in sodium loss with normal ECF volume.

Hypervolemia/hyponatremia is caused by excessive water retention. Anesthesia staff are particularly concerned with hypervolemia/hyponatremia caused by transurethral resections; oxytocin (Pitocin) administered with D_5W acts as an antidiuretic, and water is not excreted but absorbed. Treatment of hypervolemia/hyponatremia is administration of hypertonic salt. The hypertonic salt solution causes volume expansion in the extracellular space. Hypovolemia/hyponatremia often occurs when there is fluid loss through the gastrointestinal tract. This condition may be corrected by the administration of hypotonic fluids such as lactated Ringer's and 0.9 percent normal saline.

Composition abnormalities are imbalances in electrolytes and blood gases. The electrolyte disturbance most frequently encountered in the preoperative patient is hypokalemia, which can easily be corrected with the administration of potassium chloride. If the rapid addition of potassium is considered, continuous ECG monitoring should be performed. Acid–base balance is also subject to compositional disturbance and should be considered preoperatively, intraoperatively, and postoperatively.

Intraoperative Fluid Management

Preoperatively, patients require appropriate replacement of fluid and electrolytes to circumvent a hypotensive episode during the induction of anesthesia. The preoperative fluid loss can be as great as 1.5 to 2.0 mL/kg/h for an adult. (For children this loss is even greater.) The ECF loss should be replaced with hypotonic solution before the induction of anesthesia if there is no further derangement of fluid disturbances. The fluids most often considered are saline, lactated Ringer's, and dextrose and water. These fluids offer water and electrolytes in the solution. The loss of fluids during anesthesia must be assessed. Unhumidified gases, high flows, evaporation, surgical trauma, and fever all contribute to the loss of fluids in the surgical patient. Suggested methods of determining maintenance fluids are listed in Tables 18–5 and 18–6.

Because infants have a greater surface area, they also have a greater amount of insensible water and less circulat-

TABLE 18–5. TYPICAL REQUIREMENTS FOR MAINTENANCE FLUIDS

Age	Amount (mL/kg/h)
Adult	1.5–2
Child	2–4
Infant	4–6
Neonate	3

Reprinted, with permission, from Miller, RD. Anesthesia. 2nd ed. New York: Churchill Livingstone: 1986.

ing blood volume. Preoperative and intraoperative fluid maintenance for the pediatric population is a challenge.

Replacement of Blood Loss

A great deal of controversy surrounds the issue of when to initiate the replacement of blood. In normal circumstances, the average adult can tolerate a blood loss of 500 mL, or 10 percent of the estimated blood volume; however, loss of 15 percent of the blood volume should be considered the point of careful consideration for replacement. One guide used to determine the need for a blood transfusion is based on the hematocrit as a means of determining the allowable blood loss. Controversy exists today over the acceptable low hematocrit of 30 percent, which will be discussed in Chapter 19; however, a rule of thumb for estimating allowable blood loss based on this 30 percent hematocrit is presented. One could easily substitute another number for the 30 percent in this computation.

An average adult man weighs 70 kg and has a hematocrit of 40 percent and an estimated blood volume of 70 mL/kg. What is the allowable blood loss for this patient? The estimated blood volume (EBV) is obtained as

$$EBV = 70 \times 70 = 4900$$

TABLE 18–6. INTRAOPERATIVE FLUID REQUIREMENTS

1. Basic formula
   a. Deficit: baseline hourly fluid requirement

4 mL/kg/h	1–10 kg
2 mL/kg/h	11–20 kg
1 mL/kg/h	21–up

   multiplied by the number of hours NPO
   b. Maintenance: crystalloid solution such as Ringer's lactate at a rate of 5 to 15 mL/kg/h
   c. Losses: Ringer's lactate can be used if hematocrit remains above 30% at 3 mL/1 mL of blood
2. Overall formula (rough estimates)

10 mL/kg	first hour
7 mL/kg	second hour
5 mL/kg	third hour
3 mL/kg	fourth hour

   for fluid replacement
3. Surface area formula

Surface area (m²):	0.1	0.2	0.3	0.4	0.5	0.6	0.7	0.8	0.9	1.0
Weight (lb):	3	6	12	18	24	30	36	42	50	60

   Minimum rate, 60 mL/m²/h
   Maximum hourly rate, 20 mL/kg/h

Calculated estimated red cell mass (ERCM) is obtained by multiplying EBV by the patient's preoperative hematocrit:

$$ERCM = 4900 \times 0.40 = 1960$$

Estimated red cell mass desired (ERCM$_d$) is obtained by multiplying EBV by the acceptable low hematocrit (30 percent):

$$ERCM_d = 4900 \times 0.30 = 1470$$

Allowable red cell loss (ARCL) is the difference between ERCM and ERCM$_d$:

$$ARCL = 1960 - 1470 = 490$$

Allowable blood loss (ABL) is twice the ARCL:

$$ABL = 2 \times 490 = 980$$

Therefore, in this example, the allowable blood loss for this patient is 980 mL of blood, which conceivably will lower the patient's hematocrit to 30 percent.

When estimating blood loss, it is important to realize that the operative blood loss seen on the field may not be the total amount of blood lost. Some clinicians suggest that above the estimated loss observed on the field an additional 15 to 40 percent should be added.

Crystalloids are often used to replace blood lost in surgery. When replacing blood loss with crystalloids, the ratio of fluid replacement to loss is 3 mL of crystalloids to 1 mL of blood loss. Another alternative to replacement of blood loss is the use of Plasmanate-type solutions. Plasmanate is a good volume expander, but the major disadvantage of this fluid is its inability to carry oxygen.

As surgical procedures have become more complicated, the use of blood products has increased; however, particularly because of concerns about transmitting acquired immunodeficiency syndrome (AIDS) and hepatitis, there is a trend not to use blood transfusions unless necessary. Approximately 14 percent of all surgical patients receive blood transfusions, and 50 percent of all blood transfused in the hospital is given in the operating room suite.

The loss of blood during a surgical procedure is not the only fluid loss. Loss through evaporation and ECF volume depletion must be considered in the replacement of fluid in the operative course. It bears repeating that loss of ECF into the third space as a result of surgical trauma and manipulations must also be considered in the replacement of fluids.

Immediate Postoperative Period

The recovery room evaluation should include the preoperative fluid status, the amount of fluid lost and given during surgery, and clinical assessment of vital signs and urinary output. It is clinically desirable to establish normal pulse and blood pressure. Additional insidious fluid loss in the recovery room can result from bleeding at the surgical site, internal bleeding, evaporation, and loss through external draining devices. Signs of ECF deficit resulting from fluid loss are manifested primarily by circulatory instability.

The replacement of fluids in the postoperative period often requires the administration of hypotonic solutions and, as necessary, isotonic salt solution combined with packed red cells to replace surgical losses. Continuously monitoring the patient in the postoperative period includes assessing blood pressure, heart rate, urinary output, level of consciousness, pupil size, airway patency, respiratory patterns, body temperature, and skin color. Sharp observation and skilled response to the patient in the recovery room contribute to successful postoperative management.[9]

Replacement Therapy. The different types of blood and therapy with blood products are discussed in Chapter 19.

Indications for Replacement Therapy. The values obtained in the operating room when assessing blood loss are rough estimates. Therefore, vital signs, hematocrit, and all other available data are assessed to determine fluid balance. A patient who has been NPO for a long period may have an ECF deficit and often is hemoconcentrated. Such a patient may have a very high but misleading hematocrit. Hypotension occurring in a hypovolemic patient may be erroneously related to a deep stage of anesthesia. A significant fall in blood pressure may not occur until 40 percent of the patient's blood volume is lost. Therefore, the use of blood pressure as the only indicator of volume status may be a late sign. Tachycardia, another symptom of hypovolemia, may result from stimulation on intubation, surgical stimulation, or the use of pharmacologic agents and therefore may not solely be a particularly reliable sign of blood and fluid loss.

REFERENCES

1. Moore FD, Ball MR. The metabolic response to surgery. Springfield, IL: Charles C Thomas; 1952:132.
2. Metheny N, Snively WD. *Nurses' handbook of fluid balance.* Philadelphia: JB Lippincott; 1983.
3. Metheny N. *Quick reference to fluid balance.* Philadelphia: JB Lippincott; 1984.
4. Goudsouzian N, Karamanian A. *Physiology for the anesthesiologist.* 2nd ed. Norwalk, CT: Appleton-Century-Crofts; 1984:405–429.
5. Guyton A. *Textbook of Medical Physiology.* 8th ed. Philadelphia: WB Saunders; 1991.
6. Still JA, Model JH. Acute water intoxication during transurethral resection of the prostate using glycine solution for irrigation. *Anesthesiology.* 1973;38:98–99.
7. Sabiston DC. *Textbook of surgery: The biological basis of modern surgical practice.* 12th ed. Philadelphia: WB Saunders; 1991.
8. Miller RD, ed. *Anesthesia.* 3rd ed. New York: Churchill-Livingstone; 1990.
9. Jenkins MT, Gliesecke AH, Johnson ER. The postoperative patient and his fluid requirements. *Br J Anaesth.* 1975;47:143–150.

19

Coagulation and Blood Component Therapy

Lorraine M. Jordan
and Michael P. Dosch

Blood component therapy plays an important role in anesthesia practice. The principles of transfusion therapy dictate that patients be given blood products when needed. The patient is assessed and the blood products are selected based on the status and needs of the patient. The purpose of blood component therapy is to meet the needs of the patient while exposing him or her to the least amount of risk.

Selection of the blood component is not always easy. Approximately 20 different blood products are currently available to fulfill the needs of the patient. It is therefore vital that anesthesia personnel, who administer approximately 50 percent of the blood products given in the United States, be aware of the indications, contraindications, and potential side effects of the blood component chosen.

This chapter reviews the physiology of hemostasis, and describes compatibility testing of donor and recipient blood. An array of natural and synthetic blood products and related agents are presented, along with their indications and hazards. The infectivity of blood is highlighted. Finally, strategies available currently, or under investigation, to decrease the use of homologous blood are detailed.

HEMOSTASIS

When the integrity of a blood vessel wall is breached, the injured area of the vessel attracts platelets to the injured site and activates plasma coagulation proteins which leads to initial clot formation known as *primary hemostasis*. *Secondary hemostasis* refers to the formation of an insoluble fibrin clot.

During primary hemostasis many events must occur before the clot forms (Fig. 19–1). When the vessel is damaged the smooth muscle wall contracts, which alters the surface of the endothelium and facilitates the adhesive quality of the damaged membrane. Prothrombin activator is formed in response to the ruptured vessel. When the vessel is injured, collagen is exposed and offers a surface at which the platelets can adhere. As these platelets adhere to the collagen, platelet granules are formed and adenosine diphosphate (ADP) is released. ADP and other chemical agents cause the surfaces of the platelets to adhere to each other and a plug of platelets is formed at the site (Fig. 19–2).

Secondary hemostasis occurs when the insoluble fibrin clot is formed. Formation of this clot occurs when the coagulation proteins are activated to form a fibrin network. The general sequence of events in blood coagulation begins with prothrombin activator forming in response to rupture of the vessel. After the prothrombin activator is released, it acts as a catalyst to convert prothrombin to thrombin. Extrinsic or intrinsic prothrombin activator and calcium convert the prothrombin to thrombin. Thrombin then converts fibrinogen into fibrin threads to form the clot under the influence of calcium and fibrin stabilizing factors.

The extrinsic pathway for initiating clotting begins with the formation of prothrombin activator (Fig. 19–3). The intrinsic pathway begins with trauma to the vessel, initiating a cascade of events leading to activation of factor Xa (Fig. 19–4). The major difference in the pathways is their speed; the extrinsic pathway responds very rapidly (within 15 seconds of vessel damage), whereas the intrinsic pathway is much slower, responding in 2 to 6 minutes.

There are several drugs that inhibit platelet function or other aspects of the hemostatic process. Drugs may interfere with any step in this complex cascade (Table 19–1). Chronic ingestion of any of these drugs may pose a problem during the operative course for the patient. Bleeding may be difficult to control in the postoperative period as well.

There are laboratory tests that can assess a patient's degree of hemostasis. The tests listed in Table 19–2 are divided into categories based on primary or secondary hemostasis and fibrinolysis. These tests can be conducted to assess the bleeding tendency of patients, on the basis of their physical status and condition. These baseline data help to identify potential problems that may occur in the operating room, allowing for better evaluation and treatment of bleeding problems that may develop during the operative course.

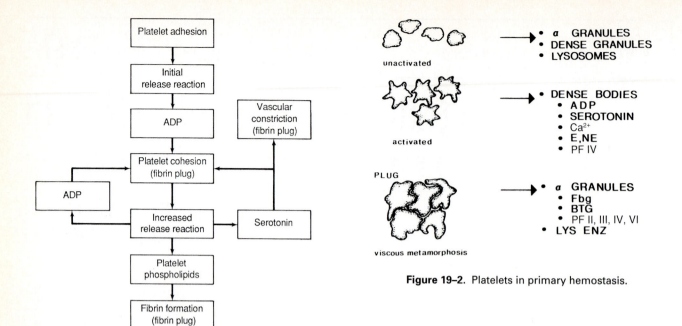

Figure 19–1. Steps in platelet activation. (*Reprinted, with permission, from Henry RL. In: Murano G, Bick RL, eds.* Basic concepts of hemostasis and thrombosis. *Boca Raton, FL: CRC Press; 1980.*)

Figure 19–2. Platelets in primary hemostasis.

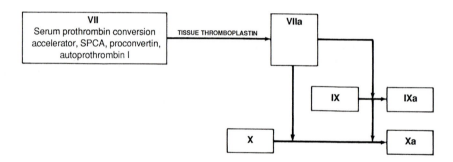

Figure 19–3. Extrinsic coagulation pathway.

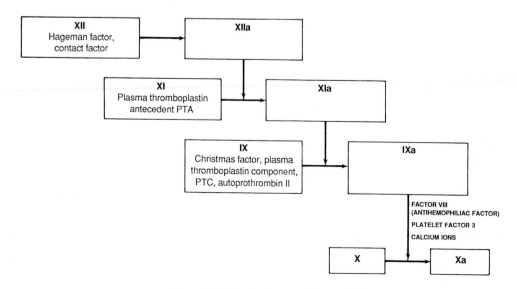

Figure 19–4. Intrinsic coagulation pathway.

TABLE 19–1. DRUGS INHIBITING HEMOSTASIS

Primary hemostasis (platelet function)
Aspirin
Penicillins
Nonsteroidal anti-inflammatory agents
Antihistamines
Secondary hemostasis
Heparin
Oral anticoagulants
Fibrinolysis
ε-Aminocaproic acid

TABLE 19–2. LABORATORY EVALUATION OF SECONDARY HEMOSTASIS AND FIBRINOLYSIS

Secondary hemostasis
Factor activities and assays
Prothrombin time (PT)
Activated partial thromboplastin time (PTT)
Thrombin time (TT)
Fibrinogen
Fibrinolysis
Thrombo-Wellco test
Protamine sulfate test

COMPATIBILITY TESTING

The extent of compatibility testing is based on the urgency of the situation. Complete testing to establish compatibility and avoid an antigen–antibody reaction is the goal whenever time permits. Establishing the patient's blood type is essential to avoid devastating agglutination and hemolysis of the donated blood. An incompatibility reaction occurs when antibodies are activated, causing hemolysis of the red blood cells. The two major antigen systems most often tested are the ABO system and the Rh or D antigen. Other blood group antigens do exist and can cause reactions; however, these reactions are usually less devastating than an ABO or Rh mismatch.

The patient's blood group (ABO) is determined by the antigens on the surface of the red blood cell. Antibodies also exist in the serum of patients with different blood types. Therefore, typing a patient's blood on the basis of the ABO blood group includes typing the surface of the red blood cell as well as the serum.

A person who has type O blood has neither A nor B antigens on the surface of the red blood cell, and may or may not have anti-A or anti-B serum antibodies. This means that type O packed cells (which lack significant amounts of the serum) can be given to type A, B, AB, and O individuals. Individuals with type O blood are thus known as *universal donors*. Individuals who have type AB blood have both A and B antigens on their red blood cells, and lack antibodies to either A or B. These individuals are known as *universal recipients*, because they are able to receive blood from any of the blood groups without having a hemolytic reaction. The typing of a blood group is illustrated in Table 19–3.

The other form of testing is Rh(D) testing. The majority (85 percent) of individuals are Rh(D)-positive. A person is classified as Rh(D)-positive when the Rh antigen on the surface is either C, D, or E. When the Rh antigen on the surface of the red blood cell is c, d, or e antigen the individual is Rh(D)-negative. Most authors agree that in emergency situations, in which blood therapy is vital, uncrossmatched group O packed red blood cells are recommended for initial resuscitation fluid therapy. This finding was confirmed in a study by Schwab et al.[1] in which 99 patients had clinical signs of class III or class IV hemorrhage and were treated with uncrossmatched group O packed cells. Schwab et al. concluded that uncrossmatched group O packed cells were a safe form of blood component therapy in the immediate resuscitative period.

When more than two units of type O uncrossmatched whole blood are given, the patient should probably not be switched back to crossmatched, type-specific blood once the blood bank determines the patient's type. Doing so could cause hemolysis of the type-specific donor red cells, as they mix with the previously transfused anti-A or anti-B from the type O whole blood.

CROSSMATCHING AND SCREENING

Crossmatching is performed to determine the potential for a blood transfusion reaction. The patient's serum and the donor's red blood cells are mixed together in vitro to detect the potential for a hemolytic transfusion reaction in vivo. Crossmatching usually takes slightly less than an hour. This technique is being used less and less in routine practice because of the limited blood supplies and to reduce the amount of time the laboratory spends on testing. Crossmatching is done for patients who are likely to receive a transfusion.

Screening is performed on both donor and recipient serum to ascertain that the most commonly found antibodies are not present. By mixing the patient's serum and panel (commercially supplied) red blood cells, it can be determined if unusual antibodies, or common antibodies that are implicated in hemolytic transfusion reactions, are present. Type and screen without a complete crossmatch does not ensure complete compatibility of the blood to less frequently found antigens.

Oberman et al.[2] studied 13,950 patients and found that only 8 had "clinically significant" antibodies following complete crossmatch that were not detected during the antibody screening. Blood screening is done when the patient may need a blood transfusion during the operative course. Blood

TABLE 19–3. ABO BLOOD GROUP ANTIGENS AND ANTIBODIES

Blood Type	Red Blood Cell Surface Antigen	Serum Antibodies
A	A	Anti-B
B	B	Anti-A
AB	A and B	No ABO antibodies
O	No ABO surface antigen	Anti-A and anti-B

will be available for transfusion if necessary, but it is not held in reserve for any one patient.

Negative antibody screening occurs when there are no irregular antibodies present to the more common red blood cell antigens. This indicates that there is little or no difficulty in crossmatching of compatible blood; however, if a positive antibody screen occurs, then the irregular antibody indicates possible difficulty in obtaining compatible blood. Additional blood screening is indicated if a positive antibody screen occurs.

If only blood typing (ABO and Rh) is performed, the possibility of transfusing incompatible blood is less than 1 in 1000. It is estimated that the chance that an antibody screen will miss potentially dangerous antibodies is less than 1 in 10,000. Thus, type and screen constitute a safe alternative to routine type and crossmatch orders.[3] As homologous blood is a scarce resource, type and screen is now more often used than type and crossmatch. Type and crossmatch dedicates units of blood to one recipient for a period. During this time, these units are unavailable for other patients, which aggravates the problem of outdated blood, particularly when more units are crossmatched than used.

BLOOD COMPONENTS AND SYNTHETIC AGENTS

The utilization of blood component therapy must be based on many factors. Military casualty studies have shown that a patient can lose up to 30 to 40 percent of blood volume without requiring red blood cell replacement, as long as blood volume is replaced by other means such as plasma substitutes and electrolyte solutions.

Blood component therapy is becoming more and more popular in the clinical arena. The advantages of component therapy include decreased cost and administration of the component that meets the needs of the patient. Whole blood can be separated into many components (Table 19–4). Many blood products are used for their red cell content; however, blood products differ in their composition and indications for use (Table 19–5).

Products Used for Red Blood Cell Count

Whole Blood. With the development of component therapy the use of whole blood has declined, because whole blood contains leukocytes, platelet, and plasma antigens which may result in a febrile or allergic transfusion reaction. Also, it is more economical to treat patients using only the component they require. There are, however, certain situations that indicate the use of whole blood as a form of treatment. The American Association of Blood Banks has stated that whole blood should be reserved for patients who are actively bleeding and have sustained a blood loss greater than 25 percent of their total blood volume.[4]

Whole blood differs from the patient's own blood by the addition of an anticoagulant–preservative solution in the bag. The anticoagulant–preservative solution most often used today is CPDA-1 (citrate–phosphate–dextrose with adenine). Citrate is an anticoagulant, phosphate is a buffer, and dextrose is a substrate for energy production. Adenine is added to allow red cells to synthesize adenosine triphosphate (ATP), which increases red cell survival. A unit of

TABLE 19–4. COMMON BLOOD COMPONENTS

Whole blood
Erythrocyte (RBC) preparations
  Packed RBCs, (plasma removed)
  Leukocyte-poor RBCs (plasma and white cells removed
  Washed RBCs (plasma and other elements removed
  Deglycerolized RBCs
  Frozen RBCs (plasma removed)
Plasma
  Stored plasma
  Fresh-frozen plasma
Platelets
Leukocyte concentration
Cryoprecipitate
Albumin
Factor concentrations

whole blood contains 513 ± 45 mL of blood of which 63 mL is CPDA-1. The hematocrit of the unit is about 40 percent. The shelf life of a unit of blood with CPDA-1 stored at 4C is 35 days, at which time 70 percent of the red blood cells present are recoverable in the circulation and survive normally. During this storage time there is a progressive loss of components and an accumulation of hydrogen and potassium ions in the plasma.

Packed Red Blood Cells. Most packed red blood cells have hematocrits between 70 and 80 percent, as the red blood cells are separated from the plasma. The high hematocrit has a high viscosity and, therefore, problems can develop with respect to flow. To alleviate the problem, 0.9 percent normal saline or other solutions compatible with blood are frequently added to the red blood cells to decrease the viscosity of the blood. The utilization of a Y-shaped blood administration set facilitates the addition of saline to the blood.

Each unit of packed red blood cells contains between 190 and 390 mL, of which 155 to 270 mL is erythrocytes. Each unit of packed red blood cells is anticipated to raise the hemoglobin 1 g/dL and the hematocrit 3 percent in a 70-kg adult man. The shelf life of packed red blood cells is 35 days if collected into CPDA-1 and stored at 4C.

Packed red blood cells (PRBCs) are effective in treating anemias when the oxygen-carrying capacity has dropped because of low hemoglobin levels and time does not permit more conventional anemia treatment such as iron replacement.

Leukocyte-Poor Red Blood Cells. Leukocyte-poor indicates red blood cell concentrates from which the leukocytes have been removed. Leukocyte-poor red blood cells are useful in those individuals who have severe febrile reactions when transfused with red blood cells or whole blood. There are different techniques to remove leukocytes from red blood cells. The most common method is inverted centrifugation, which removes more than 70 percent of all leukocytes and platelets. This method of preparation has a volume of 180 to 250 mL, with a shelf life of 35 days in CPDA-1, when stored at 4C.

TABLE 19–5. DIFFERENCES IN COMPOSITION OF MAJOR BLOOD PRODUCTS

	Normal Whole Blood	Citrated Whole Blood	Citrated PRBCs[a]	Frozen PRBCs	Fresh-Frozen Plasma
pH	7.4	6.6–6.9	6.6–6.9	6.6–7.2	6.6–6.9
Pco$_2$	35–45	180–210	180–210	0–10	180–210
Base deficit (mEq/L)	0	9–15	9–15	?	9–15
K$^+$ (mEq/L)	3.5–5.0	18–26	18–26	1–2	4–8
Citrate	None	—	—	None	—
Factors V, VIII	Normal	20–50% Normal	20–50% Normal	None	85–100% Normal
Fibrinogen	Normal	Normal	Normal	None	Normal
Platelets	240,000	None	None	None	Normal
2, 3-Diphosphoglycerate	Normal	3% Normal	3% Normal	Nearly normal	None
Hematocrit	35–45	35–45	60–70	50–95	—
Temperature	37C	4–6C	4–6C	4–6C	Cold

[a] Citrated whole blood and citrate packed red blood cells (PRBCs) have the same chemical composition, but citrated PRBCs have considerably less plasma volume.

Reprinted, with permission, from Miller RD. ASA Refresher Lecture Courses. 1973;1:101.

Washed Red Blood Cells. Washed red blood cells are indicated for patients who have febrile transfusion reactions to leukocyte-poor red blood cells or any serious allergic reaction to blood. Washed red blood cells are prepared by washing one or more liters of normal saline through red blood cells. About 93 percent of the leukocytes are removed. The shelf life of washed red blood cells is 24 hours after preparation and they should be stored at 4C.

Deglycerolized Red Blood Cells. Deglycerolized red blood cells are used to store rare donor units of blood, autologous blood, and units of blood for special purposes. The process of preparing red blood cells allows for storage of the blood in the frozen state for 3 years or more. The red blood cells are preserved and stored by adding a cryoprotective agent. The disadvantage of the process is that the units are depleted of all plasma, platelets, granulocytes, and almost all lymphocytes. Because of the preparation and purity of the blood, this product is used for intrauterine transfusions and severely immunosuppressed patients.

After the blood has been thawed and washed the glycerolized red blood cells have a shelf life of only 24 hours. The units should be stored at 4C. The product has a volume of 180 to 250 mL with a hematocrit of 50 to 70 percent.

Frozen Red Blood Cells. Frozen red blood cells (FRBCs) are a pure red cell preparation containing no citrate, white cells, platelets, or plasma. FRBCs are used for patients who have a history of febrile transfusion reactions and for those who have rare blood types. The risk of transmitting hepatitis with FRBCs is less because of the processing of the blood. The major disadvantage of FRBCs is the high cost of the product. Between 20 and 30 percent of the red blood cells are lost during preparation and in the first 24 hours posttransfusion. Once the frozen cells are reconstituted the shelf life of a unit is 24 hours. Table 19–6 highlights some of

TABLE 19–6. PRODUCTS USED FOR RED BLOOD CELL CONTENT*

Blood Component	Clinical Indications	Approximate Composition[a]			Shelf Life
		RBCs[b]	Plasma	WBCs	
Whole blood	Exchange transfusion, massive transfusion	155–270 mL	180–305 mL	25×10^8	35 d[c]
RBCs	Chronic anemia, surgical blood loss, hemorrhage	155–170 mL	40—155 mL	25×10^8	35 d[c]
Leukocyte-poor RBCs	Repeated febrile transfusion reactions and anemia, surgical blood loss, hemorrhage	125–215 mL	30—90 mL	5×10^8	35 d[c]
Saline-washed RBCs	Febrile transfusion reactions or IgA deficiency with antibody and anemia, surgical blood loss, hemorrhage	140–240 mL	Nil	1×10^8	24 h
Deglycerolized RBCs	Autologous transfusion, rare donor blood, IgA deficiency with antibody, transplant candidates, febrile transfusion reactions	140–240 mL	Nil	0.5×10^8	24 h

[a] Calculated.

[b] RBCs, erythrocytes; WBCs, leukocytes.

[c] CPD–A1: for CPD the shelf life is 21 days.

Adapted, with permission, from Kennedy MS. Essentials of immunohematology and blood therapy. In: Zuspan PF, Quilligan EJ, eds. A practical manual of obstetrical care. St. Louis MO: CV Mosby; 1982.

the clinical indications and approximate content and shelf life of blood products.

Platelet, Leukocyte, and Plasma Components

Stored Plasma. Stored plasma is obtained from whole blood during the first 72 hours of storage. Stored plasma may be kept at 4C for 35 days in the liquid state, or can be kept in the frozen state (−30C) for 12 months. Stored plasma is used to replace volume and proteins for patients. It has also been used to prime extracorporeal bypass pumps, for plasma exchange, and in patients with burns.

Fresh-Frozen Plasma. Fresh-frozen plasma (FFP) is prepared from fresh whole blood within 6 hours of collection. After preparation, the unit is stored at −18C or below to preserve the labile plasma coagulation factors. FFP contains adequate factor V and VIII levels to treat coagulation deficiencies. Each bag of FFP contains 400 mg of fibrinogen.

Fresh-frozen plasma is overused. A National Institutes of Health Consensus Conference determined that although it is efficacious in restoring plasma volume in severe hemorrhage, other alternatives are equally effective and safer.[5-7] In reference to the clinical practice of giving FFP after each 5 or more units of PRBCs, the Conference found no documentation that FFP is indicated as part of the routine management of massive hemorrhage. The indications for FFP are listed in Table 19–7.

Platelets. Platelets are necessary to maintain normal bleeding times. A platelet count above 100,000/mm^3 is usually adequate for hemostasis. Most feel that a level of 50,000 to 75,000/mm^3 is an acceptable lower level for surgery. When a platelet count of 10,000/mm^3 is reached there is a high likelihood of spontaneous bleeding (surgical wound, intravenous sites, mucous membranes) that may be life-threatening to the patient. A unit of random-donor platelet concentrate usually increases the platelet count by 5000 to 10,000/μL; however, a single unit of single-donor concentrate raises the platelet count 50,000 to 100,000/μL. The amount that the platelet count will actually increase is influenced by such factors as infection, platelet alloantibodies, splenomegaly, and fever.

During surgery, the platelet count may drop because of increased consumption, as well as dilution of the patient's blood with administered colloid and crystalloid. Platelets may be administered when treating massive hemorrhage on the basis of clinical signs and laboratory data; however, in milder blood loss, the body has adequate bone marrow reserve to respond to the small reduction in platelets. Platelets are indicated for patients who have severe aplastic anemia or thrombocytopenia and in patients undergoing cardiopulmonary bypass. Single-donor platelet concentrates may be necessary for patients who have developed antibodies that cause destruction of transfused platelets. HLA-compatible platelet concentrations are prepared by harvesting platelets from single donors by automated apheresis. Random-donor platelet concentrate can be stored for 72 hours at room temperature and 48 hours at 4C; however, single-donor platelet concentrates should be stored only 24 hours because the apheresis procedure is considered "open" and after 24 hours the incidence of contamination of the unit is increased. Platelets should be given through a standard 170-μm blood filter set.

Leukocyte Concentrates. Some chemotherapeutic agents suppress bone marrow production. Therefore, some patients on chemotherapy may develop neutropenia. Insufficient granulocytes make it difficult for the body to protect itself from infections and leukocyte therapy may help these patients. Leukapheresis removes leukocytes, granulocytes, erythrocytes, platelets, and lymphocytes from the donor.

TABLE 19–7. PLATELET, LEUKOCYTE, AND PLASMA COMPONENTS

Blood Component	Clinical Indications	Approximate Composition		Shelf Life and Storage Temperature
		Plasma	Platelets	
Random donor platelet	Thrombocytopenia with hemorrhage, severe thrombocytopenia, functional platelet disorders with hemorrhage	30 mL (4C) 50 mL (20–24C)	> 5.5 × 10^{10}	48 h at 4C 72 h at 20–24C
Single-donor platelet concentrate by apheresis	Refractory to random-donor platelet concentrate, severe thrombocytopenia, hemorrhage with thrombocytopenia or functional disorder	300–500 mL	3–8 × 10^{11}	24 h at 20–24C
Leukocyte concentrate by apheresis	Severe neutropenia, fever, and infection unresponsive to antibiotics	300–700 mL	3–8 × 10^{11} (granulocytes = 1 × 10^{10})	24 h at 4C or 20–24C
Fresh-frozen plasma	Multiple coagulation deficiencies	200–275 mL	Nil	1 y at −18C 24 h at 4C
Single-donor plasma	Plasma expansion	200–275 mL	Nil	5 y at −18C 24 h at 4C
Cryoprecipitate	Factor VIII deficiency, factor XIII deficiency, von Willebrand's disease, hypofibrinogenemia	10–15 mL	Nil	1 y at −18C 6 h at 20–24C

Adapted, with permission, from Kennedy MS. Essentials of immunohematology and blood therapy. In: Zuspan PF, Quilligan EJ, eds. A practical manual *of obstetrical care. St. Louis, MO: CV Mosby; 1982.*

The administration of leukocyte concentrates has not proven to be as effective as once thought. Leukocyte antibodies are stimulated by the transfusion. The administration of leukocyte concentrates is usually limited to some bone marrow transplants, gram-negative septicemia, and infection that is not responsive to antibiotics and in which the granulocyte count is less than $500/\mu L$. The volume of the product varies according to the apheresis technique used. As the process of apheresis is an "open" technique, the product should be discarded after 24 hours.

Cryoprecipitate. Cryoprecipitate is a major source of fibrinogen and is used in the treatment of hemophilia (factor VIII deficiency), hypofibrinogenemia, von Willebrand's disease, and rare cases of factor XIII deficiency. Cryoprecipitate contains factor I (fibrinogen), factor VIII, and factor XIII. A single unit of cryoprecipitate contains approximately 100 clotting units of factor VIII and 250 mg of fibrinogen. The volume of a bag of cryoprecipitate is 10 to 15 mL, but diluent is added resulting in a total volume of 25 to 35 mL. Cryoprecipitate is kept frozen at −18C to preserve factor VIII activity for 1 year. Transfusion of cryoprecipitate should occur within 6 hours of thawing or 4 hours of pooling. Usually, cryoprecipitate is ABO type specific whenever possible. Cryoprecipitate is the only product that contains concentrated fibrinogen. It carries a lower risk of hepatitis because it is a single-donor product.

Albumin. Albumin is used to help expand circulating blood volume when oxygen-carrying capacity is adequate. Albumin has a molecular weight of 65,000, and maintains capillary osmotic pressure. It also serves as a carrier protein for various drugs, hormones, enzymes, and metabolites. The body produces 50 g of albumin daily. The use of albumin has decreased because of the infectious complications. Hepatitis may be transmitted as the albumin is derived from a pooled sample. Abnormal liver function following administration of albumin has been reported.

Factor Concentrates. Factor VIII is used to treat patients with hemophilia A or von Willebrand's disease. Factor IX concentrate contains not only factor IX but also factors II, VII, and X. This product is used most frequently with patients who have hemophilia B (factor IX deficiency), Christmas disease, or rare congenital deficiencies of factors II, VII, and X and to reverse the effects of warfarin in life-threatening hemorrhage. The major disadvantage of factor IX administration is that there is a high risk of hepatitis transmission with this product.

The selection and successful treatment of blood derangements are based on use of appropriate blood components. In Table 19–8, coagulation factor deficiencies are listed and the component treatments indicated.

Synthetic Products

Synthetic Colloid. Synthetic colloid agents for blood volume expansion include dextran, gelatin, hydroxyethyl starch, polyvinylpyrrolidone, and stroma-free hemoglobin. These isotonic electrolyte solutions are able to act as plasma proteins to provide osmotic pressure. Colloid preparations are used as volume expanders and to treat hypovolemic shock.

Dextran and hydroxyethyl starch are nonprotein colloid volume expanders. Disadvantages of these agents include interference with ABO blood grouping because of the rouleaux formation with dextran and agglomeration of the red cells with starch. Dextran may be used for normovolemic hemodilution in major surgical procedures. Gelatin has also been used to treat polycythemia and thrombocytopenia. Hemoglobin solutions have been used for their oxygen-carrying capability and volume expansion; however, they are associated with nephrotoxicity and have an unacceptably high oxygen affinity.

All of the preparations can produce incompatibility reactions. The symptoms range from histamine release to anaphylaxis. Ennis and Lorenz[8] have reported a high incidence of adverse reactions to colloid therapy, whereas Ring and Messmer[9] have reported a relatively small number of adverse reactions to colloid therapy. Belcher and Lennox[10] reported that there were no untoward effects attributable to hydroxyethyl starch administration in 27 patients undergoing cardiac surgery. The study concluded that hydroxyethyl starch is a safe, cheap, and effective plasma substitute for volume replacement. Some of the potential side effects of colloid synthetic solutions are highlighted in Table 19–9.

Perfluorocarbons. Perfluorocarbon suspensions are inert liquids possessing high oxygen solubility. Fluosol DA initially generated enthusiasm, but it has been found to require very high partial pressures of oxygen (> 500 mm Hg) before any significant amount of oxygen is transported. It also suppresses the reticuloendothelial system. Another related compound with higher oxygen binding activity, perfluoroctyl bromide, is under investigation.

Indications for Packed Red Blood Cells, Fresh-Frozen Plasma, and Platelets

PRBCs should be used to increase oxygen-carrying capacity of circulating blood volume. They should not be used for volume expansion, in place of a hematinic, or to improve general well-being.

FFP should be used to increase the level of clotting fac-

TABLE 19–8. BLOOD PRODUCTS FOR TREATMENT OF COAGULATION FACTOR DEFICIENCIES

Fibrinogen deficiency	Cryoprecipitate
	Stored plasma
Factor V deficiency	Fresh-frozen plasma
Factor VII deficiency	Factor IX complex (II, VII, IX, X)
	Stored plasma
Factor VIII deficiency	Factor VIII concentrate (AHF)
	Cryoprecipitate
	Fresh-frozen plasma
Von Willebrand's disease	Cryoprecipitate
	Fresh-frozen plasma
Factor IX deficiency	Factor IX complex (II, VII, IX, X)
	Stored plasma
Factor XIII deficiency	Stored plasma

Reprinted, with permission, from Blajchman MA, Sheppard FA, Perrault RA. Clinical use of blood, blood components and blood products. Can Med Assoc J. 1979;121:33.

TABLE 19–9. SYNTHETIC COLLOIDS AVAILABLE FOR BLOOD VOLUME EXPANSION SIDE EFFECTS

Synthetic Colloid	Potential Side Effects
Dextran	Erythrocyte rouleaux Hemostatic abnormalities
Gelatin	Erythrocyte rouleaux
Hydroxyethyl starch	Erythrocyte rouleaux Hemostatic disorders Prolonged retention Hyperamylasemia
Polyvinylpyrrolidone	Erythrocyte rouleaux Prolonged retention in the reticuloendothelial system
Stroma-free hemoglobin	Renal damage Hypercoagulability from residual membrane lipids

Reprinted, with permission, from Blajchman MA, Sheppard FA, Perrault RA. Clinical use of blood, blood components and blood products. Can Med Assoc J. 1979;121:33.

tors in patients with demonstrated deficiency or to reverse the effect of warfarin. It should not be used for volume expansion, as a nutritional supplement, nor prophylactically in massive RBC transfusion or following cardiopulmonary bypass.

Platelets should be used to control or prevent bleeding associated with decreases in platelet count or function. They should not be used prophylactically in massive RBC transfusion or after cardiopulmonary bypass.[11–13]

HAZARDS OF TRANSFUSION THERAPY

Infectivity of Blood Products

Viral hepatitis is the disease most frequently transmitted by blood transfusions; however, the risk of acquiring hepatitis is rather low. Many viruses can be passed through blood transfusions; some of the more common are non-A, non-B (NANB) hepatitis viruses, hepatitis B virus, cytomegalovirus, and human immunodeficiency virus (HIV) (Table 19–10).

Hepatitis. The majority of transfusion recipients who become infected with viral hepatitis have NANB hepatitis (hepatitis "C"). Posttransfusion hepatitis strikes between 4 and 15 percent of those receiving transfusions.[12] The Food and Drug Administration stated the risk in 1989 as 1 : 100 per unit of blood given. Clinically patients who have NANB hepatitis may become icteric, fatigued, and anorexic; however, the majority of patients remain asymptomatic. Fifty percent will develop chronic hepatic inflammation, and 20 percent will develop cirrhosis. Thus, a significant morbidity and mortality rate is associated with posttransfusion hepatitis. Clinical diagnosis of posttransfusion hepatitis is defined as a transient twofold elevation of serum alanine aminotransferase (ALT) on at least two consecutive tests (14 days apart) performed from 2 to 26 weeks after transfusion. ALT levels may be elevated with or without jaundice. ALT levels can be elevated for reasons other than hepatitis. Therefore, the patient must have studies done to rule out other factors such as congestive heart failure and alcohol.

A viral particle for hepatitis C has been identified, and blood banks routinely test for it (since 1990)[14]; however, the test has a large false-positive rate (50 percent).[12] In addition, not all NANB hepatitis may be due to the C virus. Hepatitis B is caused by a DNA virus. The majority of patients who do develop hepatitis B are anicteric.[3] Five to ten percent of patients positive for the hepatitis B surface antigen (HBsAg) develop chronic hepatitis or become carriers. Delta hepatitis, which is a defective RNA virus that cannot replicate without the helper function of hepatitis B, is recognized as a cause of fulminant hepatitis. Screening for HBsAg helps to decrease the risk of transmitting delta hepatitis.

To help prevent the transmission of hepatitis, careful screening for HBsAg in the donated blood and use of volunteer donors are desirable. Aach et al.[15] have suggested that all blood donors be screened for ALT to reduce the risk of transmission of NANB hepatitis. The incidence of hepatitis is related to the number of units of blood products an individual receives. Therefore, unnecessary transfusions should be avoided to help decrease the transmission of viral hepatitis.

TABLE 19–10. FEATURES OF DIFFERENT TYPES OF POSTTRANSFUSION HEPATITIS[a]

Feature	B	NANB	Delta	CMV
Proportion (%)	6–15	75–90	Unknown	2–17
Donor screening tests	HBsAg	ALT (SGPT), anti-HBcAg	HBsAg	Anti-CMV
Carrier rate (%)	5–10	2–6	1	6–12
Patients at risk	Any	Any	Hepatitis B carriers, persons with hemophilia, intravenous drug abusers	Immunosuppressed, low-birth-weight premature infants
Average incubation period, wk (range)	13 (2–26)	7 (2–26)	Unknown	5 (3–6)
Clinical outcome	85–95% asymptomatic, 5–10% chronic hepatitis, 1–3% fatal	60% asymptomatic, 25–50% chronic hepatitis	Fulminant hepatitis	Usually asymptomatic, rarely fatal

[a] ALT, alanine aminotransferase; CMV, cytomegalovirus; HBcAg, hepatitis B core antigen; HBsAg, hepatitis B surface antigen; NANB, non-A, non-B.
Reprinted, with permission, from Coffin CM. Current issues in transfusion therapy. 1. Risks of infection. Postgrad Med. 1986;80(8):219–224.

Human Immunodeficiency Virus. The impact that present testing has on the transmission of human immunodeficiency virus (HIV) via transfusions may not be known for several years, as the incubation period is lengthy (> 7 years) and testing only began in 1985.[16,17] A total of 3345 cases of transfusion-related acquired immunodeficiency syndrome (AIDS) cases (excluding hemophiliacs) were reported as of April 1990, which represents approximately 3 percent of all AIDS cases.[12] Not only laboratory tests, which are reported as greater than 99 percent sensitive and specific, but also face-to-face donor screening is felt to make an important contribution to the safety of the blood supply. The current risk of acquiring AIDS by transfusion is 1 in 153,000 per donor unit exposure, or 1 in 28,000 for the average recipient exposed to 5.4 homologous units.[12]

Other Bloodborne Diseases. Cytomegalovirus (CMV) infections are spread by infected leukocytes in donor blood. The largest populations at risk for contracting CMV are immunosuppressed patients and premature, low-birth-weight infants. Epstein-Barr virus may also be transmitted, as can bacterial septicemia. Platelets are stored at room temperature and, therefore, may transmit *Streptococcus* or *Staphylococcus*. Parasites such as malaria and spirochetes such as syphilis are only rarely transmitted.

Citrate Intoxication and Hyperkalemia

Stored bank blood has three different anticoagulant preservatives: acid–citrate–dextrose (ACD), citrate–phosphate–dextrose (CPD), and citrate–phosphate–dextrose with adenine (CPDA-1). The preservative most frequently used today is CPDA-1. The purpose of the preservative is to anticoagulate the blood, maintain red cell viability, and maintain normal hemoglobin function. The anticoagulant chelates the ionized calcium and inhibits the coagulation cascade. Addition of dextrose to phosphate citrate and citric acid prolongs red cell viability by generating ATP.

Stored blood has excess acidity because of the citric acid and the lactic acid generated during ATP utilization. Massive transfusions may lead to metabolic acidosis. Most of the time this metabolic acidosis is not treated with bicarbonate. Treating metabolic acidosis may worsen the oxygen delivery (left shift of the oxyhemoglobin dissociation curve), result in large sodium loads, and impair calcium mobilization.

During massive transfusion (at rates greater than 120 mL/min) hyperkalemia may develop.[18] Plasma potassium levels are increased in stored blood; levels may be as high as 19 to 30 mEq/L in blood stored 21 days. A peaked T-wave observed on the electrocardiogram is diagnostic of hyperkalemia.

Hypocalcemia

After receiving a large amount of citrated blood, patients will exhibit a decrease in their ionized calcium level. Calcium is mobilized rather rapidly from the bones to supply the body with adequate calcium to continue physiologic functioning. Howland et al.[19] have indicated that routine empiric supplementation of calcium is not necessary during massive transfusion. The utilization of calcium should be determined by laboratory values to support the administration of the drug. Miller states that calcium administration is rarely necessary.[3] When it is, 10 percent calcium chloride can be used. Though irritating to veins, it contains three times the amount of calcium as an equal volume of 10 percent calcium gluconate.

Citrate intoxication is caused by citrate binding calcium. Therefore, the characteristics of citrate intoxication are signs of hypocalcemia. The signs of hypocalcemia are hypotension, narrow pulse pressure, and elevated left ventricular end-diastolic and central venous pressures.

Hypothermia

The potential for rendering a patient hypothermic during massive transfusion therapy is of great concern. Cold blood can cause cardiac arrhythmias as well as contribute to hypothermia. Hypothermia increases oxygen and energy requirements. The metabolism of anesthetic agents and narcotics is impaired at lower body temperature. Hypothermia impairs the metabolism of citrate and lactate, which could lead to hypocalcemia and metabolic acidosis. The cold temperature also promotes the release of potassium from the intracellular space. Therefore, the use of a blood warmer is recommended to maintain homeothermia of the patient.

The patient's exposure during the surgical procedure, especially during abdominal cases, helps to contribute to a decreased temperature. The importance of maintaining homeothermia becomes critical when large amounts of blood are being administered to a patient with a great deal of body exposure. The problem of hypothermia is especially acute during massive transfusions in cases where body cavities are opened.

One of the problems associated with administration of blood via a blood warmer is the impedance of flow rates when rapid infusion is necessary. Many different blood warmers are available on the market. Therefore, the blood warmer that offers the least amount of impedance of flow may be the best choice for rapid administration of blood.

Hemolytic Transfusion Reactions

Hemolytic transfusion reactions are difficult to assess under general anesthesia. The patient is anesthetized and unable to relate any of the symptoms of the reaction. The clinical signs a patient exhibits during a transfusion reaction may vary: fever, chills, flushing, dyspnea, pain in the back or chest, hypotension, shock, disseminated intravascular coagulation (DIC), and presence of hemoglobin in the urine and plasma (Table 19–11). During anesthesia, the symptoms that may be recognizable are hemoglobinuria, hemolysis, and hypotension.

The treatment of hemolytic transfusion focuses on stopping the transfusion and maintaining adequate renal function. A minimal urinary output of 75 mL/h is desired to maintain adequate renal function.[3] This goal is achieved by administering fluids and diuretics to facilitate renal function. The exact mechanism of decreased renal function is not certain; however, it is hypothesized that a form of acid hematin precipitates in the distal tubules and actually blocks the tubules, impairing renal function.

TABLE 19–11. HEMOLYTIC TRANSFUSION REACTION: SIGNS AND SYMPTOMS

Fever, chills, flushing

Dyspnea

Pain: chest and/or back

Hypotension, shock

Oliguria, anuria

Disseminated intravascular coagulation

Hemoglobin in plasma and urine

Reprinted, with permission, from Harrigan C, Cantrell ME. Unit VI: Anesthesia for emergency surgery; Hemostasis and blood replacement therapy. In: Current concepts in inhalation anesthesia. Philadelphia: Ted Thomas; 1986.

Treatment of a hemolytic transfusion reaction is described step-by-step in Table 19–12. The goals are to stop the infusion of the blood, maintain an adequate urinary output, alkalinize the urine, assay urinary and plasma hemoglobin, determine coagulation levels, return unused blood to the blood bank, send a sample of the patient's blood to be tested for antibodies, and avoid hypotension. Hypotension decreases renal perfusion, thus causing a decrease in renal function, potentially leading to renal failure. Therefore, adequate hydration and optimal renal function during a hemolytic transfusion reaction are absolute.

Pulmonary Dysfunction

The incidence of pulmonary dysfunction following massive transfusion is high. Many factors may be associated with the problem. Unfiltered debris found in transfused blood may cause pulmonary microvascular obstruction, which could lead to adult respiratory distress syndrome. Well-controlled human research is insufficient to justify the recommendation that microaggregate filters (40 μm) be used

TABLE 19–12. STEPS FOR THE TREATMENT OF HEMOLYTIC TRANSFUSION REACTION

1. *Stop the transfusion.*
2. Maintain the urine output at a minimum of 75 to 100 mL/h by the following methods:
   a. Generously administer fluids intravenously and possibly mannitol, 12.5 to 50 g, given over a 5- to 15-min period.
   b. If intravenously administered fluids and mannitol are ineffective, then administer furosemide, 20 to 40 mg, intravenously.
3. Alkalinize the urine; as bicarbonate is preferentially excreted in the urine, only 40 to 70 mEq/70 kg of sodium bicarbonate is usually required to raise the urine pH to 8, whereupon repeat urine pH determinations indicate the need for additional bicarbonate.
4. Assay urine and plasma hemoglobin concentrations.
5. Determine platelet count, partial thromboplastin time, and serum fibrinogen level.
6. Return unused blood to blood bank for recrossmatch.
7. Send patient blood sample to blood bank for antibody screen and direct antiglobulin test.
8. Prevent hypotension to ensure adequate renal blood flow.

Reprinted, with permission, from Miller.[3]

for all bank blood or in certain subgroups of patients, such as those receiving massive transfusions. Bank blood does not begin to develop microaggregates for at least 5 days, and possibly as long as 10 days, so there is no need for microfiltration in blood stored less than that time.[3] The other factors associated with adult respiratory distress include chest and abdominal compliance injury, circulatory overload, hypoxemia resulting from hypovolemic shock, sepsis, and extensive use of colloids rather than crystalloid for rapid volume replacement.

Hypoxemia

Transfused erythrocytes are given to improve oxygen-carrying capacity; however, stored blood is preserved in CPDA-1 which decreases 2,3-diphosphoglycerate (2,3-DPG) levels. This depletion of 2,3-DPG causes a shift in the oxygen dissociation curve to the left. The shift to the left indicates an increased affinity of hemoglobin to oxygen and a possible impairment of oxygen release to the tissues. The clinical importance of this phenomenon is not clear. To minimize the leftward shift, all blood should be warmed, and excessive bicarbonate administration should be avoided.

Sepsis

The reticuloendothelial system is depressed after trauma, major surgery, burns, and hemorrhage. The depression of the reticuloendothelial system may be related to several factors, for example, blockage of the reticuloendothelial system by debris and secretion of endogenous adrenocortical hormone in response to shock. Not only is the reticuloendothelial system depressed, but studies by Snyder et al.[20] found that fibronectin levels are also decreased under these stressful situations. Fibronectin has been identified as playing a major role in opsonization of tissue debris, soluble fibrin, and gram-positive bacteria. Mosher and Furcht[21] stated that fibronectin plays a major role in lung fluid balance during bacterial sepsis, demonstrated by an increased pulmonary vascular permeability.

Coagulopathies

Abnormal bleeding times are often attributed to massive transfusions. Many of the problems that develop, such as thrombocytopenia and decreases in labile coagulation factors, are associated with the dilutional effect of transfusion therapy. Episodes of intravascular coagulation and fibrinolysis have occurred after massive transfusions. Stored erythrocytes lack platelets, ionized calcium, and adequate levels of factors V and VIII. Therefore, during massive transfusion of red blood cells, the need for other blood component therapy should be continually assessed.

Platelets in whole blood no longer function after 48 hours when stored at 4C. Platelet function is further inhibited by depressed ionized calcium and alterations in pH and temperature. Therefore, massive transfusions may lead to dilutional thrombocytopenia, one of the most common causes of hemorrhagic diathesis in patients who receive massive transfusions. When the platelet count is less than 100,000 cells/mm^3 the likelihood of bleeding problems is increased. When bleeding problems are observed during massive transfusion, the platelet count must be assessed.

Disseminated intravascular coagulation has been reported rarely after massive transfusions. Tissue thromboplastin is released under hypoxic local conditions, such as hypovolemic shock. This activates the coagulation system, resulting in consumption of coagulation factors, with resultant uncontrolled bleeding from wounds, the gastrointestinal tract, and other sites. Heparin is seldom useful, and may worsen hemorrhage. DIC is a preterminal result of many different pathologic processes. Its presence may be assessed by testing for elevated fibrin degradation (split) products and decreased fibrinogen.

DECREASING THE USE OF HOMOLOGOUS BLOOD PRODUCTS

The AIDS epidemic has focused public and peer-review attention on transfusion practices, even though hepatitis is more prevalent and probably causes more morbidity. Any actions anesthesia personnel can take to limit the use of homologous blood products will lessen demand for a scarce resource, decrease the transmission of infectious diseases, and avoid the morbidity and mortality associated with transfusion reactions.

Decreasing the Use of Packed Cells and Whole Blood

Accept lower hemoglobin and hematocrit levels. The use of a 30 percent hematocrit (Hct) as the level at which transfusion is necessary was judged inappropriately high by the NIH Consensus Conference.[12,13] Gravelee has developed an untested set of guidelines which follow. Many patients do not need transfusion until the hemoglobin reaches 6 to 7 g/dL (Hct 18 to 21 percent), for example, patients with chronic severe anemias, those in good health (PS I or II, < 50 years) undergoing uncomplicated surgery, or those undergoing hypothermic cardiopulmonary bypass. Some patients should probably be transfused at 8 g/dL (Hct 24 percent), including those undergoing surgery in which blood loss greater than 500 mL is predicted, cardiac surgery patients in the early postoperative course, and many PS III and IV patients. Finally, a hemoglobin of 10 g/dL or higher (Hct > 30 percent) should be maintained if the patient has valvular, ischemic, or congenital heart disease and is to undergo noncardiac surgery; if complications that increase oxygen consumption (fever, infection, bronchospasm, burns, multiple trauma) or decrease cardiac reserve (ischemia, arrhythmias) are present; and critical care and mechanical ventilation are required. These guidelines assume a normovolemic state. When a patient is allowed to become hypovolemic and anemic, the oxygen extraction reserve becomes exhausted.

Increase the use of autologous transfusion. California law requires that patients be informed of alternatives to homologous transfusion, including predonation.[12] The popularity and demand for autologous predonation are increasing, yet the service remains underutilized. Over a 2- to 6-week period, weekly donations are made and a hematinic is given, as long as the patient's hematocrit remains above 35 percent. Intraoperatively, collection and salvage of shed blood are useful in intrathoracic, intraabdominal, spinal, trauma, orthopedic, vascular, cardiac, and other types of surgery.[22] Salvage of cells should be avoided when fecal, infectious, or metastatic contamination of suction aspire is likely.[12,23]

Intentional intraoperative isovolemic hemodilution (IIIH) involves phlebotomy to withdraw blood early in surgery while replacing volume. The advantage is that blood shed later will have a lower red cell mass. The withdrawn blood can be infused near the end of surgery. The practice remains controversial as it has yet to be proved that its use decreases transfusion requirements. Cardiac patients and some others may benefit from reinfusion of blood shed and salvaged postoperatively, though this is the most controversial form of autotransfusion.

Decreasing the Use of Platelets and Fresh-Frozen Plasma

Use more fresh whole blood. Studies show that the levels of factors V and VIII may exceed 50 percent of normal after 5 to 7 days of storage.[12] Platelets may exceed $100,000/mm^3$ after 5 days. A mixture of whole blood and PRBCs in massively transfused (20 to 30 units) patients greatly decreases the need for FFP and platelets. Neither platelets nor FFP should be used as routine prophylaxis in massive transfusion.

Await the onset of clinical signs of bleeding rather than administer components solely on the basis of laboratory data. Even with prothrombin and partial thromboplastin times 1.5 times control, half or more of the massively transfused patients in a prospective study exhibited no clinical coagulopathy.[7]

Use platelets before FFP in most circumstances. The rationale is that 4 to 6 units of platelet concentrate contain a plasma coagulation factor concentration equivalent to 1 unit of FFP. Also, dilutional thrombocytopenia is more often a factor in clinical bleeding than factor deficiency. Severe liver disease and injury are exceptions, as is DIC, in which FFP is needed.

Drugs That May Decrease Transfusion Requirements

Desmopressin (DDAVP) induces release of endogenous factor VIII and von Willebrand's factor, and has been investigated as a means of decreasing transfusion requirements.[3,12,24] Antifibrinolytics (ε-aminocaproic acid, tranexamic acid, aprotinin) may lessen blood loss. Perfluorocarbon suspensions may also be useful. Hemoglobin suspensions or microencapsulations show great promise as a means of eliminating the need for PRBCs, but are not a practical solution at present. Recombinant human erythropoietin has already been used to increase the yield in autologous predonation, and may have value in postoperative patients with low hemoglobin. Finally, induced hypotension has proven to decrease blood loss in many types of surgery.

MEDICOLEGAL CONSIDERATIONS

Informed consent for any transfusion must be obtained from the patient and documented in the patient's chart. This notation should specify that the hazards of transfusion were discussed, unless this is not possible.

It would seem prudent to document on the anesthesia record the indications for each transfusion. This aids retrospective review of quality care, as well as aiding the clinician in clarifying the rationale for the therapeutic intervention.

Layon et al.[25] present the rationale for refusal of blood products by Jehovah's Witnesses. Briefly, they believe that the receipt of blood is tantamount to "eating" blood, which is forbidden by Scripture. Adherents to this religion believe they will lose eternal life, and may suffer damnation on earth, if they receive transfusions. Thus, they would literally rather die than do so; however, some Jehovah's Witnesses will accept albumin, factor products, or plasma protein fractions. Refusal to accept blood products and discussion of potential consequences with the patient should be documented in the patient record by the anesthesia care provider. If anesthesia personnel agree to give care with this restriction, they should consider themselves bound by it.

In an emergency, such as unanticipated, life-threatening hemorrhage, a conflict is created between the caregiver's desire to do no harm to the patient and the patient's autonomy, that is, the patient's right to make decisions regarding his or her care. As long as the patient is a mentally competent adult who understands the consequences of the decision, it should be respected, and no blood products should be given, even if their use might be life-saving. No legal sanctions have been applied to caregivers who withheld blood products under these clearly defined preoperative conditions.

The legal system has intervened to order life-saving transfusions for minor children of Jehovah's Witnesses, as they are not of the age to make their own decisions, and for adult Jehovah's Witnesses with minor children who might become wards of the state. Thus, the state allows the individual's religious conduct (refusal of blood) when it is not in conflict with societal interests in protecting minor children.[25]

SUMMARY

As administration of blood and blood components carries risks, the advantages of therapy must outweigh the risks. Myhre[26] studied the number of fatalities caused by transfused blood and blood products reported to the Food and Drug Administration. Of those fatalities, 61 percent were due to clerical errors. The second most common problem was posttransfusion hepatitis, which led to 33 percent of the fatalities. Thus, the majority of fatalities caused by blood transfusions can be prevented by careful screening and judicious administration of blood components.

REFERENCES

1. Schwab CW, Civil I, Shayne JP. Saline-expanded group O uncrossmatched packed red blood cells as an initial resuscitation fluid in severe shock. *Ann Emerg Med.* 1986;15(11):1282–1297.

2. Oberman HA, Barnes BA, Friedman BA. The risk of abbreviating the major crossmatch in urgent or massive transfusion. *Transfusion.* 1978;18:137.

3. Miller RD. Transfusion therapy. In: Miller RD, ed. *Anesthesia.* 3rd ed. New York: Churchill-Livingstone; 1990:1467–1500.

4. *Standards for blood banks and transfusion services.* 10th ed. Washington, DC: American Association of Blood Banks; 1981.

5. Bove J. Fresh frozen plasma: Too few indications—too much use. *Anesth Analg.* 1985;64:849–850.

6. Murray DJ, Olson J, Strauss R. Packed red cells for blood replacement: When is FFP required? *Anesth Analg.* 1988;67:S155.

7. Murray DJ, Olson J, Strauss R, Tinker J. Coagulation changes during packed red cell replacement of major blood loss. *Anesthesiology.* 1988;69:839–845.

8. Ennis M, Lorenz W. Hypersensitivity reactions induced by anaesthetics and plasma substitutes. In: Dean JH, Luster M, Munson AE, Amos H, eds. *Immunotoxicology and immunopharmacology.* New York: Raven Press; 1985:457.

9. Ring J, Messmer K. Incidence and severity of anaphylactoid reactions to colloid volume substitutes. *Lancet.* 1977;1(8009):466–469.

10. Belcher P, Lennox SC. Avoidance of blood transfusion in coronary artery surgery: A trial of hydroxyethyl starch. *Ann Thorac Surg.* 1984;37(5):365–370.

11. Perez WE, Viets JL. Transfusion and coagulation: An overview and recent advances in practice modalities. Part I: Blood banking and transfusion practices. *Nurse Anesth.* 1990;1(3):149–161.

12. Gravlee GP. Blood transfusion and component therapy. In: *41st Annual Refresher Course Lectures and Clinical Update Program.* Chicago, IL: American Society of Anesthesiologists; 1990;215:1–7.

13. Stehling L, Esposito B. An analysis of the appropriateness of intraoperative transfusion. *Anesth Analg.* 1989;68:S278.

14. Stehling, L. The safe level of hemoglobin: Is anemia in? In: *41st Annual Refresher Course Lectures and Clinical Update Program.* Chicago, IL: American Society of Anesthesiologists; 1990;143:1–7.

15. Aach RD, Szmuness W, Mosley JW, et al. Serum alanine aminotransferase of donors in relation to the risk of non-A, non-B hepatitis in recipients: The transfusion-transmitted viruses study. *N Engl J Med.* 1981;304(17):989–994.

16. Scullon DI. Anesthetic implications of the acquired immunodeficiency syndrome (AIDS): Part I. *AANA J.* 1986;54(5):400–410.

17. Scullon DI. Anesthetic implications of the acquired immunodeficiency syndrome (AIDS): Part II. *AANA J.* 1986;54(6):480–485.

18. Jameson L, Popic P, Harms B. Hyperkalemic death during use of a high-capacity fluid warmer for massive transfusion. *Anesthesiology.* 1990;73:1050–1052.

19. Howland WS, Schweizer O, Carolon GC, et al. The cardiovascular effects of low levels of ionized calcium during massive transfusion. *Surg Gynecol Obstet.* 1977;145:581.

20. Snyder EL, Mosher DF, Hezzey A, et al. Effect of blood transfusion on in vivo levels of plasma fibronectin. *J Lab Clin Med.* 1981;98:336.

21. Mosher DF, Furcht LT. Fibronectin: Review of its structure and possible functions. *J Invest Dermatol.* 1981;77:175.

22. Spiess BD, Narbonr RF, Sasetti R, Truman KG, Ivankovich AD. Autologous blood donation service for high-risk patients. *Anesth Analg.* 1989;68:S272.

23. Healey TG. Intraoperative blood salvage. *AANA J.* 1989;57:429–434.

24. Viets JL, Yawn DH. Transfusion and coagulation: An overview and recent advances in practice modalities. Part II: Pharmacologic adjuncts, cell salvage mechanisms, alternations in blood donation. *Nurs Anesth.* 1990;1(4):206–220.

25. Layon AJ, D'Amico R, Caton D, Mollet C. And the patient chose: Medical ethics and the case of the Jehovah's Witness. *Anesthesiology.* 1990;73:1258–1262.

26. Myhre BA. Fatalities from blood transfusion. *JAMA.* 1980;24:1333–1335.

PART III

Applied Physiology

Cardiovascular Physiology

J. L. Reeves-Viets

Safe anesthetic practice requires the maintenance of adequate blood flow to meet the metabolic substrate and oxygen requirements of critical organs. This underscores the necessity for routine cardiovascular monitoring. The contemporary practitioners must be sophisticated in interpreting data derived from a variety of monitoring modes to ensure safe anesthetic care. This chapter introduces those principles of cardiovascular physiology that form the basis for interpretation of those data, with clinical applications.

FUNCTIONS OF THE CARDIOVASCULAR SYSTEM

The functions of the cardiovascular system may be conceptualized as incorporating four interrelated elements: conduit, pump, electrical function, and energy supplies. Each of these responds to a variety of physiologic controls that interact to maintain circulatory stability. The conduit provides a structure for transport of oxygen and metabolic substrate in the form of the vascular system. The vascular system responds to a variety of hemodynamic control mechanisms that interact to distribute adequate blood flow and maintain perfusion pressure to critical organs. The pump provides a propulsive force for movement of blood in the form of the mechanical function of the ventricles. Determinants of ventricular function include filling volume (preload), the force against which the ventricles operate (afterload), and the inotropic state (contractility). The electrical system maintains regular, synchronous atrioventricular function through a series of specialized conductive cells. The energy supply to the ventricles is distributed through the coronary circulation. Flow in the coronary circulation is autoregulated within the physiologic range by metabolic requirements.

DETERMINANTS OF CARDIAC OUTPUT

Cardiac output is determined by two primary factors: heart rate and stroke volume.[1] As only the first of these is directly measurable in the clinical setting, actual direct measurement of cardiac output is not possible in the usual practice. Calculations of cardiac output based on thermodilution technique using a Swan-Ganz catheter provide the basis for many determinations in the clinical setting; however, cardiac output calculations based on measurement of temperature gradients presume a number of external variables. As stroke volume is dynamic and dependent on a variety of physiologic factors, it is necessary to understand the basic principles controlling cardiac output.

The primary determinants of stroke volume are ventricular diastolic volume and ventricular systolic function.[1] If one assumes normal ventricular function, the primary determinant of cardiac output becomes ventricular end-diastolic volume. That relationship has been described in the Frank–Starling curve and its clinical correlates, as shown in Figure 20–1. The original Frank–Starling curve described the relationship between resting tension (preload) and peak-induced tension (contractility) in vitro, using isolated muscle strips. It demonstrated an increased peak tension as resting tension was increased. Clinical correlates typically describe the relationship between atrial pressure, central venous pressure (CVP) or pulmonary capillary wedge pressure (PCWP), and cardiac output.

The clinical counterpart to resting tension is the degree of stretch placed on myocardial sarcomeres during the resting phase of diastole. This degree of tension generally correlates with left ventricular end-diastolic pressure (LVEDP), which is determined in part by left ventricular end-diastolic volume (LVEDV).[2,3] Within the normal physiologic range, there is a direct relationship between LVEDV and LVEDP, which is determined primarily by ventricular diastolic function. Diastolic function may be separated into two elements: an active phase of ventricular relaxation termed *distensibility*, during which calcium is sequestered in an energy-dependent process, and a passive phase termed *compliance*, when the ventricle is completely relaxed immediately prior to systole.[4] LVEDP is not generally measured directly in the clinical setting. Instead, it is estimated using atrial pressure, CVP, or PCWP.

The clinical counterpart to generated tension is the con-

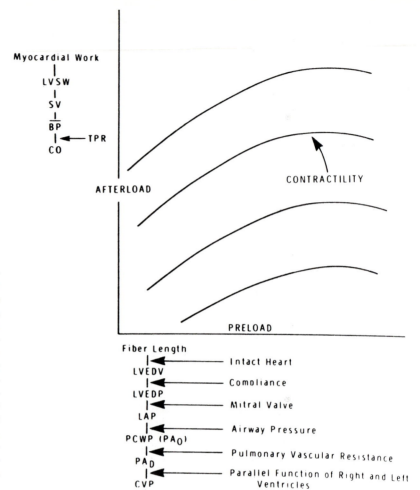

Figure 20–1. Frank–Starling curves demonstrating the relationship between preload and myocardial work. Factors estimating preload are demonstrated below the horizontal axis: factors estimating myocardial work are demonstrated alongside the vertical axis. LVSW, left ventricular stroke work; SV, stroke volume; BP, mean blood pressure; TPR, total peripheral resistance; CO, cardiac output; LVEDV, left ventricular end-diastolic volume; LVEDP, left ventricular end-diastolic pressure; LAP, left atrial pressure; PCWP, pulmonary capillary wedge pressure; PA_O, pulmonary artery occlusion pressure; PA_D, pulmonary artery diastolic pressure; CVP, central venous pressure. (*Reprinted, with permission, from Kaplan.*[1] *Adapted, with permission, from Bonner J. Anesth. Rev. 1977;7:26–29.*)

tractile force generated during ventricular systole. In the normal heart, increased ventricular end-diastolic volume produces greater stretch on myocardial fibers. This, in turn, results in increased systolic force, and yields an increased cardiac output. This physiologic relationship between filling volume and cardiac output supports the measurement of CVP or PCWP as an index of cardiac output.

Several assumptions should be recognized when applying this relationship. First, there is the statistical nature of compiled data. All physiologic data must be interpreted within the context of the individual's normal state or compensatory mechanisms that may be employed to maintain homeostasis. Second, the relationship is not absolutely linear. In fact, several portions of the curve represent hypovolemic, normovolemic, and hypervolemic states. Third, the relationship between volume and pressure is dynamic. It can be altered by agents and physiologic states affecting vascular or ventricular compliance and distensibility. Fourth, valvular dysfunction alters the interpretation of data from vascular sites in assessment of ventricular function. Valvular lesions produce characteristic physiologic changes that may necessitate higher-than-normal filling pressures to maintain adequate ventricular filling volume. Finally, atrioventricular synchrony alters interpretation of data derived from physiologic monitoring. Loss of the nor-

mal conduction mechanism may reduce ventricular filling when the normal atrial contribution to ventricular filling is lost, or when shortening the diastolic interval reduces the time available for ventricular filling.

The first assumption is based on the difference between population parameters and sample statistics. Population data describe the characteristics of large groups of individuals. Means and standard deviations provide statistical indices of the distribution of the measured parameters, and provide an estimate of the central tendency of the population. In many models, this is sufficient to make appropriate judgments. In the clinical setting, however, patients demonstrate a broad range in physiologic parameters, and measurements lying outside the typical range are not necessarily pathologic. As an example, healthy young adults may have a lower resting heart rate or CVP than described by the mean. This reflects a healthy cardiovascular system, not decreased cardiovascular function or volume. Although the values in Table 20–1 describe the tendency of large populations, those parameters cannot be stringently applied to individual patients. Therefore, it is more accurate to consider those values as typical values, rather than normal. It is important to remember that an individual may vary from the mean without being pathologic.

In the clinical setting, patients demonstrate individual-

TABLE 20–1. NORMAL CENTRAL VENOUS AND PULMONARY ARTERIAL PRESSURES IN HUMANS

Location	Abbreviation[a]	Pressure (mm Hg) Mean	Range
Central venous	CVP	6	1–10
Right atrium	RAP	4	–1 to +8
Right ventricle			
Systolic	—	24	15–28
End-diastolic	RVEDP	4	0–8
Pulmonary artery			
Systolic	PAsP	24	15–28
Diastolic	PAdP	10	5–16
Mean	PAP	16	10–22
Pulmonary artery or capillary wedge or pulmonary artery occlusion pressure	PAWP or PCWP or PAOP	9	6–15

[a] CVP, central venous pressure; RAP, right atrial pressure; RVEDP, right ventricular end diastolic pressure; PAsP, pulmonary artery systolic pressure; PAdP, pulmonary artery diastolic pressure; PAP, mean pulmonary artery pressure; PAWP/PCWP/PAOP, pulmonary artery wedge pressure. Adapted, with permission, from Miller RD, ed. Anesthesia, *2nd ed. New York: Churchill Livingstone; 1986; and Schlant RC, EH Sonnenblick, R Gorlin. Normal physiology of the cardiovascular system. In: Hurst JW, ed.* The Heart, *5th ed. New York: McGraw-Hill; 1982.*

ized pressure–volume or filling pressure–cardiac output curves, as is demonstrated in Figure 20–2. Therefore, interpretation of data obtained during anesthesia should include assessment of that patient's preoperative physiologic status, physiologic responses to anesthesia, and intervening factors that alter the pressure–volume relationship. Elevated filling pressures in the face of constant volume may be seen with the use of volatile agents or vasoconstrictors, or in the presence of hypothermia or myocardial ischemia. Thus the clinician must incorporate physiologic principles in determining

fluid and volume therapy or the use of vasoactive agents, rather than adhere to formulaic requirements.

The second assumption addresses the family of curves describing the relationship between pressure and volume. The relationship between volume and pressure remains linear only within a narrow physiologic range. In low-volume states (active continued bleeding, fluid restriction, or excessive fluid losses) the curve demonstrates a nearly flat slope: only small changes in pressure are noted with administration of comparatively large volumes. At the opposite end of the scale, in high-volume states (volume overload, congestive heart failure, reduction in fluid requirements, resorption of massive edema) the curve demonstrates a steep slope: large changes in pressure are noted with administration of comparatively small volumes.

The third assumption addresses factors that affect vascular and ventricular compliance. These factors are multiple, and affect the various circulatory systems differently. Hypoxia and hypercarbia produce peripheral arterial dilation and pulmonary arterial constriction. Thus, inadequate ventilation or compromised diffusion of gases across the alveolar membrane may produce pulmonary hypertension and systemic hypotension. During extended periods of hypoxemia, release of catecholamines may produce a late rise in systemic pressures, which is not a direct effect. Myocardial ischemia impairs the active, energy-dependent relaxation phase of ventricular diastole. This reduction in ventricular distensibility requires increased filling pressure to maintain ventricular diastolic volume. Hypoxia, ventricular hypertrophy or the use of inotropic agents may reduce ventricular compliance, likewise requiring higher filling pressure to maintain ventricular diastolic volume.

The fourth assumption includes the effects of valvular dysfunction. Valvular stenosis or insufficiency produces changes in the normal volume–pressure relationship. In the face of mitral or tricuspid stenosis, higher atrial pressures are required to generate flow across a restricted orifice. Thus to maintain normal ventricular diastolic filling vol-

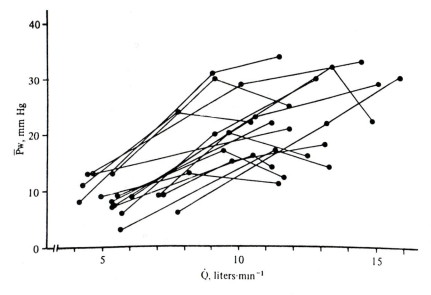

Figure 20–2. Pulmonary wedge pressure in relationship to cardiac output. (*Reprinted, with permission, from Altman PL and DS Dittmer, eds.* Respiration and circulation. *Bethesda, MD: Federation of American Societies for Experimental Biology, 1971:396–398.*)

ume, greater atrial or venous pressures (CVP or PCWP) must be maintained.[1,5] In the presence of mitral or tricuspid regurgitation, retrograde flow may be noted in the form of an exaggerated "v-wave."[5] This elevation in measured venous pressure incorporates an element of reflected ventricular systolic pressure in the upstream vascular system. Hence, CVP or PCWP may be grossly elevated to maintain adequate ventricular end-diastolic volume, whereas reductions in CVP or PCWP to "normal" values may actually result in effective ventricular hypovolemia. The effects of pulmonic and aortic valvular lesions are less prominent, provided the mitral or tricuspid valves remain competent. Patients with pulmonic or aortic stenosis need higher filling pressures based on the reduced compliance in the affected ventricle rather than a spurious gradient between measured venous or atrial pressure and the ventricular end-diastolic pressure. Aortic and pulmonic insufficiency may result in increased venous or atrial filling pressures as a reflection of the additional regurgitant volume in the affected ventricle, rather than a mismatch in corresponding ventricular diastolic pressure.

The final assumption includes the effect of atrioventricular synchroneity on the measurement of filling pressures. Loss of sinus mechanism eliminates the normal synchronous contraction that empties the atrium into a relaxed ventricle. Contraction of the atrium against a closed valve during a junctional rhythm or continuous nonphasic pressure generated in the presence of atrial fibrillation yields higher atrial or venous filling pressures that do not absolutely correspond with ventricular end-diastolic pressure.[6] Thus, when the normal atrioventricular synchronous relationship is disturbed, the absolute value of venous or atrial pressures as a guide to ventricular end-diastolic volume may be lost.

PRELOAD AND VOLUME

The term *preload* may be conceptualized as the degree of ventricular distension at the end of diastole. As previously described, diastolic ventricular volume is one primary determinant of end-diastolic pressure, which largely determines the contractile force of systole in the normal heart. Hence, in the normal heart, preload is closely related to volume, and the terms are frequently used interchangeably. A variety of factors may affect the relationship between volume per se and vascular or chamber pressures. The assumption that volume and pressure are linearly related holds true only within a relatively narrow physiologic range, determined by the individual patient's hemodynamic profile. The relationship between volume and pressure is determined by vascular or chamber compliance. Compliance is determined by the formula

$$C = \Delta V / \Delta P$$

which defines compliance as the relationship between changes in volume and changes in pressure. There are several requirements to understanding the application of this formula, however.

First, compliance is defined as an index of change. Therefore, compliance is assessed by changing volume status and measuring changes in pressure in either the chamber or the vessel. This requires serial measurements, which

means that compliance must be measured across time rather than as a periodic sample. Correctly used, it refers to an ongoing process rather than a static measurement at a single point in time.

Second, the factors determining compliance are dependent on the structure in which it is measured. Factors that determine compliance in the vascular system include vasomotor tone in the venous capacitance vessels, which contain approximately 75 percent of the intravascular volume at any point in time. Venomotor tone may be readily altered by physiologic changes such as hypoxemia and hypercarbia, or by pharmacologic intervention with vasodilators such as nitroglycerin and nitroprusside or vasoconstrictors such as phenylephrine.

The ventricle responds to a variety of additional factors, in a more complex fashion than the venous system. Although there is a reduction in ventricular compliance in response to chronic systemic hypoxemia or hypercarbia, it is equally important to appreciate the effect of acute changes in regional or subendocardial flow on compliance. That becomes more important in view of the fact that regional or subendocardial ischemia is not consistently detectable with routine electrocardiogram (ECG) monitoring. To view ventricular compliance as a singular phenomenon is furthermore an oversimplification. As previously stated, ventricular diastolic relaxation is actually composed of two phases. The first phase of relaxation is an active, energy-dependent process that involves sequestration of calcium ions. This phase is frequently termed *ventricular distensibility*. In contrast, compliance refers more accurately to the period in late diastole when the ventricle is completely relaxed, immediately prior to systole. These phases of ventricular diastole share many similar responses, although changes in distensibility may provide an early clue to ventricular diastolic function when global ventricular diastolic function is compensated by otherwise normal regions of the ventricle.[4]

Myocardial ischemia reduces ventricular distensibility in the affected regions, slowing the rate of ventricular relaxation.[7-9] This may affect only a limited region of the ventricle as occurs with occlusive coronary artery disease, or global reduction may follow subendocardial ischemia as occurs with congestive failure or ventricular hypertrophy. Neither of those events is consistently demonstrable on ECG analysis in a timely fashion. At present, only two monitoring modalities offer clues to the early appearance of ischemia. These include a discriminating analysis of waveforms from a CVP or Swan-Ganz catheter and the use of transesophageal echocardiography (TEE).[10,11]

The peak atrial pressure demonstrated in the "a"-wave obtainable from a CVP or Swan-Ganz pulmonary artery catheter tracing provides an estimate of ventricular distensibility. As it is during the period of atrial systole that the active phase of ventricular distensibility takes place, the exaggerated waveform indicates the greater peak atrial pressure required to overcome an incompletely relaxed ventricle. In fact, the presence of an exaggerated "a"-wave on the atrial waveform may represent the earliest sign of ventricular ischemia, preceding ECG changes or elevations in wedge pressure indicating global ventricular dysfunction or appearing without global indices of dysfunction.[12,13]

Physiologically significant changes in regional diastolic ventricular function may therefore be unrecognized when relying on global correlations between filling pressure and cardiac output.[14]

TEE provides an ongoing method of analyzing ventricular wall motion. This information provides a useful means of assessing ventricular function both globally and regionally, and permits the identification of small areas of dyssynergy. Additionally, the use of TEE permits assessment of right ventricular function, which may be less readily assessed by CVP waveforms because of the lower pressures generated on that side. It should be noted, however, that the standard midventricular position used for TEE does not identify the right ventricle. Selective assessment of ventricular function therefore requires sophistication in the use of modality.[6]

Ventricular compliance may likewise be altered by a variety of factors. Ventricular hypertrophy, myocardial ischemia, and the use of inotropic agents may all reduce ventricular compliance, requiring higher filling pressures to maintain ventricular end-diastolic volume. Regional reductions in ventricular compliance may not be detectable if the segment of the ventricle remains small, being compensated by otherwise normal segments of the ventricle. Thus, reductions in regional blood flow and compliance may be masked and remain undetectable by ECG or analysis of CVP or PCW, complicating assessment of ventricular function when global cardiac function demonstrates no change.

It is important to appreciate the benefits of monitoring both ventricular distensibility and compliance. Changes in regional blood flow may be insufficient to produce clinically significant changes in the filling pressure or global ventricular performance, based on compensation by well-perfused regions of the ventricle. Likewise, regional changes may escape detection with standard monitoring modalities. Although the clinical impact of these changes on long-term outcome is not determined, they should not be ignored. Further, although chronic states of subendocardial ischemia may mandate higher filling pressures to maintain LVEDV, the effects of superimposed reductions in distensibility offer a guide to acute changes in regional myocardial flow or ventricular performance that may otherwise go unappreciated.

RESISTANCE AND AFTERLOAD

The terms *resistance* and *afterload* are frequently used interchangeably. Although the two are related in the normal circulation, they are not identical, and should be recognized as separate phenomena. Resistance may be calculated for either the systemic or the pulmonary circulation, and shares a direct, linear relationship with the arterial pressure when cardiac output is held constant. Hence, within the normal physiologic range, blood pressure will increase concomitantly with increases in systemic resistance when cardiac output is maintained constant. In contrast to resistance, afterload may be conceptualized as the force that the ventricle must overcome to initiate the ejection phase of systole. As the force against which the ventricle operates increases outside the physiologic range, ventricular function may be impeded, producing a reduction in forward flow. Thus

resistance is primarily a vascular phenomenon, whereas afterload is oriented to the ventricle itself.

In the normal patient without outflow tract obstruction, the systemic vascular resistance (SVR) is the primary determinant of systemic blood pressure when cardiac output is held constant. As such, it is a primary determinant in the diastolic blood pressure, which is the force against which the ventricle must operate to initiate ejection during systole. For that reason, in the normal patient, systemic vascular resistance is a primary determinant of left ventricular afterload, as pulmonary vascular resistance (PVR) is to the right ventricle. Both of these parameters can be calculated using the mean arterial pressure, central venous pressure, cardiac output, and the formulas found in Table 20–2. When resistance increases in the systemic or pulmonary circulation, this translates as an increase in afterload. In the normal patient the ventricles adapt by increasing the inotropic state, and increased contractile state compensates for the additional workload, maintaining cardiac output. In exaggerated states, or in the patient with diminished ventricular function or reserve, the increase in afterload may lead to ventricular failure.

In contrast, afterload in the patient with outflow obstruction may be determined by the degree of valvular stenosis or outflow obstruction.[15] The degree of obstruction may be fixed as with valvular stenosis, or variable as with dynamic processes like idiopathic hypertrophic subaortic stenosis (IHSS). In the former, the ventricle operates against a static and constant afterload and can compensate only by increasing the contractile force of systole. In the latter, a band of concentric myocardium encircles the outflow tract from the ventricle just below the level of the valve. That band of myocardium is capable of contraction, effectively reducing the lumen of the outflow tract, making subaortic stenosis a dynamic dysfunction which may be treated with beta antagonists such as Inderal.

With outflow obstruction, vascular resistance no longer determines the force against which the ventricle operates. In that event, the vascular resistance becomes a primary determinant of the arterial blood pressure in the corresponding circulation. For the patient with outflow obstruction, afterload and resistance are thus separated. Systemic vascular resistance may then be viewed as a determinant of arterial pressure only, and can be presumed to have little direct impact on left ventricular performance per se; however, the necessity to maintain vascular resistance may remain paramount to maintain perfusion of the hypertrophied ventricle that typically accompanies outflow obstruction.

INOTROPIC STATE

The inotropic state defines systolic ventricular function and, with ventricular diastolic volume, determines the stroke volume and hence cardiac output. In the physiologic range, increases in LVEDV increase preload and inotropic state according to the principles demonstrated by the Starling curve. Likewise, increases in afterload will transiently increase the LVEDV and LVEDP. This relationship is demonstrated graphically in Figure 20–3. The resultant increase in ventricular volume is then compensated by increased contractile strength, thereby maintaining stroke

TABLE 20–2. NORMAL HEMODYNAMIC VALUES AVAILABLE FROM THE SWAN-GANZ CATHETER

Variable	Abbreviation	Formula	Units	Range
Cardiac output (70-kg, 1.7-m^2 man)	CO		L/min	5–6
Cardiac index	CI	$= \dfrac{CO}{BSA^a}$	L/min/m^2	2.8–4.2
Heart rate	HR		beats/min	60–90
Stroke volume	SV	$= \dfrac{CO}{HR} \times 1000$	mL/beat	60–90
Stroke index	SI	$= \dfrac{SV}{BSA}$	mL/beat/m^2	40–65
Left ventricular stroke work index	LVSWI	$= \dfrac{1.36\ BP - PAWP}{100} \times SI$	g-m/m^2	45–60
Right ventricular stroke work index	RVSWI	$= \dfrac{1.36\ PAP - CVP}{100} \times SI$	g-m/m^2	5–10
Total resistances				
Systemic vascular (total peripheral)	SVR (TPR)	$= \dfrac{BP - CVP}{CO} \times 80$	dyn-s/cm^5	900–1400
Pulmonary vascular	PVR	$= \dfrac{PAP - PAWP}{CO} \times 80$	dyn-s/cm^5	150–250

^{a} BSA, body surface area.

Reprinted, with permission, from Hug CC. Monitoring. In: Miller RD, ed. Anesthesia. *2nd ed. New York: Churchill Livingstone; 1986:453, Table 13–24.*

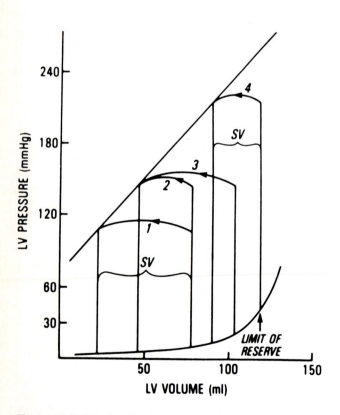

Figure 20–3. Relationship between afterload and stroke volume. The normal ventricle responds to increases in afterload with an increased stroke volume until the preload reserve is exhausted as indicated. LV, left ventricular. (*Reprinted, with permission, from DiNardo and Schwartz.[6] Adapted, with permission, from Hurst JW.* The Heart, *6th ed. New York: McGraw-Hill; 1986.*)

volume and cardiac output. Hence, within the limits of normal resting physiology, the inotropic state and volume are coordinated to maintain homeostasis. Each of these adaptations operates according to the mechanisms demonstrated by the Starling curve, which require no support from autonomic sympathetic function.

Resting myocardial tone can also be modified by input from the central vasopressor and vasodepressor centers in the brain stem. These centers operate through the intrinsic autonomic sympathetic and parasympathetic innervation of the heart. The sympathetic chain arises in the cervical and upper thoracic spinal cord[16] and terminates at receptor sites directly in the sinoatrial node, the atrioventricular node and the branches of the Purkinje system and bundles of His, all of which are diagrammed in Figure 20–4. The effects of stimulation are mediated primarily by norepinephrine. Stimulation produces an increase in the resting tone, increasing contractility and rate and enhancing arrhythmogenicity, particularly tachyarrhythmias. Parasympathetic innervation from the vagus innervates the same structures served by the intrinsic sympathetic system. The primary mediator at receptor sites is acetylcholine and stimulation produces corresponding depressant effects with a reduction in the inotropic state, chronotropism, and tachyarrhythmias. Intense parasympathetic stimulation may suppress automaticity with resulting escape rhythms.

Additional stimulation is provided through the humoral route of the autonomic sympathetic nervous system. Vasoactive catecholamines, primarily epinephrine, are released from the adrenal medulla and mediate beta-effected increases in inotropy, chronotropism, and arrhythmogenicity. Increasing the plasma level of catecholamines induces alpha-mediated vasoconstriction without completely ablating the beta-induced effects. The sympathetic nervous system can therefore maintain resting cardiac and vasomotor tone while providing augmentation of the inotropic state for the "fight or flight" stress response.

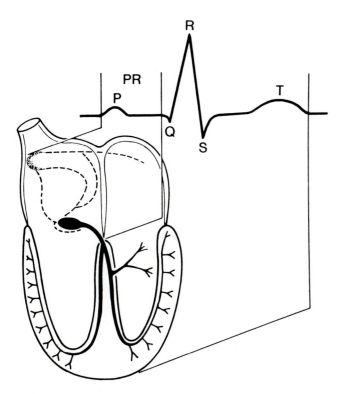

Figure 20–4. Relationship of the ECG electrical activity and the anatomy of the cardiac conduction system. (*Reprinted, with permission, from McIntyre KM, AJ Lewis, eds.* Textbook of advanced cardiac life support. *Dallas, TX: American Heart Association; 1983:64.*)

CONDUCTION SYSTEM

The conduction system is composed of the specialized tissue distributed throughout the atria and ventricles that is capable of spontaneous depolarization based on the gradual loss of electrical potential across the cell membrane, as demonstrated in Figure 20–5. The rate of spontaneous depolarization is determined by the rate of decay in membrane potential; thus the site with the most rapidly decaying membrane potential determines the heart rate. Depolarization of these conductive pathways is responsible for maintenance of a synchronous atrioventricular mechanism as demonstrated in Figure 20–6.

The conduction system includes two nodes: the sinoatrial (SA) node located at the juncture of the superior vena cava and the right atrium, and the atrioventricular (AV) node located at the juncture of the atria and ventricles. Additionally, it includes connecting pathways leading from the SA to the AV node through the level of the ventricular muscle mass via the Purkinje system and bundles of His. Several Bachmann's bundles serve to direct the impulse propagated in the SA node throughout the atria, whereas multiple pathways appear to exist for transmission of the impulse to the AV node.

The dominant pacemaker site is determined by the automaticity of the pacemaker cells. In the normal conduction system, membrane decay is most rapid in pacemaker cells in the SA node, and becomes progressively slower following the conduction pathway to the level of the ventricles. As the normal rate of decay in membrane potential declines as one proceeds down the conduction system, the dominant pacemaker site is the SA node. Failure of the dominant pacemaker site to function permits the next site to fire at the rate determined by its own intrinsic rate of depolarization. Thus, the sinus mechanism maintains a typical resting rate of about 70 beats per minute. Suppression of the sinus mechanism permits the AV node to assume dominance, with an intrinsic rate of 40 to 50 beats per minute. Progressive loss of automaticity permits the ventricles to assume dominance with an intrinsic ventricular rate around 30 to 40 beats per minute.

From the AV node, the impulse is conducted to the ventricles to initiate contraction through a single right bundle branch and dual left anterior and posterior bundle branches. Activation of the normal conduction pathway results in atrial contraction during the period of ventricular diastole, augmenting filling of a quiescent ventricle. Ventricular systole then produces a propulsive force emptying the ventricular contents from the apex toward the outflow track, which is the most efficient and least energy expensive.

A variety of dysrhythmias may occur that impact ventricular performance and cardiac output. Changes in the normal rate of automaticity of pacemaker cells may displace the site of the dominant impulse. The dominant pacemaker site may yield tachyarrhythmias when automaticity is enhanced or bradyarrhythmias when normal automaticity is depressed. Tachycardia reduces the ventricular filling time, as the reduction in diastolic time interval is proportionately greater than the reduction in systolic time interval with increases in heart rate (Fig. 20–7). That reduction in the diastolic interval may produce a significant reduction in ventricular filling at varying heart rates, depending on the individual pathology.[6] Development of a nodal mechanism reduces ventricular filling and preload, as the atria contract

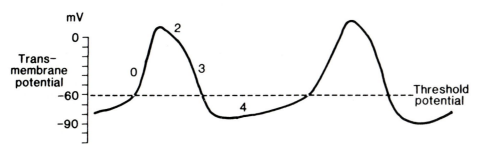

Figure 20–5. Action potential of pacemaker cells. (*Reprinted, with permission, from McIntyre KM, AJ Lewis, eds.* Textbook of advanced cardiac life support. *Dallas, TX: American Heart Association; 1983:60.*)

against a closed valve. Although "atrial kick" normally contributes only about 10 to 30 percent to the cardiac output[5,17] in the compromised ventricle atrial systole may account for 25 to 50 percent of cardiac output.[6,17] Thus, reductions in preload may produce significant reductions in stroke volume and cardiac output, particularly in the ischemic, failing, or hypertrophied ventricle. Bradyarrhythmias reduce cardiac output by rate alone if the sinus mechanism is maintained. With mild reductions in heart rate, increased ventricular filling time and increased preload may compensate by increasing stroke volume, maintaining a near-normal cardiac output. As the heart rate continues to decline, however, the effect of increased preload on stroke volume is maximized, and cardiac output begins to decline.

Ischemia also impairs ventricular function, and ischemic areas of the ventricle may demonstrate delayed depolarization or repolarization. When normal myocardium is repolarized and adjacent ischemic areas are still depolarized, an electrical gradient is established which increases the risk of developing ventricular arrhythmias. Alternately, loss of the normal conduction pathways may result in bundle branch blocks or aberrant conduction pathways. The development of aberrant pathways may increase the likelihood of developing reentry mechanisms.

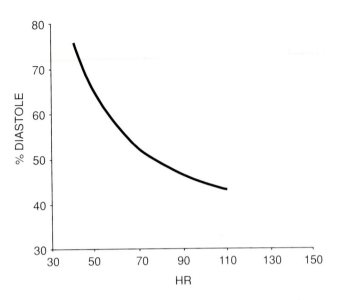

Figure 20–7. Relationship between heart rate (HR) and percentage diastole. Small changes in HR produce dramatic changes in the percentage diastole at slower HRs. (*Reprinted, with permission, from Kaplan, JA. Cardiovascular physiology. In: Miller RD, ed. Anesthesia. New York: Churchill Livingstone; 1986:1191. Adapted, with permission, from Boudoulas H, Rittgers SV, Lewis RP, et al: Changes in diastolic time with various pharmacologic agents.* Circulation *1979;60:164 and the American Heart Association, Inc.*)

CORONARY CIRCULATION

The coronary circulation is supplied by two coronary arteries which take off at the base of the aorta in the region of the sinuses of Valsalva. The distribution of circulation for both arteries is demonstrated in Table 20–3. It is useful to identify the site(s) of atherosclerotic coronary plaques as a clue to the potential effects of ischemia. Thus, lesions in the right coronary may be expected to produce more frequent right ventricular dysfunction and disturbances in normal conduction through its supply to the SA node. Lesions in the left coronary circulation may typically be expected to produce left ventricular dysfunction. Of equal importance is the presence and status of collateral flow from normal coronary arteries to regions distal to stenotic coronary arteries.

Normal coronary blood flow is 4 to 5 percent of the total cardiac output, which corresponds to about 225 cc/min or about 3.5 cc/kg/min in the adult.[1] Coronary flow is dependent on a variety of factors. At the level of origination of the left and right main coronary arteries in the sinuses of Valsalva, blood flows without impediment. Coronary blood flow at that level and through the larger vessels and their major epicardial branches is autoregulated between pressures of 60 and 140 torr.[18] At the level of the midsized intramyocardial coronary arteries, where coronary resistance is determined,[19] flow becomes dependent on a variety of factors. These may include driving force determined by systemic and chamber pressures, heart rate, coronary resistance, wall tension, and metabolic factors that mediate control of local flow.[19–21]

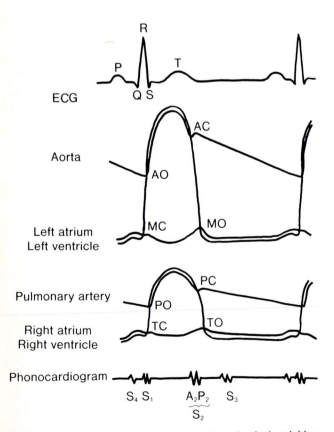

Figure 20–6. Correlation of electrical and mechanical activities of the heart. AO, aortic opening; AC, aortic closure; MO, mitral opening; MC, mitral closure; PO, pulmonic opening; PC, pulmonic closure; TO, tricuspid opening; TC, tricuspid closure. Events are demonstrated in their real time correlation. (*Reprinted, with permission, from Burnside JW. Physical diagnosis, 16th ed. Baltimore: Williams and Wilkins; 1981:154.*)

TABLE 20–3. NORMAL DISTRIBUTION OF CORONARY CIRCULATION

Area	Blood Supply
Sinus node	SA[a] nodal artery off proximal RCA (55%)[b] or circumflex (45%)
Atrioventricular node	AV nodal artery off distal RCA (90%) or distal circumflex (10%)
Right bundle branch	Septal branches of LAD and PDA
Left anterior bundle branch	Septal branches of LAD
Left posterior bundle branch	Septal branches of LAD
Left anterior papillary muscle	LAD
Left posterior papillary muscle	Distal positions of RCA and LCA
Intraventricular septum	
Anterior superior two thirds	Septal branches of LAD
Posterior inferior one third	PDA off RCA (or LCA)
Apical portion	Acute marginal branch off RCA
Left ventricle	
Anterior	LAD
Anterolateral	Anterolateral obtuse marginal off the circumflex
Posterolateral	Posterolateral obtuse marginal off the circumflex
Posterior	Posterolateral termination of circumflex
Inferior (basal)	PDA is most distal portion of RCA or circumflex artery
Apex	Most distal portion of LAD

[a] SA, sinoatrial node; RCA, right coronary artery; AV, arterioventricular node; LCA, left coronary artery; LAD, left anterior descending artery; PDA, posterior descending artery.
[b] Percentage of patients.
Reprinted, with permission, from Hug CC, Anesthesia for cardiac surgery. In: Miller RD, ed. Anesthesia, 2nd ed. New York: Churchill Livingstone; 1986.

Driving Force

The driving force for coronary flow is determined by the difference between the systemic pressure and the pressure in the chamber. The formula used for calculating the driving pressure for coronary flow, or coronary perfusion pressure (CPP), is

$$CPP = DBP - LVEDP$$

where DBP is the systemic diastolic blood pressure, and LVEDP is the left ventricular end-diastolic pressure estimated using the wedge pressure or CVP. In the normal heart, this gradient is about 50 to 60 torr. In patients with coronary atherosclerosis, it is recommended that the gradient be maintained at or above 60 torr.

The left ventricle generates high peak chamber pressures, which exceed diastolic blood pressure during systole, and flow may actually be retrograde.[20] Thus about 70 percent of coronary flow to the left ventricle occurs during diastole.[22] The right ventricle generates lower chamber pres-

sures, and flow is not demonstrably affected by ventricular systole.[20] Therefore right ventricular perfusion is probably maintained throughout the cardiac cycle in the normal patient.

Heart Rate

Heart rate is a critical factor in the maintenance of coronary flow. Increases in heart rate produce a direct increase in the metabolic demand and oxygen requirements, as well as decrease the diastolic time interval during which myocardial perfusion is maintained. The relationship between heart rate and the relative percentage of time spent in diastole is demonstrated in Figure 20–7. As increases in heart rate are affected primarily by reduction in the diastolic time interval, increases in heart rate produce disproportionate decreases in the diastolic perfusion interval of the left ventricle.

Coronary Resistance

Coronary resistance is determined primarily by the mid-sized arteries.[4] This proves important, as the majority of the branches in the left coronary circulation are proximal and the majority of branches in the right coronary circulation are distal. Similarly, lesions in the left coronary circulation are more frequently proximal, and those in the right coronary circulation are more frequently distal.

Metabolic Factors

Metabolic factors control flow in the coronary microcirculation. The primary determinants appear to be local factors, including oxygen tension and levels of metabolic by-products, particularly adenosine.[20,23] Increases in metabolic by-products such as adenosine in response to cellular hypoxia cause coronary dilation and increase local flow. These systems operate jointly to maintain a homeostatic mechanism that adjusts the microcirculation of coronary flow in the normal heart to meet immediate requirements. The normal myocardial oxygen demand extracts approximately 65 percent of the oxygen in the oxyhemoglobin complex. As the last 25 percent of oxygen in the complex is released only at the point of cell membrane dysfunction or disintegration, there is very little oxygen reserve in the normal coronary flow. Requirements for increased oxygen can be met only by increasing flow to that region.

Wall Tension

Wall tension alters coronary flow patterns. Increases in wall tension during systole and during the early relaxation phase of diastole retard flow mechanically. Wall tension is determined by three factors: pressure, diameter of the chamber, and wall thickness. The formula for estimating wall tension incorporates the pressure and diameter of the chamber divided by wall thickness. Therefore, ventricular hypertension and dilation produce an increase in wall tension, whereas ventricular hypertrophy operates as a compensatory mechanism to reduce wall tension while permitting an increase in contractile force.

CARDIOVASCULAR DISEASES AND CLINICAL MANAGEMENT

Application of the principles governing cardiac output, systemic pressure, and coronary flow should determine the management of patients with various disease states. A variety of disorders impair ventricular performance and alter the myocardial oxygen supply–demand balance. The outcome is development of myocardial ischemia with progressive ventricular dysfunction. In the extreme, this translates to myocardial infarction. Although a variety of mechanisms may produce myocardial ischemia, it can be divided conceptually into three basic forms whose characteristics determine anesthetic management. These conceptual forms follow patterns of coronary or valvular disease, and the models can be applied only to discrete pathology. Complex pathologies involving more than one mechanism require more sophisticated management based on the nature of the predominant lesion and integration of their physiologic characteristics.

The three conceptual forms of myocardial ischemia include ischemia of occlusive disease, ischemia of hypertrophy, and ischemia of failure. Each of these has a distinct pattern and physiologic characteristics that determine the cause of ischemia and the choice of management. These characteristics of distribution and management goals are summarized as follows.

Ischemia of Occlusive Disease

Ischemia of occlusive disease is found in two forms: fixed occlusive disease as found in coronary atherosclerosis, and nonfixed occlusive disease as seen in coronary spasm or Prinzmetal's variant angina. Although their characteristics are similar, the method of treatment is different. Both forms of occlusive ischemia are episodic in nature and regional in distribution and rapidly advance to transmural distribution.

Basic Physiology. First, ischemia of occlusive disease is episodic. It generally develops in response to stresses or increases in demand that cannot be met by increased flow across a vessel stenosed by atherosclerotic plaque or coronary spasm. Increased myocardial oxygen demand outstrips the ability of the coronary arteries to increase supply, at which point ischemia develops.

Second, the distribution of ischemia with occlusive disease is regional, affecting only that portion of the myocardium supplied by the stenotic vessel. In fixed atherosclerotic disease, the lesions remain static and determine the area(s) in which ischemia develops; the only means of correcting regional hypoperfusion is reduction in demand or correction of the stenosis through development of collateral flow, angioplasty, or bypass. In nonfixed spasm, ischemia follows the distribution of the vessel affected, which may vary between episodes; further, the spasm may be reversed with appropriate pharmacologic therapy. In both types of occlusive disease, the ischemia affects a discrete region rather than having a global ventricular distribution.

Finally, ischemia of occlusive disease rapidly progresses to a transmural distribution, which underscores the necessity for rapid intervention to prevent infarction. It has been estimated historically that 50 percent of those patients who suffer myocardial ischemia die within the first 2 hours unless appropriate management and therapy are instituted.[24,25]

Clinical Management. Because of the characteristics of occlusive ischemic disease, the ventricle is comparatively normal when not stressed. The goal of management in both forms of occlusive ischemia is to prevent increases in demand that exceed the limits the coronary circulation can meet by increasing flow. In the management of coronary spasm, this is achieved by the use of calcium channel blockers. Management of fixed occlusive disease is more complex. The first step is to maintain the determinants of coronary flow. Thus, cardiac output must be maintained, systemic diastolic blood pressure should be maintained, LVEDP should be maintained or decreased, and increases in heart rate and wall tension should be avoided. These can be achieved by establishing deep anesthesia prior to any stimulus and by using drugs that produce mild degrees of myocardial depression.

To achieve these goals, treatment usually includes the maintenance of cardiac output with volume and vasodilation. As these two treatments provide a less energy-expensive increase in cardiac output than increases in rate, the use of additional volume and dilators such as nitroglycerin is generally recommended. The use of drugs that provide mild vasodilation and only mild myocardial depression, such as benzodiazepines, narcotics, and low-dose volatile agents, is appropriate. An additional aim is to block the stress response to intubation, skin incision, and sternotomy. Agents such as narcotics which block the autonomic response to nociceptive impulses are again suitable for that purpose. For patients with good ventricular function, short-acting agents such as lidocaine or thiopental may also be useful for blocking brief periods of stress such as intubation. This permits the suppression of autonomic responses without prolonged ventricular depression during subsequent periods of low stress such as prepping and draping.

The most common management of patients with ischemia of occlusive disease is the use of synthetic narcotics with minimal myocardial depressant effects such as fentanyl and sufentanil, benzodiazepines such as midazolam (Versed), and muscle relaxants that produce minimal increases in heart rate and vasodilation such as vecuronium (Norcuron). Agents that produce profound arterial dilation through histamine release or ganglionic blockade (such as morphine and the curariform relaxants), myocardial depression (such as Demerol), or significant increases in heart rate (such as pancuronium when administered rapidly) find less application.

Ischemia of Hypertrophy

The prototype for ischemia of hypertrophy is the patient with aortic stenosis or outflow obstruction such as IHSS, long-standing hypertension and subsequent left ventricular hypertrophy, or aortic occlusive diseases with increased resistance which imposes additional left ventricular workload. Ischemia of hypertrophy is generally chronic, global, and subendocardial.

Basic Physiology. First, the ischemia of hypertrophy is chronic. Increases in ventricular mass require additional myocardial blood flow to meet oxygen and metabolic substrate requirements. That escalated demand outstrips the ability of the coronary arteries to compensate by increasing flow, and supply becomes essentially fixed at its upper limit. With the high myocardial oxygen extraction ratio, this leads to a chronic state of mild myocardial ischemia early in the course of the disease.

Second, ischemia follows a global pattern. The reduction in myocardial flow is not limited to discrete areas of the ventricle determined by the presence of stenotic lesions. The entire ventricle develops progressive ischemia. Worsening of ischemia rapidly becomes life-threatening and necessitates aggressive measures to prevent its development or progression.

Third, the ischemia is subendocardial. As a result of the increase in ventricular mass, and the frequent accompaniment of hypertension and ventricular dilation, subendocardial coronary flow is reduced early in the course of the disease. Additionally, the requirement for increased filling pressure to dilate the hypertrophied ventricle translates to an increase in LVEDP, which reduces the driving force for coronary flow. Hence, both the increase in wall tension and the increase in filling pressure may reduce the efficacy of subendocardial coronary perfusion.

Clinical Management. Because of the chronic nature of the disease, the ventricle is not normal in the resting state. The demand limb of the normal supply–demand relationship chronically exceeds supply. Instead of acute development of ischemia de novo in response to increased demand, preexisting ischemia worsens with increased demand. Coronary supply can be viewed as being fixed, and aggravation of the underlying ischemia is dependent on increases in demand.

Management of hypertrophic ischemia requires that coronary flow, already by definition insufficient to meet myocardial oxygen demand, be maintained scrupulously. Consequently, filling pressures must be maintained to dilate a noncompliant, hypertrophied ventricle to maintain cardiac output. As LVEDP cannot be reduced without loss of cardiac output, systemic diastolic blood pressure becomes the critical determinant in the maintenance of coronary perfusion pressure gradient. Slowing the heart rate increases the diastolic perfusion and ventricular filling time which may be beneficial, unless the stroke volume is fixed, as occurs in critical aortic stenosis or massive concentric hypertrophy with reduced chamber size. In that case, fixed stroke volume makes heart rate a primary determinant of cardiac output, and reductions in rate may reduce cardiac output. Oxygen demand may be reduced by myocardial depressants if the ventricle is not failing. The use of agents that suppress ventricular contractility may permit reductions in inotropic state without deleterious effects on the cardiac output.

To achieve these goals, the anesthetic effect should include minimal reductions in the systemic vascular resistance to maintain coronary perfusion pressure. Volume must be maintained to compensate for venodilation and venous pooling. Agents that block sympathetic activity or produce mild reductions in heart rate are appropriate if the ventricle is not failing or stroke volume is not fixed. Hence, synthetic narcotics are encouraged for their minimal reductions in SVR and induction of a mild increase in vagal tone. Volatile agents should be chosen on the basis of their myocardial depressant effect, which makes enflurane (Ethrane) popular because of its ability to reduce contractility. The use of vasoconstrictors may be appropriate to maintain SVR in the event of vasodilation and to support coronary perfusion pressure. Drugs that suppress contractility and block stress responses are useful, so lidocaine and thiopental may be employed. Beta blockers are frequently employed even during the preinduction or early induction period to reduce inotropic surges. Drugs that produce increases in heart rate or vasodilation are discouraged, so that vecuronium (Norcuron) is often preferred over pancuronium (Pavulon) or the curariform muscle relaxants. When high doses of narcotics are planned, however, pancuronium may offset the vagal tone, which would otherwise reduce heart rate in the patient with limited stroke volume.

Ischemia of Failure

The prototype for ischemia of failure is the patient with primary cardiomyopathy. The characteristics of ischemia of failure are similar in many respects to those of ischemia of hypertrophy. Ischemia of failure is chronic, global, and subendocardial; however, the causes differ. In the patient with failure, increased ventricular mass is not the primary cause for supply–demand imbalance. Ischemia of failure occurs because of chamber dilation, high LVEDP and a chronic reduction in cardiac output.

Basic Physiology. First, ischemia of failure is chronic. By definition the ventricle in failure yields a decreased cardiac output, the primary determinant of coronary flow. Chronic ventricular dysfunction also reduces left ventricular emptying, yielding an elevation in LVEDP which reduces the gradient for coronary flow. Chamber dilation, which accompanies ventricular failure, produces an increase in the wall tension generated during systole. Hence, flow across the coronary bed is limited in the resting state.

Second, as the determinants of coronary flow are not regionally affected, the ischemia of failure is global, a clinical condition requiring aggressive management. Because the entire ventricle is ischemic, management must be directed to reducing ischemia based on improvement of the myocardial oxygen supply–demand balance, rather than preventing acute ischemia in response to disturbances in the balance.

Third, ischemia of failure is subendocardial. The chronically high LVEDP, increased wall tension, and low cardiac output combine to make ischemia greater on the subendocardial surface. As subendocardial ischemia is not readily demonstrable by standard ECG analysis and the changes are chronic, ischemia may worsen without the development of new or additional clinical signs.

Clinical Management. The ventricle with ischemia of failure is not normal in the resting state. Ischemia of failure develops primarily from the limited coronary flow generated rather than from increased ventricular mass or oxygen demand. The requirement for increased cardiac output and flow across the coronary vasculature directs management. The goal is to actively increase cardiac output while improving the dynamics of coronary flow.

Management of ischemia of failure requires that systemic diastolic pressure be maintained, LVEDP be reduced, and cardiac output be increased to improve coronary flow. This can often be achieved by the use of mild arterial dilators which reduce afterload, improve ventricular emptying, and reduce LVEDP. The improvement in cardiac output often outweighs the effect of reduced systemic resistance and maintains systemic diastolic blood pressure, which further improves the gradient for flow across the coronary arteries. When dilation alone is insufficient to improve cardiac performance and coronary flow, it may be necessary to employ inotropic agents. Although maintenance of systemic diastolic pressure is indicated for improvement of coronary flow, vasoconstrictors may increase afterload and worsen the degree of failure. For that reason, the use of inotropic agents to maintain systemic pressure is preferred.

To achieve these goals, agents should be chosen on the basis of minimal myocardial depression, and mild vasodilation is encouraged. Volatile agents may be used in low doses, with particular attention to their depressant effects. Increases in the heart rate within the physiologic range are permissible. Because by definition volume is already excessive, vasodilation is required to unload the left ventricle, and increasing heart rate may permit an increase in forward flow which will result in reduced ventricular end-diastolic volume. For that reason, isoflurane (Forane) is frequently employed because of its systemic vasodilation and minimal myocardial depression. Drugs that depress ventricular function, such as thiopental and lidocaine, should be used with caution, and drugs such as etomidate, which may possess less myocardial depressant effect, are generally encouraged. Muscle relaxants that provide mild dilation or mild increases in heart rate such as the curariform relaxants are acceptable and may be employed when heart rate remains within the physiologic range.

HEMODYNAMIC MONITORING

A critical consideration in the management of patients with cardiovascular dysfunction is the use of hemodynamic monitoring. Both invasive and noninvasive monitoring is employed in the management of patients with cardiovascular disease. Routine noninvasive monitoring with continuous ECG, pulse oximetry, and auscultatory or oscillometric blood pressure cuff forms the basis for most physiologic monitoring in the otherwise healthy patient. In the patient with compromising cardiovascular disease, that basic monitoring may be supplemented with the use of invasive monitors.

Three forms of invasive vascular monitoring are employed in patients with cardiovascular dysfunction: arterial pressure monitoring, central venous pressure monitoring, and pulmonary artery pressure monitoring. In addition to directly monitoring pressures, temperature, and oxygen saturation, invasive monitoring permits the calculation of a range of parameters that can be derived only from invasive monitors such as the Swan-Ganz catheter. These include

cardiac output, systemic and pulmonary vascular resistances, and ventricular stroke work indices. All of these are covered in greater detail in the chapter on monitoring (see Chapter 12).

Arterial Monitoring

Monitoring arterial pressure with an indwelling catheter is indicated for a variety of reasons. Several of these are offered in Table 20–4. In summary, these center on surgical or anesthetic management which would be expected to affect the accuracy of routine noninvasive monitoring. As such, these would include expected wide changes in systemic pressure such as planned systemic hypotension, the need for immediate and continuous pressure assessment as required during cross-clamping of the aorta or major vessels, induction of abnormal physiologic states such as deliberate hypothermia or cardiopulmonary bypass, or the use of circulatory assist devices such as the counterpulsation aortic balloon or the atrial-to-arterial bypass with a circulatory assist device such as the Biomedicus flow device. Additionally, arterial monitoring may be indicated in the patient with severe systemic hypertension; in the patient whose surgical procedure or anesthetic management may require frequent analysis of arterial blood gases, elec-

---

TABLE 20–4. INDICATIONS FOR ARTERIAL CANNULATION

Direct measurement of arterial pressure
  Cardiac surgery, especially with cardiopulmonary bypass
  Deliberate hypothermia
  Deliberate hypotension
  Intracranial operations
  Major vascular surgery—aorta, carotid, iliac, femoral arteries, vena cava
  Extensive surgery with prospect of sudden blood loss or marked shifts of body fluids
  Extensive trauma, especially with uncontrolled hemorrhage
  Thoracic or abdominal surgery with compression of the great vessels
  Noncardiac surgery in patients with significant cardiovascular disease and hemodynamic instability
  Cardiopulmonary resuscitation
  Inability to measure blood pressure indirectly (obesity, burns of the extremities)
Arterial blood sampling (repetitive)
  Blood gas analysis
    Pulmonary disease
    Lung surgery (one-lung ventilation)
    Airway surgery (apneic oxygenation)
    Major surgery (neural, cardiac, vascular, thoracic, abdominal)
  Severe metabolic derangements
    Acid–base evaluation
    Electrolyte determinations
    Glucose analysis
    Serum osmolarity measurement
  Heparin anticoagulation and protamine antagonism
    Cardiopulmonary bypass
    Arterial shunts (Gott shunt)

Reprinted, with permission, from Hug CC. Monitoring. In: Miller RD, ed. Anesthesia. *2nd ed. New York: Churchill Livingstone: 1986:436, Table 13–14.*

trolytes, or hemoglobin concentration; or in the patient with predictable large blood losses.

Arterial catheters are typically placed in peripheral arteries, generally the radial artery at the wrist. Central arterial catheters such as femoral or axillary arterial lines may be employed when peripheral arteries are unavailable or unsuitable for cannulation or when aortic pressures are required. The latter may be appropriate when the patient is subject to extremes of temperature, such as deliberate hypothermia with cardiopulmonary bypass or deliberate hyperthermia. Augmentation of core aortic pressures by the propagation of arterial wall forces may produce elevations of peripheral systolic pressure, whereas constriction of arteries may produce reductions in flow distal to that site. Intense vasoconstriction may occur in early stages of hypothermia. Likewise, patients with occlusive vascular disease may demonstrate reductions in systemic pressure when arteries distal to the site of the obstruction are cannulated. Profound vasodilation may produce blunting of the systolic upstroke and reduction in diastolic pressure, producing erroneously low pressures distally. Profound vasodilation may occur when rewarming the deliberately cooled patient on cardiopulmonary bypass. Additionally, differences in the pressures may be seen between left and right arms either with stenotic lesions, such as coarctation of the aorta, or as a result of aortic arch aneurysms.

Finally, monitoring of systemic arterial pressure may be indicated when regional blood flow is deliberately interrupted, and supply is provided by left atrial-to-peripheral artery bypass using a Biomedicus assist device. This requirement is seen in major aortic reconstruction such as thoracoabdominal aortic resections. In those cases, the lower extremities and kidneys may be perfused by left atriofemoral bypass, and it is recommended that lower-extremity pressures be measured to assess the adequacy of perfusion pressure in the lower extremities during the period of aortic cross-clamping.

Central Venous Monitoring

Monitoring of the central venous pressure may be indicated for a variety of reasons, as indicated in Table 20–5. In the patient with an otherwise normal heart, monitoring of central venous pressure may be sufficient for estimation of ventricular preload and provides an estimate of adequate hemodynamic function when used in conjunction with the systemic blood pressure and nonvascular indices of hemodynamic function such as urine output. For cases involving expected volume shifts from surgical edema formation, deliberate diuresis, or deliberate hemodilution, monitoring the central venous pressure may be suitable and appropriate. Typical examples of the aforementioned reasons include the planned diuresis in many neurosurgical procedures, expected major blood losses as seen in selected orthopedic procedures, and cases in which blood loss cannot be accurately assessed by usual means such as transurethral resections of the prostate.

Additionally, monitoring of the central venous pressure may be indicated in the aggressive management of patients with right ventricular dysfunction or pulmonary hypertension, as a part of the value in using a Swan-Ganz

TABLE 20–5. INDICATIONS FOR PLACEMENT OF CENTRAL VENOUS CATHETER

Central venous pressure monitoring (see text)

Lack of peripheral veins for cannulation

Intravenous administration of vasopressors, potassium, and other drugs likely to injure peripheral veins and tissues; also to reduce the delay in onset of drug action

Rapid infusion of blood and fluids

Removal of blood for later reinfusion (autologous transfusion)

Frequent unmixed venous blood sampling

Aspiration of air emboli

Hyperalimentation

Transvenous insertion of temporary pacing leads

Right-sided heart catheterization studies

Insertion of a pulmonary artery catheter (Swan-Ganz)
    Pressure measurements
    Cardiac output determinations by thermodilution
    Pulmonary angiography
    Mixed venous blood sampling

Reprinted, with permission, from Hug CC. Monitoring. In: Miller RD, ed. Anesthesia. 2nd ed. New York: Churchill Livingstone; 1986:439, Table 13–15.

catheter. Although pulmonary artery pressure and wedge pressure provide valuable information regarding pulmonary vascular resistance and left ventricular preload, measurement of CVP provides an index of right ventricular filling pressure and permits a more accurate and complete assessment of biventricular cardiac function. In patients with chronic pulmonary hypertension, maintenance of right ventricular function may be the overriding concern, making right ventricular monitoring critical in case management. It should be noted that in the patient with right ventricular dysfunction, monitoring of central venous pressure is generally considered a component of the assessment of ventricular function with a Swan-Ganz catheter, rather than a singular monitor which presumes otherwise normal biventricular function.

Pulmonary Artery Monitoring

Pulmonary artery monitoring is indicated in patients with acute or chronic ventricular dysfunction and those undergoing procedures incorporating cardiopulmonary bypass and the use of cardioplegic solutions. In addition, it is indicated in those surgical procedures that would be expected to produce significant changes in left ventricular workload, such as aortic cross-clamping when occlusive disease is not a preexisting condition. In patients with aortic occlusive disease or stenosis such as Leriche's syndrome or coarctation of the aorta, the development of large collateral vessels about the site of obstruction may attenuate the increase in afterload with aortic clamping, making it possible to manage the case with only CVP monitoring if the ventricle is otherwise normal. Indications for the use of a Swan-Ganz catheter are listed in Table 20–6.

The information gained by the use of a pulmonary artery catheter is far greater than that provided by a CVP, as one can still measure central venous pressure, as well as

TABLE 20–6. INDICATIONS FOR PLACEMENT OF A PULMONARY ARTERY CATHETER

Noncardiac surgery
  Heart disease
    With suspicion or evidence of impaired left ventricular
      function (e.g., heart failure)
    Severe coronary artery disease, especially with evidence
      of left ventricular dysfunction on exertion or with an-
      gina pectoris
    Severe, uncontrolled systemic arterial hypertension, espe-
      cially with left ventricular hypertrophy
    Pulmonary hypertension (cor pulmonale)
    Valvular disease
    Pericardial disease with evidence of tamponade
  Unstable circulation
    Massive trauma
    Extensive burns
    Hypotensive shock
    Sepsis
  Suspected or diagnosed pulmonary emboli
  Aortic surgery with anticipation of crossclamping
  Portal systemic shunt surgery; severe portal hypertension
    with cirrhosis
  Severe respiratory failure
Cardiac surgery
  Coronary artery revascularization with
    Poor, left ventricular function: ejection fraction < 0.4,
      LVEDP[a] > 18 mm Hg, regional hypokinesis, dyssynergy,
      or asynergy
    Recent myocardial infarction
    Complication of myocardial infarction (e.g., ventricular
      aneurysm, septal rupture, mitral valvular insufficiency,
      papillary muscle dysfunction)
    Extensive coronary obstruction (e.g., triple-vessel disease)
      with evidence of impaired ventricular performance dur-
      ing ischemia (e.g., LVEDP increases by more than 10
      mm Hg or is greater than 18 mm Hg after injection of
      contrast medium into coronary arteries)
    Diffuse coronary atherosclerosis especially in distal ves-
      sels (anticipate impaired ventricular function after car-
      diopulmonary bypass due to poor myocardial preserva-
      tion by cold hyperkalemic perfusion of coronary arteries
      and incomplete revascularization)
    Valvular heart disease
  Mitral or aortic valvular replacement
  Pulmonary hypertension
  Hypertrophic obstructive cardiomyopathy, e.g., idiopathic
    hypertrophic subaortic stenosis (IHSS)
  Pericardiectomy with evidence of tamponade

[a] LVEDP, left ventricular end-diastolic pressure.
Reprinted, with permission, from Hug CC. Monitoring. In: Miller RD, ed.
Anesthesia. *2nd ed. New York: Churchill Livingstone; 1986:445, Table 13–18.*

pulmonary artery pressure, wedge pressure, and cardiac output, with the thermodilution Swan-Ganz catheter. The normal chamber and vascular pressures obtained by monitoring with a Swan-Ganz are given in Chapter 12. Additionally, mixed venous blood gases may be drawn from the distal tip and recent technology incorporates the capacity to measure mixed venous oxygen saturation directly. By use of the information gained from both the Swan-Ganz catheter and the arterial line, vascular resis-

tances may be calculated. Integration of further data derived from these calculations permits the derivation of indices of ventricular stroke work as well. Those calculations and their normal values are also given in Chapter 12. These permit the clinician to manage the patient with compromised cardiovascular function with greater sophistication and more precision.

REFERENCES

1. Kaplan JA. Cardiovascular physiology. In: Miller RD, ed. *Anesthesia.* New York: Churchill Livingstone; 1986.
2. Kaplan JA, ed. *Cardiac anesthesia.* New York: Grune & Stratton; 1979.
3. VandenBelt RJ, Ronan JA, et al. Cardiology: A clinical approach. Chicago: Yearbook Medical; 1979.
4. DiNardo JA. Interpreting cardiac catheterization data. In: DiNardo JA, Schwartz MJ, eds. *Anesthesia for cardiac surgery.* Norwalk, CT: Appleton & Lange; 1990.
5. DiNardo JA. Anesthesia for valve replacement in patients with acquired valvular heart disease. In: DiNardo JA, Schwartz MJ, eds. *Anesthesia for cardiac surgery.* Norwalk, CT: Appleton & Lange; 1990.
6. DiNardo JA, Schwartz MJ, eds. *Anesthesia for cardiac surgery.* Norwalk, CT: Appleton & Lange; 1990.
7. McLaurin LP, Rolet EL, Grossman W. Impaired left ventricular relaxation during pacing-induced ischemia. *Am J Cardiol.* 1973; 32:751–757.
8. Grossman W, Mann JT. Evidence for impaired left ventricular relaxation during acute ischemia in man. *Eur J Cardiol.* 1978;7:239–249.
9. Aroesty JM, McKay RG, Heller GV, et al. Simultaneous assessment of left ventricular systolic and diastolic dysfunction during pacing-induced ischemia. *Circulation.* 1983;5:889–900.
10. Kaplan JA, Wells PH. Early diagnosis of myocardial ischemia using the pulmonary artery catheter. *Anesth Analg.* 1981;60: 789–793.
11. Clements F, deBruijn NP. Perioperative evaluation of regional wall motion by transesophageal two dimensional echocardiography. *Anesth Analg.* 1987;66:249–261.
12. Rahimtoola SH. Left ventricular end-diastolic and filling pressure in assessment of ventricular function. *Chest.* 1973;63: 858–860.
13. Forsberg SH. Relationship between the pressures in the pulmonary artery, left atrium and left ventricle with special reference to the events at end diastole. *Br Heart J.* 1971;33:494–499.
14. Sasayama S, Nonogi H, Miyazake S, et al. Changes in diastolic properties of the regional myocardium during pacing-induced ischemia in human subjects. *J Am Coll Cardiol.* 1985;5:599–606.
15. Ross J. Afterload mismatch in aortic and mitral valve disease: Implications for surgical therapy. *J Am Cardiol.* 1985;4:811–826.
16. Merin RG. Pharmacology of the autonomic nervous system. In: Miller RD, ed. *Anesthesia.* New York: Churchill Livingstone; 1986.
17. Viets JL, Martin PD, Heaton DA, Biddle C. *AANA Journal* course: Advanced scientific concepts: Update for nurse anesthetists. Part I: The cardiovascular system. *AANA J.* 1987;55: 165–177.
18. Hoffman JIE. Determinants and prediction of transmural perfusion. *Circulation.* 1978;58:381.
19. Braunwald E. *A textbook of cardiovascular medicine.* 3rd ed. Philadelphia: WB Saunders; 1988.
20. Berne RM, Levy MN. Coronary circulation and cardiac metabolism. In: Berne RM, Levy MN, eds. *Cardiovascular physiology.* 4th ed. St. Louis, MO: CV Mosby; 1981.
21. Barash PG. *Clinical anesthesia.* Philadelphia: JB Lippincott; 1989.

22. Braunwald E. Control of myocardial oxygen consumption: Physiologic and clinical considerations. *Am J Cardiol.* 1971;27: 416.

23. Rubio R, Berne RM. Release of adenosine by the normal myocardium in dogs and its relationship to regulation of coronary resistance. *Circ Res.* 1969;25:407.

24. Kuller LH. Sudden death—Definition and epidemiologic considerations. *Proc Cardiovasc Disc.* 1980;23:1–12.

25. Gordon T, Kennel WB. Premature mortality from coronary heart disease: The Framingham Study. *JAMA.* 1971;215: 1617–1625.

21

Respiratory Physiology

Susan A. Ward

Homeostasis of arterial oxygen (O_2), carbon dioxide (CO_2), and acidity (pH) in the face of varying metabolic demands is maintained by a matching of the cellular consumption of O_2 and the production of CO_2 and hydrogen ions (H^+) to their whole-body exchange rates. In human beings, the lungs represent the major site at which whole-body O_2 and CO_2 exchange occurs. The elimination of metabolically produced hydrogen ions is subserved chronically by the renal system, although ventilatory compensation can elicit at least a partial correction of blood pH under more acute conditions.

The efficiency of these humoral homeostatic functions demands a respiratory-mechanical system that can generate the necessary forces for airflow generation and lung volume expansion, to accomplish an overall level of pulmonary ventilation appropriate for current humoral requirements. This requires, in turn, mechanisms to facilitate the exchange of O_2 and CO_2 between alveolar gas and pulmonary capillary blood and also to accomplish effective transport of these gases between the lungs and the peripheral tissues. Finally, control mechanisms are required to provide appropriate ventilatory responses to disturbances in the O_2, CO_2, and acidity levels of arterial blood and cerebral fluids.

MECHANICS OF VENTILATION

The respiratory tract comprises (1) the upper airway, which includes the nose, mouth, pharynx, and larynx; (2) the tracheobronchial tree, a dichotomously branching system of conducting airways through which respired air can be transported between the atmosphere and gas-exchanging regions; and (3) the acini, the major elements of which are the alveoli whose specialized structure allows local exchange of O_2 and CO_2 between gas and blood.

Air enters the respiratory tract through the upper airway (see Chapter 15 for further discussion) to pass to the tracheobronchial tree by way of the trachea. The trachea (generation 0), with a mean diameter of approximately 2 cm

and a length of about 11 cm in a normal, healthy adult, is supported by a series of transversely arranged, U-shaped cartilage "rings" whose posterior ends are linked by smooth muscle bands. The trachea bifurcates into the right and left major bronchi (generation 1), which branch successively into the lobar bronchi (generation 2) and then into the segmental bronchi (generations 3 and 4). Like the trachea, these branches are also supported by cartilage, although the U-shaped structure is progressively replaced by plates of cartilage (often irregularly arranged) contained within helically arranged bands of smooth muscle. Beyond the level of the segmental bronchi a series of small bronchi (generations 5 to 11) develop. These structures evidence progressively smaller caliber, but still receive structural support from cartilage. Further branching gives rise to smaller, unsupported airways called bronchioles (generations 12 to 16) that do, however, contain strong helical bands of smooth muscle. These small, peripheral airways are susceptible to collapse when the surrounding intrathoracic pressure exceeds the pressure inside them.

Subsequent branchings give rise to regions of the respiratory tract that become increasingly important for gas exchange. The next few generations represent the respiratory bronchioles (generations 17 to 19) which lead in turn to the alveolar ducts (generations 20 to 22), blind-ending alveolar sacs (generation 23), and finally the alveoli themselves. Some 200 to 600 million alveoli result from the progressive branching of the respiratory tract. The structures that arise from a single respiratory bronchiole are collectively referred to as an *acinus*, which represents the functional gas-exchanging unit of the respiratory tract. Gas exchange occurs by diffusion across the alveolar wall, termed the *alveolar–capillary membrane*. This is a thin structure (only about 1 µm) and, owing to the large number of alveoli, its overall area is large (some 80 m^2). These features allow for rapid exchange of respiratory and anesthetic gases.

Ventilation, the process whereby air is transported between the atmosphere and the alveoli, requires the lungs to alternately inflate (inspiration) and deflate (expiration). For inspiration to occur, it is necessary that an expanding force be generated, normally by the muscles of inspiration (primarily the diaphragm), to overcome the natural tendency for the lungs to recoil. This recoil force leads in turn to lung emptying during the subsequent expiration; when necessary, the emptying process can be speeded by activation of the expiratory muscles.

Lung Recoil Forces

The lungs have an intrinsic tendency to recoil down to a very small volume (i.e., essentially zero) at which the lung recoil force becomes zero; this volume is known as the *lung relaxation volume*. The magnitude of the lung recoil force becomes progressively greater as the lungs are inflated to higher volumes. This behavior reflects the elastic character of the lungs. The alveolar walls contain connective tissue and blood vessels which, because they contain elastin and collagen fibers, function as elastic structures. The magnitude of this tissue recoil can be significantly influenced by pulmonary diseases that affect the structure of the lungs. In *emphysema*, for example, degradation of the alveolar infrastructure results in a reduction of the fibrous tissue content, such that the tissue recoil at a given lung volume is less. Therefore, the lungs are easier to expand, and recoil more slowly. In contrast, *pulmonary fibrosis* is associated with an increased lung recoil, owing to the pathologic aggregation of fibrous tissue in the lungs; as a result, the lungs not only require a greater force for expansion, but they also recoil more forcefully.

A second important influence on lung recoil derives from surface tension forces acting at the interface between the inner surface of the alveoli, which is covered with a thin layer of liquid, and the air contained within them. Strong cohesive forces exist between molecules in the liquid phase that are essentially unopposed from the gas phase. This imbalance of forces leads to a retraction of the gas–liquid interface; the retracting force represents the surface tension force. Consequently, the alveolar volume is reduced which, in turn, compresses the gas contained within the alveoli and therefore increases the intraalveolar pressure.

The degree to which the alveoli are reduced in size and the alveolar pressure (P_{ALV}) is increased depends on the magnitude of the surface tension force (T), in accordance with Laplace's law:

$$P_{ALV} = \frac{2 \times T}{r}$$

where r is the alveolar radius. Thus, for a given surface tension force, small alveoli (with small radii) will have higher pressures than will larger alveoli. This implies that small units would tend to empty into larger units and, in the process, collapse. In reality, however, alveoli of different size are stabilized by the presence of (1) a structural fibrous "framework" within the lungs and (2) surfactant molecules at the alveolar gas–liquid interface.

The *surfactant molecule,* a lipoprotein that contains the phospholipid dipalmitoyl lecithin, is produced by specialized type II cells in the alveolar wall and secreted onto the alveolar surface. Surfactant molecules decrease the magnitude of the surface tension forces and, therefore, reduce the lung recoil. As a result, the lungs are easier to inflate than would be the case were the surface tension forces operating unopposed. Furthermore, the surface tension-reducing property of surfactant is greater at smaller alveolar volumes, as the smaller surface area causes the surfactant molecules to become relatively concentrated and therefore to exert a relatively greater effect on local surface tension forces. And as the surface tension force is reduced progressively as alveolar volume decreases, size-related variations in alveolar pressure that would occur in the absence of surfactant (see above) are effectively abolished, removing the tendency for small alveoli to empty into larger alveoli.

The absence of surfactant has important implications for lung expansion. For example, synthesis of surfactant normally starts at about the 30th week of gestation. With premature birth, lung inflation may therefore be difficult to accomplish because of abnormally high lung recoil. And as alveolar volumes are reduced in this condition, regional foci of alveolar collapse are not uncommon. This condition is known as *neonatal respiratory distress syndrome*. Similar problems are encountered in *adult respiratory distress syndrome* (ARDS). ARDS, which is the eventual outcome of a wide range of insults that include shock, septicemia, and trauma, is characterized by interstitial and alveolar edema. This, in turn, is thought to dislodge surfactant molecules from the alveolar surface and thus to increase surface tension forces at the gas–liquid interface. As a result, the lungs are difficult to inflate. Finally, although there is some evidence to suggest that anesthesia may exert a direct effect on surfactant function, such that its ability to lower surface tension forces is compromised, there is no general consensus on this issue.

Chest Wall Recoil Forces

The chest wall resembles the lungs in behaving as an elastic structure. In contrast, however, the chest wall has an intrinsic tendency to recoil outward in the normal resting volume range. This reflects the three-dimensional geometry created by the articulations between the skeletal elements constituting the chest wall (ribs, backbone, sternum), together with their fibrous and skeletal-muscle interconnections. The chest wall relaxation volume is large, about two thirds of the total lung volume, and therefore is not normally encroached on with quiet breathing. As a result, the outward chest wall recoil force decreases progressively as the lungs become larger (cf. the lungs), reaching zero at the *chest wall relaxation* volume. As lung volume is increased still further, the chest wall recoil force reverses direction to act in the inward direction, and it becomes greater as lung volume increases (i.e., as is the case for the lungs).

A Balance of Forces

At the end of a normal quiet expiration, the recoil forces of the lung and chest wall are exactly balanced. The lung volume at which this balance of recoil forces occurs is termed the *functional residual capacity* (FRC) and represents the relaxation volume of the respiratory system. This behavior reflects the structural interdependence of the lungs and the chest wall; both structures are closely apposed and thus the motion of one dictates the motion of the other (i.e., when the chest wall expands, the lungs inflate, and when the lungs retract, the chest wall follows). This structural interdependence is conferred by the subatmospheric* (or nega-tive†) pressure that exists in the intrapleural space between the lungs and the chest wall; it prevents the chest wall from recoiling freely outward during inspiration and the lungs from recoiling freely inward during expiration. The nega-tive intrapleural pressure (P_{IP}) is the simple consequence of the recoil forces of the lungs and the chest wall attempting to "pull apart" the intrapleural space by their opposing actions. A typical value for P_{IP} at the end of a quiet expira-tion is –4 cm H_2O (Fig. 21–1).‡

The intrapleural space is bounded by the parietal pleura, which lines the inner surface of the chest wall, and the visceral pleura, which covers the surface of the lungs. The space between these two pleural layers is more appar-ent than real; it contains a negligibly small volume of serous fluid that serves as a lubricant for the two layers. When the integrity of the intrapleural space is compromised, as occurs, for example, with a pneumothorax, the entry of air into this region creates a real space between the two pleural layers, and the interdependence of the lungs and chest wall is lost. This allows the recoil forces of the lungs and of the chest wall to operate unopposed; the chest wall therefore flares outward to adopt its relaxation volume and the lungs likewise collapse to a volume approaching zero.

Lung Compliance

The compliance of the lungs provides an index of lung dis-tensibility, and is defined as the increase in lung volume (V) that is achieved for a given increase of distending pressure (Fig. 21–2). The *distending pressure,* termed more specifically the *transpulmonary pressure* (P_{TP}), is given by the difference between the pressure within the lungs (intraalveolar pres-sure, P_{ALV}) and the pressure immediately outside the lungs (intrapleural pressure, P_{IP}). A normal value for lung compli-ance is 200 mL/cm H_2O. Under conditions in which lung

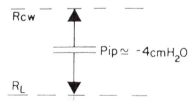

Figure 21–1. Balance of forces that determine functional resid-ual capacity (FRC). R_{CW} and R_L are the recoil forces of the chest wall and lungs, respectively; their respective magnitudes (which are equal at FRC) are indicated by the lengths of the appropriate arrows. P_{IP} is the intrapleural pressure. (*Reprinted, with permission, from Whipp BJ. The respiratory system. In: Ross G, ed.* Essentials of human physiology. *Chicago: Year Book Medical; 1982.*)

* Atmospheric pressure is normally about 760 mm Hg.
† A subatmospheric pressure may be considered to be "negative" if the barometric pressure is assumed to have a value of zero.
‡ Respiratory mechanical pressures are typically expressed as cm H_2O rather than mm Hg, in view of their small absolute magni-tude.

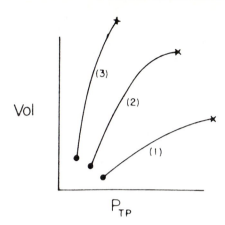

Figure 21–2. Compliance curves for normal lung (**2**), for lung with high recoil (e.g., fibrosis) (**1**), and for lung with low recoil (e.g., emphysema) (**3**). P_{TP} = transpulmonary pressure. (*Adapted, with permission, from Whipp BJ. The respiratory system. In: Ross G, ed.* Essentials of human physiology. *Chicago: Year Book Medical; 1982.*)

recoil is pathologically high (e.g., pulmonary fibrosis, neona-tal respiratory distress syndrome, ARDS), a greater increase in P_{TP} is needed to establish a given increase in lung volume; that is, the lungs are less distensible (decreased compliance). In contrast, if lung recoil is pathologically reduced (e.g., emphysema), then the opposite is the case: the lungs are more distensible (increased compliance).

Lung compliance is reduced early in the induction of anesthesia; however, the mechanisms of this effect remain conjectural. Possible candidates include alveolar collapse owing to a reduction in FRC and, possibly, a reduction in the surface-tension-reducing actions of surfactant.

It is important to recognize that the tidal volume is not distributed uniformly throughout the lungs, even in healthy individuals with no evidence of pulmonary dysfunction. This reflects the effects of gravity on the lung tissue volume (which is made up largely of water). As a consequence, the intrapleural pressure at the base of the lung (the dependent region) is greater (i.e., less negative) than at the apex, and the basal alveoli are thus smaller than are those at the apex (the nondependent region). This is shown schematically in Figure 21–3: at the end of a quiet expiration, the larger api-cal alveoli are located on the upper, flatter portion of the compliance curve (at •, **a**), whereas the smaller basal alveoli lie on the lower, steeper portion of the curve (at •, **b**). During the subsequent inspiration, both apical and basal units are exposed to identical increments of intrapleural pressure (ΔP_{IP}) and therefore expand to an extent (ΔV) dic-tated by the regional compliance. Thus, the basal alveoli, although smaller, expand more than the apical alveoli. Hence, the alveolar ventilation is distributed preferentially to the dependent portions of the lungs.

Chest Wall Compliance

As for the lungs, the compliance of the chest wall provides an index of chest wall distensibility. It is defined as the increase in the volume of the chest wall that results from a given increase in chest wall distending pressure (the pres-

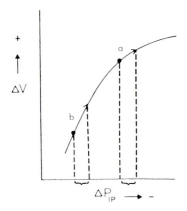

Figure 21–3. Influence of gravity on regional distribution of alveolar ventilation. Apical alveoli (**a**) have a larger volume than basal alveoli (**b**) in the upright lung; however, because the apical units normally lie on a less steep portion of the compliance curve (ΔV vs ΔP_{IP}) than the basal units, they expand from functional residual capacity (FRC = •) to a lesser extent during normal breathing in response to a given increment in P_{IP}. The apical alveoli therefore ventilate less than the basal alveoli. (*Reprinted, with permission, from Whipp BJ. The respiratory system. In: Ross G, ed. Essentials of human physiology. Chicago: Year Book Medical; 1982.*)

sure differential across the chest wall, given by the difference between atmospheric and intrapleural pressures) when the chest wall is completely relaxed (i.e., in the absence of respiratory muscle activity). Normally, the chest wall compliance has a value similar to that of the lungs (~ 200 mL/cm H_2O).* Chest wall compliance is reduced in conditions where thoracic motion is limited by skeletal abnormalities (e.g., *kyphoscoliosis, ankylosing spondylitis*), respiratory muscle rigidity, and excess adipose tissue deposition around the chest wall.

Respiratory Resistance

The expanding forces that are generated during inspiration are required not only to overcome the recoil forces of the lungs but also to overcome the resistance to airflow offered by the respiratory system. Normally, the bulk of the respiratory resistance is accounted for by the resistance of the airways.† This is defined as the ratio between the alveolar–atmospheric pressure differential (the *driving pressure*) and the airflow rate:

$$\text{airway resistance} = \frac{P_{ALV} - P_{ATM}}{\text{flow rate}}$$

---

* The compliance of the respiratory system (i.e., the lungs and chest wall) is derived from the sum of the reciprocal values for the individual components:

$$\frac{1}{\text{total compliance}} = \frac{1}{\text{lung compliance}} + \frac{1}{\text{chest wall compliance}}$$

Therefore, if the lung and chest wall compliances are each 200 mL/cm H_2O, then the total compliance is only 100 mL/cm H_2O.
† The resistance to thoracic motion offered by the tissues of the lungs and chest wall is normally negligible, although it may become significant in conditions of extreme obesity.

When flow along a simple, unbranched airway has a *laminar* (or streamlined)‡ profile, the airway resistance (R) can be defined according to *Poiseuille* as

$$R = \frac{8nl}{r^4}$$

where n is the coefficient of viscosity, and l and r are the length and radius of the airway, respectively. For a given driving pressure, flow will therefore decrease if the viscosity and/or airway length are increased, or if the airway radius is increased. The latter term is of particular functional significance: a small increase in airway radius will produce a marked increase in R (i.e., proportional to the fourth power of the radius). It is this factor that underlies the variation of airway resistance that can be demonstrated with changes in lung volume. That is, airway cross-sectional area increases when the surrounding intrathoracic pressure becomes more negative; as a result, the airways are relatively distended at high lung volumes and relatively compressed at low lung volumes.

Under certain conditions, the laminar profile of airflow is lost, and whirlpools or eddy currents are formed and, in the extreme, turbulence ensues. This results in a significant increase in the resistance to airflow, such that a greater driving pressure is required to maintain flow. Among the factors that can precipitate turbulence are multiple airway branchings, sharp turns, high velocities of flow, and irregular surface features on the inner walls of the airways.

A greater flow rate can be accomplished by increasing the driving pressure: during inspiration, with a greater lowering of alveolar pressure *below* atmospheric; during expiration, with a greater increase of alveolar pressure *above* atmospheric. Conversely, a greater driving pressure is required to sustain flow if airway resistance is increased.

Normal values for airway resistance typically lie in the range 0.5 to 2 cm H_2O/L/s. The major site of this resistance is the medium-sized bronchi, that is, the segmental bronchi and the larger-sized small bronchi. In contrast, the narrow bronchioles, which individually constitute sites of high resistance because of their very small radius, collectively contribute relatively little to the overall resistance; this reflects their very large number.

Apart from the volume dependence of airway resistance described above, several factors can affect the resistance to airflow. Contraction of the bronchial smooth muscle (*bronchoconstriction*) leads to a reduction in airway caliber and an increase in resistance. For example, stimulation of irritant receptors in the larger airways by inhaled noxious agents can reflexly activate the parasympathetic (vagal) bronchomotor innervation, via muscarinic receptors. Direct, locally mediated bronchoconstrictor effects can be induced by activation of H_1-histamine receptors, serotonin receptors, and alpha-adrenergic receptors. It is important to recognize that conditions such as asthma are often associated with airway hyperreactivity, such that exaggerated bronchoconstriction may result from provocations such as

---

‡ During laminar flow, air can be considered to be flowing along an airway as a series of concentric "cylinders," with the more central cylinders moving more rapidly than the outer ones, owing to the resistance of the walls of the airway; this generates a longitudinal profile that is parabolic or bullet-shaped.

methacholine, cold air, and histamine. Finally, physical obstruction of airways can increase the resistance to airflow; this can occur when bronchi are plugged with mucus, as is frequently the case in certain forms of *chronic obstructive pulmonary disease* (COPD), and by inhalation of foreign bodies.

In contrast, relaxation of bronchial smooth muscle (*bronchodilation*) increases airway caliber and therefore lowers airway resistance. Although reflex sympathetic stimulation can induce bronchodilation by activation of beta$_2$-adrenergic receptors, this effect is normally relatively weak. Drugs such as salbutamol and isoproterenol exert their bronchodilating actions at this receptor site.

During anesthesia, the reduced range of lung volume excursion that results from the lowering of FRC should lead to an increase in airway resistance, consequent to the reduced caliber of the airways. This may, however, be offset in the presence of inhalational anesthetics, which exert a bronchodilating influence. The functional significance of this effect is exemplified by halothane which is typically the agent of choice for asthmatic patients and for patients with a history of bronchospasm during induction and maintenance of anesthesia. Other sites that can increase resistance during anesthesia include the upper airway, as a result of obstruction or laryngospasm; the endotracheal tube, should there be accumulation of secretions, kinking of the tube, or herniation of the cuff; and the resistance of the anesthesia circuit.

Respiratory Muscles

Under normal conditions, the muscles of inspiration provide the force necessary to overcome lung recoil and therefore to expand the lungs. The principal muscle of inspiration is the *diaphragm*, a dome-shaped muscle that inserts at its peripheral border into the lower circumference of the chest wall, effectively separating the thoracic and abdominal cavities. It is innervated bilaterally by the phrenic nerves, which project from the anterior roots of the third to fifth cervical segments of the spinal cord. Contraction of the diaphragm causes its dome to descend, increasing the internal diameter of the thorax along the vertical axis and, to a lesser degree, along the transverse axis owing to the lower ribs being pulled out laterally.

The external intercostal muscles, which also have an inspiratory function, are arranged between the ribs, running down and forward. Their contraction causes the ribs to move forward, upward, and outward; this increases the internal diameter of the thorax along each of its three major axes (anteroposterior, vertical, transverse) in what have been termed the *pump handle* (forward and upward) and the *bucket handle* (lateral) movements. The external and internal intercostal muscles (see below) are innervated by the intercostal nerves which leave the spinal cord between the first and eleventh thoracic segments.

During quiet breathing, the dome of the diaphragm normally descends only a few centimeters from its relaxed position. The external intercostal muscles contract with moderate force, serving mainly to displace the upper ribs forward and up; they typically account for about 25 to 30 percent of the lung volume increase under these conditions.

A more substantial involvement of the inspiratory muscles is necessary if the breathing requirement is increased (e.g., during exercise). As a result, the diaphragm descends over a greater distance (by as much as 10 cm) and the external intercostal muscles contract with greater force than is the case for a quiet inspiration; their contribution may account for some 50 percent of the tidal volume. In addition, the accessory muscles of inspiration, typically, the scalene and the sternomastoid muscles,* may be recruited. Their action augments that of the external intercostal muscles. As a result, greater thoracic expansion occurs along all three axes, leading to further increases in lung volume.

Although the diaphragm is normally the primary muscle of inspiration, its function is supported, and can even be replaced by, the external intercostal muscles. Thus, if the chest wall structures are intact, breathing is not seriously compromised after complete denervation of the diaphragm.† Similarly, although the external intercostal muscles are normally active during inspiration, their integrity is not essential for adequate ventilation, as long as the diaphragm is intact. During anesthesia, however, diaphragmatic integrity is essential for spontaneous respiration, as the other muscles of inspiration are more susceptible to anesthesia-induced depression. The residual diaphragmatic tone that is normally evident at the end of a quiet expiration is abolished by anesthesia, and it has been argued that this action underlies the reduction in FRC that accompanies anesthetic induction.

Quiet expiration is a passive act, initiated by relaxation of the inspiratory muscles. This allows the lungs and chest wall to return to their previous end-expiratory position at FRC, under the influence of the increased lung recoil forces that were generated during the previous inspiration. Under conditions of stimulated breathing, the greater force required for expiration is largely provided by the internal intercostal muscles. These muscles run down and backward between the ribs. Their contraction pulls the ribs backward, downward, and inward; this decreases the diameter of the thorax along all three major axes. The abdominal muscles can also be recruited to assist in expiration. Their contraction forces the abdominal contents against the inferior surface of the diaphragm, pushing its dome to a higher resting position and serving to decrease the thoracic volume. Interestingly, anesthesia is often associated with increased activity in the abdominal muscles; this appears to have little or no functional significance for respiration, however.

Pressure, Volume, and Flow Fluctuations During the Respiratory Cycle

Transpulmonary pressure (P$_{TP}$) fluctuates systematically throughout the respiratory cycle. This, in turn, provides

---

* For extreme levels of ventilatory stimulation (e.g., high-intensity exercise, maximal voluntary ventilatory maneuvers), there may also be recruitment of posterior neck, trapezius, and back muscles.
† It should be noted that the relaxed diaphragm typically evidences a paradoxical upward motion during inspiration, as it passively responds to the lowering of intrathoracic pressures during inspiration.

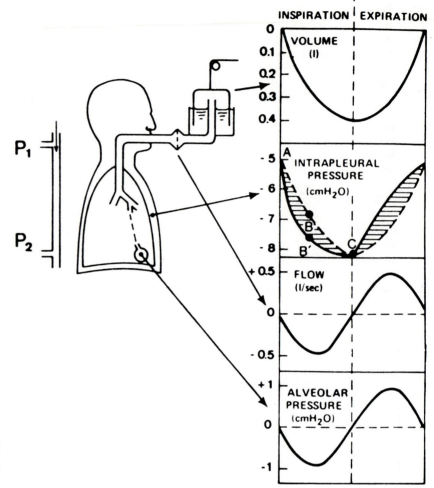

Figure 21–4. Time courses of respired volume, intrapleural pressure (with dashed profile indicating lung recoil pressure), respired flow, and alveolar pressure during inspiration and expiration for quiet breathing in a normal individual. (*Reprinted, with permission, from West JB.* Respiratory physiology: The essentials. *Baltimore: Williams & Wilkins; 1990.*)

the necessary distending pressure for the increase in lung volume during inspiration and its subsequent decline back to FRC during expiration. It should be noted that these changes in lung volume that result from the fluctuations in P_{TP} are simply predicted from the compliance curve of the lungs (Fig. 21–2). At the end of a normal quiet expiration, P_{TP} is approximately 5 cm H_2O; however, to expand the lungs during inspiration, P_{TP} must increase to overcome the greater recoil at these lung volumes (see Lung Recoil Forces) to attain a maximum at end-inspiration (about 7 cm H_2O during quiet breathing). During expiration, P_{TP} decreases back to its end-expiratory value as lung volume declines under the influence of lung recoil forces.

In the same sense that the changes in P_{TP} dictate the changes in lung volume, so the fluctuations in alveolar pressure (P_{ALV}) during the respiratory cycle dictate the profile of airflow (Fig. 21–4). Thus, at the end of a normal quiet expiration, as there is no movement of air into or out of the lungs, the driving pressure is zero (i.e., $P_{ALV} = P_{ATM}$). The thoracic expansion that ensues at the onset of inspiration causes P_{ALV} to become negative, causing air to flow into the lungs (i.e., $P_{ALV} < P_{ATM}$). Inspiratory flow reaches a peak in the midphase of inspiration, when P_{ALV} becomes most negative (about –2 or –3 cm H_2O, for a quiet inspiration). As the

end of inspiration is approached, flow ceases as P_{ALV} returns once more to zero. At the onset of expiration, P_{ALV} becomes positive as the lung recoil forces allow the lungs to collapse (i.e., $P_{ALV} > P_{ATM}$). As for inspiration, expiratory flow reaches a peak in the midphase of expiration as P_{ALV} reaches a maximum (some +2 to +3 cm H_2O, for a quiet expiration); and as the end of the expiratory phase is approached, P_{ALV} is again zero.

The intrapleural pressure (P_{IP}) reflects both lung recoil (P_{REC}) and alveolar pressure fluctuations; that is, as $P_{TP} = (P_{ALV} - P_{IP}) = P_{REC}$, then $P_{IP} = (P_{ALV} + P_{REC})$. At end-expiration, as there is no airflow, $P_{ALV} = 0$ and therefore $P_{IP} = P_{REC}$ (i.e., –5 cm H_2O); however, as P_{ALV} becomes negative and air starts to flow into the lungs, P_{IP} becomes more negative than P_{REC} (by an amount equal to P_{ALV}), again becoming equal to P_{REC} at the end of inspiration (as there is no airflow). And as P_{ALV} becomes positive during expiration, P_{IP} becomes less negative than P_{REC} (again, by an amount equal to P_{ALV}). At the end of expiration, P_{IP} once more equals P_{REC} (i.e., no airflow).

These fluctuations in intrapleural pressure become more striking when breathing becomes stimulated. During inspiration, P_{IP} may reach values of the order of –20 cm H_2O. And the large positive alveolar pressures that attend a forceful expiration can cause the intrapleural pressure to actually become positive.*

Under conditions of positive-pressure ventilation, intrapleural and alveolar pressure fluctuations during the respiratory cycle are modified. Lung expansion during inspiration still occurs because P_{TP} increases, but this increase is now accomplished by P_{ALV} becoming positive (i.e., $P_{ALV} > P_{ATM}$), such that air is "pushed" rather than "pulled" into the alveoli. And as $P_{IP} = (P_{TP} + P_{ALV})$, the intrapleural pressure now becomes less negative during inspiration and may even assume positive values, depending on the magnitude of the positive pressure applied at the airway opening.

LUNG VOLUMES AND CAPACITIES

The various volumes and capacities of the lungs provide important information about the mechanical properties of the lungs and chest wall. They are subject to alteration in conditions that are associated with abnormalities of lung recoil, chest wall recoil, and respiratory muscle function.

The major lung capacities and lung volumes (Fig. 21–5) are defined here:

- *Total lung capacity* (*TLC*): The maximal volume to which the lungs and chest wall can be expanded by volitional inspiratory effort.
- *Vital capacity* (*VC*): The maximal volume of gas that can be exhaled by volitional effort.
- *Functional residual capacity* (*FRC*): The volume of gas in the lungs at the end of a normal quiet expiration.
- *Inspiratory capacity* (*IC*): The maximal volume of gas that can be inhaled from FRC by volitional effort.

---

* If the intrapleural pressure becomes sufficiently positive during expiration so as to exceed the pressure in the small, unsupported airways, these airways are liable to collapse; this results in impaired alveolar ventilation.

- *Tidal volume* (*VT*): The volume of gas either inhaled or exhaled during a typical breath.
- *Residual volume* (*RV*): The volume of gas remaining in the lungs after a maximal volitional expiratory effort (the only volume that cannot be measured directly).
- *Inspiratory reserve volume* (*IRV*): The maximal volume of gas that can be inhaled from the normal end-inspiratory position.
- *Expiratory reserve volume* (*ERV*): The maximal volume of gas that can be exhaled from FRC.

These various volumes and capacities are clearly interrelated:

$$TLC = VC + RV \qquad VC = IC + ERV$$
$$FRC = ERV + RV \qquad IC = V_T + ERV$$

It is appropriate to consider the determinants of some of these volumes and capacities in greater detail, because of their widespread use in the formulation of functional judgments about the mechanical properties of the respiratory system.

Tidal Volume

Together with the breathing frequency, V_T is an important determinant of the level of overall ventilation and, therefore, of how well arterial blood gas and acid–base homeostasis are maintained in the face of challenges such as an increase in metabolic rate or a fall in the inspired O_2 fraction. At rest or during general anesthesia, a normal (70-kg) adult would have a V_T of about 500 mL. In response to respiratory stimuli such as hypercapnia, hypoxia, and exercise, however, values of over 2 L may commonly be attained.

Functional Residual Capacity

Functional residual capacity represents the relaxation volume of the lungs and chest wall under passive conditions, at which their respective recoil forces are balanced (Fig.

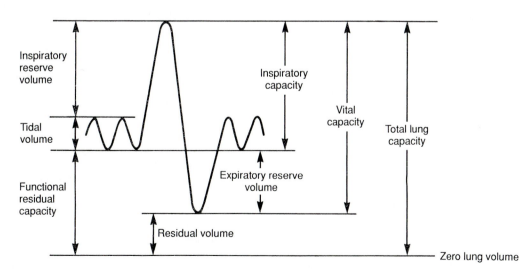

Figure 21–5. Spirogram showing static lung volumes. (*Reprinted, with permission, from Nunn JF: Applied respiratory physiology. 3rd ed. Butterworths, 1987.*)

21–1). During spontaneous quiet breathing, the end-expiratory lung volume (EEV) is usually taken as the FRC, as it is assumed that no forces are being exerted by the respiratory muscles. A value of some 2.5 to 3.0 L would be quite reasonable for a young, healthy (70-kg) individual; however, it is important to recognize that factors such as gender, body dimensions, posture, and age can influence FRC.

It is not surprising that factors affecting lung or chest wall compliance also affect FRC. For example, in emphysema the degenerative changes that take place in the lung parenchyma result in a highly compliant lung having a lower-than-normal lung recoil (Fig. 21–2). As a consequence, FRC is higher than normal. In contrast, conditions characterized by a low lung compliance and a high lung recoil (pulmonary fibrosis, neonatal respiratory distress syndrome, ARDS) are associated with a lower-than-normal FRC (Fig. 21–2).

During spontaneous breathing, the lungs do not necessarily return to FRC at the end of expiration. For example, if there is still some expiratory muscle tone at the end of expiration, EEV may well be less than FRC. This may explain in part why EEV is lower during muscular exercise than at rest. And, as discussed earlier, abolition of residual diaphragmatic tone at the end of expiration may account for the reduction in EEV with anesthesia.

Total Lung Capacity

Total lung capacity (TLC) is effectively dictated by the ability of the inspiratory muscles to override the recoil forces in both the lungs and the chest wall. (As mentioned earlier, at these high volumes, which typically exceed the relaxation volume of the chest wall, the chest wall recoil now acts to reduce rather than increase chest wall volume.) A normal value for TLC in a young, healthy (70-kg) adult would be about 6 L.

As for FRC, alterations in either lung or chest wall recoil are likely to influence TLC. For example, TLC is characteristically high in patients with emphysema, owing to the reduced lung recoil, but low in pulmonary fibrosis. Impaired function of the inspiratory muscles consequent, for example, to neuromuscular disorders will predispose to a lower-than-normal TLC.

Residual Volume

Residual volume (RV) is influenced by expiratory muscle strength. Thus, the expiratory muscles act in concert with the lung recoil force in attempting to reduce lung volume in the face of the opposing chest wall recoil force. A value of about 1.0 to 1.5 L can be regarded as a normal value for RV in a young, healthy (70-kg) adult.

Predictably, RV will be lower in conditions in which lung recoil is higher than normal (pulmonary fibrosis, neonatal respiratory distress syndrome, ARDS) and higher when lung recoil is reduced (emphysema). Expiratory muscle dysfunction will elevate RV.

Vital Capacity

A value of about 4.5 to 5.0 L can be regarded as a normal value for vital capacity (VC) in a young, healthy (70-kg)

adult; however, in making interpretations about potential sites of respiratory-mechanical impairment, it is important to recognize that, depending on the conditions under which it is measured, the VC may be subject to several interpretations. Thus, it is usual for estimates of both the *forced* VC and the *slow* VC to be made; although these are effectively equal in normal individuals, the forced VC is typically less than the slow VC in conditions such as COPD, in which small airway closure commonly occurs during forced exhalations.

Because the VC represents the difference between TLC and RV, the influence of altered recoil status will clearly depend on which of these two quantities is affected more. In the case of emphysema, for example, VC may not be greatly affected; this, of course, should not be taken as an indication of normal respiratory-mechanical function but rather of there being similar degrees of impairment in both TLC and RV.

OXYGEN TRANSPORT

Oxygen transport incorporates the sequence of mechanisms that moves O_2 molecules from the atmosphere to the mitochondria in the various organs and tissues of the body. This can be viewed as occurring along a series of O_2 partial pressure gradients—the *oxygen cascade.*

Transport to Alveoli

Oxygen (and CO_2) exchange between the atmosphere and the alveoli is brought about by the *bulk flow* of respired gas along the driving pressure gradient between the mouth and the alveolar space; however, with the progressive branching of the airways that occurs as the alveoli are approached, the overall cross-sectional area of the respiratory tree increases. As a result, the velocity within any single airway declines progressively (i.e., the overall airflow is "shared" between a greater number of airway units) and actually becomes zero in the vicinity of the respiratory bronchioles or alveolar ducts. Clearly, therefore, whereas the rate at which O_2 molecules are transported to the alveolar region depends on the overall rate of airflow, the delivery of O_2 molecules into the alveoli is dictated by diffusional flow. The rate of O_2 diffusion is governed primarily by the O_2 partial pressure gradient between the respiratory bronchioles and the interior of the alveoli.

The partial pressure (P) of a particular gas, X, in a mixture of gases is expressed as:

$$P_X = F_X \cdot P_{TOTAL}$$

where P_X is the partial pressure of X, F_X is its fractional concentration (i.e., [x]/100), and P_{TOTAL} is the total pressure of the gas mixture. For example, if an individual were to breathe pure O_2 at sea level, the partial pressure of O_2 (P_{O_2}) would be 760 mm Hg (i.e., the atmospheric pressure). Typically, however, room air (which may be supplemented with volatile anesthetics during anesthesia) is breathed. The partial pressures of the individual components are determined in accordance with *Dalton's law*. This states that in a gas mixture contained within a fixed volume, the pressure exerted by each individual gas (i.e., its partial pressure) is

independent of the pressures of the other gases in the mixture. Therefore, the total pressure of a mixture of gases is the sum of the individual partial pressures.

For example, dry atmospheric air at sea level has a total pressure of 760 mm Hg and its major constituents are O_2 (20.93%), CO_2 (0.04%), and nitrogen (79.03%). The corresponding partial pressures are P_{O_2} = 159 mm Hg, P_{CO_2} = 0.3 mm Hg, and P_{N_2} = 600 mm Hg. As an individual inspires, the incoming air is humidified during its passage through the nose, mouth, and airways. The addition of water vapor to the inspired gas serves to lower the partial pressures of the remaining components (Dalton's law). That is, as, at a normal body temperature of 37C, fully humidified gas will have a water vapor pressure of 47 mm Hg, this leaves a pressure of (760 – 47) mm Hg or 713 mm Hg available for N_2, O_2, and CO_2. Consequently, the P_{O_2} of moist inspired air (P_{IO_2}) is 149 mm Hg (i.e., $20.93/100 \times 713$), P_{ICO_2} is 0.3 mm Hg, and P_{IN_2} is 563 mm Hg.

In the alveoli, however, the P_{O_2} (i.e., alveolar, P_{AO_2}) is only about 100 mm Hg. This decrease in P_{O_2} reflects the uptake of O_2 molecules into the pulmonary capillary blood perfusing the alveoli. It should be emphasized that the volume of gas resident in the alveolar volume serves as a potential reservoir of O_2.

Although the greater proportion of the inspired tidal volume reaches the alveolar space and participates in the exchange of O_2 (and CO_2), the final 150 mL or so remains in the conducting airways, also known as the *anatomic dead space*, where no significant gas exchange can take place; it therefore retains its inspiratory composition. The dead-space gas is the first gas to be exhaled, followed only later by gas from the alveolar space. As a result, the P_{O_2} of the exhaled tidal volume (the mixed expired P_{O_2}, $P_{\bar{E}O_2}$) is greater than P_{AO_2}, and $P_{\bar{E}CO_2}$ is less than P_{ACO_2}. Typical normal values for $P_{\bar{E}O_2}$ and $P_{\bar{E}CO_2}$ at rest are approximately 120 and 30 mm Hg, respectively.

The alveolar P_{O_2} can be estimated from the alveolar air equation

$$P_{AO_2} = P_{IO_2} - \frac{P_{ACO_2}}{R} + F$$

where P_{AO_2} and P_{IO_2} represent the alveolar and inspired P_{O_2}, respectively; P_{ACO_2} is the alveolar P_{CO_2} (usually assumed to equal the arterial P_{CO_2}); R is the respiratory exchange ratio (i.e., the ratio of pulmonary CO_2 output to O_2 uptake), which, under steady-state conditions, equals the respiratory quotient; and F is a correction factor that, for practical purposes, can be ignored.* It is important to note that the P_{AO_2} obtained in this manner is the ideal P_{AO_2}, or the P_{AO_2} that would prevail were there to be no impairment to pulmonary O_2 exchange.

This, in turn, provides the basis for estimation of the *alveolar–arterial P_{O_2} difference* or P_{AO_2}–P_{aO_2} difference. The P_{AO_2}–P_{aO_2} difference is a widely used clinical index of impaired pulmonary gas exchange. The contributions of diffusional impairment, dead space, shunt, and ventilation–

perfusion maldistribution to the P_{AO_2}–P_{aO_2} difference are discussed later. In healthy young adults at sea level, the P_{AO_2}–P_{aO_2} difference normally does not exceed 15 mm Hg, although it may increase to as much as 35 mm Hg in the elderly who are otherwise healthy. As will become evident later, however, the P_{AO_2}–P_{aO_2} difference cannot be predicted from readily measurable quantities; rather, arterial P_{O_2} must be measured directly.

Gas is transported from the alveolar gas to pulmonary capillary blood by diffusion across the alveolar capillary membrane, with diffusion equilibrium between the blood and gas phases being normally reached well before blood leaves the capillary circulation (i.e., the P_{O_2} of pulmonary end-capillary blood equals P_{AO_2}, typically about 100 mm Hg); however, venous blood from the larger airways and from the myocardium drains into the arterialized blood downstream of the lungs (anatomic shunt), to provide a systemic arterial P_{O_2} (P_{aO_2}) that is slightly lower than P_{AO_2} (see Shunt). In healthy young adults at sea level, P_{aO_2} typically lies in the range 90 to 95 mm Hg, although with increasing age, this value is likely to be lower.

Transport in Blood

The amount of O_2 dissolved in the plasma is governed by *Henry's law*, which states that the amount of a gas that can be dissolved in a liquid is proportional to the partial pressure of the gas to which the liquid is exposed. For example, 1 mL of plasma at 37C carries 0.00003 mL of O_2/mm Hg P_{O_2}. Therefore, arterial blood with a P_{O_2} of 100 mm Hg carries 0.3 mL of O_2 per 100 mL of blood. For a resting individual with a normal cardiac output and a normal tissue O_2 consumption of 250 mL/min, a minimum of 5 mL of O_2/100 mL of blood would have to be dissolved in the blood to meet the body's metabolic demands. Clearly, therefore, the carriage of O_2 in a chemically bound form with hemoglobin is needed to ensure adequate rates of tissue O_2 delivery.

Hemoglobin (Hb), which is contained within the red blood cells, has a molecular weight of about 65,000. Each molecule has four subunits; each subunit consists of a polypeptide chain having a complex three-dimensional structure and incorporating an iron-containing heme group, to which a single O_2 molecule can combine reversibly (as long as the iron remains in the ferrous form). This process of oxygenation (not to be confused with oxidation) is governed by the affinity of the hemoglobin subunit for O_2; this depends, in turn, on the three-dimensional structure of the particular subunit and that of the surrounding three subunits in the hemoglobin molecule.

The process of oxygenation (and deoxygenation) of the hemoglobin molecule is described by the following general equation, which indicates that four steps are involved (one for each subunit):

$$Hb_4 + 4O_2 \rightleftharpoons Hb_4(O_2)_4$$

This can be simplified, however:

$$Hb + O_2 \rightleftharpoons HbO_2$$

The complete oxygenation of hemoglobin to oxyhemoglobin (HbO_2) requires 1.34 mL of O_2/g of hemoglobin (values as high as 1.39 may be cited). This corresponds to 20.1 mL

---

* The correction factor, $F = P_{ACO_2} \cdot F_{IO_2} \cdot \{(1 - R)/R\}$. For example, in a healthy, air-breathing subject at sea level (i.e., P_{ACO_2} = 40 mm Hg, F_{IO_2} = 0.2093 and R = 0.8), F equals only 2 mm Hg.

O_2/100 mL blood for a normal blood hemoglobin concentration of 15 g/100 mL blood, and is termed the O_2 *capacity*. Clearly, therefore, in conditions that are characterized by increased levels of circulating hemoglobin (e.g., polycythemia), the O_2 capacity will be greater than normal; this provides an increased potential for tissue O_2 delivery at a given cardiac output. In contrast, the O_2 capacity is reduced when hemoglobin levels are lower than normal, as in anemia. It is possible to allow for such alterations in O_2 capacity by expressing the amount of O_2 combined with hemoglobin as O_2 *saturation* (SO_2). Thus, at a particular PO_2,

$$SO_2\ (\%) = \frac{O_2 \text{ bound to Hb}}{O_2 \text{ capacity}} \times 100$$

The amount of O_2 carried by the blood both in physical solution and in combination with hemoglobin is termed the O_2 *content*. Owing to the combining characteristics of the hemoglobin molecule, the relationship between the O_2 content (or the O_2 saturation) and the PO_2 of blood—the O_2 dissociation curve—is not linear but rather is S-shaped, or sigmoid (Fig. 21–6). When the hemoglobin molecule is in the deoxygenated form, it has a relatively low affinity for O_2. Thus, as PO_2 is increased from zero, only a small proportion of hemoglobin subunits become oxygenated; this is reflected in the shallow slope of the O_2 dissociation curve in this low-PO_2 range. Once a single combination occurs in a hemoglobin molecule, however, small conformational changes in the three-dimensional structure of the polypeptide chains result that facilitate O_2 combination at the remaining three binding sites (termed *cooperative interaction*). As a result, the dissociation curve is steep over the PO_2 range 10 to 50 mm Hg; however, as PO_2 increases further to approach the normal arterial value of 90 to 100 mm Hg,

fewer and fewer vacant sites remain for O_2 binding, and thus the O_2 dissociation curve starts to plateau.

The sigmoid shape of the O_2 dissociation curve has important functional implications for O_2 transport. A consequence of the flat, upper portion of the dissociation curve is that the amount of O_2 bound to hemoglobin is scarcely affected by moderate reductions in PaO_2 that would result from conditions such as ascent to altitude or pulmonary disease. For example, arterial blood having a PO_2 of 95 mm Hg and an SO_2 of 97 percent will have an O_2 content of 19.79 mL O_2/100 mL blood, that is, 19.5 mL bound to hemoglobin ($20.1 \times 97/1000$) and 0.29 mL in physical solution (0.003×95). If PaO_2 falls to 60 mm Hg (i.e., $SaO_2 = 90$ percent), the O_2 content is reduced only by 1.52 mL O_2/100 mL blood; that is, 18.09 mL O_2 is bound to hemoglobin and 0.18 mL is dissolved in plasma, giving a total of 18.27 mL O_2/100 mL blood.

In contrast, when arterial blood enters the capillary beds of the peripheral tissues and PO_2 starts to fall in response to the diffusion of O_2 molecules from the blood toward the mitochondria, a modest fall will lead to considerable unloading of O_2 from hemoglobin as a result of the steep slope of the dissociation curve in this lower PO_2 range. Thus, while a 30 mm Hg fall in PO_2 from the normal arterial point is required to unload 1.52 mL O_2/100 mL blood, the same amount of O_2 can be released from the normal resting venous point ($PO_2 = 40$ mm Hg and $SO_2 = 75$ percent) merely by a 5 mm Hg reduction in PO_2. Likewise, when mixed venous blood reaches the lungs, substantial loading of O_2 from the alveolar gas into the blood can occur as the PO_2 of pulmonary capillary blood starts to increase.

It is important to recognize that the shape and position of the O_2 dissociation curve can be affected by a variety of factors. Increases in blood PCO_2, [H^+] (i.e., a decrease in pH), and temperature, such as occur in metabolically active tissues (e.g., skeletal muscle during exercise or *malignant hyperthermia*), cause a rightward shift of the dissociation curve. As a result, less O_2 will be bound to hemoglobin at a particular PO_2. This unloading action is thought to facilitate the delivery of O_2 to sites having increased metabolic O_2 requirements. Conversely, at the lungs, where blood PCO_2 and [H^+] are lower as a result of CO_2 exchange, the O_2 dissociation curve is shifted to the left. This should enhance the combination of O_2 with hemoglobin at a given PO_2.

An index of the magnitude of such shifts in the O_2 dissociation curve is provided by the P_{50}, or the PO_2 at which the blood O_2 saturation is 50 percent. Under standard conditions (pH 7.4, $PCO_2 = 40$ mm Hg, temperature = 37C), the P_{50} is normally about 27 mm Hg. A rightward shift of the dissociation curve will result in an increased P_{50}, and a leftward shift in a decreased P_{50}.

The actions of CO_2 and [H^+] on the O_2 dissociation curve, referred to collectively as the *Bohr effect*, are thought to reflect the action of [H^+] ions (formed by hydration, in the case of CO_2) combining with basic amino acid residues on the hemoglobin polypeptide chains. This, in turn, influences the affinity of the hemoglobin subunits for O_2.

The blood levels of *2,3-diphosphoglycerate* (2,3-DPG) also may affect the position of the O_2 dissociation curve. An end product of red blood cell glycolysis, 2,3-DPG levels are

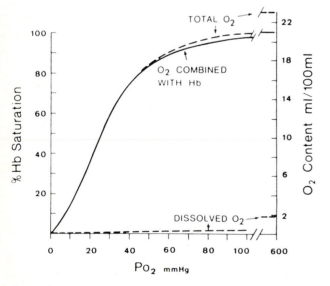

Figure 21–6. Oxygen dissociation curve, expressing O_2 saturation and O_2 content as a function of PO_2. (*Reprinted, with permission, from West JB.* Respiratory physiology: The essentials. *Baltimore: Williams & Wilkins; 1990.*)

increased during conditions of chronic hypoxemia,* as would be encountered with an extended sojourn at altitude or in COPD, for example. An elevated 2,3-DPG concentration has been shown to shift the O_2 dissociation curve to the right (i.e., increasing the P_{50}); the reduced affinity of hemoglobin for O_2 is thought to improve tissue O_2 delivery in the face of hypoxemic conditions. Therefore, in a clinical context, it is crucial to recognize that blood that has been stored in a blood bank with acid–citrate–dextrose (ACD) has a low [2,3-DPG] and thus a relatively high affinity for O_2; however, this effect is less marked if blood is stored with citrate–phosphate–dextrose (CPD). The transfusion of such blood could therefore be expected initially to impair O_2 delivery to vital organs; within a few hours, the 2,3-DPG concentration of transfused blood typically returns to normal.

Other factors influence Hb–O_2 binding through effects on the shape of the O_2 dissociation curve, rather than simply on its position. Carbon monoxide (CO), for example, resembles O_2 in being able to combine reversibly at the heme groups of the hemoglobin molecule. Thus, O_2 and CO compete for available binding sites; and as the affinity of hemoglobin for CO is about 210 times greater than for O_2, a substantial proportion of the binding sites will be occupied by CO, even at low P_{CO}. At a blood P_{CO} of 1 mm Hg and a P_{O_2} of 100 mm Hg, for example, hemoglobin is almost completely saturated with CO. Furthermore, the inhalation of automobile exhaust fumes or cigarette smoke may lead to binding of more than 5 percent of the circulating hemoglobin to CO. The influence of CO on O_2 delivery is further exacerbated by the O_2 dissociation curve becoming less sigmoid, which also effectively moves the curve to the left. Thus, at a given blood P_{O_2}, less of the bound O_2 (already at a lower-than-normal level because of CO–Hb combination) will be released from the hemoglobin.

Certain drugs, including nitrites, nitroglycerine, sulfonamides, and prilocaine, oxidize the ferrous irons in hemoglobin to the ferric form, which renders the hemoglobin molecule unable to carry O_2. This form of hemoglobin is called *methemoglobin*.

Anesthetics such as halothane, methoxyflurane, and cyclopropane are able to bind to hemoglobin. However, it appears unlikely that the binding of such agents occurs at the O_2 binding sites, as the P_{50} is not affected.

Transport to Tissues

Oxygen delivery to the peripheral tissues is dictated by the cardiac output and the arterial O_2 content, and thus may be compromised under conditions in which one or the other (or both) of these variables is inappropriately low. This, in turn, has the potential to lead to tissue hypoxia. Three major types of tissue hypoxia are conventionally recognized: stagnant hypoxia, in which the blood supply to the tissues is impaired; hypoxic hypoxia, in which arterial P_{O_2} is abnor-

mally low; and anemic hypoxia, in which blood has a reduced ability to carry O_2.

Stagnant hypoxia may be generalized if it results from a decrease in cardiac output, or localized if it results from partial or complete vascular occlusion within a particular tissue or organ. Typically, P_{aO_2} can be normal, whereas $P_{\bar{v}O_2}$ is reduced. The predisposition to stagnant hypoxia can be exacerbated in hypermetabolic conditions associated with anesthesia (e.g., surgical stimulation; reversal agents, such as doxapram and ethamivan; shivering; "thyroid storm" in hyperthyroid patients; and, rarely, malignant hyperthermia), where cardiac output may not increase appropriately owing to depression of cardiovascular control mechanisms and myocardial function.

Treatment of stagnant hypoxia demands correction of the underlying cardiovascular impairment; administration of 100 percent O_2 will have little effect, owing to the already high arterial O_2 saturation.

Hypoxic hypoxia can occur in the absence of impaired pulmonary function or ventilatory control as a result of a reduced inspired P_{O_2}. This results when individuals ascend in altitude. Also, inadvertent reduction of F_{IO_2} during anesthesia can occur consequent to the diluting effects of anesthetic gases (e.g., nitrous oxide) on the inspired gas mixture. Mechanical failure of the O_2 supply system for the anesthesia machine and inappropriate setting of the O_2 flowmeter can have a similar effect. In such situations, administration of 100 percent O_2 should restore arterial P_{O_2} toward normal levels.

Alveolar hypoventilation, unaccompanied by impaired pulmonary gas exchange, can also lead to a lowered P_{aO_2}; in this case, however, inspired P_{O_2} may be normal. During anesthesia, mechanical obstruction of the airway will lead to hypoventilation (e.g., laryngospasm, obstruction of the posterior pharynx by the tongue, obstruction of the endotracheal tube, aspiration of foreign material), as will any substantial increase in apparatus dead space. Central nervous system depressant drugs (e.g., barbiturates, narcotics, volatile anesthetics) lead to hypoventilation through their depressant actions on ventilatory control mechanisms. Again, in the absence of a gas-exchange impairment, arterial P_{O_2} can generally be corrected by O_2 inhalation.

In contrast, the reduction in P_{aO_2} that results from diffusion impairment, shunt, and ventilation–perfusion maldistribution cannot be so readily corrected by administration of 100 percent O_2. This is discussed in greater detail in the appropriate sections.

Anemic hypoxia may occur either because there is an insufficient amount of hemoglobin or there is an inability of the hemoglobin to actually transport O_2, owing to a diminished availability of O_2 binding sites on hemoglobin or a reduced affinity of the hemoglobin for O_2. Anemia is the most frequent cause of this type of hypoxia and may result from hemorrhage, hemolysis, or decreased formation of red cells. In this condition, the arterial O_2 content is low owing to reduced levels of circulating hemoglobin, even though P_{aO_2} may be normal. Minor reductions in the hemoglobin available for O_2 combination may not have serious consequences in healthy individuals, at least under resting conditions; however, they may pose a problem in patients with

---

* Hypoxemia is a special case of *hypoxia* (a condition in which the P_{O_2} of a particular region, such as alveolar gas, arterial blood or the peripheral tissues, is below the normal air-breathing value at sea level) and is defined as a decrease in blood P_{O_2} below normal.

borderline O_2 supply resulting from coronary or cerebro-vascular insufficiency.

If an anemic individual is also hypoxemic (i.e., low Pa_{O_2}), arterial O_2 content may fall to levels that would likely cause tissue P_{O_2} to encroach on the critical levels for sustained aerobic metabolism. Thus, with a Pa_{O_2} of 100 mm Hg but a hemoglobin concentration of only 10 g/100 mL blood, a resting individual would have an arterial O_2 content of 13.35 mL/100 mL blood and, with a normal peripheral O_2 extraction of 5 mL/100 mL blood, a mixed venous O_2 content of 8.35 mL/100 mL blood. This corresponds to a mixed venous and, therefore, tissue P_{O_2} of less than 35 mm Hg. With even mild hypoxia, tissue P_{O_2} would fall even lower were it not for the increased cardiac output that is often seen in such conditions. This is the primary reason that elective surgery is typically not considered for patients whose hemoglobin concentration is less than 8 to 10 g/100 mL blood. The impact of these effects is likely to be exacerbated during hypermetabolic conditions.

Although the anemic patient may be treated by O_2 inhalation, it is preferable to correct the cause of the anemia.

CARBON DIOXIDE TRANSPORT

Carbon dioxide transport can also be viewed as a cascade of steps that resemble those making up the O_2 cascade but that operates in the reverse direction, from tissues to the atmosphere.

Transport from Tissues

The demand for the removal of metabolically produced CO_2 from tissues is challenged by increases in metabolic rate (see previous section) and also by alterations in the dietary substrate undergoing oxidation. During aerobic metabolism, carbohydrate and fat are oxidized to yield ATP, together with the end products CO_2 and water. For example, a resting individual with an O_2 consumption of 250 mL/min who is metabolizing solely carbohydrate will produce CO_2 also at a rate of 250 mL/min (giving a respiratory quotient [RQ] of 1.0); in contrast, the metabolism of fatty acids will result in a CO_2 production of about 175 mL/min (i.e., RQ ~ 0.7). Normally, however, the dietary substrate is a mixture of fat and carbohydrate (RQ ~ 0.8); this yields a resting CO_2 production of ~ 200 mL/min.

Intravenous nutritional support involving administration of high concentrations of glucose can also influence substrate utilization. This will cause an increase in the RQ and, therefore, in tissue CO_2 production.

Under conditions in which aerobic mechanisms cannot satisfy tissue demands for energy production (e.g., skeletal muscle during heavy exercise or malignant hyperthermia, the brain during cerebral hypoxia), anaerobic mechanisms of ATP production (i.e., not requiring O_2) come into play; these involve the breakdown of carbohydrate to lactic acid. A significant proportion of the lactic acid so produced is buffered, or neutralized, by sodium bicarbonate in both tissue fluids and blood; this yields CO_2 and sodium lactate. Hence, the CO_2 produced by metabolism is supplemented by that resulting from the buffering of lactic acid. This

increases the demands for the transport of CO_2 to, and its subsequent clearance from, the lungs.

Because of tissue CO_2 production, the P_{CO_2} within the peripheral tissues is high relative to that in the capillary blood. CO_2 molecules diffuse down this partial pressure gradient into the capillary circulation. At rest, this yields a P_{CO_2} of 46 mm Hg in mixed venous blood; this value is higher during exercise and other hypermetabolic states, as a result of increased CO_2 production rates in the tissues.

Transport in Blood

The rate of CO_2 delivery to the lungs is dictated by the venous return and the CO_2 content of mixed venous blood. As is the case for O_2, CO_2 is transported by blood both in physical solution and in chemical combination. The amount of dissolved CO_2 is governed by the P_{CO_2} in plasma and by the solubility coefficient for CO_2 (0.03 mmol/L/mm Hg), as defined by Henry's law (see above). As CO_2 is some 24 times more soluble in plasma than O_2, a greater proportion is transported in this form (i.e., ~ 5 percent). For example, at a normal Pa_{CO_2} of 40 mm Hg, 1.2 mmol/L CO_2 is carried in physical solution, compared with 1.38 mmol/L in mixed venous blood at rest (P_{CO_2} = 46 mm Hg).

The chemical combination of CO_2 in blood is more complex than that of O_2 and involves three different forms: carbonic acid (H_2CO_3), bicarbonate ions (HCO_3^-), and carbamino compounds.

Carbonic acid (H_2CO_3) is formed from the hydration of CO_2 molecules:

$$CO_2 + H_2O \rightleftharpoons H_2CO_3$$

This reaction takes place slowly in plasma but is catalyzed within the red blood cells by the enzyme carbonic anhydrase. Once formed, carbonic acid dissociates readily into H^+ and HCO_3^- ions, and therefore only a very small amount of CO_2 is transported as carbonic acid:

$$H_2CO_3 \rightleftharpoons H^+ + HCO_3^-$$

The full reaction sequence is given by

$$CO_2 + H_2O \rightleftharpoons H_2CO_3 \rightleftharpoons H^+ + HCO_3^-$$

Bicarbonate formation takes place largely in the red blood cells and proceeds according to the law of mass action with a dissociation constant (K):

$$K = \frac{[H^+] [HCO_3^-]}{[H_2CO_3]}$$

As $[H_2CO_3]$ is proportional to the concentration of dissolved CO_2, the dissociation constant may be redefined as:

$$K' = \frac{[H^+] [HCO_3^-]}{[CO_2]_{\text{DISSOLVED}}}$$

$$= \frac{[H^+] [HCO_3^-]}{\alpha \cdot P_{CO_2}}$$

where α is the solubility coefficient for CO_2. At a given P_{CO_2}, the extent to which the hydration of CO_2 and the subsequent dissociation of carbonic acid proceed is limited by the concentrations of H^+ and HCO_3^-. If the means exist to remove one or both of these reaction products, the formation of HCO_3^- can be maintained as P_{CO_2} increases. For example, newly formed H^+ ions are buffered within the red blood cells (RBCs) largely by imidazole residues of the hemoglobin molecules. In addition, HCO_3^- ions diffuse across the red cell membrane into the plasma, where $[HCO_3^-]$ is lower owing to the slower rate of HCO_3^- formation in this phase.

The equation defining the dissociation constant K' can be reformulated by taking logarithms of both sides,

$$\log K' = \log[H^+] + \frac{\log[HCO_3^-]}{\alpha \cdot P_{CO_2}}$$

and rearranging:

$$-\log[H^+] = -\log K' + \frac{\log[HCO_3^-]}{\alpha \cdot P_{CO_2}}$$

As -log $[H^+]$ is pH and -log K' is pK' (equal to 6.1 in plasma),

$$pH = pK' + \frac{\log[HCO_3^-]}{\alpha \cdot P_{CO_2}}$$

This important relationship between pH, P_{CO_2}, and $[HCO_3^-]$ is known as the *Henderson–Hasselbalch* equation and is widely used in the analysis of primary respiratory and metabolic acid–base disturbances and the secondary consequences of the compensatory mechanisms they invoke.

To preserve electrical neutrality across the red cell membrane in the face of the flux of HCO_3^- ions from the red blood cells, there is a corresponding influx of anions (the cell membrane being largely impermeable to cations) principally in the form of chloride (Cl^-) ions, according to the *Gibbs–Donnan equilibrium:*

$$\frac{[HCO_3^-]_{PLASMA}}{[HCO_3^-]_{RBC}} = \frac{[Cl^-]_{PLASMA}}{[Cl^-]_{RBC}}$$

This is termed the *chloride shift* or the Hamburger shift.

These reactions result in approximately 90 percent of the total transported CO_2 being in the form of HCO_3^- ions and carried mostly in the plasma (although formed largely within the red cells).

Carbamino-CO_2 compounds represent the remaining 5 percent of the CO_2 that is carried in blood. These compounds are formed from the combination of CO_2 molecules with amino (—NH_2) groups of the hemoglobin molecules in the red cells, together with an additional small amount in association with plasma proteins. Thus,

$$R=NH_2 + CO_2 \rightleftharpoons R—NH \cdot COO^- + H^+$$

It is possible to construct a CO_2 dissociation curve (Fig. 21–7) that is analogous to the O_2–hemoglobin dissociation curve (Fig. 21–6), which relates the total CO_2 content of blood (i.e., physically dissolved and chemically combined forms) to the P_{CO_2}. In contrast to the O_2 dissociation curve, the CO_2 dissociation curve is essentially linear over the physiologic range. As a result, the capacity for the blood to

load and unload CO_2 is reasonably independent of the prevailing P_{CO_2}. That is, there are no significant changes in the slope of the dissociation curve between the normal arterial and mixed venous points (cf. Fig. 21–6).

As is the case for O_2, the ability of blood to transport CO_2 is not merely a function of the P_{CO_2}. The oxygenation status of hemoglobin also exerts an influence: at a given P_{CO_2}, deoxygenated blood can carry more CO_2 than can fully oxygenated blood (Fig. 21–7). This is termed the *Haldane effect*. It reflects the greater H^+-buffering power of the deoxygenated hemoglobin molecule; this allows greater HCO_3^- formation, and also the greater availability of amino side chains on hemoglobin for carbamino-CO_2 formation. The contributions of the various chemically combined forms of CO_2 to the total amount of CO_2 *transported* in blood at a particular level of oxygenation are therefore not the same as those that relate to the total amount of CO_2 *exchanged* at the lungs with concomitant loading of O_2 into the blood: in the lung 30 percent of the exchanged CO_2 comes from carbamino-CO_2, 60 percent from HCO_3^- ions, and 10 percent from dissolved CO_2.

As blood flowing through the pulmonary capillary bed changes its composition from mixed venous to arterialized, the oxygenation of hemoglobin encourages the unloading of CO_2. Conversely, as discussed in the preceding section, the unloading of CO_2 (which lowers blood P_{CO_2} and $[H^+]$ to their arterial values) encourages the loading of O_2 onto hemoglobin. Hence, the transport of O_2 and the transport of CO_2 in blood are mutually dependent.

Transport from Alveoli

Within the pulmonary capillary bed, CO_2 molecules diffuse down a partial pressure gradient from blood to alveolar gas. The bulk flow of gas during expiration subsequently clears CO_2 from the respiratory tree, completing the final step in the carbon dioxide cascade.

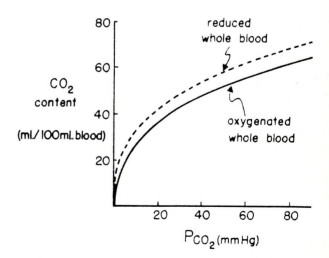

Figure 21–7. Carbon dioxide dissociation curve, expressing CO_2 content as a function of P_{CO_2} for oxygenated (—) and deoxygenated (---) blood. (*Reprinted, with permission, from Whipp BJ. The respiratory system. In: Ross G, ed. Essentials of human physiology. Chicago: Year Book Medical; 1982.*)

DIFFUSION

The movement of O_2 and CO_2 molecules within the alveoli and across the alveolar–capillary membrane relies on diffusion. Diffusion is a passive process (i.e., with no energy expenditure) that requires only a partial pressure difference (or driving pressure). Gas molecules will therefore move from an area of high partial pressure to an area that has a lower partial pressure, consequent to their random motion. That is, as molecules collide more frequently in a region of high partial pressure, the net effect is for molecules to move toward the region of low partial pressure until there is no longer a difference in partial pressure between the two regions. The rate of diffusion therefore depends on the magnitude of the driving pressure.

The rate of diffusion of a gas x is defined as

$$V_x = D_x \cdot \frac{A}{l} \cdot \Delta P_x$$

where D_x is the diffusion coefficient of the gas, ΔP_x is the partial pressure difference across the interface, A is the surface area of the interface, and l is the path length for diffusion. Factors that speed the rate of diffusion lead to a more rapid attainment of diffusion equilibrium across the interface; factors slowing the rate of diffusion will prolong the time required for equilibrium to occur.

The density of the gas also influences its rate of diffusion. *Graham's law* states that, for a given partial pressure difference, a light gas will diffuse more readily through a gaseous medium than will a dense gas, in inverse proportion to the square root of the density. For example, O_2 (with a molecular weight [MW] of 32) is relatively more diffusible than CO_2 (MW = 44):

$$\frac{\text{rate of } O_2 \text{ diffusion}}{\text{rate of } CO_2 \text{ diffusion}} = \frac{\sqrt{MW\ CO_2}}{\sqrt{MW\ O_2}} = \frac{\sqrt{44}}{\sqrt{32}} = \frac{6.6}{5.6} = 1.18$$

Oxygen therefore diffuses some 18 percent more rapidly than CO_2 in alveolar gas.

Relative to the duration of the respiratory cycle, the diffusion of O_2 and CO_2 between the alveolar ducts and the alveolar–capillary interface is sufficiently rapid that there are negligible differences in both P_{O_2} and P_{CO_2} within the alveolar gas volume. For example, diffusion of gas in a normal alveolus (diameter approximately 100 µm) is thought to be 80 percent complete in 0.002 second, assuming the average diffusion distance to be 0.5 mm; however, in conditions such as emphysema, where destruction of alveolar walls results in the formation of large air sacs, the distance required for diffusion of gas molecules between the alveolar duct and the gas-exchanging surface may be too great to allow diffusion equilibrium to occur in the time available. As a result, P_{O_2} and P_{CO_2} gradients will be present within the alveolar gas, leading to inefficient exchange of O_2 and CO_2 and thus to arterial hypoxemia and hypercapnia.

In diffusing from alveolar gas to pulmonary capillary blood, O_2 molecules must cross a series of anatomic barriers (and likewise for CO_2, which diffuses in the opposite direction): the alveolar epithelium, the interstitial tissue volume between the alveolar epithelium and capillary endothelium, the capillary endothelial membrane, plasma in the pulmonary capillary, the red blood cell membrane, and, finally, the interior of the red blood cell for ultimate binding to the hemoglobin molecule. Despite the number of structures involved, the alveolar–capillary membrane is very thin (normally, about 0.2 µm).

In a liquid medium, such as plasma, an important determinant of the diffusion coefficient is the solubility (α) of the gas in the medium. Defining solubility as the number of molecules of gas that can be dissolved in 1 mL of water at 37C for a partial pressure of 1 atm (or 760 mm Hg), the solubilities for CO_2 and O_2 are 0.5920 and 0.0244, respectively. Thus, CO_2 is approximately 24 times more soluble than O_2. The other major determinant of the diffusion coefficient is the gas density, that is, $D_x = \alpha_x / \sqrt{MW_x}$. Therefore,

$$\frac{\text{rate of } CO_2 \text{ diffusion}}{\text{rate of } O_2 \text{ diffusion}} = \frac{\alpha_{CO_2}}{\alpha_{O_2}} \cdot \frac{\sqrt{MW_{O_2}}}{\sqrt{MW_{CO_2}}}$$

$$= \frac{0.5920}{0.0244} \cdot \frac{5.6}{6.6}$$

$$= 20.7$$

Thus, in contrast to the gas phase, CO_2 diffuses 20 times more rapidly across the alveolar–capillary membrane than does O_2, for a given partial pressure difference between blood and gas.

The difference between the P_{O_2} of the mixed venous blood (normally about 40 mm Hg at rest) entering the pulmonary capillary bed from the pulmonary artery and the P_{O_2} of alveolar gas (normally 100 mm Hg) provides the initial driving pressure for diffusion of O_2 into the blood (in this case, 60 mm Hg). As O_2 molecules diffuse into the pulmonary capillary blood, the blood P_{O_2} rises progressively and normally reaches the alveolar value (i.e., 100 mm Hg) within 0.25 to 0.30 second (Fig. 21–8). Thus, diffusion equilibrium between alveolar gas and pulmonary capillary blood is established well before the blood reaches the end of the pulmonary capillary bed (at rest, the vascular transit time is normally about 0.8 second). Most of the O_2 that enters the pulmonary capillary blood does so at the beginning of the capillary bed, where the difference between P_{O_2} in the gas and blood phases is greatest; this is evident in the rapid rate of blood P_{O_2} increase in the early stages of the gas-exchange process (Fig. 21–8). As the capillary P_{O_2} rises and the P_{O_2} difference between gas and blood becomes narrower, the rate of O_2 diffusion slows progressively until, beyond the point of diffusion equilibrium, no more O_2 is taken up (i.e., as the alveolar and pulmonary capillary O_2 pressures are now equal, there is no longer a driving pressure for diffusion).

For CO_2, diffusion equilibrium between the blood and gas phases is normally also attained reasonably rapidly. At rest, the initial driving pressure for exchange, given by the difference between mixed venous P_{CO_2} and alveolar P_{CO_2}, is about 6 mm Hg (i.e., 46 mm Hg – 40 mm Hg, normally). This is an order of magnitude less than the corresponding driving pressure for O_2. The small CO_2 driving pressure, however, is more than offset by the substantially greater diffusibility of CO_2 relative to O_2. As a result, impairments that influence gaseous diffusion across the alveolar–capillary interface are likely to affect O_2 exchange before CO_2 exchange, leading in turn to arterial hypoxemia.

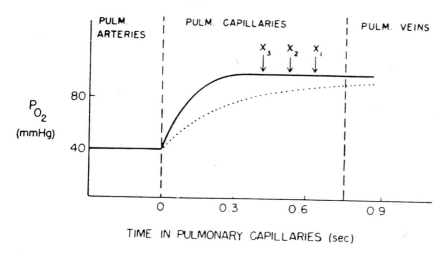

Figure 21–8. Time course of pulmonary capillary P_{O_2} in a normal lung (—) and a lung with a diffusion impairment (---). Shown is the effect of progressive increases in cardiac output, which reduce pulmonary capillary transit time (to X_1, X_2, and X_3) but do not normally encroach on time required for attainment of diffusion equilibrium. (*Reprinted, with permission, from Whipp BJ. The respiratory system. In: Ross G, ed. Essentials of human physiology.* Chicago: *Year Book Medical; 1982.*)

Diffusion equilibrium will be attained sooner in conditions that are associated with rapid rates of O_2 or CO_2 diffusion across the alveolar–capillary interface. In contrast, factors that cause a slowing of O_2 or CO_2 diffusion will delay the attainment of diffusion equilibrium. If these effects are sufficiently marked, blood will reach the end of the pulmonary capillary bed before equilibrium can occur. That is,

$$\text{pulmonary end-capillary } P_{O_2} < \text{alveolar } P_{O_2}$$

and

$$\text{pulmonary end-capillary } P_{CO_2} > \text{alveolar } P_{CO_2}$$

Diffusion impairment therefore predisposes to both arterial hypoxemia and arterial hypercapnia (or CO_2 retention).

With increased metabolic rate, the mixed venous P_{O_2} falls and the mixed venous P_{CO_2} rises because of the increased rates of tissue O_2 consumption and CO_2 production. This serves to widen the O_2 and CO_2 driving pressures for diffusion across the alveolar–capillary membrane and, in turn, causes more rapid rates of gas exchange. Conversely, when the driving pressure is reduced, the rate of diffusion is slowed. This can occur in hypoxemic conditions (altitude, inhalation of hypoxic gas mixtures, pulmonary disease) where, because of the sigmoid shape of the O_2 dissociation curve (Fig. 21–6), a given arteriovenous O_2 content difference (at rest, this is normally ~ 5 mL O_2/100 mL blood or 5 volume percent) will be associated with a smaller corresponding arteriovenous P_{O_2} difference if the arterial point falls on the lower, steeper portion of the dissociation curve. Therefore, the difference between mixed venous and alveolar O_2 pressures will also be smaller.

Alterations in both the surface area of the alveolar–capillary interface and the path length for diffusion between gas and blood phases can affect the rates of O_2 and CO_2 diffusion. The surface area for gas exchange can be increased under conditions in which the efficiency of regional gas exchange in the lungs is improved. This may occur on going from rest to exercise in the upright posture, as the increased cardiac output results in a more uniform perfusion of the pulmonary capillary bed (at rest in the upright posture, gravitational influences lead to a pooling of pulmonary blood toward the base of the lungs) and therefore a greater homogeneity of the regional alveolar ventilation-to-pul-

monary blood flow ($\dot{V}_A/\dot{Q}$) (see Ventilation–Perfusion Distribution). In contrast, pathologic conditions that increase the heterogeneity of the regional $\dot{V}_A/\dot{Q}$ matching (e.g., COPD) or that lead to a reduction in the number of functioning pulmonary capillaries (e.g., *pulmonary vascular occlusive disease*) compromise the surface area available for diffusion of O_2 and CO_2 between alveolar gas and pulmonary capillary blood.

Several pathologic conditions can lead to an increased path length for diffusion of O_2 and CO_2 across the alveolar-capillary interface. For example, in *pulmonary alveolar proteinosis*, an extrusion of proteinaceous material into the alveolar space occurs, limiting the alveolar volume and increasing the diffusion distance across the alveolar–capillary interface. The formation of edema in the lungs has a similar consequence.

It is important to recognize that, although factors such as the initial driving pressure for diffusion and the geometry of the alveolar–capillary interface may be normal, diffusion impairment can result under conditions in which the pulmonary capillary transit time is shortened. Modest progressive reductions in transit time, as schematized in Figure 21–8 (i.e., from X_1 to X_2 to X_3), as might be encountered in conditions that increase cardiac output, will not affect the P_{O_2} of pulmonary end-capillary blood as long as the transit time does not encroach on the time required for diffusion equilibrium to be attained. Should such encroachment occur, however, the blood P_{O_2} will not have sufficient time to attain the alveolar value and arterial hypoxemia will ensue.

This form of diffusion impairment may occur in response to marked increases in cardiac output (e.g., during severe exercise in highly fit athletes) or in conditions such as pulmonary vascular occlusive disease, in which the pulmonary capillary bed is compromised to such a degree that blood at a given cardiac output must traverse a fewer number of competent capillaries in a shorter period. More importantly, diffusion impairment may occur despite only a modest increase in cardiac output (and, therefore, a modest decrease in pulmonary capillary transit time) when this is accompanied by a decreased driving pressure for diffusion, a decreased surface area for exchange, or an increased path length for diffusion.

In the context of anesthesia, relatively soluble inhalational agents can influence O_2 and CO_2 diffusion. At the start of nitrous oxide anesthesia, relatively large quantities of N_2O initially will enter pulmonary capillary blood from alveolar gas. And as N_2O is more soluble than N_2, a smaller quantity of N_2 is displaced from the blood into the gas phase. This reduces the alveolar volume transiently and therefore concentrates both O_2 and CO_2 in the alveolar gas—the *concentration effect*. The converse occurs at the cessation of nitrous oxide anesthesia, leading to a temporary dilution of alveolar O_2 and CO_2. The reduction in P_{AO_2} that occurs at the end of N_2O administration narrows the driving pressure for O_2 diffusion across the alveolar–capillary membrane, slowing the rate of O_2 diffusion into blood; this predisposes to arterial hypoxemia or to its exacerbation should it be preexisting. This phenomenon has therefore been termed *diffusion hypoxia*.

Diffusion impairments are therefore characterized by arterial hypoxemia and a widened P_{AO_2}–P_{aO_2} difference, reflecting the lack of diffusion equilibrium between alveolar gas and pulmonary end-capillary blood. Inhalation of 100 percent O_2 can effectively abolish the diffusion component of the P_{AO_2}–P_{aO_2} difference. By increasing P_{AO_2} substantially and thus widening the initial driving pressure for diffusion from the gas phase to the blood phase, the rate of O_2 diffusion is speeded; the P_{O_2} in pulmonary capillary blood therefore rises more rapidly.

DEAD SPACE

The dead space refers to those regions of the respiratory tract and lungs in which no gas exchange takes place. The ventilation of these regions can therefore be regarded as wasted ventilation. The total respiratory dead space is called the physiologic dead space. This has two major components: the *anatomic dead space*, which comprises the respiratory tract, and the *alveolar dead space*, which represents those alveoli that are ventilated but not perfused and in which, therefore, gas exchange cannot occur.

Anatomic Dead Space

The anatomic dead space ($V_{DS_{ANAT}}$) is normally about 150 mL in a normal healthy adult. A variety of factors can influence the volume of the anatomic dead space. For example, body size influences $V_{DS_{ANAT}}$ through an effect on the dimensions of the respiratory tract. It is useful to note that $V_{DS_{ANAT}}$ (in milliliters) is approximately equal to the weight of an individual (in pounds). Posture also affects $V_{DS_{ANAT}}$. Changing from the sitting position to a semireclining posture, and likewise to the supine posture, typically causes $V_{DS_{ANAT}}$ to decrease. These effects can amount to as much as ~ 15 percent of $V_{DS_{ANAT}}$.

Lung volume can influence $V_{DS_{ANAT}}$: it is larger at the end of inspiration than at the end of expiration. This reflects the greater traction exerted on the airways by the surrounding lung parenchyma at higher lung volumes. Because of the poor distensibility of the less compliant upper and conducting airways, however, the magnitude of this effect is not large (i.e., ~ 20 mL/L of lung volume). As a result,

under conditions in which tidal volume is increased (most usually because of ventilatory stimulation), the bulk of the increased volume occurs at the alveolar level and, consequently, the ratio of $V_{DS_{ANAT}}$ to V_T decreases.

The anatomic dead space can be affected by the position of the head. An increase in $V_{DS_{ANAT}}$ of as much as 20 percent may occur with hyperextension. Bronchoconstrictor agents (e.g., histamine) may decrease $V_{DS_{ANAT}}$, whereas bronchodilators (e.g., aminophylline, hexamethonium, atropine) would be expected to have the opposite effect.

Intubation leads to a reduction in the anatomic dead space, as some 50 percent of the volume of the conducting airways is typically bypassed. Apparatus dead space in an anesthesia circuit (i.e., the volume of the face mask, endotracheal tube, and connectors up to the level of the Y-piece*) increases $V_{DS_{ANAT}}$. This can be kept to a minimum during anesthesia by not placing extensions between the face mask or endotracheal tube and the Y-piece.

Several techniques may be used to measure the anatomic dead space. The *single-breath technique* developed by Fowler uses the profile of exhaled $[N_2]$ which obtains during the expiration that immediately follows the single inspiration of a nitrogen-free gas, such as 100 percent O_2. In an ideal situation, $[N_2]$ would be expected to remain at zero from the onset of expiration until such time as the entire volume of the anatomic dead space (which contains 100 percent O_2 in this instance) had been exhaled. Thereafter, $[N_2]$ would rise abruptly and instantaneously to reach the alveolar value (this reflecting the composition of gas in the alveolar volume during the previous breath, influenced by the inhalation of the O_2 and the simultaneous uptake of O_2 by the blood), at which it would remain until the start of the next inspiration.

In reality, however, the transition between the anatomic-dead-space and alveolar phases is not instantaneous (although it is normally reasonably rapid) (Fig. 21–9). This is predominantly a result of some alveoli having shorter airways and therefore smaller regional dead spaces than others; alveolar gas from these alveoli will thus start to "contaminate" the dead-space gas that is still being exhaled from other regions. It is necessary to correct for the $V_{DS_{ANAT}}$ contribution to this transitional phase. This is accomplished by assigning the volume exhaled during the transitional phase equally to the dead-space and alveolar phases; that is, as shown in Fig. 21–9, such that the areas of region A (assigned to the dead-space phase) and region B (assigned to the alveolar phase) are exactly equal. In other words, it is assumed that all the exhaled N_2 has come from an alveolar compartment with uniform exchange characteristics.

A second approach is the CO_2 *proportion technique* pioneered by Bohr. This CO_2-based method assumes that the total amount of CO_2 exhaled during a complete exhalation derives solely from the alveolar phase. That is, the tidal volume can be empirically subdivided into dead-space and alveolar phases, with the exhaled CO_2 being confined to the latter. The total volume of CO_2 exhaled (V_{CO_2}) is easily measured as the product of the tidal volume (V_T) and its frac-

---

* The Y-piece is the point in an anesthesia circuit where the inhaled gas and the exhaled gas no longer traverse the same pathway.

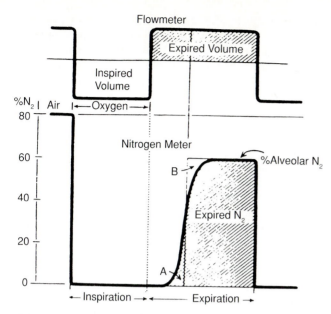

Figure 21–9. Single-breath analysis for measurement of anatomic dead space. Upper panel: idealized airflow profile, which for simplicity indicates a constant flow rate in inspiration and expiration (cf. Fig. 21–4). Lower panel: corresponding profile for 100 percent oxygen. See text for further details. (*Reprinted, with permission, from Comroe JH Jr. Physiology of respiration. 2nd ed. Chicago: Year Book Medical; 1974.*)

tional concentration of CO_2, which is termed the *mixed expired CO_2 fraction* ($F\bar{E}CO_2$):

$$V_{CO_2} = V_T \cdot F\bar{E}CO_2$$

As this volume of CO_2 actually originated from the alveoli, it can also be expressed in terms of the portion of the tidal volume that is alveolar gas (V_A) and the fractional concentration of CO_2 in alveolar gas (F_{ACO_2}):

$$V_{CO_2} = V_A \cdot F_{ACO_2}$$

Combining these two expressions,

$$V_T \cdot F\bar{E}CO_2 = V_A \cdot F_{ACO_2}$$

Substituting for V_A (i.e., $= [V_T - V_{DS_{ANAT}}]$) and rearranging,

$$V_{DS_{ANAT}}/V_T = \frac{F_{ACO_2} - F\bar{E}CO_2}{F_{ACO_2}}$$

Then, transforming fractional concentration to partial pressure by multiplying by (barometric pressure – 47),

$$V_{DS_{ANAT}}/V_T = \frac{P_{ACO_2} - P\bar{E}CO_2}{P_{ACO_2}}$$

The volume of the anatomic dead space is important in determining how effective a particular level of total or minute ventilation ($\dot{V}_E$) is in promoting gas exchange. Given that the volume of inspired air that actually enters the alveolar compartment each breath is

$$V_A = V_T - V_{DS_{ANAT}}$$

then the alveolar ventilation is given by

$$(V_A \times f) = (V_T \times f) - (V_{DS_{ANAT}} \times f)$$

or

$$\dot{V}_A = \dot{V}_E - \dot{V}_{DS_{ANAT}}$$

where f is the breathing frequency, $\dot{V}_A$ is the alveolar ventilation, and $\dot{V}_{DS_{ANAT}}$ is the ventilation of the anatomic dead space.

In the face of an increase in the anatomic dead space, the alveolar ventilation can be preserved (and appropriate levels of O_2 and CO_2 exchange therefore maintained) if $\dot{V}_E$ is caused to increase; this can be accomplished by an increase in V_T, f, or both. It is important to recognize that although an increase in the volume of the anatomic dead space can lead to hypoventilation of the alveolar compartment and hence a fall in alveolar PO_2 (P_{AO_2}) and an increase in alveolar PCO_2 (P_{ACO_2}), this of itself will not impair the gas-exchanging characteristics of the lungs. Any fall in P_{AO_2} will be reflected in the arterial PO_2. As a result, arterial hypoxemia prevails, but the P_{AO_2}–Pa_{O_2} difference is not widened.

Physiologic Dead Space

Because the physiologic dead space ($V_{DS_{PHYS}}$) reflects not only the volume of the anatomic dead space but also that of the alveolar dead space ($V_{DS_{ALV}}$), which is susceptible to increase in many cardiopulmonary disease states, it generally receives more attention.

In healthy individuals, as $V_{DS_{ALV}}$ is negligible, the volumes of the physiologic and anatomic dead space are similar. At rest, the physiologic dead space typically represents about 30 percent of the tidal volume. This fraction decreases somewhat under conditions in which cardiac output is increased, providing a more even perfusion of the lungs and therefore reducing the (already low) alveolar dead space (see Ventilation–Perfusion Distribution). A similar distribution improvement can be accomplished by adopting the supine posture, which reduces the influence of gravity on the lungs (i.e., their vertical height may be reduced by as much as 30 percent). Hence, perfusion of the nondependent regions of the supine lung does not require such a high pulmonary artery pressure as in the upright lung.

Conversely, conditions that lead to reduced pulmonary artery pressures (e.g., hemorrhage, administration of atropine, nitroglycerin, or sodium nitroprusside) accentuate the alveolar dead space, owing to reduced perfusion of the nondependent regions of the lungs (see Ventilation–Perfusion Distribution). In COPD, $V_{DS_{ALV}}$ may be substantially increased, owing to regions of $\dot{V}_A/\dot{Q}$ mismatching which develop as a result of regional pulmonary tissue destruction and airway obstruction. Pulmonary embolism has a similar effect because of regional obstruction in the pulmonary capillary bed.

Anesthesia leads to an increase in the volume of the alveolar dead space. The underlying causes are unclear, however. Pulmonary hypotension appears to be an unlikely factor. There may, however, be an involvement of $\dot{V}_A/\dot{Q}$ maldistribution. Artificial ventilation in the lateral decubitus position may increase $V_{DS_{ALV}}$, as there is likely to be a preferential distribution of ventilation to the nondependent lung (especially when the pleural membranes are opened in thoracotomy), whereas the pulmonary blood flow is distributed primarily to the dependent lung. The $\dot{V}_A/\dot{Q}$ ratio will therefore be low in the dependent lung and high in the nondependent lung.

The most widely used approach for estimating the volume of the physiologic dead space is the *modified* Bohr method (see above). It relies on the assumption that the alveolar volume (V_A) is not homogeneous, and can be viewed as a dead-space component ($V_{DS_{ALV}}$) and a gas-exchanging component ($V_{A_{EX}}$). Thus,

$$V_{DS_{PHYS}} = V_{DS_{ANAT}} + V_{DS_{ALV}}$$

and

$$V_T = V_{A_{EX}} + V_{DS_{PHYS}}$$

As discussed earlier, the total volume of CO_2 exhaled is given by

$$V_{CO_2} = V_T \cdot F\overline{E}_{CO_2}$$

As this volume of CO_2 originated in the *exchanging* alveoli, it can also be expressed in terms of the portion of the tidal volume that derives from the exchanging alveoli ($V_{A_{EX}}$) and the associated fractional CO_2 concentration ($F_{A_{EX}CO_2}$):

$$V_{CO_2}V_{A_{EX}} \cdot F_{A_{EX}CO_2}$$

Therefore,

$$V_T \cdot F\overline{E}_{CO_2} = V_{A_{EX}} \cdot F_{A_{EX}CO_2}$$

Using a development similar to that presented earlier,

$$V_{DS_{PHYS}}/V_T = \frac{P_{A_{EX}CO_2} - P\overline{E}_{CO_2}}{P_{A_{EX}CO_2}}$$

Making the further assumption that the P_{CO_2} in arterial blood equals $P_{A_{EX}CO_2}$,

$$V_{DS_{PHYS}}/V_T = \frac{Pa_{CO_2} - P\overline{E}_{CO_2}}{Pa_{CO_2}}$$

The quantity $V_{DS_{PHYS}}/V_T$ (or, more usually, V_D/V_T) is termed the *physiologic dead-space fraction of the breath* and is widely used as a means of quantitating gas-exchange impairments in terms of dead-space abnormality. Such impairment is characterized by arterial hypoxemia and (in contrast to increases in the anatomic dead space) a widened $P_{AO_2}–Pa_{O_2}$ difference (see Ventilation–Perfusion Distribution).

SHUNT

By analogy with dead space, shunt may be regarded as that portion of the cardiac output that does not participate in gas exchange. Likewise, the total or physiologic shunt may be viewed as the sum of an anatomic shunt and an alveolar shunt.

Not all tissues and organs contribute blood to the common venous return, however. A few, such as the larger airways of the respiratory tree (bronchial veins) and the myocardium (thebesian veins), drain into the circulation downstream of the pulmonary capillary bed (i.e., after gas exchange has taken place). This component constitutes the anatomic shunt, and normally amounts to less than 5 percent of the total cardiac output. The addition of this venous blood to the arterialized stream causes a small reduction in P_{O_2} between the end of the pulmonary capillary bed and the systemic arterial circulation (typically, no more than about 5 mm Hg). The prominence of the anatomic shunt can be increased substantially in clinical conditions characterized by the presence of an intracardiac right-to-left shunt (e.g., atrial or ventricular septal defects).

The alveolar shunt represents the fraction of the cardiac output that perfuses the pulmonary capillary bed but is directed to nonventilated alveoli. In the normal individual, the alveolar shunt is negligible. It can, however, assume considerable significance in pulmonary disease states where factors such as regional airway obstruction can lead to collapse (*atelectasis*).

During anesthesia, there is evidence of an increased shunt (typically, about 10 percent of the cardiac output). Although the precise reasons for this are not clear, development of $\dot{V}_A/\dot{Q}$ mismatching may be involved, as a result of factors such as airway and alveolar collapse and possibly an impaired hypoxicpulmonary vasoconstrictor response (see Ventilation–Perfusion Distribution).

The magnitude of the physiologic shunt can be estimated in a fashion analogous to that used for dead-space estimation, except that oxygen is the gas of reference. The cardiac output ($\dot{Q}_T$) is assumed to be made up of two components: a *shunt component* ($\dot{Q}_S$) composed of anatomic and alveolar shunt, which contains blood having a mixed venous content ($C\overline{v}_{O_2}$), and an *alveolar component* ($\dot{Q}_{A_{EX}}$), which perfuses the exchanging alveoli and has an O_2 content equal to that of pulmonary end-capillary blood (Cc'_{O_2}). Thus,

$$\dot{Q}_T = \dot{Q}_S + \dot{Q}_{A_{EX}}$$

The rate at which O_2 is transported by the cardiac output into the systemic arterial circulation is given by

$$\dot{Q}_{O_2} = \dot{Q}_T \cdot Ca_{O_2}$$

where Ca_{O_2} is the arterial O_2 content. And as the O_2 entering the systemic arterial circulation derives from the shunt and the exchanging alveoli, this can also be expressed as

$$\dot{Q}_{O_2} = (\dot{Q}_S \cdot C\overline{v}_{O_2}) + (\dot{Q}_{A_{EX}} \cdot Cc'_{O_2})$$

Thus,

$$(\dot{Q}_T \cdot Ca_{O_2}) = (\dot{Q}_S \cdot C\overline{v}_{O_2}) + (\dot{Q}_{A_{EX}} \cdot Cc'_{O_2})$$

Rearranging this yields the shunt fraction of the cardiac output:

$$\frac{\dot{Q}_S}{\dot{Q}_T} = \frac{Cc'_{O_2} - Ca_{O_2}}{Cc'_{O_2} - C\overline{v}_{O_2}}$$

The arterial and mixed venous O_2 contents can be measured by means of direct blood sampling. An indirect estimate of the Cc'_{O_2} is obtained by assuming that the alveolar P_{O_2}

(which can be measured directly or derived from the alveolar air equation, as described under Oxygen Transport) equals the P_{O_2} of pulmonary end-capillary blood, and then using a standard O_2 dissociation curve to obtain the corresponding O_2 content.

The isoshunt diagram developed by Nunn is a useful alternative for estimating $\dot{Q}_S/\dot{Q}_T$ when pulmonary artery catheterization is not available for the sampling of mixed venous blood (Fig. 21–10). This diagram depicts the relationship between arterial P_{O_2} and the inspired O_2 fraction (F_{IO_2}) for a series of isoshunt bands, which are sufficiently wide to accommodate variations of Pa_{CO_2} (25 to 40 mm Hg) and hemoglobin concentration (10 to 14 mg/100 mL blood), assuming a constant value for the arteriovenous O_2 content difference of 5 mL O_2/100 mL blood.*

Hence, from knowledge of the Pa_{O_2} and F_{IO_2}, it is possible to predict the magnitude of the shunt fraction, $\dot{Q}_S/\dot{Q}_T$. This, in turn, allows prediction of the level of F_{IO_2} required to establish a particular level of Pa_{O_2}. It is important to emphasize that such predictions rely on the assumption that shunt is the primary gas-exchange defect and that the magnitude of the shunt is independent of Pa_{O_2}. It is also crucial to recognize that the isoshunt technique should *not* be used under conditions in which the arteriovenous O_2 content difference is likely to change, as would occur if tissue O_2 consumption or cardiac output were to change.

The degree to which arterial P_{O_2} is reduced in the presence of a shunt depends primarily on the size of the shunt.

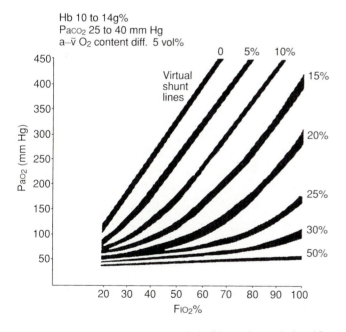

Figure 21–10. Isoshunt chart describing the relationship between arterial P_{O_2} and inspired O_2 fraction for a range of shunt fractions (0 to 50 percent). (*Reprinted, with permission, from Benatar SR, Hewlett AM, Nunn JF. The Use of Iso-Shunt Lines for Control of Oxygen Therapy. Br J Anaesth. 1973;45:713.*)

* As the arteriovenous O_2 content difference is not measured directly in this approach, it is usual to refer to the shunt as the "virtual shunt."

Also important is the location of the pulmonary end-capillary and mixed venous points on the O_2 dissociation curve. For example, assuming that the gas-exchanging portion of the lungs is operating effectively, the end-capillary point will be on the upper, flat portion of the curve (e.g., Pc'_{O_2} = 100 mm Hg, Cc'_{O_2} = 20 mL O_2/100 mL blood), whereas the mixed venous point (e.g., $P\bar{v}_{O_2}$ = 40 mm Hg, $C\bar{v}_{O_2}$ = 15 mL O_2/100 mL blood) will lie on the lower, steep portion (Fig. 21–6). Admixture of blood from these two sources yields arterial blood of an intermediate O_2 content.

For example, assuming that 20 percent of the cardiac output is shunt, the resulting Ca_{O_2} is given by $(20 \cdot C\bar{v}_{O_2} + 80 \cdot Cc'_{O_2})/100$, that is, 19 mL O_2/100 mL blood; however, because of the curvature of the dissociation curve, the corresponding arterial P_{O_2} is weighted toward $P\bar{v}_{O_2}$.

The presence of a shunt is characterized by arterial hypoxemia and a widened PA_{O_2}–Pa_{O_2} difference, even though pulmonary end-capillary P_{O_2} may be normal. Oxygen administration increases Pa_{O_2} in the presence of a shunt. On occasion, the magnitude of a shunt may actually be increased in the face of sustained O_2 breathing, thus causing further widening of the PA_{O_2}–Pa_{O_2} difference. This is the consequence of *absorption atelectasis*, a condition in which O_2 molecules are absorbed by pulmonary capillary blood at a greater rate than they can be delivered to the alveoli from the inspirate. It is often seen in COPD. Alveolar collapse results and the magnitude of the alveolar shunt is increased.

VENTILATION–PERFUSION DISTRIBUTION

Considerations of effective pulmonary gas exchange and therefore the provision of a normal arterial P_{O_2} and P_{CO_2} should also incorporate the regional distribution of alveolar ventilation to pulmonary capillary perfusion (i.e., $\dot{V}_A/\dot{Q}$) throughout the lungs. It is not sufficient that the *overall* levels of $\dot{V}_A$ and $\dot{Q}$ are approximately equal (i.e., yielding an overall $\dot{V}_A/\dot{Q}\sim1.0$); the *regional* rates of alveolar ventilation and perfusion should also be well matched.

The consequences of variations in $\dot{V}_A$ and $\dot{Q}$ on Pa_{O_2} and Pa_{CO_2} can be illustrated by the following simple example, in which the lungs are described as a single uniform compartment. Let us assume that at rest $\dot{V}_A$ and $\dot{Q}$ both equal 5 L/min. This yields a $\dot{V}_A/\dot{Q}$ of 1.0, and normal values for Pa_{O_2} and Pa_{CO_2} of 100 and 40 mm Hg, respectively.

Now assume that the airway is abruptly and completely obstructed so that no fresh air enters the alveoli during the subsequent inspiration. The uptake of O_2 into blood from, and the release of CO_2 into, the trapped gas of the alveolar compartment continues by diffusion until the respective O_2 and CO_2 driving pressures for diffusion between the gas the blood phases are abolished. Therefore, alveolar P_{O_2} falls progressively and alveolar P_{CO_2} rises, to eventually attain their respective mixed venous values; PA_{O_2} = 40 mm Hg and PA_{CO_2} = 46 mm Hg. And as $\dot{V}_A$ is now zero, $\dot{V}_A/\dot{Q} = 0/5 = 0$. This situation corresponds to a total alveolar shunt (see above).

At the other extreme, we can assume that the pulmonary capillary bed is completely obstructed. Thus, although the alveoli are ventilated normally (i.e., $\dot{V}_A$ = 5 L/min), there can be no exchange of O_2 or CO_2 with blood.

Thus, $\dot{V}_A/\dot{Q} = 5/0 = \infty$, with the alveolar gas tensions now being equal to the inspiratory gas tensions; that is, $P_{AO_2} = 149$ mm Hg and $P_{ACO_2} = 0$. This condition represents a total alveolar dead space.

Clearly, all possible combinations of $\dot{V}_A/\dot{Q}$ between total shunt ($\dot{V}_A/\dot{Q} = 0$) and total dead space ($\dot{V}_A/\dot{Q} = \infty$) could exist regionally within the lungs. For example, a condition characterized by a lower-than-normal $\dot{V}_A$ (i.e., hypoventilation) would yield a $\dot{V}_A/\dot{Q}$ less than 1.0 (but greater than zero), P_{AO_2} between 100 and 40 mm Hg, and P_{ACO_2} between 40 and 46 mm Hg. Conversely, with a greater-than-normal $\dot{V}_A$ (i.e., hyperventilation), $\dot{V}_A/\dot{Q}$ would be greater than 1.0 but less than infinity, P_{AO_2} would lie between 100 and 149 mm Hg, and P_{ACO_2} would lie between 40 and 0 mm Hg.

In conditions where alveolar P_{O_2} is low (e.g., inadequate alveolar ventilation or low inspired P_{O_2}), pulmonary arterioles typically become constricted. This phenomenon, known as *hypoxic pulmonary vasoconstriction* (HPV), can lead to significant elevation of pulmonary arterial pressures if the alveolar hypoxia is widespread (e.g., COPD, sleep apnea syndromes, residence at altitude), predisposing to pulmonary edema and right-sided heart failure (or cor pulmonale). Administration of oxygen can often ameliorate the pressor response in such conditions.

When alveolar hypoxia is localized to particular regions of the lungs, such as occurs with regional impairments of alveolar ventilation (e.g., COPD, atelectasis), HPV serves to divert much of blood flow away from these under-ventilated regions (having a low P_{AO_2}) to areas of the lungs that are better ventilated and thus have a higher P_{AO_2}. In this way, perfusion is more evenly matched with ventilation. This mechanism therefore reduces the degree of alveolar shunt and minimizes local deviations in $\dot{V}_A/\dot{Q}$.

HPV represents a direct vasoconstrictive effect on the smooth muscle of adjacent pulmonary vessels (i.e., mediated independently of autonomic nervous system innervation). It has been proposed that alveolar hypoxia initiates the release of vasoactive substances (e.g., histamine, serotonin, catecholamines, prostaglandins, leukotrines) which, in turn, induce contraction of pulmonary arteriolar smooth muscle.

Inhalational anesthetic agents have been reported to inhibit HPV, though this is not the case for intravenous anesthetics. This inhibitory action might be expected to increase the perfusion of poorly ventilated regions of the lungs. The inappropriately high perfusion (relative to ventilation) leads to a lowering of both alveolar and pulmonary end-capillary P_{O_2} in these regions, predisposing toward arterial hypoxemia. It has been suggested that inhibition of HPV may contribute to the increased alveolar shunt, $\dot{V}_A/\dot{Q}$ maldistribution, and $P_{AO_2}-P_{aO_2}$ difference that occur during anesthesia.

Owing to the effect of gravity, blood entering the lungs is not evenly distributed to all of the pulmonary capillaries. In the sitting or standing posture, the perfusion of the apices of the lungs is less than to the middle or basal segments because the pulmonary artery pressure is not normally sufficiently high—at least, at rest—to propel blood against the force of gravity. As a result, even the lungs of a healthy individual show evidence of an uneven regional distribution of both alveolar ventilation (see Mechanics of Ventilation) and perfusion, owing to the influence of gravity.

Therefore, as shown in Figure 21–11, both $\dot{V}_A$ and $\dot{Q}$ are distributed preferentially to the dependent regions of the lungs (the base in the upright posture). This effect, however, is more striking for $\dot{Q}$ than for $\dot{V}_A$: although the nondependent regions have a low $\dot{V}_A$ and a low $\dot{Q}$, the $\dot{V}_A/\dot{Q}$ is higher than the average value for the whole lung. These hyperventilated areas therefore have a P_{O_2} in alveolar gas and pulmonary end-capillary blood that is higher than normal and a corresponding P_{CO_2} that is lower than normal. Conversely, the dependent regions of the lungs have higher $\dot{V}_A$ and $\dot{Q}$ relative to the rest of the lungs, resulting in a low $\dot{V}_A/\dot{Q}$. These areas are thus hypoventilated, having a lower-than-normal P_{O_2} and a higher-than-normal P_{CO_2} in both alveolar gas and pulmonary end-capillary blood.

The mean alveolar P_{O_2} and P_{CO_2} are determined by the arithmetic mean of their regional partial pressures, weighted by regional volume. (Because regional volume variations are far less prominent than the corresponding perfusion changes in normal lungs, their influence is assumed to be relatively minor in the present context.) Thus, although P_{AO_2} at the base of the lungs is low and that at the apex is high (and conversely for P_{ACO_2}), admixture of alveolar gas from these different regions of the lungs will normally yield typical average values of about 100 mm Hg for P_{AO_2} and 40 mm Hg for P_{ACO_2}.

Prediction of the mean arterial P_{O_2} and P_{CO_2}, however, is complicated by the more marked differences in regional perfusion and, in the case of O_2, the sigmoid character of the O_2 dissociation curve (see Shunt) (Fig. 21–6). The composition of the arterial blood will therefore be biased in favor of the relatively highly perfused dependent regions. These regions have a relatively high CO_2 content and a low O_2 content, which, in turn, yield an arterial P_{CO_2} that is slightly higher than the average P_{ACO_2} and an arterial P_{O_2} that is

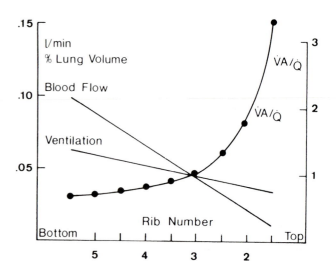

Figure 21–11. Distribution of ventilation, perfusion, and ventilation–perfusion ratios in the upright lung. (*Reprinted, with permission, from West JB. Respiratory physiology: The essentials. Baltimore: Williams & Wilkins; 1990.*)

somewhat less than the average $P_{A_{O_2}}$. This effect is exacerbated for O_2 where the arterialized (i.e., end-capillary) blood from the hyperventilated nondependent regions lies on the upper, flat portion of the O_2 dissociation curve whereas that from the dependent regions lies on the lower, steeper portion. The arterial O_2 content resulting from their admixture thus yields a P_{O_2} that is biased toward the lower, basal value (i.e., the average arterial point, of necessity, also lies on a steeper portion of the dissociation curve) (see Shunt).

In cardiorespiratory disease states, the degree of regional maldistribution of both $\dot{V}_A$ and $\dot{Q}$ can be quite striking, leading to wide regional variations in $\dot{V}_A/\dot{Q}$, characteristic, for example, of COPD and pulmonary vascular occlusive disease. This situation can result in extreme degrees of arterial hypoxemia, together with a substantial widening of the $P_{A_{O_2}}$–$P_{a_{O_2}}$ difference.

During anesthesia, there is evidence of development of $\dot{V}_A/\dot{Q}$ mismatching. The exact causes remain unclear, although the functional consequences for pulmonary gas exchange are well recognized: small airway collapse in the dependent regions of the lung, collapse of involved alveoli owing to absorption of O_2 from the alveolar space into the pulmonary capillary blood (i.e., absorption atelectasis), and therefore alveolar vascular shunting. In addition, it has been proposed that anesthesia may impair the hypoxic pulmonary vasoconstrictor response (see above).

The presence of $\dot{V}_A/\dot{Q}$ maldistribution is therefore characterized by arterial hypoxemia and a widened $P_{A_{O_2}}$–$P_{a_{O_2}}$ difference. The arterial hypoxemia that results from regional mismatching of $\dot{V}_A$ and $\dot{Q}$ is typically abolished by O_2 inhalation. This reflects a far more rapid rate of delivery of individual O_2 molecules to the poorly ventilated regions (i.e., regions with a low $\dot{V}_A/\dot{Q}$).

CONTROL OF VENTILATION

Spontaneous ventilation is produced by the rhythmic discharge of the motor neurons that innervate the respiratory muscles. The muscles of respiration do not have the property of inherent rhythmicity possessed by heart muscle, but rather are dependent on their nerve supply to bring about contraction. The periodic nature of inspiration and expiration is initiated and controlled by diffuse collections of neurons located in the medulla and pons, whose functions appear to be closely integrated. These regions receive neural and chemical inputs from sensing elements placed strategically in the body and also from higher centers such as the hypothalamus, the limbic system, and the cerebral cortex.

Considerable capability normally exists for influencing breathing volitionally (or consciously), even to the extent of overriding the more fundamental control processes. This is demonstrated by activities such as breath holding while swimming underwater and by speaking. Furthermore, the maximal level of ventilation that a normal individual can generate volitionally typically exceeds the highest level observed during the severest exercise. Also, on emerging from anesthesia, patients are often able to breathe quite forcefully in response to instruction, even though arterial P_{CO_2} may be very low (and therefore presumably restraining the activity of the central and peripheral chemoreceptors).

Brainstem Mechanisms

Considerable insight into the role of the brainstem in the control of breathing has derived from studies employing sequential brainstem transections in anesthetized animals (Fig. 21–12). If the brainstem is sectioned at the junction of the pons and the midbrain, there is no effect on breathing pattern. In contrast, transection at the junction of the pons and medulla is associated with a pattern of breathing that, although rhythmic, is less smooth in the transition between inspiration and expiration (and vice versa) and is also more rapid. All breathing movements are completely abolished with transection at the junction of the medulla and the spinal cord. On the basis of these observations, it was concluded that the medulla was responsible for the generation of respiratory rhythmicity, with the pons exerting a modulating influence.

Further insight into the involvement of the pons was indicated by means of a midpontine transection which, when coupled with bilateral cervical vagotomy, caused a sustained inspiratory effort (also termed *apneusis*). With the vagi intact, however, the transection resulted in a slower rhythmic pattern of breathing characterized by a longer-than-normal inspiratory duration (i.e., apneustic breathing). Thus, the fundamental rhythmogenic mechanisms of the medulla appear to be subject to a strong inspiratory drive from the caudal pons; the periodic interruption of this drive by either rostral pontine or vagal afferent influences ensures that breathing retains its rhythmic character.

More recent techniques involving the identification and mapping of respiratory-related cells within the brainstem have provided a more precise picture of the neuronal basis for the generation and modulation of respiratory rhythm. The medulla contains both inspiratory and expiratory neurons, which are located in the reticular formation beneath the floor of the fourth ventricle. It is thought that the rhythmic discharges of these neurons produce the rhythmic pat-

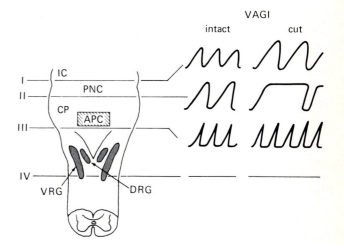

Figure 21–12. Effects of transections at various brainstem levels. APC, apneustic center; CP, cerebellar peduncle; DRG, dorsal respiratory group; IC, inferior colliculus; PNC, pneumotaxic center; VRG, ventral respiratory group. (*Reprinted, with permission, from Berger AJ, Mitchell RA, et al. Regulation of respiration.* N Engl J Med. *1977;297:140.*)

tern of breathing. These neurons are not located in discrete areas, but are anatomically intermingled; however, two dense bilateral concentrations of respiratory neurons have now been identified in the medulla: the dorsal respiratory group and the ventral respiratory group.

The *dorsal respiratory group* (DRG) is located in the nucleus of the tractus solitarius. It is composed primarily of inspiratory cells, which project to the spinal cord and stimulate the contralateral phrenic neurons to initiate contraction of the diaphragm. DRG cells also project to the ventral respiratory group and the pons. The DRG receives afferent projections from sources such as the glossopharyngeal and vagus nerves. It is thought that the DRG plays a primary role in respiratory motor control and respiratory phase switching and may be the site of medullary respiratory rhythmogenesis.

The *ventral respiratory group* (VRG) is composed of both inspiratory and expiratory neurons, which project to phrenic, intercostal, and abdominal motoneurons. The VRG has two divisions, the cranial division and the caudal division. The cranial division, composed of neurons in the nucleus ambiguus, innervates primarily the laryngeal musculature by way of the recurrent laryngeal nerves. The caudal division, composed of neurons in the nucleus retroambigualis, has various projections: to the contralateral nucleus retroambigualis and to spinal respiratory motoneurons, for example. The VRG is thought to be the final integrating site for respiratory-related activity in the brainstem.

Two pontine areas are recognized in the context of brainstem respiratory control: the *apneustic center* and the *pneumotaxic center*. The apneustic center is located in the caudal pons and is thought to be responsible for the generation of the sustained inspiratory activity that leads to apneusis. This activity of the *apneustic center* appears to be restrained by influences from the more rostral pneumotaxic center and from the vagus nerves. The apneustic center therefore appears to represent an important integrating site for mechanisms involved in inspiratory termination.

The *pneumotaxic center* is located in the rostral pons within the nucleus parabrachialis medialis. Consistent with the postulated role of the pneumotaxic center as a modulator of respiratory rhythm, electrical stimulation of its dorsal region can hasten the onset of inspiration, whereas stimulation in the ventral region hastens expiration.

Modulation of Brainstem Mechanisms

A variety of regions are able to influence the level and pattern of ventilation. As mentioned earlier, these include higher centers of the nervous system as well as reflex inputs. Their precise contribution to ventilatory control will vary with the prevailing conditions.

Central Chemoreceptors. Central chemoreceptors are located superficially on the ventral medullary surface within bilateral rostral and caudal regions. They are thought to be stimulated by increases in the P_{CO_2} or $[H^+]$ of the local extracellular fluid; it is the hydrogen ion, however, that is thought to represent the primary stimulus to the receptor, with the CO_2 molecule exerting its effect via its hydration to H^+ and HCO_3^-. Because CO_2 molecules can dif-

fuse freely between cerebral extracellular fluids and cerebral capillary blood (by way of the blood–brain barrier), the central chemoreceptors are also responsive to increases in arterial P_{CO_2}. As the blood–brain barrier is relatively impermeable to hydrogen ions, however, the central chemoreceptors are unable to respond to metabolically induced alterations in arterial pH. It is important to point out that the central chemoreceptors are anatomically and functionally distinct from the medullary respiratory centers; the latter are located more deeply within the medullary tissue and have no chemosensory properties. The primary reflex consequence of central chemoreceptor stimulation is hyperpnea.*

Carotid Body Chemoreceptors. The carotid bodies are paired structures located at the bifurcation of the common carotid arteries. Chemoreceptors contained within the carotid bodies project to the brainstem respiratory centers by way of the carotid sinus nerve (nerve of Hering), a branch of the glossopharyngeal nerve (IXth cranial nerve). Analogous chemosensory structures, the *aortic bodies,* are located in the region of the aortic arch and innervated by the vagus nerve; however, their primary reflex function in humans involves cardiovascular rather than ventilatory control.

The carotid receptors are responsive to increases in arterial P_{CO_2} and $[H^+]$ and (unlike the central chemoreceptors) to decreases in arterial P_{O_2}. As for the central chemoreceptors, the stimulatory action of the CO_2 molecule is thought to be exerted via the hydrogen ion formed in its hydration. The presence of arterial hypoxemia normally potentiates carotid chemoreceptor responsiveness, resulting in a larger increase in discharge frequency for a given increment in arterial P_{CO_2} or $[H^+]$.

The reflex action of the carotid chemoreceptors is primarily to increase ventilation. In humans, the carotid bodies appear less important than the central chemoreceptors in establishing resting levels of ventilation. The integrity of the carotid bodies is, however, essential if a compensatory hyperpnea is to accompany either arterial hypoxemia or arterial metabolic acidosis.

Pulmonary Mechanoreceptors. Three major categories of vagally innervated pulmonary mechanoreceptors are recognized with regard to the control of ventilation and, in particular, its pattern: the pulmonary stretch receptor, the irritant receptor, and the juxtapulmonary-capillary (or J) receptor.

Stretch Receptors. Stretch receptors are located in the smooth muscle of the airways and respond to lung inflation, evidencing slowly adapting discharge characteristics. Their major reflex action is to inhibit inspiration, that is, the *Hering–Breuer inflation reflex.* As the lungs inflate during inspiration, these receptors become activated to terminate the inspiration (they may also induce bronchodilation, tachycardia, and vasoconstriction). There is some controversy concerning the significance of this reflex during quiet breathing in humans, as the strength of the reflex is weak in the tidal range; however, it may assume greater importance

---

* Hyperpnea refers to a condition of increased minute ventilation.

at the higher tidal volumes characteristic of stimulated breathing. The role of the inflation reflex may therefore be to prevent overinflation of the lungs.

Common inhaled anesthetics, such as halothane, appear to sensitize pulmonary stretch receptors, increasing discharge at a given lung volume. It has been proposed that this effect underlies the relatively rapid, shallow breathing pattern typically seen with administration of inhaled anesthetics.

Irritant Receptors. Irritant receptors are so called because they are stimulated by inhaled dust, smoke, cold air, histamine, and irritant gases (including diethyl ether, but not halothane). They are also stimulated by mechanical influences, including rapid changes in lung volume. These receptors are located in the airway epithelium, particularly of the larger airways; they exhibit rapidly adapting discharge characteristics. The reflex consequences of irritant receptor stimulation range from cough, bronchoconstriction, and laryngeal constriction to hyperpnea. It has been argued that they are involved in the *Hering–Breuer deflation reflex*, whereby a decrease in lung volume may evoke hyperpnea, and *Head's paradoxical reflex*, whereby lung inflation prolongs an inspiratory effort rather than terminates it.

Juxtapulmonary–Capillary Receptors. Juxtapulmonary-capillary receptors, so called because of their location within the alveolar–capillary interstitial space, are stimulated by pulmonary congestion and pulmonary edema, possibly through an increase in the interstitial fluid volume. Their reflex actions include tachypnea, hypotension, and bradycardia. The J-receptors are not thought to contribute significantly to the normal control of breathing.

Ventilatory Response to Carbon Dioxide

Carbon dioxide is a potent stimulus to ventilation. The CO_2 responsiveness of the ventilatory control system can be assessed by means of controlled CO_2-inhalation procedures. For example, an individual may inhale a series of gas mixtures, each having a different F_{ICO_2}, until a steady state is reached. The ensuing relationship between ventilation ($\dot{V}_E$) and arterial P_{CO_2} (Pa_{CO_2}) is essentially linear over a substantial range of Pa_{CO_2} (although the response may start to plateau because of a depressant effect of severe hypercapnia on neural function at high values of Pa_{CO_2}) (Fig. 21–13). The slope of this relationship, $\Delta\dot{V}_E/\Delta Pa_{CO_2}$, represents the ventilatory CO_2 responsiveness. A normal value for a healthy, normoxic individual (i.e., $Pa_{O_2} \sim 90$ to 100 mm Hg) is about 3 L/min/mm Hg.

The value of the CO_2 responsiveness depends crucially on the background level of arterial P_{O_2}. Figure 21–13 indicates that the slope of the ventilatory response to inhaled CO_2 is least during hyperoxia and greatest during hypoxia. This hypoxia-induced potentiation of ventilatory CO_2 responsiveness is generally ascribed to the carotid chemoreceptors, recalling that hypoxia serves to potentiate (or increase) their CO_2 responsiveness. Furthermore, in humans, hyperoxia (when sufficiently extreme) is thought to actually silence the carotid chemoreceptors, so that they

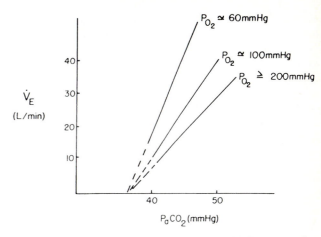

Figure 21–13. Ventilatory response to arterial P_{CO_2} at various levels of arterial P_{O_2}. (*Reprinted, with permission, from Whipp BJ. The respiratory system. In: Ross G, ed.* Essentials of human physiology. *Chicago: Year Book Medical; 1982.*)

no longer respond to the imposed CO_2 stimulus; the ventilatory CO_2 responsiveness is then thought to represent solely that of the central chemoreceptors.

Administration of many anesthetics results in hypoventilation (i.e., Pa_{CO_2} is increased, while Pa_{O_2} is reduced). This is reflected in a shift of the $\dot{V}_E$–Pa_{CO_2} relationship to the right (i.e., increased Pa_{CO_2} intercept). Typically, the relationship is also less steep (i.e., decreased $\Delta\dot{V}_E/\Delta Pa_{CO_2}$); as a result, $\dot{V}_E$ does not increase as much as normal in response to a given increase in Pa_{CO_2}. These effects often occur in a dose-dependent fashion, such that $\Delta\dot{V}_E/\Delta Pa_{CO_2}$ decreases and the Pa_{CO_2} intercept increases with increasing multiples of the *minimum alveolar concentration* (MAC).

It is important to recognize that the interpretation of a reduced ventilation during anesthesia should take account not only of anesthetic actions at the level of the participating chemoreceptors, but also of possible actions at the level of effector structures. For example, were an increase in the resistance to airflow or a decrease in lung compliance to develop during anesthesia, ventilation could be lower despite maintained levels of neural efferent output to the muscles of respiration. This could assume some importance in patients with respiratory impairments (e.g., COPD, fibrosis).

Finally, after a period of assisted ventilation that is characterized by inadvertent overventilation of the patient, there is a possibility that apnea* may occur as a result of the low Pa_{CO_2}. Such an effect could well be exacerbated during anesthesia, consequent to anesthetic-induced depression of ventilatory CO_2 responsiveness.

Ventilatory Response to Hypoxia

Inhalation of a hypoxic gas mixture normally causes an increase in ventilation, owing to the fall in Pa_{O_2}. As was the case for CO_2, it is possible to define the $\dot{V}_E$–Pa_{O_2} relationship by having an individual breathe a series of gas mixtures,

---

* Apnea is a condition in which breathing has ceased.

each with a different F_{IO_2}, until a steady state is attained. Recognizing that the hypoxia-induced hyperpnea will also cause a fall in Pa_{CO_2} and therefore interfere with the full expression of the hypoxic stimulus (i.e., the low Pa_{CO_2} will reduce the extent of the potentiation between CO_2 and hypoxia at the carotid bodies and also reduce the degree of central chemoreceptor stimulation), it is important to maintain Pa_{CO_2} during the hypoxic exposures by adding an appropriate amount of CO_2 to the inspirate.

The relationship between $\dot{V}_E$ and Pa_{O_2} is curvilinear (and well described by a hyperbola) (Fig. 21–14). It is taken to represent the hypoxic responsiveness of the carotid chemoreceptors: after surgical removal or inactivation of the carotid bodies, the ventilatory response to hypoxia is absent. Three aspects of the $\dot{V}_E$–Pa_{O_2} relationship deserve attention: (1) there is little ventilatory response to decreasing arterial P_{O_2} until a substantial level of hypoxia has been achieved; (2) the hypoxic responsiveness increases progressively as arterial P_{O_2} falls; (3) the hypoxic responsiveness that obtains over a particular range of arterial P_{O_2} is potentiated (or increased) by arterial hypercapnia (a manifestation of the complex interaction that occurs between CO_2 and hypoxia at the carotid chemoreceptors). Therefore, in clinical conditions where a patient's CO_2 responsiveness is abnormally low (e.g., COPD), care should be taken when O_2 is administered: if the Pa_{O_2} is raised excessively, the carotid chemoreceptors will be silenced and ventilation will fall to very low levels (in the extreme, the patient would become apneic).

A wide range of inhalational anesthetics have been shown to depress the ventilatory response to hypoxia, in some cases at subanesthetic doses. This effect appears to be localized to the carotid body chemoreceptors. Caution should therefore be employed when administering anesthesia to an individual who has little or no ventilatory CO_2 responsiveness (e.g., the blue bloater or type B COPD patient); the reduction of hypoxic responsiveness with anesthesia may lead to apnea.

NONRESPIRATORY FUNCTIONS OF THE LUNGS

Air Conditioning

The extremely vascular mucosal linings of the nose, mouth, and portions of the pharynx serve to warm and moisten inhaled air (only a minor contribution comes from the tracheobronchial tree). As a result, when inspired air arrives in the alveolar region, it approximates body temperature and 100 percent relative humidity. The mucosal vessels can, in turn, conserve heat and moisture by extraction from the air as it is exhaled. This process continues to function in the face of wide variations in the temperature and moisture content of the inspirate.

Filtration and Cleansing

Many diseases of the lungs result from the inhalation of particulate matter, such as dusts, cigarette smoke, microorganisms, and allergens. It is therefore of some importance that the tracheobronchial tree serves as a filter for removing particulate matter from the inhaled air.

Large particles (> 10 μm in diameter) are filtered by the large, stiff hairs (vibria) within the vestibule just inside each side of the nose and also by the mucous lining of the airway (*mucociliary clearance*). As the inhaled air moves into the nasopharynx and larynx, abrupt changes in the direction of airflow caused by the complex geometry of these regions lead to further deposition as particles impact against the airway walls. Smaller particles are deposited in the tracheobronchial tree (~ 5 to 8 μm in diameter) and the alveoli (~ 3 μm in diameter).

Mucociliary clearance of particulate matter from the upper and lower airways relies on the sustained beating of cilia that project from the ciliated epithelium, which lines the respiratory tract within the nose and nasopharynx in the upper airway, and from the larynx to the respiratory bronchioles in the lower airways. Within the nose, ciliary action

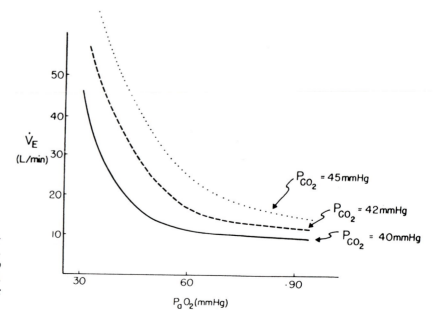

Figure 21–14. Ventilatory response to arterial P_{O_2} at various levels of arterial P_{CO_2}. (*Reprinted, with permission, from Whipp BJ. The respiratory system. In: Ross G, ed. Essentials of human physiology. Chicago: Year Book Medical; 1982.*)

moves mucus backward either to be swallowed or to be expectorated. For regions distal to the larynx, secretions are moved up the respiratory tract toward the larynx.

Cilia are complex, hairlike structures that beat spontaneously in a methodical, wavelike fashion; they appear to have no innervation. The energy for ciliary beating derives from adenosine triphosphate (ATP). The normal rate of beating is ~ 12 to 14 beats/min. Alterations in the rate of ciliary beating influence the rate of mucociliary clearance (see below).

Mucus is produced by tracheobronchial mucous glands and goblet cells, and released by exocytosis. It is composed mainly of a mixture of water (~ 95%), glycoproteins (~ 3%), proteoglycans (~ 0.5%), and lesser amounts of proteins and lipids.

The normal rate of mucociliary clearance is ~ 100 $\mu m/s$, although it can be affected by many factors. For example, dehydration and low inspired humidity can reduce mucociliary clearance by increasing the viscosity of the mucous layer and by slowing the rate at which the cilia beat. Cholinergic drugs and beta-adrenergic agonists increase the rate of mucociliary clearance, presumably through stimulation of mucus secretion (and, in the case of beta agonists, stimulation of ciliary beating). Conversely, beta-adrenergic blocking agents slow the rate of mucociliary clearance. Chronic cigarette smoking is associated with a slowed rate of ciliary beating and the replacement of ciliated cells by goblet cells; this results in depressed mucociliary clearance. Although this effect may be reversed on cessation of smoking in asymptomatic individuals, this is typically not the case in patients with chronic bronchitis. General anesthetics reversibly impair mucociliary clearance, probably as a result of impaired ciliary beating.

Coughing and Sneezing

Another protective function of the upper airway is the cough–sneeze reflex. This is preceded by a forceful expiration against a closed glottis. After pressure builds up behind the glottis, it suddenly opens to permit an explosive expulsion of air at velocities that approach supersonic.

Smell and Taste

The senses of smell and taste also reside in the upper airway. In humans, these special senses are probably more aesthetic than protective in character.

Vascular Reservoir

The lungs function as one of several blood reservoirs in the body, representing a volume of blood that can be quickly mobilized into the general circulation in case of an immediate need. The potential significance of any particular reservoir is directly related to the volume of blood it contains and to the ease or promptness with which it can be mobilized. About 50 percent of the pulmonary vessels do not function in gas exchange at rest and may therefore be classified as reserve units; these constitute a volume of about 30 mL of blood which can be immediately furnished to the left ventricle to buffer transient discrepancies between venous return and cardiac output.

Blood Filtering

An ancillary function of the pulmonary vascular system is to filter the blood. Substances filtered by the pulmonary capillaries include cancer cells, fat cells, gas bubbles, fibrin clots, bone marrow cells, damaged red blood cells, platelets, and white cells. The capillary serves as the filter, and is often sacrificed in the process. The loss of capillaries from this source is normally not a problem for gas-exchange function, in view of the considerable reserve of units available. Moreover, the patency of some of these capillary "filters" may actually be restored after a time.

Besides acting as a filter for the systemic circulation, the lungs also protect themselves. Phagocytes (including leukocytes and macrophages) can engulf both particulate matter and bacteria that escape the mucociliary boundary that normally defends the respiratory tract.

Metabolic Functions

Considerable metabolic activity occurs within the lungs. For example, the type II alveolar epithelial cells synthesize pulmonary surfactant. Other substances synthesized within the lungs include histamine, serotonin, bradykinins, prostaglandins, proteins, mucopolysaccharides, hydroxytryptamine, and acetylcholine. Many of these are vasoactive. Finally, enzymes in the lungs catalyze the conversion of angiotensin I to angiotensin II.

These actions lead to several important consequences. For example (neglecting pulmonary O_2 and CO_2 exchange), the composition of arterialized blood within the pulmonary veins cannot be assumed to provide an accurate reflection of systemic venous blood composition. Furthermore, a given drug may exert different effects, depending on whether it is administered intravenously or intraarterially.

BIBLIOGRAPHY

Bates DV, Macklem PT, Christie RV. *Respiratory function in disease.* Philadelphia: WB Saunders; 1971.

Benumof JL. Respiratory physiology and respiratory function during anesthesia. In: Miller RD, ed. *Anesthesia.* New York: Churchill Livingstone; 1990;1:505–549.

Berger AJ, Mitchell RA, et al. Regulation of respiration. *N Engl J Med.* 1977;297:92–97, 138–143, 194–201.

Biebuyck JF, Stene JK. Nutritional aspects of anesthesia. In: Miller RD, ed. *Anesthesia.* New York: Churchill Livingstone; 1990;2:2277–2306.

Churchill-Davidson HC. *A practice of anaesthesia.* 5th ed. Chicago: Year Book Medical; 1984.

Clarke SW, Pavia D. Mucociliary clearance. In: Crystal RG, West JB, eds. *The Lung: Scientific foundations.* New York: Raven Press; 1991;2:1845–1859.

Comroe JH Jr. *Physiology of respiration.* 2nd ed. Chicago: Year Book Medical; 1974.

Cunningham DJC. The control system regulating breathing in man. *Q Rev Biophys.* 1974;6:433–483.

Gilman AG, Goodman LS, et al. *The pharmacological basis of therapeutics.* 7th ed. New York: Macmillan; 1985.

Gronert GA, Schulman SR, Mott J. Malignant hyperthermia. In: Miller RD, ed. *Anesthesia.* New York: Churchill Livingstone; 1990;1:935–956.

Hickey RF, Severinghaus JW. Regulation of breathing: Drug effects. In: Hornbein TF, ed. *Regulation of breathing, part 2.* New York: Dekker; 1982:1251–1312.

Hyatt RE, Black LF. The flow–volume curve: A current perspective. *Am Rev Respir Dis.* 1973;107:191.

Loeschcke HH. Central chemosensitivity and the reaction theory. *J Physiol [Lond]* 1982;332:1–24.

Macklem PT, Mead J. The physiological basis of common pulmonary function tests. *Arch Environ Health.* 1967;14:5.

McDonald DM. Peripheral chemoreceptors: Structure–function relationships of the carotid body. In: Hornbein TF, ed. *Regulation of breathing.* New York: Marcel Dekker; 1981:105–319.

Mitchell RA, Berger AJ. Neural regulation of respiration. *Am Rev Respir Dis.* 1975;111:206–224.

Murphy TM, Brown DL, Wedel DJ. Spinal, epidural, and caudal anesthesia. In: Miller RD, ed. *Anesthesia.* New York: Churchill Livingstone; 1990;2:1377–1406.

Newsom Davis J. Control of the muscles of breathing. In: Widdicombe JG, ed. *Respiratory physiology.* MTP International Review of Science—Physiology Series. Baltimore: University Park Press; 1974;2:221–245.

Nunn JF. *Applied respiratory physiology.* London: Butterworths; 1987.

Otis AB. Quantitative relationships in steady-state gas exchange. In: Fenn WO, Rahn H, eds. *Handbook of physiology.* Washington, DC: American Physiological Society; 1964:681–698.

Otis AB. The work of breathing. In: Fenn WO, Rahn H, eds. *Handbook of physiology.* Washington, DC: American Physiological Society; 1964:463–766.

Paintal AS. Vagal sensory receptors and their reflex effects. *Physiol Rev.* 1973;53:159–227.

Pavlin EG, Hornbein TF. Anesthesia and the control of ventilation. In: Cherniack NS, Widdicombe JG, eds. *Handbook of physiology.* Section 3: *The respiratory system.* Washington, DC: American Physiological Society; 1986;2:793–813.

Rahn H, Farhi LE. Ventilation, perfusion, and gas exchange—The $\dot{V}_A/\dot{Q}$ concept. In: Fenn WO, Rahn H, eds. *Handbook of physiology.* Washington, DC: American Physiological Society; 1964:735–766.

Rebuck AS, Slutsky AS. Control of breathing in diseases of the respiratory tract and lungs. In: Cherniack NS, Widdicombe JG, eds. *Handbook of Physiology.* Section 3: *The respiratory system.* Washington, DC: American Physiological Society; 1986; 2:771–791.

Rehder K. Anesthesia and the respiratory system. *Can Anaesth Soc J.* 1979;26:451–462.

Roizen MF. Anesthetic implications of concurrent diseases. In: Miller RD, ed. *Anesthesia.* New York: Churchill Livingstone; 1990;1:793–893.

St. John WM. Central nervous system regulation of ventilation. In: Davies DG, Barnes CD, eds. *Regulation of ventilation and gas exchange.* New York: Academic Press; 1978:1–30.

Torrance RW. Prolegomena. In: Torrance RW, ed. *Arterial chemoreceptors.* Oxford: Blackwell Scientific; 1968:1–40.

Ward SA. Ventilatory requirements during general anesthesia: The determinants of an "appropriate" response. *Nurse Anesth.* 1990; 1:134–148.

West JB. *Pulmonary pathophysiology: The essentials.* Baltimore: Williams & Wilkins; 1987.

West JB. *Ventilation/blood flow and gas exchange.* Oxford: Blackwell Scientific; 1977.

West JB. *Respiratory physiology: The essentials.* Baltimore: Williams & Wilkins; 1990.

Whipp BJ. The respiratory system. In: Ross G, ed. *Essentials of human physiology.* Chicago: Year Book Medical; 1982:287–357.

Whipp BJ, Ward SA, et al. Reflex control of ventilation by peripheral arterial chemoreceptors in man. In: Acker H, O'Regan RG, eds. *Physiology of the peripheral arterial chemoreceptors.* Amsterdam: Elsevier; 1983:299–324.

Widdicombe JG. Reflex control of breathing. In: Widdicombe JG, ed. *Respiratory physiology.* MTP International Review of Science—Physiology Series. Baltimore: University Park Press; 1974;2: 273–301.

Neurophysiology

Joseph T. Rando

The human nervous system is an extensive network of billions of interconnected neurons supported by glial cells. The inherent complexity of this system presents an overwhelming number of details. Many components of anesthesia practice are dependent on a thorough understanding of nervous system physiology. This chapter describes the role that the nervous system plays in the function of the entire human organism.

GROWTH AND DEVELOPMENT OF THE NERVOUS SYSTEM

Embryonic Formation

The embryonic formation of the human brain requires the production of 45,000 neurons per minute, assuming a typical human gestation period of 40 weeks. Neuron formation occurs by mitosis throughout gestation, ending shortly before parturition. It has been demonstrated that the human nervous system is functional by the end of the second month of gestation. Activity is manifested by the avoidance reflex, which the fetus expresses by moving the head when stimulated. Although all of the neurons are formed at birth, there are noticeable changes that will be elaborated in this chapter.

The brain develops from the ectodermal layer of the neural plate. As the ectoderm thickens along what will become the back, it begins to curl into a neural tube. The first part of the neural tube to fuse (the neural folds) is located in the cervical region. As the fusion continues caudad and cephalad, additional areas of the ectoderm develop to form primordial structures of the sense organs, that is, ears, nose, and eyes. The cephalic portion of the neural tube enlarges as it fuses and becomes the brain. The neural tube is completely fused by the 24th gestational day, leaving a lumen down its center which becomes the ventricular system of the brain and the central canal of the spinal cord.

Adjacent to the neural tube, as it develops, are 31 pairs of somites (blocklike masses of mesoderm) arranged in sequence from the first cervical to the coccygeal level. Each of these pairs of somites differentiates into muscles, bones,

and connective tissues. They are each innervated by one pair of spinal nerves. As these somite structures grow and develop, they take their innervation along. This is exemplified by the diaphragm which originates at the cervical level and pulls the innervation from C-3, C-4, and C-5 to its final location in the abdomen.

As the neural tube continues to develop, the spinal cord portion differentiates into three distinct cell layers. The inner layer of cells lining the central canal is made up of columnar epithelial cells and is called the matrix. It is the source of origin of the other two layers through mitosis. The middle layer of cells is called the mantle layer and is high in neuron content. It becomes the gray matter of the spinal cord. The cells in the outer layer of cells are also formed from the matrix and migrate to their final position, where they become the white matter of the spinal cord. These cells constitute the marginal layer of the cord.

Sensory and motor neurons form from the matrix cells of the neural tube as the tube becomes grooved by the sulcus limitans, an indentation on the lateral aspects of the entire length of the spinal cord. The area posterior to the sulcus limitans is called the *dorsal* or *alar plate* and becomes the sensory nuclei associated with input from the peripheral, spinal, and cranial nerves. The alar plate also forms the telencephalon and diencephalon of the brain. The area anterior to the sulcus limitans is known as the *ventral* or *basal plate* and becomes the motor nuclei. It is also associated with the functions of cranial and spinal nerves and forms the lobes of the brain known as the metencephalon, rhombencephalon, and myelencephalon. This developmental anatomy helps us understand the premise of the Bell–Magendie law, which states that sensory nerve fibers enter the posterior cells of the spinal cord and motor neurons exit the anterior spinal segments.

Until the third prenatal month, the spinal cord extends the entire length of the vertebral column and the nerves entering and leaving the cord exit the vertebral column at right angles. After the third gestational month, the vertebral column elongates faster than the spinal cord. At birth the spinal cord ends at the level of the third lumbar vertebra. This disproportionate elongation of spinal cord and vertebral column results in the nerves leaving the lumbar, sacral, and coccygeal areas at an acute angle caudally. Additionally, the subarachnoid space below the first lumbar area is occupied by multiple nerves making up the cauda equina.

The brain is a three-vesicle organ prior to the second gestational month. It consists of a prosencephalon, mesencephalon, and rhombencephalon. At about the 36th day of gestation the prosencephalon subdivides into telencephalon and diencephalon and the rhombencephalon subdivides into metencephalon and myelencephalon (Fig. 22–1). From this point the brain continues to grow in size by becoming more contorted through the formation of flexures and enlarged segments. The surface area of the brain is increased by the formation of sulci and gyri, which are generally present by the seventh gestational month. Each person's brain is patterned individually and continues to maintain these unique patterns throughout life.

Postnatal Development

It is well recognized that the brain of the newborn is proportionately larger than that of the adult (10 percent of body weight and 2 percent of body weight, respectively). The newborn's brain continues to develop rapidly and by the end of the second year of life the relative size and proportion of all parts of this organ are similar to those in the adult. From an average weight at birth of 350 g, the newborn brain triples in size during the first year of life, reaching approximately 1000 g by 1 year. At puberty it reaches the adult size of 1375 g in the male and 1250 g in the female.

The "avoidance" reflex has been documented at 8 weeks of gestation wherein the fetus withdraws the head in response to stimulation of the upper lip. There is also evidence of intercostal muscle activity by 13 weeks. A well-developed sense of touch has been documented at birth. Although the newborn can only distinguish light from dark, vision develops rapidly after delivery. By 1 month of age the newborn can follow an object placed in front of the eyes, although he or she is usually farsighted. Hearing is not developed at birth because the structures in the middle ear are not fully developed. In addition, there is no air in the eustachian tube at birth to help with the transmission of sound. The senses of taste and smell are present at birth and become well developed in the first months of life. Pain sensations are also present at birth, although the infant cannot localize pain. It is thought that an infant is less sensitive to pain than an older child. It has been established that infants are easily distracted from painful stimuli by stronger reflexes such as sucking.

There are changes in the brain and nervous system with age, although neurons are essentially formed and differentiated at birth. The number of neurons decreases with age because neurons that die are not replaced by new ones—a loss generally not noticeable for several years as humans have an excess and the remaining neurons compensate for these slight losses. One estimate places the rate of neuron loss between 20 and 70 years of age at 100,000 neurons per day, or a 10 percent total loss over a half-century of aging, a rate that may be increased through abuse.

As neurons age, there is an increase in pigmentation, especially up to 40 years. This is the result of an accumulation of ribonucleic acid (RNA) within the neurons. By contrast, there is a decrease in Nissl's substance, which has been identified as ribosomes. There is a decrease in RNA after about 60 years of age, as well as a decrease in total brain weight with age. Cerebral blood flow decreases approximately 20 percent by age 75. There is a 66 percent decrease in the number of taste buds and a 10 percent decrease in the velocity of neuronal impulse conduction in the aged. In addition, meningeal calcification, increased ventricular size, and atrophic changes in the rhinencephalon, insula, frontal, and parietal lobes are observed.

Developmental Abnormalities

A number of developmental abnormalities affect the nervous system. Noback (1980) has classified them into genetic and environmental categories. Among the developmental

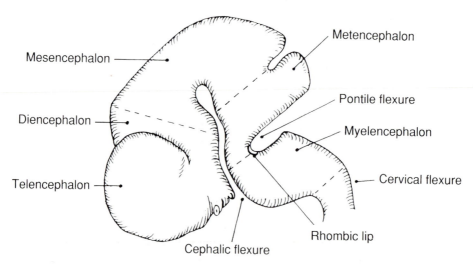

Figure 22–1. Flexures and secondary vesicles in the brain of a human embryo. (*Reprinted, with permission, from Buchanan AR. Functional neuroanatomy. Malvern, PA: Lea & Febiger; 1961:6.*)

abnormalities of the nervous system of genetic origin is Down syndrome, which occurs in 1 out of every 800 births. Over 90 percent of these defects are due to extra material present at chromosome 21. Another genetic abnormality is phenylketonuria, which results in an accumulation of phenylalanine in the brain as a result of a lack of phenylalanine hydroxylase.

Environmental factors can also influence central nervous system formation. German measles, syphilis, increased irradiation, birth trauma, or chemical exposure can result in abnormalities of the nervous system. Infection of the mother by the cytomegalovirus in the second trimester of pregnancy is most detrimental to the fetus, with an incidence of 4 to 10 infected infants per thousand live births. Mental retardation, microencephaly, and deafness may result. Maternal HIV is universally transmitted to the fetus. Nutritional deficiencies, such as protein deficiency of the mother, may affect the infant. Infant or childhood nutritional deficiencies can manifest as marasmus or kwashiorkor syndrome, especially during the first 2 years of life. Cretinism may result in the infant whose mother had decreased thyroid function during the last trimester of pregnancy. Hypoxia during the last half of pregnancy or the first month of life may lead to cerebral palsy, mental retardation, cortical atrophy, or sclerosis of white matter. Finally, developmental abnormalities of the neural tube can lead to a number of central nervous system anomalies including anencephaly, spina bifida, and meningomyelocele. Their occurrence is more frequent in female infants and the overall combined incidence is approximately 5 per 1000 live births.

NEURONS AND REFLEX ARCS

Structure, Function, and Classification of Neurons

The neuron is recognized as the basic structural and functional unit of the nervous system (Fig. 22–2). Along with connective tissue it makes up the sum of the nervous system. Neurons interconnect across synapses, which are described in more detail later in this chapter.

The cell body is an important component of a neuron; without it, the neuron would die. The cell body is also called the *soma* or the *perikaryon*. Most cell bodies are visible with a light microscope. They are polymorphologic and surrounded by a cell membrane of the typical sugar–fat–protein configuration. Within the cell membrane are several organelles. Along with the typical nucleus, nucleolus, and endoplasmic reticulum, there are large numbers of mitochondria, especially at synapses and nodes of Ranvier, which are described later. The cell bodies contain structures called *Nissl bodies*, which are large granules of ribonucleoprotein that are also found in the ribosomes of other cells. They are located on the endoplasmic reticulum as well as freely distributed in the cytoplasm of the cell body. Nissl bodies are critical to normal cell function, protein synthesis, and neuronal repair and increase in amount as these processes are carried out. Very little chromatin (a deoxyribonucleic acid) is found within the cell body, possibly reflecting its inability to regenerate. Neurofibrils made up of strands of protein can be seen throughout the cytoplasm, especially if neuronal regeneration is occurring. Golgi bod-

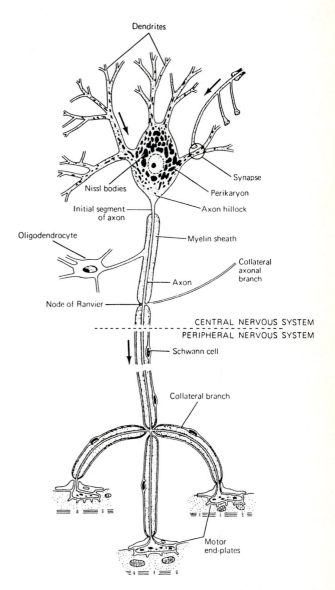

Figure 22–2. Schematic drawing of Nissl-stained motor neuron. (*Reprinted, with permission, from Junqueria LC, Carneiro J, Long JA. Basic histology. 5th ed. Norwalk, CT: Appleton & Lange; 1986.*)

ies and lysosomes typically exist in the cell body and conduct functions similar to those seen in other cells. The cell body varies in size from 0.1 to 13.5 nm. Cell bodies are found in the gray matter of the brain and in the peripheral nervous system as automatic nervous system ganglia, dorsal root ganglia, and sensory ganglia of the cranial nerves.

The functions of the cell body are to receive nerve endings that convey excitatory or inhibitory stimuli generated in other nerve cells and to transmit these stimuli to the remainder of the neuron. In addition, the cell body contains the organelles essential for the overall functioning of the neuron as a viable unit.

Another component of the neuron is the dendrite. The dendrite is usually short, seldom extending more than 700 nm from the cell body. As many as 4000 dendrites have been identified in some neurons. This widespread arborization allows an extensive relay of stimuli. In addition, the dendrites have small, spinelike projections called gemmules that increase the surface area for contact. Dendrites lack a Golgi apparatus but do have Nissl bodies, mitochondria, and neurofibrils. The function of a dendrite is to conduct excitatory or inhibitory impulses to the cell body.

A third component of the neuron is the axon. It originates from a broadened area of the cell body known as the hillock. Only one axon arises from a cell body, and it enlarges slightly in diameter beyond the first 100 μm of the hillock. This portion of the axon (from the hillock to where the axon begins to enlarge) is called the *initial segment*. The axon is longer and narrower than the dendrite and constitutes the bulk of the white matter in the nervous system. Axons have terminal branches that arborize; each of these branches is known as a telodendron. The end of each telodendron has an enlarged knob called a *bouton*. It is these boutons that liberate a neurohumoral transmitter substance to aid in the transmission of a message from one neuron to another. Many of the axons are covered by a layer of fat and protein material known as myelin, which is secreted by the neurilemma, lies inferior to it in a "jelly-roll" fashion, and is avascular, thereby giving the axon a white appearance. The myelin is secreted by cells that surround all peripheral axons. Schwann cells originate from an outer layer that covers the axon, also known as the neurilemma. In contrast to myelin, the neurilemma is a thin, delicate, nucleated, fatty substance. Axons with a diameter greater than 2 μm are usually myelinated; those smaller than 2 μm are not. The myelination of axons occurs in an intermittent fashion, with each portion of myelin sheath being 80 to 100 μm long. The gap between two adjacent Schwann cells wrapped around the axon is called the *node of Ranvier*. It is from these gaps, or nodes of Ranvier, that collateral axons extend from the main axon, usually at a 90-degree angle.

The axon functions to conduct stimuli away from the cell body of its neuron. Because of the elaborate array of telodendrons and collateral axons, impulses can be conducted (1) to the dendrite of an adjacent neuron, called *axondendritic conduction*; (2) to the cell body of an adjacent neuron, called *axosomatic conduction*; or (3) to the axon of another neuron, called *axoaxonal conduction*.

Generally, no neuronal covering exists around the cell body or dendrites of a neuron; nor does it exist around the telodendrons or boutons. The situation is different, however, with regard to the covering around the axon. Peripheral axons are encircled by the neurilemma consisting of a sheath of Schwann cells. Axons smaller than 2 μm in diameter have only a single layer of covering and are therefore said to be unmyelinated. Larger axons of the peripheral nervous system have a thicker layer of myelin as described earlier. The amount of myelinization of nerves differs, but all peripheral nerves contain this covering with the exception of some postganglionic autonomic nerves and some afferent nerves transmitting pain sensation (slow pain fibers). Although the myelinization of nerves is incomplete at birth, sensory fibers are almost completely myelinated. Motor nerves require 2 to 3 years for complete myelinization to occur. Several functions and advantages are provided by myelinization. This covering prevents cross-talk or interference between impulse conduction among adjacent axons. Myelinated nerves are less susceptible to damage

and have a faster rate of impulse conduction, in addition to requiring less ion flux because they only depolarize at the node of Ranvier. In the central nervous system, myelin is secreted by connective tissue cells known as oligodendroglia, as there is no neurilemma covering these axons. Myelin does cover those central nerves outside the gray matter and accounts for the white appearance of white matter of the brain and spinal cord.

In looking at the organization of nerves, the axon is central to what is often called a nerve fiber. The axon is surrounded immediately by myelin, which is then covered by neurilemma. An additional covering known as *endoneurium* closely surrounds the neurilemma. Several fibers thus invested are surrounded by *perineurium*, a thicker connective tissue covering, collecting these fibers into fascicles. The fascicles in turn are joined together by a similar covering of connective tissue known as *epineurium*. Finally, nerves are often grouped together into fascial compartments separating them from muscles and blood vessels.

Neurons have been typically classified in three ways: (1) by the number of processes, (2) by the diameter of the axon, and (3) by the length of the axon. Bipolar neurons have dendrites on one end and an axon on the other, and the cell body is interposed between the dendrite and axon. The unipolar neuron is called a modified bipolar neuron in that a common pathway is shared by the axon and dendrite connecting the cell body. A multipolar neuron has many short dendrites and one long axon, which may have collateral branches coming off the axon at a 90-degree angle near the cell body.

Classification of neurons based on the diameter of the axon is somewhat more complex, but it is commonly referred to by clinicians and academicians alike. The first group of neurons is referred to as *A type*. They are myelinated and are the axons with the largest diameter, ranging from 2 to 22 μm. Because the velocity of neuron conduction varies directly with the diameter of the axon, this group has the greatest velocity of conduction, 12 to 120 m/s. A-type neurons are further subdivided into (1) alpha, conducting impulses of proprioception and somatic motor innervation; (2) beta, conducting impulses of touch and pressure; and (3) gamma, innervating muscle spindles and delta fibers and conducting temperature and fast pain impulses. The second group of neurons classified according to axonal diameter is known as *B type*. They are also myelinated, having a diameter of 1 to 3 μm and a conduction velocity of 3 to 14 m/s, and function as preganglionic autonomic fibers. The third classification is the *C type*. These neurons are usually unmyelinated or only lightly myelinated with a diameter of 0.3 to 1.3 μm and a conduction velocity of 0.2 to 2 m/s. These fibers serve two functions: to conduct slow pain impulses and to make up the postganglionic autonomic fibers.

A third method of classifying neurons is according to axonal length. This method is older and less frequently used. Golgi I neurons have long axons and make up spinal and peripheral neurons. Golgi II neurons have short axons and are found in the brain and the interneurons of the spinal cord.

Neuronal Degeneration and Regeneration

In the process of degeneration, the entire neuron responds to an injury (the injury acts as a stimulus to the neuron), and the whole neuron irreversibly degenerates if there is no neurilemma or if the cell body is destroyed. If the axon is cut, the distal portion and the myelin covering degenerate. Macrophages consume the debris left by this degeneration. This is termed *Wallerian degeneration of the neuron*, and neural innervation is interrupted to the area. If the neuron conducted motor impulses, the muscle undergoes atrophic changes; if it is a sensory neuron, the sensory modality is impaired. The proximal segment of the axon may show retrograde degeneration, stopping short of the cell body. If the cell body is involved, no regeneration occurs.

The process of regeneration depends on the presence of neurilemma, an undamaged cell body, and a minimal gap between the proximal and distal segments of the axon. Regeneration occurs as the proximal end of the axon grows toward the neurilemma sheath or shell of the distal portion of injured neuron. The neurilemma does not secrete a new axon, however. As the axon grows, if the distal portion of the neurilemma sheath has not shifted or become distorted in any way, the growing axon recannulates the distal portion of axon and functional integrity is reestablished. There is no proven chemical attraction between the two ends of the injured axon. The axon regenerates at the rate of approximately 3 to 4 mm per day.

Reflex Arcs

Functionally integrated neuronal units incorporate the principles of the Bell–Magendie law, which states that in the spinal cord the posterior roots are sensory and the anterior roots are motor. Reflexes are traditionally classified into three types according to the components of the neuronal unit. The monosynaptic reflex is the simplest and has one synapse. It includes a sensory receptor and a sensory neuron that conduct afferent impulses into the dorsal horn of the spinal cord. This apparatus synapses in the cord, with a motor neuron carrying efferent impulses to an effector unit, usually a skeletal muscle. In response to stretching of the sense organ in the muscle (namely, the muscle spindle intrafusal fibers lying parallel to the regular muscle contractile unit), activation causes the efferent limb of the reflex arc to produce motor activity. This is typified by the well-known knee jerk.

The disynaptic reflex arc has the same components as described above plus one interneuron interposed in the spinal cord between the afferent and efferent neurons, which allows further nervous system integration as exemplified by the reflex withdrawal from a noxious stimulus. And finally, the polysynaptic reflex arc is the most complex and has multiple interneurons all linked through collateral branches arranged in parallel chains. This branching is variable and causes prolonged responses. The complexity of this reflex system allows for coordinated flexion and extension of muscles to allow smoother reflex activity of the organism as a whole.

MEMBRANE EXCITATION AND IMPULSE TRANSMISSION

Characteristics of a Stable Membrane

Typically, the distribution of electrolytes inside and outside cells of the nervous system is similar to the makeup of other cells. The extracellular environment contains 10 to 14 times more sodium than is found inside the cell. Sodium is also present in much greater concentrations than is seen for extracellular potassium. The principal extracellular anion is the chloride ion. Within the cell there is far more potassium—some 30 to 40 times more than extracellular potassium. There is considerably less sodium within the cell in the resting state. The intracellular anions consist of proteins, organic phosphates, and sulfates as well as bicarbonate.

Factors Maintaining the Polarized State

In the resting state there exists a potential charge across the cell membrane. The charge is always measured on the inside and is negative relative to the outside. This is referred to as the *transmembrane potential*, or the *resting membrane potential*. Its actual value differs with the type of cell measured, but for most neurons it is −90 mV when measured on the inside of the cell. This transmembrane potential requires some basic conditions to maintain it. First, the cell membrane must be selectively permeable, allowing for more rapid diffusion of some ions over others. A concentration gradient is thereby established for various anions and cations on either side of the cell membrane, providing the membrane with the potential to react. This reaction depends on the tissue type: muscle tissue contracts, glandular tissue secretes, and nervous tissue conducts impulses.

Because of the differences in concentration of the ions on either side of the cell membrane, there is a natural tendency for ions to diffuse to equilibrium. Sodium ions therefore enter the cell and potassium ions exit. This "leak" is thought to occur through pores or sodium channels. This selective permeability of the cell membrane is far less for sodium than it is for potassium. There is perhaps 50 to 100 times more potassium leaking out of the cell than sodium leaking into the cell. The explanation for this is that the hydrated potassium ion is smaller than the sodium ion and can therefore more freely pass through the cell pore. Only a minimal amount of chloride ions enters the cell because there is a relatively small gradient on the two sides of the cell membrane for this anion. The intracellular anions are generally too large to diffuse out of the cell and are therefore said to be nondiffusible. In addition to the minimal permeability of the cell membrane to sodium and potassium ions, there is an ATP-utilizing carrier system that keeps ahead of the diffusion by carrying much of the sodium that diffuses into the cell back out and the potassium back into the intracellular cytoplasm.

Sequence of Depolarizing Events

Before the activity of depolarization begins, the resting membrane potential must increase from −90 mV to −65 mV, which is called the threshold. When the threshold is reached, selective permeability is lost, sodium ions rush into the cell causing the development of an action potential, and depolarization of the cell occurs. The cell thus performs its designated function as indicated above. With the development of an action potential, the intracellular electrical potential changes from −90 mV at rest to +45 mV during the initial period of depolarization. Stimuli can be of a chemical, mechanical, thermal, or electrical nature. Irrespective of the type of stimulus, the common result is a change in membrane permeability, making it much more permeable first to sodium and then later to potassium. It is postulated that the pores of the cell membrane are lined with calcium ions. This bound calcium alters the pore diameter and tends to decrease its permeability. The stimulus displaces the calcium from its membrane binding sites, thereby increasing cell membrane permeability. Sodium ions rapidly diffuse into the cell at a rate hundreds of times greater than during the resting state, overpowering the active transport mechanism which attempts to move excess sodium ions into the extracellular environment. Potassium ion flux changes very little. There also occurs some movement of chloride ions into the cell, but this is minimal and not instrumental in affecting depolarization of the cell. The net gain of intracellular cations causes the intracellular membrane potential to go from –90 mV to +45 mV. This is referred to as a reversal potential. As a consequence of this action potential and with the achievement of the reversal potential, cells are excited and perform their characteristic function by contracting, transmitting impulses, secreting their contents, and so on. This process of depolarization takes approximately 0.4 millisecond. The process is terminated by the diffusion of potassium out of the cell. This movement of potassium begins approximately 0.3 millisecond after stimulation of the cell and continues for another 0.4 millisecond, ending when the resting membrane potential reaches –94 mV. The state of hyperpolarization is due to the outpouring of potassium and the slight influx of chloride ions into the cell. The period of hyperpolarization lasts from 50 milliseconds to a few seconds and is called a positive afterpotential, a confusing term because it is even more negative than the resting membrane potential.

Once a cell has depolarized, it is said to be refractory or resistant to subsequent stimuli while it reestablishes the ionic distribution that exists at rest. This refractory period is divided into an initial one third of the repolarization period in which the cell is completely resistant to further stimuli irrespective of their strength or duration. This is referred to as the absolute refractory period. It is followed by the last two thirds of the repolarization period in which a stimulus of greater-than-normal magnitude or duration may cause subsequent depolarization of the cell. This is called the relative refractory period.

Several characteristics of the stimulus should be considered. As mentioned earlier, the stimulus can be chemical, mechanical, thermal, or electrical in nature. It must be of sufficient magnitude to cause depolarization of a cell. It is thus said to be of rheobase strength. The stimulus must also be applied for a sufficient length of time to cause depolarization. This is known as the utilization time. The term *chronaxy* applies to the length of time a stimulus of two rheobase intensity must be applied to produce depolarization action of a cell.

SYNAPSE AND MUSCLE CONTRACTION

General Description and Location

A synapse is defined as a functional connection between neurons, neurons and receptors, or neuron and effector organs. There is considerable morphologic and physiologic variation between synapses, and in general, all are involved in impulse transmission. As the average axon terminates in 1000 synapses and as dendrites can receive synaptic contact from 100,000 axons, there is a tremendous proliferation of synapses throughout the body.

Structural and Functional Characteristics

The most frequently studied synapse is found between the motor efferent neuron and the skeletal muscle effector. It is large in size, having the dendrites and cell body of the efferent neuron in the anterior horn of the spinal cord. The axon emerges from the anterior horn, forms a spinal nerve, and terminates by synapsing at the sarcolemma of a skeletal muscle fiber. The axonal ending forms a bouton or knoblike terminal at the telodendron. The end of the neuron is called the *presynaptic terminal* or *endplate*. The membrane around these terminal ends of the neuron is the presynaptic membrane. A space separates the presynaptic membrane from the skeletal muscle. This space is known as the synaptic cleft or space and varies in synapses from 2 to 12 nm. The membrane of skeletal muscle lying across from the presynaptic membrane is the postsynaptic membrane or sole plate. This postsynaptic membrane is specialized tissue that differs from adjacent areas of skeletal muscle in that it is specifically adapted to receive and react to chemical substances released from the presynaptic terminal.

Mechanism of Impulse Transmission

Within the boutons of the telodendron, concentrations of mitochondria are high, producing a great deal of adenosine triphosphate, the high-energy source of the body. There are also several vesicles containing the chemical neurohumoral transmitter substance specific for that neuron. In the specific effector neuron–skeletal muscle unit, the chemical is acetylcholine, the transmitter we discuss in detail here.

The depolarization wave passes down the axon to the terminal bouton and causes the vesicles adjacent to the synaptic cleft to rupture and exocytose their contents into the cleft. Approximately 200 to 300 such vesicles release their contents in this process. The exact mechanism by which the depolarization wave causes the vesicles to rupture is unclear, but it has been determined that the impulse causes an inrushing of calcium ions through the terminal knob at the time of the action potential. The liberated acetylcholine transits the synaptic cleft and attaches to the specific receptor site on the postsynaptic membrane. It alters the permeability of the postsynaptic membrane, increasing the permeability of sodium and therefore causing depolarization of the sarcolemma. This depolarization next spreads in all directions to the skeletal muscle.

Before repolarization can occur and the muscle can respond to another stimulus, the acetylcholine must be removed from the receptor sites. This occurs by two processes. A small amount is reabsorbed into the presynaptic terminal and back into the vesicles where it is in the inactive state. The predominant amount of acetylcholine is chemically inactivated by the enzyme acetylcholinesterase, which is present along the synaptic cleft. This enzyme is specific for the hydrolysis of acetylcholine. Another esterase found in the brain, liver, and plasma is pseudo-cholinesterase or nonspecific cholesterase and is effective in hydrolyzing succinyldicholine into succinylmonocholine. Acetylcholinesterase breaks acetylcholine down into choline and acetate, which are reabsorbed back into the presynaptic terminal where they are acted on by cholineacetylase, an enzyme found in that terminal. Once synthesized, the newly formed acetylcholine is taken into vesicles and stored. These vesicles have been alternately called packets and quanta.

Synaptic Transmitter Substances

The postsynaptic membrane is specifically adapted to receive and react to the substance released by the presynaptic terminal. There are two general categories of neurohumoral transmitters. Some excite the postsynaptic membrane causing depolarization; these include acetylcholine, norepinephrine and epinephrine. Others are limited to the central nervous system and include dopamine, serotonin, histamine, and a number of hypothalamus-stimulating hormones, as well as enkephalins/endorphins. There are also inhibitory neurohumoral transmitters released at some synapses. These are said to stabilize or inhibit depolarization of the postsynaptic membrane. Examples of such inhibitory substances include glycine and γ-aminobutyric acid. In addition, the excitatory neurohumoral transmitters can stimulate inhibitory fibers that act to produce negative feedback inhibition of neurons.

Muscle Contraction and Relaxation

In considering the activity of muscle we must first understand the makeup of a muscle fiber. The typical muscle fiber comprises hundreds of actin and myosin filaments attached end-to-end the entire length of the fiber. The actin filaments are thin, double-helical strands of protein extending on either side of a so-called Z-band, much as the fingers extend from the hand. Interdigitating with the actin are thicker protein molecules known as myosin. There are generally twice as many actin as myosin filaments in a myofibril. The Z-bands pass between myofibrils all along the muscle fiber. The part of the muscle lying between two successive parallel Z membranes, including the projections of actin from each and the interdigitating myosin filaments, is referred to as a sarcomere. The sarcomere is approximately 2 μm in length when completely relaxed. Thus, a myofibril when viewed in transverse cross section will appear as one myosin filament surrounded by six actin filaments in a regular hexagonal pattern. This pattern of actin and myosin filaments continues repeatedly up to approximately 3000 actin and 1500 myosin filaments over the entire length of each myofibril. As mentioned previously, hundreds to thousands of these myofibrils lie parallel to each other to form a muscle fiber and many muscle fibers constitute a muscle. The muscle fiber is distinguished by a surrounding cell membrane known as sarcolemma. Interweaving around the individual myofibrils is a lacelike structure of sarcoplasmic reticulum. This consists of complex channels that connect with a transverse tubular system running the length of the myofibril and connecting the sarcoplasmic reticulum with the extracellular environment. The T-tube system, as it is called, contains extracellular fluid. Several mitochondria are found between the myofibrils. The sarcoplasmic reticulum also has enlarged areas or terminal cisterns near the junction with the T-tube system. These terminal cisterns contain numerous calcium ions.

The interdigitating makeup of actin and myosin molecules gives skeletal muscle its typical striated appearance. In addition to the Z-band, several other anatomic demarcations of the myofibril are evidenced. The portion of the sarcomere where the actin overlaps with the myosin is termed the *A-band*, the portion where the actin does not overlap with myosin is the *I-band*, and, finally, the central portion of the myosin where there is no overlapping actin is the *H-band*.

Arranged and recessed in the cleft of the double-helical actin strand is a double strand of tropomyosin that contains regularly spaced subunits of troponin. Both tropomyosin and troponin are proteins, the latter being made up of three differing subunits (I, T, and C). The tropomyosin–troponin complex prevents muscle contraction and is therefore known as an inhibitory complex. Tropomyosin covers the receptor sites on the actin filament and prevents the interaction of actin and myosin.

With this background of the anatomy of the muscle unit, we now move on to the process of excitation–contraction coupling. When an action potential occurs in muscles, the impulse spreads throughout the muscle by way of the transverse tubular system. As the action potential moves past the terminal cisterns of the sarcoplasmic reticulum, calcium is released into the vicinity of the myofibril. This calcium binds with troponin C and moves the tropomyosin–troponin complex away from the receptor sites on the actin. This then sets the stage for muscle contraction. Excitation–contraction coupling occurs between the actin and myosin filaments. The myosin filament consists of a single strand of protein with shorter projections extending along the filament, much as feathers extend from the shaft of an arrow. These extensions are meromyosin cross-bridges protruding every 120 degrees around the myosin filament and spaced every few nanometers the entire length of the myosin filament. The meromyosin strands extend from the center of the myosin filament toward the ends in both directions. The meromyosin strands characteristically are slender and have a bulbous "head" at the end opposite that which attaches to the myosin filament. The meromyosin strands generally lie closely arranged around the myosin. There are two areas of the meromyosin strands that "hinge," allowing it to move further away from the myosin filament and the head portion to attach to the receptor sites of the actin. No meromyosin strands extend from the very center of the myosin filament.

When the calcium released from the terminal cistern moves the inhibitory proteins away from the receptor sites of the actin, the heads for the meromyosin attach to these sites and swivel in unison in a "cocking" motion, moving the two opposing actin filaments of the sarcomere closer to each other and interdigitating over a greater portion of the myosin. Once the meromyosin head has swiveled, moving the actin filament, the receptor site on the actin is exposed and the head detaches from the actin receptor site. Adenosine triphosphate binds with the head, causing it to detach from the actin. Once the head becomes detached from the actin, the enzyme ATPase, found in the meromyosin molecule, causes the ATP to be split from the meromyosin head. This splitting causes the head to be recocked into position to once more reattach to a receptor site on the actin filament and move the actin again along the myosin filament. This process occurs repeatedly in a cogwheel fashion and is called the *ratchet theory of muscle contraction*.

Relaxation of the muscle occurs when the calcium ions are pumped back into the sarcoplasmic reticulum. This process occurs by active transport using ATP. The inhibitory bonds between the actin, troponin, and tropomyosin are reestablished. Energy for the process of contraction and relaxation of muscle uses oxygen to supply ATP and phosphocreatine to furnish anaerobic supplies of energy.

Comparison of Muscle Types

Skeletal muscle makes up about 40 percent of the body weight; smooth muscle and cardiac muscle constitute another 10 percent. Although skeletal muscle has regularly occurring cross-striations as a result of organized, recurring actin and myosin filaments, the same characteristic is not evidenced by smooth muscle, which is arranged in an irregular pattern. There are two types of smooth muscle. The first, visceral, is found in the walls of hollow organs such as intestines, ureters, urinary bladder, and the uterus. Visceral muscle has a tightly connected border between cells which allows inherent, rhythmic contractions without extraneous innervation. These cells have an unstable resting membrane potential because of a greater sodium and potassium leak than found in skeletal muscle. There is, therefore, continuous depolarization, a summation of repetitive action, and a rippling of action potentials which result in tonic contractions lasting several seconds. The second type of smooth muscle is a multiunit type consisting of discrete muscle fibers in which each fiber has a nerve ending. This fiber contracts only when directly stimulated. Multiunit smooth muscle is found in blood vessels and in the iris of the eye.

Smooth muscle has a poorly developed sarcoplasmic reticulum and no transverse tubule system. It also differs from skeletal muscle in that it has autonomic nervous system innervation instead of spinal nerve innervation. The fibers of smooth muscle are smaller in diameter and shorter in length compared with those of skeletal muscle.

Cardiac muscle has some of the characteristics of both smooth and skeletal muscle. There are visible cross-striations and a well-developed sarcoplasmic reticulum. The T-tubule system opens at the Z-lines rather than at the A-band/I-band junction as occurs in skeletal muscle. The duration of action potentials in cardiac muscle is 15 to 30 times longer than in skeletal muscle. Cardiac muscle is also intrinsically self-excitable as is smooth muscle because of a greater sodium ion permeability. Cardiac muscle has intercalated disks, areas where the ends of muscle fibers abut each other through an extensive series of folds, forming a strong union. Because of the intercalated disks and tight cell junctions or borders, cardiac muscle cells contract when denervated; however, they are generally innervated by the autonomic nervous system.

SPINAL CORD, MENINGES, AND CEREBRAL SPINAL FLUID

Spinal Cord Structure

The spinal cord appears as an elongated cylindrical structure approximately 1 cm in diameter and 42 to 45 cm long. The cranial end of the cord extends to the medulla oblongata at the upper border of the atlas. The caudal end terminates at the body of the second lumbar vertebra in the adult. The spinal cord tapers to a blunt end caudally and is called the *conus medullaris*. It is suspended and supported laterally by the dentate ligament and is surrounded by meninges, which are discussed later. *Filum terminale* is the term given to the delicate filament continuing down the vertebral canal from the conus medullaris to the first coccygeal vertebra. It is approximately 20 cm long. The first 15 cm is contained within the dura mater and surrounded by nerves of the cauda equina. This section is called the *filum terminali internum* because it is invested by dura mater. The lower 5 cm, called *filum terminali externum*, has dura mater adherent to it and extends to the dorsal border of the first coccygeal vertebra, where it attaches to become the periosteum of the coccyx. The blood supply to the spinal cord consists of spinal branches arising from the vertebral, deep cervical, intercostal, and lumbar arteries with branches of the anterior and posterior spinal arteries. There is an extensive array of spinal vasculature. The venous drainage of the spinal cord collects into venous plexuses and empties into the vena cava. The external configuration of the cord shows it to be slightly flattened anteroposteriorly, with a cervical enlargement from the third cervical vertebra to the second thoracic vertebra corresponding with the large nerves supplying the upper extremities. A similar enlargement corresponding with the nerves supplying the lower extremities is found in the lumbar region.

A cross-sectional view (Fig. 22–3) shows the gross appearance of the spinal cord, with a central area of gray matter immediately surrounding the central canal. The gray matter is made up primarily of dendrites, cell bodies, unmyelinated axons, and neuroglia arranged horizontally. The H-shaped distribution of gray matter varies with the amount of tissues innervated by the different segments. The thoracic segment of the cord has a smaller amount of gray matter, compared with the cervical, lumbar and sacral segments. The gray matter of the thoracic and upper lumbar areas shows small lateral projections (lateral horns) giving rise to the sympathetic preganglionic fibers. The horns of the gray matter are arranged so that they divide the gray matter into anterior, lateral, and posterior columns. Each of these columns is further subdivided, carrying nerve fibers to and from respective areas of the body. A transverse commissure of gray matter connects the right and left columns, forming a central gray isthmus. A hole can be seen in the middle of the gray commissure extending from the fourth ventricle of the brain and traveling the length of the spinal cord; it contains cerebrospinal fluid and is called the central canal. The gray matter is the area of synapse of afferent,

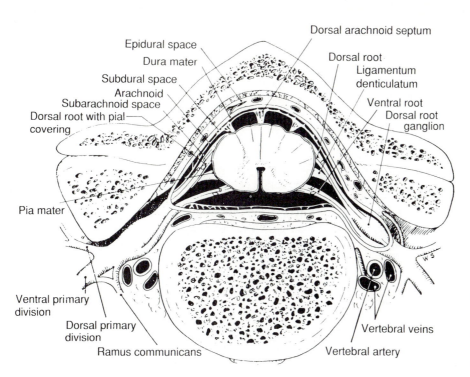

Epidural space
Dura mater
Subdural space
Arachnoid
Subarachnoid space
Dorsal root with pial covering
Pia mater
Ventral primary division
Dorsal primary division
Ramus communicans

Dorsal arachnoid septum
Dorsal root
Ligamentum denticulatum
Ventral root
Dorsal root ganglion
Vertebral veins
Vertebral artery

Figure 22–3. Cross section of the spinal cord in the spinal canal. (*Reprinted, with permission, from Buchanan AR.* Functional neuroanatomy. *Malvern, PA: Lea & Febiger; 1961:25.*)

internuncial, and efferent neurons. The posterior horn is the point of synapse for most somatic afferent fibers and the anterior horn, the area where impulses are relayed for voluntary movement, as well as effector neurons of spinal reflex arcs.

The white matter of the spinal cord generally surrounds the gray. It consists primarily of myelinated afferent and efferent axons vertically arranged as projection tracts. The white matter in each half of the cord is divided into three columns or funiculi, namely, the anterior, lateral, and posterior. Each funiculus is subdivided into fascicles or tracts representing groups of axons carrying similar sensory or motor impulses. The specific tracts are covered elsewhere in this chapter.

Spinal Cord Coverings

The coverings of the brain and spinal cord are almost identical. They generally consist of nonneuronal connective tissue arranged in three separate but continuous layers around the brain and spinal cord. The meninges are innervated by somatic and visceral afferent fibers from spinal and autonomic nerves.

Beginning with the outermost layer, we find the dura mater a tough, nonelastic, fibrous layer of connective tissues. Around the brain, the dura is composed of two layers. The outer endosteal layer is the same as the periosteum of the skull and is adherent to the inner tablet of the skull. It sends many fine fibrous and vascular projections into the bone, which gives it a fuzzy appearance when peeled off from the bone. There is no real space between this outer layer and the skull; however, hemorrhage may occur in this area separating the outer dura from the skull. This extradural hemorrhage usually occurs from tearing of the

middle meningeal artery, most commonly in the temporoparietal area.

The inner layer of dura is the meningeal layer and is generally adherent to the outer layer, forming one membrane. The meningeal layer does separate from the endosteal layer to follow large fissures between the cerebral hemispheres to form the falx cerebri, extending down to the corpus callosum and from the cristi galli anteriorly to the occipital tuberance posteriorly. The cerebellar hemispheres are similarly separated by a fold of dura known as falx cerebelli. In addition, the dura forms a tent separating the occipital lobe from the cerebellum and is called the tentorium cerebelli. The two layers of dura mater also separate to form large dural sinuses that are venous channels draining blood from the brain into the internal jugular veins. These veins have no valves and are situated between the two layers of dura. There are two such groups of sinuses. The anterior–inferior group drains that portion, and the posterior–superior group, including the largest superior sagittal sinus, drains the upper posterior brain. There is a potential space below the inner layer of dura that contains a few milliliters of lubricating fluid in immediate contact with the dura. This subdural space exists around the brain, but it does not follow the fissures or sulci except for the falx and tentorium.

Around the spinal cord the dura mater loses its double-layered configuration, which ends at the foramen magnum. The endosteal layer is represented below the foramen magnum as the periosteum of the vertebrae. The subdural space continues in the same manner as around the brain. In addition, there is an epidural space around the spinal cord as the cord does not completely fill the cerebral canal. This space contains adipose and areolar tissue, blood vessels, and nerve roots. The dura continues caudally below the conus medullaris to form a sac called the *lumbar cistern* extending to the second sacral vertebra. Below this, the dura attaches to the coccygeal vertebrae, becoming the periosteum of the coccyx.

The arachnoid mater is a single-layered avascular covering around the brain and spinal cord. It lies below the dura and dips into the fissures and sulci of the brain as do the falx and tentorium. It is separated from the dura mater by the subdural space. The space below the arachnoid mater, known as the *subarachnoid space*, contains cerebrospinal fluid and is continuous with the ventricular system.

The arachnoid mater does not follow the contours of the brain but rather bridges over portions of the brain that do not fill the cranial vault. This bridging effect varies in different areas of the brain. Two areas are of great interest: the cisterna magna lying below the cerebellum and the lumbar cistern lying below the conus medullaris at the caudal end of the spinal cord. These cisterns are filled with cerebrospinal fluid.

The arachnoid mater has the unusual characteristic of thin vertically arranged filaments that traverse the subarachnoid space, attaching it to the underlying pia mater. These filaments have no known function but are known as *trabeculae* and give the arachnoid mater a weblike appearance. The arachnoid continues below the level of the conus medullaris and terminates at the level of the second sacral vertebra along with the dura after forming the lumbar cistern.

Arachnoid villi or granulations are extensions of the arachnoid membrane into the venous sinuses. They appear as berrylike tufts and usually are not found before the age of 3 years; however, they increase in number and size with age. These granulations push against the dura mater and eventually cause the absorption of bone, leaving a depression in the inner table of the skull. More will be said about these arachnoid villi when we discuss cerebrospinal fluid absorption.

The pia mater is a thin delicate layer of connective tissue adherent to the brain and spinal cord following all fissures and sulci and contains the blood supply for the brain and spinal cord, with the spinal portion being somewhat less vascular. The pia mater extends into the transverse cerebral fissure to contribute to the formation of the choroid plexus of the lateral, third and fourth ventricles. Pia mater continues as a fibrous thread at the conus medullaris into the filum terminale. The pia also forms the denticulate ligament which extends laterally on either side of the spinal cord and attaches to the vertebral bodies, providing support and stability to the spinal cord.

Cerebrospinal Fluid

A discussion of cerebrospinal fluid formation, circulation, and absorption must be preceded by the anatomy of the cerebral ventricular system. The lateral (right and left) ventricles are found lying within each cerebral hemisphere, in the midbrain, below the corpus callosum. Each lateral ventricle connects to the centrally located third ventricle by a foramen of Monro. The third ventricle is located in the midbrain above the area of the brainstem. The cerebral aqueduct or aqueduct of Sylvius connects the third and fourth ventricles. The fourth ventricle is in the area of the brainstem anterior to the cerebellum and drains into the cisterna magna via three

openings. One foramen of Magendie opens posteromedially and two foramina of Luschka open laterally into the cisterna magna. From there, the cerebrospinal fluid normally circulates freely around the spinal cord and brain.

The formation of cerebrospinal fluid (CSF) occurs primarily with the action of the choroid plexus in each ventricle and, to a much lesser extent, by an identical process in the perivascular spaces of the brain. The process begins with the secretion of sodium ions by the cuboidal cells of the choroid plexus, resulting in a positively charged cerebrospinal fluid. This positively charged fluid, in turn, attracts negatively charged chloride ions. The excessive concentration of ions causes osmotic pressure in the ventricular fluid to increase, exerting a pressure up to 160 torr greater than the plasma osmotic pressure. Water and dissolved substances therefore move through the choroidal membrane into the CSF. The fluid circulates through the subarachnoid space around the brain and spinal cord by virtue of this pressure.

Cerebrospinal fluid is absorbed into the large venous sinuses because of the pressure gradient within the subarachnoid space. When the pressure of the CSF is greater than venous sinus pressure, leaflike unidirectional valves in the arachnoid villi open, allowing CSF to drain into the dural sinuses. When the venous pressure is greater than the CSF pressure, the valves close and prevent the backflow of blood into the subarachnoid space.

Although figures from different sources may vary, the body of an average adult man has approximately 150 mL of CSF. Approximately one third of this is in the ventricular system and two thirds in the subarachnoid space. Cerebrospinal fluid is formed at the rate of 0.50 mL per minute or 750 mL per day. Obviously, a similar amount must be absorbed into the venous sinuses each day as well. This formation of CSF produces a pressure ranging from 6 to 18 cm H_2O (mean 13 cm H_2O). The mean opening pressure for the arachnoid granulations is 6.8 cm H_2O. These figures can be converted to milliliters of mercury by dividing by 1.36.

Examining the chemistry of CSF reveals a composition similar to that of plasma because of the intimate contact between CSF and plasma. Sodium concentration is 145 mEq/L; chloride, 113 mEq/L; potassium, 2.8 mEq/L; magnesium, 2.3 mEq/L; and calcium, 2.45 mEq/L. There is slightly less glucose in CSF than in plasma and considerably less protein. Few red or white blood cells are found in CSF. When they are present, red cells indicate frank hemorrhage and white cells point to viral or bacterial infections. The specific gravity of CSF ranges from 1.003 to 1.009 and the pH from 7.32 to 7.35.

The overall functions of CSF are protective. The brain floats in CSF which decreases its relative weight. The fluid also acts as a shock absorber, reducing trauma to the brain when rapid movement occurs. Finally, the CSF regulates the composition of the neuronal environment within the narrow limits required for normal functioning.

SPINAL NERVE ACTIVITY

General Description of Spinal Nerves

Each spinal nerve is composed of an afferent sensory component and an efferent motor component. The afferent neurons enter the spinal cord by the posterior horn and the efferent neurons exit the anterior horn. The sensory and motor axons are termed *rootlets*. These rootlets meet at the point of exit from the vertebral column to form one spinal nerve. All of the sensory rootlets are axons entering into formation of one spinal nerve and called the sensory roots of that nerve. The same makeup is seen in the motor roots of spinal nerves.

With the exception of the first cervical spinal nerve, which has only motor fibers, all spinal nerves have both sensory and motor components. The sensory and motor roots join to become one nerve from the vertebral column to the areas of receptor and effector innervation. The roots of the spinal nerve traverse the space between the cord and inner wall of the vertebral canal. The anterior and posterior roots unite in the area of the intervertebral foramen to form the common spinal nerve. The intervertebral foramen is a hole formed by the inferior vertebral notch located on the inferior surface of one vertebra and the superior vertebral notch of the vertebra below it. Most of the spinal nerves exit the vertebral column by way of the intervertebral foramen.

Prior to entering into formation of the common spinal nerve, each sensory neuron has its cell body. The cell body is located at a point just before the spinal roots become one common spinal nerve and leave the vertebral column. The cell body, which is within the bony framework of the vertebra, is known as a dorsal root ganglion.

The common spinal nerve runs only a short distance before dividing into a larger and more important anterior primary ramus and a generally smaller posterior primary ramus. Each ramus carries sensory and motor fibers. The anterior primary ramus sends off the lateral cutaneous and anterior cutaneous branches. It is the anterior primary ramus that connects with the sympathetic paravertebral ganglia. The posterior primary ramus divides into a medial branch and a lateral branch. Before branching into primary rami, the spinal nerve sends off a meningeal branch carrying sensory and motor fibers back into the intervertebral foramen to supply the meningeal vessels.

The anterior primary rami leave the numbered spinal nerves, with some entering into plexus formation. The nerves exiting the plexuses are named for the specific areas they supply. These nerves supply sensory and motor innervation to the arms, legs, front and sides of the neck, thorax, and abdomen. The larger of these plexuses are discussed later in this section. The posterior primary rami do not enter into plexus formation and do not extend into the extremities, but rather are limited to sensory and motor innervation of the muscles and skin of the back and neck.

Origin and Nomenclature of Spinal Nerves

The naming/numbering of spinal nerves occurs with the distribution of the 31 pairs into 8 cervical, 12 thoracic, 5 lumbar, 5 sacral, and 1 coccygeal nerve. With the exception of the first pair of cervical spinal nerves, which are strictly motor, all have sensory and motor fibers. In general, a spinal nerve is named for the vertebra above or below its point of exit through the intervertebral foramen. The human vertebral column has 7 cervical, 12 thoracic, 5 lumbar, 5 sacral, and 4 to 5 fused coccygeal vertebrae. The first pair of

cervical spinal nerves exits between the first vertebra or atlas and the occiput. The second through seventh pairs exit through the intervertebral foramen and are named for the cervical vertebrae below their points of exit. The eighth pair of cervical spinal nerves exits below the seventh cervical vertebra. The thoracic, lumbar, and sacral spinal nerves are named for the vertebrae above their points of exit from the vertebral column (Fig. 22–4).

Each pair of spinal nerves innervates a specific area of the body with its sensory, motor, and accompanying autonomic nerve components. The areas overlap considerably, any specific area of the body being innervated by more than one pair of spinal nerves. Because the nerves below the thoracic level do not exit the intervertebral foramen corresponding to their level of origin off the spinal cord, the area of the body that these nerves innervate is not transversed to the level from which the nerves originated. Named in reference to their point of origin, the cervical spinal nerves extend at a more or less right angle off the spinal cord and exit the intervertebral foramen at about the same level. These nerves are the most horizontal of all spinal nerves. Beginning with the thoracic level, the nerves run down from the point of origin and exit the vertebral column approximately one vertebral body lower. Below the level of the second lumbar vertebrae, the spinal nerves extend below the end of the spinal cord and exit the vertebral column much lower than their point of origin off the cord. This forms a network of loosely arranged spinal nerves referred to as the *cauda equina* because, like the horse's tail, the central mass ends much higher with many fibers extending downward to the end.

As the spinal nerve roots pass through the subarachnoid space surrounding the spinal cord, they first pierce the pia mater and arachnoid mater, which form a sleeve around the roots known as the *perineurium*. When these roots reach the outer dural membrane, an outer sleeve of dura mater, known as the *epineurium*, surrounds the roots and common spinal nerve.

Functional Anatomy of the Brachial Plexus

The brachial plexus is often instrumented by the nurse anesthetist. It is therefore imperative that nurse anesthetists have a thorough understanding of the anatomy of this plexus. The brachial plexus includes all nerve structures arising from the fifth cervical spinal nerve, through and including the first thoracic spinal nerve. This plexus furnishes almost total somatic, autonomic, sensory, and motor innervation to the upper extremities. The anterior primary rami of the fifth, sixth, seventh, and eighth cervical and the first thoracic spinal nerves intertwine after exiting the intervertebral foramina. They next pass through the posterior triangle of the neck, which is formed by the trapezius and sternocleidomastoid muscles, and the middle third of the clavicle between the anterior and middle scalene muscles.

Occasionally the roots from the fourth cervical and second thoracic spinal nerves contribute to the makeup of the brachial plexus. The subclavian artery accompanies the roots as they pass between the scalene muscles. The roots of the above-mentioned spinal nerves collect between the scalene muscles into three trunks and are named with refer-

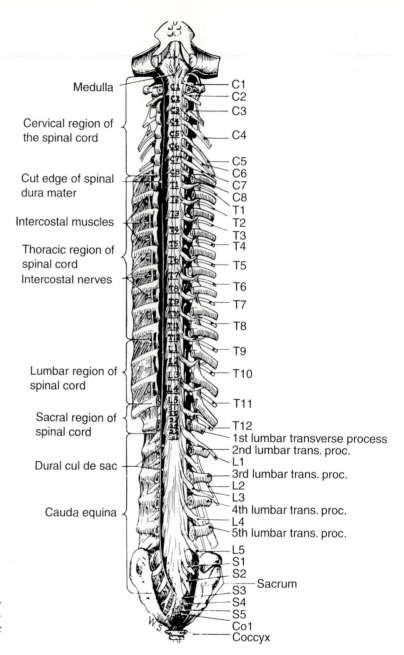

Medulla

Cervical region of
the spinal cord

Cut edge of spinal
dura mater

Intercostal muscles

Thoracic region of
spinal cord
Intercostal nerves

Lumbar region of
spinal cord

Sacral region of
spinal cord

Dural cul de sac

Cauda equina

C1
C2
C3
C4
C5
C6
C7
C8
T1
T2
T3
T4
T5
T6
T7
T8
T9
T10
T11
T12
1st lumbar transverse process
2nd lumbar trans. proc.
L1
3rd lumbar trans. proc.
L2
L3
4th lumbar trans. proc.
L4
5th lumbar trans. proc.
L5
S1
S2
S3   Sacrum
S4
S5
Co1
Coccyx

Figure 22–4. Dorsal view of the spinal cord. (*Reprinted, with permission, from Buchanan AR.* Functional neuroanatomy. *Malvern, PA: Lea & Febiger; 1961:24.*)

ence to their position. They are the superior trunk, made up of fibers from the fifth and sixth cervical spinal nerves; the middle trunk, made up of fibers from the seventh cervical spinal nerve; and the inferior trunk, made up of fibers from the eighth cervical and first thoracic spinal nerves. These three trunks exit from between the scalene muscles and run behind the clavicle to extend to the lateral aspect of the first rib. There they divide into six divisions, each trunk forming an anterior and a posterior division at the lateral border of the first rib. These divisions lie behind the clavicle and subclavius muscle, descending into the axilla with the axillary artery.

The brachial plexus divisions then collect into three cords, which are named in relation to their position around the axillary artery. The lateral cord is formed by the union of anterior divisions of the superior and middle trunks and carries fibers from the fifth, sixth, and seventh cervical spinal nerves. The medial cord arises from the anterior division of the inferior trunk and carries fibers from the eighth cervical and first thoracic spinal nerves. The posterior cord is a combination of the posterior divisions of all three trunks and has fibers from all five spinal nerves of this plexus. The cord gives rise to several branches and terminal nerves. We discuss the origin and termination of six of the peripheral nerves of the brachial plexus.

The musculocutaneous nerve is one of two nerves resulting from the bifurcation of the lateral cord. The other branch of the lateral cord makes up a part of the median nerve discussed later in this section. Motor fibers innervate the muscles that flex and adduct the upper and lower arm, as well as supinate the hand. Sensory components innervate the skin over the radial half of the forearm from just above the antecubital fossa to the wrist, anteriorly and posteriorly.

The radial nerve originates as a continuation of the posterior cord. It supplies motor activity to the muscles flexing, extending, adducting, and abducting the arm. The radial nerve also provides sensory innervation posteriorly, over the middle aspect of the forearm, the dorsal surface of the hand to the lateral half of the ring finger, excluding the tips of the thumb, index, middle, and ring fingers. Anteriorly, the radial nerve supplies the lateral margins of the thumb and hand.

The median nerve is made up of roots from the lateral and medial cords. Its motor fibers innervate muscles that serve to flex, adduct, and abduct the thumb and first two fingers and to pronate the hand. Sensory fibers go to the anterior palmar surface from a line running through the ring finger to the wrist just short of the extreme lateral aspect of the thumb and palm. On the posterior aspect of the hand, the median nerve supplies the tips of the thumb, index and middle fingers as well as the lateral aspects of the tip of the ring finger.

The ulnar nerve originates as a continuation of the medial cord after the cord makes its contribution to the median nerve. Motor fibers innervate all the intrinsic hand muscles, providing flexion and extension to the fingers and extension and adduction of the hand. The sensory fibers innervate the medial aspect of the hand, anteriorly and posteriorly, from the middle of the ring finger to and including the little finger.

The medial cutaneous nerve of the arm originates off the medial cord prior to the formation of the ulnar nerve. It terminates in sensory fibers only to the medial aspect of the upper arm from the axilla to the antecubital space.

Finally, the medial cutaneous nerve of the forearm originates off the medial cord and also has only sensory fibers which, in this case, innervate the medial aspect of the forearm from the wrist to above the antecubital space and elbow, anteriorly and posteriorly.

SPINAL TRACTS AND SPECIAL RECEPTORS

Cross Section of the Spinal Cord

The ascending and descending spinal tracts travel in the anterior, lateral, or posterior columns bilaterally. Each of these columns (funiculi) is further subdivided into tracts (fascicles) that represent groups of axons carrying similar sensory or motor information to or from the brain. Detailed anatomy texts describe more then 20 spinal cord tracts transferring information to and from the brain. Discussion of each is beyond the scope of this text, but several of the more commonly understood are presented here.

Ascending Spinal Tracts

Sensory input to the central nervous system occurs by a series of three afferent neurons. The first-order neuron originates in receptors widely distributed in the periphery. This neuron commonly terminates in the medulla. Sensory neuron I, as it is referred to, synapses in the posterior horn with sensory neuron II. This second-order neuron ascends the spinal cord in a named tract of fibers located in the white matter to the thalamus. Some of the second-order sensory neurons travel up the cord in a tract on the same side that the first-order neuron entered. These fibers are said to be traveling in ipsilateral named tracts. Some of the second-order neurons cross the spinal cord in the anterior commissure or isthmus and ascend the cord in the contralateral spinal tract to the thalamus. In the thalamus, these neurons synapse with sensory neuron III, which has axons extending through the corona radiata and internal capsule, and terminate in the sensory area of the postcentral gyrus of the parietal lobe.

Most of the sensory neurons form synapses with many other neurons located at various spinal cord and brain levels (Fig. 22–5). This is referred to as the *principle of divergence*. There are major ascending pathways for the transmission of pain, temperature, touch, pressure, proprioception and kinesthesia; these should be well understood by the anesthetist.

The lateral spinothalamic tract carries sensations of pain and temperature from the periphery to the brain. Sensory neuron I originates in the skin, muscles, tendons, and viscera and terminates in the posterior horn of the cord. Fibers making up sensory neuron II of this tract originate in the posterior horn, and the axons decussate before ascending in the lateral spinothalamic tract and finally terminating in the thalamus. Sensory neuron III originates in the ventrolateral nucleus of the thalamus, and the axons radiate to the cerebral cortex by way of the thalamocortical tract via the internal capsule.

The ventral spinothalamic tract functions to transmit sensations of touch and pressure from the periphery to the postcentral gyrus. Although the receptors are different from those for pain and temperature and the tracts in which the fibers of the second-order sensory neurons travel are different, the route of each of the fibers of this tract is similar to that traveled by fibers of the dorsal spinothalamic tract to the postcentral gyrus.

A third ascending tract is made up of fibers from the funiculus gracilis, which carries impulses from below the sixth thoracic spinal level, and the funiculus cuneatus, which carries fibers above the sixth thoracic level. Together these fibers make up the medial lemniscal tract, which transmits sensations of conscious kinesthesia, vibration, stereognosis, deep touch, pressure, and two-point discrimination. Sensory neuron I for this tract originates at the peripheral receptors. It enters the posterior horn of the cord, decussates at its level of entry, and extends up the spinal cord to the nuclei of gracilis and cuneatus in the medulla instead of terminating in the posterior columns of the cord. Sensory neuron II originates in these nuclei of the medulla and extends through the midbrain to the thalamus. Sensory neuron III of this tract extends from the thalamus to the cerebral cortex, as have the previously mentioned radiating fibers.

The dorsal spinocerebellar tract carries sensations of unconscious kinesthesia from cord levels of the sixth cervical through second lumbar regions. The fibers making up this tract originate in Golgi apparatus and muscle spindles and travel to the posterior horns of the gray matter. Sensory neuron II extends up the cord ipsilaterally as the dorsal spinocerebellar tract to the cerebellar cortex, which has a homunculus similar to that of the cerebrum. This homunculus is described under The Brain: General Organization and

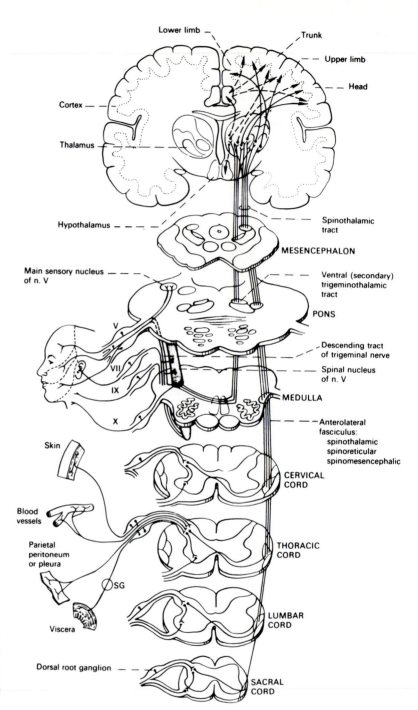

Figure 22–5. Schema of the primary neural pathways for transmission of nociceptive information from various body structures to the brain. (*Reprinted, with permission, from Bonica JJ. The management of pain, 2nd ed. Malvern, PA: Lea & Febiger; 1990;1:29.*)

Functions. There are no third-order sensory neurons for the spinocerebellar tract.

The fibers of the ventral spinocerebellar tract array unconscious kinesthetic sensations from below the second lumbar level into the cerebellum as uncrossed fibers. The second- and third-order sensory neurons originate and terminate in the same areas as those for the dorsal spinocerebellar tracts.

Descending Tracts

Four major descending tracts are presented here. They consist of fibers traveling in either pyramidal or extrapyramidal tracts. The pyramidal tracts are phylogenetically newer and have fibers that converge in the medulla to form pyramids. Their axons originate from cell bodies located in the cerebral cortex cells of Betz in the precentral gyrus of the frontal lobe. These tracts are necessary for skilled, voluntary movements or coordination. The fibers terminate at various levels of the cord by synapsing with interneurons, which in turn synapse with anterior horn neurons. Approximately 80 percent of the fibers of the pyramidal tracts decussate in the medulla and extend down the cord in named tracts. Impulses traveling over these tracts stimulate individual muscles to contract.

Extrapyramidal tracts are phylogenetically older and more complex. They consist of all pathways between the motor cortex and the anterior horn cells except those of the pyramidal system, and they conduct impulses important to muscle tone, automatic movements, and facial expression (see Fig. 22–5). The extrapyramidal fibers originate from areas of the brain other than the cerebral cortex. Many of the fibers of the extrapyramidal tracts project directly from the motor cortex into several components of the basal ganglia.

Specific descending motor tracts include two pyramidal and two extrapyramidal tracts. The lateral corticospinal tract carries crossed pyramidal fibers, and it controls voluntary movement and contraction of individual or small groups of muscles, particularly those moving hands, fingers, feet, and toes of the opposite side of the body. Dendrites and cell bodies of these neurons originate in areas 1 to 6 of the precentral gyrus. The axons descend through the cerebrum and brainstem, decussate in the medulla, and continue down the cord in the lateral corticospinal tract prior to terminating in the internuncial neurons of the gray matter. The roots then go to the spinal nerves and terminate in somatic effectors such as skeletal muscles.

The ventral corticospinal tract is a direct pyramidal tract and its functions are the same as those of the lateral corticospinal tract except that it controls the muscles on the same side of the body. The dendrites, cell bodies, and axons are the same as those for the lateral corticospinal tract, except that the fibers descend uncrossed in the ventral corticospinal tract in the anterior white column and then into spinal nerves to somatic effectors.

The lateral reticulospinal tract is an extrapyramidal tract consisting of fibers facilitating flexor activity and inhibiting extensor activity. These fibers influence motor neurons to skeletal muscles controlling posture and expression. The fibers originate in the lateral reticular formation of the brainstem and terminate in the internuncial neurons sending fibers to the spinal nerves supplying flexor and extensor muscles contralaterally.

Fibers of the medial reticulospinal tract facilitate extension activity and inhibit flexor activity of skeletal muscles. They originate in the reticular formation of the medulla and descend in the medial reticulospinal tract, controlling flexion and extension ipsilaterally.

Special Receptors

Special receptors are structures responsible for responding to stimuli and are intermediate transducers between the stimulus and the sensory neuron. These receptors are sensory nerve endings or dendrites and are modified in two ways. First, the peripheral fiber loses both myelin and neurilemma near its end; the remaining free or naked nerve ending then becomes the receptor. The second means of modification occurs where the peripheral portion of the dendrite loses its covering as above and becomes encased in a special capsule or end organ; with this modification it is said to have formed an accessory structure.

There are several systems for classifying special sensory receptors. The one used here is related to the nature of the stimulus and categorizes receptors as mechanorecep-

tors, thermoreceptors, chemoreceptors, and electromagnetic receptors.

The mechanoreceptors respond to stimuli that distort specific accessory organs or free nerve endings. There are three receptors in this category that respond to light touch. Meissner's corpuscles are accessory structures with widespread, uneven distribution under the epidermis. They are most numerous in hairless areas such as hands, feet, forearms, tongue, lips, and nipples. These receptors are useful in defining texture and movement of light objects over the skin as well as in detecting low-frequency vibrations. Merkel's disks are a second type of touch receptor and are distributed similarly to Meissner's corpuscles. They initially transmit strong but adapting touch sensations of objects on the skin such as occurs when putting on clothing. The last type of touch receptor is the free nerve ending located around the base of hair follicles that serves to sense movement along the surface of the body. Pressure receptors respond to a mechanical force greater then touch and are known as Pacinian corpuscles. They are located deeper than touch receptors and are anatomically separate from other receptors. Pacinian corpuscles are found in the mesentery, periosteum, and subcutaneous, submucous, and subserous connective tissue, as well as in the palms, soles, and genitalia.

There are many kinds of stretch receptors in the body. Those known as proprioceptors provide information with regard to position or orientation of the body in space or body movement. They are stimulated as muscles become stretched, preceding or during movement. There are muscle spindles attached in parallel to skeletal muscles, Golgi tendon organs, which detect the stretching of tendons and free nerve endings located in joint capsules. Other stretch receptors are termed *baroreceptors* and are located at the bifurcation of the common and internal carotid arteries, and are called the carotid sinus. In addition, similar stretch receptors in the arch of the aorta make up the aortic sinuses. These receptors respond to the stretch of vascular smooth muscle as occurs with a change in blood volume. They help to maintain blood pressure. Hering–Breuer stretch receptors located in the smooth muscles of the bronchi and bronchioles respond to stretch of the airways during inflation of the lungs and help to prevent overinflation. Finally, stretch receptors located in the wall of the right atrium are stimulated by increased venous return to the right side of the heart and cause an increase in heart rate; these are called *Bainbridge receptors*.

Another example of mechanoreceptors is found in the inner ear. The vestibular receptors function to maintain equilibrium, knowledge of body position, and movement. The stimulus is a fluid wave in the semicircular canals of the inner ear. Changes in this fluid level are sensed by the otoliths of that vestibular apparatus. Additionally, in the inner ear there are receptors known as organs of Corti that perceive sound and are stimulated by fluid waves secondary to vibration of the tympanic membrane.

The last example of a mechanoreceptor is found in skin and deeper structures and responds to tissue damage from any cause. These free nerve endings transmit painful stimuli to the spinal cord and the higher centers to provide basic protective responses for the organism.

A second category of receptors according to our classification is the thermoreceptors. They are specific accessory organs sparsely located in the skin and mucosa of the lips, tongue, and genitalia. Cold receptors are also called Krause end bulbs and respond to a negative quantity or lack of heat. They are typically stimulated at temperatures less than 25C down to about 15C. Below this level Krause end bulbs are nonfunctioning and pain receptors are stimulated. Interestingly, physiologists have found that these Krause end bulbs are again stimulated at approximately 45C, as are pain receptors. Ruffini corpuscles are specific receptors stimulated between 25C and 45C. They are therefore responsive to heat. The distribution of Ruffini corpuscles is similar to that of cold receptors.

The next category of receptors is chemoreceptors and includes five types. Central receptors are diffusely located in the medulla, aiding in the regulation of respirations. They are stimulated by hydrogen ion and carbon dioxide concentrations in the arterial blood and cerebrospinal fluid. Likewise, peripheral receptors located in the carotid bodies and aortic bodies respond to low arterial oxygen tensions and stimulate the respiratory center. Another chemoreceptor is located in the mucous membrane of the roof of the nasal cavity. Specific rods and cilia are responsive to inhaled vapors and initiate the sense of smell. Taste buds located in the tongue respond to salt, sour, bitter, and sweet stimuli and osmolality of the arterial blood. These receptors have not been specifically identified but are theorized to be in the anterior hypothalamus.

The final category of receptors is termed electromagnetic, and they are involved in visual perception. Light is the stimulus and the receptors are the rods and cones of the retina. Light acts to decompose the chemical composition of opsins, which in turn stimulate the specific receptors. The rods act to detect shape and the cones distinguish color.

Stimuli, applied to receptors in sufficient magnitude, will produce receptor depolarization. This is referred to as *generator* or *receptor potential*. The generator potential in turn acts as a stimulus to depolarize the peripheral sensory fiber. If encapsulated in a corpuscle, the peripheral fiber depolarizes at the first node of Ranvier and elicits an action potential. Generator potentials differ from action potentials in that they do not self-propagate. Instead, the magnitude of the receptor potential is determined by the magnitude of the stimulus. It does not follow the "all or none" law of the action potential.

Another characteristic of special sensory receptors is receptor specificity. A specific stimulus for which a receptor is adapted will most readily cause depolarization of that receptor. That is, the threshold is lowest for the specific stimulus for which the receptor is adapted. Nonspecific stimuli can cause receptor depolarization but must be of greater intensity than the specific stimulus.

Modality specificity is another characteristic of sensory receptors. The sensations perceived will be those for which the receptor is adapted, regardless of the type of stimulus or where along the neuron it is applied. These receptors also exhibit a phenomenon of adaption: the frequency of receptor response or depolarization decreases in the presence of continued application of the stimulus. The degree of adaptivity varies with the receptors. For example, pain receptors, muscle spindles, Golgi tendon apparatus, Hering–Breuer receptors, pressoreceptors, and chemoreceptors are poorly adaptive; thermoreceptors are moderately adaptive; and touch and pressure receptors are readily adaptive.

AUTONOMIC NERVOUS SYSTEM

General Concept

The autonomic nervous system has been referred to by many other names. It has been called the visceral nervous system because it influences visceral function by innervating smooth muscle, cardiac muscle, and glands. It has been called the involuntary/automatic nervous system because most responses and actions occur automatically and on an unconscious level. It has been called the vegetative nervous system because of the basic or primitive effects of the hypothalamus on its activities. Finally, it has been most often, and perhaps erroneously, referred to as the autonomic nervous system, because it was felt to function independently and to be uninfluenced by other components of the nervous system. This name can be shown to be fallacious if one tries to imagine a "fight-or-flight response" without skeletal muscle integration.

In its overall placement within the nervous system, we see that the autonomic system is a subunit of the peripheral nervous system along with the spinal cord and cranial nerves (Fig. 22–6).

Sensory and Motor Components

There are no inherent sensory components to the autonomic nervous system per se; however, sensory input from the viscera occurs by way of neurons arising from sensors in smooth muscles, cardiac muscles, or glands. The afferent fibers travel from these sensors back to the spinal cord with spinal nerve afferent fibers. These visceral afferent fibers, as the autonomic nerves are sometimes referred to, have their cell body in the dorsal root ganglia as do spinal (somatic) afferent neurons. The visceral fibers terminate in the lateral horn of the gray matter of the spinal cord where they synapse with the nuclei of visceral efferent neurons. These efferent autonomic fibers involve two efferent neurons and a synapse that occurs at a ganglion. The efferent fibers then terminate in smooth muscle, cardiac muscle, and glandular epithelium. The efferent fiber originating in the lateral horn of the spinal cord exits the anterior horn of the cord and travels a short distance with the spinal nerve roots and common spinal nerve. The function of the autonomic nervous system involves primarily monitoring, via visceral efferent fibers, the body's internal activities through coordination efforts of the central nervous system.

Sympathetic Division

The autonomic nervous system is divided into two divisions based on structural and functional differences. These differences become evident as the makeup of each is discussed.

Beginning with the anatomy of the sympathetic division, the cell body and dendrites of the preganglionic effer-

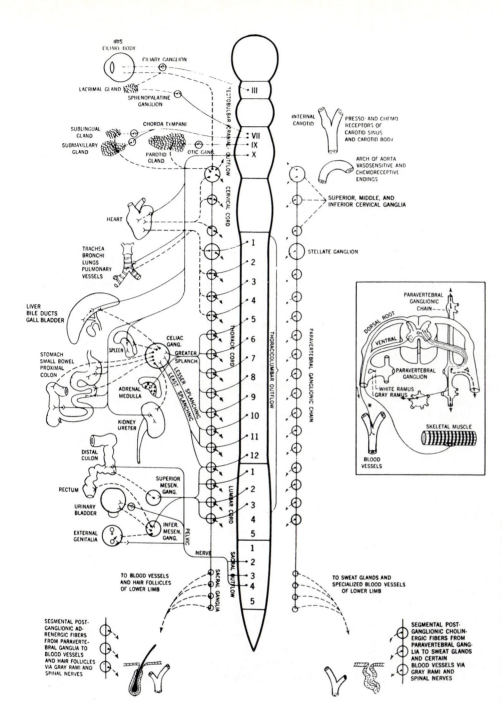

Figure 22–6. Autonomic nervous system. Schematic representation of autonomic nerves and effector organs on the basis of the chemical mediation of nerve impulses. (*Reprinted, with permission, from Lefkowitz RJ, Hoffman BB, Taylor P. The autonomic and somatic nervous systems. In: Gilman AG, Rall TW, Nies AS, Taylor P, eds. Goodman and Gilman's the pharmacological basis of therapeutics. 8th ed. Elmsford, NY: Pergamon Press; 1990:86, 87.*)

ent fibers originate in the lateral horn of the spinal cord from cord levels of the first thoracic spinal nerve through the second lumbar spinal nerve. The sympathetic division is therefore also referred to as the thoracolumbar division of the autonomic nervous system. The preganglionic sympathetic fibers are multipolar, B-type, lightly myelinated fibers.

As mentioned earlier, the preganglionic fiber exits the cord with the spinal nerve through the intervertebral foramen and follows the anterior primary ramus of the spinal nerve for a short distance. The sympathetic efferent fiber then leaves the common spinal nerve and enters a ganglion located approximately 1 in. lateral to the vertebral body.

There it meets the dendrites and cell body of the postganglionic sympathetic fiber. The portion of nerve fiber running from the common spinal nerve out to the paravertebral ganglion is known as a white ramus communicans. Although several routes or "fates" are evidenced by sympathetic postganglionic fibers, one very common route is back to the common spinal nerve from the paravertebral ganglion by a separate track called the gray ramus communicans. These are loops in which the white ramus occurs distal to the gray along the spinal nerve. The postganglionic fiber then travels with the anterior primary ramus of the spinal nerve, leaving it at some more distal point to innervate its intended viscera.

Explanation of sympathetic paravertebral ganglia seems in order as they are involved in all of the "fates" of the efferent fibers. The sympathetic paravertebral ganglia consist of a chain of 20 to 24 pairs of ganglia found 1 in. lateral to either side of the vertebral column, extending from the level of the second cervical vertebra to the coccygeal vertebra. At each vertebral level, there are 3 pairs of ganglia at the cervical level, 10 to 12 pairs at the thoracic level, 2 to 4 pairs at the lumbar level, 4 pairs at the sacral level, and 1 pair at the coccygeal level. The ganglia appear as polymorphic nodular beads strung on a chain, with the string being represented by nerve fibers interconnecting one bead to the next. At the coccygeal end of the chain of ganglia, a single ganglion, the coccygeal impar, joins the right and left chains together.

There is some added complexity to the sympathetic division because there are four distinctly different "fates" in addition to the one already described. A second fate of the preganglionic fiber is that it enters the paravertebral ganglion but does not synapse therein. Instead, it passes to a different ganglion, up or down the chain, and synapses at that level. The postganglionic fiber then travels back to the spinal nerve by way of the gray ramus communicans and travels with the anterior primary ramus of that spinal nerve. By this method, sympathetic nerve fibers can come off at one spinal cord level and innervate a higher or lower level of the body. It is by this method, for example, that structures above T-1 and below T-2 receive sympathetic innervation. A third fate has the preganglionic fiber entering the paravertebral ganglion at its level of origin from the cord, synapsing within the ganglion, and then sending the postganglionic fiber not back to the spinal nerve, but rather to exit the ganglion as a postganglionic fiber to an effector organ. Another fate has the preganglionic sympathetic fiber passing through the paravertebral fiber and traveling to the periphery to synapse in a prevertebral ganglion. The fiber synapses within the prevertebral ganglion and sends a postvertebral fiber to the effector organ, namely, the adrenal medulla, the adrenal being referred to as a postganglionic sympathetic fiber.

Parasympathetic Division

The parasympathetic division of the autonomic nervous system has its origin from cranial and sacral outflow tracts. The nuclei of the cranial outflow lie near the nuclei of cranial nerves III, VII, IX, and X. Their fibers extend along with fibers of the respective cranial nerves to the effector. The cell body of the parasympathetic fibers traveling with the oculomotor nerve arises in the Edinger–Westphal nucleus near the aqueduct of Sylvius. As is characteristic of the preganglionic parasympathetic fibers, they are lightly myelinated type C fibers of similar length to the postganglionic parasympathetic fibers. The preganglionic fiber synapses just behind the globe of the eye in the ciliary ganglion, and the postganglionic fiber innervates the intrinsic eye muscles. The fibers traveling with the facial nerve originate in the upper medulla and synapse in the sphenopalatine ganglion near the lacrimal gland and in the submandibular ganglion near the parotid gland. The postganglionic parasympathetic fibers of this nerve innervate the nasal mucosa, lacrimal

glands and salivary glands. The nuclei of the parasympathetic preganglionic outflow traveling with the glossopharyngeal nerve originate in the upper medulla and synapse in the otic ganglion. The postganglionic fiber innervates the parotid glands. Finally, the vagus nerve has parasympathetic nuclei in the medulla and synapses in the thorax and abdomen, with the postganglionic fibers innervating the thoracic and abdominal viscera excluding the distal half of the large bowel.

The sacral portion of the parasympathetic division originates in the lateral horn of gray matter of spinal cord levels S-2, S-3, and S-4. The preganglionic fibers exit with the spinal roots, follow the anterior primary rami to peripheral ganglia, and there synapse with postganglionic fibers that innervate the distal half of the colon, rectum, bladder musculature and sphincter, uterus, uterine tubes, and genitalia.

Transmitter Substances

The hallmark of the sympathetic division of the autonomic nervous system is diffuse mass action and effects on several organs and systems simultaneously. Several anatomic and physiologic parameters support this diffuse action. The paravertebral chain affords the sympathetic division a method of spreading influence to various levels above and below the actual point of origin off the cord. One preganglionic neuron can synapse with an average of 30 postganglionic neurons, and one postganglionic neuron synapses with several effector sites. Splanchnic nerves provide additional divergence to the sympathetic division. The adrenal medulla is directly innervated by splanchnic fibers, which pass through the celiac plexus causing the adrenal medulla to liberate epinephrine and, to a lesser degree, norepinephrine into the bloodstream. These sympathetic neurohumoral transmitters are inactivated more slowly than the parasympathetic transmitters. The sympathetic system is involved with the control of fight-or-flight mechanisms, which bring about coordinated changes controlling the internal environment during stress. These processes are catabolic in nature, requiring the breakdown of energy stores.

The parasympathetic division, by contrast, functions in a discrete manner, controlling one organ or system. This system lacks chain ganglia or adrenal medulla. There is less divergence between the pre- and postganglionic parasympathetic neurons and between postganglionic neuron and effectors. The parasympathetic neurons liberate acetylcholine at the preganglionic fibers, just as occurs in the sympathetic preganglionic parasympathetic fibers. Acetylcholine is also the neurohumoral transmitter liberated by the postganglionic parasympathetic fibers. The predominant response caused by parasympathetic stimulation is anabolism—building up body energy stores. The parasympathetic system dominates the control of visceral activities under basal conditions and is responsible for long-term, day-to-day regulation of visceral functions.

Muscarinic and Nicotinic Effects

Muscarine is a parasympathetic substance derived from a poisonous mushroom. This substance exhibits a cholinergic effect on smooth muscle, cardiac muscle, and glands but has essentially no effect at the ganglionic synapses or at the motor endplates of skeletal muscles. Muscarinic responses occur by stimulating visceral effectors innervated by cholinergic postganglionic neurons. The agents included in this category include acetylcholine and congeners of acetylcholine esterase. Diisopropyl fluorophosphate, organophosphates, and other anticholinesterase are examples of these substances. Atropine-like drugs block the muscarinic actions of acetylcholine by preventing it from acting at visceral effector organs.

Nicotine has a dual effect on autonomic ganglia and skeletal muscles but no direct effect on smooth muscle, cardiac muscle, or glands. It initially stimulates and then inhibits the excitation of postsynaptic neurons or muscles. The initial effect is depolarization of the postsynaptic membrane, which results in postganglionic neuron depolarization. The subsequent effect is maintenance of depolarization so the postsynaptic membrane cannot be further stimulated.

Actions of the Autonomic Nervous System

Prior to embarking on a discussion of specific organ effects of autonomic stimulation the reader should be familiar with the concept of alpha and beta receptor sites. This concept is applicable only to the sympathetic division and applies because the idea that sympathetic stimulation produces strictly excitatory responses does not hold true. Researchers of physiologic processes found that when sympathetic fibers were stimulated, the responses of effector organs could be excitatory or inhibitory. On inspection of the effectors the postganglionic neurons were found to be identical, each liberating epinephrine and norepinephrine. If the neurons and the neurohumoral transmitters are the same then the difference in response must be the result of some difference in the effector. As the receptors could not be identified anatomically but could be separately identified by physiologic response to pharmacologic agents, Ahlquist termed the responses *alpha* and *beta* and named the receptors, located on the effector organ, *alpha* and *beta*.

Generally speaking, one type of receptor is present on an effector; however, some have both alpha and beta receptors, with a balance being maintained between the two. In some effectors one receptor type predominates. It can be said that stimulation of alpha receptors causes effector excitation and that stimulation of beta receptors causes inhibition. There are two exceptions to this concept. First, the myocardium is innervated by beta receptors but stimulation of these receptors causes positive chronotropic and positive inotropic activity. Second, the bowel has alpha receptors that, when stimulated, result in decreased peristalsis and tone.

An additional subdivision of the beta receptors exists as determined by the effects of certain drugs on some but not all beta receptors. These receptors are designated beta-1 and beta-2. Beta-1 receptors are found in the heart and beta-2 receptors in the coronary vessels, ciliary muscle of the eye, bronchi, urinary bladder, and uterus.

Two alpha-adrenergic receptor subtypes have been identified. Presynaptic alpha receptors differ in pharmacologic properties from postsynaptic alpha receptors. They are designated alpha-1 and alpha-2 receptors and are sites on the cell membrane where pharmacologic substances are bound, leading to mediation of smooth muscle contraction by postsynaptic receptors. Alpha-2 receptors are located in the presynaptic bulb and to a lesser extent in postsynaptic receptors. Stimulation of presynaptic alpha-2 receptors inhibits norepinephrine release. Alpha-1 stimulation causes smooth muscle contraction. The physiologic response of alpha receptors is currently under extensive pharmacodynamic investigation as is evaluation of the agonist–antagonist response of drugs through these receptors. The result will be a clearer understanding of their mechanisms.

In considering the autonomic responses it should be kept in mind that the preganglionic fibers, both sympathetic and parasympathetic, liberate acetylcholine and are known as cholinergic neurons. The postganglionic parasympathetic fibers likewise release acetylcholine to the effector organ. The postganglionic sympathetic fibers, however, are adrenergic; that is, they liberate norepinephrine, which stimulates alpha receptors, and to a lesser extent epinephrine, which stimulates both alpha and beta receptors.

The organ effects of autonomic nervous system stimulation usually involve dual innervation. Few structures have only one division innervating an effector. Where there is dual innervation both divisions exert tone as is seen in blood vessels. Under basal conditions, the parasympathetic division usually predominates and during stress states the sympathetic division usually dominates. The actions of the two autonomic divisions are synergistic.

Looking at specific organ response, when the sympathetic fibers supplying the iris of the eye are stimulated; this causes contraction of the radial muscle and results in dilation of the pupil, or mydriasis. Parasympathetic stimulation causes contraction of the sphincter muscle of the iris and constriction of the pupil, or miosis. The lens of the eye is held in a flattened configuration by the tension on radial ligaments. Stimulation of the parasympathetic fibers causes the lens to become increasingly convex to accommodate for near vision. There is little or no sympathetic effect on the lens of the eye.

Sympathetic stimulation of the myocardium consists of beta-1 stimulation, but, as an exception to the rule, the result is an increase in heart rate and contractile force leading to increased cardiac output. Parasympathetic stimulation causes negative inotropism and negative chronotropism. If we look at autonomic innervation of blood vessels, we see that sympathetic stimulation causes constriction of coronary, skin, cerebral, skeletal muscle, and pulmonary and abdominal vessels. Parasympathetic stimulation, by contrast, causes vasodilation.

Glandular secretions follow the expected pattern of autonomic responses. Sympathetic stimulation of sweat glands results in copious sweating; parasympathetic stimulation has no effect. Sympathetic stimulation causes inhibition of gastric secretions and parasympathetic stimulation causes increased secretion. Nasal, lacrimal, and salivary glands produce sparse, thick secretions when stimulated by sympathetic fibers and produce profuse, watery secretions when stimulated by parasympathetic fibers.

Bronchial smooth muscle relaxes when its sympathetic innervation is stimulated. Parasympathetic stimulation causes bronchiolar constriction. The latter effect is due to vagal stimulation to the bronchiolar smooth muscle. The smooth muscle of the bowel is the second exception to the rule that alpha-receptor stimulation causes excitation because, although alpha receptors predominate, sympathetic stimulation causes a decrease in intestinal tone and a decrease in peristaltic activity. Parasympathetic stimulation, on the other hand, causes increases in tone and peristalsis. The smooth muscle of the urinary bladder relaxes with sympathetic contraction and contracts with parasympathetic stimulation. The action on the bladder sphincter is just the opposite, however. Sympathetic stimulation contracts the sphincter to prevent urination; parasympathetic stimulation relaxes it, allowing urination.

The autonomic influence on the liver results in glycogenolysis with sympathetic stimulation, thereby releasing more glucose for ready access as a source of energy to meet the additional demands during stressful circumstances. Pancreatic secretions decrease and the gallbladder relaxes which prevents emptying. Parasympathetic stimulation produces the opposite effects, resulting in glycogen synthesis by the liver, as well as secretion by the pancreas and gallbladder.

The response of autonomic stimulation of the kidneys is unique. Sympathetic stimulation causes a decrease in urinary output by decreasing renal blood flow. The mechanism by which this occurs is through increased renin secretion by the juxtaglomerular cells of the kidneys. Parasympathetic system stimulation results in no clinically significant effects on renal function.

THE BRAIN: GENERAL ORGANIZATION AND FUNCTIONS

Telencephalon

The cortex is the convoluted outer gray mantle of brain tissue made up of multiple layers of neuronal cell bodies. It ranges in thickness from 2 to 5 mm, representing recent phylogenetic development. The cortex appears gray because of the dense concentration of unmyelinated cell bodies. The convoluted pattern is typical, providing a large surface area of approximately 2 square feet. Examination shows that two thirds of the surface area lies within the convolutions and therefore is not grossly visible in the intact human brain. The cortex makes up about one third of the brain's weight.

The white matter of the brain lies below the cortical layer and above the diencephalon. It consists of myelinated axons from sensory and motor fibers arranged as tracts interconnecting different areas of the brain with one another or with the spinal cord. There are commonly three pathways taken by these fibers. Projection tracts interconnect higher centers of the cortex with more caudal areas of the brain and cord. Commissural tracts interconnect the right and left hemispheres. Association tracts connect anterior with posterior portions of the brain.

The telencephalon (or forebrain) is the larger portion of the prosencephalon. It is divided into six lobes by fissures or sulci. The frontal lobe is the largest of these lobes and is located anterior to the central sulcus, above the lateral fissure, and medially, anterior to the central sulcus and above the cingulate sulcus. In 1909, Bordmann, a German neurolo-

gist, mapped out 47 areas of localized functions of the cortex. This map is referred to as Bordmann's cytoarchitectural graph. Bordmann found that several areas of specialization are ascribed to the frontal lobe. The area of the precentral gyrus just anterior to the central sulcus is termed the primary motor area. This area, numbered 4 and 6, extends from the lateral surface of the frontal lobe to the medial surface. Areas of the body have representation in a *motor homunculus*, a disproportioned human figure whose toes stand in the cingulate sulcus medially with hips extending to the top of the longitudinal fissure and then draped laterally extending toward the lateral fissure. Areas more important in reacting or responding to the external environment, such as the head, hands, and thumbs, are represented by larger areas of distribution on the cortex of each hemisphere. This is also the area of origin of corticospinal tracts carrying motor impulses from the cortex to the spinal cord.

Broca's area, numbered 44 and 45, is the motor area controlling speech. It lies on the inferior lateral aspect of the frontal lobe bilaterally. It is dominant in the dominant hemisphere and, its destruction or damage leads to the inability to articulate speech (motor aphasia).

There is also a secondary or associative motor area, numbered 8, located anterior to the primary motor strip and with a homunculus similar to that of the primary motor area. This secondary motor area has a higher response threshold, but the result is a less refined motor response.

The prefrontal area, numbered 9 to 12, is located anterior to areas 44, 45, and 46 and operates in the formulation of abstract thinking, in the ability to plan or predict, and in judgment. It is also involved in the appreciation of and reaction to pain. It was thought by previous investigators to be the seat of intellect, but present researchers have indicated that intellect is not isolated to the cortex of any single lobe but rather involves cortical activity of the whole brain.

The parietal lobe of the telencephalon consists of the area of the brain posterior to the central sulcus and anterior to the parietooccipital sulcus. Medially it is bounded by the longitudinal fissure down to the cingulate sulcus. The parietal lobe houses the primary sensory area, numbered 1, 2, and 3, also known as the postcentral gyrus. The homunculus is the same as that of the primary motor area, again with larger areas devoted to parts of the body that have the most importance in interpreting stimuli. This sensory area is the point of termination of all third-order neurons, which carry sensory impulses from peripheral receptors to the cortex of the telencephalon.

The temporal lobe is located inferior to the lateral fissure and anterior to the parietooccipital sulcus. It is responsible for audition, and the posterior portion is involved in the visual interpretation of lines, borders, and angles. Disease affecting this lobe may lead to the inability to identify objects and marked distractibility. Olfactory areas are also associated with temporal lobe control.

The occipital lobe extends posterior to the parietooccipital sulcus and is the primary visual area, numbered 17. This is also a bilateral area, as are all the areas discussed in the telencephalon. Part of the visual cortex is located within the calcarine fissure of the occipital lobe.

Another lobe of the telencephalon, the limbic lobe, is central to the cingulate sulcus, forming a ring of cortical tissue visible on the medial surface only. *Limbic lobe* is the older name for the cingulate gyrus, parahippocampus, and uncus. This area of the brain controls functions associated with aggression, arousal, and primitive drives related to self-preservation including feeding behavior, sexual behavior, range, fear, and motivation.

The insula lies within the lateral sulcus and cannot be seen in a lateral view of the telencephalon until the temporal lobe is retracted downward at the lateral sulcus and the tissue of the frontal and parietal lobes is retracted upward at the sulcus. The insula therefore lies medial to the temporal, frontal, and parietal lobes and lateral to the lentiform nucleus. Functions of the insula include the communication of sensory and motor impulses to and from the viscera. Stimulation of the cortex of the insula evokes an epileptic type of motor activity and visceral sensations.

Diencephalon

The diencephalon or interbrain lies deep in the ventromedial aspect of the cerebrum, connecting the cerebrum with the midbrain. It lies above the mesencephalon and below the white matter surrounding the third ventricle. Five principal divisions of gray matter make up the diencephalon.

The epithalamus is the narrow band of tissue at the roof of the diencephalon that houses the pineal gland. Once considered a vestigial structure with a possible role in hypothalamic and endocrine functions in growth and development, more recently, the pineal gland has been identified as a neurosecretory structure analogous to the adrenal medullae and neurohypophysis. Sympathetic stimulation leads to secretion of melatonin, a hormone that acts on the ovaries to inhibit ovulation.

Another structure of the diencephalon, the subthalamus, lies lateral and inferior to the thalamus. It contains some extrapyramidal fibers and has a stabilizing role in extrapyramidal motor activities because it receives fibers from the basal ganglia prior to the descent of these fibers into the spinal cord.

The thalamus consists of 1-cm-wide, 3-cm-long bilateral egg-shaped masses of gray matter, one lying in each hemisphere beside the third ventricle. Fibers from numerous corticospinal tracts synapse in the thalamus as do fibers from the basal ganglia. The thalamus also acts to relay impulses to and from the hypothalamus and various areas of the cerebral cortex. A number of functions are recognized as being mediated by the thalamus. As mentioned, it is a relay point for impulses traveling between the cortex and cord. The thalamus provides the first conscious awareness of sensory impulses. Interpretation is crude and localization is poor, however. The thalamus aids in arousal and alerting of the organism and is linked to the reticular activating and limbic systems. Finally, the thalamus monitors and influences voluntary and involuntary motor activities.

The hypothalamus is an area lying below the thalamus, on either side of the third ventricle, above the midbrain and optic chiasm. Anatomically, it comprises four parts: the optic chiasm, the tuber cinereum, mamillary bodies, and the infundibulum. The hypothalamus receives input from almost every area of the nervous system. It acts as a moderator or clearinghouse for impulses, coordinating critical vegetative functions. The hypothalamus regulates autonomic nervous system excitation or inhibition and controls the release of hormones from the pituitary gland.

The hypothalamus functions to influence heart rate, force of contraction, and vessel diameter through autonomic nervous system control. The hypothalamus monitors the temperature of the blood perfusing thermoreceptors and promotes heat loss, through vasodilation and decreases in basal metabolic rate, or heat gain, through vasoconstriction and increases in metabolic rate and shivering. It also secretes or controls secretions for the neurohypophysis and the adenohypophysis. The regulation of body water is controlled by the hypophysis which monitors blood osmolality via osmoreceptors and adjusts thirst through the secretion of antidiuretic hormone by the posterior pituitary. Gastrointestinal activity and feeding action are stimulated through the monitoring of blood sugar by the hypothalamus.

The hypothalamus houses areas of rage, docility, pleasure, and punishment. Rage and docility are moderated and expressed as blushing, palpitations, tears, and other physical responses. The lateral and medial hypothalamus houses areas of pleasure and punishment, respectively. In addition, it integrates sleep and awake states with input from the reticular activating system.

The basal ganglia is another division of the diencephalon and is made up of several small areas of gray matter. There are three major subdivisions. The corpus striatum is made up of the lentiform nucleus, the globus pallidus, the putamen, and the caudate nucleus. The second subdivision is termed the *amygdala*, and the third, the *claustrum*. All of these areas of the basal ganglia are interconnected and act to coordinate voluntary motor activity to prevent purposeless movements. Recent studies show that the basal ganglia appears to be involved in the planning and programming of voluntary movement. Disorders such as chorea, athetosis, and Parkinson's disease are seated in the basal ganglia.

Mesencephalon

The midbrain is located below the thalamus, above the metencephalon and in front of the cerebellum. The mesencephalon interconnects these three areas with higher centers. These fibers are made of myelinated tracts passing between the spinal cord and higher centers. There are also nuclei for the oculomotor, trochlear, and trigeminal nerves. The mesencephalon functions to interconnect the higher centers with the spinal cord and cerebellum. It is also the location of reflex centers for hearing and sight.

Metencephalon

The mentencephalon is made up of the pons varolii and the cerebellum. The myelencephalon and metencephalon constitute the rhombencephalon.

The pons is a bulbous enlargement on the anterior, superior surface of the brainstem. It forms one continuous structure with the mesencephalon and the medulla. The nuclei for cranial nerves VI, VII, and VIII are located in the pons. In addition to acting as interconnecting pathways between the brainstem and higher centers, the pons also houses the pneumotaxic and apneustic centers which influence respiratory activity.

The cerebellum is located posterior to the pons, medulla oblongata, and the fourth ventricle. It lies in the posterior fossa of the occipital bone and is connected to the pons and midbrain by three stalks of white matter known as peduncles. The cerebellum consists of two hemispheres separated by the falx cerebelli. They have regularly spaced furrows, a cortex, and white matter, similar to the telencephalon. The tentorium cerebelli is a fold of dura mater separating the cerebellum from the occipital lobe above. The cerebellum derives sensory input from spinocerebellar tracts and contributes to the control of auditory and visual responses, motion sickness, equilibrium, stretch reflexes, and adjustments for posture and movement. Cerebellar lesions lead to scanning speech, intention tremors, and inability to stop movement promptly.

Myelencephalon

The medulla oblongata is separated superiorly from the pons by a transverse sulcus. It is cone-shaped with the apex pointed toward the spinal cord. The inferior border is the area where the highest rootlet of the first cervical spinal nerve emerges. The medulla is slightly longer than 2 cm. The rootlets of cranial nerves IX, X, and XI emerge from the dorsal lateral sulcus of the medulla. The rootlet of the hypoglossal nerve emerges from the ventrolateral sulcus. Internally, the medulla is mixed white and gray matter.

The medulla oblongata has three major functions. First, it contains vital reflex centers for the control of heart action, blood vessel diameter, and respirations. Second, it is also the control center for such nonvital reflexes as vomiting, sneezing, coughing, hiccoughing, and swallowing. Finally, the medulla houses projection tracts interconnecting the brain with the spinal cord. Those fibers that decussate do so in the medulla.

CEREBRAL CIRCULATION

Vascular Circuits

The entire blood supply to the brain arises from the internal carotid and vertebral arteries (Fig. 22–7). Venous drainage is completed by the superior sagittal sinus and the sigmoid sinuses into the internal jugular veins.

The internal carotid arteries extend up the neck, entering the cranial vault by way of the posterior portion of the foramen of Lacerum and the petros portion of the temporal bone (Fig. 22–8). The carotid artery enters the area of the temporal bone without branching, generally supplying the anterior portions of the brain, especially the cerebrum. After ascending to the area of the temporal lobe, it gives rise to three main branches. The first, the middle cerebral artery,

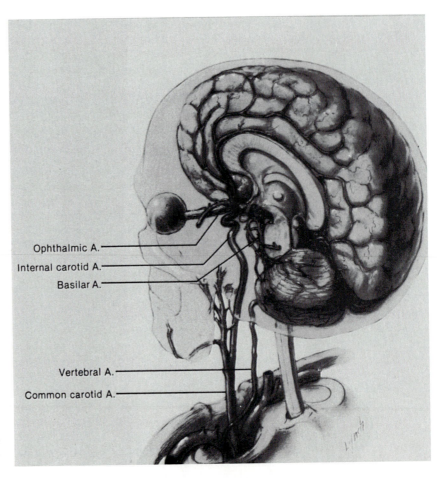

Ophthalmic A.
Internal carotid A.
Basilar A.
Vertebral A.
Common carotid A.

Figure 22–7. Normal cerebral circulation (lateral view). (*Reprinted, with permission, from Toole JF. Cerebrovascular disorders. 4th ed. New York: Raven Press; 1990:4.*)

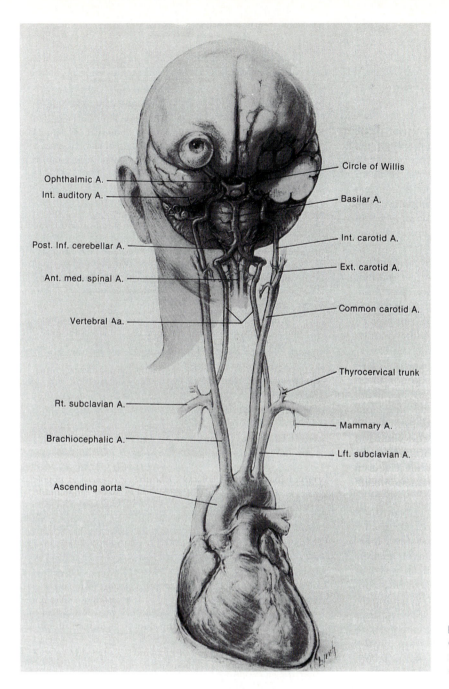

Ophthalmic A.

Int. auditory A.

Post. Inf. cerebellar A.

Ant. med. spinal A.

Vertebral Aa.

Rt. subclavian A.

Brachiocephalic A.

Ascending aorta

Circle of Willis

Basilar A.

Int. carotid A.

Ext. carotid A.

Common carotid A.

Thyrocervical trunk

Mammary A.

Lft. subclavian A.

Figure 22–8. Normal cerebral circulation (frontal view). (*Reprinted, with permission, from Toole JF. Cerebrovascular disorders. 4th ed. New York: Raven Press; 1990:2.*)

the largest of the three, extends laterally along the lateral sulcus and continues posteriorly. The middle meningeal artery supplies portions of the temporal, parietal, and frontal lobes, including portions for the primary motor and sensory areas. The anterior cerebral artery branches from the internal carotid, enters the basal portion of the superior longitudinal fissure, and extends medially and anteriorly. It supplies portions of the frontal and parietal lobes as well as the medial aspects of the primary sensory and motor gyri. The anterior cerebral artery ends in an anastomosis with the posterior cerebral artery coming off from the vertebral artery circuitry. The right and left anterior cerebral arteries are joined by the anterior communicating artery, which is approximately 4 mm long. Finally, the third branching of the internal carotid arteries becomes the right and left poste-

rior communicating arteries. These vessels pass posteriorly to supply portions of the thalamus, the internal capsule, and the walls of the third ventricle. They terminate by joining with posterior cerebral arteries.

The vertebral artery network is somewhat less complex. The vertebral arteries also arise as bilateral structures from the brachiocephalic artery on the right and directly from the aorta on the left. The vertebral arteries ascend through the foramina of the transverse processes for the upper six cervical vertebrae. Before entering the cranium the vertebral arteries give rise to the posterior inferior cerebellar arteries. Entering the cranial vault via the foramen magnum, the vertebral arteries next anastomose to form a single basilar artery. The basilar artery runs a short distance along the pons, giving off several small branches along its route which supply the cerebellum, pons, and middle ear. It then divides into two main branches: the right and left posterior cerebral arteries. These arteries supply the lateral portions for the temporal and occipital lobes and end by anastomosing with the posterior communicating arteries.

The network of anastomosing blood vessels at the base of the brain surrounding the optic chiasm allows for collateral circulation of the brain. It provides union of blood vessels supplying the brain by way of the carotid and vertebral arteries. This network of vessels is known as the circle of Willis and includes the anterior and posterior cerebral arteries and the anterior and posterior communicating arteries.

Physiology

Cerebral blood flow is maintained relatively constant at the rate of 45 to 50 mL per 100 g of tissue weight per minute. The average adult male brain weighs 1450 g, and the female brain, 1350 g. Cerebral blood flow therefore is approximately 665 mL per minute, or 15 percent of the cardiac output. The regional distribution of cerebral blood flow results in the white matter receiving only 20 mL/100 g of tissue, and the gray matter, 80 mL/100 g. This obviously shows that gray matter receives a proportionately greater amount of blood flow owing to its greater metabolic rate. The overall oxygen consumption in the brain is 3.3 mL of oxygen per 100 g of tissue weight per minute. We see that the ratio of cerebral blood flow to cerebral metabolic rate of oxygen is approximately 15:1. Despite this disproportionately high ratio, there is little basal oxygen reserve in the brain, and interruption of adequate blood flow for as little as 10 seconds can lead to loss of consciousness.

The constancy of cerebral blood flow is ensured by maintaining a stable, effective perfusion pressure to the brain. The perfusion pressure is the mean pressure difference between the veins and arteries. Venous pressure is relatively low and constant, typically being less than 10 torr in the internal jugular veins. The mean arterial blood pressure, therefore, generally ranges between 85 and 90 torr, keeping cerebral blood flow relatively constant. In addition to the perfusion pressure constancy, we find that the cerebral vasculature is extremely sensitive to changes in tissue oxygen and carbon dioxide tensions. These vessels have the ability to constrict and dilate to autoregulate cerebral blood flow within certain limits of perfusion pressures, thereby helping to ensure adequate cerebral perfusion. The limits spoken of above include mean arterial blood pressure between 60 and 180 torr, which encompasses most normal fluxes of systemic blood pressures. Above mean arterial blood pressures of 180 torr, the cerebral vasculature can no longer constrict to keep cerebral blood flow within normal limits and flow increases. This results in increased intracranial pressure and may lead to intracranial hemorrhage. Below a mean pressure of 60 torr, cerebral vessels cannot dilate further to keep blood flow constant and flow begins to decline. At this point, an additional mechanism ensures adequate cerebral tissue oxygenation. Below a mean pressure of 60 torr and down to a pressure of 35 torr, the cerebral tissue can extract more oxygen from hemoglobin to keep tissue oxygenation adequate. Below arterial pressures of 35 torr, signs of cerebral hypoxia are seen and irreversible brain damage may occur.

In addition to perfusion pressures, other factors maintain normal cerebral blood flow. There appears to be no evidence of direct action of the autonomic nervous system on human cerebral blood flow. Carbon dioxide and oxygen do effect changes in blood flow by acting to dilate or constrict arterial diameter, however. Carbon dioxide is the most potent dilator and constrictor, exerting its effect directly on the vascular smooth muscle, which results in a direct relationship between Pa_{CO_2} and cerebral blood flow (CBF) and an inverse relation between Pa_{CO_2} and CBF. Between Pa_{CO_2} values of 25 and 115 torr, there is a 1 mL/100 g/min change in cerebral blood flow. The influence of Pa_{CO_2} on cerebral flow is narrower, in the range 25 to 50 torr. At a Pa_{CO_2} of 50 torr, cerebral flow is approximately 50 mL/100 g/min, and at a Pa_{CO_2} of 25 torr, CBF is approximately 25 mL/100 g/min. This gives a ratio of change of 1 mL decrease in CBF for each 1 torr decrease in Pa_{CO_2} between 25 and 50 torr Pa_{CO_2}.

It is important for the anesthetist to have some understanding of the effects of anesthetics on cerebral blood flow and cerebral metabolic rate (Table 22–1). The agents listed in Table 22–1 relate to either 1 MAC level of inhalation agents or clinically effective levels of anesthesia. The plus symbols represent increases and the minus symbols represent decreases in the parameter reported.

Blood–Brain Barrier

The blood–brain barrier was conceived in an attempt to explain the different rates of permeability of most substances between the capillary bed and interstitial fluids of the brain compared with the more rapid equilibration between these two compartments, as seen in other organ systems. It was noted that water, carbon dioxide, oxygen, and glucose move rapidly from the blood into brain tissue. In general, the rapidity of the movement of all substances follows the specifics of Graham's law. Although many substances require a longer time to equilibrate, very few, if any, substances are totally prohibited entry. The cerebral capillaries are more permeable in the newborn, with the blood–brain barrier developing in the first few years of life. This explains why in jaundiced infants bile pigments may enter the nervous system and produce damage to the basal ganglia, resulting in kernicterus.

Some areas of the brain are more impregnable than

TABLE 22–1. EFFECTS OF ANESTHESIA ON CEREBRAL BLOOD FLOW

Agent	Cerebral Blood Flow	Cerebral Metabolic Rate
Halothane	+++	−−−
Enflurane	0	−−−−
Isoflurane	0	0
Ketamine	+++	−−−
Thiobarbiturates	−−−−	−−−−
Fentanyl/droperidol	−−	−
Diazepam + N₂O	−−−−	−−−−

others. The pineal gland, the posterior pituitary, and areas surrounding the ventricular structures are more susceptible to substances circulating in the plasma. Ions such as Na^+, K^+, Mg^{2+}, Cl^-, HCO_3^-, and HPO_4^{2-} equilibrate with cerebrospinal fluid but may require up to 30 times longer than water. Bile salts, catecholamines, and proteins have very limited access to the adult brain. Acid substances and cations penetrate more slowly than bases and anions. Finally, there is a very high correlation between lipid solubility and penetrability.

The clinical implication associated with knowledge of the permeability of the blood–brain barrier to drugs is that those anesthetics with a high solubility coefficient generally cause unconsciousness more quickly. Drugs enter the brain at differing rates; sulfadiazine and erythromycin enter readily, whereas penicillin and aureomycin enter slowly. Atropine readily crosses the blood–brain barrier, whereas glycopyrrolate does not. In addition to this information, the clinician should also be aware that the blood–brain barrier breaks down as the result of irradiation, local infection, and tumor growth.

CRANIAL NERVES

Categorization

The cranial nerves can be thought of as peripheral nerves arising from the brain. They consist of 12 pairs of nerves numbered in reference to their points of origin on the brainstem, anteriorly to posteriorly or superiorly to inferiorly. Each nerve is represented by a name and a Roman numeral. Cranial nerves enter or exit the brain by way of foramina in the base of the cranium. Because of the higher level of development of cephalic structures, cranial nerves are more complex than spinal nerves. Cranial nerves are involved primarily in innervation of structures of the head and neck and are further differentiated on the basis of input or output to special senses. The cranial nerves consist of either sensory or motor fibers, with some nerves containing both types. The commonly learned mnemonic represents the first letter of each named nerve: "On Old Olympus Towering Tops, A Finn and German Viewed Some Hops." Another mnemonic indicates whether the nerve is sensory, motor, or both: "Some Say Marry Money But Brothers Say Bad Business Marry Money." Creative students have devised a number of variations over the years.

Specific Cranial Nerves

All of the cranial nerves are now summarized with respect to type, course, function, and pathology

I. Olfactory Nerves
  A. Type: Sensory.
  B. Course: Receptors are modified exposed dendrites located in the nasal cavity and sensitive to a variety of vapors. Cell bodies are embedded in respiratory mucosa covering the cribriform plate of the ethmoid bone. Axons terminate in the primary area for smell (area 36) in the temporal lobe.

  C. Function: Sense of smell is relatively poorly developed in humans compared with lower animals.
  D. Pathology: Usually, local dysfunction is due to respiratory mucosal inflammation leading to anosmia. Pathology may be caused by intracranial tumors or head injuries which can present as olfactory hallucinations or anosmia.

II. Optic Nerves
  A. Type: Sensory.
  B. Course: The dendrites and cell bodies are in the retina and are not directly stimulated by light; rather, the stimulus causes a release of chemical transmitters, rhodopsin in the rods and iodopsin and photospsin in cones. From the retina the optic nerve travels to the optic chiasm, where medial fibers from each eye decussate. Each tract from the optic chiasm to the visual cortex (area 17) of the occipital lobe carries fibers from both eyes. The visual cortex is necessary for conscious perception of an upright image. Collateral fibers of this nerve also extend to the cranial nerves involved in extraocular movement to coordinate globe movement with visual perception.
  C. Function: Vision.
  D. Pathology: Prechiasmic involvement produces ipsilateral blindness; chiasm or postchiasm pathology produces varieties of hemianopsia.

III. Oculomotor Nerves
  A. Type: Somatic and visceral motor.
  B. Course: Somatic fibers originate in the Edinger–Westphal nucleus of the midbrain and synapse with all extraocular muscles except superior oblique and lateral rectus muscles, in addition to muscles elevating eyelids. Visceral fibers share their origin with the preganglionic fibers terminating in the ciliary muscle of the lens and the sphincter muscle of the iris.
  C. Function: Somatic fibers innervate levator palpebral, inferior oblique, inferior rectus, medial rectus, and superior rectus extraocular muscles to provide conjugate globe movement. The visceral nerves provide accommodation for far vision and for constriction of the iris.
  D. Pathology: Disjunctive eye movements, ptosis, and loss of accommodation.

IV. Trochlear Nerves
  A. Type: Somatic motor.
  B. Course: Fibers originate in the midbrain at the floor of the cerebral aqueduct, at the junction of the upper pons and cerebellar peduncles. These fibers terminate in the superior oblique extraocular muscle.
  C. Function: Allow conjugate globe movement medially.
  D. Pathology: Inability to turn eyes downward and outward with vertical diplopia.

V. Trigeminal Nerves
  A. Type: Sensory and somatic motor.
  B. Course: Sensory receptors for touch, pressure, pain, and temperature originate in the anterior half of the head. The cell body is in the gasserian ganglion and fibers terminate in the pons. The somatic motor fibers originate in the pons and terminate in the muscles of mastication and the tympanic membrane.
  C. Function: General sensation to the anterior half of the face with three divisions. The ophthalmic division is sensory, the maxillary division is sensory, and the mandibular division is both sensory and motor. The motor components control mastication, swallowing, movement for the soft palate, and eardrum tension.
  D. Pathology: Injury to the sensory root results in anesthesia to the anterior half of the face, dryness of the nose, and loss of sense of taste. Motor root involvement results in loss of mastication and paralysis of facial muscles, as well as tic douloureux.

VI. Abducens Nerves
  A. Type: Somatic motor.
  B. Course: The multipolar neurons of this nerve originate in the pons and innervate the lateral rectus extraocular muscle.
  C. Function: Operate conjugate globe movement temporally.
  D. Pathology: Internal or convergent squint.

VII. Facial Nerves
  A. Type: Sensory and somatic and visceral motor.
  B. Course: Sensory unipolar neurons have their receptors in the taste buds of the anterior two thirds of the tongue. Somatic motor fibers course from the pons to the facial muscles. Visceral fibers synapse in parasympathetic ganglia and terminate in salivary glands.
  C. Function: Sensory—taste to the anterior two thirds for the tongue; somatic motor—facial expressions; visceral motor—salivary, nasal, lacrimal, oral secretions.
  D. Pathology: Loss of sensation of taste to anterior two thirds of tongue, Bell's palsy, and inability to grimace.

VIII. Vestibulocochlear Nerves
  A. Type: Sensory.
  B. Course: The vestibular portion has receptors and cell bodies in the otoliths and semicircular canal of the inner ear and terminates in the cerebellum. The dendrites of the cochlear portion of this nerve originate as dendrites in the organ of Corti of the inner ear and terminate in the primary auditory area (area 41) of the temporal lobe.
  C. Function: The vestibular division ensures equilibrium, and the cochlear division, hearing.
  D. Pathology: Results in vertigo and perceptive deafness.

IX. Glossopharyngeal Nerves
  A. Type: Sensory and somatic and visceral motor.
  B. Course: Sensory neurons originate in the taste buds in the posterior third of the tongue, the chemoreceptors in the carotid bodies, the pressoreceptors in the carotid sinuses, as well as general sensory receptors in the oropharynx, hypopharynx, and middle ear. They terminate in the medulla oblongata. Somatic and visceral motor fibers originate in the medulla, with somatic efferent fibers innervating the pharyngeal constrictor muscles and the visceral efferent fibers terminating in the salivary glands.
  C. Function: Taste, general sensation to the throat, swallowing salivation, and monitoring of blood pressure, Pao_2, and $Paco_2$.
  D. Pathology: Loss of taste in posterior third of tongue, inability to swallow, loss of gag reflex.

X. Vagus Nerves
  A. Type: Visceral sensory and motor.
  B. Course: Sensory fibers originate in abdominal and thoracic viscera, as well as in chemoreceptors and pressoreceptors. They terminate in the medulla. The motor fibers originate as preganglionic parasympathetic fibers in the medulla and, after synapsing, innervate smooth muscles, cardiac muscle, and glands.
  C. Function: Sensory components provide general visceral afferent sensations and monitor blood pressure, Pao_2, and $Paco_2$, left-sided heart filling, and lung inflation. Motor components provide the characteristic parasympathetic autonomic excitatory effects.
  D. Pathology: Sensory dysfunction ranges from anesthesia of the larynx to overdistension of the lungs. Motor dysfunction results in paralysis of laryngeal function, absence of bowel activities, and generalized decrease in daily anabolic functions.

XI. Spinal Accessory Nerves
  A. Type: Somatic motor.
  B. Course: The cell bodies originate in the medulla and the anterior horn gray matter of the first five cervical spinal cord segments. The cranial fibers terminate in pharyngeal and laryngeal muscles; the spinal fibers innervate muscles of the neck and shoulders.
  C. Function: The cranial segment aids in swallowing and phonation; the spinal segments in movement of head and shoulders.
  D. Pathology: Dysphagia, hoarseness, and weakness of head and shoulder muscles.

XII. Hypoglossal Nerves
  A. Type: Somatic motor.
  B. Course: Cell bodies originate in the medulla and terminate in the tongue.
  C. Function: Movement of the tongue.
  D. Pathology: Inability to extend the tongue or weakness in movement of the tongue.

BIBLIOGRAPHY

Anthony CP, Thibodeau LC. *Structure and function of the body.* 11th ed. St. Louis, MO: CV Mosby; 1987.

Barr L, Kiernan JA. *The human nervous system.* 5th ed. Philadelphia: JB Lippincott; 1988.

Bates B, Hoeckelman RA. *A guide to physical examination.* 4th ed. Philadelphia: JB Lippincott; 1987.

Carpenter MB. *Human neuro-anatomy.* 8th ed. Baltimore: Williams & Wilkins; 1982.

Collins VJ. *Principles of anesthesiology.* 3rd ed. Philadelphia: Lea & Febiger; 1989.

Cousins MJ, Bridenbaugh PO, eds. *Neural blockage in clinical anesthesia and management of pain.* Philadelphia: JB Lippincott; 1980.

Crelin ES. *Clinical symposia: Development of the nervous system.* Summit, NJ: CIBA-Geigy; 1974;26:No. 2.

Cucchiara RF, Michenfelder JD. *Clinical neuroanesthesia.* New York: Churchill Livingstone; 1990.

Eliasson SC, Prensky BH Jr. *Neurological pathophysiology.* 2nd ed. Oxford: Oxford Press; 1978.

Ganong WF. *Review of medical physiology.* 14th ed. Los Altos, CA: Lange Medical; 1989.

Goodman AG, Gilman A. *The pharmacological basis of therapeutics.* 8th ed. New York: Macmillan; 1990.

Gray TC, Nunn JF, Utting JE. *General anesthesia.* 4th ed. London: Butterworths; 1986.

Guyton AC. *Textbook of medical physiology.* 8th ed. Philadelphia: WB Saunders; 1991.

Hoffman BB, Lefkowitz RJ. Alpha-adrenergic receptor subtypes. *N Engl J Med.* 1980;302:1390.

Johnson K. *Human developmental anatomy.* Media, PA: Harwal; 1988.

Junqueirra LC, Carneiros J. *Basic histology.* 6th ed. Los Altos, CA: Lange Medical; 1989.

Kandel ER, Schwartz JH. *Principles of neural science.* 2nd ed. New York: Elsevier/North-Holland; 1985.

Katz J, Benumof J, Kadis LB. *Anesthesia and uncommon diseases.* 3rd ed. Philadelphia: WB Saunders; 1990.

Merritt HH, ed. *A textbook of neurology.* 6th ed. Philadelphia: Lea & Febiger; 1979.

Miller RD, ed. *Anesthesia.* 3rd ed. New York: Churchill Livingstone; 1990.

Murray JM, Weber A. The cooperative action of muscle proteins. *Sci Am.* 1974;230(2).

Netter FH. *Atlas of human anatomy.* Summit, NJ: Ciba-Geigy; 1989.

Noback CR, Demarest RJ. *The human nervous system, basic principles of neurobiology.* 3rd ed. New York: McGraw-Hill; 1980.

Pansky B, Allen DJ. *Review of gross anatomy.* 6th ed. New York: Macmillan; 1989.

Rosenberg H. *Skeletal muscle structure and function. ASA Refresher Courses Anesthesiol.* 1977;5:149–160.

Shapiro HM. *Physiologic and pharmacologic regulation of cerebral blood flow. ASA Refresher Courses Anesthesiol.* Philadelphia, 1977;5: 161–178.

Warwick R, Williams PL. *Gray's anatomy.* 35th ed. Philadelphia: WB Saunders; 1973.

23

Hepatic and Renal Physiology

Nancy Bruton-Maree

Biodegradation and excretion of drugs, although not always consciously acknowledged, plays a major role in every anesthetic given. As the kidney and the liver are the major organs for metabolism and elimination of drugs, disease of either or both will have tremendous impact on anesthetic management. Successful anesthetic management is best accomplished when consideration is given to changes in hepatic and renal blood flow that can accompany anesthesia and surgery. In addition, fluid and electrolyte status and the nutritional well-being of the patient depend on both of these systems. Therefore, knowledge of basic hepatic and renal physiology is paramount for comprehension of the effects of pathophysiologic changes in either of these two systems and on perioperative management of patients.

HEPATIC SYSTEM

In the last three decades, mortality from liver disease has almost doubled in the United States and is increasing rapidly in other countries.[1] Alcohol consumption appears to be the major culprit, resulting in more patients with hepatic pathology presenting for anesthesia and surgery. For appropriate management a thorough understanding of hepatic function and the impact of pathophysiologic changes is important.

Anatomic Considerations

The liver, located in the upper right quadrant of the abdomen, is the largest visceral organ. In adults it weighs between 1.2 and 1.5 kg. It is divided into two lobes, with the right lobe being six times as large as the left. All of the major structures (i.e., ducts, portal vein, hepatic artery) enter the liver at an area known as the porta hepatis. The functional unit of the liver is the lobule and the most abundant liver cell is the hepatocyte. The liver lobules are cylindrical in shape, several millimeters in length, and 0.8 to 2

mm in diameter. About 50,000 to 100,000 lobules compose the total organ.

Each liver lobule is composed of hepatic cellular plates radiating from a central vein, much like the spokes of a wheel. The hepatic cellular plates are only one to two cells thick. Between adjacent cells that form the cellular plates lie the bile canaliculi, which drain bile from hepatocytes into the bile ducts located in septa separating adjacent liver lobules. The portal vein and the hepatic artery provide the major blood supply to the liver. Small portal venules, which are found in the septa, receive blood from the gastrointestinal tract, spleen, pancreas, and gallbladder via the portal vein. Blood in the hepatic artery, a branch of the celiac axis, merges with blood in the portal system in hepatic capillaries called sinusoids. The blood in the sinusoids flows through the liver lobules, ultimately emptying into the central veins, the hepatic veins, and finally the vena cava.

The venous sinusoids are composed of two types of cells, the endothelial cells, which line the sinusoids, and the Kupffer cells, which are phagocytic for bacteria and other foreign matter carried in the blood. The endothelial lining of the sinusoids is highly porous, allowing substances in the plasma to move through into spaces between the endothelial cells and the hepatocytes called *spaces of Disse*. These spaces connect with the lymphatic vessels in the interlobular septa and drain excess fluid through the lymphatics. The nerve supply to the liver is thought to be predominantly sympathetic, arising from the celiac plexus. These fibers are thought to control blood vessel caliber and bile duct sphincter tone.

Hepatic Blood Flow

The liver is the only major organ that receives a dual afferent blood supply.[2] The total hepatic blood flow is 1450 mL min^{-1}, with 1100 mL supplied by the portal vein and the remainder by the hepatic artery. Overall, about 25 to 30 percent of the cardiac output moves through the liver per minute. Hepatic arterial blood supplies the structural elements of the liver and then empties into the venous sinuses and mixes with portal blood. The combination of portal venous blood and hepatic arterial blood supplies nutrients, including oxygen, to the hepatocytes. Because of this mixing of arterial and venous blood prior to perfusion of the vital hepatocytes, oxygen delivery to the liver may be marginal, and the cells adjacent to the hepatic venules are extremely susceptible to hypoxia.

Hepatic blood flow is determined by perfusion pressure (mean arterial or portal vein pressure minus hepatic vein pressure) and splanchnic vascular resistance.[2] Normal mean portal venous pressure is 10 mm Hg; normal hepatic venous pressure is 5 mm Hg. Both alpha and beta sympathetic innervation are present in hepatic vessels and stimulation or blockade of either influences hepatic blood flow. The sympathetic stimulation is via sympathetic fibers arising at T-3 to T-11. Sympathetic stimulation from hypercarbia, arterial hypoxemia, or catecholamines will result in reduced blood flow through both of these vessels. Beta blockade, congestive heart failure, and positive-pressure ventilation with high inspiratory pressures also decrease hepatic blood flow. The presence of autoregulation of hepatic vessels is controversial.[3]

Physiologic Considerations

The major physiologic functions of the hepatocytes include glucose and fat metabolism, protein synthesis, drug and hormone biotransformation, bilirubin formation and synthesis, and phagocytosis of bacteria in the portal blood by the Kupffer cells.

Glucose Metabolism. Glucose homeostasis is maintained by the liver through complex biochemical mechanisms. Glycogenesis is the storage of glucose as glycogen. Hepatocytes form glycogen when glucose levels are high and exceed the cellular needs. Conversely, glycogenolysis is the conversion of glycogen to glucose when blood glucose levels are insufficient to meet cellular demand. In addition, hepatocytes can further ensure glucose homeostasis by converting fat and proteins to glucose, a process called *gluconeogenesis*.

Much of glucose homeostasis is controlled by hormones such as insulin, epinephrine, and glucagon. Insulin stimulates glycogenesis but inhibits gluconeogenesis. Glucagon and epinephrine stimulate gluconeogenesis and glycogenolysis and inhibit glycogenesis. The liver can store only approximately 75 g of glycogen, an amount that can be depleted in 24 to 48 hours of starvation. Once glycogen stores are depleted, gluconeogenesis is responsible for glucose homeostasis. Anesthesia may inhibit gluconeogenesis, as evidenced by dose-related decreases in the formation of glucose from lactate production by halothane.[4]

Fat Metabolism. Hepatocytes are the primary site for the conversion of chylomicrons to fatty acids and glycerol. These fatty acids, when influenced by glucagon, are then converted to ketone bodies and used as an energy source by cells in other body organs. If fatty acids are in excess, triglycerides are formed by the liver and used to synthesize lipoproteins and cholesterol. Excess accumulation of triglycerides in the liver can be a consequence of diseases such as diabetes mellitus, obesity, and Reye's syndrome.

Protein Synthesis. All proteins except gamma globulin and antihemophilic factor are produced by the liver.

Approximately 10 to 15 g of albumin is produced daily by hepatocytes.[2] Because the liver is so important for synthesis of albumin, liver disease often results in decreased albumin production and hypoalbuminemia. Hepatocytes are responsible for the synthesis of many of the protein clotting factors, among them prothrombin, fibrinogen, and factors V, VII, IX, and X. Pseudocholinesterase, an enzyme required for hydrolysis of drugs, is also metabolized in the liver. Predominant among these drugs are succinylcholine and ester local anesthetics.

Drug Metabolism. Hepatocytes have an abundance of smooth endoplasmic reticulum. These cellular organelles contain many enzymes for biotransformation of lipid-soluble drugs into water-soluble agents which can be eliminated by the kidney and the biliary system.

Bile Formation and Excretion. Bilirubin, in amounts of 250 to 350 mg per day, is produced from the breakdown of heme-containing compounds in the reticuloendothelial system.[2] This bilirubin is bound to albumin in the plasma, transported to the hepatocytes, and conjugated with glucuronic acid into a water-soluble form of bilirubin. The enzyme responsible for this conjugation is glucuronyl transferase. The majority of conjugated bilirubin is then excreted into the biliary canaliculi and eventually into the small intestine. In the intestine, bilirubin is converted to urobilinogen and urobilin. The urobilinogen can be reabsorbed and recirculated to the liver or excreted by the kidney.

Pathophysiology of the Liver

Liver disease is usually classified as acute or chronic. The most common types of hepatic pathology are hepatitis and cirrhosis. Both of these are parenchymal liver diseases that can result in hepatic failure and death.

Hepatitis. Hepatitis is a global inflammatory process of the liver.[5] The major forms of hepatitis are acute viral hepatitis, chronic active hepatitis, chronic persistent hepatitis, alcoholic hepatitis, and drug-induced hepatitis. Sometimes, patients who have chronic active, chronic persistent, or alcoholic hepatitis are scheduled for surgery. The various causes of hepatitis are listed in Table 23–1.

Hepatitis A virus is spread by fecal–oral contact, although transmission via blood and saliva has been documented. The virus does not persist in humans, and many cases of hepatitis are subclinical and anicteric. It is estimated that 50 percent of the U.S. adult population has serologic evidence of past infections.[6] Pertinent data for hepatitis A are summarized in Table 23–2.

TABLE 23–1. ETIOLOGIES OF HEPATITIS

Hepatitis A virus
Hepatitis B virus
Non-A, non-B hepatitis virus
Cytomegalovirus
Herpes simplex virus
Coxsackie virus
Epstein-Barr virus

TABLE 23–2. HEPATITIS A

Significant Features

Incubation period 20–45 days; often subclinical and anicteric
Affects primarily a young age group, median age 15 years
Carrier state: rare
First abdominal liver function test: increased transaminase
No chronic form of the disease
Mortality < 1:1000
Immunologic diagnosis
    Early: serum anti-HAAg IgM[a]
    Late: serum anti-HAAg IgG
Recovery usually occurs within 1–2 months
Occurrence of liver failure rare

Risk Factors

Contact with infected person
Foreign travel
Male homosexual
Exposure through day-care center participation

Diagnostic Features

History indicative of exposure to virus
Presence of serum anti-HAV IgM alone or in combination with anti-HAV IgG
IgM decreases over time IgG persists as an indication of developing immunity
With the appropriate equipment, HAAg (HAV) can be confirmed during the acute phase (This virus can be found only in the acute phase because there is no long-term carrier state.)
SGOT and SGPT can be very high
Abnormal liver enzyme levels do not always correlate with severity
Icteric phase usually begins with dark urine, followed by jaundice; bilirubinemia peaks in 1–2 weeks

[a] HAAg, hepatitis A antigen; HAV, hepatitis A virus; Ig, immunoglobulin; SGOT, serum glutamic–oxaloacetic transaminase; SGPT, serum glutamic–pyruvic transaminase.

The more important features of hepatitis B are listed in Table 23–3. This disease is more serious, from an anesthesia perspective, than hepatitis A. The disease can progress from an acute illness to a chronic disease. Patients can develop posthepatic cirrhosis and, although rare, hepatocellular carcinoma. Patients who develop subclinical hepatitis B have a higher incidence of chronic active and chronic persistent hepatitis, are more likely to be carriers of the virus, and are at greater risk for developing hepatocellular carcinoma.

Chronic hepatitis is defined as an inflammatory condition of the liver persisting beyond the acute episode, usually beyond 10 to 12 weeks from onset of illness.[3] Chronic persistent hepatitis carries a reasonably good prognosis. It is an immune-mediated disease that occurs in 6 to 12 percent of patients who have had icteric hepatitis B.[5] Transaminases demonstrate a fluctuating pattern, and the only indication of liver disease is occasional hepatomegaly. Absolute diagnosis of chronic persistent hepatitis is by liver biopsy, which

reveals inflammation but no fibrosis. Serologic markers are hepatitis B surface antigen (HBsAg) and antibody to hepatitis B core antigen (anti-HBc); the presence of hepatitis B e antigen (HbeAg) is variable. Although cases have been reported to continue for long periods, the usual time to recovery after acute hepatitis is 24 months. There are no clotting abnormalities accompanying chronic persistent hepatitis; nonetheless, anesthesia should be attempted only for nonelective procedures.

About 3 percent of patients with hepatitis B develop chronic active hepatitis and the prognosis of this disease is poor. These patients may be asymptomatic or have evidence of varying degrees of liver disease. All cases are positive for HBsAg and anti-HBc. HBeAg may be positive as well. Diagnosis is confirmed by liver biopsy which indicates bridging necrosis with disruption of limiting liver plates.[5] As the disease progresses, bilirubinemia may exist, prothrombin time may be abnormal, and anemia and thrombo-

TABLE 23–3. HEPATITIS B

Significant Features

Usually affects people between the ages of 15 and 44
Mortality may approach 5%
Carrier state does exist; asymptomatic carriers possible
Benign persistent hepatitis or chronic active hepatitis may develop

Risk Factors

Drug abuser
Homosexual
Contact with an infected person
Health care professional
Institutionalized person
Infant of mother with hepatitis B
Recipient of blood transfusions

Serologic Markers for Hepatitis B

HBsAg[a]: indicates active infection
Anti-HBs: implies immunity
(HBeAg)e antigen: may indicate chronic hepatitis
Anti-HBe: indicates benign infectivity

Diagnostic Features

Mutation phase can be from 30 to 120 days
Many vague symptoms, i.e., malaise, nausea, vomiting, anorexia, headaches
Right upper quadrant pain
Liver enlargement
Onset signaled by extreme elevations of serum transaminase
Usually icterus develops but anicterus is possible
Icteric phase begins within 3 to 10 days of onset of disease and is characterized by jaundice, gastrointestinal sequelae, pruritus, and hepatomegaly; acute liver failure can result
Convalescent phase is characterized by disappearance of jaundice over 1–6 weeks, gradual recovery from gastrointestinal symptoms, and full recovery within 3 months

[a] HBsAg, hepatitis B surface antigen; HBeAg, hepatitis B e antigen; anti-HBs(e), antibody to hepatitis B surface (e) antigen.

TABLE 23–4. NON-A, NON-B HEPATITIS

Significant Features	Risk Factors
Mortality rate 1–3%, > 20% if contracted during pregnancy	Drug abuse
Carriers do develop	Recipient of blood transfusions
At least three viral types have been isolated	Contact with an infected person
Cannot be detected by serum testing	Recent hospitalization
70% of cases may be asymptomatic and anicteric	**Diagnostic Features**
Sequelae are similar to those of hepatitis B, but occurrence of more serious sequelae is higher with non-A, non-B hepatitis	Diagnosis made through exclusion of hepatitis A and B

cytopenia occur. Anesthesia and surgery should be reserved for nonelective situations, as surgical and anesthetic risks become extremely high with progressive liver involvement.

The third type, non-A, non-B hepatitis, has been referred to as hepatitis C. Pertinent facts about non-A, non-B hepatitis are given in Table 23–4. Non-A, non-B hepatitis may be responsible for 40 to 50 percent of all patients hospitalized with hepatitis.[6] Again, only nonelective anesthesia and surgery should be performed on patients with known disease.

Cholestasis. Cholestasis means stagnation of bile.[7] Both extrahepatic impediments to bile flow in the extrahepatic biliary tree and intrahepatic obstruction of bile flow in the hepatocyte occur. Extrahepatic cholestasis is the easiest to cure surgically.[7,8] Clinical features distinguishing cholestasis from parenchymal liver disease are hyperbilirubinemia, increased alkaline phosphatase with minimal to moderate elevation in transaminases, and elevation of bile acids.[7]

Complications of cholestasis are proportional to the intensity and duration of the jaundice.[8] Biliary obstruction may result in ascending infection of the biliary tree, septic cholangitis, and secondary biliary cirrhosis which can result in liver cell failure and portal hypertension. Vitamin K, a fat-soluble vitamin, may not be absorbed from the intestine, leading to a decrease in vitamin K-dependent coagulation factors which manifests as prolonged prothrombin time. Patients with biliary obstruction who undergo biliary tract surgery may develop postoperative acute oliguric renal failure.[8]

Cirrhosis. Cirrhosis of the liver is a chronic process in which hepatic parenchyma is destroyed and replaced by collagen. This destruction of the organization of the liver lobules interferes with normal hepatic function. The most frequent cause of cirrhosis in the United States is alcoholism; other causes include congestive heart failure, Wilson's disease, hemochromatosis, primary biliary cirrhosis, and hepatitis.

The sequelae of cirrhosis include reductions in the number of hepatocytes, resulting in impairment in hepatic physiologic functions. The fibrotic process associated with cirrhosis results in increased intrahepatic resistance to portal vein flow and resultant portal hypertension. As the bulk of the blood flow through the liver is shunted to the hepatic artery, decreased perfusion pressure and arterial oxygenation are more likely to compromise hepatic blood flow and delivery of oxygen to liver cells. Alcoholic cirrhosis usually progresses from acute alcoholic hepatitis to portal vein hypertension. The diagnostic features of portal hypertension are listed in Table 23–5. Extrahepatic complications of cirrhosis can be dramatic (Table 23–6).

Preoperative Assessment

All patients with known or suspected liver disease should have a thoroughly documented history and physical. It is through these types of assessment that suspected liver disease may be confirmed and acute disease distinguished from chronic disease. In reviewing the history of patients with suspected hepatic or biliary disease, symptoms of jaundice, dark urine, pale stools, high fever, chills, anorexia, nausea and vomiting, weight loss, abdominal pain, hemorrhoids, fatty food intolerance, ascites, edema, nosebleeds, and bruises should be noted. In addition, patients should be questioned concerning possible exposure to hepatotoxic environmental factors, alcohol and drug abuse, and hepatitis. Routine examination of all organs and systems with par-

TABLE 23–5 DIAGNOSTIC FEATURES OF PORTAL HYPERTENSION

Anorexia and loss of skeletal mass, particularly of the head, neck, and arms
Hepatomegaly, splenomegaly, and ascites
Palmar erythema
Subcutaneous bleeding with minor trauma
Hematocrit 30–35%
Hyponatremia
With normal renal function, BUN[a] < 10 mg dL^{-1}
With renal insufficiency, BUN > 20
Mild to moderate elevation in alkaline phosphatase, plasma bilirubin, and transaminases

[a] BUN, blood urea nitrogen.

TABLE 23–6. EXTRAHEPATIC COMPLICATIONS OF CIRRHOSIS

Hyperdynamic circulation
Cardiomyopathy manifested as congestive failure
Megaloblastic anemia
Arterial hypoxemia
Renal failure
Hypoglycemia
Gallstones
Duodenal ulcers
Esophageal varices
Hepatic encephalopathy
Impaired immune defenses

ticular emphasis on the liver and spleen should be performed. The patient's appearance, including observation and evaluation of ascites, jaundice and degree of encephalopathy, hepatomegaly, and splenomegaly should be scrutinized.

Blood tests are important for diagnosing the presence, etiology, or degree of severity of hepatic disease. Patients may feel and look better than the laboratory values portray. Liver function tests useful for evaluation of hepatic disease are listed in Table 23–7. Other tests that are beneficial include hemoglobin/hematocrit, platelet count, serum electrolytes, prothrombin time, arterial blood gases, blood urea nitrogen, serum proteins, and blood glucose concentration. In addition, state of hydration and adequacy of renal output should be assessed.

Anesthetic Management of the Patient with Liver Disease

Patients with acute hepatitis or chronic active hepatitis, regardless of viral type, should not undergo surgery except in life-threatening situations. Because of the increased mortality/morbidity that anesthesia and surgery impose for patients with acute hepatitis, as well as the risk of infection to anesthesia and surgical personnel, every effort should be made to secure an accurate diagnosis in patients with liver disease of unknown etiology. Mortality associated with surgery has been reported as high as 9.5 percent in patients with acute hepatitis, and a 12 percent morbidity has been reported in those who survived.[9] As gloves are not fully protective against hepatitis B, the Centers for Disease Control strongly recommends all anesthesia personnel be vaccinated against this disease.[10]

Surgery on patients with chronic persistent hepatitis or other forms of chronic liver disease, such as cirrhosis, is usually reserved for nonelective procedures, as anesthetic drugs and surgical stress can further compromise hepatic function. If a patient with liver disease must have surgery, the amount of preoperative intervention depends on the severity of the hepatic disease. Some patients require no treatment; others require extensive interventions such as correction of clotting factors with vitamin K, fresh-frozen plasma, or both; correction of acid–base disturbances; hydration with appropriate fluid therapy; administration of diuretics to ensure adequate diuresis; treatment of hypoglycemia, prophylactic use of antibiotics; and stabilization of electrolyte abnormalities.

Whenever surgery permits, anesthetic management should include local infiltration, with or without sedation. Midazolam and small doses of fentanyl have been used successfully with hepatic disease, but it is important to remember that midazolam, like all highly protein bound drugs,

may have an enhanced effect if plasma protein levels are low. It has also been demonstrated that an increased number of benzodiazepine receptors may be present in advanced hepatic disease, which can result in a relative overdose from both receptor proliferation and greater drug affinity.[11] Careful drug titration of all intravenous agents is required in this patient population.

Regional techniques, including spinal anesthesia, may be considered for more extensive surgical procedures if clotting problems have not been identified. Any drugs used to control the disease should be given prior to surgery. Premedications should be administered with caution and in reduced doses. Premedication with an H_2-histamine blocker or metoclopramide may be considered to offset the sequelae of aspiration prior to a general anesthetic, as many of these patients have hiatal hernia, decreased gastric and intestinal motility, and ascites.

Routine monitors should be used on all hepatic disease patients regardless of the anesthetic technique chosen. Other more invasive monitors should be considered according to the severity of the disease and the extent of surgery. Induction of general anesthesia should include rapid sequence techniques if there is any suspicion of a full stomach. Intravenous barbiturates and benzodiazepines have been used successfully as induction agents in patients with liver disease, but careful titration is recommended as increased sensitivity is possible. Intubation has been facilitated by both depolarizing and nondepolarizing muscle relaxants without significant adverse sequelae even though liver dysfunction may be severe. The duration of action of succinylcholine may be prolonged with hepatic pathology if plasma cholinesterase levels are decreased. The volume of distribution may be increased for curare if elevated levels of gamma globulin are present because of increased protein binding of this drug. The volume of distribution is increased for pancuronium for unknown reasons and for atracurium because of increased extracellular fluid.[12,13] The clearance and elimination half-life for atracurium remain normal.[13] In small doses, there appears to be no alteration in pharmacokinetics for vecuronium.[14] As pharmacokinetic differences between muscle relaxants exist, a peripheral nerve stimulator facilitates titration of drugs according to patient need.

Further injury to the liver can occur during anesthesia if oxygen supplies are jeopardized as perfusion pressures are already minimal. Therefore, inspired oxygen tension should be adequate and oxygen carrying capacity should be maintained. Circulating volume, arterial blood pressure, cardiac output, and regional perfusion pressures should be optimized. Anesthesia-induced hypotension must be avoided and deliberate hypotension should not be used. Isoflurane and enflurane appear to be the best volatile

TABLE 23–7. LIVER FUNCTION TESTS AND DIFFERENTIAL DIAGNOSIS

Hepatic Dysfunction	Bilirubin	Transaminase Enzyme	Alkaline Phosphatase
Prehepatic	Unconjugated	Normal	Normal
Intrahepatic	Conjugated	Elevated	Normal to elevated
Extrahepatic	Conjugated	Normal to elevated	Elevated

agents to maintain perfusion pressure; isoflurane may be preferable. Nitrous oxide has been used extensively in liver disease, but this agent may stimulate sympathetic activity which may decrease hepatic blood flow. Adequate levels of anesthesia should be maintained to avoid endogenous release of catecholamines, renin–angiotension hormone, or antidiuretic hormone, all of which can decrease hepatic blood flow and potentially decrease oxygen delivery. Positive-pressure ventilation should be optimized to prevent increased thoracic pressure, which would decrease venous return to the right side of the heart and ultimately decrease cardiac output.

Studies support fentanyl as the best opioid for use in hepatic disease. This drug does not decrease oxygen supply or hepatic perfusion and does not increase oxygen delivery.[15] One possible anesthetic technique for the patient with hepatic disease is to decrease the concentration of isoflurane by using fentanyl as an adjunct agent. This may maintain better perfusion pressure and heart rate.

As renal dysfunction may accompany hepatic disease, existing renal function should be preserved during anesthesia. Patients with significant hepatocellular disease should have a urinary catheter and, depending on the type and duration of surgery, a pulmonary artery catheter and central venous pressure monitor. Furosemide and mannitol are both advocated as diuretics of choice to maintain urine flow.[16] In addition, dopamine, 2 to 4 μg kg^{-1} min^{-1}, may be infused to encourage renal function.[17] In severe liver dysfunction, coagulation factors should be monitored and replaced as indicated with platelets, fresh-frozen plasma, and cryoprecipitate.

Patients with biliary disease who require surgery, in the absence of severe hepatic dysfunction, have no absolute contraindications to any anesthetic agents. Careful use of opioids is recommended as these drugs can increase the tone of the sphincter of Oddi. This increase in tone, however, does not contraindicate the use of the drugs during anesthesia or for pain management. Drugs such as atropine, naloxone, glucagon, and nitroglycerine can reverse the increased sphincter tone caused by the analgesics.[17–19]

EXCRETORY SYSTEM

The kidney is important for the maintenance of body fluid and electrolyte homeostasis, acid–base balance, and elimination of metabolic by-products. In addition, this system has a major responsibility for excretion of drugs and their metabolites. The incidence of end-stage renal failure is estimated to be 91 per million people per year.[20,21] There is a striking difference in the occurrence of this disease relative to race: 188 per million for blacks and 44 per million for caucasians.[20,21] Renal disease, therefore, has a significant incidence in the general population and an important effect on homeostasis, which will influence selection of anesthetic agents as well as actual management.

Anatomy

The kidneys are paired organs located retroperitoneally on either side of the vertebral column against the posterior abdominal wall. The anatomic zones of the kidney are the cortex, the outer medulla, and the inner medulla. All major structures such as the ureters, renal artery, and renal vein enter through the renal pelvis.

The functional unit of the kidney is the nephron. Approximately 1 million nephrons compose one kidney. Anatomically, this microscopic unit is composed of Bowman's capsule, a proximal convoluted tubule, Henle's loop, a distal convoluted tubule, and a collecting duct. Each collecting duct is the conduit for 3000 to 5000 distal convoluted tubules. Nephrons are classified as cortical and juxtaglomerular of which 85 percent are cortical nephrons. Juxtaglomerular nephrons have loops of Henle that dip deep into the inner medullary portion of the kidney and participate significantly in concentrating urine prior to excretion. The loops of Henle of cortical nephrons penetrate only into the outer medullary surface.

The amount of total cardiac output circulating through the kidney varies from 12 to 30 percent in the resting normal person. The blood supply to the nephron flows progressively through the arcuate artery, the afferent arteriole, the glomerulus, the efferent arteriole, the peritubular capillaries, the venules, and then into the arcuate vein. A special portion of the peritubular capillaries, the vasa recti, descends into the medulla around the loops of Henle of the juxtamedullary nephrons. The renal vasculature is unique in that it has two capillary beds: (1) the glomeruli and (2) the peritubular capillaries. The glomeruli are considered high-pressure beds, whereas the peritubular capillaries are low-pressure beds.

Renal Vascular Physiology

The pressures in the renal vasculature are compatible with filtration of fluid into the structures of the nephron, reabsorption of fluid and electrolytes into the capillaries, and secretion and excretion of metabolic end products. The two major areas of vascular resistance are the small renal arteries and afferent arteriole and the efferent arterioles. The high-pressure capillary bed in the glomerulus operates at a mean of 50 mm Hg, causing rapid filtration of fluid into Bowman's capsule. The low-pressure capillary bed in the peritubular capillaries operates at a mean pressure of 13 mm Hg, allowing rapid reabsorption of fluid because of the higher osmotic pressure of plasma.

About 180 L of fluid is filtered through the glomeruli each day. The rate at which fluid is filtered is called the *glomerular filtration rate (GFR)*. Of this filtrate, only 1 to 1.5 L becomes urine. The remainder is reabsorbed into the renal interstitial fluid and then into the peritubular capillaries. Factors that influence the GFR are listed in Table 23–8.

Formation of Urine. The nephron has a blind end called *Bowman's capsule* which is surrounded by the glomerulus. Fluid is filtered from the glomerulus into Bowman's capsule and then into the proximal convoluted tubule, a direct continuation of the capsule. Eighty-five percent of sodium, chloride, and water reabsorption occurs from this tubule into the peritubular capillaries. Calcium ions, glucose, phosphate, and potassium are reabsorbed from these same

TABLE 23–8. FACTORS THAT INFLUENCE THE GLOMERULAR FILTRATION RATE

Decreased systemic arterial pressure	Creates a decreased hydrostatic pressure in the glomeruli and, consequently, outward filtration into Bowman's capsule
Hemorrhage/dehydration	Causes an increase in oncotic pressure of plasma; results in decreased filtration pressure
Ureteral obstruction	Results in increased hydrostatic pressure in Bowman's capsule and opposed glomerular filtration

tubules. About 25 percent of the total sodium is reabsorbed from Henle's loops into the medullary interstitium. The majority is absorbed from the ascending limbs of Henle's loops via active transport processes. In comparison to sodium reabsorption, water reabsorption from these loops is less, creating a tubular filtrate hypotonic to plasma. A hypertonic medullary interstitium is created by the loops of Henle via the countercurrent mechanism.

The distal convoluted tubules reabsorb sodium, chloride, and water and do this maximally when influenced by aldosterone. Secretion of hydrogen, potassium, and ammonia also occurs into these areas of the nephron. Free water reabsorption into the peritubular capillaries can occur dramatically in the presence of antidiuretic hormone (ADH), a pituitary hormone that increases the permeability of both the distal convoluted tubules and the collecting ducts. Without ADH, the urine will contain a high volume of free water. Hydrogen ion secretion and excretion of ammonium ions (formed by a combination of hydrogen and ammonia) facilitate the elimination of acid metabolites and the maintenance of acid–base balance.

Hormonal Function. Insulin is deactivated by the kidney. As renal failure can interfere with this deactivation, patients with a glucose intolerance who develop renal failure may improve in this respect. Some afferent arterioles and segments of distal convoluted tubules have special smooth muscle cells called macula densa. It is in the macula densa that renin is synthesized and secreted. This area of specialized cells is also known as a juxtaglomerular apparatus. Renin is secreted in response to beta-adrenergic stimulation, decreased perfusion pressure in afferent arterioles, and reductions in sodium load delivered to distal convoluted tubules.[22] Renin acts on α_2-globulins in plasma to form angiotensin I. Angiotensin I is converted in the lungs to angiotensin II, a potent vasoconstrictor. The vasoconstrictive response of the renal artery to angiotensin II decreases both renal blood flow and glomerular filtration rate. Aldosterone secretion is also increased if circulating levels of angiotensin II are high.

Prostaglandins E_2 and I_2 (PGE_2 and PGI_2) are released by the renal medulla in response to increased sympathetic nervous system activity and increased levels of angiotensin II. These hormones cause renal artery vasodilation. Prostaglandin F_2 is a potent vasoconstrictor that increases renal artery vascular tone. An optimal effect of ADH appears lacking without prostaglandins.

Renal Pathophysiology

Acute Renal Failure. Acute renal failure (ARF) can be defined as an abrupt deterioration of renal function resulting in accumulation of nitrogenous waste products in the blood and various fluid, electrolyte, and acid–base imbalances.[23] The usual etiology is ischemic or toxic injuries to the kidney.[23] Acute renal failure is a collective term used to refer most often to acute tubular necrosis (ATN) and lower nephron nephrosis.[24] The three types of ARF classified by etiology are listed in Table 23–9.[24] Prerenal failure usually reverses if circulation is restored promptly. Postrenal failure reverses if obstruction is alleviated without delay. Acute renal failure may also be described as oliguric, nonoliguric, and polyuric renal failure. Acute renal failure resulting from primary disease is the most serious and often requires hemodialysis.[25]

The major problems associated with ARF are the inability to maintain a normal intake of necessary nutrients and excrete the by-products associated with their utilization. The resulting symptoms for ARF are listed in Table 23–10. Acute renal failure usually progresses through three phases: (1) oliguria, (2) diuresis, and (3) return of total function. Hemodialysis is required during the oliguria phase, and diuresis following oliguria usually signals the beginning of recovery. As urine volume increases, fluids and electrolytes must be replaced and maintained as the renal concentrating ability is restored late in renal recovery.[24] About 50 to 60 percent of patients with ARF either do not survive or develop chronic renal failure; about two thirds of the patients who survive ARF recover all parameters of renal function.

Chronic Renal Failure. Chronic renal failure (CRF) is characterized by a progressive loss of functioning nephrons.[22] This loss leads to irreversible reduction in the GFR, hemodialysis, and possibly renal transplantation. Diseases that can lead to CRF are diabetic nephropathy, polycystic kidneys, chronic glomerulonephritis, and tubulointerstitial disease. The changes characteristic of CRF are listed in Table 23–11. In CRF, hemoglobin concentrations range from 5 to 8 g dl^{-1}. The degree of anemia usually parallels the decrease in renal dysfunction but remains relatively constant after end-stage renal failure has occurred.[22] Anemia is

TABLE 23–9. ACUTE RENAL FAILURE

Type	Etiology
Prerenal	Circulatory problems that severely impair perfusion
Renal	Primary or secondary renal disease, toxins, and pigments
Postrenal	Obstruction of the urinary tract

TABLE 23–10. SYMPTOMS OF ACUTE RENAL FAILURE

Progressive elevation in blood chemistries (i.e., blood urea nitrogen, creatinine, uric acid, magnesium, sulfate)

Daily rise in potassium

Decreased serum Na^+ and Ca^{2+}

Decreased serum proteins

Metabolic acidosis

Increased total lipids, cholesterol, phosphorus, and triglycerides

Hyperglycemia

Disorders of aldosterone and renin–angiotensin secretion

Decreased erythropoietin resulting in anemia

Heart failure, coagulation abnormalities, and abnormalities in liver function

the direct result of decreased erythropoietin. The major complication associated with anemia is decreased oxygen carrying capacity. The patient with CRF increases cardiac output and shifts the oxygen dissociation curve to the right as compensatory mechanisms. The predominant coagulopathy observed in CRF is platelet dysfunction. Other factors that may contribute to coagulopathies are heparinization required for patency of vascular shunts needed for dialysis and a decrease in coagulation factors caused by associated liver dysfunction.

Patients with CRF have an unpredictable hydration status often complicated by hyperkalemia, hypermagnesemia, and hypocalcemia. In addition, the incidence of congestive heart failure is increased in CRF. Abnormal central and peripheral nervous system function can lead to fatigue, insomnia, and mental depression. Peripheral neuropathies precipitated by uremia are not uncommon. Compensatory responses to changes in blood volume are often adversely altered. Gastric volume is often increased along with a decrease in gastric pH when uremia is present. In addition, the incidence of diabetes mellitus is increased in CRF.

Preoperative Assessment

History and Physical. A thorough history and physical are important preoperatively for renal patients, with special emphasis placed on a comprehensive medical history.[24] If renal disease is suspected, laboratory tests more specific for diagnosis are needed (Table 23–12). A urinalysis can be examined for bacteria, evidence of bleeding, urinary pH,

protein content, and glucose. Hematuria is suggestive of glomerular disease or trauma to the kidney or lower urinary tract. Presence of white blood cells, pyuria, or both may indicate renal infection such as pyelonephritis. Determination of urinary pH may assist in diagnosing acid–base disturbances. Proteinuria is another indicator of glomerular disease. The best indicator for GFR dysfunction is an elevated creatinine clearance. Exercise tolerance can be as important as hemoglobin in assessing the need for preoperative transfusion. Transfusion should be performed prior to surgery and can be done concomitantly with dialysis to prevent unnecessary increases in intravascular volume. A preoperative electrocardiogram can reflect elevated potassium, digitalis toxicity, and hypocalcemia. Preoperative findings that differentiate between renal insufficiency and renal failure are listed in Table 23–13.

Anesthetic Management. Monitors and monitoring techniques are selected according to the severity of the renal pathology and the type of surgery planned. Routine monitors to monitor blood pressure, heart rate and rhythm, adequacy of oxygenation, and temperature and, if possible, capnography should be employed. Arterial cannulation may be desirable for evaluation of blood gases, serum electrolytes, and coagulation factors. Urinary catheterization is the only indirect measure of urinary function. In high-risk patients, monitoring of cardiovascular status via central venous pressure, pulmonary artery pressure, or both may be desirable. Functioning arteriovenous shunts should be protected by correct patient positioning and checked routinely for patency. Chronic antihypertensive and cardiac drugs should be continued up to time of surgery.[22] As increased gastric volume and decreased gastric pH are problematic, premedication to decrease volume and increase pH may be desirable. Central nervous system premedication should be used cautiously as increased sensitivity is not unusual.

Drugs should be carefully selected for anesthetic management. Renal disease patients may have hypoalbuminemia, an acidic pH, or an altered blood–brain barrier, all of which may increase sensitivity to drugs usually selected for intravenous induction. The initial dose of thiopental should be lower and given more cautiously than that administered to a nonrenal patient; however, the overall total dose needed may be the same.[27] Ketamine and benzodiazepines are less affected by decreases in plasma albumin levels, although ketamine may have a deleterious effect on blood

TABLE 23–11. CHARACTERISTICS OF CHRONIC RENAL FAILURE

Chronic anemia

Coagulopathies

Altered hydration

Electrolyte imbalance

Systemic hypertension

Metabolic acidosis

Increased incidence of infection

TABLE 23–12. LABORATORY TESTS FOR RENAL DISEASE

Urinalysis

Complete blood count

Serum creatinine and creatinine clearance

Blood urea nitrogen

Serum electrolytes

Arterial blood gases

Chest x-ray

Electrocardiogram

TABLE 23–13. RENAL INSUFFICIENCY VERSUS RENAL FAILURE

Renal insufficiency	Mild azotemia
	Nocturia
	Slight anemia
	Decreased maximum urinary concentrating ability
Renal failure	Moderate to severe anemia
	Hypocalcemia
	Hyperphosphatemia
	Inability to concentrate and dilute urine
	Possibly hyponatremia, polyuria, and hyperchloremia
	Creatinine 2.5–4.0 mg/100 mL
	Creatinine clearance 15–20 mL/min

pressure and cardiac output. Debilitated renal patients may have exaggerated respiratory and cardiovascular effects from benzodiazepines.[28]

Morphine-induced respiratory depression is prolonged in patients with renal failure.[29] Additionally, fentanyl, alfentanil, and sufentanil are all metabolized by the liver and have metabolites that are excreted by the kidney. Sufentanil has been shown to cause prolonged respiratory depression in renal disease, and cautious use of both fentanyl and alfentanil is recommended in this patient population as well. Low doses of drugs should be carefully titrated to the effect desired.

Most popular inhalation agents appear to have minimal impact on patients with renal disease as their elimination does not rely on renal function. If some degree of renal function is present, consideration should be given to not using agents that produce metabolites excreted by the kidney. If the patient is anephric, nephrotoxic inhalation agents are not a major consideration. Of the major agents, isoflurane undergoes the least metabolism. Other advantages of the inhalation agents are the ability to deliver a high concentration of oxygen during administration and the inherent muscle relaxation afforded by their use.

Muscle relaxants of choice for the patient with renal disease are atracurium and vecuronium.[30,31] Atracurium has an elimination half-life of 30 minutes with and without renal failure.[30] Ester hydrolysis and Hoffmann elimination are responsible for clearance of atracurium from the blood, and neither of these metabolic pathways relies on renal function for effect. All of the longer-acting muscle relaxants rely on renal elimination of unchanged drug to some degree and have prolonged durations of action in the presence of decreased renal function. Succinylcholine has been used for many years in patients with renal disease, even those with elevated serum potassium levels. Although succinylcholine increases serum potassium levels in patients with renal failure, its use does not increase the incidence of serious cardiac dysrhythmias. It would, however, appear prudent to eliminate this risk by using an intermediate-acting nondepolarizing muscle relaxant.

Reversal agents for neuromuscular blockade such as neostigmine, pyridostigmine, and edrophonium are heavily

dependent on renal elimination, and renal failure prolongs their duration of action.[32–34] This fact has little effect on their use in this patient population, as prolonged duration results in less chance of recurarization from lingering nondepolarizing muscle relaxant drugs. Peripheral nerve stimulators can facilitate the safe use of muscle relaxants as well as the reversal of neuromuscular blockade with the anticholinesterase agents.

Perioperative Oliguria

Oliguria is defined as a urinary output of less than 0.5 mL $kg^{-1} h^{-1}$ and the causes can be categorized as prerenal, renal, and postrenal.[22] Aggressive and early treatment of oliguria in the perioperative period is imperative, particularly in patients at great risk for developing renal failure (Table 23–14). Occurrence of transient oliguria during elective operations in young patients without evidence of renal disease does not require the aggressive treatment required in the groups at risk for development of renal failure.[22]

The initial treatment of oliguria when risk of renal failure is high is rapid infusion of 500 mL of a balanced salt solution. This is preferable to diuretics, which can worsen cardiovascular parameters if the cause of oliguria is hypovolemia. Further fluid may be infused without response to the initial challenge if the patient is not at risk for cardiovascular decompensation. In the patient at risk for cardiovascular complications or the patient who does not respond to an additional fluid load, drug therapy must be considered. If decreased renal blood flow from decreased cardiac output is suspected and pulmonary capillary wedge pressure is high, dopamine, 1 to 5 $\mu g \; kg^{-1} \; min^{-1}$, may be useful. If dopamine fails to produce urine, a diuretic such as furosemide can be added. Recommended doses of furosemide for perioperative oliguria range from 1 to 15 mg kg^{-1}.[22]

SUMMARY

Patients with hepatic disease or renal disease present a challenge to the anesthetist when they appear for anesthesia and surgery. A careful history and physical followed by further diagnostic tests are required for the development of an appropriate plan of management. Additionally, information gleaned from the preoperative assessment must be related to changes in pharmacokinetics and pharmacodynamics of current drugs to ensure the best perioperative care is provided for the patient with either or both of these disease processes.

TABLE 23–14. PATIENTS AT RISK FOR OLIGURIA

Geriatric patients

Patients with sepsis

Patients with coexisting cardiac and renal disease

Patients undergoing surgical procedures carrying a high risk of postoperative renal compromise

REFERENCES

1. Schmidt W. The epidemiology of cirrhosis of the liver. In: Fisher MM, Rankin JG, eds. *Alcohol and the liver.* New York: Plenum Press; 1979:1.

2. Stoelting RK, Dierdorf SF, McCammon RL. Diseases of the liver and biliary tract. In: Stoelting RK, Dierdorf SF, McCammon RL, eds. *Anesthesia and Co-existing disease.* New York: Churchill Livingstone; 1988;19:355–389.

3. Norris CP, Barnes GE, Smith EE. Autoregulation of superior mesenteric blood flow in fasted and fed dogs. *Am J Physiol.* 1979;237:H1174.

4. Biebuyck JF. Effects of anesthetic agents on metabolic pathways: Fuel utilization and supply during anesthesia. *Br J Anaesth.* 1973;45:263–268.

5. Brown BR. Hepatitis. In: Brown BR, ed. *Anesthesia in hepatic and biliary tract disease.* Philadelphia: FA Davis; 1988;14:183–200.

6. Krugman S, Ward R, Giles JP. The natural history of infectious hepatitis. *Am J Med.* 1962;32:717.

7. Brown BR. Obstructive (cholestatic) jaundice. In: Brown BR, ed. *Anesthesia in hepatic and biliary tract disease.* Philadelphia: FA Davis; 1988;20:253–261.

8. Mervyn M, Marie CP. Anesthesia and the liver. In: Miller RD, Cucchiara RF, Miller ED Jr, Reves JG, Roizen MF, Savarese JJ, eds. *Anesthesia.* 3rd ed. New York: Churchill Livingstone; 1990;56:1809–1824.

9. Harville DD, Dummerskill WHJ. Surgery in acute hepatitis. Causes and effects. *JAMA.* 1963;184:257.

10. Reingold AL, Kane MA, Hightower AW. Failure of gloves and other protective devices to prevent transmission of hepatitis B virus to oral surgeons. *JAMA.* 1988;259:2558.

11. Samson Y, Bernuau J. Cerebral uptake of benzodiazepine measured by positron emission tomography in hepatic encephalopathy. *N Engl J Med.* 1987;316Z:414.

12. Duvaldestin P, Agoston S, Henzel D, et al. Pancuronium pharmacokinetics in patients with liver cirrhosis. *Br J Anaesth.* 1978;50:1131.

13. Ward S, Neill EAM. Pharmacokinetics of atracurium in acute hepatic failure (with acute renal failure). *Surv Anesth.* 1984;28:364.

14. Arden JR, Cannon JC, Lynam DP, et al. Vecuronium pharmacokinetics and pharmacodynamics in hepatocellular disease. *Anesth Analg.* 1987;66:S3.

15. Gelman S, Dillard E, Bradley EL Jr. Hepatic circulation during surgical stress and anesthesia with halothane, isoflurane, or fentanyl. *Anesth Analg.* 1987;66:936.

16. Gelman S. Anesthesia and the liver. In: Barash PG, Cullen BF, Stoelting RK, eds. *Clinical anesthesia.* Philadelphia: JB Lippincott; 1989;42:1133–1159.

17. Arguelles JE, Franatovic Y, Romo-Salas F, et al. Interbiliary pressure changes produced by narcotic drugs and inhalation anesthetics in guinea pigs. *Anesth Analg.* 1979;58:120.

18. McCammon RL, Viegas OJ, Stoelting RK, et al. Naloxone reversal of choledochoduodenal sphincter spasm associated with narcotic administration. *Anesthesiology.* 1978;48:437.

19. Jones RM, Fiddian-Green R, Knight PR. Narcotic-induced choledochoduodenal sphincter spasm reversed by glucagon. *Anesth Analg.* 1978;48:437.

20. Easterling RE. Racial factors in the incidence and causation of endstage renal disease. *Trans Am Soc Artif Intern Organs.* 1977;23:28.

21. Rostand SG, Kirk KA, Rutsky EA, et al. Racial differences in the incidence of treatment for end-stage renal disease. *N Engl J Med.* 1982;306:1276.

22. Stoelting RK, Dierdorf SF, McCammon RL. Renal disease. In: Stoelting RK, Dierdorf SF, McCammon RL, eds. *Anesthesia and co-existing disease.* New York: Churchill Livingstone; 1988;21:409–441.

23. Torrente AD. Acute renal failure. *Int Anesthesiol Clin.* 1984;22(1):83–100.

24. Mazze RI. Anesthesia and the renal and genitourinary systems. In: Miller RD, Cucchiara RF, Miller ED Jr, Reves JG, Roizen MF, Savares JJ, eds. *Anesthesia.* 3rd ed. New York: Churchill Livingstone; 1990;55:1791–1805.

25. Mazze RL. Critical care of the patient with acute renal failure. *Anesthesiology.* 1977;47:138.

26. Brown CB, Cameron JS, Ogg CS, et al. Established acute renal failure following surgical operations. In: Friedman EA, Eliahue HE, eds. *Proceedings of the conference on acute renal failure.* DHEW Publication No. (NIH) 74-608. Washington, DC: U.S. Government Printing Office; 1973.

27. Burch PG, Stanski DR. Decreased protein binding and thiopental kinetics. *Clin Pharmacol Ther.* 1982;32:212.

28. Prough DS, Foreman AS. Anesthesia and the renal system. In: Barash PG, Cullen BF, Stoelting RK, eds. *Clinical anesthesia.* Philadelphia: JB Lippincott; 1989;39:1079–1099.

29. Don HF, Dieppa RA, Taylor P. Narcotic analgesics in anuric patients. *Anesthesiology.* 1975;42:745.

30. Fahey MR, Rupp SM, Fisher DM, et al. Dose-response of tubocurarine in patients with and without renal failure. *Anesthesiology.* 1984;61:699.

31. Fahey MR, Morris RB, Miller RD, et al. Pharmacokinetics of OrgNC45 (Norcuron) in patients with and without renal failure. *Br J Anaesth.* 1981;53:1049.

32. Cronnelly R, Stanski DR, Miller RD, et al. Renal function and the pharmacokinetics of neostigmine in anesthetized man. *Anesthesiology.* 1979;51:222.

33. Cronnelly R, Stanski DR, Miller RD, et al. Pyridostigmine kinetics with and without renal function. *Clin Pharmacol Ther.* 1980;28:78.

34. Morris RB, Cronnelly R, Miller RD, et al. Pharmacokinetics of edrophonium in anephric and renal transplant patients. *Br J Anaesth.* 1981;53:1311.

Endocrine Physiology

Bruce Skolnick

The study of hormones and the glands that secrete them is known as endocrinology. Endocrine glands are distinct from exocrine glands, because their chemical products pass into the bloodstream rather than into ducts, as do the secretions of the exocrine glands; however, the point should not be missed that some glands, such as the pancreas, are properly considered to be both endocrine and exocrine in function. Insulin and glucagon, the most important of the pancreatic hormones, are secreted by the islets of Langerhans into the portal venous blood. The acinar cells of the pancreas, the exocrine portion, secrete bicarbonate and digestive enzymes into the pancreatic duct.

Despite the fact that the individual endocrine glands are scattered over numerous locations, they collectively are considered to be a single system. This is because it is the rule rather than the exception that, if a given physiologic function is controlled by one endocrine gland, it is almost always also controlled by at least one other gland. An example would be endocrine regulation of blood pressure, which is directly or indirectly influenced by the pituitary, the hypothalamus, the kidney, and the thyroid. Other physiologic functions that are of importance to the anesthetist and that are controlled by multiple endocrine glands include temperature regulation, metabolism, and the blood concentrations of glucose, calcium, sodium, and potassium.

This chapter is divided into two portions. The first deals with certain topics common to the understanding of the endocrine system in general. The second portion is devoted to a more thorough discussion of those endocrine glands that are the most important to the anesthetist.

CHEMICAL CLASSIFICATION OF HORMONES

Hormones can be grouped into three main categories according to their chemical composition: (1) proteins or polypeptides, (2) amino acids or amino acid derivatives, and (3) steroids.

Proteins and Polypeptides

Most of the hormones in the body are composed of proteins or polypeptides. A peptide bond is a special junction formed between two amino acids, and when several amino acids are joined together by such bonds, the resulting molecule is called a polypeptide. Most biochemists restrict the use of the term *polypeptide* to chains of only a few amino acids, leaving the designation *protein* to refer to much longer chains of amino acids. The two terms are often used to refer to the same molecule, however. In this chapter, *polypeptide* refers to hormones of 10 or fewer amino acids, whereas *protein* refers to larger hormones.

About 20 different amino acids are used in the synthesis of the protein hormones in the body. Each such hormone has a unique sequence of these amino acids, and it is in part this uniqueness that allows hormones made of the same building blocks to influence different physiologic parameters. Some protein hormones share similar sequences of amino acids in a portion of their molecules, and the result is that in certain circumstances they may cause similar responses. A good example would be the pituitary hormones adrenocorticotropic hormone (ACTH) and melanocyte-stimulating hormone (MSH), both of which share an identical sequence of seven amino acids and, when secreted in excess, can cause pigmentation of the skin.

The same hormone in different species often has slight differences in the amino acid sequence. These differences become important when hormone deficiencies are treated by replacement therapy with the hormone from another species. A difference of only a single amino acid can lead to an immune response against the exogenous hormone, particularly if extended treatment is necessary, as in insulin replacement in diabetics. Because the chemical synthesis of a large protein is at present both costly and time consuming, the solution to the problem of immune response lies in the tremendous advances that have been made in genetic engineering. It has now become possible to produce in the laboratory strains of microorganisms that synthesize large protein hormones with the identical amino acid sequence found in humans. Human insulin produced by bacteria has been the first such hormone to become commercially available, but other such products are certain to follow. The easy availability of more hormones will make the treatment of endocrine disorders infinitely easier.

Chemical synthesis of a hormone with an altered amino acid sequence is sometimes used to provide an inhibitor of an endogenous hormone. The idea is that the resulting hormone resembles the natural hormone closely enough so that it can competitively bind to the receptor sites on the target organ, preventing attachment of the normal hormone. If the altered molecule has been prepared properly, it may bind to the receptor sites without stimulating the target organ cells. Such inhibitors have been prepared for blocking angiotensin II receptors and may become available for other hormone systems in the future.

Amino Acids and Amino Acid Derivatives

Although only a few hormones are classified as amino acids or amino acid derivatives, some are of utmost importance to the anesthetist. These hormones include thyroid hormone and the adrenal catecholamines epinephrine and norepinephrine. Because of the small size of these hormones, it has been relatively easy to prepare blockers for some of them, particularly for the catecholamines. Similarly, it has been possible to prepare physiologically active analogs of these hormones. In some cases, it has been possible to prepare analogs that have only a selected number of the normal physiologic effects of the original hormone. An example is the compound phenylephrine, which stimulates alpha-adrenergic receptors but has little effect on beta-adrenergic receptors.

Steroid Hormones

The steroid hormones are compound ring structures (Fig. 24–1) with slight modifications such as a ketone or hydroxyl group here or there. The steroid hormones include the adrenal glucocorticoids and mineralocorticoids and the sex steroids estrogen, progesterone, and testosterone. The physiologically active form of vitamin D, 1,25-dihydroxycholecalciferol, is actually a hormone and is similar in structure to the steroids. As a result of their hydrocarbon skeleton, the steroids are very lipid soluble, which makes it easy for them to cross cell membranes. The steroids are another class of compounds that have been synthesized in the laboratory. This has been particularly important for the glucocorticoids, which are so widely used in many areas of medicine. In addition, it has been possible in some instances, by producing small structural differences, to increase the potency of a steroid hormone with regard to one of its physiologic actions and at the same time either not affect or decrease its potency with regard to other actions. An example is the adrenal steroids, for which *both* glucocorticoid activity and mineralocorticoid activity are a feature of several of the secreted compounds. It has been possible with slight alterations to accentuate one or the other of these activities. Such an increase in potency has obvious clinical advantages because it allows a more specific attack to be made in correcting hormonal deficiencies.

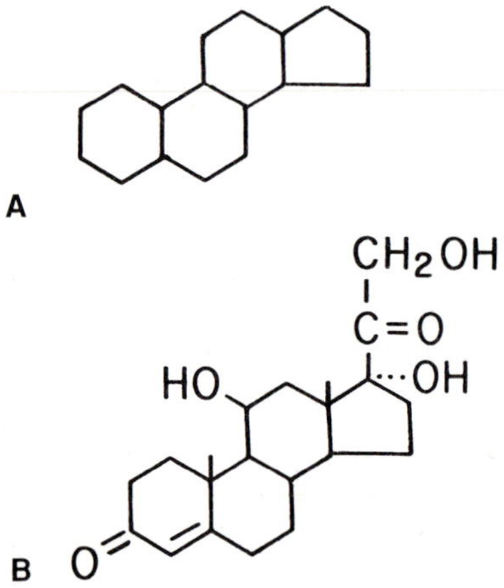

PROTEIN BINDING OF HORMONES IN THE PLASMA

Many hormones, including all of the steroids and some of the amino acid-derived hormones, are carried in the plasma bound to carrier proteins. There are a number of advantages to such binding. Particularly in the case of a steroid hormone, the hydrophobic nature of the molecule makes it difficult for an adequate concentration of the hormone to be dissolved in the plasma; however, a steroid easily attaches to the hydrophobic portion of the binding proteins, increasing the plasma concentration of the hormone. A second advantage of protein binding relates to the fact that it is the free hormone in the plasma that stimulates the target organ and that hormones are constantly being metabolized in the target organ, in the liver, or in other organs. The amount of the free hormone is maintained by the equilibrium that exists between the protein-bound hormone and the free hormone in the plasma. As the free hormone concentration is decreased by metabolism, it is quickly replaced by bound hormone diffusing away from the protein.

Another advantage of having hormones bound to carrier proteins in the plasma lies in the prevention of excretion of the hormones in the urine. The smaller hormones in the free form are small enough to be filtered across the glomerular capillaries in the kidneys. Large proteins, however, cannot be filtered across the capillaries. If a small hormone is bound to a large carrier protein, then it too is protected from being filtered in the glomerulus. The larger protein hormones are by themselves too big to be filtered in the glomerulus, so with regard to handling by the kidneys it is inconsequential that the large protein hormones are not bound to carrier proteins.

MEASUREMENT OF HORMONE CONCENTRATIONS

In the early days of endocrinology, the only type of assay available for measuring the concentration of a hormone in a

Figure 24–1. A. Carbon skeleton of the steroid hormone. **B.** Complete structure of cortisol.

blood or tissue sample was the bioassay. A bioassay involves observation of some type of biologic response after treatment of a living organism or excised tissue with an aliquot of the sample being examined. Examples of bioassays are the measurement of blood glucose concentration after injection into an animal of a sample containing insulin and the observation of cornification of the vaginal epithelium in rats after treatment with a sample containing estrogen. Bioassays are in most cases much less sensitive than the competitive binding and radioassays now available for most of the common hormones. Therefore, bioassays are used infrequently today.

The basic features of a radioassay are quite simple. First, a binding protein or antibody is prepared against a hormone. Then a radioactive preparation of the hormone is produced and a known amount is mixed with the binding protein in such a way that the degree of radioactivity of the solution is known. Finally, a sample of fluid containing an unknown concentration of the hormone is mixed with the solution containing the binding protein–radioactive hormone complex. The hormone in the unknown solution then competes for binding sites on the protein and decreases the radioactivity found on the protein in direct proportion to the concentration of the hormone in the unknown. From the decreased radioactivity, it is possible to calculate the concentration of the hormone in the unknown. Such radioassays are exquisitely sensitive and have been prepared for most of the known hormones.

HORMONE METABOLISM

Hormones are continuously being secreted (although not always at the same rate). What prevents a buildup of hormone concentration in the blood over a period of time? Such an event is avoided because of mechanisms for the metabolism or breakdown of hormones. Although each hormone is metabolized in a distinct way, a few generalizations can be made regarding this aspect of endocrine physiology. The organs that are most active in the breakdown of hormones are the liver and the kidneys. Other organs, including the target organs of some hormones, may be involved to a lesser extent.

The protein hormones are inactivated by enzymatic cleavage of the polypeptide chain. Thyroid hormone is inactivated by deiodination and deamination. It may also be converted in the liver to inactive sulfate and glucuronide conjugates (glucuronide is a slightly modified glucose molecule). Metabolism of steroids takes place primarily in the liver and generally involves a two-step process: (1) a slight alteration of the steroid molecule itself and (2) conjugation of the steroid to either sulfate or glucuronic acid. The significance of this alteration and conjugation is that the molecule is more polar and dissolves to a greater degree in the plasma without being bound to plasma protein. Consequently, the conjugates can be filtered and excreted more easily by the kidneys.

An understanding of the metabolism of catecholamines is particularly important for the anesthetist; however, because this topic is discussed in detail in most pharmacology texts, only the basics are given here. The catecholamines are inactivated by two different enzymes, mon-

amine oxidase (MAO) and catechol-*O*-methyltransferase (COMT). MAO catalyzes the oxidation of the catecholamines and is found in high levels in the liver, the kidneys, and the ends of neurons that use catecholamines as neurotransmitters. COMT attaches a methyl group to a catecholamine and is found primarily in the liver and kidneys. The oxidized and methylated catecholamines may then be further oxidized or conjugated to sulfate or glucuronic acid. These metabolites are excreted by the kidneys.

An understanding of hormone metabolism is important in the diagnosis of endocrine disease, particularly with regard to the steroids and catecholamines. As a consequence of the metabolism of these hormones, a certain normal pattern of the metabolites appears in the urine. By observing changes in this pattern, the locus of a disease may be pinpointed.

The epinephrine secreted by the adrenal medulla increases the contractility of cardiac muscle, yet it has no such effect on skeletal muscle. Angiotensin II is a hormone that stimulates the secretion of aldosterone from the adrenal cortex, whereas the same angiotensin II is a potent stimulating agent for the contraction of vascular smooth muscle. How can a given hormone such as epinephrine have a certain effect on one tissue and have no effect on other tissues? How can a hormone such as angiotensin II have one effect on a given tissue and an entirely different effect elsewhere? The answers to these questions lie in the specificity of hormone action brought about by the presence or absence of specific receptors in the target organs. If no receptors for a hormone are present in an organ, any action by the hormone is impossible. The situation is analogous to a key needed to unlock a door. If a key fits into the keyhole and it is the right key, the door may be unlocked. If there is no keyhole, the key is useless in unlocking the door. Epinephrine excites the heart because there are receptors for the hormone on cardiac muscle cells. Epinephrine has no effect on skeletal muscle because no receptors are present in that tissue. The situation of a single hormone having different effects on different target organs can be likened to the same key fitting into similar locks on doors opening into different rooms. Thus, angiotensin II can have one effect on the adrenal cortex and an entirely different effect on vascular smooth muscle.

MECHANISMS OF HORMONE ACTION

Once a hormone has interacted with a receptor, how does it influence the function of the cell? The topic addressed here is the mechanism of hormone action. Although other mechanisms probably exist, the two most common mechanisms of action of hormones are referred to as the second-messenger hypothesis and the mobile receptor hypothesis.

Second-Messenger Hypothesis

Most of the protein hormones and the amino acid or amino acid-derived hormones exert their influence according to the second-messenger hypothesis (Fig. 24–2). Most of these hormones are either too large or too polar to pass through the cell membrane. The result is that the only way such hormones can affect a cell is if they bind to a receptor molecule

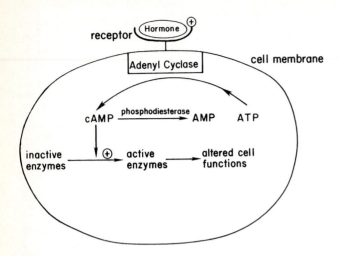

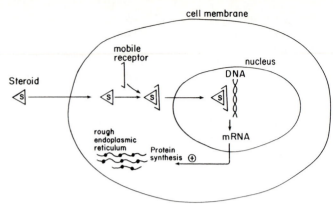

Figure 24–2. Second-messenger hypothesis. The hormone binds to the receptor on the cell membrane, activating adenyl cyclase, which in turn alters cellular functions. Adenyl cyclase converts ATP to cAMP, which activates cellular enzymes. cAMP is destroyed by the enzyme phosphodiesterase.

Figure 24–3. Mobile receptor hypothesis. The steroid hormone passes across the cell membrane and binds to the "mobile receptor." This hormone–receptor complex then passes into the nucleus, stimulating mRNA synthesis. The mRNA goes back out to the cytoplasm and calls for synthesis of specific proteins.

on the surface of the cell membrane. Activation of the receptor increases the activity of an enzyme known as adenyl cyclase, which converts adenosine triphosphate (ATP) into cyclic adenosine monophosphate (cAMP). In most cases, cAMP then changes the activity of enzymes within the cell, thereby altering cellular metabolism. The hormone can therefore be considered a "first messenger," bringing a signal from a distant endocrine gland, and the cAMP is the "second messenger," relaying the signal within the cell. The cAMP that is formed remains as an influence on cellular metabolism unless it is broken down by the enzyme phosphodiesterase. Phosphodiesterase activity is physiologically altered by hormones and can also be affected by certain drugs, such as the methylxanthines (caffeine falls into this category).

Mobile Receptor Hypothesis

Because the steroid hormones are quite lipid soluble, they readily cross the cell membrane, alleviating the need for a receptor located on the outer surface of the membrane (Fig. 24–3). Instead, a steroid hormone binds to a receptor protein in the cytoplasm, and the hormone–receptor complex then moves into the nucleus. The movement of the complex is the basis of the name *mobile* receptor hypothesis. Once in the nucleus, the steroid binds to DNA, stimulating the synthesis of a particular messenger RNA (mRNA) molecule (or set of molecules). The mRNA passes back out into the cytoplasm, where it becomes associated with rough endoplasmic reticulum and calls for the synthesis of a particular protein or group of proteins. The synthesized proteins may be structural proteins or enzymes, but whatever the particular proteins synthesized in a given cell under steroid stimulation, the change in cell structure or metabolism is specifically dependent on which proteins are synthesized. All of the steroid hormones are believed to act via the mobile receptor hypothesis.

CONTROL OF ENDOCRINE SECRETION

What factors control the secretion of hormones? In the case of most hormones, secretion is prominently (in some instances exclusively) influenced by other hormones. All of the anterior pituitary hormones are controlled by releasing hormones or release-inhibiting hormones, which are secreted by cells in the hypothalamus into the hypothalamohypophyseal portal vessel. The releasing hormones then pass down to the pituitary gland to stimulate or inhibit the secretion of the appropriate hormones. Of the six anterior pituitary hormones—growth hormone, adrenocorticotropic hormone, thyroid-stimulating hormone, follicle-stimulating hormone, luteinizing hormone, and prolactin—all but prolactin in turn are important regulators of the secretion of hormones from their target organs. Secretion of the releasing hormones and the anterior pituitary hormones is controlled in a feedback fashion (usually negatively) by the hormones of the pituitary target organs. Further examples of control of hormonal secretion by other hormones include stimulation of aldosterone secretion from the adrenal cortex by angiotensin II and regulation of secretion of insulin and glucagon by gastrointestinal hormones. The adrenal medullary catecholamines affect secretion of a number of other hormones and may be either excitatory or inhibitory, depending on the target organ and whether alpha- or beta-adrenergic receptors are stimulated.

Another major method of control of hormonal secretion is by intermediary metabolites in the blood. Perhaps the best-known example is the stimulation of insulin secretion from the pancreas in response to a rising blood glucose concentration. Glucose inhibits the secretion of glucagon from the pancreas and of growth hormone from the anterior pituitary. Amino acids stimulate the secretion of insulin, glucagon, and growth hormone. Free fatty acids inhibit the secretion of glucagon and growth hormone. Ketone bodies stimulate the secretion of insulin and inhibit secretion of glucagon. It is likely that secretion of other hormones is also affected by intermediary metabolites such as glucose, amino acids, and fatty acids.

The concentrations of inorganic ions in the blood are key factors controlling a number of hormones. High potassium (within the physiologic range) and low sodium (probably not within the physiologic range) stimulate secretion of aldosterone by the adrenal cortex. The total osmotic pressure of the plasma is monitored by osmoreceptors in the hypothalamus, and when this pressure is elevated, secretion of antidiuretic hormone (ADH) increases. Renin secretion by the juxtaglomerular apparatus is inversely proportional to the rate of transport of Na^+ or Cl^- out of the distal convoluted tubule. The secretion of parathyroid hormone and calcitonin, two hormones responsible for calcium metabolism, is regulated by Ca^{2+}. Parathyroid hormone secretion is inversely proportional to plasma Ca^{2+} concentration, whereas the secretion of calcitonin is proportional to plasma Ca^{2+}. 1,25-Dihydroxycholecalciferol (commonly referred to as vitamin D), which is secreted by the kidneys and is involved in control of plasma Ca^{2+} and PO_4^{3-} concentrations, is secreted in response to low PO_4^{3-} concentrations. Finally, acid in the lumen of the duodenum increases the secretion of the hormone secretin, which among other actions stimulates the secretion of bicarbonate by the pancreas to neutralize the acid in the duodenum.

Direct neural control of hormone secretion is of importance with regard to regulation of some hormones. The adrenal medulla secretes epinephrine and norepinephrine in response to neural activity in the preganglionic sympathetic axons reaching the gland. The adrenal medulla can therefore be considered a part of the sympathetic nervous system, functioning as a mass of postganglionic sympathetic neurons that release epinephrine and norepinephrine into the bloodstream as hormones to act on target organs rather than as neurotransmitters to act on postsynaptic cells. Other hormones that have secretion regulated by the nervous system include renin, the hypothalamic releasing hormones, and the posterior pituitary hormones oxytocin and vasopressin.

Effects of a Hormone: Physiologic versus Pharmacologic

In a discussion of the effects of a hormone, it is very important to distinguish whether the concentration being considered is within the normal range found in the body, which would be a physiologic concentration, or at a level far in excess of what might be found, which would be a pharmacologic concentration. This knowledge is important because a hormone may not have the same effects at different concentrations. Several of the hormones frequently dealt with by anesthetists have different effects at physiologic and pharmacologic concentrations. At physiologic concentrations, ADH has as its major effect the stimulation of water reabsorption in excess of solute in the collecting ducts of the kidney. The result is that a smaller volume of more concentrated urine is produced. Another action that has been attributed to ADH is constriction of blood vessels, and for this reason ADH has also been called *vasopressin*. Constriction of blood vessels is an effect of ADH at pharmaco-

logic concentrations, and it is questionable whether such an effect ever occurs at concentrations within the physiologic range. Nonetheless, vasoconstriction as a result of exogenous ADH must be kept in mind and may be a contraindication to use if a patient has coronary artery or other vascular disease.

Another group of hormones of which physiologic and pharmacologic effects are frequently confused is the glucocorticoids. Glucocorticoids are among the most prescribed drugs, but they are given most often because of their effects at pharmacologic doses. At physiologic concentrations, the glucocorticoids have such effects as increased glycogenesis and gluconeogenesis in the liver, a permissive action for many of the effects of glucagon and the catecholamines, inhibition of ACTH secretion by the pituitary, maintenance of the ability to excrete a water load by the kidneys, alterations of lymphatic organs and of blood cells, and provision of a resistance to stress. Although treatment with glucocorticoids is often necessary for maintenance of these functions, glucocorticoids are also frequently given at higher, pharmacologic doses to inhibit an inflammatory response.

STRESS AND HORMONES

We are all familiar with the word *stress* and the unpleasant connotations it conjures up. Physiologists sometimes describe stress as those stimuli that increase the secretion of ACTH. Although the ability to secrete ACTH and the glucocorticoids that are secreted in response to ACTH is essential for life, we have very little understanding of exactly why these hormones are necessary for the response to stress. Many other hormones are secreted in response to stress, including ADH, GH, glucagon, and the adrenal catecholamines. Again, the benefit of increasing the plasma concentrations of these hormones is not fully understood. Perhaps the changes in the endocrine environment confer on the individual some metabolic advantage that is beneficial in combating the effects of stress.

TYPES OF ENDOCRINE DISEASE

Endocrine disease is quite simply manifested in two forms: excess or deficiency; however, the underlying pathologic condition may stem from several sources. Tumors are a common cause of hormonal excess, and symptoms may be directly or indirectly an indication of the site of the tumor. For example, an excess of glucocorticoids may result directly from an adrenal tumor or indirectly from an ACTH-secreting pituitary tumor. If a particular endocrine gland secretes more than one hormone, a tumor of that gland may secrete excess amounts of one or any combination of the hormones normally secreted, depending on the particular cell type involved.

Some endocrine disorders are autoimmune diseases. In Graves' disease of the thyroid gland, antibodies are produced against the thyroid-stimulating hormone receptors on the follicular epithelial cells in the thyroid, resulting in stimulation of the cells and the ensuing hyperthyroidism. Autoimmune diseases are known to exist for other endocrine glands, and they may result in either hormonal excess or deficiency, depending on the exact component against which the antibodies are formed. It has been suggested that diabetes mellitus (the juvenile form) may be an autoimmune disease.

Congenital enzyme deficiencies are the basis of another important category of endocrine pathology. An example is congenital adrenal hyperplasia. Androgens may be secreted by the same cells of the adrenal cortex that secrete the glucocorticoids, and the androgens are in fact intermediates in the pathway for glucocorticoid synthesis. The major regulator of both androgen and glucocorticoid secretion by the adrenal cortex is ACTH from the pituitary. When the glucocorticoid concentration of the blood reaches a certain level, there is a negative feedback effect on the hypothalamus–pituitary axis, shutting down the secretion of ACTH; however, the adrenal androgens do not inhibit ACTH secretion, even when present in high concentrations. If there is an enzymatic deficiency in the adrenal cortex in the synthetic pathway between the androgens and the glucocorticoids, secretion of glucocorticoids will be low and ACTH secretion will rise. The increased ACTH will stimulate the adrenal cortex, but because glucocorticoids cannot be formed, the androgens will be secreted in excess and a deficiency in the glucocorticoids will remain. There are a number of such enzyme deficiency diseases in the adrenal cortex, and the patient's symptoms depend on which enzyme in the synthetic pathway is inadequate.

Another form of endocrine disease is the result of target organ insensitivity to a hormone. In nephrogenic diabetes insipidus, ADH is present but does not increase the uptake of water from the collecting ducts because these structures do not respond to ADH as they should. As a result, a large volume of dilute urine is formed. In maturity-onset diabetes, the β cells that secrete insulin from the pancreas may have normal morphology and insulin content and may secrete the hormone, but the number of receptors for insulin on the cell membranes of target organ tissues may be decreased. This paucity of receptors may account for the inability to handle a glucose load.

Dietary problems can also contribute to endocrine disease. Perhaps the best known of such diseases is hypothyroidism caused by insufficient dietary iodine. The dietary iodine is needed for the synthesis of thyroid hormone, and if it is lacking, the thyroid gland cannot produce enough hormone for normal thyroid function to occur. The gland may hypertrophy in an attempt to bring hormone synthesis back to normal levels. Simply supplementing the diet with iodine alleviates this type of hypothyroidism.

HORMONES AS NEUROTRANSMITTERS

The student should be aware that several hormones are also found as neurotransmitters. By definition, to be a hormone a compound must be released by a cell and then pass into the bloodstream to act on a target organ some distance away. To be a neurotransmitter, a compound must be released by a neuron and diffuse across a synaptic gap to act on a postsynaptic cell, usually another neuron, a muscle cell, or a glandular cell. The terms *hormone* and *neurotransmitter* are functional terms and do not place a limit on the chemical nature of the compound involved. The most widely known example of a hormone working double duty

as a neurotransmitter is norepinephrine, which is secreted as a hormone by the adrenal medulla and is found as the neurotransmitter of most postganglionic sympathetic neurons and in several locations in the central nervous system. Epinephrine and to a much lesser extent dopamine are also secreted by the adrenal medulla and are found as well as neurotransmitters in the brain. Dopamine also serves as a hormone released by the hypothalamus into the hypothalamohypophyseal portal vessel to inhibit secretion of the hormone prolactin from the pituitary. Somatostatin is a polypeptide that acts as a hormone in two locations. It is found in the islets of Langerhans in the pancreas, where it may be involved in the control of insulin and glucagon secretion, and it is secreted by the hypothalamus, from which it passes to the pituitary to inhibit the secretion of growth hormone. Somatostatin is also found as a neurotransmitter in the pain pathway in the spinal cord and elsewhere in the brain. Finally, a great deal of attention has in recent years been given to a family of compounds known collectively as opioid peptides. These compounds, which include the enkephalins, are known to be secreted as hormones by the pituitary gland, and they are found in neuronal endings in many parts of the brain and spinal cord, where they may act as neurotransmitters. Although the enkephalins are known to have an analgesic effect when injected into certain parts of the brain and are found in high concentrations in pain pathways in the spinal cord and brain, their significance is not yet fully understood. The enkephalins may be found to play an important role in controlling pain, so anesthetists may expect to hear more about these compounds in the future.

THE THYROID GLAND

The thyroid gland consists of two elongated lobes (right and left) joined close to their inferior poles by an isthmus (Fig. 24–4A). Occasionally, a pyramidal lobe is seen extending upward from the isthmus toward the thyroglossal duct and foramen cecum of the tongue. Wrapped around the junction between the larynx and the trachea, the thyroid has an important anatomic relationship with the recurrent laryn-

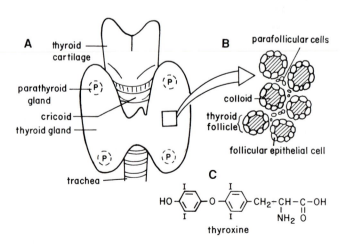

Figure 24–4. A. Gross anatomy of the thyroid gland. **B.** Histology of the thyroid gland. **C.** Thyroxine.

geal nerves, the major nerves controlling laryngeal function. The recurrent laryngeal nerves are located on either side, between the thyroid and the trachea. This anatomic relationship is important to keep in mind when the thyroid is manipulated during surgery, as physical trauma to the recurrent laryngeal nerves may result in laryngeal dysfunction.

Histologically the thyroid gland is composed of fluid-filled spheres called *follicles*, each of which is covered by a single layer of follicular epithelial cells (Fig. 24–4B). The fluid of the follicles, which is known as thyroid colloid, contains "extracellularly" stored thyroid hormone. The quantity of extracellularly stored thyroid hormone is great enough that handling of a hyperactive gland during surgery may cause enough release of the hormone to produce the systemic hyperthyroid state described as thyroid storm (discussed below).

Thyroid hormone can be classified chemically as an amino acid that has been iodinated (Fig. 24–4C). Four or three atoms of iodine may be added to the molecule, resulting in tetraiodothyronine (T_4) or triiodothyronine (T_3), respectively. Eighty percent of the hormone secreted is in the tetraiodinated form, and this is the molecule commonly known as thyroxine. It should be noted, however, that T_3 may be the physiologically active form of the hormone and that T_4 is converted to T_3 peripherally before any effect is seen.

An important aspect of thyroid physiology is that the gland avidly concentrates iodide from the plasma for synthesis into thyroid hormone. Secretion of thyroid hormone is in part regulated by the availability of iodide from the diet. If a dietary deficiency of iodide exists, the thyroid gland will enlarge in an attempt to accumulate more iodide to produce an adequate amount of hormone. Such an enlargement constitutes an iodine-deficient goiter. The term *goiter* implies only that the thyroid is enlarged and denotes nothing regarding the thyroid state of an individual. In the presence of a goiter, an individual can be hypothyroid, euthyroid, or hyperthyroid with respect to the normal physiologic state.

The main regulator of thyroid gland function is thyroid-stimulating hormone (TSH) from the anterior pituitary (Fig. 24–5). TSH stimulates both the synthesis and the secretion of thyroid hormone. The radioimmunoassay currently available for measuring TSH levels in the blood is very accurate, and a knowledge of the concentration of TSH acting on the thyroid gland is important in being able to make an informed diagnosis regarding thyroid function. Thyrotropin-releasing hormone (TRH) is secreted by the hypothalamus into the hypothalamohypophyseal portal vessel and stimulates the secretion of TSH. Both TRH and TSH are controlled in a negative feedback fashion by thyroid hormone in the blood.

It should be noted that most of the thyroid hormone in the blood is bound to a carrier protein, thyroid-binding globulin (TBG), which is produced in the liver; however, it is the unbound thyroid hormone that is responsible for the physiologic effects and for the feedback control over TRH and TSH secretion. For unknown reasons, when the concentration of estrogen in the blood increases, such as in women who are taking contraceptives or who are pregnant, the liver responds by producing more TBG. More thyroid hor-

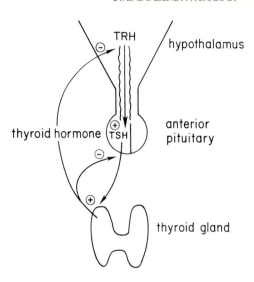

Figure 24–5. Regulation of thyroid hormone secretion. TRH, thyrotropin-releasing hormone.

mone then becomes associated with the carrier protein, and the concentration of free thyroid hormone drops. This drop results in release of the negative feedback on the pituitary and hypothalamus, resulting in increased TSH secretion. The rise in TSH stimulates secretion of thyroid hormone until the free thyroid hormone concentration in the blood has risen enough so that a new feedback effect can be exerted on the pituitary–hypothalamus system. What has happened is that the total amount of thyroid hormone in the blood has increased; however, it is only the protein-bound fraction that has actually risen. The free thyroid hormone concentration is restored to its previous level. It is therefore important when measuring thyroid hormone clinically to distinguish between total thyroid hormone and free thyroid hormone. Again, it is the free thyroid hormone in the blood that is physiologically active and exerts the negative feedback effects on the pituitary–hypothalamus system.

Although the thyroid hormone is not a steroid, it acts by entering the cell and binding to receptors associated with the DNA in the nucleus. New mRNA is synthesized, calling for the synthesis of protein in the cytoplasm. It is the specific enzymatic action of the thyroid-induced proteins that is responsible for the effects of the hormone. A well-known action of thyroid hormone is the stimulatory effect it has on the metabolic rate. This effect may in part be the result of an increase in the activity of Na^+, K^+-ATPase. The energy released when the ATP is hydrolyzed may be responsible for the increased generation of heat caused by thyroid hormone. Thyroid hormone is also involved in regulation of carbohydrate and lipid metabolism and is important in normal growth and development.

Hypothyroidism

Symptoms. Most of the symptoms of hypothyroidism can be traced directly to the effects of the decreased metabolic state on the particular organ involved. The overall metabolic rate is often decreased. Neurologic symptoms of hypothyroidism may include slowing of mental function, slowing of stretch reflexes, loss of motivation, depression, poor memory, and somnolence. The accumulation of osmotically active proteins and mucopolysaccharides in the skin and elsewhere results in the condition known as myxedema, a nonpitting edema that is particularly evident externally as puffiness around the eyes and on the dorsa of the hands and feet. The skin may be dry, cold, and pale, although hypercarotenemia may cause yellowing. Internally the myxedema may cause thickening of the mucous membranes of the larynx and pharynx, as well as enlargement of the tongue. These features lead to a husky voice, which when added to slow motor control of the laryngeal muscles make the slow speech of a myxedema patient very characteristic. Gastrointestinal function is often slowed, resulting in constipation. Gastric emptying may be delayed, and segments of intestine may be impacted with stool. Significant changes may also be seen in cardiovascular function. Cardiac output and contractility may be decreased, possibly because of the myxedematous infiltration that occurs. The heart sounds may be muffled, and low voltage and repolarization abnormalities may be seen in the electrocardiogram (ECG). The response of the heart to circulatory stress may be insufficient, and stress may put further strain on the already diseased organ. Total blood volume may be decreased, making hypothyroid patients vulnerable to hypovolemic shock.

Younger patients may be hypotensive, but older patients may exhibit diastolic hypertension. Cardiovascular reflexes may be defective, including decreased heart rate, blood pressure responses to the Valsalva maneuver, and baroreceptor dysfunction. Respiratory abnormalities may include depressed hypercapnic and hypoxic ventilatory drives, decreased maximum breathing capacity, and decreased diffusion capacity for carbon monoxide. Pleural effusions are also common. There are many more symptoms of hypothyroidism, and it should be stressed that those symptoms described above are for overt hypothyroidism. In less severe cases, the symptoms may not be quite as dramatic. The most advanced state of hypothyroidism is myxedema coma, which can develop as a result of undiagnosed or neglected hypothyroidism. A patient with myxedema coma exhibits hypoventilation, respiratory acidosis, hypothermia, hypoglycemia, low serum sodium, high serum lactate, cachexia, inappropriate ADH secretion, and progressive stupor ending in a comatose state.[1]

Early detection and treatment of hypothyroidism in infants or children who are hypothyroid is critical to avoid permanent brain damage caused by abnormal development. In adults, early hypothyroidism is often misdiagnosed as a psychiatric problem. Treatment of hypothyroidism basically involves replacement of the thyroid hormone.

Anesthetic Management. Whenever possible, treatment with thyroid hormone at a daily dose of 100 to 200 mg should be initiated before bringing a patient with mild hypothyroidism to surgery. The more severe the hypothyroid state, the greater the danger of increased sensitivity to a number of drugs. Patients who are overtly hypothyroid may metabolize drugs at a slower rate, so a given dose may act longer. Because of the potential for the development of

hypothyroid coma after general anesthesia, elective surgery should be postponed until severely hypothyroid patients have been made euthyroid. Thyroid hormone replacement in hypothyroid patients who have ischemic heart disease carries the risk of exacerbating angina or even precipitating myocardial infarction, perhaps by increasing the metabolic demands of the heart. In such patients, incomplete thyroid hormone replacement may have to be accepted.[2]

The increased incidence of adrenocortical insufficiency in hypothyroid patients is the basis for steroid replacement with hydrocortisone in preparation of such a patient for surgery.

Prudent anesthetic management of hypothyroid patients requires close attention to the underlying pathologic condition. Because of the decreased rate of drug metabolism and an already depressed central nervous system, preoperative sedation should not be given. When feasible, regional nerve blocks are preferable over general anesthesia. As a result of the delayed gastric emptying that may be present in a hypothyroid patient, endotracheal intubation should be performed with cuffed tubes, and in severe cases awake intubation may be preferable.[3] Because of the hypovolemic state of hypothyroid patients, central venous pressure should be monitored during any major surgery. Possible decreases in blood volume should be considered when deciding on an induction agent. A controlled induction, with smaller incremental doses, is preferable to large bolus injections. The agent of choice for anesthesia is nitrous oxide and oxygen under controlled ventilation.[4] Hypocapnia should be avoided. Because of the danger of prolonged recovery from anesthesia or even hypothyroid coma, narcotics including fentanyl and morphine are contraindicated. As for muscle relaxants, succinylcholine has been found to have a normal duration of action in hypothyroid patients.[5] Because of the underlying defects in metabolism, hypothyroid patients may be particularly prone to develop hypothermia. As hypothermia increases mortality in hypothyroid patients, body temperature should be monitored throughout anesthesia and postoperatively. Warming blankets, peritoneal lavage, increased operating room temperature, and warmed intravenous solutions can all be used to maintain body temperature. Care must be taken to avoid hypovolemic shock, which may result from peripheral vasodilation when warming blankets are used.

After surgery, respiration must be closely watched in hypothyroid patients; respiratory failure may develop as a result of hypothermia or because of the use of narcotics.

Hyperthyroidism

Symptoms. Hyperthyroidism is generally expressed as a hypermetabolic state of both individual organs and the body as a whole. The basal metabolic rate (BMR) is often increased, and a slight increase in body temperature may be seen, perhaps because of the increased BMR. Many hyperthyroid patients show heat intolerance. If the caloric intake is not increased to keep pace with the increased BMR, metabolism of endogenous protein and fat will occur, and weight loss results. Another consequence of the increased metabolic rate is the possibility of vitamin deficiencies because the need for vitamins exceeds the intake. The chronic depletion of liver glycogen in hyperthyroid patients leads to abnormal susceptibility to liver failure. Because the liver is a site of thyroid hormone metabolism, hepatic failure resulting from hyperthyroidism may actually worsen the hyperthyroid state. A change may occur in bowel habits (including diarrhea), and increased thirst and urination may also be seen. Nervous system changes in hyperthyroidism include nervousness, irritability, restlessness, emotional instability, depression, and difficulty in sleeping. Reflexes may be brisk, and a fine tremor of the extended hands or a coarse tremor and jerking of the trunk may be seen. Movements may be rapid and jerky, and muscle weakness is sometimes present. The skin temperature is usually elevated, and the skin is often soft and moist as a result of excess sweating. Reticuloendothelial involvement may be seen as a relative lymphocytosis, neutropenia, palpable spleen, and hyperplasia of lymphatic tissue. One form of hyperthyroidism, Graves' disease, is thought by some to be an autoimmune condition and is sometimes associated with other autoimmune disorders. Mild anemia is also a common finding in hyperthyroidism.

Ocular involvement in hyperthyroidism is often apparent in the form of exophthalmos as a result of swelling of the orbital contents. The underlying cause of exophthalmos is not clearly understood. It seems unlikely that thyroid hormone itself is directly responsible for exophthalmos, as this manifestation of hyperthyroidism sometimes worsens after the thyroid gland is removed. It has been suggested that a breakdown product of TSH from the pituitary may be the compound directly responsible. In addition to the protrusion of the eyes that is most characteristic of exophthalmos, pain, infection of the conjunctivae, tearing, sensation of a foreign body in the eye, diplopia, loss of visual acuity, and discordant extraocular muscles may also be part of the ocular symptoms of a hyperthyroid patient.

An understanding of the cardiovascular consequences of hyperthyroidism is of utmost importance for the anesthetist. The increased metabolic state of the tissues of the body requires an increased supply of oxygen and hence an increased blood flow. This is one factor increasing the demands made on the heart. A second factor is that vasodilation occurs in the skin because of the increased body temperature, approximating an arteriovenous fistula. Thus, cardiac output in hyperthyroidism must increase even in the resting state to keep pace with the increased metabolic demands of the tissues and the increased blood flow to the skin. The cardiac output may not increase sufficiently, leading to a condition known as high-output failure. Excess thyroid hormone has direct effects on the heart, including tachycardia and a tendency to create dysrhythmias. There is likely an interaction between the effects of thyroid hormone on the heart and those of the catecholamines, and it has been well documented that beta-adrenergic blockers are of tremendous value in reducing the cardiac problems in hyperthyroidism.

Anesthetic Management. The most important consideration in the anesthetic management of a hyperthyroid patient is, whenever possible, to bring the patient back to the euthyroid state before surgery is begun. There is great risk involved in anesthetizing a hyperthyroid individual, and it

is only in emergencies that surgery should be performed on such patients. The drugs used to bring about the euthyroid state function in three basic ways:

1. To suppress uptake of iodine by the thyroid gland and decrease synthesis of thyroid hormone
2. To decrease secretion of thyroid hormone by the gland
3. To interfere with the peripheral action of the hormone on the tissues of the body

The thionamides are the most frequently used antithyroid agents. Carbimazole (given at an initial dose of 30 mg/d) is generally preferred over propylthiouracil (initial dose 300 mg/d). Both of these compounds prevent the incorporation of iodine into thyroid hormone and inhibit later stages in thyroid hormone synthesis. Potassium perchlorate, which blocks uptake of iodine by the gland, has been used when problems develop with other drugs; however, the perchlorate treatment may lead to anemia, and it is not the drug of choice. The main problem encountered in suppression of thyroid hormone synthesis with the thionamides is that it may take up to 8 weeks for the euthyroid state to be reached. In addition, these antithyroid drugs may cause an increase in the size of a goiter. Thus, it may be preferable to stop treatment with these antithyroid drugs 2 weeks before the surgery and switch the patient to iodide tablets (60 mg/d). The iodide prevents secretion of thyroid hormone by the gland and, as an added benefit, also decreases the size and vascularity of the gland. Radioiodine may also be used to decrease the size of the thyroid. A subtotal thyroidectomy may be performed as an alternative to the drug treatments described above. If insufficient time is available to bring the patient to a euthyroid state, the beta-adrenergic blocking drug propranolol should be used to decrease the risks inherent in performing surgery on a hyperthyroid individual. The propranolol helps to control tachycardia and dysrhythmias, and its use should be continued into the postoperative period.

Because anxiety is a prominent characteristic of hyperthyroid patients, premedication is very useful, and in the absence of airway obstruction any premedication can be used. If the patient has been brought to the euthyroid state, the anesthetic agent may be chosen on general medical grounds. Particularly if the patient still shows signs of hyperthyroidism, there may be an increase in the requirement for the anesthetic agent. Such a situation may result from the faster metabolic clearance of the anesthetic by the hypermetabolic tissues. If exophthalmos is present, special care should be taken to keep the patient's eyes from becoming too dry during surgery. This may be done by applying protective drops or by maintaining the eyelids in the closed position.

Thyroid Storm. The most severe manifestation of hyperthyroidism is the condition referred to as *thyroid storm* or *thyrotoxic crisis*. This relatively rare condition arises as a result of excess thyroid hormone acting on the tissues and is characterized by the presence of the previously described signs of hyperthyroidism pushed to the extreme. The body temperature may rise to 41C (106F). Profuse sweating may occur, leading to severe dehydration. Cardiovascular problems include sinus tachycardia, tachyarrhythmias, and large increases in systolic and pulse pressures. Particularly in patients with preexisting heart disease, signs of congestive heart failure may appear. Other signs of thyrotoxicosis include nausea, vomiting, tremor, restlessness, and delirium. A comatose state with hypotension develops as the condition worsens. Thyroid storm frequently occurs in a patient who is hyperthyroid but has not been diagnosed as such. The episode of thyroid storm can be brought on by stress such as surgery or infection.

If not treated vigorously, thyroid storm is frequently fatal. The proper treatment must consist of combating the symptoms of the excess thyroid hormone already present, as well as attempting to prevent further release of hormone. Administration of propranolol may be useful in alleviating some of the cardiovascular problems.

A vigorous attempt should be made to lower the body temperature, and fluid balance and respiratory parameters should be closely watched. Thionamides and iodide should be given to prevent further production of thyroid hormone. A patient who undergoes thyroid storm during surgery should be watched carefully during the postoperative period.

CALCIUM METABOLISM AND THE PARATHYROID GLAND

Ionized calcium is essential for the normal function of many physiologic processes, including muscle contraction, nerve function, secretory activity by endocrine and exocrine glands, and blood clotting. It is important that the total plasma Ca^{2+} level (ionized plus protein-bound) be maintained in the normal range of 9 to 10.5 mg/100 mL. If the Ca^{2+} concentration falls, muscle cell membranes become hyperexcitable and there is an increased tendency for tetany to develop. Latent tetany may be seen at a plasma $[Ca^{2+}]$ less than 8 mg/100 mL. Should plasma $[Ca^{2+}]$ fall to less than 7 mg/100 mL, tonic contractions may occur. Tetany of the laryngeal muscles, known as laryngospasm, is particularly likely to occur when plasma $[Ca^{2+}]$ falls. The asphyxia that results from laryngospasm underscores the need to maintain plasma $[Ca^{2+}]$. Acute hypercalcemia can also develop into an emergency situation, with symptoms that may include nausea, vomiting, polyuria, and coma. Moderate but chronic elevation of plasma $[Ca^{2+}]$ may lead to kidney failure and kidney stones.

The regulation of plasma $[Ca^{2+}]$ concentration on a day-to-day basis is coordinated primarily by two hormones,

parathyroid hormone and 1,25-dihydroxycholecalciferol. A third hormone, calcitonin, may be involved to a lesser extent. Other hormones that may play a role in calcium metabolism in special situations include growth hormone, glucocorticoids, estrogen, and thyroxine. The discussion that follows is concerned primarily with the effects of parathyroid hormone, 1,25-dihydroxycholecalciferol, and calcitonin on plasma $[Ca^{2+}]$. The major actions of these hormones are summarized in Table 24–1.

Parathyroid Hormone

Parathyroid hormone (PTH) is a polypeptide secreted by the chief cells of the parathyroid glands. The main action of PTH is to increase plasma $[Ca^{2+}]$ by mobilizing Ca^{2+} from bone stores and by increasing the reabsorption of filtered Ca^{2+} by the kidney tubules. PTH also increases the formation of 1,25-dihydroxycholecalciferol by the kidneys, and the actions of this hormone (discussed below) increase the plasma $[Ca^{2+}]$. PTH also decreases plasma phosphate by increasing the excretion of phosphate in the urine.

Secretion of PTH is regulated in a negative feedback fashion by Ca^{2+}. When the plasma $[Ca^{2+}]$ drops, secretion of PTH by the parathyroid glands is increased, and this PTH then restores the plasma $[Ca^{2+}]$ to normal. As the plasma $[Ca^{2+}]$ rises, the secretion of PTH is decreased, thereby limiting the level reached by plasma $[Ca^{2+}]$. Magnesium ions also exert an effect on PTH secretion, with low plasma $[Mg^{2+}]$ inhibiting it.

One of the consequences of hypoparathyroidism is hypocalcemic tetany, which is due to hyperexcitability of muscle cell membranes. The condition is demonstrated by contraction of the facial muscles after a tap on the facial nerve in front of the ear—Chvostek's sign. Additional evidence of hypocalcemic tetany is Trousseau's sign, which consists of extension of the fingers and flexion of the wrist and thumb (carpopedal spasm). It may be necessary to occlude the blood supply to the limb for 3 minutes to demonstrate Trousseau's sign. The greatest danger of hypocalcemic tetany is the occurrence of laryngospasm, which can lead to asphyxia.

Hypoparathyroidism occurs frequently after thyroidectomy because the parathyroid glands were unintentionally removed. Hypoparathyroidism also occurs after the parathyroids have been removed to treat *hyper*parathyroidism. Treatment of acute hypocalcemia after parathyroidectomy is by intravenous injection of 10 mL of 10 percent calcium gluconate over a 5- to 10-minute period. If the plasma magnesium concentration is low, it may also be necessary to give

TABLE 24–1. SUMMARY OF ENDOCRINE REGULATION OF Ca²⁺ METABOLISM

Hormone	Bone	Kidney	Intestines
Parathyroid hormone (PTH)	↑ Mobilization of Ca^{2+}	↑ Reabsorption of Ca^{2+} ↑ Formation of 1,25-dihydroxycholecalciferol ↑ Excretion of PO_4^{3-}	
1,25-Dihydroxycholecalciferol	↑ Mobilization of Ca^{2+} ↑ Mobilization of PO_4^{3-}		↑ Transport of Ca^{2+} into blood
Calcitonin	↓ Mobilization of Ca^{2+}		

magnesium to eliminate tetany. Chronic hypocalcemia is treated by a combination of oral calcium salts and vitamin D.

The most common type of hyperparathyroidism is primary hyperparathyroidism caused by increased secretion in the chief cells in the parathyroid gland. Hypercalcemia is generally produced in response to primary hyperparathyroidism. Ectopic hyperparathyroidism, such as seen in carcinoma of the breast, lung, and pancreas, is also accompanied by hypercalcemia. Hyperparathyroidism secondary to chronically low plasma $[Ca^{2+}]$, as seen in chronic renal failure or intestinal malabsorption, is not accompanied by hypercalcemia. The untoward effects of hyperparathyroidism are due to the hypercalcemia that is produced. These effects may include renal failure and calculi, hypertension, ECG abnormalities (prolonged P-R interval and shortened Q-T interval), vomiting, peptic ulcer, pancreatitis, muscle weakness, bone pain and demineralization, gout, lethargy, and coma. The treatment of acute hypercalcemia resulting from hyperparathyroidism includes hydration and the administration of a diuretic and electrolytes. At present, however, parathyroidectomy is the only feasible permanent treatment for hyperparathyroidism. Before parathyroidectomy is performed to relieve hypercalcemia, causes other than hyperparathyroidism must be ruled out. Other potential causes of hypercalcemia include malignancies, vitamin D intoxication, and adrenal insufficiency.

1,25-Dihydroxycholecalciferol

1,25-Dihydroxycholecalciferol is a sterol-derived compound properly considered to be a hormone secreted by the kidneys. It is formed in the kidneys by hydroxylation of 25-hydroxycholecalciferol, a compound produced in the liver from cholecalciferol. Cholecalciferol, also known as vitamin D_3, is ingested in the diet and is formed in the skin by the influence of sunlight on 7-dehydrocholesterol. This sequence of reactions is summarized in Figure 24–6. Note that 25-hydroxycholecalciferol is actually converted into two different dihydroxy compounds, 1,25 and 24,25. The 1,25 compound is the physiologically active form that influences calcium and phosphorus metabolism. The 24,25 form is an inactive metabolite. The amount of 1,25 compound produced is increased under the direct influence of PTH and low plasma $[PO_4^{3-}]$.

1,25-Dihydroxycholecalciferol acts primarily on intestine and bone, and its overall effect is to increase plasma $[Ca^{2+}]$ and $[PO_4^{3-}]$. The action on the intestine is to increase the transport of Ca^{2+} from the lumen into the blood. The action of 1,25-dihydroxycholecalciferol on bone is to increase the mobilization of Ca^{2+} and PO_4^{3-} from bone stores. As will be recalled from the previous discussion, PTH also has a direct effect on bone to mobilize Ca^{2+}. Thus, both 1,25-dihydroxycholecalciferol and PTH increase plasma $[Ca^{2+}]$.

What is commonly known as a dietary deficiency of vitamin D is actually a deficiency of one of the precursors of 1,25-dihydroxycholecalciferol; however, the pathologic condition that develops is expressed as a decreased secretion of 1,25-dihydroxycholecalciferol by the kidneys. Such a deficiency may also be caused by a lack of exposure to sunlight and is made worse by a diet low in calcium. Whatever the cause of decreased secretion of 1,25-hydroxycholecalciferol, the result is a softening of the bones. The condition is known as rickets in children and osteomalacia in adults. It should be noted that there are many other causes of rickets and osteomalacia besides a dietary deficiency, for example, renal disease and vitamin D resistance. In children, a lack of 1,25-dihydroxycholecalciferol decreases absorption of Ca^{2+} from the intestine, which in turn leads to poor mineralization of bone. In adults, because the amount of Ca^{2+} brought in from the intestine is insufficient to maintain plasma Ca^{2+}, existing bone is demineralized. In both rickets and osteomalacia, plasma $[Ca^{2+}]$ is maintained by mobilization of bone Ca^{2+} under the influence of PTH. The anesthetist, however, should be aware that a patient with rickets or osteomalacia is prone to develop hypocalcemic tetany. In addition, problems in airway management may be encountered as a result of bone abnormalities consequent to demineralization.

Calcitonin

Calcitonin is a protein hormone secreted by the parafollicular cells of the thyroid gland, the cells surrounding the follicular epithelial cells that secrete thyroid hormone (see Fig. 24–4B). Calcitonin is secreted in response to high plasma $[Ca^{2+}]$. The action of calcitonin is to decrease mobilization of Ca^{2+} from existing bone. Although it would make a complete picture to say that the physiologic role of calcitonin is to oppose the ability of PTH and 1,25-dihydroxycholecalciferol to raise plasma $[Ca^{2+}]$, the evidence for such a role does not exist. A calcitonin deficiency condition has yet to be identified, and patients with an excess of calcitonin secretion do not have problems in calcium metabolism. Thus, the true role (if one exists) of calcitonin in calcium metabolism is not known at present.

Parathyroidectomy

Symptoms. Parathyroidectomy is the only long-term treatment presently available for primary hyperparathyroidism. Normally, four parathyroid glands are present, but about 10 percent of the population is believed to have fewer or more than four. The parathyroid glands are small, commonly described individually as being the size of a split pea. Each gland measures only about $1 \times 3 \times 5$ mm and weighs about 35 mg. In most cases, the four parathyroids are located one

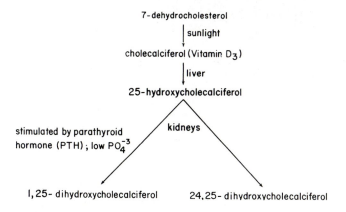

Figure 24–6. Formation of 1,25-dihydroxycholecalciferol.

each behind the two upper and two lower poles of the thyroid gland (see Fig. 24–4A). The parathyroids may lie on or within the substance of the thyroid gland; however, parathyroid tissue may be located elsewhere, including as low as the superior mediastinum. The anesthetist should be prepared to cope with a pneumothorax during a parathyroidectomy, particularly if mediastinal exploration is performed. A parathyroidectomy may be a prolonged surgical procedure for any of four reasons:

1. The small size of the glands
2. The difficulty in distinguishing the parathyroid glands from surrounding tissue in a surgical field
3. The variation in location of the glands
4. The need to identify and examine all four parathyroid glands to determine possible involvement in hyperparathyroidism

Anesthetic Management. Preoperative care of a patient scheduled for parathyroidectomy should include careful management of fluid and electrolyte balance. Prior to surgery the vocal cords should be examined. There is no particular agent of choice for the anesthetic; however, because of the common occurrence of renal problems in hyperparathyroidism, agents such as enflurane, which may have adverse effects on the kidneys, may be contraindicated. Despite the presence of hypercalcemia in hyperparathyroid patients, the use of muscle relaxants generally has not been reported as causing any particular problems. Because of its effects on calcium in the heart, digitalis, if necessary, should be used with caution.

Endotracheal intubation should be carefully established so that the traction of the neck tissues may be performed without compromising the airway. Because physical trauma to the recurrent laryngeal nerves is possible during surgery, the vocal cords should be carefully examined at the end of a parathyroidectomy. The hyperparathyroid patient may have osteoporosis, so special care should be taken when the patient is positioned. The head-up position, although it increases the possibility of air embolism, may be preferable to maintain a surgical field free of blood.

The major postoperative problem after parathyroidectomy is hypoparathyroidism, manifested by hypocalcemia. Such hypocalcemia is initially demonstrated by the neuromuscular hyperexcitability encountered in Chvostek's and Trousseau's signs and paresthesias located circumorally or in the extremities. The hypocalcemia is usually noticed 24 to 28 hours postoperatively. Treatment must be initiated to avoid frank tetany and laryngospasm. Treatment consists of administration of calcium gluconate, which may be necessary for several days until parathyroid tissue left after the surgery resumes function. If hypoparathyroidism persists, treatment is maintained with calcium salts and vitamin D therapy.

THE PANCREAS AND DIABETES

The pancreas is a flattened, elongated organ extending from the concavity of the duodenum on the right to the hilum of the spleen on the left. The pancreas is both an exocrine

gland and an endocrine gland. Approximately 98 to 99 percent of the weight of the pancreas is composed of the acinar cells, which serve an exocrine function by secreting enzymes and bicarbonate into the pancreatic duct. These secretions then pass into the duodenum, where they play an important role in digestive processes. The 1 to 2 percent of pancreatic cells with an endocrine function exist as clusters of cells known as the islets of Langerhans. The most important hormones secreted by these cells are insulin (from the B cells), glucagon (from the A cells), and somatostatin (from the D cells). As discussed in detail below, insulin and glucagon are intimately involved in control of intermediary metabolism. Somatostatin has been proposed to have a regulatory role in the secretion of insulin and glucagon.

It has been estimated that almost 5 percent of the U.S. population has diabetes, a disease characterized by a real or relative lack of insulin. As discussed later in this section, the pathology behind the diabetes is not always the same. Because the disease is so common and because it complicates the administration of anesthesia, an understanding of the actions of insulin and the consequences of an insulin deficiency is of utmost importance for the anesthetist. Knowledge of certain basic aspects of intermediary metabolism is necessary for understanding the pathology involved in diabetes. Therefore, the following three topics are discussed to give the student the ability to administer anesthesia in an informed fashion to diabetic patients:

1. The major events of intermediary metabolism and the effects of insulin and other hormones on these events
2. Diabetes and control of blood glucose
3. Anesthesia for diabetic patients

Metabolism and Its Control by Hormones

In a discussion of the subject of metabolism, three groups of substrates must be considered: carbohydrates, lipids (fats), and proteins. A knowledge of carbohydrate metabolism and lipid metabolism is important for understanding the development of hyperglycemia and ketoacidosis, respectively. Because knowledge of these conditions is important in proper anesthetic management of diabetic patients, carbohydrate and lipid metabolism are discussed in some detail below. A few relevant points regarding amino acid and protein metabolism are interspersed in this discussion.

The entry of substrates into the cell is the initial event in all metabolic pathways. Carbohydrates are generally transported into the cell as monosaccharides (i.e., glucose), fats as free fatty acids, and proteins as single amino acids. Insulin stimulates the transport into the cell of all three substrate types in many organs. An absolute or relative lack of insulin and the resulting decrease in glucose transport into the cells constitute the main event producing hyperglycemia in diabetes. It should be noted that other hormones, particularly growth hormone and the glucocorticoids, inhibit glucose transport into the cells, and an excess of these hormones may cause hyperglycemia. Once inside the cell, a substrate may be stored for later use, metabolized for energy, or converted into another type of substrate.

Carbohydrate Metabolism. In many tissues, particularly liver and muscle, glucose can be stored in a polymerized form as glycogen (Fig. 24–7). Glycogen synthesis is stimulated by insulin. Breakdown of glycogen back to glucose is stimulated by other hormones, notably glucagon, epinephrine, and norepinephrine. The lack of insulin in diabetes decreases glycogen synthesis and allows glycogen breakdown to occur unopposed. Most of the glucose produced in this fashion in the liver diffuses out of the cells and adds to the hyperglycemia already present because of decreased transport of glucose into the cells.

Glucose can be metabolized by two pathways, the hexose monophosphate shunt and glycolysis. The hexose monophosphate shunt produces ribose for nucleic acid synthesis and coenzymes for lipid metabolism. As this pathway is relatively unimportant in the present discussion, it will not receive further attention.

Glycolysis is the pathway by which glucose is converted to pyruvate (aerobically) or lactate (anaerobically). The pyruvate is converted to acetyl-CoA and runs through the tricarboxylic acid (TCA) cycle for production of the reduced form of nicotinamide–adenine dinucleotide (NADH). Oxidation of NADH in the electron transport chain then yields ATP. An alternative use for the acetyl-CoA produced from glucose is the synthesis of fatty acids, which are in turn synthesized into triglycerides (see Fig. 24–7). This pathway, which is particularly important in liver and adipose tissue, is stimulated by insulin. Thus, insulin

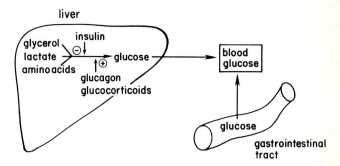

Figure 24–8. Gluconeogenesis and sources of blood glucose.

can be considered a hormone of storage, promoting synthesis of both glycogen and triglycerides from glucose. Insulin also promotes protein synthesis from amino acids in muscle and other tissues.

Most of the glucose in the blood comes directly from food that has been digested in the gastrointestinal tract. An additional source of glucose in the blood is that produced by the liver via gluconeogenesis (Fig. 24–8). Gluconeogenesis is the synthesis of "new glucose" from glycerol, lactate, and amino acids. This additional output of glucose becomes important in starvation, particularly as the brain relies on glucose as its primary energy source. Gluconeogenesis also increases in uncontrolled diabetes, and the glucose released into the blood adds to the hyperglycemia caused by the lack of glucose transport into the cells. Gluconeogenesis is inhibited by insulin and stimulated by glucagon and the glucocorticoids.

Lipid Metabolism. The triglycerides are carried in the blood as part of a lipoprotein complex. They are split into their component glycerol and fatty acids by the enzyme lipoprotein lipase. This enzyme is found in the endothelial cells of the capillaries and is particularly active in adipose tissue (Fig. 24–9). The activity of the enzyme is increased by insulin.

Depending on the tissue and the nutritional state of the individual, once inside the cell fatty acids are either resynthesized into triglycerides for intracellular storage or metabolized for energy (see Fig. 24–9). The enzymatic pathways leading to the synthesis of triglycerides for storage are particularly important in adipose tissue and liver and are activated by insulin. Triglyceride synthesis is increased in the nourished state if insulin is present and is decreased in starvation and in uncontrolled diabetes.

Those tissues that store triglycerides, such as adipose and liver, also have the capability of breaking down the triglycerides into the component fatty acids and glycerol. This process is known as lipolysis. The enzyme responsible for lipolysis, hormone-sensitive lipase, is stimulated by epinephrine, norepinephrine, and growth hormone. In adipose tissue, the enzyme is also stimulated by increased sympathetic activity, which may be the main mechanism for lipolysis under physiologic conditions. Lipolysis via hormone-sensitive lipase is *blocked* by insulin (see Fig. 24–9). This fact is demonstrated by the release of fatty acids that can occur when there is a lack of insulin, such as in diabetes. As will be discussed below, it is the body's failure to properly

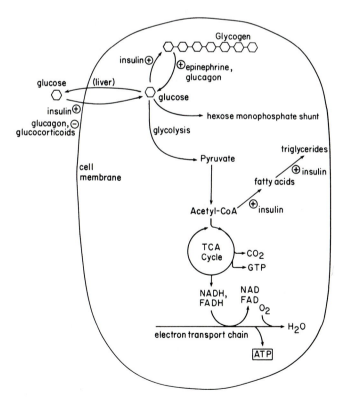

Figure 24–7. Summary of carbohydrate metabolism. TCA, tricarboxylic acid; GTP, glutamine triphosphate; FAD, flavin–adenine dinucleotide; NAD, nicotinamide–adenine dinucleotide; FADH and NADH, reduced forms of FAD and NAD.

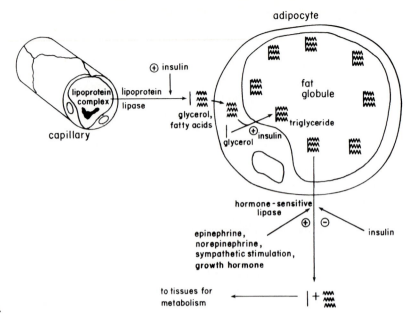

Figure 24–9. Metabolism in adipose tissue.

metabolize large numbers of fatty acids that leads to ketoacidosis in diabetes.

In summary, the amount of lipids held in storage is controlled by two opposing enzyme systems, lipoprotein lipase and hormone-sensitive lipase. (The student should not be confused by the poor choice used in naming hormone-sensitive lipase; both enzymes are "sensitive" to hormones, but in different ways.) Lipoprotein lipase facilitates storage of triglycerides by providing the cells with a source of free fatty acids, and hormone-sensitive lipase breaks down the triglycerides, releasing the glycerol and the fatty acids into the blood. Lipoprotein lipase activity is increased by insulin. Hormone-sensitive lipase activity is increased by the catecholamines, glucagon, and growth hormone and is decreased by insulin. It can therefore be seen that by promoting storage and preventing breakdown, insulin plays a key role in regulating the fat stores of the body.

Fat is an important component in the typical American diet, providing about 35 percent of the daily caloric requirement. Fatty acids are metabolized two carbons at a time to acetyl-CoA, which is then run through the TCA cycle. In certain situations, such as in uncontrolled diabetes, there is an excess of fatty acids and the ability of the cells to burn all of the acetyl-CoA is overcome. Particularly in the liver, the acetyl-CoA is converted into ketone bodies. Small amounts of ketone bodies can be metabolized by the tissues, but when the supply exceeds this capability the ketone concentration in the blood increases. Two of the three "ketone" bodies, β-hydroxybutyric acid and acetoacetic acid, contain a carboxylic acid group (Fig. 24–10). If the H^+ released from these compounds is not adequately buffered, ketoacidosis results. Ketoacidosis is a severe complication of diabetes, and its treatment in relationship to anesthesia is discussed below.

Diabetes Mellitus and Control of Blood Glucose

The disease known as diabetes mellitus has classically been subdivided into two separate forms, juvenile-onset and maturity-onset. Although the average age of onset of the juvenile form is 12 years and most maturity-onset cases appear after the age of 35, there is some crossover in occurrence between the two forms. It is therefore better to categorize the types of diabetes as either insulin dependent (most juvenile-onset diabetics are of this type) and insulin independent (most maturity-onset diabetics are of this type).

Insulin-dependent diabetes is characterized by pathologic changes in the β cells of the pancreatic islets that decrease the amount of insulin secreted. Insulin-dependent diabetics are more prone to develop ketoacidosis when the disease goes out of control. There are suggestions that at least some cases of insulin-dependent diabetes may be characterized as an autoimmune response resulting in the destruction of the β cells.[6,7] Control of insulin-dependent diabetes is simplified by a regulated diet; however, the key distinguishing feature of insulin-*dependent* diabetes is that exogenous insulin is required for controlling the disease.

Insulin-independent diabetics are commonly obese.

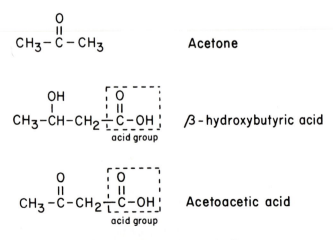

Figure 24–10. The ketone bodies.

Their plasma insulin concentration may be normal or even elevated. These individuals show a decreased sensitivity to insulin that may be related to a reduced number of insulin receptors on cell membranes, particularly in adipocytes. Insulin-independent diabetics are prone to hyperglycemia but do not usually proceed into ketoacidosis, possibly because the amount of insulin present is sufficient to prevent lipolysis. Many insulin-independent diabetics can bring their disease under control by losing weight and continuing dietary regulation; however, many insulin-independent diabetics must also take an oral hypoglycemic agent such as a sulfonylurea. The sulfonylureas, which include tolbutamide, stimulate insulin secretion (remember that in insulin-independent diabetics the pancreas may still have the ability to secrete normal amounts of insulin). Less commonly used are the phenethylbiguanides, which increase the utilization of glucose by the tissues. Although many insulin-independent diabetics rely on the oral hypoglycemic agents, these drugs have fallen into disfavor. The sulfonylureas can have adverse cardiovascular effects, and the biguanides cause lactic acidosis.

The goal in the control of diabetes is to keep the blood glucose concentration within normal limits as much as possible, because both hyperglycemia and hypoglycemia have adverse effects on the patient. Except in an absolute emergency, surgery should not be performed on a patient in hyperglycemia (with or without ketoacidosis) or hypoglycemia. Administration of anesthesia itself is greatly complicated by these conditions and should not be attempted until the patient's metabolism has been brought under control. The sequelae and treatment of hyperglycemia (with and without ketoacidosis) and hypoglycemia in the awake patient are discussed next. Special problems encountered in controlling blood glucose in the perioperative period are considered in a subsequent section.

Hyperglycemia. Hyperglycemia may occur in any situation in which there is a relative or actual deficiency of insulin in the blood. The prime cause of the hyperglycemia is the failure of glucose to be transported into the cells; however, further increases in blood glucose occur because of the increased breakdown of glycogen and gluconeogenesis, which can occur in the liver when not enough insulin is available.

As the blood glucose concentration increases, the amount of glucose filtered in the glomeruli of the kidneys also increases, and eventually the ability of the tubules to reabsorb the glucose is exceeded. The result is an osmotic diuresis and glycosuria (diabetes mellitus is derived from the Greek words *diabetes*, "a siphon," and *mali*, "honey"). More than just glucose is lost in the urine, however. As the urine flow increases, electrolytes, including sodium and potassium, are also excreted in increasing amounts. An additional consequence of the diuresis is hypovolemia, and when the plasma volume becomes very low renal function is further impaired. The patient attempts to replace the lost water by increasing the intake of water (polydipsia).

Hyperglycemia can become so severe that the extreme hyperosmolality that results may draw water out of the neurons in the brain, inducing neurologic abnormalities. Initial signs include altered mentation, areflexia, and hallu-

cinations. The neurologic signs may proceed to seizures and ultimately coma, a condition known as hyperglycemic, hyperosmolar, nonketotic coma (HHNKC). HHNKC is more likely to occur in older insulin-independent diabetics and is rare in insulin-dependent patients. HHNKC is often preceded by an infection or dehydration and frequently occurs in nondiabetic patients, particularly the elderly.

Treatment of hyperglycemia requires insulin to move glucose into the cells. Because K^+ may have been lost in the diuresis and because insulin directly stimulates movement of K^+ into the cells, it is advisable to give K^+ when treating hyperglycemia with insulin. If K^+ is not given, hypokalemia may be an unwanted result of the insulin treatment. If full-blown HHNKC has developed and hypotension has occurred, it will also be necessary to replace the lost fluids, preferably with 0.45 percent saline. The blood glucose concentration in HHNKC is often greater than 600 mg/mL, and serum osmolality may exceed 330 mosm/L. Small doses (10 to 20 U/h) of intravenous regular insulin will initially be effective toward lowering the blood glucose to 300 mg/100mL; 300 to 400 units may be required in the first 24 hours in the average patient.[8] To avoid cerebral edema and other problems, the osmolality should be brought down slowly to below 320 mosm/L in approximately 4 to 6 hours.[9,10]

Hyperglycemia as a result of anxiety and the stress of surgery itself is difficult to avoid. Surgery increases the secretion of GH, ACTH, the glucocorticoids, epinephrine, norepinephrine, and glucagon. These hormones collectively act to increase blood glucose by antagonizing the utilization of glucose normally stimulated by insulin, by increasing gluconeogenesis, or by increasing glycogen breakdown in the liver. Sympathetic nervous system stimulation during surgery also increases glycogen breakdown. The degree of increase of blood glucose as a result of these endocrine and neural processes is proportional to the length and severity of the surgery.

Development of Ketoacidosis. Ketoacidosis in diabetics is almost always preceded and accompanied by hyperglycemia. Although there is an overabundance of glucose extracellularly in hyperglycemia, there is a paucity inside the cells. More commonly in insulin-dependent diabetics than in insulin-independent diabetics, other metabolic events begin to take place as the blood glucose rises. Perhaps as a means of supplying an alternate source of substrate for energy produced through metabolism, lipolysis is increased in adipose tissue. The large number of fatty acids released into the blood cannot be completely metabolized by the other tissues, and an excess of ketone bodies is generated in the liver and released into the blood. Ketoacidosis will ensue if the lipolysis and ketone body generation continue. The lipolysis that occurs is a direct consequence of the absence of insulin, and insulin replacement returns fat metabolism to normal. It is not fully understood why insulin-independent diabetics are less prone to develop ketoacidosis than insulin-dependent diabetics. It may be that the amount of insulin present in the insulin-independent individual is sufficient to prevent lipolysis (even though it may not be sufficient to prevent hyperglycemia).

Of the three types of ketone bodies produced, one, acetone, is very volatile and may be detected on the breath of a patient in ketoacidosis. The other two ketone bodies, β-hydroxybutyric acid and acetoacetic acid, contain carboxylic acid groups and must be buffered to prevent the blood pH from dropping (see Fig. 24–10). As the ketones increase in concentration, the ability to buffer the acids is exceeded and the plasma pH may drop to 7.2 or below. This may produce the deep, rapid pattern of respiratory movements known as Kussmaul's breathing. Below a plasma pH of 7.1, ventilation decreases.

The way in which the kidneys handle the ketoacidosis adds to the seriousness of the situation. The excess of ketone bodies is filtered in the glomeruli of the kidneys. Initially, the ketone bodies are excreted in the urine accompanied by either H^+ or NH_4^+. However, as more ketones are filtered, Na^+ and K^+ are also used as accompanying cations and are lost in the urine in increasing amounts. Despite the loss of K^+ in the urine, hyperkalemia may be present. The hyperkalemia is due to a movement of K^+ from inside to outside the cells as a result of insufficient insulin. The ketonuria contributes to the osmotic diuresis caused by the hyperglycemia that may be present and thus increases the degree of dehydration, hypovolemia, and hypotension.

Recognition. A patient in ketoacidosis presents with thirst, polyuria, glycosuria, ketonuria, dehydration, hypovolemia, and hypotension. The patient may experience nausea and vomiting, and bowel sounds may be sparse or even absent. There may be severe abdominal pain that may mimic an acute abdomen as encountered in appendicitis; however, when the abdominal pain is caused purely by ketoacidosis, it will disappear completely with appropriate treatment of the ketoacidosis.[11] Muscle tone is decreased and reflexes are depressed. Central nervous system signs may include headache, drowsiness, stupor, and coma.

Treatment. Treatment of ketoacidosis includes a three-pronged attack: (I) insulin replacement, (II) fluid replacement, and (III) potassium replacement.

  I. The need for treatment with insulin in a patient in ketoacidosis is paramount, as only insulin can bring the underlying metabolic abnormality under control. Insulin has the following effects in returning the patient to a physiologic state:
    A. Insulin brings blood glucose down to normal levels by
      1. stimulating glucose transport into the cells
      2. increasing glucose metabolism by the cells
      3. decreasing gluconeogenesis in the liver
      4. increasing glycogen synthesis and decreasing glycogen breakdown in the liver
    B. Insulin lowers the plasma concentration of ketone bodies by
      1. increasing uptake of ketones by the cells
      2. decreasing ketogenesis in the liver
      3. decreasing lipolysis in adipose tissue
      4. increasing lipid synthesis in adipose tissue and liver
    C. Insulin moves K^+ into the cells, alleviating the hyperkalemia that may be present (this is also the rea-

son why K^+ must be given to prevent *hypo*kalemia).

The preferred route of administration of insulin to treat ketoacidosis is a continuous intravenous infusion of short-acting insulin at a rate of 5 to 6 U/h. Administration via a syringe pump is much preferable to a drip, as insulin adheres to plastic tubing and the amount of tubing is minimized by using a syringe pump. Alternative plans for administration of insulin in ketoacidosis combine intravenous infusion with intramuscular injections.[12] The effectiveness of the insulin should be monitored by hourly analysis using reagent strips to measure blood glucose (Dextrostix) and ketone bodies (Ketostix). The dose of insulin given can be adjusted according to the results of these tests. The results obtained from the reagent strips should be compared periodically with determinations made from blood sent to the clinical laboratory. Monitoring hyperglycemia and ketoacidosis by measurement of urine glucose and ketones is unwise, because catheterization is necessary to obtain freshly formed urine for accurate determinations. Diabetics are particularly prone to urinary tract infections, especially after catheterization. In addition, the hypoglycemia that may occur as a result of excess insulin administration cannot be detected by urine glucose measurements.

  II. Fluid replacement is best achieved using isotonic saline. Rapid replacement of fluids should be avoided.[9,10] A recommended rate of replacement is to give the first liter in 30 minutes, the second liter in 1 hour, a third liter in the next 2 hours, and 500 mL every 4 hours.[13]

  III. As indicated above, potassium must be given when treating ketoacidosis because of the amount lost in the urine and to avoid the hypokalemia that would result from movement of the ion into the cells. A recommended rate of administration of potassium is 15 mEq in the first liter of intravenous fluid. This should be doubled if the plasma potassium falls below 4 mmol/L, and it should be stopped if the level rises above 6 mmol/L.[13] Monitoring the ECG is useful in following the course of the potassium treatment.

As treatment with insulin and fluids usually corrects the acidosis, administration of bicarbonate is generally unnecessary. Bicarbonate may even be detrimental because it may cause alkalosis some time into the recovery from the acidosis; however, if the blood pH is less than 7.0, 50 mmol of bicarbonate may be given with potassium.[12]

Hypoglycemia. Hypoglycemia among diabetics occurs most often in insulin-dependent patients and in insulin-independent patients taking long-acting oral hypoglycemic agents (the sulfonylureas). The basic cause of hypoglycemia in either case is an excess of insulin relative to the needs of the individual. The result is an increase in movement of glucose into the cells and a decrease in the concentration of glucose in the blood. In the case of insulin-dependent diabetics, hypoglycemia may result from too strong an insulin injection, an unusual alteration in dietary habit, or participation in unanticipated exercise. Among insulin-independent diabetics, hypoglycemia is most likely to occur as a result of altered food intake or an incorrect dosage of the oral hypoglycemic agent. These factors are particularly prevalent in elderly patients who are chronically malnourished, have existing arteriosclerosis, have underlying renal or hepatic disease, or are taking drugs (such as alcohol and propranolol) that by themselves may cause hypoglycemia. Patients with arteriosclerosis are prone to hypoglycemic episodes as they may already have marginal cerebral blood flow. Renal and hepatic diseases contribute to hypoglycemia because the kidneys and the liver are very important in the degradation of insulin. If these organs are diseased, the insulin that is in the blood will be effective longer and thus the possibility of hypoglycemia developing is increased. In addition, the liver stores a large amount of glycogen. If the amount of glycogen stored is decreased (as it often is in hepatic disease), the ability of the liver to break down glycogen into glucose and release it into the blood is decreased. Thus, one of the key homeostatic mechanisms for maintaining the blood glucose concentration and preventing hypoglycemia will have been lost.

The student should be aware that there are many other causes of hypoglycemia other than those discussed here. Additional potential causes include abnormal gastric function, the presence of an insulin-secreting tumor, and hypofunction of endocrine organs (deficiencies of glucocorticoids, glucagon, and catecholamines). A more detailed discussion of hypoglycemia and its causes may be found in a textbook of clinical endocrinology.

Recognition. The symptoms of hypoglycemia generally first appear when the blood glucose concentration falls below 45 mg/100 mL. The blood glucose level at which a given patient shows signs of hypoglycemia is, however, variable and is influenced by such factors as the rate at which the blood glucose falls and the actual level and duration of hypoglycemia.

The clinical signs of hypoglycemia are initially neurologic. The brain is heavily dependent on glucose as an energy source, so any deprivation will affect neural function. The initial signs may include tremor, sweating, nervousness, weakness, hunger, palpitations, tachycardia, diaphoresis, blurred vision, diplopia, mental confusion, violent behavior, and inappropriate affect. If the hypoglycemic episode continues, coma may ensue. Death may result from failure of the cardiorespiratory control centers in the brainstem.

Treatment. If the individual is conscious and cooperative, hypoglycemia can be treated by simply having the person swallow some glucose (which may be given in the form of juice or a couple of sugar cubes); 10 to 20 g of glucose should be sufficient. In a patient who is unable to swallow, 25 g of glucose should be given intravenously. In a violent patient, 1 mg of glucagon may be injected subcutaneously for initial treatment, followed by oral or intravenous glucose.

If the hypoglycemia was not too long in duration, in most cases a return to normoglycemia will reverse the patient's signs and symptoms. The recovery may be immediate, as in mild cases of hypoglycemia, or it may take days if the hypoglycemia was severe. Particularly in patients taking long-acting oral hypoglycemic agents, care must be taken that there is not an immediate recurrence of hypoglycemia. Because prolonged hypoglycemia may cause neuronal death and thus permanent brain damage, it is extremely important to initiate treatment of hypoglycemia as soon as the condition is recognized. If a patient remains unconscious even after treatment for hypoglycemia, it may be that cerebral edema has developed. In such a case, mannitol may be given intravenously to reduce the edema.

Except when the urgency of the situation demands it, patients who are hypoglycemic should not be anesthetized for surgery until the blood glucose has been normalized. There are two reasons why hypoglycemia should be corrected before administering anesthesia. The first and most important reason is that prolonged hypoglycemia can cause permanent brain damage. The second reason is that most of the neurologic and behavioral symptoms present in the awake individual are not present in an anesthetized patient. This makes the diagnosis of hypoglycemia much more difficult and therefore increases the risk of brain damage if a hypoglycemic episode occurs intraoperatively.

If a patient is in need of emergency surgery, hypoglycemia can be treated by an intravenous bolus of up to 50 mL of 50 percent dextrose, followed by establishment of an intravenous line of 10 percent dextrose. Although reversal of symptoms should occur quickly, a second bolus injection may be needed. Because the hypoglycemia was most likely caused by an excess of insulin or of an oral hypoglycemic agent, the patient should be monitored closely in case the hypoglycemia recurs. Because of the inherent difficulty of recognizing hypoglycemia under anesthesia, the optimal intraoperative blood glucose concentration range has been set at 150 to 250 mg/mL. This is slightly higher than the normal blood glucose of 100 mg/mL, but it decreases the possibility of a hypoglycemic episode. Should the blood glucose fall below 150 mg/100 mL intraoperatively, more glucose can be given (or if insulin is being administered, the amount of insulin given can be decreased). If the blood glucose exceeds 250 mg/100 mL, the delivery of glucose to the patient should be decreased or the administration of insulin increased or both.

Control of Blood Glucose Perioperatively. The key to proper metabolic management of a diabetic patient undergoing surgery is frequent measurement of blood glucose, with insulin and glucose being given to the patient as needed to maintain the blood glucose within the desired range. Blood glucose measurement should be made before surgery, hourly during surgery, and hourly postoperatively until oral feeding has been resumed. The importance of carefully monitoring the patient postoperatively cannot be overemphasized. Any prolonged abnormal blood glucose level after surgery will make intraoperative vigilance totally meaningless.

Glucose oxidase (Dextrostix) is suitable for glucose measurement, although care must be taken that the determinations are accurate. This may be done by periodically comparing the glucose oxidase values with those derived from blood samples sent to the clinical laboratory. The amount of insulin or glucose that must be administered to maintain blood glucose can then be based in confidence on the glucose oxidase measurements. Should hyperglycemia occur, testing for ketone bodies with ketone oxidase (Ketostix) should also be performed. Periodically in the past, the recommendation has been made that insulin and glucose administration during surgery be based on a sliding scale dependent on urinary glucose; however, the urinary glucose concentration is at best a late reflection of blood glucose and, therefore, an unreliable basis on which to manage a patient.

The two most important factors to be considered in determining the best means of management of blood glucose in a diabetic patient undergoing surgery are (1) the patient's history with regard to means of blood glucose control and (2) the duration and nature of the surgery. A variety of regimens for managing diabetics during anesthesia have been postulated. A few possible guidelines for blood glucose management are offered here.

Insulin-Independent Diabetics. A patient whose diabetes is successfully controlled by diet alone needs no special metabolic management for minor surgery.[12] A patient whose diabetes is treated by long-acting oral hypoglycemic agents should be switched to short-acting agents a few days before minor surgery. No hypoglycemic agent should be given the morning of the operation, and treatment should be resumed when the patient is able to eat. If it should become necessary to give a carbohydrate-containing infusion during the surgery, then insulin should also be given to prevent hyperglycemia from developing.

An insulin-independent diabetic patient scheduled for a major surgical procedure should be switched from oral hypoglycemic agents to regular insulin several days before surgery. Such a patient should then be treated in the same manner as an insulin-dependent patient undergoing major surgery (discussed next).

Insulin-Dependent Diabetics. In managing an insulin-dependent diabetic patient during surgery, it is important for the anesthetist to have as much control over the blood glucose as possible. This is particularly true with respect to the ability to respond quickly to changes in blood glucose. It is important to be as certain as possible about the length of action of any administered insulin. No intermediate- or long-acting insulin should be given before or during surgery, as a hypoglycemic episode that occurs perioperatively may be prolonged.

It is important that the route by which insulin is administered be the most reliable with respect to time of action. Because many factors may influence cutaneous blood flow during and after surgery (i.e., stress, temperature regulatory mechanisms, anesthetics, and other drugs), it is inadvisable to administer insulin subcutaneously. For example, a sudden increase in cutaneous blood flow may cause an increased release of insulin from a subcutaneous insulin depot, resulting in a hypoglycemic episode. Therefore, the best route by which to give insulin is the intravenous route, either done through a regular intravenous line or via a syringe pump. There has been some concern about the fact that some insulin adheres to the administration tubing. Obviously, the shorter the tubing used the less adhesion will occur. A delivery of up to 90 percent of the available insulin has been demonstrated when a constant infusion pump with a plastic syringe is used.[14]

It is preferable to use separate intravenous delivery systems for insulin and glucose so that adjustments of the two to maintain blood glucose can be made independently. Unless it is necessary to combat severe hyperglycemia, it is best not to use large bolus injections of insulin. Such injections result in uncertainty in blood glucose management by increasing the likelihood of hypoglycemia in the short run. In addition, because the half-life of insulin in the circulation is only 5 minutes, there may be a need for further injections when the insulin from the first injection is no longer effective.

The actual amounts of glucose and insulin that should be given vary from patient to patient. Miller and Walts have suggested a glucose infusion of 2 mL/kg/h of 5 percent dextrose (which is approximately 100 mg/kg/h) piggy-backed into a non–dextrose-containing fluid.[10] These authors recommend not giving insulin preoperatively and, if blood glucose exceeds 250 mg/dL, administering single intravenous injections of insulin, 1 to 2 U/h. If blood glucose drops below 150 mg/dL, more glucose can be given.

Another recommended plan[12] for treating insulin-dependent diabetics perioperatively is to begin glucose and insulin administration at the time of the first missed meal at the following rates: 5 percent dextrose infusion delivering 1 L/8 h and an infusion (syringe pump recommended) of short-acting insulin at the rate of 1 to 3 U/h.

Another recommendation (based on a study of insulin-dependent patients undergoing orthopedic procedures) is to give 5 percent dextrose at the rate of 500 mL during the first hour after induction and at 125 mL/h during the following 4 hours.[14] In this study, insulin was administered either preoperatively as two thirds of the regular dose of neutral protamine Hagedorn (NPH) insulin given subcutaneously or via an infusion pump at the rate of 1 or 2 U/h (1 U/h if the patient normally received 20 U/d or less and 2 U/h if the normal dose was greater than 20 U/d). For those patients receiving 2 U/h, diabetic control was better (on average) than for those receiving the subcutaneous shot. In those patients receiving 1 U/h, diabetic control was equivalent to that of patients receiving the subcutaneous treatment.

Although recommendations regarding perioperative management of diabetics have been made and some specific examples of treatment have been cited, it is important to remember that the insulin and glucose needs of every patient are unique. These needs are a function of the normal means of metabolic control and are influenced by the nature of the surgery. Trouble can best be avoided by paying close attention to the metabolism of the patients as monitored by frequent determinations of blood glucose and appropriate adjustments in the amounts of insulin and glucose given.

Anesthesia for Diabetic Patients. The most important consideration in the handling of a diabetic patient in the perioperative period is the maintenance of the metabolic state. If the blood glucose is maintained within normal limits and ketoacidosis is avoided, anesthesia may in most cases be handled as it would be for a nondiabetic patient. Some general anesthetics themselves have hyperglycemic effects, but the degree is relatively minor compared with the hyperglycemia caused by the surgical intervention. Thus, if a general anesthetic is needed, the choice of which one to use can be made on general medical grounds. Spinal and local anesthesia have very little effect on blood glucose. Therefore, with regard to consideration of the metabolic management of a diabetic patient in surgery, spinal or local anesthesia may be preferable to general anesthesia when possible. Muscle relaxants and premedications generally have little effect on blood glucose. It should be noted that a major part of the physiologic response to combat hypoglycemia involves a sympathetically mediated breakdown of glycogen in the liver. Any diabetic who is taking beta blockers such as propranolol may show a deficient response to a declining blood glucose and be more inclined to develop hypoglycemia when an excess of insulin has been given perioperatively.

THE ADRENAL GLANDS

The adrenal glands comprise two embryologically and functionally distinct glands, the adrenal cortex and the adrenal medulla. The adrenal cortex is derived from mesoderm and secretes three types of steroid hormones: mineralocorticoids, glucocorticoids, and androgens. The adrenal medulla is derived from ectoderm and is functionally an important part of the sympathetic nervous system, secreting the catecholamines norepinephrine and epinephrine. The adrenal cortex is wrapped around the medulla like a shell.

The adrenal glands sit one atop each kidney. The right adrenal has a close relationship with the inferior vena cava, the right crus of the diaphragm, and the liver. The left gland is close to the tail of the pancreas, the peritoneum, the stomach, and the left crus of the diaphragm. The adrenals have a very rich blood supply, receiving from branches of the phrenic and renal arteries and from branches directly off of the aorta. The venous return is to the inferior vena cava on the right and the renal vein on the left. A unique aspect of the venous drainage of the adrenal cortex is that the blood drains through sinusoids into the adrenal medulla before passing into the adrenal vein. This fact is functionally important because the glucocorticoids secreted by the adrenal cortex are necessary for the synthesis of epinephrine from norepinephrine by the adrenal medulla.

Although they are anatomically related, the adrenal cortex and adrenal medulla are quite distinct in the physiologic parameters each affects in the body.

The Adrenal Cortex

The adrenal cortex consists of three histologically distinct layers, which from the outer surface inward are the zona glomerulosa, the zona fasciculata, and the zona reticularis. The zona glomerulosa secretes primarily mineralocorticoids, whereas the inner two zones secrete both glucocorticoids and androgens. Although many other hormones are secreted in lesser amounts, the major hormones secreted by

the adrenal cortex are aldosterone, cortisol, corticosterone, and dehydroepiandrosterone. Aldosterone is a mineralocorticoid, cortisol and corticosterone are glucocorticoids, and dehydroepiandrosterone is an androgen. Small amounts of estrogen may also be secreted by the adrenal cortex.

Aldosterone. The major action of aldosterone is on the kidney, where it increases the reabsorption of Na^+ in exchange for K^+ and H^+ in the distal convoluted tubules and collecting ducts. Water is reabsorbed with the sodium, thereby expanding the extracellular fluid volume. The amounts of K^+ and H^+ in the urine increase under the influence of aldosterone. It should be noted that aldosterone has no effect on Na^+ reabsorption in the proximal convoluted tubule or loop of Henle of the nephron.

Aldosterone also affects the ionic composition of saliva, gastric secretions, and sweat, although these actions are minor compared with the actions on the kidneys.

Secretion of Aldosterone. Four factors regulate the secretion of aldosterone: ACTH, the plasma concentrations of Na^+ and K^+ and the renin–angiotensin system. The role of ACTH in the regulation of aldosterone secretion is of some importance, but it is not the major factor. Low plasma Na^+ concentrations increase the secretion of aldosterone, although it is doubtful that the low level of Na^+ needed for the secretion is reached under physiologic conditions. Increased plasma K^+, within levels reached on a normal diet, increases aldosterone secretion in the renin–angiotensin system.

Renin is a protein hormone secreted by the juxtaglomerular cells of the kidney. These cells are located in the afferent arterioles, in close association with the distal convoluted tubules. Renin is secreted in response to (1) decreased pressure in the afferent arteriole such as might occur in hypotension, hemorrhage, dehydration, or renal artery stenosis; (2) decreased passage of Na^+ and Cl^- in the distal tubules; (3) stimulation of the sympathetic nerves to the kidneys; and (4) prostaglandins.

Renin acts on a globulin secreted by the liver to produce angiotensin I (Fig. 24–11). Angiotensin I is a decapeptide and

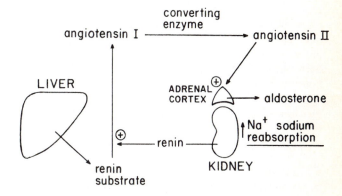

Figure 24–11. Control of aldosterone secretion by the renin–angiotensin system. Renin increases production of angiotensin I from renin substrate, which is converted to angiotensin II. Angiotensin II increases aldosterone secretion from the adrenal cortex.

is shortened to angiotensin II by converting enzyme, which exhibits high activity in the lungs. Angiotensin II is the physiologic endpoint of the renin–angiotensin system, acting to increase the secretion of aldosterone from the adrenal cortex (angiotensin II also causes constriction of arterioles, increasing blood pressure). The aldosterone that is secreted then acts on the kidney to increase sodium resorption, restoring the blood pressure or state of hydration to normal and shutting off the original stimulus for renin secretion.

Excess Aldosterone Secretion. An excess of aldosterone (or other adrenal cortex hormones with mineralocorticoid activity) leads to an elevation of diastolic blood pressure because of the extracellular fluid volume expansion that occurs. Because of the exchange of K^+ for Na^+ when the resorption of Na^+ increases in the kidney, the excretion of K^+ increases and hypokalemia develops. A metabolic alkalosis develops both because of increased H^+ excretion by the kidney (in exchange for Na^+ reabsorption) and because of movement of H^+ into the cells to replace K^+ that has been lost. In addition to diastolic hypertension, hypokalemia, and alkalosis, other signs and symptoms of hyperaldosteronism may include muscle weakness, fatigue, tetany (as a result of the lowering of plasma $[Ca^{2+}]$ by the alkalosis), paralytic ileus, and headache. The hypokalemia may cause impaired renal function leading to polyuria and polydipsia. The hypokalemia may also contribute to the appearance of cardiac arrhythmias, including flattened T-waves, prominent U-waves, prolongation of Q-T intervals, and depression of ST segments.[15] The hypokalemia also results in altered insulin secretion in many patients, and glucose tolerance may be impaired.

For unknown reasons, an excess of aldosterone is in most cases self-limiting in its effect on Na^+ reabsorption, an occurrence known as the escape phenomenon. The significance of the escape phenomenon is that many patients with hyperaldosteronism will develop hypertension, but fewer than 10 percent of the patients develop edema.[16]

Hyperaldosteronism may be primary, usually as a result of adrenal hyperplasia or adenoma, or secondary, as a result of activation of the renin–angiotensin system. Primary hyperaldosteronism is known as Conn's syndrome. Primary and secondary hyperaldosteronism can be distinguished from each other in part by considering the plasma levels of aldosterone, renin, and angiotensin. In primary hyperaldosteronism, the plasma level of aldosterone is high but the levels of renin and angiotensin are not. In secondary hyperaldosteronism, the plasma levels of all three of these hormones are elevated. In either primary or secondary hyperaldosteronism, measurement of the excretion of metabolites of aldosterone in the urine may be more useful than determination of the plasma concentration of the hormone itself.

Treatment of Hyperaldosteronism. Primary hyperaldosteronism may be managed medically with spironolactone, an aldosterone antagonist that inhibits the Na^+–K^+ exchange mechanism in the kidney. It may also be necessary to administer potassium supplements to correct the hypokalemia. Medical treatment of secondary hyperaldosteronism can be achieved with a drug such as indomethacin,

which inhibits the synthesis of prostaglandins and thus decreases the secretion of renin by the kidney. An alternative medical treatment for secondary hyperaldosteronism involves administration of potassium and triamterene (which inhibits the secretion of K^+ by the kidneys). Spironolactone may be given, and propranolol has been used to block the secretion of renin.[17]

The value of surgery for treatment of hyperaldosteronism depends on the specific pathology involved. Surgical removal is called for in the presence of an adenoma or carcinoma secreting aldosterone. After removal of an adenoma, blood pressure is significantly reduced in most patients[18,19] and the electrolyte abnormalities are reversed in virtually all patients.[20] In patients with idiopathic hyperaldosteronism or hyperplasia, the results of surgery are poor. If bilateral adrenalectomy is being considered, it should be recognized that the problems involved in total replacement of all the adrenal hormones may be worse than medical management of the isolated aldosterone excess.[21]

Anesthesia for Primary Hyperaldosteronism. The key preoperative consideration in preparing a patient with primary hyperaldosteronism for surgery is correction of any existing hypokalemia and hypertension. The acid–base status of the condition should also be carefully considered. The choice of anesthetic may be made on general medical grounds. Because of the proximity of the adrenal glands to the pleural cavity, respiratory management should include tracheal intubation and controlled respiration. Right atrial pressure or pulmonary artery pressure should be monitored by an appropriately placed catheter to assess intravascular fluid volume.

After surgery for hyperaldosteronism, it may be necessary for the patient to receive a mineralocorticoid such as fludrocortisone. If extensive manipulation of the adrenals was necessary during surgery or if a considerable amount of adrenal tissue was removed, a glucocorticoid may also be necessary postoperatively.

Additional considerations regarding adrenal surgery may be found later in this section under Excess Secretion of Glucocorticoids: Cushing's Syndrome.

The Glucocorticoids. The two major glucocorticoids secreted by the adrenal cortex are cortisol and corticosterone. The amount of cortisol secreted is about seven times greater than the amount of corticosterone secreted. Because the effects of cortisol and corticosterone are fairly similar, in this section of the chapter the more general term *glucocorticoid* is used to describe the actions of both hormones. The term *glucocorticoid* is appropriate as these hormones are involved in the control of intermediary metabolism; however, as discussed in the following paragraphs, the glucocorticoids also affect many other functions.

Effects on Intermediary Metabolism. The glucocorticoids have a number of important effects on the metabolism of carbohydrates, fat, and protein. The overall action the glucocorticoids have on carbohydrate metabolism is to increase the blood glucose concentration, acting in opposition to insulin. The glucocorticoids decrease utilization of glucose by many peripheral tissues. In the liver, glucocorticoids increase the formation of glucose from amino acids and glycerol by the process known as gluconeogenesis. Although the glucocorticoids increase the amount of glycogen stored in the liver, the extent of the decreased utilization of glucose in other tissues and the gluconeogenesis in the liver is such that the blood glucose concentration rises. Patients with an excess of glucocorticoids may show altered glucose tolerance curves and may even be classified as diabetic because of the glucocorticoids.

The glucocorticoids increase the breakdown of proteins in a number of tissues. Many of the amino acids released are converted to glucose in the liver (gluconeogenesis). An excess breakdown of protein may be deleterious, causing wasting and weakness in skeletal muscle, osteoporosis in bone, creatinuria, and a negative nitrogen balance.

Glucocorticoids promote deposition of fat, but in excess a characteristic redistribution known as truncal obesity occurs. In this condition, the fat depots in the abdomen, trunk, shoulders, and cheeks are enlarged but those in the extremities are smaller.

Effects on Water and Electrolyte Metabolism. The glucocorticoids have important actions on the kidney, facilitating the excretion of a water load. The glucocorticoids increase glomerular filtration and decrease reabsorption of water by the renal tubules; both actions increase the volume of urine formed. A patient who has adrenal cortical insufficiency will be unable to excrete a water load in the same amount of time as a normal person and may develop water intoxication. The glucocorticoids also exert a weak mineralocorticoid activity on the kidney, increasing the reabsorption of sodium and increasing potassium excretion.

Permissive Actions and the Cardiovascular System. To comprehend the effects of the glucocorticoids on the cardiovascular system, a phenomenon known as the "permissive" actions of the glucocorticoids must be understood. There are a group of physiologic functions that are not directly controlled by the glucocorticoids but, in the presence of other stimulatory factors (such as other hormones), are "permitted" to occur by the glucocorticoids. The permissive actions of the glucocorticoids include many of the functions stimulated by the catecholamines, some gastrointestinal functions, and nervous system activity.

Perhaps the most important permissive actions of the glucocorticoids are those involved in cardiovascular function. The glucocorticoids maintain vascular reactivity to the catecholamines and are thereby important in blood pressure regulation.

Effects on Hematologic and Lymphatic Tissue. Glucocorticoids decrease the number of circulating basophils, eosinophils, and lymphocytes but increase the number of erythrocytes, platelets, and neutrophils.

Pharmacologic Effects of the Glucocorticoids. Many of the more familiar effects of the glucocorticoids on the inflammatory response and the immune system occur only at pharmacologic doses of the hormones. The glucocorticoids decrease the amount of histamine released by mast cells in response to antigen–antibody complexes. As hista-

mine is responsible for many of the unpleasant manifestations of allergic reactions, this action of the glucocorticoids is very important.

The glucocorticoids are believed to stabilize lysosomal membranes. Lysosomes are cellular organelles that basically are membrane-lined bags of very powerful proteolytic enzymes. Release of these enzymes may cause damage in the tissues, so by stabilizing lysosomal membranes the glucocorticoids help prevent such damage.

The glucocorticoids decrease the activity of fibroblasts and thus may be of use in the prevention of keloid formation and adhesions after surgery.

A note of caution is necessary in the consideration of the use of glucocorticoids in any situation in which a bacterial infection may be present. Although the glucocorticoids may in some cases relieve many of the symptoms of such infections, including fever, toxin effects, and effects of released histamine, the hormones do not have bactericidal actions. Thus, inappropriate use of glucocorticoids in the presence of a bacterial infection may relieve the symptoms but allow the infection to spread.

Regulation of Secretion of the Glucocorticoids. Secretion of the glucocorticoids is under the control of ACTH, which is secreted by the anterior pituitary (Fig. 24–12). Under the influence of ACTH, the adrenal cortex (the zona fasciculata and the zona reticularis) secretes increasing amounts of glucocorticoids. In the absence of ACTH, the secretion of glucocorticoids is decreased. In a situation in which ACTH is absent for a prolonged period, the adrenal cortex atrophies and fails to secrete an adequate amount of glucocorticoids when ACTH is again present. After a period of absence of ACTH stimulation, it may take some time for the adrenal cortex to readapt the appropriate responsiveness to ACTH.

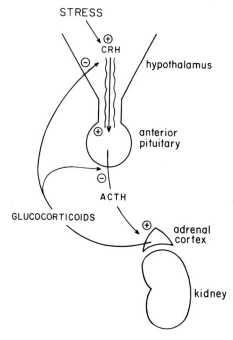

Figure 24–12. Regulation of glucocorticoid secretion.

Secretion of ACTH is increased by corticotropin-releasing hormone (CRH). CRH is produced in the hypothalamus and secreted into the hypothalamohypophyseal portal vessel, down which it passes to the anterior pituitary, where it increases ACTH secretion (see Fig. 24–12). Secretion of CRH is increased in a number of stressful situations by neural inputs that act on the hypothalamus.

The glucocorticoids exert feedback to directly inhibit the secretion of both CRH from the hypothalamus and ACTH from the pituitary (the decrease of CRH secretion further decreases the secretion of ACTH). This situation is a classic negative feedback cycle. It should be clear that a problem in the secretion of glucocorticoids may be primary, as in the case of adrenal disease, or secondary, as a result of a problem in the hypothalamus or pituitary. For example, hyposecretion of glucocorticoids in the presence of normal or high levels of ACTH is a sign of adrenal disease. On the other hand, hyposecretion of glucocorticoids accompanied by low levels of ACTH is an indication of pituitary or hypothalamic disease.

Circadian Rhythm of Glucocorticoid Secretion. The secretion in stressful situations of CRH, then ACTH, and finally the glucocorticoids is superimposed on a basal level of secretion. A characteristic of this basal level of secretion is the circadian rhythm that exists. The peak secretion of glucocorticoids with respect to the circadian rhythm occurs in the early morning hours. In determining the status of adrenal function, it is important to take the circadian rhythm into account.

Excess Secretion of Glucocorticoids: Cushing's Syndrome. An excess secretion of glucocorticoids from the adrenal cortex causes a characteristic condition known as Cushing's syndrome. Many of the clinical findings in Cushing's syndrome can be described as an exaggeration of the normal actions of the hormones.

The protein catabolism encountered in Cushing's syndrome leads to skeletal muscle weakness and wasting, osteoporosis, purpura, and ecchymoses. Wound healing is very poor. Because of the decreased peripheral utilization of glucose and increased gluconeogenesis in the liver, glucose tolerance may be abnormal in about 20 percent of cases and characteristic of diabetes in 10 percent of cases. Alterations in fat metabolism lead to truncal obesity, with a characteristic moon face, pendulous abdomen, and fat hump on the back (sometimes described as a buffalo hump).

Arterial hypertension is present in most patients with Cushing's syndrome, and heart failure and other circulatory problems may result. The glucocorticoids may cause hypertension because of effects on blood vessels or because of mineralocorticoid effects that may be exerted. Sodium is retained, and hypokalemia may also be present.

Other abnormalities encountered in Cushing's syndrome include hirsutism, menstrual abnormalities, acceleration of encephalographic rhythms, mental disturbances, and an increased incidence of infections.

TREATMENT OF CUSHING'S SYNDROME. Treatment of Cushing's syndrome depends on the type of pathology involved. If the cause is excess ACTH secretion by the pituitary, radiation

therapy or partial transsphenoidal hypophysectomy would be the appropriate treatment. If the pathology is in the adrenal gland, removal of the involved gland (or glands) is the only long-term treatment that has been successful. Medical suppression of hypersecreting adrenals with agents such as aminoglutethimide has not been very successful.

ANESTHESIA FOR PATIENTS WITH CUSHING'S SYNDROME. Careful attention must be paid to preoperative treatment of a number of the medical problems that may exist in a patient with excess secretion of glucocorticoids. The underlying abnormalities in intermediary metabolism may necessitate treatment with insulin and glucose in the perioperative period. Existing hypertension may be treated with diuretics. The patient may be hypokalemic as a consequence of some mineralocorticoid action of the excess adrenal hormones, so potassium supplementation should be given preoperatively. The acid–base status of the patient should be evaluated and corrected, if necessary. Osteoporosis is a common occurrence in patients with Cushing's syndrome, and evidence of this condition should be sought preoperatively from radiographs. Awareness of the possibility of existing osteoporosis underscores the care that should be taken in positioning a patient with Cushing's syndrome to avoid fractures.

Preoperative medications and the anesthetic agent may be chosen on general medical grounds. Because muscle weakness and hypokalemia are characteristic of Cushing's syndrome, the dose of muscle relaxant used should initially be low.[22] The status of the neuromuscular block should be monitored periodically with a nerve stimulator.

Mechanical ventilation is recommended during adrenal surgery for two major reasons. First, the combination of muscle weakness and truncal obesity in Cushing's syndrome may make spontaneous respiration difficult during surgery. The second reason is related to the position of the adrenal glands in front of the posterior diaphragmatic recess of the pleura. The possibility of pneumothorax is increased, and mechanical ventilation will be necessary to deal with the situation intraoperatively. It is advisable to examine a chest x-ray in the recovery room to be sure that a pneumothorax has not occurred.

Even if some adrenal tissue is left intact after adrenal surgery (as it would be in partial or unilateral adrenalectomy), it will be necessary to begin treating the patient with glucocorticoids intraoperatively. The reason for this is that the remaining adrenal cortical tissue becomes hypoactive in the presence of the hyperactive tissue secretions during the long period preceding diagnosis of the disease. For the same reason, immediate treatment with glucocorticoids will be necessary postoperatively. It may also be necessary to administer a mineralocorticoid postoperatively.

Adrenal Androgens. Steroid hormones classified as androgens are secreted by the adrenal cortex in both males and females. The adrenal androgen secreted in the largest amount is dehydroepiandrosterone, although this hormone has less than 20 percent of the activity of the gonadal androgen testosterone. The function of the adrenal androgens is not clearly understood. Androgens are generally referred to as the "male" sex hormones; however, this categorization may be inappropriate in the case of the adrenal androgens, as the amount of hormones secreted in females is normally as high as two thirds of what it is in males. Thus, it seems unlikely that the adrenal androgens are serving an exclusively male function. It is possible that the adrenal androgens have a predominantly metabolic function in both sexes, promoting actions such as protein synthesis and growth. The adrenal androgens may also be involved in sexual maturation at puberty.

When the adrenal androgens are secreted in excess, problems arise and the androgenic nature of the hormones becomes most apparent. Excess adrenal androgens result in a condition known as the androgenital syndrome. In females, this condition is characterized by an increasingly masculine appearance, including clitoral enlargement, development of a masculine distribution of body hair, and baldness. Excess adrenal androgens cause accentuation of male secondary characteristics in adult males and precocious development of these characteristics in prepubertal males.

The adrenogenital syndrome may be a result of an adrenal tumor or an enzyme deficiency in the pathway for synthesis of the adrenal hormones. An understanding of how the condition develops in the presence of an enzyme deficiency is based on a knowledge of the synthetic pathway for adrenal hormone synthesis and of the control of adrenal cortex secretion by ACTH from the pituitary. As discussed earlier in this section, secretion of glucocorticoids from the adrenal cortex is stimulated by ACTH, and the glucocorticoids in turn exert feedback to inhibit the secretion of ACTH. If glucocorticoids are not secreted by the adrenals, ACTH secretion remains elevated. If an enzyme deficiency exists in the synthetic pathway for the glucocorticoids, the continuous stimulation by ACTH that results from a lack of feedback inhibition causes a buildup of the intermediates in the synthetic pathway for the glucocorticoids. In the normal state, some of these intermediates are synthesized into androgens. If there is a buildup of the intermediates, as would occur in the presence of an enzyme deficiency, there is increased production of the adrenal androgens and the adrenogenital syndrome may result (Fig. 24–13). Such an enzyme deficiency is treated by the administration of cortisol. As cortisol inhibits the secretion of ACTH, the buildup of synthetic intermediates in the adrenal cortex declines and the secretion of androgens also drops.

The adrenogenital syndrome may be accompanied by either an excess or a deficiency of mineralocorticoid secretion, and if a deficiency exists, it may be necessary to treat the patient with a mineralocorticoid as well as cortisol.

Adrenal Cortical Hypofunction. Adrenal cortical hypofunction, a condition known as Addison's disease, may potentially involve any or all of the hormones normally secreted. The situation demands attention when there is a deficiency of glucocorticoids or mineralocorticoids or both. Adrenal hypofunction may be a result of any of the following conditions:

1. Primary adrenal disease resulting from such factors as enzyme deficiencies, physical trauma, infection, and adrenalectomy.

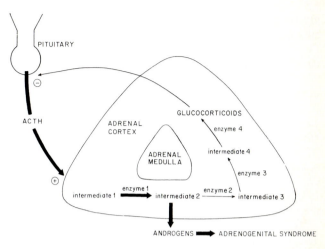

Figure 24–13. Adrenogenital syndrome. A deficiency in enzyme 2, 3, or 4 leads to a buildup of synthesis intermediates and decreased production of glucocorticoids. The lack of glucocorticoids removes the inhibition of secretion of adrenocorticotropin (ACTH) from the pituitary. The increased secretion of ACTH stimulates the adrenal cortex, and the ensuing increased secretion of androgens causes the adrenogenital syndrome.

2. Secondary involvement resulting from hypothalamic or pituitary hypofunction. If CRH is secreted in insufficient quantities from the hypothalamus or if ACTH secretion from the pituitary is lacking, glucocorticoids are not secreted from the adrenal cortex. Atrophy of the zona fasciculata and zona reticularis (the areas secreting the glucocorticoids and androgens) occurs, and the adrenal becomes insensitive to stimulation by ACTH at a later time.

3. Suppression of the adrenal cortex secondary to prolonged treatment with exogenous glucocorticoids used for anti-inflammatory or anti-immune system actions. Exogenous glucocorticoids inhibit secretion of CRH and ACTH, and, as described above, when ACTH is low for a prolonged period the adrenal cortex becomes insensitive to stimulation by ACTH when administration of exogenous glucocorticoids is discontinued. Even while exogenous glucocorticoids are being given, suppression of the adrenal gland will result in an inadequate secretory response in stressful situations.

Signs and Symptoms of Adrenal Hypofunction. A major concern in patients with adrenal hypofunction is hypotension. Although a deficiency of aldosterone may cause hypotension as a result of loss of fluids and electrolytes in the kidneys, a lack of glucocorticoids plays an important but poorly understood role in the ability to maintain blood pressure. Faintness and dizziness are consequences of the hypotension. If aldosterone is deficient, hyponatremia and hyperkalemia are likely to occur and metabolic acidosis may develop.

Weight loss, anorexia, weakness, and anemia are common complaints in adrenal hypofunction. Depression and fatigue are accompanying mental symptoms. Glucocorticoid deficiency will result in a tendency to develop hypoglycemia because of decreased gluconeogenesis in the liver and anti-insulin activity in other tissues. If there is a deficient secretion of adrenal androgens, loss of body hair may be seen.

If the adrenal hypofunction is primary in nature, an increase in ACTH secretion will occur because of a release from the negative feedback normally mediated by the glucocorticoids. ACTH has a certain degree of MSH activity, and abnormal, spotty pigmentation results.

Anesthesia for Patients with Adrenal Hypofunction. Provided that adrenal hormone replacement is adequate to compensate for the surgical stress, there are no special instructions regarding anesthetic management of a patient with adrenal hypofunction; however, hormone replacement is of immense concern because of the potentially fatal consequences of inadequate coverage.

The normal adrenal gland responds to the stress of surgery by increasing secretion of glucocorticoids. The exact ways by which the glucocorticoids benefit the patient are unknown, but it is known that hypotension, cardiovascular collapse, and ultimately death may ensue if glucocorticoids are not present. That is why if there is any doubt about whether or not to give glucocorticoids to a patient who may have adrenal hypofunction, it is better to err on the side of too much than too little.

Because treatment with glucocorticoids for anti-inflammatory or immunosuppressive purposes depresses the pituitary–adrenal system, glucocorticoids should be given preoperatively to a patient who has been on steroid therapy. Agreement on what degree of previous treatment calls for supplementation in the perioperative period is not universal, however. One opinion is that supplemental corticosteroids should be given to any patient who has been treated for more than 1 month in the past 6 to 12 months.[23] Another opinion is that supplementation should be given to patients who have been treated with steroids within the previous 2 months.[24] Still another opinion is that supplementation should be given to surgical patients who have received adrenal steroid treatment for a period of 4 days or longer during the preceding 6 months.[25] In patients already on a glucocorticoid regimen at the time of surgery, the hormone replacement should be continued. A recent study has indicated that an increase in the dose of corticosteroids at the time of surgery in patients already on a low-dose regimen seems unnecessary and is undesirable because of possible side effects.[26]

REFERENCES

1. Werner SC. Myxedema coma. In: Werner SC, Ingar SH, eds. *The thyroid: A fundamental and clinical text.* New York: Harper & Row; 1978:970–973.
2. Murkin JM. Anesthesia and hypothyroidism: A review of thyroxine physiology, pharmacology, and anesthetic implications. *Anesth Analg.* 1982;61:371.
3. Abbott TR. Anaesthesia in untreated myxoedema: Report of two cases. *Br J Anaesth.* 1967;39:510.
4. Pender JW, Fox M, Basso LV. Disease of the endocrine system. In: Katz J, Benumof J, Kadis LB, eds. *Anesthesia and uncommon diseases.* Philadelphia: WB Saunders; 1981:155–220.
5. Kim JM, Hackman L. Anesthesia for untreated hypothyroidism: Report of three cases. *Anesth Analg.* 1977;56:299.
6. Walker A, Cudwoith, AG. Type I (insulin dependent) diabetes multiplex families: Mode of genetic transmission. *Diabetes.* 1980;29:1036.
7. Palmers JP, Asplin CM. Insulin antibodies in insulin-dependent diabetics before insulin treatment. *Science.* 1983;222:1337.
8. Moorthy SS. Metabolism and nutrition. In: Stoelting RK, Dierdorf SF, eds. *Anesthesia and co-existing disease.* New York: Churchill Livingstone; 1983:485–521.
9. Maw DSJ. Emergency management of diabetes mellitus. *Anaesthesia.* 1975;30:520.
10. Miller J, Walts LF. Perioperative management of diabetes mellitus. In: Brown BR, ed. *Anesthesia and the patient with endocrine disease.* Philadelphia: FA Davis; 1980:91–103.
11. Campbell JW, Duncan LJP, Innes JA, et al. Abdominal pain in diabetic metabolic decompensation. Clinical significance. *JAMA.* 1975;233:166.
12. Hayes TM. The endocrine pancreas. In: Vickers MD, ed. *Medicine for anaesthetists.* 2nd ed. Oxford: Blackwell Scientific; 1982:497–514.
13. Ahern RS, Walker BA. Diabetes in relation to anaesthesia. In: Gray TC, Nunn JF, Utting JE, eds. *General anaesthesia.* 4th ed. London: Butterworths; 1980:797–806.
14. Taitelman V, Reece EA, Bessman AN. Insulin in the management of the diabetic surgical patient, continuous intravenous infusion vs. subcutaneous administration. *JAMA.* 1977;237:658.
15. Maddi R, Gabel RA. Anesthetic considerations for adrenalectomy. In: Brown BB, ed. *Anesthesia and the patient with endocrine disease.* Philadelphia: FA Davis; 1980:1–9.
16. Weinberg MH, Clarence EG, Hollifield JW, et al. Primary aldosteronism: Diagnosis, localization, and treatment. *Ann Intern Med.* 1979;90:386.
17. Block GW, Montgomery AD. Adrenal disease. In: Vickers MD, ed. *Medicine for anaesthetists.* 2nd ed. Oxford: Blackwell Scientific; 1982:451–496.
18. Biglieri EG, Schambelan M, Slaton PE, et al. The intercurrent hypertension of primary aldosteronism. *Circ Res.* 1970;27:195.
19. Hunt TK, Schambelan M, Biglieri EG. Selection of patients and operative approach in primary aldosteronism. *Ann Surg.* 1975;182:353.
20. Ferris JB, Beeves DG, Brown JJ, et al. Low-renin (primary) hyperaldosteronism: Differential diagnosis and distinction of the subgroups within the syndrome. *Ann Heart J.* 1978;95:641.
21. Shipton EA, Hugo JM. Primary aldosteronism and its importance to the anaesthetics. *S Afr Med J.* 1982;62:60.
22. Tasch MD. Endocrine diseases. In: Stoelting RK, Dierdorf SF, eds. *Anesthesia and co-existing disease.* New York: Churchill Livingstone; 1983:437–483.
23. White VA, Kumagai LF. Preoperative and metabolic considerations. *Med Clinic North Am.* 1979;63:1321.
24. Millar RA. Pituitary and adrenal glands in relation to anaesthesia. In: Gray TC, Nunn JF, Utting JE, eds. *General anaesthesia.* 4th ed. London: Butterworths; 1980:807–824.
25. Vandam LD, Moore FD. Adrenocortical mechanisms related to anesthesia. *Anesthesiology.* 1960;21:531.
26. Symreng T, Karlberg BE, Kagedal B, et al. Physiological cortisol substitution of long-term steroid-treated patients undergoing major surgery. *Br J Anaesth.* 1981;53:949.

BIBLIOGRAPHY

Brown BR, ed. *Anesthesia and the patient with endocrine disease.* Philadelphia: Davis; 1980.

Ezrin C, Gadden JO, Volpe R, eds. *Systemic Endocrinology.* 2nd ed. New York: Harper & Row; 1979.

Friesen SR, Boliner RE, ed. *Surgical endocrinology, clinical syndromes.* Philadelphia: JB Lippincott; 1978.

Ganong WR. *Review of medical physiology.* 14th ed. Los Altos, CA: Lange Medical; 1989.

Gray TC, Nunn JF, Utting JE, eds. *General anaesthesia.* 4th ed. London: Butterworths; 1980.

Katz J, Kadis LB, Benumof J, eds. *Anesthesia and uncommon diseases: Pathophysiologic and clinical correlations.* 3rd ed. Philadelphia: WB Saunders; 1990.

Oyama T. *Anesthetic management of endocrine disease.* 2nd ed. New York: Springer-Verlag; 1973.

Stoelting RK, Dierdorf SF, McCannon AL, eds. *Anesthesia and co-existing disease.* 2nd ed. New York: Churchill Livingstone; 1983.

Traynor C, Hall GM. Endocrine and metabolic changes during surgery: Anaesthetic implications. *Br J Anaesth.* 1981;53:153.

Vickers MD, ed. *Medicine for anaesthetists.* 2nd ed. Oxford: Blackwell Scientific; 1982.

Wilson JD, Foster DN, eds. *Williams textbook of endocrinology.* 7th ed. Philadelphia: WB Saunders; 1985.

Yao FF, Artusio JF, eds. *Anesthesiology, problem-oriented patient management.* Philadelphia: JB Lippincott; 1988.

PART IV

Applied Pharmacology

Pharmacologic Principles, Uptake and Distribution, and Pharmacology of Inhalational Anesthetics

Michele E. Gold and Linda S. Finander

The intravenous and inhalational anesthetic drugs used in the delivery of anesthesia are potent, rapid-acting agents with distinct pharmacologic properties. The first part of this chapter outlines the basic pharmacologic principles of drug action pertaining to those intravenous agents used in anesthesia. These principles include the absorption, distribution, biotransformation, and elimination of drugs, the time course of drug effect, and the mechanisms of drug action. The pharmacologic properties of the inhalational anesthetics are distinct from those of the intravenous agents. Molecular theories of inhalational anesthetic action and the principles of uptake and distribution, minimum alveolar concentration, and physical properties of the inhalational anesthetics are discussed.

The second part of this chapter describes the effects of nitrous oxide, halothane, enflurane, and isoflurane on specific organs, providing the anesthetist with the information needed to make a rational choice of agent for any surgical procedure. The pharmacology of two investigational anesthetics, sevoflurane and desflurane, is also presented. A detailed knowledge of the pharmacologic principles of anesthetic agents is vital to the safe practice of anesthesia.

BASIC PHARMACOLOGIC PRINCIPLES OF DRUG ACTION

The selection and administration of drugs used in anesthesia must encompass a knowledge of the pharmacodynamic and pharmacokinetic principles of these agents. Pharmacodynamics is the study of the actions of chemicals or drugs in producing biologic effects, whereas pharmacokinetic principles identify the factors that determine the time course and the amount of drug reaching the site of action to produce a biologic effect. One of the goals of anesthesia delivery is the administration of drugs within the proper dosage range and time interval that will ensure appropriate drug concentrations in the organ, tissue, or cellular site of drug action. The determinants of pharmacodynamic and pharmacokinetic principles include (1) drug bioavailability, a consequence of the absorption, distribution, biotransformation and elimination of drugs; (2) time course of drug effects; and (3) mechanisms of drug action.

Drug Bioavailability

The absorption of drugs across biologic membranes is necessary to produce a drug effect. The more classic routes of anesthesia delivery are the inhalation, intravenous, and rectal routes; however, new routes of administration that are increasing in popularity include the intranasal,[1,2] aerosol,[3] and transmucosal routes.[4] The bioactive form of a drug is generally the un-ionized form which is lipid soluble and readily permeates lipid membranes. Ionized drugs are hydrophilic and do not easily permeate lipid membranes. Most therapeutic drugs are weak acids or bases, and the percentage of drug that is un-ionized can be determined by the Henderson–Hasselbalch equation.[5] This equation defines the relationship between the pK_a of the drug and the pH gradient across a particular membrane. The pK_a of a drug is a constant, determined by the pH at which the drug is 50 percent ionized. This suggests that the local pH surrounding the drug molecule influences the degree of ionization, drug absorption, and bioavailability.

Drug distribution involves the transfer of a drug to its central or peripheral sites of action. Drugs are more rapidly distributed to those organs that are well perfused, such as the brain, heart, and liver, and less rapidly distributed to smooth muscle and fat. Binding of drugs to various circulating plasma proteins, such as albumin and globulin, affects the concentration of the bioactive drug. The degree of protein binding of a particular drug is dependent on the affinity of the drug for plasma proteins, the pH of the plasma, and temperature. Another influencing factor is the plasma protein concentration which is altered in many disease states.[6,7] The concept of redistribution is important in that it may affect certain anesthetic agents. Redistribution involves the removal of a drug from its site of action. For example, rapid recovery from sodium pentothal is due to its redistribution from the brain to smooth muscle and fat.

The absorption of drugs across biologic membranes and the distribution to active sites may be limited by the physical and chemical characteristics of the drug and the cellular barriers. The concentration gradient of the drug and its molecular size determine whether a drug can passively diffuse across membranes. In addition, drugs may be transported by facilitated diffusion, which is also dependent on the concentration gradient, or active transport processes using energy for passage across membranes. Specialized membranes, such as the blood–brain barrier and placenta, provide some protection against drug delivery to the central nervous system and the fetus, respectively; however, because of the high lipophilicity of anesthetic agents, some drugs used in anesthesia can penetrate these protective membranes.[8,9]

Bioactive, lipophilic substances are not readily eliminated in the urine and must be metabolized to water-soluble substances. The liver is the predominant metabolic organ and drug biotransformation occurs here through two distinct metabolic pathways. Phase I processes include oxidative, reductive, and hydrolytic reactions that enzymatically convert the parent compound into more polar metabolites. The cytochrome P450 system, found in the hepatic microsomal fraction, is responsible for enzymatic catalysis of the oxidative and reductive reactions. The benzodiazepines, for example, are substrates for this microsomal enzyme system.[10] Hydrolytic enzymes, found in most organs, plasma, and tissue, catalyze the metabolism of drugs containing ester or amide linkages.[11] The depolarizing muscle relaxant succinylcholine is rapidly hydrolyzed by plasma esterases to an inactive metabolite, succinyl-monocholine. Conjugation reactions constitute phase II processes and involve the chemical combination of a reactive group on the drug molecule with a variety of endogenous substrates. Glucuronide conjugation is the most common reaction undergone by drugs, but conjugation with sulfate, glycine, and acetate is possible.[11] At times, hepatic metabolism is necessary in the enzymatic conversion of a drug into a more pharmacologically active species. The actual drug administered serves as a prodrug, which in itself has little or no biologic activity. Extensive metabolism of some orally administered drugs (i.e., lidocaine) can limit the bioavailability of these agents. This first-pass metabolism can be prevented by intravenous drug administration.

The rate at which biotransformation of drugs takes place is affected by hepatic blood flow and enzyme induction or inhibition. Alterations in hepatic blood flow by drugs, congestive heart failure, or shock can impair the metabolic rate. The cytochrome P450 enzyme system is subject to enzyme induction, which may increase the amount of metabolic enzyme 25-fold and result in a marked increase in the metabolic rate. A variety of drugs such as phenobarbital and alcohol are capable of enzyme induction. Enzyme inhibition leads to a decrease in the rate of drug metabolism and can occur after cimetidine administration.[12]

Drug elimination most commonly occurs through renal excretion. Most eliminated substances are polar metabolites, but excretion of unchanged drug can also account for the termination of drug action. The renal tubular system depends on the processes of filtration, passive diffusion, and active tubular secretion.[13] Ionized unbound drug molecules of low molecular weight pass through the glomerular filtrate into the renal tubular fluid. Within the renal tubules, the size of the concentration gradient, the molecular size of the ionized drug, and the urinary pH influence passive diffusion. In addition, a number of drugs are substrates for active secretory systems located in the renal tubule cells and are actively transported into the urine. Metabolites formed by conjugation reactions are most likely eliminated by active secretion. Morphine is one of many compounds using active secretory processes for elimination.

Other excretory routes include the hepatobiliary system and the lungs. Drugs can pass easily into the liver, but movement into the bile necessitates diffusion mechanisms and active transport systems. Intestinal reabsorption of drugs can occur, and such recycling is referred to as the *enterohepatic cycle*. The recycled drug may ultimately be further metabolized and excreted in the urine. Inhalational anesthetic agents are eliminated essentially unchanged in the lung. (See Metabolism of Inhalational Agents.) The concentration gradient, the solubility, and the alveolar ventilation determine the rate of drug elimination.

Time–Response Effects of Drugs

The time course of drug effects can be divided into three phases: (1) time to onset of action, (2) time to peak effect, and (3) duration of action.[14] The onset of drug action is the length of time from drug administration to the first measurable drug effect; the duration of action is the length of time from drug administration to the cessation of drug effect. Peak effect occurs at the maximal drug concentration. The factors described previously—absorption, distribution, biotransformation, and elimination—influence the time in which a critical concentration of a drug has access to its site of action. Half-life ($t\frac{1}{2}$), volume of distribution, and clearance can be derived by mathematical principles based on measurements of the drug concentration that occur over time.

The half-life of a drug is the time required for the plasma concentration of the drug to be reduced by 50 percent and indicates the time required for drug elimination from the body. The clearance of a drug refers to the rate of elimination by the kidneys, liver, or other routes. Volume of distribution relates the amount of drug in the body with the same concentration measured in the plasma. Large volumes of distribution indicate the presence of drug in tissues or fluids outside the plasma compartment. Half-life, rate of clearance, and volume of distribution are interrelated. For instance, a decrease in the rate of clearance secondary to renal disease increases the half-life of a drug and possibly intensifies the drug effect. A decrease in plasma protein binding raises the level of free drug in the plasma, increasing the volume of distribution and the rate of drug clearance.[6,14]

Mechanisms of Drug Action

General anesthesia can be induced using either intravenous or inhalational anesthetic agents. The mechanisms of action of these two groups of anesthetics are markedly different.

Drug–receptor interactions have been described for most of the intravenous agents used in the administration of anesthesia. Inhalational anesthetics are considered to elicit a drug response following a nonspecific interaction with cellular membranes.

Intravenous agents used in anesthesia, such as the barbiturates, the benzodiazepines, the neuromuscular blockers, and the narcotics, interact reversibly with specific macromolecular proteins to elicit a response. The physicochemical interaction between a drug and a specific receptor triggers a cellular response, resulting in a measurable drug effect. The cellular response can be an alteration in ion transport, the generation of second messengers such as cyclic AMP and calcium, or inhibition of the physiologic drug–receptor interaction. For instance, there is strong evidence linking the mechanism of action of the benzodiazepines to a protein receptor within the central nervous system. Binding of a benzodiazepine to the γ-aminobutyric acid (GABA) receptor increases the affinity of the inhibitory neurotransmitter, GABA, to a specific site on the protein receptor. GABA binding results in an inward flux of chloride ion and a decrease in cellular excitability.[15,16] On the other hand, drugs such as the neuromuscular blockers do not directly interfere with cellular function. Rather, they occupy the nicotinic cholinergic postsynaptic receptor to inhibit the acetylcholine transmission necessary in membrane depolarization and repolarization for neuromuscular activity.

The relationship between the concentration of drug and the magnitude of drug effect is important in the administration of either intravenous or inhalational anesthetics. Concentration–response curves evaluate the clinical effects of drugs and provide information about a drug's potency, efficacy, 50 percent effective concentration (EC50), 50 percent lethal concentration (LC50), and therapeutic index. Potency refers to the concentration of drug required to produce a maximum response. A relatively potent drug will elicit an effect at a low concentration. Efficacy is related to the intrinsic ability of the drug to elicit a response. An agonist has maximum efficacy, whereas an antagonist has zero efficacy. The EC50 is the concentration of drug necessary to elicit a response in 50 percent of individuals and the LC50 is the concentration of drug that results in death in 50 percent of individuals. The therapeutic index represents the relative safety of a drug and is determined by the ratio between LC50 and EC50.[17] It is relatively easy to determine these drug parameters for the intravenous anesthetic agents, most of which produce a response through interaction with specific receptors. The inhalational anesthetics are less amenable to interpretation by these parameters because of the nonspecific nature of their actions and their not fully identifiable receptors.

Drug–Drug Interactions

Current clinical anesthetic practice incorporates the use of many pharmacologic agents that act generally to induce hypnosis, skeletal muscle relaxation, and analgesia and to block reflex responses. Not only do these drugs have specific actions, but often the administration of a combination of these drugs produces a variety of different actions and interactions.

A number of pharmacologic principles are relevant to a discussion of drug interactions. Summation, or an additive dose effect, is seen when the combined effect of two or more drugs acting simultaneously is the same as the arithmetic sum (S) of the effects of the individual drugs (A + B) in their selected doses, or A + B = S. Synergism indicates that the simultaneous total effect of drugs A and B is greater than the effect of either drug A or drug B alone, provided that both drugs evoke a similar response (A + B > A or B). Potentiation, often considered a special type of synergism, is the augmentation of an effect of drug A by drug B even though drug B may not have any discernible effect on its own (A + B > A, B = 0). Antagonism is the effect observed when administration of drug A in the presence of drug B decreases the effectiveness of drug B (A + B < B). Agonism can be seen when an exogenously administered drug mimics the effects observed with endogenous drugs. An exogenously administered drug displays intrinsic activity if it can produce an effect usually seen with an endogenous substance. Drug allergy is due to an altered state of reaction to a specific drug or class of drugs produced by a prior sensitization. Anaphylaxis is a life-threatening allergic response to a drug that may or may not follow prior drug sensitization. An idiosyncratic response is an untoward or abnormal response to a given drug. Another spectrum of responses includes tolerance, which occurs when there is a decreased physiologic response with repeated drug administration of the same or chemically related drug. Tachyphylaxis is that special case of tolerance that occurs rapidly with repeated frequent drug administration. Cumulation is seen when the body does not completely metabolize one dose of a drug prior to administration of a second dose. Drug dependence may be physical, psychologic, or both. Physical dependence refers to an altered physiologic state that produces profound physiologic symptoms when the drug is suddenly withdrawn. Psychologic dependency denotes emotional reliance on certain drugs. Psychologic dependency often occurs concurrently with physiologic dependency.

Drug interactions may be separated in three categories; however, these categories are strictly a didactic tool. Some drugs, like phenothiazines, exhibit interactions that encompass all three categories.

1. *Category 1* includes pharmacologic interactions that occur in vitro and in vivo. These drug–drug interactions may be the result of chemical, physical, or physiologic influences. For example, penicillin G is incompatible with heparin when mixed together in a single tube or infusion bag for administration; thiopental and opiates cannot be combined together in the same syringe because precipitation will occur; agents that alter gastric pH influence the absorption of acetylsalicylic acid by the gut; opiate administration alters gastric motility and slows the drug absorption processes.
2. *Category 2* includes pharmacokinetic factors that may be attributed to the physiologic state by the patient or the influence of other drugs. For example, the presence of lipids slows the absorption of alcohol from the gut; alcohol and phenylbutazone alter the plasma protein binding of warfarin; kidney disease

prolongs the duration of action of those drugs requiring the kidney as the primary route for elimination; the interaction between succinylcholine and atypical pseudocholinesterase is well documented and is discussed in detail in Chapter 28; propranolol administration produces bronchoconstriction and increases airway resistance, thereby decreasing the ventilation/perfusion ratio in patients; sulfonamides inhibit and barbiturates stimulate the hepatic microsomal drug-metabolizing enzyme system.

3. *Category 3* includes pharmacodynamic interactions resulting from the ongoing effects of endogenous and exogenous drugs as associated with active or silent receptors. For example, halothane produces cardiac arrhythmias when endogenous catecholamine levels are elevated or when exogenous catecholamines are administered simultaneously; administration of a therapeutic concentration of potassium modifies the influence of digitalis on cardiac muscle; and neostigmine alters the effects of succinylcholine.

As drug effects can be strictly quantified only in a mathematical sense, the clinician is constrained to deal with mean distributions for normal and abnormal responses. In the clinical setting, however, this information may not be readily available and the anesthetist must be aware of and prepared to treat any possible untoward drug interaction response.

Molecular Theories of Anesthetic Action

Several theories of molecular mechanisms of action have been proposed for the inhalational anesthetics. The inhalational anesthetics used in clinical practice (halothane, enflurane, and isoflurane) or those under current investigation (sevoflurane and desflurane) are all halogenated compounds. They are not structurally similar (Fig. 25–1) and it is unlikely that a specific protein receptor is responsible for the anesthetic effect. Inhalational anesthetics cause an alteration in synaptic transmission. Whether the dysfunction

occurs in the release of a neurotransmitter from the presynaptic terminal or at the postsynaptic receptor is unknown.[18] Theories of anesthesia mechanisms include (1) the lipid theory, (2) the physicochemical theory, and (3) the molecular mechanism theory.

The lipid theory, described in 1901 by Meyer and Overton, is based on the affinity of an anesthetic molecule for lipid, specifically nerve cell membranes composed of a lipid matrix. The potency of an anesthetic correlates with its degree of lipid solubility. Oil:gas coefficients (Table 25–1) for the inhalational anesthetics are a measure of the lipid solubility of these agents. According to the second theory of anesthesia, the lipid component of the nerve cell membrane expands and thereby increases fluidity or perturbs the membrane. This can lead to an alteration in the membrane channels and result in an anesthetic action. This expansion in the physicochemical properties of the nerve cells can be reversed at high hydrostatic pressures.[19]

More recently, advances in molecular pharmacology have led to investigations into molecular mechanisms of anesthetic action. Currently, the molecular theory of anesthetic action is focused on the inhibitory neurotransmitter (GABA).[20–24] As mentioned previously, the mechanism of action of benzodiazepines may also be linked to GABA transmission, as well as the mechanism of action of the barbiturates.[15,16] Clinical concentrations of halothane, enflurane, and isoflurane enhance the GABA-induced ionic current, resulting in postsynaptic membrane hyperpolarization.[24] 4,5,6,7-Tetrahydroisoxazolo[5,4-c]pyridin-3-ol (THIP), a GABA analog, was found to induce general anesthesia,[21] and the use of GABA agonists and antagonists caused an increase or decrease, respectively, in the amount of sleep induced by halothane anesthesia.[23] These "receptor-specific" actions suggest that general anesthetic action may occur directly on a specific target site.

Another possible mechanism of anesthetic action is also a result of cellular hyperpolarization with a decrease in central nervous system excitability.[25,26] It is proposed that anesthetic molecules bind to potassium channels and stabilize them in the open state. An increase in potassium conductance correlates with the anesthetic potency of general anes-

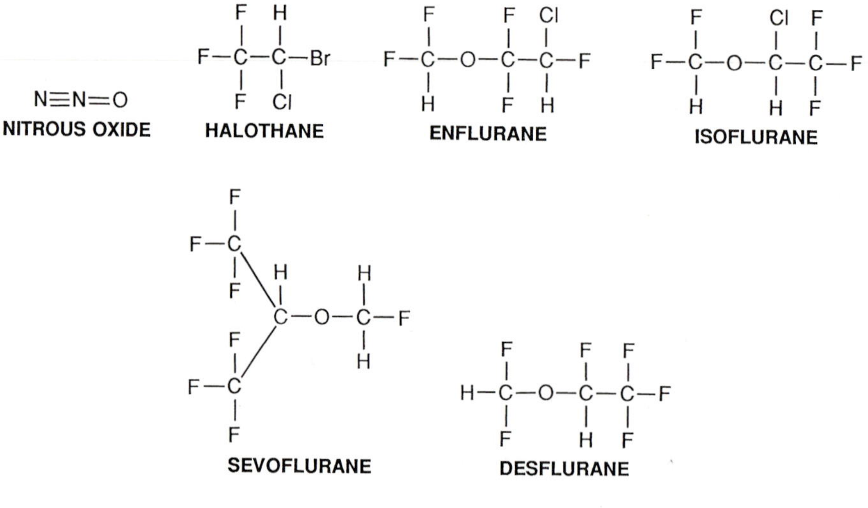

Figure 25–1. Molecular structures of inhalational anesthetics.

TABLE 25–1. PHYSICAL PROPERTIES OF INHALATIONAL ANESTHETICS

	Halothane	Enflurane	Isoflurane	Desflurane	Sevoflurane	Nitrous Oxide
Molecular weight (g)	197.4	184.5	184.0	168.0	200	44.0
Boiling point (C)	50.2	56.5	48.5		58.5	−88.0
Vapor pressure at 20C	243.0	175.0	250.0		160.0	39,000
Partition coefficient at 37C						
Blood:gas	2.3	1.9	1.4	0.42	0.60	0.47
Oil:gas	224.0	98.5	97.8	18.7	53.4	1.4
Water:gas	0.7	0.8	0.61			0.47
Brain:blood	2.0	1.4	1.6	1.3	1.7	1.1
Fat:blood	62.0	36.0	52.0	30.0	55.0	2.3
Minimum alveolar concentration (%)	0.75	1.7	1.3	5.72[a]	1.71	110
% Metabolites (approximate)	15–20	2.4–9	0.2	Minimal	1.5–2	

[a] In rats.

Sources. *Wallin WF, Regan BM, Napoli MD, et al.* Anesth Analg. *1975;54:758. Wade JG, Stevens WC.* Anesth Analg. *1981;60:666. Eger EI.* Anesth Analg. *1987;66:971. Eger EI, Johnson BH.* Anesth Analg. *1987;66:974. Koblin OD, Weiskopf RB, Holmes MA.* Anesth Analg. *1989;68:147.*

thetics, including halothane and enflurane. The potassium channel may be an alternate site of anesthetic action, but further investigation is necessary.

UPTAKE AND DISTRIBUTION OF INHALATION AGENTS

The pharmacologic properties of the inhalational agents used in anesthesia differ significantly from those of the intravenous agents. The most striking difference is the unique mechanism of action of the inhalation agents, as discussed previously. As the inhalation agents are gaseous molecules that can interact with particular nerve cell membranes to cause an alteration in synaptic transmission, distinct pharmacodynamic and pharmacokinetic properties including uptake and distribution, metabolism, and recovery apply to these anesthetics.

Minimum Alveolar Concentration

The minimum alveolar concentration (MAC) of an inhaled anesthetic relates the inhalational anesthetic concentration to the observed effect and is a measure of anesthetic potency. MAC is defined by the concentration of anesthetic that produces immobility in 50 percent of those patients or animals exposed to a noxious stimulus.[27] Therefore, MAC indicates the relative concentration of anesthetic necessary to achieve surgical anesthesia. MAC is measured as the alveolar partial pressure of anesthetic, which reflects the partial pressure of anesthetic at the active site, the brain, at equilibrium. Clinical measurements of intraoperative anesthetic concentrations have been made easy by the advent of

mass spectrometry. MAC values of the inhalational anesthetics are noted in Table 25–1. The MAC values of the various anesthetic agents are used as the basis for comparison among agents; 1-MAC levels of these agents produce equivalent anesthetic states. In addition, MAC values of the anesthetics are additive; combination of 0.5 MAC of nitrous oxide with 0.5 MAC of halothane produces the same anesthetic effect as each agent when used separately. Although conflicting data have been reported,[28] the simultaneous use of other anesthetic agents such as intrathecal morphine with inhalational anesthetics has also been shown to cause a reduction in the anesthetic requirements of the inhalational anesthetics.[29,30]

Many factors are known to alter anesthetic requirements, necessitating an increase or decrease in the MAC. For example, hyperthermia, chronic alcohol abuse, and young age (i.e., neonates), may increase the anesthetic requirement whereas hypothermia, pregnancy, preoperative medication, hypotension, and advancing age may decrease MAC.[27,31]

Partial Pressure of Inhaled Anesthetics

The principal objective of inhalational anesthesia is delivery of an optimal concentration of drug to the site of anesthesia action, the brain. Administration of an inhalational anesthetic results in a partial pressure gradient of anesthetic at the alveolar–arterial membrane. The desired anesthetic effect occurs when the partial pressure at the alveolar–arterial membrane is equal to the partial pressure in the brain. The partial pressure at the alveolar membrane is an indirect measure of the concentration of anesthetic in the brain. The partial pressure of a gas is described by Dalton's law which states that the tension (pressure) of an individual gas in a mixture of gases is proportional to its concentration.[32] Development of the alveolar partial pressure is dependent on the concentration of the inspired anesthetic (concentration effect), the presence of a second gas (second gas effect), the ventilatory rate, and the solubility of the gas in blood. An increase in these parameters affects the speed of induction of anesthesia.

The concentration effect describes the impact of the inspired concentration of anesthetic on the rate at which the alveolar partial pressure can equilibrate with the inspired concentration.[27(pp113–121)] A high inspired concentration of anesthetic will accelerate the rate of rise of the alveolar partial pressure. This principle is demonstrated during the induction of an anesthetic, as the initial concentration of anesthetic delivered to the patient is above the MAC of that anesthetic (Fig. 25–2). The use of nitrous oxide during the induction of anesthesia also influences the rate of equilibration of the alveolar partial pressure with the inspired partial pressure. In the presence of high inspired concentrations of nitrous oxide, a second, more potent anesthetic agent, such as halothane, is delivered at a higher concentration because of the augmentation of inspiratory inflow of halothane (see Fig. 25–2).[33,34] It is important to recognize, however, that the effect of delivery of a high initial concentration of an anesthetic or concurrent administration of a high concentration of nitrous oxide on the rate of anesthetic equilibration in the lung is dependent on ventilation. The inhalation anesthetics are respiratory depressants that impair the inflow of anesthesia and slow induction. This can be overcome by mechanical ventilation of the patient to provide an adequate anesthetic depth.

Uptake and Distribution

The inspired partial pressure of an inhalational anesthetic influences the rate of equilibration of the anesthetic and therefore influences the induction of anesthesia. The inspired concentration of anesthetic is offset by the uptake of inhalational agent from the alveolus into the bloodstream. Anesthetic uptake is dependent on (1) the solubility of the anesthetic in blood, (2) the circulatory system (i.e., cardiac output), and (3) tissue uptake of anesthesia.

Anesthetic solubility is a physical property of the individual drug and is measured as the degree to which the drug can partition itself between a gaseous phase and a liquid phase at equilibrium. Blood:gas partition coefficients have been determined for the inhalational anesthetics in clinical use and those under investigation (see Table 25–1) and are used as relative index of solubility. The more insoluble an anesthetic agent (i.e., nitrous oxide), the sooner equilibrium of the alveolar partial pressure gradient is reached. The more potent inhalational anesthetics—halothane, enflurane, and isoflurane—are moderately soluble, indicating that a larger amount of anesthetic needs to be dissolved in the blood before an equilibrium state is reached and an anesthetic effect observed (Fig. 25–3). Again, the use of high inspired initial concentrations of these anesthetics (greater than the MAC) will overcome the solubility factor and speed induction.

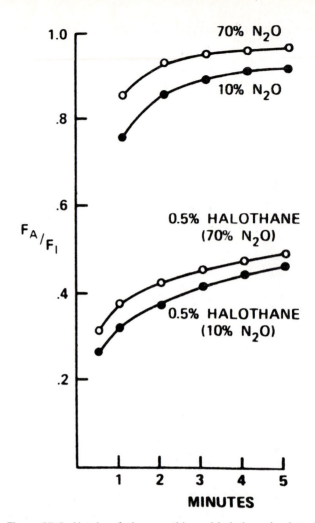

Figure 25–2. Uptake of nitrous oxide and halothane is plotted as the ratio of the alveolar anesthetic concentration (F_A) to inspired concentration (F_I) for each agent. High inspired concentrations of nitrous oxide can augment the inspiratory inflow of halothane. (*Reprinted, with permission, from Epstein et al.*[33(p367)])

The cardiac output carries blood away from the lung and increases the uptake of anesthetic into the blood from the alveolus. This results in a decrease in the alveolar concentration of the anesthetic. An increase in cardiac output, therefore, slows the rate of induction of anesthesia, because the larger blood volume perfusing the lung effectively dilutes the concentration of anesthetic in the arterial blood. Although the anesthetic agent is taken up more rapidly and may be delivered to the blood circulation faster, a lower arterial blood concentration limits the onset of an anesthetic state. Conversely, a decrease in cardiac output may result in an excessive anesthetic depth. As a lowered cardiac output may be present in the elderly, debilitated, or trauma patients, slow, cautious induction of anesthesia is necessary.

Tissue uptake of the inhalational anesthetics influences the uptake of anesthetic at the alveolus by creating an alveolar-to-venous anesthetic partial pressure difference.[34] The amount of anesthetic removed from the bloodstream to the tissues is dependent on the tissue solubility of the anesthetic agent, the tissue blood flow, and the partial pressure

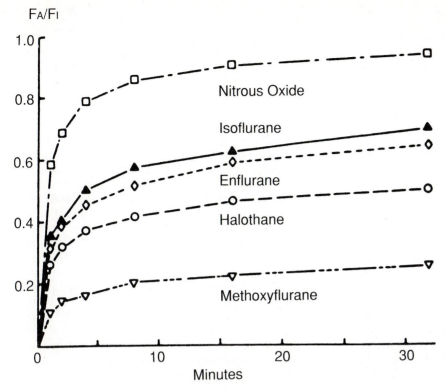

Figure 25–3. The rise in alveolar (FA) anesthetic concentration toward the inspired (FI) concentration is most rapid with the least soluble anesthetic agent, nitrous oxide. The moderately soluble anesthetic agents, halothane, enflurane, and isoflurane, have a slower rate of rise in the ratio of alveolar to inspired concentration. (*Reprinted, with permission, from Eger EI II. Isoflurane (Forane): A compendium and reference. 2nd ed. Madison, WI: Anaquest, BOC; 1985.*)

difference between the arterial blood and the tissue. Tissue solubility is influenced by the amount of blood flow to a particular tissue. Four tissue groups have been identified (Table 25–2) based on their solubility and perfusion characteristics. The vessel-rich group includes the brain, heart, liver, and kidney, which receive 75 percent of the cardiac output. Tissue solubility of these organs is high, resulting in rapid equilibration of anesthetic. Tissues in the muscle group (muscle and skin) and fat group are poorly perfused. Anesthetic partial pressure in the muscle group equilibrates slowly with the blood, but because fat has a very high affinity for the inhalational anesthetics, equilibration usually does not occur. The fat group can continue to take up the anesthetic for several hours. The vessel-poor group includes ligaments, tendons, cartilage, and bone. Blood perfusion to this group is insignificant and does not influence tissue uptake.

Anesthetic uptake can be limited by ventilation/perfusion abnormalities that may occur in the healthy patient or in patients with problems such as emphysema, atelectasis, and cardiac anomalies. Ventilation/perfusion abnormalities

result in an increase in the alveolar partial pressure of anesthetic and a decrease in the arterial partial pressure of anesthetic. A partial pressure difference develops between the alveolus and arterial blood that influences the induction of anesthesia. Perfusion of an unventilated alveolus prevents the uptake of anesthetic. The blood leaving this area mixes with blood from ventilated areas and lowers the arterial partial pressure. In a well-ventilated alveolus with poor perfusion, the arterial partial pressure in the blood may increase and compensate for the diminished arterial partial pressure emerging from a poorly ventilated area.[35]

Recovery from Inhalational Anesthetics

Recovery of anesthesia occurs after the elimination of anesthetic from its site of action, the brain. The concentration, duration, and solubility of the inhalational anesthetic are all involved in the time to recovery from anesthesia.[36] On termination of the inspired anesthetic, the inspired partial pressure is zero, creating a partial pressure gradient between the tissue and the blood. The anesthetic will be

TABLE 25–2. TISSUE GROUP CHARACTERISTICS

	Group			
	Vessel-Rich	**Muscle**	**Fat**	**Vessel-Poor**
Body mass (%)	9	50	19	22
Perfusion (% cardiac output)	75	18.1	5.4	1.5

Adapted, with permission, from Eger EI. Anesthetic uptake and action. Baltimore: Williams & Wilkins; 1974.

rapidly eliminated from vessel-rich tissues; however, depending on the duration of anesthesia, the muscle and fat group tissues most likely will not have reached equilibrium. Anesthetic elimination from these tissues is thereby prolonged, although the continued uptake of anesthetic into fat may contribute to recovery. Recovery from anesthesia is prolonged with the more soluble anesthetics, that is, halothane, enflurane, and isoflurane. Use of the insoluble anesthetics, nitrous oxide, sevoflurane, and desflurane, the blood:gas solubility coefficients of which are significantly lower (see Table 25–1), results in more rapid recovery.

Diffusion hypoxia can occur during recovery from anesthesia secondary to the discontinuation of nitrous oxide. The rapid elimination of nitrous oxide from the tissues and blood into the lung causes a dilution of the other gases present and a relative hypoxemia. Oxygen saturation decreases but can be prevented by the administration of 100 percent oxygen.[37]

Hepatic metabolism of the anesthetics is not a contributing factor during the maintenance of anesthesia. The high concentrations of drug present during anesthesia appear to saturate the hepatic microsomal enzymes responsible for metabolism, preventing metabolic breakdown. As the anesthetic concentration falls, metabolic breakdown then contributes to the recovery from anesthesia.[38] The impact of metabolism on recovery may be significant only with the anesthetic halothane, as this agent is more highly subject to hepatic metabolism than enflurane or isoflurane (see Table 25–1).

Nitrous Oxide Special Considerations

The low solubility of nitrous oxide is advantageous in the delivery, maintenance, and emergence from anesthesia; however, its low solubility is also responsible for the diffusion of nitrous oxide into hollow bodily cavities, for example, closed bowel loops and emphysematous bullae. The rapid diffusion of nitrous oxide can interfere with certain surgical procedures. Nitrous oxide should be discontinued in prolonged gastrointestinal surgery, during placement of a tympanic membrane graft, or in ophthalmologic procedures involving air–fluid exchanges in enclosed spaces. Nitrous oxide must also be discontinued when sudden air emboli occur as in neurosurgery and when pneumothorax is present or suspected. Diffusion of nitrous oxide into endotracheal tube cuffs can exert pressure on tracheal mucosa, resulting in local ischemia. Endotracheal tube cuff pressures should be routinely monitored during anesthesia.

PHARMACOLOGY OF INHALATIONAL AGENTS

Overview

History. Because of many disagreeable properties of commercially available anesthetics, including nausea and vomiting, flammability, and slow induction, the search for better and safer agents proliferated after World War II. The discovery that addition of a halogenated atom decreased flammability and increased potency led to the exploration of many chemical compounds for possible use in anesthesia. Halothane, enflurane, and isoflurane are in widespread use today.

Halothane was released in the United States in 1957, enflurane in 1972, and isoflurane in 1981. Other agents, such as ether and methoxyflurane, released during these years are virtually not used in current clinical practice. Present scientific investigations are screening newer inhalational agents (i.e., sevoflurane and desflurane) that may be available in the near future.

Physical Properties. The physical properties of the inhalational anesthetics are summarized in Table 25–1. Nitrous oxide is the most commonly used inhalational agent, either as a primary anesthetic or as an adjuvant to other anesthetic agents. Nitrous oxide is a colorless, odorless gas stored in liquid form in cylinders at 50 atm of pressure. The volatile anesthetics—halothane, enflurane, and isoflurane—are liquids at room temperature and are readily vaporized by passing a carrier gas, that is, oxygen, through the liquid. These agents are nonflammable and nonexplosive. Halothane is a halogenated hydrocarbon that differs from enflurane and isoflurane. The latter inhalational agents are isomers and possess an ether linkage. Sevoflurane and desflurane are experimental anesthetics. Sevoflurane is a liquid at room temperature, whereas desflurane is a gas at room temperature. Both agents have ether linkages. The molecular structures of these inhalational anesthetics are shown in Figure 25–1.

Preservatives. Halothane is the only inhalational anesthetic that contains a preservative. Addition of 0.01 percent thymol helps stabilize halothane and prevents its decomposition on exposure to light. A high concentration of thymol may coat the rotary valves on anesthesia vaporizers, causing stickiness, which may affect the accuracy of the halothane vaporizer.

Respiratory Effects

With the exception of nitrous oxide, all of the inhalational anesthetics are respiratory depressants as measured by arterial P_{CO_2} response during spontaneous ventilation in unstimulated volunteers (Fig. 25–4). Substitution of nitrous oxide for a portion of the anesthesia supplied by the other inhalational agents reduces their respiratory depressant effects.

Nitrous Oxide. The respiratory effects of 50 to 67 percent and even 1 MAC (110 percent) of nitrous oxide include a decrease in tidal volume with an increase in respiratory rate and minute ventilation, keeping Pa_{CO_2} normal. Although nitrous oxide causes minimal respiratory depression, it does predispose the patient to atelectasis in isolated alveoli because of its ease of absorption. Indeed, postoperative Pa_{O_2} is lower when nitrous oxide has been used.[39]

Halothane. Halothane produces less respiratory depression than isoflurane or enflurane. Tidal volume and minute ventilation are decreased whereas respiratory rate is increased at 1 MAC. This tachypnea is probably due to an increase in the discharge of pulmonary stretch receptors.[40]

Halothane does not stimulate secretions but does depress mucociliary flow in a dose-related fashion. Like enflurane and isoflurane, halothane is a bronchial smooth

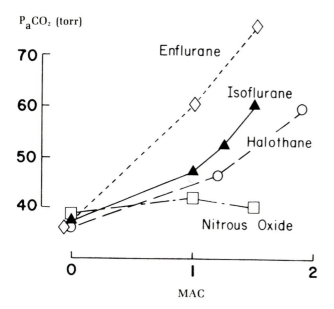

Figure 25–4. $Paco_2$ increases with all the anesthetic agents, but enflurane is the most potent respiratory depressant. Nitrous oxide causes minimal respiratory depression with a normal $Paco_2$. MAC, minimum alveolar concentration. (*Reprinted, with permission, from Eger El II. Isoflurane: A review. Anesthesiology. 1981;55:559.*)

muscle dilator. It is the most potent of the three inhalational agents in its ability to relax constricted airways. Halothane is often the choice for use in patients with asthma or chronic obstructive pulmonary disease.

Enflurane. Enflurane is the most potent respiratory depressant of all the inhalational agents (see Fig. 25–4). Unstimulated volunteers have a $Paco_2$ of 61 at 1 MAC and become apneic at 2 MAC.

Enflurane's pungent odor may stimulate secretions and limits the inspired concentration that can be given without eliciting coughing or laryngospasm. This characteristic limits its use for inhalation induction in children. Patients allowed to breathe spontaneously during enflurane anesthesia may elicit an occasional sigh from an unknown mechanism.

Isoflurane. Isoflurane depresses ventilation in a dose-related fashion, falling between enflurane and halothane in its respiratory depressant effects (see Fig. 25–4). Pulmonary compliance is slightly decreased at 1 MAC and returns to normal at 2 MAC. Isoflurane is also a bronchodilator and may be an alternative to halothane when halothane administration is not possible in an asthmatic patient.

Cardiovascular Effects

To varying degrees, all of the inhalational anesthetic agents are cardiovascular depressants, as measured by indices of stroke volume, cardiac output, mean arterial pressure, and myocardial contractility (Figs. 25–5 and 25–6). Substitution of nitrous oxide for an equivalent dose of a potent inhaled

anesthetic may decrease the cardiovascular depressant effect of that agent.

Nitrous Oxide. Contrary to long-held beliefs, nitrous oxide is a direct myocardial depressant. This cardiovascular depression is counterbalanced by the ability of nitrous oxide to increase sympathetic outflow from the brain and inhibit removal of norepinephrine by the lung. These actions together usually result in comparatively little cardiovascular depression at 1 MAC; however, addition of nitrous oxide to a narcotic anesthetic may depress cardiovascular function, exceeding the depression seen with nitrous oxide or the narcotic alone. The probable mechanism of action for this occurrence is the ability of narcotics to block sympathetic stimulation. Thus, the overall cardiovascular depressant effects of nitrous oxide must be evaluated in terms of resting sympathetic tone, presence of cardiopulmonary disease, and presence of other analgesic and anesthetic drugs.

Nitrous oxide causes a slight increase in pulmonary vascular resistance. This may be detrimental in patients with increased pulmonary blood flow and may result in increased ventilation/perfusion abnormalities and impaired oxygenation.

Halothane. Halothane is a direct myocardial depressant, decreasing all cardiovascular variables including cardiac output, stroke volume, and myocardial contractility by at least 20 percent at 1 MAC (see Figs. 25–5 and 25–6). This cardiovascular depression parallels the decrease in mean arterial pressure and is dose related. The elevation in mean right atrial pressure seen with halothane administration is due to a decrease in stroke volume.

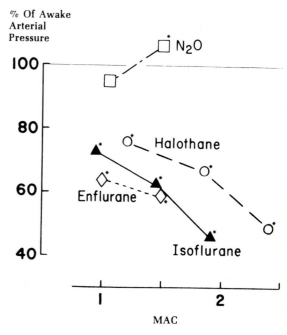

Figure 25–5. The anesthetic agents are cardiovascular depressants and thus cause a decrease in mean arterial blood pressure in anesthetized, normocapnic volunteers. MAC, minimal alveolar concentration. (*Reprinted, with permission, from Eger El II. Isoflurane: A review. Anesthesiology. 1981;55:559.*)

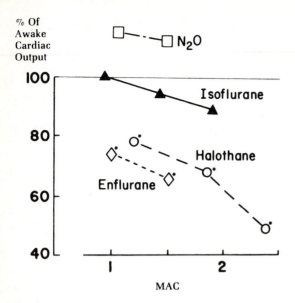

Figure 25–6. The anesthetic agents produce a decrease in cardiac output in anesthetized, normocapnic volunteers. MAC, minimum alveolar concentration. (*Reprinted, with permission, from Eger El II. Isoflurane: A review.* Anesthesiology. *1981;55:559.*)

Halothane is unique in its sensitization of the myocardium to catecholamines, producing premature ventricular contractions. The amount of epinephrine that can be administered to a patient anesthetized with halothane is limited to 1 to 3 µg/kg over 10 minutes, but this may be repeated up to three times in 1 hour.[41]

Halothane causes depression of sympathetic nervous system outflow and may decrease conduction time in atrioventricular nodal pathways.

Enflurane. Enflurane is the most potent myocardial depressant of the inhalational agents (see Figs. 25–5 and 25–6). Depression of cardiovascular variables is proportional to its anesthetic concentration. The mechanism of action for the direct myocardial depressant effects of enflurane may be a reduction in free calcium ion concentration or an alteration in the sensitivity of contractile proteins to available calcium.[42]

Enflurane decreases systemic vascular resistance to a greater extent than halothane but to a much smaller extent than isoflurane. Enflurane provides a stable heart rhythm and allows for greater than twice the dose of injectable epinephrine as halothane.

Isoflurane. Isoflurane depresses the contractility of isolated cardiac muscle, though this depression is significantly less in vivo. In volunteers, myocardial contractility and cardiac output are only mildly affected by 1 to 1.8 MAC of isoflurane (see Fig. 25–6).

Isoflurane produces a large decrease in systemic vascular resistance and has a tendency to cause an increase in heart rate. This increase in heart rate may be the result of a greater depression in vagal activity than in beta sympathetic activity.[43] Isoflurane provides a stable cardiac rhythm and does not sensitize the heart to catecholamines. Admin-

istration of 7 to 10 µg/kg epinephrine will not result in cardiac arrhythmias.

Much controversy surrounds the actions of isoflurane on the coronary vasculature. Isoflurane in the dog model dilates small coronary resistance vessels. In patients with coronary artery disease, this action may potentially divert blood flow away from collateral dependent areas of borderline perfusion toward areas that are already adequately perfused. This coronary steal phenomenon has been extensively investigated since Reiz et al[44] reported that almost one half of their study patients exhibited evidence of inadequate coronary perfusion (ischemic electrocardiographic changes) when anesthetized with isoflurane and nitrous oxide.[44] This is more pronounced in patients with reduced systemic vascular resistance (SVR). Subsequent researchers have failed to encounter as high an incidence of myocardial ischemia[45,46] but have demonstrated isoflurane's capacity to cause coronary steal. Patients at high risk for isoflurane-induced ischemia are those with multivessel coronary artery disease.[47] The safest course at present appears to be the avoidance of isoflurane in these patients or the use of less than 5 percent isoflurane with narcotic supplementation. These recommendations await further support from future scientific investigations.

Central Nervous System Effects

Nitrous Oxide. Changes in the central nervous system (CNS) with administration of nitrous oxide are often inconsistent and probably reflect the limited potency and the need for nitrous oxide to be combined with other anesthetic agents. Fifty to seventy-five percent nitrous oxide appears to dilate cerebral blood vessels and cause an increase in intracranial pressure. These changes may be decreased or prevented by hyperventilation and administration of barbiturates.[48] Unlike the other inhalational anesthetics, nitrous oxide does not protect the brain by decreasing cerebral oxygen consumption.

Nitrous oxide also has variable effects on the electroencephalogram (EEG). At 30 percent nitrous oxide, there is an increase in EEG frequency with lower voltage, and at higher nitrous oxide concentrations an increase in voltage is observed. Somatosensory evoked potentials remain essentially unchanged with nitrous oxide.

Halothane. Halothane is the most potent cerebral vasodilator of all the inhalational agents. Cerebral blood flow increases dramatically with 0.6 to 1.6 MAC of halothane and increases almost 200 percent at 2 MAC (Fig. 25–7). This drastic cerebral blood flow increase and, hence, increase in intracranial pressure can be prevented or greatly attenuated by hyperventilation and the establishment of hypocapnia prior to halothane administration.

Enflurane. Enflurane also causes cerebral vasodilation, although less than 50 percent of the amount produced by halothane (see Fig. 25–7). Cerebral blood flow is increased while cerebral metabolic rate is decreased. Enflurane is unique in its ability to promote epileptogenic activity in the anesthetized patient. An increase in the depth of anesthesia

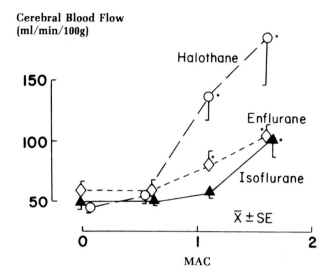

Figure 25–7. Cerebral blood flow increases during halothane, enflurane, and isoflurane anesthesia. Systemic blood pressure and Paco$_2$ were held at normal levels. MAC, minimum alveolar concentration. (*Reprinted, with permission, from Eger El II. Isoflurane [Forane]: A compendium and reference. 2nd ed. Madison, WI: Anaquest, BOC; 1985.*)

with greater than 1.5 MAC of enflurane is accompanied by the appearance of slow EEG waves with increased voltage, progressing to burst suppression at 3 percent. These EEG effects are more pronounced in the presence of hypocapnia. As seizure activity can greatly increase cerebral metabolism, the use of enflurane in high doses and in combination with a decreased Paco$_2$ should be avoided in patients with seizure disorders or occlusive cerebrovascular disease.

Isoflurane. Isoflurane produces the least cerebral vasodilation of the inhalational agents (see Fig. 25–7). One MAC of isoflurane produces only small increases in cerebral blood flow. Isoflurane can cause EEG spiking but is not associated with the epileptogenic activity produced by enflurane. It is currently favored as the inhalation agent of choice for neurosurgical procedures.

Neuromuscular Effects

Nitrous Oxide. Nitrous oxide may increase skeletal muscle activity and can be associated with rigidity and increased muscle tone when combined with narcotics. The precise mechanism for this skeletal activity enhancement has not been established. Nitrous oxide appears to have minimal effect on the neuromuscular block produced by nondepolarizing muscle relaxants.

Halothane, Enflurane, and Isoflurane. These inhalational agents potentiate the neuromuscular block produced by nondepolarizing muscle relaxants. Isoflurane produces the most potentiation, followed by enflurane and halothane, in a dose-dependent fashion (Fig. 25–8). Probable mechanisms of action for this augmentation are a decrease in the respon-

siveness of the motor endplate to acetylcholine and a rise in the threshold for depolarization.[49] There is minimal alteration of blockade when the inhalational agents are used with the depolarizing muscle relaxant succinylcholine.

Renal Effects

The effects of the inhalational anesthetics on the kidney result from their effects on the renal circulation. Renal blood flow, glomerular filtration rate, and urinary flow rate are decreased as a result of the reduction in cardiac output or arterial pressure or the increase in renal vascular resistance. There is no histologic evidence of renal injury in animals after prolonged administration of halothane or isoflurane[43]; however, patients with preexisting renal dysfunction may experience a transient increase in renal impairment after enflurane administration. This topic is discussed further under Metabolism of Inhalational Agents.

Hepatic Effects

Hepatic dysfunction and histologic changes following the administration of enflurane and isoflurane are rare; however, all anesthetic agents that decrease cardiac output produce a proportional reduction in total hepatic blood flow. Isoflurane has been shown to increase hepatic artery blood flow at 1 and 2 MAC.[50]

Halothane is distinct from the other inhalational agents in that it actually may decrease hepatic flow to a greater extent by increasing hepatic arterial resistance.[51] Halothane-associated hepatic dysfunction has an incidence of 1 in 35,000 and may be caused by hypoxic liver injury from reduced blood flow or may reflect a genetic predisposition, allergic reaction, or immunologically mediated injury. Clinical recommendations include avoidance of halothane in patients with preexisting liver dysfunction, in patients undergoing liver or biliary surgeries, in adult patients in whom halothane has been used within the preceding 6 months.

Metabolism of Inhalational Agents

Nitrous Oxide. Nitrous oxide is not metabolized in the liver. Anaerobic bacteria in human intestinal contents metabolize nitrous oxide through a reductive pathway, forming free radicals that can produce toxic lipids.[48] Yet, only 0.004 ± 0.005 percent of the nitrous oxide may be metabolized, and this amount is reduced when antibiotics are given. The clinical importance of this metabolic pathway is unclear at present.

Halothane. Fifteen to twenty percent of inhaled halothane may be metabolized by oxidative and reductive metabolism to trifluoroacetic acid (TFA), Cl$^-$, F$^-$, Br$^-$, and other volatile metabolites detectable in urine or exhaled air.[52] Patients taking drugs known to induce cytochrome P450 activity of liver microsomes (i.e., phenobarbital) tend to metabolize halothane at a higher-than-normal rate.

Enflurane. Metabolism of enflurane occurs in the liver, and the metabolites, 2.4 to 9 percent of absorbed enflurane, are

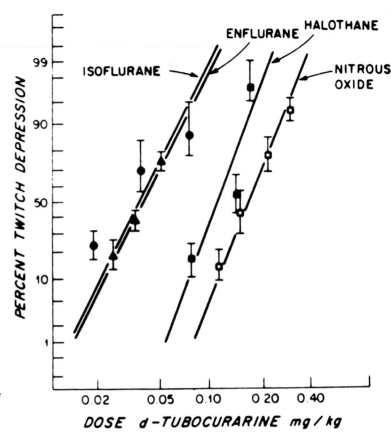

Figure 25–8. The anesthetic agents halothane, enflurane, and isoflurane potentiate the neuromuscular block produced by D-tubocurarine. (*Reprinted, with permission, from Ali HH, Savarese JJ. Monitoring of neuromuscular function.* Anesthesiology. *1976;45: 216.*)

excreted in the urine. Equal amounts of organic and inorganic fluoride ions are excreted. Peak serum fluoride levels depend on the number of MAC hours and the concentration of enflurane administered. Peak levels occur 4 to 12 hours after anesthesia and may cause temporary renal dysfunction. Clinical recommendations are to avoid use of enflurane in patients with known renal disease.

Isoflurane. Minimal oxidative metabolism of isoflurane results in the formation of TFA and F⁻. Less than 0.2% of isoflurane is metabolized, and this amount is insufficient to cause any effects on renal function and other organ systems of the body.[53]

Miscellaneous Effects

Nitrous Oxide. Nitrous oxide may not be the benign agent it was once thought to be. In addition to the previously discussed effects on the myocardium, cerebrum, and skeletal muscle, nitrous oxide is known to inactivate a component of methionine synthetase, an enzyme involved in the metabolism of folate.[54] This inactivation can impair DNA synthesis and produce a condition similar to vitamin B_{12} deficiency. This enzyme inactivation has been shown to occur after prolonged exposure to nitrous oxide inhalation (> 24 hours in normal patients and shorter periods in ill patients).[55] Very recent investigations have, however, failed to show a clinically relevant effect of nitrous oxide on folate and vitamin B_{12} metabolism.[56,57]

No teratogenic, carcinogenic, and mutagenic effects of

nitrous oxide have been reported in the scientific literature. The most consistent finding is an increased incidence of spontaneous abortion among women exposed to waste anesthetic gases, specifically nitrous oxide.[58]

Conflicting reports also exist concerning the relationship between nitrous oxide and the incidence of postoperative nausea and vomiting.[59–61] Nitrous oxide may cause nausea and vomiting because its diffusion into the gastrointestinal tract is faster than the outward diffusion of nitrogen, leading to bowel distention, or the nausea and vomiting may result from an interaction with endogenous opioid receptors. Many other factors, including postoperative pain, perioperative narcotics, and variations in surgical site and technique, may obscure the influence of nitrous oxide on nausea and vomiting. Patient age, gender, and a history of prior postoperative nausea and vomiting may be more important determinants in predicting the incidence of nausea and vomiting after surgery.

Halothane, Enflurane, and Isoflurane. Halothane, enflurane, and isoflurane produce similar dose-related depressions in uterine tone and contractility and a decrease in the uterine response to oxytocic agents by relaxation of uterine smooth muscle. These agents must be used cautiously in patients undergoing therapeutic abortion and dilation and curettage.

The effects of the inhalational anesthetics on various biochemical processes have been examined. Halothane, enflurane, and isoflurane have been shown to inhibit the secretion of epinephrine and norepinephrine from bovine adrenal chromaffin cells.[62] This action can lead to depression of excitatory synaptic transmission, which may account for the general anesthetic effects of these agents. The inhalational agents do not cause release of antidiuretic hormone (ADH). Radioimmunoassay techniques for ADH measurement show that an increase in ADH and, ultimately, a decrease in urine output are due to a secondary stress response that can be attenuated with deeper levels of anesthesia and positive-pressure ventilation for long periods.[63]

Significant decreases in body temperature are frequently recorded during general anesthesia. Thermal stresses are associated with low ambient temperatures in the operating room, cold intravenous and irrigation fluids, dry anesthetic gases, and exposure of body surfaces and viscera.[64] In addition, general anesthetics inhibit normal thermoregulatory responses.[65] In an anesthetized patient, hypothermia results in intense peripheral vasoconstriction. The most effective means of minimizing heat loss are covering exposed body parts, using a warming mattress and placing a heated humidifier in the anesthetic circuitry.

Several reports in the literature[66–68] describe patient recall or awareness under general anesthesia. Recall can occur when either inhalational or intravenous anesthetics are used. The auditory pathway is very active within the central nervous system and recall of conversations and operating room sounds is most commonly described. Pain sensations are also reported yet clinical signs of light anesthesia, such as changes in blood pressure or heart rate, are not correlated with recall.

Recall under general anesthesia can result in emotional trauma; therefore, the prevention of recall is important. Rigid protocols for the delivery of anesthesia are not feasible as individual patients' needs can vary significantly. Premedication with benzodiazepines may decrease the likelihood of recall. Extraneous noise and conversation within the operating room should be minimized. If recall does occur, an honest explanation of the incident should be given along with a referral for follow-up care.

New Agents

Sevoflurane. Sevoflurane, first detailed in 1971, is an experimental inhalational anesthetic. It has recently been released for clinical use in Japan. Sevoflurane's low blood:gas partition coefficient, 0.68, is an attractive feature for the rapid induction of and emergence from general anesthesia. At 1.1 MAC, sevoflurane produces almost the same amount of respiratory depression as seen with halothane.[69] Its cardiovascular depression capabilities parallel those effects seen with isoflurane; however, at 1.2 MAC heart rate may be increased to a degree even greater than that observed with isoflurane.[70] Sevoflurane does not sensitize the myocardium to the arrhythmic effects of catecholamines.[71]

Sevoflurane undergoes some hydrolytic degradation in the presence of soda lime. The biologic significance of this small amount of reaction products is unknown. More importantly, approximately 1.5 to 2 percent of sevoflurane is metabolized to free fluoride ions. Peak serum fluoride ion concentration 1 hour after administration of 1 to 1.5 MAC of sevoflurane is roughly comparable to that produced by enflurane.[72]

Desflurane (I-653). Desflurane is the newest of the experimental inhalational agents currently undergoing extensive scientific investigations. It is a gas at room temperature. Desflurane has an even lower blood:gas partition coefficient than sevoflurane, 0.42, indicating shorter induction and emergence times. Desflurane strongly resists biodegradation in the presence of soda lime, exhibiting greater stability than any current inhalational agent.[73] It is relatively free of hepatotoxic, pneumotoxic, and nephrotoxic effects in enzyme-induced hypoxic rats.[74]

Desflurane is minimally biotransformed in various animal species. Serum fluoride ion concentrations 4 hours after termination of desflurane anesthesia are much lower than those found with isoflurane.[75]

The cardiovascular depressant properties of desflurane are similar to those of isoflurane. Systemic vascular resistance and mean arterial pressure are depressed at 0.8, 1.2, and 1.6 MAC and are accompanied by small increases in heart rate.[76] More human subject studies need to be carried out to verify these animal data. Presently, desflurane appears to have safe cardiovascular actions at clinical anesthetic concentrations.

REFERENCES

1. Henderson JM, Brodsky DA, Fisher DM, Brett CM, Hertzka RE. Pre-induction of anesthesia in pediatric patients with nasally administered sufentanil. *Anesthesiology.* 1988;68:671–675.
2. Aldrete JA, Roman-de-Jesus JC, Russell LJ, D'Cruz O. Intranasal ketamine as induction adjunct in children: Preliminary report. *Anesthesiology.* 1987;67:A514. Abstract.
3. Sinclair R, Cassuto J, Hogstrom S, et al. Topical anesthesia with lidocaine aerosol in the control of postoperative pain. *Anesthesiology.* 1988;68:895–901.
4. Mock DL, Streisand JB, Hague B, Dzelzkalns RR, Bailey PL, et al. Transmucosal narcotic delivery: An evaluation of fentanyl (lollipop) premedication in man. *Anesth Analg.* 1986;65:S102. Abstract.
5. Smith EL, Hill RL, Lehman IR, et al. *Principles of biochemistry.* 7th ed. New York: McGraw-Hill; 1983:289–315.
6. Winter ME, Katcher BS, Koda-Kimble MA. *Basic clinical pharmacokinetics.* Spokane, WA: Applied Therapeutics; 1980:5–67.
7. Wood M. Plasma drug binding: Implications for anesthesiologists. *Anesth Analg.* 1986;65:786–804.
8. Pardridge WM. Recent advances in blood brain barrier transport. *Annu Rev Pharmacol Toxicol.* 1988;28:25–39.
9. Kanto J. Obstetric analgesia: Clinical pharmacokinetic considerations. *Clin Pharmacokin.* 1986;11:283–298.
10. Rall TW. Hypnotics and sedatives: Ethanol. In: Gilman AG, Rall TW, Nies AS, Taylor P, eds. *The pharmacological basis of therapeutics.* 8th ed. New York: Pergamon Press; 1990:345–382.
11. Gram TE. Metabolism of drugs. In: Craig CR, Stitzel RE, eds. *Modern pharmacology.* 2nd ed. St. Louis, MO: Little, Brown; 1986:41–64.
12. Brunton LL. Drugs affecting gastrointestinal function. In: Gilman AG, Rall TW, Nies AS, Taylor P, eds. *The pharmacologic basis of therapeutics.* 8th ed. New York: Pergamon Press; 1990:897–913.
13. Stitzel R. Excretion of drugs. In: Craig CR, Stitzel RE, eds. *Modern pharmacology.* 2nd ed. St. Louis, MO: Little, Brown; 1986:65–74.
14. Levine RR. *Pharmacology: Drug actions and reactions.* 3rd ed. Boston: Little, Brown; 1983:211–247.
15. Richter JJ. Current theories about the mechanisms of benzodiazepines and neuroleptic drugs. *Anesthesiology.* 1981;54:66–72.

16. Olsen RW, Stauber GB, King RG, Yang J, Dilber A. Structure and function of the barbiturate-modulated benzodiazepine/GABA receptor protein complex. In: Biggio G, Costa E, eds. *GABAergic transmission and anxiety.* New York: Raven Press; 1986:21–49.

17. Kenakin TP. The classification of drugs and drug receptors in isolated tissues. *Pharmacol Rev.* 1984;36:165–222.

18. Judge SE. Effect of general anaesthetics on synaptic ion channels. *Br J Anaesth.* 1983;55:191–200.

19. Miller KW, Paton WD, Smith RA, Smith EB. The pressure reversal of general anesthesia and the critical volume hypothesis. *Mol Pharmacol.* 1973;9:131–143.

20. Cheng SC, Brunner EA. A neurochemical hypothesis for halothane anesthesia. *Anesth Analg.* 1975;54:242–246.

21. Cheng SC, Brunner EA. Inducing anesthesia with a GABA analog, THIP. *Anesthesiology.* 1985;63:147–151.

22. Cheng SC, Brunner EA. Anesthetic effects on GABA binding. *Anesthesiology.* 1984;61:A326. Abstract.

23. Fontenot HJ, Wilson RD, Norris JC, Ho IK. The GABA system: New evidence of neurotransmitter involvement in the mechanism of anesthesia. *Anesthesiology.* 1984;61:A327.

24. Nakahiro M, Yeh JZ, Brunner E, Narahashi T. General anesthetics modulate GABA receptor channel complex in rat dorsal root ganglion neurons. *FASEB J.* 1989;3:1850–1854.

25. Nicoll RA, Madison DV. General anesthetics hyperpolarize neurons in the vertebrate central nervous system. *Science.* 1982;217:1055–1057.

26. Franks NP, Lieb WR. Volatile general anesthetics activate a novel neuronal K$^+$ current. *Nature.* 1988;333:662–664.

27. Eger EI. *Anesthetic uptake and action.* Baltimore: Williams & Wilkins; 1974.

28. Licina MG, Schubert A, Tobin J, et al. Intrathecal morphine does not reduce the MAC of halothane in humans: Results of a double blind study. *Anesthesiology.* 1988;69:A643.

29. Drasner K, Bernards C, Ozanne GM. Intrathecal morphine reduces the minimal alveolar concentration of halothane in man. *Anesth Analg.* 1988;67:S52.

30. Valverde A, Dyson DH, McDonnell WN. Epidural morphine reduces halothane MAC in the dog. *Can J Anesth.* 1989;36:629–633.

31. Stoelting RK, Miller RD. *Basics of anesthesia,* 2nd ed. New York: Churchill Livingstone; 1989:9–23.

32. Dale O, Brown BR. Clinical pharmacokinetics of the inhalational anesthetics. *Clin Pharmacokinet.* 1987;12:145–167.

33. Epstein RM, Rackow H, Salanitre E, Wolf GL. Influence of the concentration effect on the uptake of anesthetic mixtures: The second gas effect. *Anesthesiology.* 1964;25:364–371.

34. Eger EI. Uptake and distribution. In: Miller RD, ed. *Anesthesia.* 3rd ed. New York: Churchill Livingstone; 1990:85–104.

35. Eger EI, Severinghaus JW. Effect of uneven pulmonary distribution of blood and gas on induction with inhalation anesthetics. *Anesthesiology.* 1964;25:620–626.

36. Eger EI, Johnson BH. Rates of awakening from anesthesia with I-653, halothane, isoflurane, and sevoflurane. *Anesth Analg.* 1987;66:977–982.

37. Brodsky JB, McKlveen RE, Zelcer J, Margary JJ. Diffusion hypoxia: A reappraisal using pulse oximetry. *J Clin Monit.* 1988;4:244–246.

38. Sawyer DC, Eger EI, Bahlman SH, Cullen BF, Impelman D. Concentration dependence of hepatic halothane metabolism. *Anesthesiology.* 1971;34:230–234.

39. Gawley TF, Dundee JW. Attempts to reduce respiratory complications following upper abdominal operations. *Br J Anaesth.* 1981;53:1073–1078.

40. Eger EI II. Respiratory effects of nitrous oxide. In: Eger EI II, ed. *Nitrous oxide.* New York: Elsevier Science; 1985:111.

41. Katz RL, Bigger JT. Cardiac arrhythmias during anesthesia and operation. *Anesthesiology.* 1970;33:193–213.

42. Pavlin EG, Su JY. Cardiopulmonary pharmacology. In: Miller RD, ed. *Anesthesia.* 3rd ed. New York: Churchill Livingstone; 1990:127.

43. Eger EI II. The pharmacology of isoflurane. *Br J Anaesth.* 1984;56(suppl):71–99.

44. Reiz S, Balfors E, Sorensen MB, Ariola S, Friedman A, Truedsson H. Isoflurane: A powerful coronary vasodilator in patients with coronary artery disease. *Anesthesiology.* 1983;59:91–97.

45. Hess W, Arnold B, Schulte-Sasse U, Tarnow J. Comparison of isoflurane and halothane when used to control intraoperative hypertension in patients undergoing coronary artery bypass surgery. *Anesth Analg.* 1983;62:15–20.

46. Moffitt EA, Barker RA, Glenn JJ, et al. Myocardial metabolism and hemodynamic responses with isoflurane anesthesia for coronary artery surgery. *Anesth Analg.* 1986;65:53–61.

47. Becker LC. Is isoflurane dangerous for the patient with coronary artery disease? *Anesthesiology.* 1987;66:259–261.

48. Frost EAM. Central nervous system effects of nitrous oxide. In: Eger EI II, ed. *Nitrous oxide.* New York: Elsevier Science Publishing; 1985:157–176.

49. Viby-Mogensen J. Interaction of other drugs with muscle relaxants. In: Katz RL, ed. *Muscle relaxants: Basic and clinical aspects.* Orlando, FL: Grune & Stratton; 1985:249.

50. Gelman S, Fowler KC, Smith LR. Liver circulation and function during isoflurane and halothane anesthesia. *Anesthesiology.* 1984;61:726–730.

51. Thulin L, Andreen M, Irestedt L. Effect of controlled halothane anesthesia on splanchnic blood flow and cardiac output in the dog. *Acta Anaesthesiol Scand.* 1975;19:146–153.

52. Sharp TH, Trudell JR, Cohen EN. Volatile metabolites and decomposition products of halothane in man. *Anesthesiology.* 1979;50:2–8.

53. Holaday DA, Fiserova-Bergerova V, Latto IP, Zumbiel MA. Resistance of isoflurane to biotransformation in man. *Anesthesiology.* 1975;43:325–332.

54. Koblin DD, Waskell L, Watson JE, Stokstad ELR, Eger EI II. Nitrous oxide inactivates methionine synthetase in human liver. *Anesth Analg.* 1982;61:75–78.

55. Skacel PO, Hewlett AM, Lewis JD, Lumb M, Nunn JF, Chanarin I. Studies on the haemopoietic toxicity of nitrous oxide in man. *Br J Haematol.* 1983;53:189–200.

56. Koblin DD, Tomerson MS, Waldman FM, Lampe GH, Wauk LZ, Eger EI II. Effect of nitrous oxide on folate and vitamin B$_{12}$ metabolism in patients. *Anesth Analg.* 1990;71:610–617.

57. Waldman FM, Koblin DD, Lampe GH, Wauk LZ, Eger EI II. Hematologic effects of nitrous oxide in surgical patients. *Anesth Analg.* 1990;71:618–624.

58. Colton T. Report to the ASA Annual General Meeting. New Orleans, 1981.

59. Melnick BM, Johnson LS. Effects of eliminating nitrous oxide in outpatient anesthesia. *Anesthesiology.* 1987;67:982–984.

60. Korttila K, Hovorka J, Erkola O. Nitrous oxide does not increase the incidence of nausea and vomiting after isoflurane anesthesia. *Anesth Analg.* 1987;66:761–765.

61. Eger EI II, Lampe GH, Wauk LZ, Whitendale P, Calahan MK, Donegan JH. Clinical pharmacology of nitrous oxide: An argument for its continued use. *Anesth Analg.* 1990;71:575–585.

62. Pocock G, Richards CD. The action of volatile anesthetics on stimulus–secretion coupling in bovine adrenal chromaffin cells. *Br J Pharmacol.* 1988;95:209–217.

63. Mazze RI, Cousins MJ. Renal diseases. In: Katz J, Benumof J, Kadis LB, eds., Anesthesia and Uncommon Diseases, 2nd ed. Philadelphia, PA: WB Saunders Co., 1981:464.

64. Imrie MM, Hall GM. Body temperature and anaesthesia. *Br J Anaesth*. 1990;64:346–354.

65. Sessler DI, McGuire J, Moayeri A, Hynson J. Isoflurane-induced vasodilation minimally increases cutaneous heat loss. *Anesthesiology*. 1991;74:226–232.

66. Wilson SL, Vaughan RW, Stephen CR. Awareness, dreams, and hallucinations associated with general anesthesia. *Anesth Analg*. 1975;54:609–617.

67. Dosch MR. On being aware: Patient recall of intraoperative events. *AANA J*. 1988;56:238–245.

68. Lyons G, Macdonald R. Awareness during cesarean section. *Anaesthesia*. 1991;46:62–64.

69. Doi M, Kazuyuki I. Respiratory effects of sevoflurane. *Anesth Analg*. 1987;66:241–244.

70. Bernard JM, Wouters PF, Doursout MF, Florence B, Chelly JE, Merin RG. Effects of sevoflurane and isoflurane on cardiac and coronary dynamics in chronically instrumented dogs. *Anesthesiology*. 1990;72:659–662.

71. Wallin RF, Regan BM, Napoli MD, Stern IJ. Sevoflurane: A new inhalational anesthetic agent. *Anesth Analg*. 1975;54:758–765.

72. Holaday DA, Smith FR. Clinical characteristics and biotransformation of sevoflurane in healthy human volunteers. *Anesthesiology*. 1981;54:100–106.

73. Eger EI II. Solubility of I-653 in soda lime. *Anesth Analg*. 1987;66:983–985.

74. Eger EI, Johnson BH, Strum DP, Ferell LD. Studies of the toxicity of I-653, halothane and isoflurane in enzyme-induced hypoxic rats. *Anesth Analg*. 1987;66:1227–1229.

75. Koblin DD, Weiskopf RB, Holmes MA, et al. Metabolism of I-653 and isoflurane in swine. *Anesth Analg*. 1989;68:147–149.

76. Weiskopf RB, Holmes MA, Eger EI II, Johnson BH, Rampil IJ, Brown JG. Cardiovascular effects of I-653 in swine. *Anesthesiology*. 1988;69:303–309.

Pharmacology of Intravenous Anesthetics and Adjuncts

Doris J. Tanaka

The most efficient and most commonly used routes of administration of anesthetics are the inhalation and intravenous routes. This chapter reviews the pharmacokinetics and pharmacology involved in the actions of intravenously administered drugs. Pharmacokinetics describes the fate of drugs in the body, including the processes of absorption from sites, distribution to body tissues and fluids, biotransformation, and excretion from the body. A knowledge of the pharmacokinetics of a drug can be used to control the intensity and duration of its action and to understand the variable responses of individuals to the drug.

PHARMACOKINETICS OF INTRAVENOUSLY ADMINISTERED DRUGS

Absorption

Intravenously administered drugs bypass the absorption phase and therefore have an onset and intensity of action more rapid and more predictable compared with drugs administered by other routes.

Distribution

After intravenous injection, a dilution occurs because the drug mixes with the blood volume. An injected drug is mixed within 30 seconds and is distributed almost immediately. The blood plasma is the medium in which drugs are distributed and transported to their sites of action. The concentration of drug delivered to these sites is therefore proportional to its concentration in the plasma.

The rate of tissue uptake of the intravenously administered drugs is determined by the rate of drug delivery to the tissue (cardiac output or blood flow) as well as the ability of the drug to enter the tissue (permeability). For those drugs that are able to pass rapidly through cell membranes, permeability can be the rate-limiting factor.[1]

Variables that affect drug permeability are (1) lipid solubility, (2) ionization, (3) molecular size, and (4) protein binding. Lipid solubility is probably the most important property. The greater the lipid solubility, the more quickly a drug will penetrate the biologic membranes. Ionization of a drug will limit permeability by reducing its lipid solubility and also by causing it to be repelled by similarly charged parts of the membrane or attracted and bound by oppositely charged portions of the membrane. Ionization affects entry into cell membranes but does not seem to affect diffusion across capillary membranes. Molecular size affects penetration of the membrane via pores. Most intravenously administered anesthetic drugs are small enough to pass through the pores of vascular capillary membranes but are too large to penetrate the pores of cellular membranes.[2]

Protein-bound drugs cannot cross capillary or cellular membranes because of the nature of protein. Proteins are large molecules, are ionized, and have low lipid solubility. Protein binding also reduces tissue uptake by reducing the concentration of diffusable, free drug in the plasma. Only the unbound, free drug is able to reach the site of action.

Changes occurring in blood volume, cardiac output, and distribution of blood flow alter the distribution and concentration of the drug. A decrease in blood volume decreases dilution and results in an increased blood concentration of the drug. A lowered blood volume also alters distribution of blood flow, decreasing blood flow to skin and muscle while preserving perfusion to the vital organs. Consequently, a greater portion of the administered drug reaches the brain and heart, which may cause an increase in both central nervous system and cardiac depression. Febrile state, apprehension, and sympathetic stimulation results in increased cardiac output and, subsequently, increased skin and muscle blood flow, which divert the drug from the brain and may result in a lighter-than-expected level of anesthesia.

Organs receiving a higher percentage of the cardiac output initially receive the bulk of the active drug. The normal distribution of blood flow to various organs is outlined in Table 26–1. Each group is differentiated from the others on the basis of the volume of blood flow to the tissues and the tissue:blood partition coefficient. The rate at which each tissue equilibrates with the drug depends on the capacity of

TABLE 26–1. DISTRIBUTION OF BLOOD VOLUME TO VARIOUS ORGANS AND TISSUES

Organs/Tissues	Body Weight (%)	Cardiac Output (%)
Vessel-rich group (70–75% of cardiac output)		
Brain	2.0	14
Heart	0.5	5
Liver	4.0	28
Kidney	0.5	23
Total	7.0	70
Intermediate group		
Skeletal muscle	49	15
Skin	6	8
Total	55	23
Fat group	19	6
Vessel-poor group (ligaments, tendons, bone)	19	1

the tissue for the drug (volume of tissue multiplied by tissue:blood partition coefficient) relative to the tissue perfusion.

Because of its high blood flow, the vessel-rich group of tissues initially receives the major portion of the drug. As the drug penetrates the vessel-rich group, the plasma concentration of the drug declines, and the partial pressure of the drug in the vessel-rich group exceeds that in the plasma now coming to it. The drug then reenters the blood and accumulates in fat and muscle at a rate dependent on solubility, tissue volume, and blood flow.

Biotransformation

Biotransformation of a drug to its metabolites usually terminates its action; however, this is not always true. Drug metabolites may be "active" or "inactive." The active metabolites may be more or less potent than the parent drug, and it is also possible for the metabolite to possess similar or dissimilar actions. The rate of biotransformation of most drugs is determined by the concentrations of the drug at the site of metabolism. This is dependent on the concentration in the plasma as well as the volume of blood flow to the liver. Biotransformation of some drugs can occur to a small extent in the brain, kidneys, and other tissues as well. Other factors that determine the rate of biotransformation are the numerous variables that affect enzyme activity, the particular chemical means by which the enzymes metabolize the individual drug, and the genetic, nutritional, physiologic, and pharmacologic status of the body.

Elimination

The kidneys and gastrointestinal tract are the major routes of drug excretion for intravenously administered drugs. Drugs may be excreted either in the unchanged form or after biotransformation. The rate of renal excretion of drugs is determined by glomerular filtration, tubular secretion, and tubular reabsorption.

Glomerular filtration depends on molecular weight, the

plasma concentration of the unbound drug, and the volume of glomerular filtrate.

Tubular secretion involves a selective active transport mechanism that removes drugs from the renal tubular plasma. The process is selective for certain drugs and metabolites and can affect free as well as protein-bound forms of the drugs.

Tubular reabsorption removes from the renal tubules drugs that entered by glomerular filtration and tubular secretion. The ability of a drug to be reabsorbed is determined by its ability to penetrate cellular membranes. Some drugs are reabsorbed very easily and therefore only small amounts of the unchanged drugs are lost in the urine. Biotransformation frequently produces more polar metabolites, which have less ability to penetrate the cell membranes, and therefore results in less tubular reabsorption and greater excretion in the urine. The rate of reabsorption may be altered by the degree of ionization, rate of tubular urine flow, and pH of the urine.[1]

Intestinal excretion of drugs usually occurs to a much lesser extent than renal excretion. The biliary system acts as a transport mechanism for the intestinal excretion of drugs. The same factors that determine drugs' rate of absorption and ability to be absorbed from the gastrointestinal tract also affect the elimination of drugs and their metabolites via the biliary system. Specialized transport mechanisms resemble those of the renal system.

BARBITURATES

Barbiturates are the most popular anesthetic induction agents in use today. Historically the first successfully and extensively used intravenous anesthetic was a barbiturate known as hexobarbital introduced in 1932. Hexobarbital remained popular until the introduction of thiopental in 1934. Thiopental still remains the most widely used of all intravenous anesthetics. Intravenous methohexital, introduced in 1956, has been the only serious rival to thiopental. Thiamylal has limited popularity in the United States but has not been a serious challenge to thiopental. Clinically, thiopental and thiamylal are very similar in action and their effects are almost indistinguishable. Methohexital is two to three times more potent than thiopental but has a shorter duration of action and rate of metabolism.

Thiopental and methohexital are probably the two most commonly used intravenous agents in anesthesia practice. Both drugs have been traditionally classified among the "ultrashort-acting" barbiturates. The classic grouping of barbiturates into long-, intermediate-, short-, and ultrashort-acting drugs is misleading. It is now known that the elimination half-lives do not coincide with the apparent duration of action[3]; however, a more accurate classification has not yet been universally adopted.

Chemistry. The term *barbiturate* refers to any derivative of barbituric acid. Barbituric acid, 2,4,6-trioxohexahydropyrimidine, is formed by the condensation of malonic acid with urea. Barbituric acid itself lacks central depressant activity. Barbiturates are formed by certain substitutions made on the parent molecule of barbituric acid (Fig. 26–1).[3]

There are three chemical groups of barbiturates of clini-

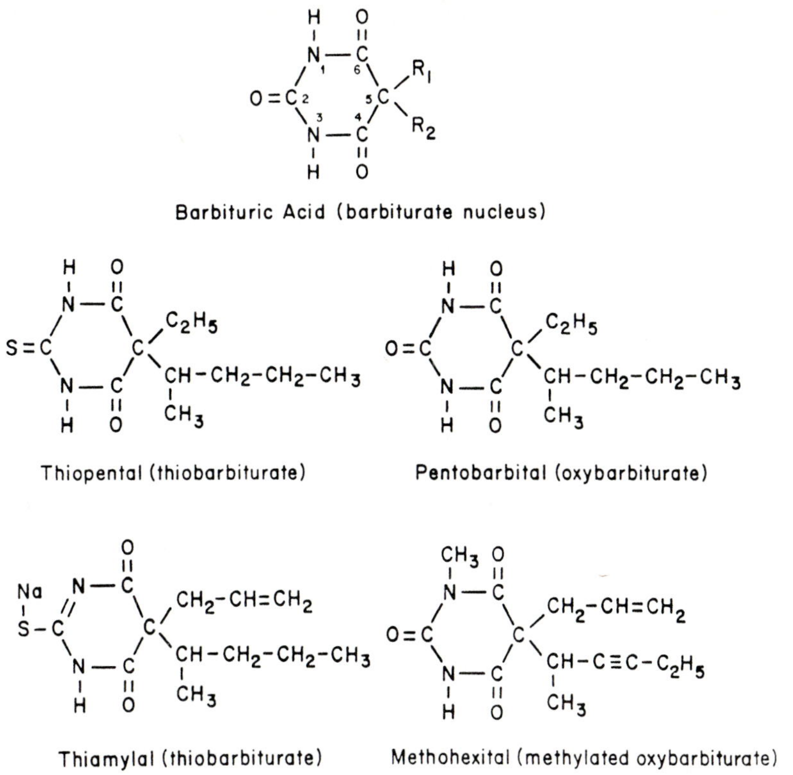

Figure 26–1. The barbiturate nucleus and four different barbiturates resulting from various substitutions.

cal use: oxybarbiturates, thiobarbiturates, and methylbarbiturates. Oxybarbiturates, such as pentobarbital, are used commonly as hypnotics for sleep or intramuscularly as anesthetic premedication. Oxybarbiturates are not routinely used for intravenous anesthesia, but the N-methylated oxybarbiturates, such as methohexital, are popular anesthesia induction agents for outpatients. Thiobarbiturates, such as thiopental and thiamylal, are used as anesthesia induction agents.

Substitutions at the carbon 5 position R_1 or R_2 affect potency.[4,5] Both positions must be occupied by alkyl, straight saturated or unsaturated, branched or cycled, or aromatic groups to produce a sedative-hypnotic effect. An increase in length of one of these side chains will progressively increase the potency and decrease the duration of action. There are normally no more than eight or less than four carbon atoms in the two chains. One side chain must remain short and simple, and together the two side chains should not number more than eight carbons. Potency reaches a maximum when there are seven or eight carbon atoms. Beyond this, toxicity increases more rapidly than potency. Branching or unsaturated chains also tend to increase potency and provide greater hypnotic activity. An aromatic nucleus in an alkyl group that is directly attached to the carbon 5 position produces a compound with convulsant properties; however, direct substitution with a phenyl group confers anticonvulsant properties.[4,5]

In position 1, a methyl (CH_3) or ethyl (C_2H_5) group often results in a compound that has a more rapid onset and recovery but is also associated with a high incidence of excitatory phenomena such as tremor, hypertonus, and spontaneous involuntary muscle movements.[5,6]

When position 2 is occupied by an oxygen atom, the oxybarbiturates are formed. A sulfur atom in this position forms the thiobarbiturate group, which is highly fat soluble and is responsible for rapid onset and very short duration of action.[4–6] The thiobarbiturates also increase vagal activity (Table 26–2).

Physical Properties. The barbiturates supplied for clinical use are in the form of sodium salts. Barbituric acid derivatives do not readily dissolve in water, but the sodium salts of barbiturates will dissolve in water, forming an alkaline and unstable solution.

Thiopental is supplied for clinical use as thiopental sodium for injection, U.S.P. Each gram of thiopental sodium contains 60 mg of anhydrous sodium carbonate. The mixture is strongly alkaline (pH 11). Once in the circulation, the sodium carbonate becomes neutralized and the thiopental is converted to its acidic, nonionized form. Approximately 80 percent of the drug is bound to plasma proteins, mainly albumin, in an inactive form. The alkaline pH makes the solution bacteriostatic but also makes it incompatible with acid solutions. Unused solutions of thiopental should be dis-

TABLE 26–2. SUBSTITUTIONS ON THE BARBITURIC ACID MOLECULE THAT DISTINGUISH THE THREE MAJOR BARBITURATE GROUPS

Group	Substitution	
	Position 1	*Position 2*
Oxybarbiturate	H	0
Methylbarbiturate	CH_3	0
Thiobarbiturate	H	S

carded after 24 hours. Thiopental should be administered separately from other drugs to prevent precipitation in the intravenous line.

Clinical concentrations used for intravenous administration vary between 2.0 and 5.0 percent. The 2.0 or 2.5 percent solution is most commonly used. Concentrations greater than 2.5 percent are more likely to cause serious problems if extravasation or intraarterial injection should occur. A 3.4 percent concentration in sterile water for injection is isotonic. Concentrations less than 2.0 percent in sterile water may cause hemolysis.

Methohexital, U.S.P., is supplied for use as methohexital sodium for injection. Each 500-mg ampule of methohexital contains 30 mg of anhydrous sodium carbonate. Sterile water for injection is the preferred diluent; however, D_5W or 0.9 percent sodium chloride injection may be used. Methohexital sodium is not compatible with lactated Ringer's injection. The pH of the aqueous solution is 11. A 1 percent solution is recommended for induction of anesthesia.

Thiamylal is supplied as thiamylal sodium for injection, U.S.P. The pH of its aqueous solution is 11. The recommended diluents are sterile water, D_5W, and 0.9 percent sodium chloride for injection. A 2.5 percent solution is the recommended concentration for induction of anesthesia.

Pharmacokinetics

Distribution. Physical redistribution plays a crucial role in the termination of action of the ultrashort-acting, highly lipid-soluble barbiturates. The role of redistribution of drugs from the brain to other tissues has been studied most thoroughly using thiopental.[3,7] The same principles apply to thiamylal and methohexital.

An intravenous injection of a barbiturate is initially distributed to the central blood volume of the body. Dilution of the drug by the blood establishes an initial concentration, which is then further decreased by distribution to the tissues. Plasma levels of intravenous thiopental 400 mg were studied.[8,9] An initial rapid decline occurred within the first 5 minutes, representing drug distribution and establishment of plasma–tissue equilibrium. Within 15 minutes the plasma levels were less than one-half the initial concentration and the patient regained consciousness. A slower rate of decline in the plasma thiopental level occurs during the next 20 minutes and an even slower decline after 30 minutes, until a plateau is reached at 120 minutes. The peak concentration in the muscles occurs within 20 to 30 minutes; the fat and vessel-poor groups may take up to 6 hours before reaching peak concentration. Intravenous barbiturates are highly lipid soluble, but they are absorbed more slowly by fat because of the lower blood supply to these tissues (Fig. 26–2).

Clinical effects can be seen as the barbiturates undergo a rapid, flow-limited uptake into the most vascular areas of the central nervous system. Unconsciousness occurs in one arm-to-brain circulation time (10 to 20 seconds) after a single intravenous anesthetic dose. The depth of anesthesia may increase for up to 40 seconds and then progressively decrease. Excessive or prolonged administration leads to drug accumulation in all tissue compartments and may cause excessive drowsiness or unconsciousness in the postoperative period. That thiopental remains in the body after it ceases to be active explains the cumulative effects of re-

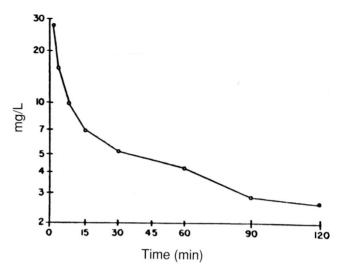

Figure 26–2. Thiopental levels after a single intravenous dose of 400 mg. Note that patients regain consciousness in a few minutes while blood levels are still high. (*Reprinted, with permission, from Brodie BB, Mark LC, et al. The fate of thiopental in man and a method of estimation in biological material.* J Pharmacol Exp Ther. *1950;98:85–96.*)

peated doses.[6,9,10] The rate of equilibration is determined not only by blood flow and cardiac output but also by the ability of the active drug to penetrate cell membranes. Three important factors governing the ability of barbiturates to cross cellular membranes are (1) lipid solubility, (2) degree of ionization, and (3) plasma protein binding[2]:

1. The greater the lipid solubility, the more rapid is the redistribution and equilibration process. The less lipid-soluble oxybarbiturates equilibrate much more slowly than the thiobarbiturates because uptake is limited more by the drug's cell membrane permeability than by blood flow.
2. The extent of dissociation of the intravenous barbiturates into an ionized form depends largely on the pH of the blood and tissues. There is greater ionization with alkalosis and less with acidosis. The nonionized active form crosses membranes more rapidly than the ionized form.
3. Barbiturates are bound to plasma proteins, mostly albumin. Approximately 75 to 80 percent of the injected barbiturate binds with proteins. The unbound active form of the drug is available to penetrate cell membranes.

Keeping all of these variables in mind, the anesthetist can make sound judgments regarding dose, duration, and effect of the barbiturates. A patient who presents in an acidotic state with low plasma protein and blood volume can be expected to respond more dramatically to the usual doses of barbiturates. The patient's physiologic state can alter the normal kinetics of the drug.

Metabolism. The biotransformation of barbiturates is mediated by the microsomal enzyme systems, located primarily in the liver. The thiobarbiturates are also transformed to a small extent in the brain and kidneys. Methohexital is metabolized only by the liver.

Barbiturates are transformed by three main routes: (1) oxidation of radicals at carbon 5; (2) nitrogen dealkylation (methohexital undergoes N-demethylation to a very slight extent, but the rate of oxidation of the carbon 5 substitutes is so rapid that N-demethylation products make up only a minute fraction of the metabolites); and (3) desulfuration of thiobarbiturates.[11]

The ultrashort-acting barbiturates are almost completely transformed in the body to an inactive form. The rate of transformation of thiopental is slow, approximately 10 to 15 percent per hour; 3 percent of the original dose may remain after 24 hours.[10] Metabolism of methohexital is slightly more rapid and accounts for the more rapid recovery. Methohexital has been found to have a short half-life of 75 to 125 minutes.[12]

The duration of action of intravenous barbiturate anesthesia is short and patients regain consciousness fairly quickly; however, the duration of action of intravenous barbiturates has no correlation with the rate of biotransformation of the drugs. Patients awaken with a large amount of unmetabolized drug in the body. Although they may behave and speak normally, patients who have received intravenous barbiturates, especially outpatients, should be advised against taking alcohol or other drugs on the same day. The effects of these substances may be enhanced by the subclinical levels of barbiturate still present in the body. This caution also applies to methohexital, although it is metabolized slightly more rapidly than thiopental.[13]

Excretion. The transformed products of the intravenous barbiturates are excreted primarily by the kidneys; however, a small fraction may appear in the feces by way of the biliary system. Only minute traces (0.3 percent) of these drugs are excreted unchanged in the urine.

Pharmacologic Effects

Central Nervous System. The intravenous barbiturates rapidly cross the blood–brain barrier to produce a progressive central nervous system depression ranging from mild sedation to coma, depending on the dose injected and the rate of injection. The depth of anesthesia produced depends on the plasma concentration of the barbiturate but can be evaluated in terms of the initial dose and rate of administration.[4]

General anesthesia with thiopental is believed to result primarily from the suppression of the cerebral cortex and the reticular activating system.[14] In large enough doses, it can also affect medullary, respiratory, and cardiovascular centers. The mechanism of action is now believed to involve the ability of barbiturates to enhance and mimic GABA action.[15]

Central nervous system depression occurs in the same pattern as with inhalation anesthetics, but the clinical state may not bear a precise relationship because the anesthetic state is reached more rapidly with intravenous agents. A patient given an intravenous barbiturate will go through the classic "stages of anesthesia," but at a much faster rate so that each stage may not be clearly appreciated by the ob-

server. Stage I, consciousness, is lost first. The patient falls asleep suddenly. If there is conversation during induction, the patient's words may suddenly become jumbled and slurred, and he or she may take a few deep breaths or yawn before the eyelids close. Stage II, the excitement stage, is passed so quickly that it is usually not seen. Stage III is achieved very quickly: superficial and deep reflexes diminish and disappear. Pupils constrict and the eyes become fixed at midline. The eyelid reflex is lost and there is profound relaxation of the pharyngeal and masseter muscles. This relaxation is most profound in the first minutes of anesthesia and is transient. Planes III and IV of this stage can be obtained only when extremely large, toxic doses are administered.

As with the inhalational anesthetics, the cerebral cortex is depressed first, followed by the subcortex (in stage II and stage III–plane I), and then the midbrain in the latter planes of stage III. Stage IV is reached when brainstem depression or failure occurs.

The intravenous barbiturates, in doses insufficient to cause unconsciousness, can cause amnesia for events occurring during the time of sedation. This effect correlates well with the plasma levels of the drug.[11]

The lower doses of barbiturates are also capable of increasing sensitivity to painful stimuli. Barbiturates have little or no direct effect on pain relief. Subhypnotic doses increase the sensitivity to deep somatic pain, especially visceral pain, while decreasing the sensitivity to pain from mild, superficial skin stimulation. The latter phenomenon is explained as a result of diminished apprehension and fear, not an analgesic effect. The hyperalgesia to deep somatic and visceral pain appears to result from depression of the inhibitory system in the ascending reticular activating system, which then permits facilitation of secondary slow pain impulses.[14,16,17]

Clinically, small doses of thiopental can antagonize the analgesic actions of nitrous oxide or narcotic. Even large doses of thiopental appear to be lacking analgesic effects. The clinical level of anesthesia is related to the intensity of surgical stimulus. A patient may appear to be in a surgical plane of anesthesia and may even be apneic, but with surgical stimulation, he or she may reflexly initiate movement and respirations. Doses of thiopental sufficient to produce surgical anesthesia in the presence of strong stimulation may cause prolonged respiratory depression and unconsciousness when the stimulation ceases.

Cerebral blood flow and oxygen utilization are reduced with thiopental and the other barbiturates. This decrease in cerebral blood flow decreases intracranial pressure and this effect is frequently used in anesthesia for neurosurgery.

Thiopental and thiamylal produce a rapid, smooth, and quiet induction of anesthesia. Methohexital induction is followed by an appreciable incidence of excitatory phenomena such as tremor, hypertonus, and spontaneous involuntary muscle movements. The methyl group added to position 1 on the oxybarbiturate molecule is believed to be responsible for the excitatory phenomena. The incidence of these effects is reduced by narcotic premedication but increased by preoperative phenothiazines or anticholinergics.[14,18] Methohexital is more likely to induce seizures in susceptible patients than the other intravenous induction agents.[19]

Cardiovascular System. Clinical doses of thiopental, thiamylal, or methohexital generally depress myocardial function (hemodynamic changes are usually fewer with methohexital than with the thiobarbiturates).[5,14] The medullary vasomotor center is depressed as are the hypothalamic centers.[1] A transient fall in the mean arterial pressure can be noted. There is a redistribution of the blood volume, with pooling in the systemic capacitance vessels.[20] This shift causes a decrease in venous return and a reduction in left ventricular diastolic filling pressure, leading to reduced stroke volume and cardiac output. An increase in total calculated peripheral resistance occurs over a period and is believed to be compensatory to decreased cardiac output; however, a cause of central origin cannot be ruled out.[11] The heart rate is usually slightly increased or unchanged as is myocardial oxygen consumption and increases are noted in coronary artery blood flow.[21] Arrhythmias are uncommon, and there is no evidence of myocardial sensitization to catecholamines.

The recommended induction doses of the ultrashort-acting barbiturates given to healthy individuals will cause only a minor and transient change in blood pressure and heart rate; however, the same "normal" dose given to hypovolemic, septic, hypertensive, or debilitated patients or to those with an already compromised hemodynamic state can produce exaggerated effects. Severe and prolonged hypotension or cardiovascular collapse may result. Even very small doses of intravenous barbiturates have been known to produce hypotension in these patients and should be used with caution. Cardiovascular depression resulting from barbiturate administration in healthy individuals is usually the result of rapid injection of very large doses (Table 26–3).

The redistribution of blood increases blood flow to the muscles and extremities while decreasing blood flow to the brain, renal, and splanchnic bed. A decrease in renal plasma flow and glomerular filtration occurring even in small doses has been reported, but recovery is rapid once the anesthetic is terminated.[22] The release of antidiuretic hormone (ADH) by the barbiturates produces an antidiuretic effect.

Some histamine is released with the intravenous barbiturates, especially thiopental, but it does not appear to be significant in altering hemodynamics.[23]

Respiratory System. The ultrashort-acting barbiturates depress respirations by direct action on the medullary and pontine centers. The sensitivity of these centers to respond to carbon dioxide levels is minimally affected.[14]

TABLE 26–3. HEMODYNAMIC EFFECTS OF INTRAVENOUS BARBITURATES

Stroke volume	Decreased
Cardiac output	Decreased
Mean arterial pressure	Decreased
Total peripheral resistance	Increased
Cerebral vascular resistance	Increased
Cerebral blood flow	Decreased
Cerebral oxygen consumption	Decreased
Renal and splanchnic blood flow	Decreased

The extent of respiratory depression depends on dose, rate of administration, and narcotic premedication. Small doses in patients without premedication cause only a transient and minimal decrease in minute ventilation, affecting primarily the tidal volume. Arterial P_{CO_2} is minimally elevated. A larger dose depresses minute ventilation to an even greater extent and can transiently produce apnea. The period of apnea is brief and is attributed to the rapid rate of redistribution of the drug out of the central nervous system. After narcotic premedication, respiratory depression is more marked at all levels of barbiturate anesthesia.

The usual sequence of events after slow administration of thiopental in recommended doses is a few deep breaths or yawning, followed by reduction in ventilation or transient apnea. The surgical stimulus can stimulate respiration and offset the respiratory depression to a certain degree. A patient may breathe adequately during surgical manipulation but become apneic or subside into shallow respirations when the stimulus is removed. The respiratory depression and apnea produced by methohexital are usually not as prolonged as with the thiobarbiturates.

Laryngeal and pharyngeal protective reflexes are not completely obtunded by barbiturates until deep levels of anesthesia are reached. Laryngospasm can occur during barbiturate anesthesia, caused by surgical stimulation and by stimulation of the vagal nerve endings in the larynx by mucus, blood, or secretions.[24] A light level of anesthesia combined with any one or more of the various stimuli can produce laryngospasm.

Coughing, sneezing, and hiccoughing can occur with any of the intravenous barbiturates but seem to occur more frequently with methohexital.[11] These side effects can be minimized by the use of a small total dose and slow injection. Premedication with narcotics and anticholinergics has been noted to be helpful in this respect.

Intravenous thiobarbiturates appear to have a parasympathetic effect, which has been implicated in the bronchoconstriction and bronchospasms that are sometimes seen.[14,20] Although bronchospasm after administration of thiopental is infrequent, clinical use of this drug in asthmatics or patients with increased bronchiolar tone is often avoided.

Indications and Contraindications. Induction of anesthesia using a barbiturate is simple, rapid, and pleasant for the patient. For the majority of the general anesthetics administered, anesthesia is induced with an intravenous barbiturate regardless of the agent to be used for maintenance; however, the clinical use of intravenous barbiturates is not suitable for all patients.

When the adequacy of an airway is in doubt, intravenous barbiturates should not be used. Patients with head and neck tumors or gross anatomic abnormalities or patients who may lose a patent airway with loss of consciousness should not be induced with barbiturates until the airway is secured.

Patients in hypovolemic shock or impending shock and dehydrated or debilitated patients will not react normally to barbiturates, and thus these drugs should be used with extreme caution. Caution must be exercised with severe asthmatics and patients with other bronchospastic disorders.

Patients with acute intermittent porphyria may experience exacerbation of symptoms after barbiturate administration. This can sometimes be fatal; barbiturates are therefore a definite contraindication in these patients.

Complications. Laryngospasm is not an uncommon problem during barbiturate anesthesia. Secretions or blood in the pharynx, stimulation of the pharynx with an airway, or peripheral stimulation during a light plane of anesthesia will induce a laryngospasm. Coughing, sneezing, and hiccoughing can also occur with barbiturate anesthesia, most frequently with methohexital.

Barbiturate solutions are very irritating to the tissues. If large amounts of the drug are placed extravascularly, necrosis of the subcutaneous tissue can result. The higher the concentration of the solution, the greater the danger of a serious problem. Methohexital is usually used in a 1 percent solution and carries a low risk of tissue damage with extravasation. Thiopental and thiamylal in a 2.5 percent solution are also unlikely to cause serious damage, and no permanent sequelae have been reported after use of this concentration. Extravasation of the 5.0 percent solutions of thiopental has been reported to cause serious damage.

Intraarterial injections of barbiturates have been reported when the antecubital site has been selected for the intravenous injection. Intraarterial injection in the awake patient always results in severe pain, described as hot or scalding. Arterial spasm occurs and a chemical endarteritis destroys the endothelial and subendothelial layers of the vessels. Muscle layers may also be involved and thrombosis can occur. The degree of damage depends on the amount and concentration of the solution injected.

Arterial spasms are believed to be caused by the local release of norepinephrine. Necrosis and gangrene are believed to result from thrombosis and crystallization of the drug, leading to vascular occlusion.

Clinical Uses. The intravenous barbiturates have a number of clinical uses. The most popular use is for the induction of anesthesia. A bolus of the barbiturate is administered to supply sufficient depth of anesthesia and sufficient time for endotracheal intubation and to introduce an inhalation agent or narcotic for maintenance. The induction dose can be preceded by a 50-mg test dose to determine the pharmacologic effect before the bolus of barbiturate is administered. Adequate time should be allowed for the test dose to exert an effect, if any, before proceeding with the induction. Blood pressure should be measured and the patient's consciousness assessed about 1 minute after the test dose. Patients who are hemodynamically unstable may show an exaggerated fall in blood pressure in response to the test dose, whereas patients who are less tolerant of the effects of hypnotics may become very sedate and drowsy. Pain on injection may indicate extravasation, and the intravenous site should be checked before proceeding with the injection.

The induction dose of the barbiturate must be tailored to the individual patient. The patient's size, the premedication used and its effect, and the patient's physical status (i.e., state of hydration and nutrition, metabolic and acid–base status, previous drug therapy) must be assessed to determine the proper dose. The amount of barbiturate given for induction may also vary with the technique or method of anesthesia to be employed. Table 26–4 lists the usual required doses for induction of anesthesia for healthy patients.

Thiopental is the most widely used induction agent for all types of procedures; however, methohexital, because of its more rapid rate of metabolism and recovery, is frequently used for dental and other outpatient procedures of shorter duration. Methohexital also appears to be less toxic to the cardiovascular system and has found popularity for use in cardioversions and electroconvulsive therapy.

Barbiturates have been used as the sole anesthetic agent for short surgical procedures by either intermittent bolus injections or continuous drip. These techniques can be used in conjunction with nitrous oxide or an intravenous narcotic premedication. A barbiturate alone is usually not sufficient for most surgical procedures, even with the addition of nitrous oxide, but can be used successfully for very short procedures that do not require relaxation. When doses greater than 500 to 1000 mg are required, or if the procedure lasts longer than 45 minutes to 1 hour, another anesthetic technique should be considered. These techniques should always be performed with supplemental oxygen, and resuscitative equipment should be available. The technique is usually as follows: Intermittent bolus injections of 25 to 75 mg are administered after a sleep dose of the barbiturate is given according to clinical signs of anesthetic depth. An attempt is made to correlate dose and time of administration to the degree of surgical stimulus. Hypoventilation or apnea can occur at any time, and therefore the anesthetist must always be prepared to ventilate the patient. These procedures are frequently done as "mask" cases. Narcotic premedication usually decreases the amount of barbiturate required to produce the desired effects and the respiratory depressant effects can be expected to be greater. For very brief procedures such as a closed reduction of a fracture or dislocation, one bolus injection of the barbiturate may be all that is required. Continuous barbiturate infusion is rarely used for anesthesia today and, when used, is usually limited to procedures of short duration. A dilute concentration should be prepared. A 0.1 percent concentration in D_5W with no more than 500 mg in the solution is a fairly safe mixture. Barbiturate infusion carries a risk of overdosage and prolonged depression, but use of a dilute solution and a fixed amount of the drug affords some protection. If it appears that the entire amount is required, an alternative method should be considered.

The barbiturate infusion is started after a small sleep dose of the barbiturate is injected. The infusion is used to maintain the patient in a consistent plane of anesthesia. This

TABLE 26–4. TYPICAL DOSES FOR INDUCTION OF HEALTHY PATIENTS

Agent	Induction Dose (mg/kg body weight)
Thiopental	3–5
Methohexital	1
Thiamylal	2–3

method usually requires nitrous oxide supplementation, and premedication is very helpful in maintaining a smooth course. The infusion rate can be increased, decreased, or stopped during the procedure according to the surgical stimulus and clinical signs of the depth of anesthesia. To repeat, when an intravenous barbiturate is used, resuscitative equipment should be available.

ETOMIDATE

Etomidate is a relatively new hypnotic induction agent approved for clinical use in the United States in the 1980s. It was first synthesized in 1965 in the laboratories of Janssen Pharmaceutica at Beerse, Belgium.

Chemistry and Physical Properties. Etomidate, (R)-(+)-ethyl-1-(1-phenylethyl)-1H-imidazole-5-carboxylate is a carboxylated imidazole (Fig. 26–3). It is available as a water-soluble compound in 35 percent propylene glycol, with a pH of 5.6. Only the dextroisomer is anesthetically active. Etomidate is available in a 0.2 percent solution. This solution is very stable and can be left at room temperature for more than 2 years.

On a milligram-per-milligram basis, etomidate is approximately 25 times more potent than thiopental and approximately 6 times more potent than methohexital. It has a wider margin of safety than thiopental or methohexital. Its therapeutic index (LD50/ED50) is 26.0, whereas that of thiopental is 4.6.

Distribution, Metabolism, and Excretion. Intravenous injections of etomidate 0.3 mg/kg produce unconsciousness in one arm-to-brain circulation time. Etomidate is highly lipid soluble and has a pK_a of 4.2. Recovery from a single dose of etomidate is very rapid, approximately 3 to 5 minutes for responsiveness. It both enters and leaves the brain quickly because of rapid redistribution. The distribution half-life is just over 2 minutes. Much of the drug is distributed to fat and muscle. The duration of action is dose dependent, usually about 3 minutes for a 0.3 mg/kg dose, and the duration of action is doubled when the dose is doubled. Etomidate is approximately 78 percent protein bound.[5]

Etomidate is metabolized through hydrolysis by esterases in both the liver and plasma. The compound is metabolized into pharmacologically inactive forms. Plasma levels of etomidate decrease rapidly during the first 30 minutes and less rapidly over the next 3 to 6 hours. Detectable amounts of etomidate can be found in the plasma for at least 6 hours. The elimination half-life is approximately 3 hours. Eighty-seven percent of the administered drug is excreted in the urine, 3 percent in an unchanged form. The remaining 13 percent is excreted in the bile. Seventy-five percent of the drug is excreted in 24 hours.[5]

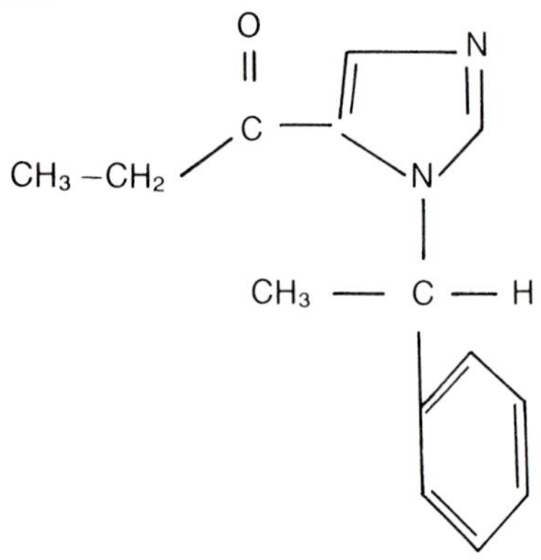

Pharmacologic Effects

Central Nervous System. Etomidate is a hypnotic agent and does not provide analgesia. It appears to exert its central nervous system depressant actions on the brainstem reticular formation by a γ-aminobutyric acid (GABA)-mimetic mechanism.[25]

Electroencephalographic changes noted after etomidate administration are similar to those reported for other intravenous anesthetics.[26] Etomidate has effects on cerebral blood flow and cerebral metabolism similar to those of barbiturate anesthetics. Studies indicate that both cerebral blood flow and cerebral oxygen use are reduced.[27]

A major problem associated with etomidate administration is myoclonic movements.[28] These movements are involuntary, irregular contractions of individual or groups of skeletal muscles and are usually seen during anesthesia induction with etomidate. Electroencephalographic patterns during these movements have not been indicative of seizure activity. The incidence of myoclonus has been reported to be between 10 and 60 percent. Premedication with fentanyl or diazepam appears to reduce the incidence of these movements.

Cardiovascular System. One of the major advantages of etomidate use is that it appears to have minimal effects on the cardiovascular system.[29–31] Arrhythmias are not usually seen when this drug is used. When compared with other intravenous induction agents, etomidate produces fewer and milder consequences in the cardiovascular system.

In patients without cardiopulmonary disease, a dose of 0.3 mg/kg etomidate does not produce significant alterations in cardiovascular parameters. Heart rate and cardiac output are not significantly affected. The mean arterial pressure decreases slightly, as does peripheral vascular resistance and myocardial oxygen consumption. Similar findings have been published for patients with significant cardiovascular disease.

In contrast to some other drugs used in anesthesia, etomidate does not have significant histamine-releasing properties.[32]

Respiratory System. Etomidate has minimal effects on blood gases and pulmonary function. Tidal volume and minute ventilation are reduced, whereas respiratory rate is increased.[33] Transient apnea has been reported with 0.3 mg/kg, especially in debilitated or geriatric patients. The incidence of apnea varies with premedications, but it is considerably less when compared with thiopental.

Endocrine System. The primary effect of etomidate on the endocrine system is its ability to inhibit corticosteroid syn-

Figure 26–3. Chemical structure of etomidate (Amidate).

thesis. The resultant effects are low plasma cortisol and aldosterone levels. Etomidate and the other structurally related imidazole drugs inhibit the adrenal mitochondrial cytochrome P450-dependent enzymes.[34] Etomidate produces a dose-dependent and reversible inhibition of 11β-hydroxylase with subanesthetic and induction doses[35,36]; higher doses also inhibit 17α-hydroxylase.[37]

Following anesthetic induction doses of etomidate, the cortisol response to adrenocorticotropic hormone usually returns to normal within 6 to 8 hours, whereas prolonged infusions (20 hours) produce inhibition for at least 4 days.[38,39] Prolonged infusion of etomidate is not recommended by the manufacturer.

Clinical Uses. Etomidate has been used in many clinical situations and with various techniques. It is probably most commonly used as an induction agent for outpatient surgery, short diagnostic procedures, in the elderly, or in patients with some cardiovascular compromise. Because of the short duration of action and also the relatively hangover-free effect, it is suitable for outpatient use. Etomidate is used in the elderly and in those who may not tolerate other agents because of its minimal effect on the cardiovascular system. In such patients, the induction dose should be administered slowly and cautiously to avoid undesirable cardiovascular changes. Because etomidate does not appear to release histamine, it has been used in patients who are inclined to asthma and other forms of bronchospastic disorders. Etomidate may be useful in neurosurgical and ophthalmic procedures because of its ability to reduce cerebral blood flow, cerebral metabolism, and intraocular pressure. The administration of etomidate to patients with increased intracranial pressure (ICP) or open eye injuries for induction or maintenance may be very useful.

The use of etomidate in a continuous infusion for anesthetic maintenance is gaining popularity, especially when it is administered with fentanyl and nitrous oxide. The recommended infusion rate for maintenance of general anesthesia is 10 μg/kg/min. Infusion rates for short periods of sedation are between 5 and 8 μg/kg/min.

Undesired Effects and Side Effects. Pain on injection is a distinct side effect of etomidate. The average incidence of pain on injection appears to be approximately 20 to 30 percent, although reported incidences vary from 30 to 80 percent.[40] The incidence and severity of pain can be reduced by premedication or pretreatment of a vein with fentanyl or lidocaine or by use of a larger vein.[41] Pain occurs most frequently from injections given into small veins in the wrist or dorsum of the hand and when no premedication was given. Thrombophlebitis has been reported as a side effect of etomidate injection, and appears to have an incidence of approximately 23 percent.[42]

Another major disadvantage of etomidate is the myoclonic movements produced on induction. The incidence ranges from 10 to 60 percent and can sometimes be severe.[40] The myoclonic movements are reduced by premedication with diazepam or fentanyl.[43] A second injection of etomidate may precipitate new myoclonic movements; external stimuli have also been implicated in causing these movements.

Nausea and vomiting can occur postoperatively after the administration of etomidate. The incidence is greater when etomidate is used for both induction and maintenance.

Precautions. Etomidate probably should be avoided in patients with a history of seizure disorder or in patients who require higher levels of cortisol and aldosterone during anesthesia and in the postoperative period.

KETAMINE

Ketamine was introduced into clinical anesthesia by Corssen and Domino in 1966. It was first approved for human use in 1970.

Chemistry and Physical Properties. Ketamine hydrochloride is a phencyclidine derivative used to produce a state of "dissociative" anesthesia. It is sometimes referred to as a cyclohexylamine (Fig. 26–4). Ketamine is a water-soluble solution and can be administered intravenously or intramuscularly. Ketamine is acidic, with a pH between 3.5 and 5.5, and is available in 10, 50, or 100 mg/mL solutions. Benzethonium chloride (Phemerol) 1:10,000 is added as a preservative. Ketamine is nonirritating on injection. It is recommended that the higher concentrations of ketamine be diluted and administered slowly over 60 seconds.

Intravenous administration of 1 to 2 mg/kg produces surgical anesthesia in one circulation time, lasting about 5 to 10 minutes. Repeated doses may be given for a prolonged effect without significant cumulative effects. Intramuscular doses of 5 to 10 mg/kg of the 10 percent solution produce surgical anesthesia within 3 to 4 minutes and last approximately 15 to 30 minutes.

Metabolism and Excretion. Ketamine undergoes N-demethylation and hydroxylation of the cyclohexane ring, resulting in the formation of conjugates, which are then excreted through the kidneys. Ninety-three percent of the metabolites can be found in the urine and approximately 3 percent in the feces. The metabolites have very weak anesthetic potency. Adverse effects on the hepatic or renal systems have not been reported.

Pharmacologic Effects
Central Nervous System. Ketamine produces unconsciousness, analgesia, and amnesia; however, the patient does not appear to be anesthetized but is "dissociated" from

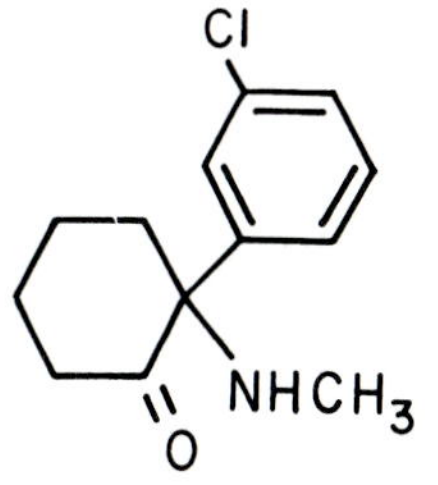

Figure 26–4. Chemical structure of the phencyclidine ketamine hydrochloride (Ketalar).

the environment. *Dissociative anesthesia*, as it is termed, is characterized by catalepsy, catatonia, hypertonus, surgical anesthesia, and amnesia.[45] On entry into the dissociative state, the eyes may remain open, and nystagmus occurs. Deep anesthetic levels may be reached even though the eyes remain open.

Ketamine is believed to exert its effects by depressing the neocorticothalamic system, especially the association areas and the sensory and motor cortex; at the same time it stimulates areas of the limbic system.[46] Both visual and somatosensory impulses travel unimpaired from the periphery to the primary sensory cortex, but under the effects of ketamine the cortex is unable to interpret the afferent impulses and make appropriate responses.

Ketamine greatly increases cerebral blood flow and cerebral metabolic rate and is not recommended for use in patients with cerebral vascular disease or space-occupying lesions. Ketamine also increases intraocular pressure and is contraindicated in open-globe eye injuries.

Cardiovascular System. Unlike most other anesthetic agents, ketamine produces cardiovascular stimulation that affects cardiac output, blood pressure, and heart rate. Cardiac output is increased because of the rise in heart rate rather than because of an increase in stroke volume.[5] This is associated with increased work and myocardial oxygen consumption. In unpremedicated patients, the rise in blood pressure after an intravenous dose of 1 to 2 mg/kg ranges from 20 to 40 mm Hg, with a slightly lower rise in the diastolic pressure. The rise in blood pressure occurs over the first 3 to 5 minutes and declines to normal values within 10 to 20 minutes. A rise in heart rate of approximately 15 beats per minute occurs immediately after intravenous injection (Fig. 26–5).[47]

After ketamine administration there is an increase in the circulating norepinephrine level. The hypertension and tachycardia are probably due to sympathetic stimulation, increased norepinephrine levels, and depression of baroreceptors.[5,44,47] An effect similar to that seen with cocaine occurs: the reuptake of norepinephrine at the adrenergic nerve terminals is prevented.[48] As ketamine causes depression of the isolated myocardium, the cardiostimulatory actions would appear to be caused primarily by sympathetic overactivity.[5]

There is wide individual variation in the blood pressure response to ketamine. There is very little evidence of a dose-related hypertensive effect and the rate of injection does not appear to affect the degree of hypertension.[5,13]

Respiratory System. After intravenous injection, ketamine can produce a transient period of apnea.[22] Slight respiratory depression without apnea may also occur and this is usually most pronounced 1 to 2 minutes after injection.[49] The tidal volume is affected more than the respiratory rate. The initial period of apnea or respiratory depression is dose dependent; larger doses appear to produce greater respiratory depression. Within a few minutes of induction, respiration is restored to normal or, on many occasions, mildly stimulated.

The protective reflexes usually remain intact. Coughing, gagging, and swallowing can be seen with stimulation.

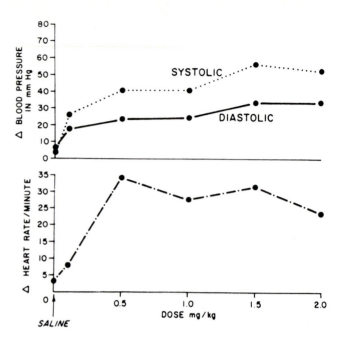

Figure 26–5. Cardiovascular changes in response to ketamine administration. (*Reprinted, with permission, from Zsigmond, Domino. In: Aldrete JA, Stanley TH, eds.* Trends in intravenous anesthesia. *Chicago: Year Book Medical; 1980. Courtesy of the authors.*)

Because both pharyngeal and laryngeal reflexes remain intact, ketamine was at one time used for anesthetizing patients with full stomachs. It is now known that despite the presence of protective reflexes, aspiration can and has occurred.[22,50] The incidence of aspiration is increased by narcotic premedication or preoperative sedation. Benzodiazepines, droperidol, and narcotics all depress laryngeal reflexes. Ketamine should be used with the same precautions taken with any other general anesthetic agents.

In patients with bronchospastic disorders, including asthma, ketamine appears to offer protection and even reduce symptoms of an acute attack.[51,52] The mechanism of action is believed to be the sympathetic stimulation (and consequent increased plasma catecholamine levels).

Ketamine produces an increase in salivation and tracheal mucus formation. An anticholinergic agent should be administered prior to the use of ketamine. Laryngospasm can occur with stimulation of the larynx by saliva or mucus, especially because reflex activity remains intact.

Clinical Uses. Ketamine can be used as the sole anesthetic agent for minor procedures or as an induction agent. Indications for use as the sole agent are (1) relatively short procedures that do not require muscle relaxation, such as minor orthopedic surgery (closed reductions of fractures), gynecologic procedures, diagnostic procedures, ophthalmic examinations, or radiotherapy in small children; (2) mass casualty situations; (3) procedures where there is difficulty maintaining an airway, especially for burns and trauma that affect the face, neck, or upper airway; and (4) dressing changes in severely burned patients.

Ketamine can be used as an induction agent before general anesthesia followed by conventional anesthetic techniques. Because of its effects on blood pressure, it is frequently used for poor-risk patients, such as patients suffering from shock or hypovolemia or patients who might be at risk for severe hypotension should a barbiturate be used. Anesthetic induction in the asthmatic patient can be managed with ketamine if thiopental is to be avoided. Patients with porphyria who cannot receive barbiturate induction agents do well with ketamine.

Intramuscular ketamine is often very useful in young children who are uncooperative or unmanageable. A dose of 5 to 10 mg/kg or less administered intramuscularly to the pediatric patient will produce a manageable state within 5 minutes. Nystagmus will occur as the child enters the dissociative state. The anesthetist can then apply monitors, place an intravenous line, and continue the anesthetic with another technique or continue with intravenous doses of ketamine.

Undesired Effects and Complications. A commonly reported feature of ketamine anesthesia is the occurrence of an "emergence delirium" consisting of vivid, unpleasant dreams and bizarre hallucinations.[5,13] Emergence delirium or excitement usually occurs in the immediate postoperative period and is characterized by restlessness, agitation, disorientation, moaning, or crying. The incidence of hallucinations in adults receiving ketamine anesthesia has been reported to be as high as 50 to 77 percent.[5] Hallucinations have been experienced by approximately 50 percent of unpremedicated patients. Women appear to have a higher incidence of hallucinations than do men or children. Hallucinations seem to be less of a problem in short procedures (5 to 10 minutes) than in long procedures (30 to 40 minutes) but are uncommon in prolonged procedures.[5,13] It has also been suggested that emergence disturbances may be caused by stimulation during the arousal or emergency period.

Dreams and hallucinations can occur up to 24 hours after administration of ketamine.[5] Amnesia persists for about an hour after the apparent recovery from anesthesia and the emergence delirium and excitement are usually not remembered. The dreams and hallucinations, however, are upsetting to the patient.

Medication with benzodiazepines appears to be most effective in reducing the incidence of emergence delirium.[53] Intravenous diazepam appears to decrease the incidence of unpleasant dreams, although it has little effect on emergence delirium.[5] Physostigmine has also been used for emergence delirium with success.

Precautions and Contraindications. Ketamine is contraindicated in patients with coronary artery disease or angina. The increase in heart rate and blood pressure caused by this agent may increase myocardial oxygen demand while decreasing supply. Patients with a history of hypertension or cerebrovascular accident and patients at risk from increased intracranial or intraocular pressure should not be given this drug. Patients having a history of or suffering from neuropsychiatric disturbance should not be given this drug.

The major disadvantages associated with ketamine administration have been the postoperative hallucinations,

dreams, and delirium seen even in patients without psychiatric disturbances. Another disadvantage of this agent is the slow recovery. Patients are usually in full control of their reflexes, but it is often very difficult to determine the exact moment of emergence from the dissociative state. Patients should be left in an environment without a great deal of sensory stimulation to avoid emergence delirium and excitement. To prevent unpleasant reactions, the anesthetist should take care to select appropriate patients, order adequate premedications, be certain that the procedure is short, and avoid use of high doses of ketamine.

PROPOFOL

Propofol (Diprivan) is the most recently marketed intravenous anesthetic available for clinical use. This drug was introduced into practice in 1989 and is classified as a sedative-hypnotic that produces a dose-dependent depression of central nervous system function.[54]

Chemistry and Physical Properties. Propofol is an alkylphenol derivative and is chemically known as 2,6-diisopropylphenol. This compound (Fig. 26–6) is insoluble in an aqueous solution. It is therefore prepared as a 1 percent isotonic emulsion of soybean oil (10 percent), glycerol (2.25 percent), and purified egg phosphatide (1.2 percent) with a pH range of 7 to 8.5.[54,55]

Distribution, Metabolism, and Excretion. Propofol is a highly lipophilic compound distributed rapidly to the vessel-rich tissues and subsequently redistributed to other vessel groups, analogous to the thiobarbiturates used for induction of anesthesia. Blood concentrations of propofol decline rapidly because of the rapid distribution and elimination of this drug.[54] Awakening is more rapid and complete after propofol when contrasted with thiopental or methohexital for induction.[56] Propofol is metabolized in the liver to water-soluble conjugates which are excreted primarily in the urine. The elimination half-life is 0.5 to 1.5 hours.[56] Although metabolism occurs in the liver, patients with cirrhosis exhibit no evidence of impaired or prolonged elimination. Elimination of propofol does not appear to be affected by renal dysfunction; however, elderly patients exhibit a reduced rate of plasma clearance when compared with younger patients.[56] Propofol crosses the placental barrier, but clears rapidly from neonatal circulation.[57]

Induction and Maintenance Doses. Propofol is useful for both induction and maintenance of anesthesia. The induction dose varies from 1.5 to 2.5 mg/kg. Most healthy adults

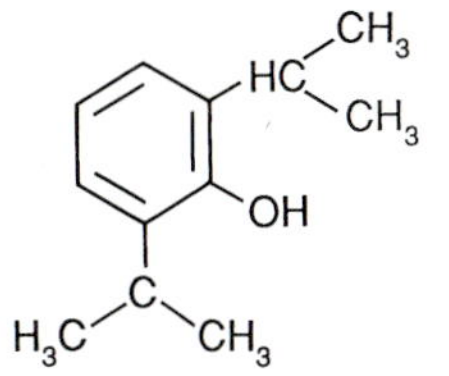

Figure 26–6. Chemical structure of propofol.

require doses between 2 and 2.5 mg/kg.[58] The induction dose should be titrated 40 mg every 10 seconds until clinical signs of anesthesia appear.[54] Elderly and debilitated patients may be more sensitive to the physiologic drug effects and should receive an induction dose reduced by approximately 50 percent (1 to 1.5 mg/kg, administered 20 mg every 10 seconds).[54] Propofol has been used for pediatric anesthesia with similar results.[59] The ease of control of anesthetic depth coupled with the rapid recovery rate seem to make propofol superior to barbiturates and equal to inhaled agents for maintenance of anesthesia.[59,60] Propofol can be administered in intermittent boluses or as a continuous infusion for maintenance of anesthesia.[61] A continuous propofol infusion of 100 to 150 µg/kg/min generally produces a propofol blood level of 3 to 6 µg/mL, which is suitable for major surgery. Infusions of 50 to 100 µg/kg/min are adequate for nonmajor superficial surgeries.[54] Continuous intravenous infusion rates seem to decrease with long operations which suggests a cumulative effect.

Pharmacologic Effects

Central Nervous System. Although the effect of propofol on cerebral dynamics has not been studied extensively, it would appear to produce cerebral hemodynamic effects similar to those of other sedative-hypnotics. Propofol-induced excitatory activity, such as movements and muscle tremors, have been reported occasionally during induction of anesthesia. Such activity appears to be attenuated by small doses of potent rapid-acting opioid analgesics.[54]

Cardiovascular System. Propofol administration causes a decrease in blood pressure greater than that seen with thiopental in equipotent doses. Concurrent administration of narcotic analgesics may further intensify the hypotensive episode. Hypotension may be exaggerated in patients who are hypovolemic, who have compromised left ventricular function due as a result of coronary artery disease, or who are elderly; however, despite the decrease in blood pressure, no corresponding increase in pulse rate has been noted.[56] Occasionally bradycardia and heart block have been observed after induction of anesthesia. Because of this, James et al[62] recommend the prophylactic use of anticholinergic drugs in those patients in whom vagal stimulation is anticipated.

Respiratory System. Like the thiobarbiturates, propofol is a profound respiratory depressant. Opioids administered preoperatively may enhance this ventilatory depression. Therefore, caution should be exercised when using a combination of agents such as propofol and alfentanil for monitored anesthesia care to avoid respiratory depression.

Endocrine and Excretory Systems. As mentioned previously, propofol does not affect hepatic or renal function adversely. Although renal function is not affected, patients who receive prolonged intravenous infusions of propofol should be advised that green urine may be excreted for a period because of the presence of phenols in the urine.[56]

Clinical Uses. Propofol, because of its rapid onset and elimination, is an ideal anesthetic agent for the outpatient surgical setting and for other short procedures such as cardioversion and electroshock therapy. Propofol has been studied extensively with a number of surgical procedures, particularly gynecologic surgeries and strabismus surgery, where a high incidence of postoperative nausea and vomiting is often reported. Watcha et al[63] found that maintenance of anesthesia with a total intravenous regimen using propofol resulted in a more rapid recovery and less postoperative emesis than maintenance with a halothane–N_2O–droperidol regimen. Similar results have been reported in other studies. Because of its central nervous system depressant effects, propofol appears to reduce intracranial and intraocular pressures and would appear to be an appropriate anesthetic choice for patients exhibiting these symptoms.

Undesired Effects, Side Effects, and Complications. The emulsion of propofol itself appears to lack any propensity for initiation of an allergic response. Propofol has been associated with a number of side effects. Most bothersome to the patient is pain on injection. The incidence of this effect can be reduced by administering the drug through a large-bore intravenous catheter into a large vessel such as the antecubital vein. A bolus dose of lidocaine preceding the propofol may reduce the incidence of venous irritation.[58] Other reported side effects such as hypotension and myoclonic movements have already been discussed.

BENZODIAZEPINES

Diazepam

Benzodiazepines were first synthesized in 1933. Chlordiazepoxide was the first compound introduced for clinical use. At present, a number of benzodiazepines are available and they are primarily used as antianxiety agents and central-acting muscle relaxants. Of the benzodiazepines, diazepam was at one time the most widely used and accepted. More recently, a new benzodiazepine, midazolam, has gained popularity in anesthesia as an intravenous sedative. Diazepam is considered the prototype drug for the benzodiazepines (Fig. 26–7).

Chemistry and Physical Properties. Diazepam is a benzodiazepine derivative; it is a colorless crystalline compound that is insoluble in water. It contains propylene glycol, ethyl alcohol, 5 percent sodium benzoate, and benzoic acid as

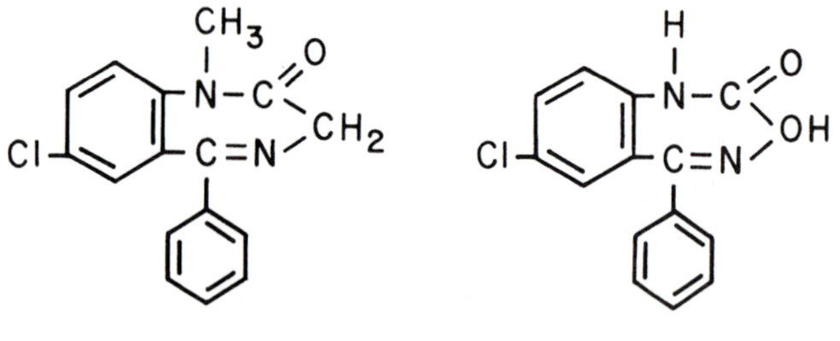

Diazepam   **Lorazepam**

Figure 26–7. Chemical structures of diazepam and lorazepam.

buffers and benzyl alcohol as a preservative. Each milliliter contains 5 mg of diazepam. The pH of the solution ranges from 6.4 to 6.9. A transient cloudiness occurs when diazepam is diluted with water or saline, but this does not affect the potency. The manufacturer does not recommend dilution because it produces an emulsion of small, particulate matter. Diazepam should not be mixed with other drugs.

Metabolism and Excretion. After intravenous administration, redistribution is rapid and follows kinetics similar to those of highly lipid-soluble agents. Diazepam is 80 to 90 percent bound to plasma proteins. After distribution is complete, elimination proceeds at a slow rate because of a relatively long half-life.

The major metabolic pathway involves *N*-demethylation by hepatic microsomal enzymes. This process yields a pharmacologically active product, *N*-desmethyldiazepam, which is only slightly less potent than the parent compound. There is a constant rise in *N*-desmethyldiazepam levels over the first 24 hours, which is mirrored by the steady decline in diazepam levels.[11] After 24 hours, levels of both the metabolite and diazepam decline at approximately the same rate. There is an increase in plasma diazepam levels 6 to 8 hours after administration and then a second smaller rise at approximately 10 to 12 hours.[5,11,13] This is believed to result from enterohepatic recirculation but this has not been substantiated. The rise in plasma levels at 6 to 8 hours is of clinical significance because patients may become sedate and sleepy again at this time. Oxazepam, another active metabolite of diazepam, reaches a peak plasma concentration in 4 hours and is excreted as the glucuronide conjugate in the urine.[1]

Approximately 70 percent of the drug is excreted in the urine as glucuronide and other inactive metabolites. The elimination half-life of diazepam is approximately 1 to 3 days.[1,13] To date, there has been no evidence of impairment of liver or renal function in patients receiving diazepam.

Pharmacologic Effects

Central Nervous System. Benzodiazepines are believed to exert their central nervous system effects by occupying the benzodiazepine receptor that modulates GABA neurotransmission. The binding of benzodiazepines at these receptor sites offers resistance to excitatory neurotransmitters.[64] The effects of benzodiazepines can vary from tranquility to sedation and, with larger doses, sleep. Diazepam also produces relaxation of striated muscles by a central action. Intravenous administration produces anterograde but not retrograde amnesia.[5,13,65]

When diazepam is administered intravenously, there is a delay of approximately 60 to 90 seconds before maximum depression occurs; however, there is a great deal of individual variation in response to diazepam.

The amnesic action is rare after oral or intramuscular administration, but after intravenous injection of 10 mg diazepam, the peak effect occurs in approximately 2 minutes and persists about 5 minutes, declining over the next 30 to 40 minutes. The amnesic actions of benzodiazepines are most marked when sedation is produced.[5] Patients may respond appropriately to questions or commands but recall for these events is suppressed (Fig. 26–8).

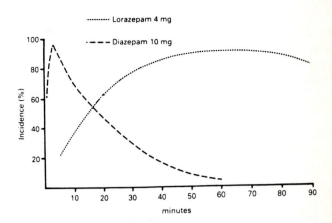

Figure 26–8. Comparison of the amnesic actions of diazepam and lorazepam. Percentage incidence of patients who could not recall being shown objects at various times after the intravenous administration of diazepam and lorazepam. (*Adapted, with permission, from Dundee JW. In: Feldman HS, Scurr E, eds.* Current topics in anesthesia: Intravenous anesthetic agents. *Chicago: Year Book Medical; 1979.*)

Diazepam is frequently used in anesthesia for purposes of sedation, reduction of anxiety, and amnesia. The level of sedation achieved is dose related. Most patients are heavily sedated with 10 to 20 mg. Thickened, slurred speech and nystagmus often precede the onset of sleep. Narcotics administered concomitantly often reduce the amount of diazepam required to produce the desired effect, as do alcohol ingestion, shock, and debilitation.

Benzodiazepines are not analgesic and do not enhance the action of narcotics. The antianxiety effect combined with the narcotic action may sometimes appear to produce analgesia.

It is well known that diazepam possesses anticonvulsant properties that can promptly control seizure activity by abolishing seizure discharge within a few seconds of injection. It is often used as the drug of choice in status epilepticus. The anticonvulsant properties and the elevation of the seizure threshold by diazepam may be of clinical importance in patients who are to receive large doses of local anesthetics. Diazepam can be administered intramuscularly or intravenously for seizure control. Intravenous diazepam controls seizures within seconds of intravenous injection, and intramuscular injection, within a few minutes.

Benzodiazepines have a centrally mediated muscle-relaxant property, which is effective in the treatment of muscle spasms of varying etiology. This effect is believed to result from the action of these drugs on the polysynaptic pathways within the spinal cord or on supraspinal structures.[13] Diazepam has been used successfully for control of rigidity and muscle spasms caused by tetanus. Although diazepam produces a significant amount of relaxation of muscle rigidity and spasm, it does not produce adequate muscle relaxation for abdominal surgical procedures.

Cardiovascular System. The cardiovascular changes occurring with diazepam injection appear to be minimal. There is little change in ventricular contractility, heart rate, or pressures even with large doses (0.5 to 1.0 mg/kg).[13,66] Although the cardiovascular depressant effects of diazepam appear to be minimal in most patients, the drug must be used with caution in patients in hypovolemic shock, of advanced age, or in a debilitated state of health. Wide variations in the response to diazepam should always be kept in mind.

Diazepam has been used for cardioversions in poor-risk and emergency situations. When compared with thiopental, diazepam produces a significantly lower incidence of ventricular arrhythmias and hypotension with this procedure.

Respiratory System. Clinical doses of diazepam cause a slight degree of respiratory depression. The hypoventilation is due primarily to a decrease in tidal volume, resulting in a slight reduction in P_{O_2} and a slight rise in P_{CO_2}.[13] Even small doses of diazepam administered intravenously have been reported to cause a transient period of apnea, especially if given with a narcotic.

Large doses of diazepam should be given with caution in patients with respiratory impairment, those receiving other central nervous system depressants such as barbiturates, and those who may have recently ingested alcohol. All these factors can lead to respiratory compromise or an exaggerated response.

Clinical Uses. Clinical uses of intravenous diazepam include the following:

1. Preoperative medication
2. Induction of anesthesia
3. Sedation and amnesia for local or regional anesthesia
4. Cardioversion
5. Long-term sedation and amnesia for intensive care patients
6. Control of seizures and tetanus
7. Treatment of severe delirium tremens

In anesthesia, diazepam is used most often for the first three purposes listed.

Diazepam is an excellent premedicant because of its efficacy in relieving anxiety and, at the same time, producing sedation and amnesia. Intravenous diazepam can be administered in doses of 2.5 to 10 mg with or without a narcotic. If both narcotic and benzodiazepines are to be given, the doses should be adjusted accordingly. Oral diazepam is also very effective as a premedicant in doses of 5 to 10 mg. Gastrointestinal absorption of diazepam is rapid and complete, with plasma levels peaking shortly after administration. Intramuscular injections of diazepam are not as reliable in terms of absorption and distribution. The oral and intramuscular routes do not produce amnesia. If amnesia is to be a desired effect of premedication, diazepam must be injected intravenously.

Intravenous diazepam in doses of 0.2 to 0.6 mg/kg (in 5- to 10-mg increments at 1- to 2-minute intervals) may be required to induce general anesthesia. The dose may vary according to the degree of preoperative sedation. The onset of sleep occurs 1 to 2 minutes after diazepam injection.

Diazepam induction is an alternative to the use of barbiturates in patients with porphyria, asthma, or bronchospastic disorders and in poor-risk patients. Because of the long half-life and the active metabolites present, patients may be sleepier after the large doses of diazepam used for induction.

Intravenous diazepam had been used extensively for sedation for endoscopic procedures under local anesthesia and other minor surgical procedures carried out with local anesthesia, such as dental procedures and plastic surgery. Diazepam is also used in conjunction with a regional anesthetic technique to relieve anxiety and provide sedation and amnesia. Because diazepam does not provide analgesia, it can be given together with a narcotic to achieve a desired effect. Both the narcotic and the diazepam should be titrated carefully to avoid loss of consciousness or loss of airway because of upper airway obstruction. It must be remembered that under local anesthesia, with "sedation," the patient should be arousable, cooperative, and comfortable.

Contraindications and Complications. Injectable diazepam is contraindicated in patients with acute narrow-angle glaucoma and open-angle glaucoma unless patients are receiving appropriate therapy.

When administered intravenously, diazepam must be injected slowly to reduce the possibility of venous thrombosis, phlebitis, local irritation, and swelling. In a study conducted to investigate venous sequelae after diazepam and lorazepam injection, it was found that there was a significantly higher incidence of sequelae after intravenous diazepam than after lorazepam.[12] Both thrombosis and phlebitis were found on the second and third days after injection, with an incidence of 23 percent for diazepam and 8 percent for lorazepam. Painless thrombosis that extended to the upper arm and axilla was noted at 7 to 10 days. Very long thrombosed segments of vein were found more often after diazepam; the incidence was 39 percent with diazepam and 15 percent with lorazepam at 7 to 10 days[67] (Table 26–5).

The complications occur most frequently when smaller vessels are selected for use. Venous thrombosis after diazepam is related to age.[5] The incidence increases with age and increases sharply after age 60. Patients who are 70 years or older have almost a 100 percent chance of a venous thrombosis sequela (Fig. 26–9).

Hypotension and apnea are always possible complica-

TABLE 26–5. INCIDENCE OF VENOUS SEQUELAE AFTER ADMINISTRATION OF INTRAVENOUS BENZODIAZEPINES

Drug	Dose (mg)	No.	Total Venous Sequelae (%)	
			2–3 days	7–10 days
Diazepam	10	44	23	39
Lorazepam	4	40	8	15

Reprinted, with permission, from Dundee JW. In: Feldman HS, Scurr E, eds. Current topics in anesthesia: Intravenous anesthetic agents. Chicago: Year Book Medical; 1979.

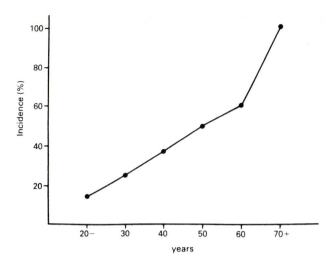

Figure 26–9. Incidence of venous thrombosis after intravenous administration of 10 mg diazepam, relative to age of patients. (*Reprinted, with permission, from Dundee JW. In: Feldman HS, Scurr E, eds.* Current topics in anesthesia: Intravenous anesthetic agents. *Chicago: Year Book Medical; 1979.*)

tions of intravenously administered central nervous system depressants. Resuscitative equipment should be available when moderate-to-large doses are administered. Diazepam must be administered with caution to patients in shock, patients taking barbiturates, phenothiazines, narcotics, monoamine oxidase inhibitors, or alcohol, and elderly or debilitated patients.

Lorazepam

Chemistry and Physical Properties. Lorazepam is a benzodiazepine derivative with actions very similar to those of diazepam. It is a white powder that is insoluble in water. Each milliliter contains polyethylene glycol in propylene glycol with benzyl alcohol as a preservative. Each milliliter of sterile injection contains 2.0 or 4.0 mg of lorazepam.

Absorption, Metabolism, and Excretion. Lorazepam is rapidly and virtually completely absorbed by the intramuscular route. Peak plasma concentrations are reached in 60 to 90 minutes. Maximum depressant effects after intravenous administration of lorazepam do not occur for 10 to 20 minutes. After oral administration, peak plasma levels are reached within 2 hours. Absorption from the gastrointestinal tract is essentially complete. The mean half-life for intravenous or intramuscular lorazepam is approximately 16 hours. It is 85 percent bound to plasma proteins.

Lorazepam is conjugated in the liver into its major metabolite, lorazepam glucuronide. The metabolite is inactive and is excreted in the urine. The extent of drug accumulation with multiple-dose therapy is considerably less than that seen with diazepam. Dilution of lorazepam with an equal volume of compatible solution is recommended before intravenous use.

Pharmacologic Effects. Lorazepam and diazepam have basically very similar effects on the central nervous, cardio-

vascular, and respiratory systems. Lorazepam has a much slower onset of action and a longer amnesic action.[68] If lorazepam is to be given for sedation or relief of preoperative anxiety, it must be given earlier than most preoperative medications.[5] The effects of a clinical dose of lorazepam usually last 6 to 8 hours. The amnesic action peaks at 15 to 20 minutes intravenously and 2 hours intramuscularly and can continue for 4 to 8 hours. The degree of sedative and anxiety-relieving effects is similar for both diazepam and lorazepam. The amnesic effects occur more rapidly and also subside more rapidly with diazepam. Lorazepam is indicated when a longer period of sedation and amnesia is desired.

Lorazepam can be diluted with sterile water, sodium chloride, or D_5W for injection. The drug should be administered slowly. The incidence of venous sequelae is much lower than with diazepam, probably because of the lower concentration of propylene glycol contained in the lorazepam.

Clinical Uses. Premedication and sedation for local or regional procedures can be accomplished quite nicely with lorazepam; however, induction of anesthesia with lorazepam is not recommended because of the slow onset of action. Other situations indicating benzodiazepines and requiring rapid onset of action would best be handled with diazepam or midazolam. On the other hand, sedation and amnesia for intensive care patients on a respirator may best be accomplished with lorazepam.

The suggested dose for intramuscular premedication with lorazepam is 0.05 mg/kg up to 4 mg. For optimum amnesic effects, intramuscular lorazepam should be administered 2 hours before the anticipated procedure. For intravenous sedation and relief of anxiety, 0.04 mg/kg up to a total dose of 2 mg may be given. If optimum amnesic effects are required and would be beneficial, 0.05 mg/kg up to 4 mg may be administered intravenously.

Precautions. As with diazepam, caution must be exercised when administering intravenous lorazepam. The same precautions should be taken regarding drug interactions, selection of patients, and availability of resuscitative equipment. The manufacturer does not recommend the use of lorazepam in persons under 18 years of age. Table 26–6 compares diazepam, lorazepam, and midazolam.

Midazolam

Midazolam is a relatively new benzodiazepine with actions very similar to those of diazepam. The principal differences between the two drugs are (1) the shorter duration of action, (2) the rapid metabolism, and (3) the water solubility. Midazolam is approximately three times more potent than diazepam.

Chemistry and Physical Properties. Midazolam, imidazole-1,4-benzodiazepine (Fig. 26–10), is water soluble in an acidic aqueous medium (pH < 4.0). At physiologic pH, midazolam becomes highly lipid soluble and is one of the most lipid soluble benzodiazepines. The high lipid solubility promotes rapid entry of the drug into brain tissue.

TABLE 26–6. COMPARISON OF DIAZEPAM, LORAZEPAM AND MIDAZOLAM

	Diazepam	Lorazepam	Midazolam
1. Equivalent dose	10 mg	2.0–2.5 mg	2–4 mg
2. Intravenous administration			
Peak effect	2–5 min	30–40 min	1–2 min
Duration of sedation	30 min–1 h	3–6 h	30 min–1 h
Duration of amnesia	3–30 min	30 min–4 h	20–45 min
3. Active metabolites	Desmethyldiazepam 3-Hyroxydiazepam Oxazepam	None	1–Hydroxymidazolam (minimal activity)
4. Half-life	36 h (20–50)	12 h	1–4 h
5. Half-life of active metabolites	Desmethyldiazepam: 48–96 h 3-Hydroxydiazepam: 15–20 h Oxazepam: 6–8 h	— — —	1–4 h (clinically insignificant)

Studies have indicated that in an acid medium, the benzodiazepine ring opens and creates the desired water-soluble solution. At a pH_a close to 7.4 the ring closes, and the drug becomes lipid soluble and readily crosses the blood–brain barrier.[14] Each milliliter contains midazolam hydrochloride equivalent to 1.0 or 5.0 mg. The compound contains sodium chloride and disodium edetate with benzyl alcohol as preservative.

Distribution, Metabolism, and Excretion. Intravenous administration of midazolam at physiologic pH produces a rapid onset of activity. Entry into brain tissue and clinical activity occur within 30 to 90 seconds. Midazolam's high lipid solubility and its rapid distribution and metabolism contribute to the drug's short duration of action. Midazolam is the shortest-acting benzodiazepine available. The initial phase of drug disappearance is a result of drug distribution. This is followed by the less rapid phase, which is attributed mainly to biotransformation. After distribution and equilibration, midazolam is rapidly eliminated. The half-life ranges from 1 to 4 hours.

Midazolam is approximately 96 to 97 percent protein bound. The biotransformation involves hydroxylation by hepatic microsomal enzymes. The major metabolite is 1-hydroxymethyl midazolam. Two other metabolites are formed in very small amounts, 4-hydroxymidazolam and 1,4-dehydroxymidazolam. The metabolites are excreted in the urine in the form of glucuronide conjugates. Both the 1-

hydroxy and 4-hydroxy metabolites possess less pharmacologic activity than the parent compound; this is not believed to be a significant factor in the overall clinical effects.

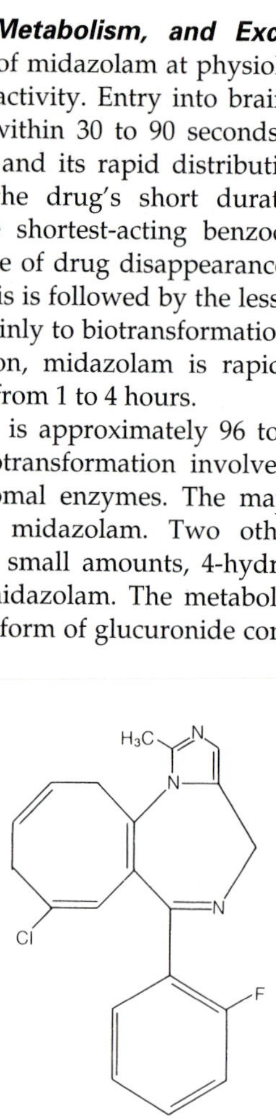

Pharmacologic Effects

Central Nervous System. Once midazolam has crossed the blood–brain barrier, it works at the level of the central nervous system benzodiazepine receptors. Midazolam appears to have three to four times the affinity for these receptors as has diazepam; thus there are estimates of approximately three to four times the potency of diazepam.[69]

Midazolam has clinical effects similar to those of diazepam. Premedicated patients usually lose consciousness after an intravenous dose of 0.2 mg/kg. Unpremedicated patients may require 0.3 mg/kg or higher doses. These doses sufficient to cause loss of consciousness are recommended for induction of anesthesia. Midazolam is an excellent hypnotic, anxiolytic, and amnesic. Anterograde amnesia can be obtained by both the intravenous and intramuscular routes of administration; the duration of amnesia is dose related. Sedation and reduction in the level of anxiety are easily achieved with intravenous doses of approximately 1.0 to 2.5 mg. Intramuscular doses for adequate sedation range from 0.07 to 0.08 mg/kg.

Midazolam possesses anticonvulsant actions similar to those of diazepam. The electroencephalographic changes produced by midazolam are also similar to those observed with diazepam. Cerebral blood flow and cerebral oxygen consumption are reduced much more effectively by midazolam than by diazepam. Intraocular pressures are reduced to a degree similar to that achieved with diazepam.

Cardiovascular System. Midazolam's cardiovascular actions are very similar to those of diazepam. The decrease in blood pressure occurs by two mechanisms: (1) systemic vascular resistance is reduced, and (2) venous return is therefore reduced.[70]

When pulmonary artery occlusion pressures are initially high, midazolam has been shown to reduce them. Midazolam appears to maintain hemodynamic values in patients with ischemic heart disease.[71] Samuelson et al[72] reported a small increase in heart rate; small decreases in blood pressure, pulmonary artery pressure, and pulmonary artery occlusion pressure; and no change in cardiac output

Figure 26–10. Chemical structure of midazolam.

after induction with 0.5 mg/kg of midazolam. Cardiac arrhythmias have not been reported to be a problem.

Elderly patients and other poor-risk patients are more sensitive to midazolam. Volume-depleted patients may respond to midazolam with serious decreases in blood pressure; it would therefore be wise to reduce the dose and to use caution. Although midazolam appears to produce only minimal cardiovascular depression, it has not been proven to be a safe agent for induction in hemodynamically unstable patients.

Respiratory System. Intravenous induction doses of midazolam cause a transient respiratory depression (tidal volume reduction), apnea, or both. Ventilatory depression peaks at about 3 minutes and can last up to 15 minutes after doses of 0.2 mg/kg.[73] The respiratory depression and apnea appear to occur most frequently in patients premedicated with narcotics. Recovery from this depression corresponds with recovery from unconsciousness.

In patients with chronic obstructive pulmonary disease, there is a more profound and persistent depression of ventilation.[74] This probably is true for elderly and poor-risk patients, who are more sensitive to drugs. Sedation and respiratory depression can be reversed with physostigmine.[75] Coughing, breath holding, and laryngospasms occur less frequently with midazolam than with thiopental.

Sedative doses of midazolam given intravenously may in some patients causes transient respiratory depression; therefore, patients should be observed closely whenever intravenous midazolam is used.

Renal System. Midazolam induction produces a reduction in renal blood flow and glomerular filtration rate (GFR), while increasing renal vascular resistance. These results are comparable to those observed with thiopental, with the exception of GFR reduction: a smaller reduction occurred in patients who received midazolam.[76]

Patients with chronic renal failure had shorter induction times and longer recovery times. These findings can be related to the lower degree of binding of midazolam to albumin and the greater availability of the active, unbound drug in these patients, who also showed a reduction of free drug clearance when compared with normal subjects.[77]

Clinical Uses. Intravenous midazolam can be used for many of the same indications as diazepam: (1) induction agent, (2) maintenance agent, (3) sedation for local anesthesia or regional techniques, and (4) premedication.

Induction doses for midazolam range from 0.2 to 0.34 mg/kg. The dose is influenced by premedication, age, physical status, speed of injection, and serum albumin concentration. Narcotic premedication appears to decrease the dose of midazolam required and shortens the induction time. Sedatives and hypnotic premedications do not have the same ability to reduce dosage or induction times.

Induction times vary from 30 seconds to almost 5 minutes depending on the speed of injection. When compared with thiopental, midazolam induction and emergence are considerably slower. Patients regained consciousness after midazolam in approximately 15 minutes. Although this is prolonged compared with thiopental, patients were considered street fit 3 to 4 hours after induction with either midazolam or thiopental induction. Induction and emergence times may be abnormal in patients with chronic renal failure.

Midazolam offers no advantage over thiopental for speed of induction and is not more effective in maintaining cardiovascular dynamics than etomidate. The advantages of midazolam as an induction agent are its increased reliability, speed of induction, and duration of action when compared with diazepam.

Midazolam can be used during anesthetic maintenance in the same manner as diazepam. Midazolam lacks analgesic properties, so it must be used in combination with narcotics in a balanced technique or as an adjunct to an inhalation anesthetic. For short procedures, midazolam may be used similarly to thiopental by infusion after induction, supplemented by nitrous oxide and a narcotic premedication.

To supplement a regional or local anesthetic, small doses of intravenous midazolam in combination with small doses of narcotics will produce hypnosis, sedation, and amnesia. Both midazolam and narcotic should be carefully titrated to obtain the desired effect. Close observation of blood pressure and respirations is crucial when any intravenous agent is administered for sedation.

Premedication with midazolam can be accomplished intravenously, intramuscularly, or orally. Intravenous premedication may supplement previously administered oral or intramuscular drugs or may be used for acute sedation in an unpremedicated patient. When used for sedation, intravenous midazolam should be titrated to obtain the desired effect. Intramuscular premedication with midazolam produces much of the same effects obtained by the intravenous route, namely, hypnosis, amnesia, and anxiolysis. The recommended intramuscular dose is 0.07 to 0.08 mg/kg approximately 1 hour before surgery. Oral midazolam is rapidly absorbed from the gastrointestinal tract. Peak plasma concentrations and clinical effects are noted within 1 hour. After oral administration, only 40 to 50 percent of the dose is available in the systematic circulation in the intact form.[78] This is due to extensive first-pass hepatic extraction and necessitates oral doses approximately twice the intravenous dose to achieve the same effect. The elimination half-lives of oral and intravenous midazolam are similar and are independent of the route of administration.

Advantages over Diazepam. Midazolam causes minimal local irritation and pain after intravenous or intramuscular administration. Intravenous midazolam has not been associated with the venous sequelae common with diazepam. Other advantages are the rapid onset of action, metabolism, and half-life. Midazolam has superiority over diazepam in outpatient use and in short surgical or diagnostic procedures requiring sedation and amnesia.

NEUROLEPTANALGESIA

Neurolepsis is a term coined by Delay and his colleagues in 1959 to describe a drug-induced behavioral syndrome consisting of diminished aggression, indifference to surroundings, and somnolence with easy arousability to full rational attention. *Neuroleptic* is the term used to describe drugs that produce neurolepsis or a neuroleptic state and is synonymous with the term *major tranquilizer.*[79]

In the same year that Delay defined neurolepsis, DeCastro and Mundeleer introduced *neuroleptanalgesia* at the French Anesthesia Congress in Lyon. Neuroleptanalgesia has since become an extremely popular and useful anesthetic technique. As the name suggests, it is a state produced by combining a potent neuroleptic drug with a potent narcotic. DeCastro and Mundeleer emphasized the uniqueness of this technique with respect to "balanced anesthesia" techniques in that the patients were neither asleep nor awake but in a state of profound analgesia and psychomotor sedation. DeCastro and Mundeleer originally used haloperidol with a narcotic, muscle relaxant, and oxygen. With the introduction of the potent narcotic fentanyl and the neuroleptic droperidol in 1963, use of the previously mentioned drugs was discontinued and Innovar, a mixture of these two drugs, came into frequent use. The effects produced by Innovar are the result of each component exerting its own pharmacologic effect independently of the other. The combination contains fentanyl and droperidol in a fixed ratio of 1:50; each milliliter of Innovar contains 0.05 mg fentanyl and 2.5 mg droperidol.

Neuroleptanalgesia has been described as a state of tranquilization and intense analgesia with little or no hypnosis. The technique affects the subcortical areas of the brain—the thalamus, hypothalamus, and reticular system—to provide analgesia and sedation, leaving cortical functions intact. Central nervous system characteristics of this state include somnolence without loss of consciousness, psychologic detachment from the environment, inhibition of learned behavioral activity and reflexes, and analgesia.[69]

From an anesthetic viewpoint, neuroleptanalgesia offers several advantages: (1) mental withdrawal from the immediate situation with an ability to respond and cooperate when the need arises, (2) a disinclination to move, (3) potent antiemetic effects, (4) analgesia, and (5) cardiovascular stability. When undisturbed, the patient remains in a state of calm detachment. The technique has been especially useful for diagnostic or surgical procedures requiring consciousness and cooperation of the patient. If an anesthetic agent is added to produce unconsciousness and amnesia, the technique is termed *neuroleptanesthesia.* If required, a muscle relaxant can be added, and this technique then becomes a balanced anesthesia technique.

Droperidol

Droperidol is a potent butyrophenone, a fluorinated derivative of phenothiazine (Fig. 26–11). Droperidol is available alone or in combination with fentanyl as Innovar. Whether alone or in combination with fentanyl, 2.5 mg droperidol is contained in each milliliter. The pH of the clear, colorless solution is adjusted to 3.5. The 10-ml vial contains methylparaben and propylparaben as preservatives. The onset of action after intravenous injection is 3 to 5 minutes. The full effect may not be apparent for 30 minutes. The duration of action is generally 2 to 4 hours, but the effects of the drug may be noted for up to 12 hours.

Metabolism and Excretion. Droperidol is metabolized in the liver. Excretion of the drug occurs by way of urine and

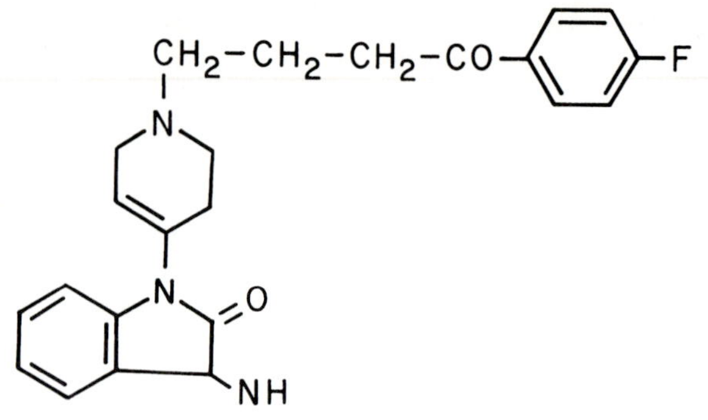

Figure 26–11. Chemical structure of droperidol (Inapsine).

feces, with the majority of the metabolites being excreted within 24 hours. Approximately 10 percent of the drug is excreted intact through the kidneys. No untoward effects on the liver or kidneys have been noted.

Pharmacologic Effects

Central Nervous System. The droperidol component of Innovar contributes most to the state of neurolepsis. Droperidol produces marked tranquilization and inhibits operant (learned) behavior. The butyrophenones are able to induce cataleptic immobility, in which patients appear tranquil and dissociated from the environment but are readily accessible when spoken to. Neuroleptics also inhibit symptoms of delusions, hallucinations, paranoia, and mania.

The ability of the neuroleptics to exert these effects on the central nervous system result from their ability to competitively antagonize the norepinephrine-, serotonin-, and dopamine-mediated synapses in the brain. The action is on the postsynaptic neuron, where dopamine is the neurotransmitter. At certain synapses, GABA is the inhibitory transmitter and dopamine the stimulatory transmitter. It is believed that neuroleptics compete for the dopaminergic receptors to decrease transmission.[80]

Neuroleptics have a predilection for areas in the brain that are high in dopaminergic receptors, including the chemoreceptor trigger zone (CTZ) and the nigrostriatum. The marked antiemetic activity of droperidol is due to its action on the CTZ in the medulla. Droperidol does not antagonize motion sickness originating in the labyrinth. Extrapyramidal symptoms sometimes occur in a small percentage of patients as a result of dopamine blockade at the extrapyramidal nigrostriatum, and pseudoparkinsonian effects can be noted, though they may sometimes be delayed up to 24 hours. Such effects are usually associated with high doses but have also been reported with low doses administered intramuscularly. These effects respond to anticholinergics or antiparkinson therapy.

Droperidol can potentiate the effects of other central nervous system depressants such as thiopental, other tranquilizers, narcotics, and general anesthetics. Dosage adjustments should be made accordingly.

Cardiovascular System. Droperidol has little or no effect on the myocardium, heart rate, or cardiac output. The systemic blood pressure falls slightly (in a normovolemic patient) because of the alpha-adrenergic blocking activity.[81] This action is usually very mild, but marked hypotension can occur in a hypovolemic patient. There is also a small decrease in pulmonary vascular pressures caused by decreased resistance. In general, the cardiovascular hemodynamics are well maintained. There has been some evidence that droperidol may reduce the incidence of epinephrine-induced arrhythmias, but it does not appear to prevent other cardiac arrhythmias.[81]

Respiratory System. Droperidol has not been found to produce any significant degree of respiratory depression. The respiratory depression occurring with the administration of Innovar is due to the narcotic component, fentanyl.

Fentanyl

Fentanyl is the narcotic component in Innovar. It is a synthetic narcotic that is structurally related to meperidine. Fentanyl is approximately 100 times more potent than morphine and 1000 times more potent than meperidine. Fentanyl 0.1 mg is roughly equal to 10 mg of morphine or 75 mg of meperidine (Fig. 26–12).

Fentanyl is available alone or in combination with droperidol as Innovar. Each milliliter contains 0.05 mg of fentanyl. The pH is adjusted to 4.0 to 7.5 with sodium hydroxide. Ten percent of fentanyl is excreted unchanged; the remainder is degraded in the liver. Liver function and renal function are unaltered by fentanyl.

Pharmacologic Effects

Central Nervous System. Fentanyl is a potent analgesic. After intravenous administration, there is an immediate onset of action, with the peak effect occurring at about 4 to 5 minutes. The analgesic effect lasts 30 to 60 minutes after a single dose.

The primary sites of action appear to be the thalamus, hypothalamus, cerebral cortex, limbic system, midbrain, extrapyramidal area, substantia gelatinosa, and sympathetic preganglionic neurons.[82] At the cortical level, an indifference to pain is noted. Fentanyl alone has very little hypnotic or sedative action. Fentanyl also possesses typical narcotic features, such as stimulation of miosis, euphoria, and depression of the ventilatory control centers.

Fentanyl appears to have less emetic activity than the other narcotic analgesics.

Cardiovascular System. Fentanyl has minor effects on the cardiovascular system. Cardiac output usually remains unchanged. Myocardial function is not depressed nor is the vascular system affected. A slight decrease in systemic blood pressure is sometimes seen. This is consistent with the effects of sedation and analgesia. Bradycardia may occur because of fentanyl's central vagotonic effect. This is easily reversed with anticholinergics.[83]

Respiratory System. Fentanyl is a potent respiratory depressant; the degree of depression is directly related to dosage. Respiratory frequency and tidal volume are both affected. There is a lowered sensitivity of the ventilatory control centers to carbon dioxide levels. Larger doses may produce total apnea. The peak respiratory depressant effect of a single intravenous dose of fentanyl appears between 5 and 10 minutes after injection. The ventilatory status is usually returned to normal by approximately 30 minutes; however, altered responses to carbon dioxide have been noted up to 4 hours after a single dose.[84] This depression of carbon diox-

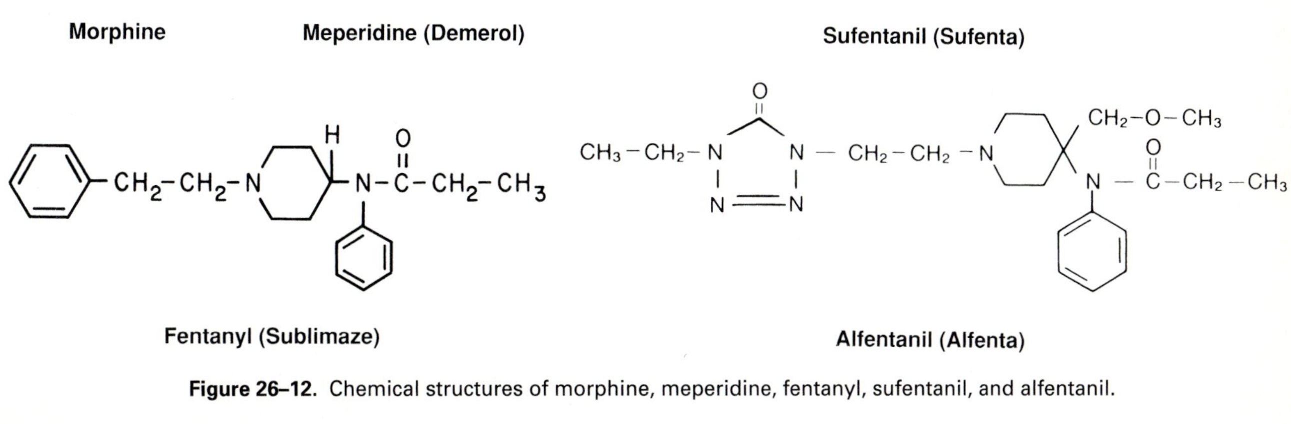

Figure 26–12. Chemical structures of morphine, meperidine, fentanyl, sufentanil, and alfentanil.

ide sensitivity may persist longer than the depression of respiratory rate or the analgesic effect.

Histamine release rarely occurs with fentanyl, but bronchoconstriction caused by histamine is always a possibility.

Occasionally, there is difficulty ventilating a patient who has been given intravenous fentanyl. This is usually a result of muscle rigidity of the thorax and abdomen. The severity seems to be related to the dose and speed of injection. The exact mechanism of this rigidity is not clearly defined. This phenomenon has been referred to as the "stiff chest" syndrome and can be overcome with a small dose of succinylcholine. Slow intravenous injections or pretreatment with nondepolarizing muscle relaxants usually prevents this occurrence.

Innovar

Clinical Uses. Innovar has been used clinically for many procedures with great success and effectiveness. It has been especially useful when a sedated but cooperative patient was required. Patients undergoing diagnostic procedures, such as angiography, esophagoscopy, or bronchoscopy, who are given Innovar with local anesthesia appear to tolerate it well. The drug is also useful in providing sedation for surgical procedures under local or regional anesthesia.

An awake intubation is usually well tolerated by patients under neuroleptanalgesia, especially when cooperation is essential, as in an awake blind nasal intubation.

Innovar has been used for cardiopulmonary bypass surgery to avoid the depressant effects of volatile agents. It has also been used in neurosurgical procedures, such as stereotactic surgery, where conscious cooperation is required, and for craniotomies in combination with nitrous oxide and muscle relaxant. An advantage of neuroleptanesthesia using Innovar for neurosurgical procedures is that it reduces both cerebral blood flow and cerebral oxygen consumption.

Contraindications and Precautions. Innovar is contraindicated in patients with Parkinson's disease. The droperidol component can cause an increase in the symptoms caused by action on the dopaminergic synapses. Innovar is not recommended for use in outpatients because of the prolonged duration of action of droperidol. The safety of Innovar in children under 2 years of age and in pregnancy has not been established.

Innovar must be used with caution in elderly, debilitated, or hypovolemic individuals. Dosages should be titrated slowly. Caution must be exercised when administering this drug to patients who have compromised ventilatory reserve. The narcotic component may additionally reduce respiratory drive and increase airway resistance. The doses of other central nervous system depressants must be adjusted for patients who have received Innovar.

The advantages of neuroleptanalgesia are many and include (1) lowered incidence of nausea and vomiting, (2) profound sedation with easy arousability, (3) profound analgesia, and (4) cardiovascular stability. There are, however, certain disadvantages that must be considered as well when selecting an anesthetic technique. It must be remembered

that Innovar can cause extrapyramidal side effects. The effects of droperidol outlast the analgesic effects and may be prolonged, and the respiratory depressant effects often far outlast the analgesic effects.

NARCOTICS: MORPHINE, MEPERIDINE, FENTANYL, SUFENTANIL, AND ALFENTANIL

Opium is a Greek word meaning "juice" and describes the drug obtained from the milky exudate of the incised unripe seed capsules of the poppy plant, *Papaver somniferum*, which is indigenous to Asia Minor. The term *opioid* refers to any natural or synthetic drug with pharmacologic properties similar to those of morphine. The term is synonymous with narcotic analgesics.

Opium has been used as a narcotic for a long time. Greek history contains records of opium use that date back to 300 B.C. It has been used for various purposes including pain relief and control of dysenteries. When opium was first used in connection with surgery is difficult to determine. The earliest known soporific sponge dates back to the 9th century. Soporific sponges were sponges filled with opium, *Mandragora*, *Cicuta*, and *Hyoscyamus* that were used to relieve pain during operations in the 14th century. The first attempt to administer opiates intravenously for anesthesia was made by Elscholtz in 1665. In 1778, Boerhaave used opium for anesthesia as a vapor by inhalation and as a powder. The extreme variability of the opium in terms of doses and absorption rate often resulted in inadequate analgesia, coma, and death. Pravaz in 1853 invented the syringe, and Alexander Wood developed the hollow needle in the same year. It was not until this time that accurate means of administering opioids became feasible.

In 1805, Serturner described a pure alkaloid base isolated from opium. In 1817, he published this report and called the compound *morphine* after Morpheus, the Greek god of dreams.

Opium in the form of dried powder contains a number of alkaloids. About 25 different alkaloids have been identified and placed into two groups. Alkaloids in the phenanthrene group possess narcotic properties; morphine and codeine are two clinically significant opioids in this group. The benzylisoquinoline group yields drugs such as papaverine and noscapine that lack narcotic activity but are used as antitussives and smooth muscle relaxants.

Morphine constitutes approximately 10 percent of the opium powder and is the oldest narcotic in use at present. It is also the standard with which all other narcotics are compared.

The following information about this class of drugs pertains to morphine as well as the others unless otherwise specified. The narcotics to be discussed are morphine, meperidine, fentanyl, sufentanil, and alfentanil (Fig. 26–12).

Morphine and the other naturally occurring analgesic alkaloids are phenanthrene derivatives, so called because of the tricyclic system they contain. Meperidine, fentanyl, sufentanil, and alfentanil are chemically dissimilar to morphine and are phenylpiperidine derivatives (Fig. 26–13).

The analgesic activity of the opiates is highly stereospecific in that the levoisomer produces the analgesic effects.[85,86] A tertiary nitrogen, a quaternary carbon separated from the

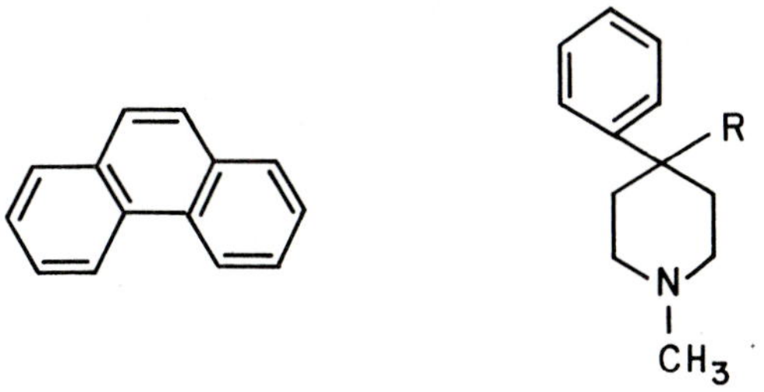

Phenanthrene   **α-Phenyl-N-methyl piperidine**

Figure 26–13. Chemical structures of phenanthrene and piperidine. The phenanthrene rings are evident in the structure of morphine; the piperidine structure is contained in meperidine.

nitrogen by an ethane chain, and an electrophilic carbon that attaches a phenylic or ketone group appear to be common structural characteristics.[86]

Meperidine is a totally synthetic opiate introduced in 1939 by Eisleb and Schaumann in Germany. It was originally studied because of its atropine-like effect and the similarity of its chemical structure to that of atropine. Initial tests demonstrated a narcotic analgesic property and subsequent studies verified this effect.

Like meperidine, fentanyl is a synthetic piperidine derivative. It was introduced in 1963 by Janssen as the narcotic component of Innovar. Sufentanil and alfentanil are the newest of the available synthetic opioids used in anesthesia. Both are chemical analogs of fentanyl with very similar effects.

Absorption, Metabolism, and Excretion. Narcotics are absorbed completely from all routes of administration. Those used for anesthesia are usually administered by intravenous injection and therefore the pharmacokinetics of absorption is not a major consideration.

With respect to tissue uptake and distribution, narcotics follow the same pharmacokinetic principles as other drugs injected intravenously. Plasma levels of narcotics fall rapidly after injection, and only a small percentage of the injected drug actually reaches the central nervous system tissues (Table 26–7). Plasma concentrations of narcotics have been noted to be higher in older individuals.[87] The elderly are also more sensitive to the respiratory depressant effects of narcotics.

Narcotics are metabolized in the liver and their primary route of excretion is the kidneys. Approximately 5 percent of morphine is N-demethylated and almost all of this is excreted as normorphine in the urine. Only about 5 to 10 percent of free morphine or any of its metabolites can be detected in the feces. Respiratory depression after morphine anesthesia has been found to be inversely related to urinary flow rate and excretion of morphine. Patients with low urine outputs have been shown to have a longer period of respiratory depression after high-dose morphine anesthesia.[88]

Meperidine is N-demethylated to normeperidine and hydrolyzed to meperidinic acid. N-demethylation of the meperidinic acid occurs, forming normeperidinic acid. The liver conjugates these metabolites with glucuronide before they are excreted in the urine.[89]

A hydrolytic reaction in the liver metabolizes 80 to 90 percent of fentanyl and produces 4-*n*-(N-proprionyl-anilino)piperidine and proprionic acid. An oxidative reaction also occurs but to a much smaller extent. Only about 10 percent of fentanyl is excreted unchanged. Approximately 70 percent of the administered drug is excreted in 4 days, with the greatest concentration detected between 8 and 24 hours after administration. The brevity of action of fentanyl is due primarily to rapid redistribution rather than to rapid metabolism and excretion.

The major sites of sufentanil biotransformation are the liver and small bowel. Approximately 80 percent of the drug is excreted in the urine and feces within 24 hours; 20 percent of the drug is excreted unchanged.

Alfentanil is classified as an ultrashort-acting narcotic (as opposed to fentanyl and sufentanyl, which are short-acting). Alfentanil has a duration of action approximately one-third that of fentanyl. The shorter duration of action of alfentanil reflects its kinetic profile. Alfentanil is less lipid soluble than sufentanil and fentanyl. Its volume of distribution and clearance are lower, and its elimination half-life is much shorter. The lower volume of distribution results in greater access of the drug to clearing organs and a shorter elimination half-life despite the low clearance. In contrast to fentanyl, the clinical duration may be more dependent on metabolism than redistribution. There is less of a cumulative effect when compared with fentanyl.

The liver is the major site of biotransformation of alfentanil. Approximately 81 percent of the administered dose is excreted within 24 hours; 0.2 percent of the dose is eliminated unchanged. Excretion is primarily by the renal route.[90]

Pharmacologic Effects
Central Nervous System. Narcotic effects on the central nervous system include analgesia, drowsiness, mood changes, and mental clouding.

The site and mechanism of analgesic action are be-

TABLE 26–7. COMPARISON OF FENTANYL, SUFENTANIL, ALFENTANIL, AND MORPHINE

	Fentanyl	Sufentanil	Alfentanil	Morphine
Potency	130	1,250	30	1
Therapeutic index	277	26,000	1080	70
Elimination half-life (min)	219	164	94	180
Volume of distribution (L/kg)	4	3	1	3
Clearance (L/kg/min)	13.0	12.7	5.0	14.7

lieved to be the result of stimulation of the opioid receptors. The receptors of this system are excited by narcotics, endorphins, enkephalins, and electrical stimulation and are located around the third ventricle, the cerebral aqueduct, and the rostral areas of the fourth ventricle. Stimulation of this system is believed to cause descending inhibition of transmission of nociceptive information through the spinal cord. Narcotics also induce an alteration in the limbic system response to painful stimuli without significant alteration of the sensory pathways. The narcotics do not alter the threshold or responsiveness of the nerve endings to painful stimuli, nor do they affect peripheral nerve conduction.

Clinically, pain threshold is raised and the perception of response to pain is blunted. The painful stimulus may be noted but not perceived as painful. Patients often report that the pain is present but tolerable.

Dull, continuous pain can be relieved more effectively than sharp intermittent pain, but most types of pain can be relieved by narcotics if sufficient doses are administered. Analgesia usually occurs without loss of consciousness but sedation, drowsiness, and mental clouding become more prominent as the dose is increased. Therapeutic doses usually produce minimal sedative effects, but increasingly larger doses produce effects that range from sedation to coma.

When an appropriate amount of narcotic is administered to a patient with pain, discomfort, fear, anxiety, or tension, the patient reports that he or she is less distressed. Drowsiness, euphoria, or sleep may ensue. The onset of sedation is slower than that of the analgesic effect but its duration is greater. Narcotics given to patients who are without pain may cause dysphoria rather than euphoria and unnecessary anxiety or fear.

Although narcotics provide excellent analgesia, they do not always provide amnesia when used alone. Amnesia may be associated with loss of consciousness after large doses of narcotics. Narcotics combined with nitrous oxide will produce amnesia during general anesthesia but narcotic-with-oxygen techniques should not be relied on to produce amnesia.

Nausea and vomiting are due primarily to the ability of narcotics to directly stimulate the CTZ located in the medulla.[1] A vestibular component may be involved as well, because there appears to be a greater incidence of emesis in ambulatory patients. Other causes of nausea and vomiting after narcotic administration include delayed emptying of gastrointestinal contents, increased tone of smooth muscle and sphincters, and increased volume of pancreatic and biliary secretions. Hypotension and inadequate cerebral perfusion may also stimulate the CTZ. Very large doses of narcotics may depress it. The emetic effect is counteracted by narcotic antagonists, phenothiazines, droperidol, and drugs used for motion sickness.

Cardiovascular System. Myocardial depression is not a feature of intravenously administered fentanyl, sufentanil, or alfentanil. Morphine has a positive inotropic effect on dogs that is dependent on the release of endogenous catecholamines[91]; this effect can be blocked by beta blockers. Plasma and urine catecholamine levels are usually elevated after meperidine or morphine administration as in plasma histamine.[92] Morphine, fentanyl, sufentanil, and alfentanil are benign with respect to myocardial function, whereas meperidine has been found to cause significant depression.[93]

Morphine is thought to depress intraatrial and atrioventricular nodal conduction.[94] Intravenous administration of meperidine often causes a significant increase in heart rate as a result of a vagolytic effect. With the exception of meperidine, all narcotics can cause a vagal-induced bradycardia. The decrease in heart rate may be related to the dose, the rate of injection, or both.

All narcotics produce a certain degree of arterial and venodilating effects. Morphine is believed to possess an alpha-blocking property, and its effects on the capacitance vessels are much more profound and prolonged than on the arterial system.[95] The venodilating effects appear to be dose dependent and usually are not significant at lower doses.[96] Histamine release also plays a role in vasodilation after morphine or meperidine administration. This effect is rarely seen with fentanyl, sufentanil, or alfentanil.

Hypotension after narcotic injections may be caused by a number of factors. Hypotension after morphine administration is usually attributed to increased plasma histamine resulting in lowered vascular resistance or to a direct effect of morphine on vascular smooth muscle. Meperidine is a myocardial depressant and it also releases histamine, and hypotension after meperidine is usually attributed to these factors. Administration of fentanyl, sufentanil, or alfentanil may cause hypotension because of an accompanying bradycardia. Sufentanil may also have a direct effect on vascular smooth muscle that contributes to hypotension.[97] Hypotension can occur with any narcotic and is usually related to the rate of injection and the volume status of the patient. Fluid administration and a slight Trendelenburg position usually correct the hypotensive episode.

Intravenous narcotics combined with nitrous oxide produce cardiovascular effects quite different from the effects of the narcotic alone. The meperidine–nitrous oxide combination produces a reduction in the arterial pressure and a significant lowering of cardiac output and stroke volume with an increase in peripheral vascular resistance. Combinations of nitrous oxide with other narcotics also produce a similar effect. The reduction in cardiac output is usually greater than the reduction in mean arterial pressure caused by the increase in systemic vascular resistance and may not be evident during routine cardiovascular monitoring.

Cerebral blood flow is not directly affected by narcotics. Respiratory depression and carbon dioxide retention caused by large doses of narcotics will produce cerebral vasodilation and an increase in intracranial and cerebrospinal fluid pressure. Artificial ventilation that maintains $Paco_2$ at normal levels will maintain a normal cerebral blood flow despite large doses of narcotics.

Respiratory System. Therapeutic doses of narcotics produce respiratory depression that can be detected without other apparent signs of central nervous system depression. The respiratory depression is dose related and can proceed to apnea with large doses.

The mechanism of respiratory depression involves direct depression of the medullary centers involved in ventilatory control.[98] There is a reduction in the response of the central chemoreceptors to carbon dioxide levels as well as a decrease in response of the carotid and aortic chemoreceptors to hypoxia. The carbon dioxide threshold is elevated and the P_{CO_2}–alveolar ventilation curve is shifted to the right. The pontine and medullary centers involved in ventilatory rhythmicity are also depressed, which may result in irregular and periodic breathing. Often, the inspiratory phase is prolonged and the expiratory phase is delayed.

Respiratory rate, minute volume, and tidal volume are all depressed. Small doses of narcotics decrease the respiratory rate without significantly affecting tidal exchange, whereas anesthetic doses may terminate involuntary respirations. Voluntary mechanisms for ventilation remain intact and the patients are able to respond to commands to breathe. The respiratory rate is greatly depressed but at this stage the tidal volume is markedly increased to compensate. Narcotic overdoses and deaths usually result from profound respiratory depression and respiratory arrest.

Other effects of narcotics on respiration include depression of ciliary action within the bronchial tree, inhibition of the cough reflex caused by action on the cough center located in the medulla, and increased bronchial tone. It is not clear whether the last effect is mainly a direct effect on smooth muscle or an indirect action caused by histamine liberation or elevation of the Pa_{CO_2}.

Miscellaneous Effects. Opiates decrease gastric and intestinal secretions and motility and decrease lower esophageal sphincter tone.[99] There is a delay in gastric emptying and the passage of bowel contents. Because of the delay, water is more completely absorbed. This is believed to contribute to the constipating effects of narcotics. Propulsive contractions of the bowel are virtually abolished, and the tone may be increased to the point of spasm. Atropine partially antagonizes the spasmogenic action but has little effect on the decreased propulsive activity.

Opiates tend to stimulate smooth muscle of the gastrointestinal and genitourinary tracts, and the resulting spasms can create increased pressure within these tracts, producing pain or rupturing smooth muscle that has been weakened by surgery or disease. Biliary colic and spasm are intensified by morphine. Meperidine and fentanyl can also precipitate biliary colic but to a lesser degree than morphine. It has been noted that patients who are already suffering from colic can obtain relief of their pain from opiates even though these do increase the intensity of the spasm.

The opiates cause pupillary constriction, which occurs even in total darkness. The exact mechanism by which narcotics induce miosis is uncertain but is believed to be a central effect via the Edinger–Westphal nucleus of the oculomotor nerve rather than an effect on the pupillary sphincter. Anticholinergics can counteract the opioid-induced miosis. Tolerance to the miotic effect is not usually seen, and miosis can be detected even in heroin addicts.

Renal System. It was previously thought that the antidiuretic effect of morphine was due to the release of ADH. The decrease in urine output noted with the use of morphine anesthesia is now believed to be related to renal hemodynamics.[100] Rapid administration of the drug and the addition of nitrous oxide may decrease hemodynamic function enough that the GFR and urine output are markedly diminished. Fentanyl, sufentanil, and alfentanil are believed to cause only minimal changes in renal function.

Uncatheterized patients may have decreased urine output caused by the increased detrusor tone and contraction of muscles and urethral sphincters, which makes urination difficult.[89] The central effects of the drugs may render the patient inattentive to the stimuli arising in the bladder.

Clinical Uses. In anesthesia, narcotics are often used (1) for premedication, (2) as adjuncts to regional or local anesthesia, (3) for postoperative analgesia, and (4) as anesthetic agents.

Premedication. Narcotic premedications should not be used routinely but are usually reserved for the patient with pain or patients who may require some analgesia before the induction of anesthesia. There are also those who believe that narcotic premedications lower the anesthetic requirements during general anesthesia and that certain narcotics in themselves provide tranquilizing effects. Most anesthetists ordering a narcotic premedication will order a combination with a benzodiazepine, phenothiazine, barbiturate, or other major tranquilizer. This combination is often used for patients about to undergo surgery with regional or local anesthesia or narcotic–nitrous oxide general anesthesia. Narcotic premedication can often provide some postoperative analgesia after inhalation anesthesia for a short surgical procedure.

Narcotic premedication should be avoided in patients who cannot tolerate even mild respiratory depression (e.g., those at risk of increasing intracranial pressure or with severe pulmonary compromise). Although histamine release from premedicant doses of narcotics is rarely a problem, this should be kept in mind when ordering morphine or meperidine for asthmatics. Administration of morphine to patients with biliary colic or some history of significant biliary tract disease is contraindicated.

Adjunct to Regional or Local Anesthesia. For this purpose, intravenous narcotics are used in conjunction with tranquilizers such as midazolam, diazepam, lorazepam, and droperidol to provide sedation and analgesia. Some patients receiving a regional or local anesthetic are very anxious and will request sedation, amnesia, or both. The narcotic and tranquilizer must be titrated to achieve the desired effect. The desired effect is usually a calm, sedate but responsive and cooperative patient. Care should be taken not to oversedate and render the patient apneic or unresponsive.

Immediate Postoperative Analgesia. Anesthetists often administer analgesics in the recovery room for postoperative pain. The intravenous route is the route of choice because the effects are immediate and the uncertainty of the rate of absorption is not a problem. The drug must be titrated, starting with small doses. It must be remembered that the postoperative patient is frequently still depressed from the anesthetic agents received during the surgery. These patients usually require very small doses of narcotics to obtain analgesia. The respiratory rate should be monitored closely in patients receiving intravenous analgesics in the recovery room.

Narcotic Anesthesia. Narcotics are often used with nitrous oxide, oxygen, and a muscle relaxant for a technique known as balanced anesthesia or with oxygen and muscle relaxants without nitrous oxide. The narcotic provides analgesia; the nitrous oxide supplements the analgesic effect and provides amnesia. Muscle relaxation can be achieved by any nondepolarizing relaxant or a succinylcholine drip.

The aim of balanced anesthesia is to maintain a consistent level of narcosis during the anesthetic. This can be accomplished by titrating the narcotic by intermittent doses or by continuous infusion. The advantages of the narcotic–nitrous oxide technique are that it (1) produces very little alteration in cardiovascular dynamics; (2) decreases laryngeal, tracheal, and cough reflexes; (3) does not cause myocardial sensitization to catecholamines; (4) permits a smooth emergence; (5) provides postoperative analgesia; and (6) decreases metabolic rate. The technique does, however, have disadvantages, including (1) possible cardiovascular depression in the susceptible patient, especially if nitrous oxide is added; (2) chest wall rigidity with rapid administration; (3) no muscle relaxation; (4) requirement of at least 50 percent nitrous oxide (thus it may not be a wise choice for middle ear surgery or bowel obstruction); (5) possible renarcotization after reversal; and (6) decreased cough reflex postoperatively.

REFERENCES

1. Benet LZ, Mitchell JR, Sheiner LB. Pharmacokinetics: The dynamics of drug absorption, distribution and elimination. In: Goodman GA, Rall TW, Nies AS, Taylor P, eds. *The pharmacological basis of therapeutics.* New York: Pergamon Press; 1990:3.
2. Hug CC Jr. Pharmacokinetics of drugs administered intravenously. *Anesth Analg.* 1978;57:704–723.
3. Breimer DD. Clinical pharmacokinetics of hypnotics. *Clin Pharmacokinet.* 1977;2:93–109.
4. Stanley TH. Pharmacology of intravenous non-narcotic anesthetics. In: Miller R, ed. *Anesthesia.* New York: Churchill Livingstone; 1981:451–459.
5. Dundee JW. Intravenous anesthetic agents. In: Feldman HS, Scurr E, eds. *Current topics in anesthesia.* Chicago: Yearbook Medical; 1979.
6. Dundee JW. Comparative analysis of intravenous anesthetics. *Anesthesiology.* 1971;35:137–148.
7. Price HL, Kovnat PJ, Safer JN, Conner EH, Price ML. The uptake of thiopental by body tissues and its relation to the duration of hypnosis. *Clin Pharmacol Ther.* 1960;1:16–22.
8. Collins, VJ. *Principles of anesthesiology.* 2nd ed. Philadelphia: Lea & Febiger; 1976;chaps 21–23.
9. Brooks LM, Bollman JL, Flock EV, et al. Tissue distribution with time following single intravenous administration of sodium pentothal. *Am J Physiol.* 1948;155:429.
10. Brodie BB. Physiological disposition and chemical fate of thiobarbiturates in the body. *Fed Proc.* 1952;11:632.
11. Rall TW. Hypnotics and sedatives: Ethanol. In: Goodman GA, Rall TW, Nies AS, Taylor P, eds. *The pharmacological basis of therapeutics.* New York: Pergamon Press; 1990:345.
12. Breimer DD. Pharmacokinetics of methohexitone following intravenous infusion in humans. *Br J Anaesth.* 1976;48:643–648.
13. Dundee JW, Wyatt GM. *Intravenous anesthesia.* Edinburgh: Churchill Livingstone; 1974:64–127.
14. Aldrete JA, Stanley TH, eds. *Trends in intravenous anesthesia.* Chicago: Year Book Medical; 1980.
15. Olson RW. Barbiturates. *Int Anesthesiol Clin.* 1988;26:254.
16. Clutton-Brock J. Pain and the barbiturates. *Anaesthesia.* 1961;16:80–88.
17. Dundee JW. Alterations in response to somatic pain. II. The effect of thiopentone and pentobarbitone. *Br J Anaesth.* 1960;32:407–414.
18. Dundee JW. Some effects of premedication on the induction characteristics of intravenous anaesthetics. *Anaesthesia.* 1965;20:299–314.
19. Barron DW. Methohexital. *Int. Anesthesiol Clin.* 1969;7:33.
20. Eckstein JW, Hamilton WK, McCammond JM. The effect of thiopental on peripheral venous tone. *Anesthesiology.* 1961;22:252.
21. Sonntag H, Hellberg K, Schenk HD, et al. Effects of thiopental on coronary blood flow and myocardial metabolism in man. *Acta Anesthesiol Scand.* 1975;19:69.
22. Habif DV, Papper EM, Fitzpatrick HF, et al. The renal and hepatic blood flow, glomerular filtration rate, and urinary output of electrolytes during cyclopropane, ether and thiopental anesthesia and the immediate post operative period. *Surgery.* 1951;30:241.
23. Lorenz W, Doenicke A, et al. Histamine release in man by propanidid and thiopentone: Pharmacologic effects and clinical consequences. *Br J Anaesth.* 1972;44:355.
24. Harrison GA. The influence of different anesthetic agents in the response to respiratory tract infection. *Br J Anaesth.* 1962;34:804.
25. Evans RH, Hill RG. GABA-mimetic action of etomidate. *Br J Pharmacol.* 1977;61:484.
26. Ghoneim MM, Yamada T. Etomidate: A clinical and electrographic comparison with thiopental. *Anesth Analg.* 1977;56:479.
27. Renou AM, Vemhiet J, Macrez P. Cerebral blood flow and metabolism during etomidate anesthesia in man. *Br J Anaesth.* 1978;50:1047.
28. Giese JL, Stockham RJ, Stanley TH, et al. Etomidate versus thiopental for induction of anesthesia. *Anesth Analg.* 1985;64:871.
29. Lamalle D. Cardiovascular effects of various anesthetics in man. Four short-acting intravenous anesthetics: Althesin, etomidate, methohexital, and propanidid. *Acta Anaesthesiol Belg.* 1976;27:208–224.
30. Kettler D, Sonntag H. Dontah M, et al. Hemodynamics, myocardial mechanics, oxygen requirements and oxygen consumption of the human heart during etomidate induction into anaesthesia. *Anaesthetist.* 1974;23:116.
31. Gooding J, Corssen G. Effect of etomidate on the cardiovascular system. *Anesth Analg.* 1977;56:717.
32. Guldager H, Sodergaard I, Jensen FM, Cold G. Basophil histamine release in asthma patients after in vitro provocation with althesin and etomidate. *Acta Anaesthesiol Scand.* 1985;29:352.
33. Morgan M, Lumley J, Whitwan JG. Respiratory effects of etomidate. *Br J Anaesth.* 1977;49:233.
34. Ledingham IM, Findlay WE, et al. Etomidate and adrenocortical function. *Lancet.* 1983;1:1434.
35. Diago MC, Amado JA, Otero M, Lopez-Cordovilla JJ. Antiadrenal action of a subanesthetic dose of etomidate. *Anaesthesia.* 1988;43:644–645.
36. Schulte HM, Benker G, Reinwein D, Sippell WG, Allolio B. Infusion of low dose etomidate: Correction of hypercortisolemia in patients with Cushing's syndrome and dose–response relationship in normal subjects. *J Clin Endocrinol Metab.* 1989;70:1426–1430.
37. Sear JW, Edwards CRW, Atherden SM. Dual effect of etomidate on mineralocorticoid biosynthesis. *Acta Anaesthesiol Belg.* 1988;39:87–94.

38. Wagner RL, White PF, Kan PB, Rosenthal MH, Feldman D. Inhibition of adrenal steroidogenesis by the anesthetic etomidate. *N Engl J Med.* 1984;310:1415–1421.

39. Crozier TA, Beck D, Schlaeger M, Wultke W, Kettler D. Endocrinological changes following etomidate, midazolam, or methohexital for minor surgery. *Anesthesiology.* 1987;66:628–635.

40. Holdcraft A, Morgan M, Whitwan JG, et al. Effect of dose and premedication on induction complications with etomidate. *Br J Anesth.* 1976;48:199.

41. Giese JL, Stockham RJ, Stanley TH, et al. Etomidate versus thiopental for induction of anesthesia. *Anesth Analg.* 1985;64:871.

42. Zacharias M, Clark RS, Dundee JW, Johnston SB. Venous sequelae following etomidate. *Br J Anaesth.* 1979;51:779.

43. Zacharias M, Dundee JW, Clark PS, Hegarty JE. Effect of preanesthetic medication on etomidate. *Br J Anaesth.* 1979;51:127.

44. Boill JG, Clark RSJ, Davis EA, Dundee JW. Some cardiovascular effects of ketamine. *Br J Pharmacol.* 1971;41:411.

45. Corssen G, Domino EF. Dissociative anesthesia: Further pharmacologic studies and first clinical experience with the phencyclidine derivative CI-581. *Anesth Analg.* 1966;45:29.

46. Miyasaka M, Domino EF. Neural mechanisms of ketamine-induced anesthesia. *Int J Neuropharmacol.* 1968;7:557.

47. Dowdy EG, Kaya K. Studies of the mechanisms of cardiovascular responses to CI-581. *Anesthesiology.* 1968;29:931.

48. Flacke JW, Flacke WE, Mehmed H, Seifen EE. A peripheral cocaine-like effect of ketamine. In: *Abstracts of science papers, ASA Meeting, New York, 1971.*

49. Stanley V, Hunt J, Willis KW, Stephen CR. Cardiovascular and respiratory function with CI-581. *Anesth Analg.* 1968;47:760.

50. Taylor PA, Towey RM. Depression of laryngeal reflexes during ketamine anesthesia. *Br Med J.* 1971;2:688.

51. Huber FC, Reves JC, Gutierrez J, Corssen G. Ketamine: Its effect on airway resistance in man. *South Med J.* 1972;65:1176.

52. Corssen G, Gutierrez J, Reves JC, Huber FC. Ketamine in the anesthetic management of asthmatic patients. *Anesth Analg.* 1972;51:588.

53. Dundee JW, Lilbum JK. Ketamine–lorazepam: Attenuation of the psychic sequelae of ketamine by lorazepam. *Anaesthesia.* 1977;37:312.

54. White PF. Propofol: Pharmacokinetics and pharmacodynamics. *Semin Anesth.* 1988;7:4–20.

55. Sebel PS, Lowdon JD. Propofol: A new intravenous anesthetic. *Anesthesiology.* 1989;71:260–277.

56. Stoelting RK. Nonbarbiturate induction drugs. In: *Pharmacology and physiology of anesthetic practice.* 2nd ed. Philadelphia: JB Lippincott; 1991:143–147.

57. Dailland P, Cockshott ID, Lirzin JD, et al. Intravenous propofol during cesarean section: Placental transfer, concentrations in breast milk and neonatal effects. A preliminary study. *Anesthesiology.* 1989;71:827–834.

58. Waugaman WR, Foster SD. New advances in anesthesia. *Nurs Clin North Am.* 1991;26:451–461.

59. Mirakhur RK. Induction characteristics of propofol in children: Comparison with thiopentone. *Anaesthesia.* 1988;43:593.

60. Purcell-Jones G, Yates A, Baker JR, et al. Comparison of the induction characteristics of thiopentone and propofol in children. *Br J Anaesth.* 1987;59:1431.

61. Robinson FP. Propofol (Diprivan®) by intermittent bolus with nitrous oxide in oxygen for body surface operations. *Postgrad Med J.* 1985;61:116.

62. James MFM, Reyneke CJ, Whiffler K. Heart block following propofol: A case report. *Br J Anaesth.* 1989;62:213–215.

63. Watcha MF, Simeon RM, White PF, Stevens JL. Effect of propofol on the incidence of postoperative vomiting after strabismus surgery in pediatric outpatients. *Anesthesiology.* 1991;75:204–209.

64. Mohler H, Richards JG. The benzodiazepine receptor: A pharmacological control element of brain function. *Eur J Anaesthesiol.* 1988;2:15.

65. Heisterkamp DV, Cohen PJ. The effect of intravenous premedication with lorazepam (Ativan), pentobarbitone or diazepam on recall. *Br J Anaesth.* 1975;47:79–81.

66. Rao S, Sherbaniuk RW, Prasad K, et al. Cardiopulmonary effects of diazepam. *Clin Pharmacol Ther.* 1973;14:182.

67. Hegarty JE, Dundee JW. Sequelae after the intravenous injection of three benzodiazepines—Diazepam, lorazepam and flunitrazepam. *Br Med J.* 1977;2:1384–1385.

68. Blitt CD, Petty WC, et al. Clinical evaluation of injectable lorazepam as a premedicant: The effect on recall. *Anesth Analg.* 1976;55:522–525.

69. Reves, JG, Glass PSA. Non-barbiturate intravenous anesthetics. In: Miller RD, ed. *Anesthesia.* New York: Churchill Livingstone; 1990:243–279.

70. Dundee JW, Halliday NJ, Harper KW, Brogden RN. Midazolam—A review of its pharmacological properties and therapeutic uses. *Drugs.* 1984;28:519–543.

71. Reves JG, Samuelson PN, Linnan M. Effects of midazolam maleate in patients with elevated pulmonary artery occluded pressure. In: Aldrete JA, Stanley TH, eds. *Trends in intravenous anesthesia.* Chicago: Year Book Medical; 1980:253–257.

72. Samuelson PN, Reves JG, Kouchoukos NT, Smith LR, Dole KM. Hemodynamic responses to anesthetic induction with midazolam or diazepam in patients with ischemic heart disease. *Anesth Analg.* 1981;60:802.

73. Gross JB, Zebrowski ME, Carel WO, et al. Time course of ventilatory depression after thiopental and midazolam in normal subjects and in patients with chronic obstructive pulmonary disease. *Anesthesiology.* 1983;58:540.

74. Gross JB, Smith TC. Ventilation after midazolam and thiopental in subjects with COPD. *Anesthesiology.* 1981;55:A384.

75. Caldwell CB, Gross JB. Physostigmine reversal of midazolam-induced sedation. *Anesthesiology.* 1982;57:125.

76. Lebowitz PW, Cote ME, Daniels AL, Bonventive J. Comparative renal effects of midazolam and thiopental. *Anesthesiology.* 1982;57:35.

77. Vinik HR, Reves JG, Greenblatt DJ, Abernethy DR. Pharmacokinetics of midazolam in chronic renal failure patients. *Anesthesiology.* 1983;59:390–394.

78. Allonen H, Ziegler G, Klotz U. Midazolam kinetics. *Clin Pharmacol Ther.* 1981;30:653.

79. Fox JWC, Fox E. Neuroleptanalgesia: A review. *NC Med J.* 1966;27:471.

80. Corssen G, Reves JG, Stanley TH. Neuroleptanalgesia and neuroleptanesthesia. In: Corssen G, et al., eds. *Intravenous anesthesia and analgesia.* Philadelphia: Lea & Febiger; 1988:175.

81. Yelnosky J, Katz R, Dietrich EV. A study of some pharmacologic actions of droperidol. *Toxicol Appl Pharmacol.* 1964;6:37.

82. Bailey PL, Stanley TH. Narcotic intravenous anesthetics. In: Miller RD. *Anesthesia.* New York: Churchill Livingstone; 1990:287.

83. Stanley TH, Webster LR. Anesthetic requirements and cardiovascular effects of fentanyl–oxygen and fentanyl–diazepam–oxygen anesthesia in man. *Anesth Analg.* 1978;57:411.

84. Cartwright P, Prys-Roberts C, Gill K, et al. Ventilatory depression related to plasma fentanyl concentrations during and after anesthesia in humans. *Anesth Analg.* 1983;62:966.

85. Thorpe AH. Opiate structure and activity: A guide to understanding the receptor. *Anesth Analg.* 1984;63:143.

86. Beckett AH, Casey AF. Synthetic analgesics, stereochemical considerations. *J Pharm Pharmacol.* 1954;6:986.

87. Berkowitz BA, Ngai SH, Yang JC, et al. The disposition of morphine in surgical patients. *Clin Pharmacol Ther*. 1975;17:629.

88. Stanley TH, Lathrup GD. Urinary excretion of morphine during and after valvular and coronary-artery surgery. *Anesthesiology*. 1977;46:166.

89. Jaffe JH, Martin WR. Opioid analgesics and antagonists. In: Goodman GA, Rall TW, Nies AS, Taylor P, eds. *The pharmacological basis of therapeutics*. New York: Pergamon Press; 1990:485.

90. Hull CJ. The pharmacokinetics of alfentanil in man. *Br J Anaesth*. 1983;55:1575–1645.

91. Vasko JS, Henney RP, Brawley RK, et al. Effects of morphine on ventricular function and myocardial contractile force. *Am J Physiol*. 1966;210:329.

92. Flacke JW, Van Etton AP, Bloor BC, et al. Histamine release by four narcotics: A double blind study in humans. *Anesth Analg*. 1987;66:723.

93. Sugioka K, Boniface KJ, Davis DA. The influence of meperidine on myocardial contractility in the intact dog. *Anesthesiology*. 1957; 18:623.

94. Kennedy BL, West TC. Effect of morphine on electrically-induced release of autonomic mediators in the rabbit sinoatrial node. *J Pharmacol Exp Ther*. 1967;157:149.

95. Hsu HO, Hickey RF, Forbes AR. Morphine decreases peripheral vascular resistance and increases capacitance in man. *Anesthesiology*. 1979;50:98.

96. Stanley TH, Gray NJ, Staford W, Armstrong R. The effects of high-dose morphine on fluid and blood requirements in open heart operations. *Anesthesiology*. 1973;38:536.

97. Starck T, Hall D, Freas W, et al. Peripheral vascular depression with sufentanil in the dog. *Anesth Analg*. 1989;68:S277.

98. Tabatabai M, Kitahata LM, Collins JG. Disruption of the rhythmic activity of the medullary respiratory neurons and phrenic nerve by fentanyl and reversal with nalbuphine. *Anesthesiology*. 1989;70:489.

99. Dowlatshahi K, Evander A, Walther B, Skinner DB. Influence of morphine on the distal oesophagus and the lower oesophageal sphincter—A manometric study. *Gut*. 1985;26:802.

100. Deutsch S, Bastron RD, Pierce EC, Vandam LD. The effects of anaesthesia with thiopentone, nitrous oxide, narcotics and neuromuscular blocking drugs on renal function in normal man. *Br J Anaesth*. 1969;4:807.

Pharmacology of Local Anesthesia

Michael D. Stanton-Hicks

Local anesthetics are chemical substances that can, by definition, cause the temporary loss of sensation in a circumscribed area of the body. This loss of sensation, or anesthesia, results from a reversible depression of the process of nervous conduction. Though such a state can be produced in nervous tissues by many physical and chemical agents, this discussion is confined to those compounds that temporarily interrupt nerve conduction by preventing the process of depolarization (omitting those neurolytic substances that act in a different manner and are more commonly used in the treatment of intractable pain).

HISTORY OF LOCAL ANESTHESIA

Local anesthesia began with the isolation of cocaine from the *Erythroxylon coca* bush, a plant indigenous to Peru, by Niemann in 1860, but any clinical application had to await the revelation by Koller, a pupil of Freud, of its use as a topical anesthetic for surgery on the eye. Soon after this discovery, cocaine was used for spinal anesthesia by Bier in Germany and within a year, in 1898, by Halstead in the United States for blocks of the brachial plexus. After its chemical identification as an ester of benzoic acid, many similar compounds were synthesized, among them the topical anesthetic benzocaine. Unfortunately, because of its addictive qualities, cocaine was very quickly relegated to the historical shelf; however, because of its unique propensity among local anesthetics to produce vasoconstriction, it still has a limited but specific use to this day as a topical anesthetic for mucous membranes. Benzocaine was poorly soluble in water, but procaine, another ester of *para*-aminobenzoic acid, synthesized by Einhorn and Braun in 1905, proved to be sufficiently water soluble and to have such a satisfactory margin of safety that its clinical use as an injectable agent was ensured. Of the many hundreds of ester local anesthetics synthesized in the ensuing half-century, tetracaine, discovered in 1930, and chloroprocaine, in 1952, have remained clinically important. More of these ester-type local anesthetics would have been developed but for the fact that they are associated with the production of endogenous hypersensitivity.

A major departure from this class occurred when, in 1943, Löfgren synthesized lidocaine. This became the forerunner of a completely new type of chemical compound, the amino amides. Fortunately, the amino amides seem to be practically free from any tendency to produce allergic reactions and, in addition, possess other kinds of local anesthetic action that are an improvement over the esters. Most recently interest has centered around a group of biologically related substances called guanidines, which are extremely potent inhibitors of nerve function. At this time, however, these are still experimental curiosities; this account concerns itself with a description of the two main classes of local anesthetics already mentioned, the amino esters and the amino amides.

PHYSIOLOGY OF NERVE CONDUCTION

To understand the principles of local anesthetic pharmacology a description of neural anatomy and physiology is necessary.

Anatomy

All peripheral nerves contain a mixture of sensory and motor elements, the size and histology of which vary with their particular function. The principal element, or *axon*, is surrounded by a connective tissue sheath called the *endoneurium*; groups of axons are bound together by more connective tissue, forming an external sheath known as the *perineurium*. The perineurium then binds these groups of axons into what is seen as a peripheral nerve fiber (Fig. 27–1). The axon itself is encased in myelin and, depending on whether the myelin is in a single or multiple layers, the axon is referred to as unmyelinated (C fiber) or myelinated (A and B fibers) nerve, respectively. The myelin is produced by Schwann cells; the nuclei of these cells can be seen in histologic sections (Fig. 27–2). Although it consists primarily of lipid, the myelin sheath does contain some protein, which,

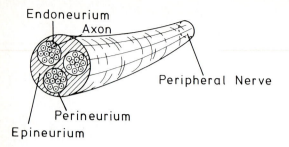

Figure 27–1. Schematic drawing of a peripheral nerve fiber in which the principal structures are illustrated.

when added to the cell membrane (axolemma), functionally alters the characteristics of the nerve fiber. Conceptually, the cell membrane consists of a bilaminar lipoprotein matrix with the lipoid and protein arranged in a heterogenous fashion as shown in Figure 27–3. The physicochemical properties of local anesthetics (i.e., water solubility, lipid solubility, and protein binding properties) not only determine the manner in which they interact with the cell membrane but also dictate the particular characteristics of the resulting nerve block.

Nerve Conduction

The nerve membrane behaves like a semipermeable structure that separates an electrolyte solution high in potassium concentration on the inside of the cell from one high in sodium on the outside. This lipoprotein membrane has small channels, or *pores*, that under certain conditions allow the passage of ions in either direction (although the potassium ion, which is smaller than sodium, can move freely even when the cell is at rest). The selective permeability of this membrane is under the influence of tiny electrical fields. The analogy to small "gates" that control the transit of ions through these channels has been suggested.

Because of the ionic asymmetry across the membrane, an electrochemical potential is created that, at rest, is about − 70 mV in mammalian nerves, the inside being negative with respect to the outside of the cell (Fig. 27–4). During this resting state the cell is said to be polarized, the opposite of

which is depolarization. The electrochemical process of depolarization that results from the increase in ionic permeability occurs only when the nerve has been excited by a stimulus sufficient to achieve what is termed the *depolarization threshold*.

During the process of depolarization, the influx of sodium ions into the cell through the so-called sodium channel is so great that not only is the original electrical potential neutralized, but there is also a slight overshoot as can be seen in Figure 27–5. The "gates" close at this point and potassium ions now move out of the cell. The electrical disturbance created by depolarization spreads along the cell axon, initiating a "wave" of depolarization that travels along the length of the fiber. Repolarization commences in each segment of a nerve immediately after the impulse or wave has been propagated along the complete length of the nerve. This process is initiated by closure of the sodium gates, thereby preventing any further influx of sodium. Potassium, which has until now leaked outside of the membrane, commences its return into the cell, under the influence of both a concentration gradient and the pull of electrostatic forces within the cell. The ionic imbalance caused by sodium influx is now restored by an active metabolic process termed the *sodium pump*, which continuously transports these ions out of the cell to satisfy the previous resting ionic equilibrium. Without such a mechanism requiring metabolic activity, the nerve cell would ultimately become exhausted and cease to develop the ionic gradients necessary for the creation of the electrochemical potential across the membrane.

The foregoing description of impulse propagation along a nerve by the creation of an electrochemical disturbance across its membranes applies only to unmyelinated nerves, which have a thin unilaminar covering of myelin. Propagation in myelinated nerves is different. Here, the electrical impulse jumps from node to node instead of propagating slowly and continuously along the membrane (Fig. 27–6). This saltatory (jumping) action is possible because the nerve membrane at each node of Ranvier is in direct contact with the extracellular fluid and consequently is more excitable than a membrane covered thinly but continuously with myelin. The speed of conduction in such nerves is about 100 m/s, whereas in the smallest unmyelinated nerves (C fibers) the conduction speed is between 1 and 2 m/s.

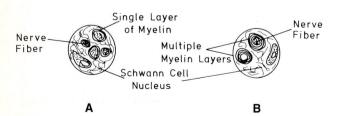

A　　　　**B**

Figure 27–2. Cross sections of a peripheral nerve showing the basic differences between (**A**) unmyelinated and (**B**) myelinated nerves. Schwann cell nuclei, from which myelin is produced, can also be seen.

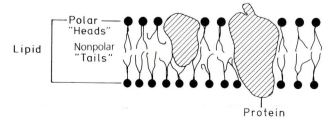

Figure 27–3. The concept of the nerve cell membrane as a bilaminar lipoprotein matrix is illustrated. Note that the protein molecules can "bridge" the entire membrane thickness in places.

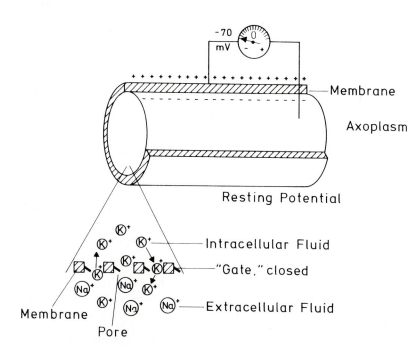

Resting Potential

Intracellular Fluid

"Gate," closed

Extracellular Fluid

Membrane

Pore

Figure 27–4. Diagram of an unmyelinated nerve fiber at rest. Note the resting potential of –70 mV, the inside of the cell being negative with respect to the outside. The magnified section of the nerve membrane illustrates the ionic relationships during this resting phase. Note that ionic passage through the pores is controlled by "gates," which when closed allow free passage to potassium ions (K⁺) but prevent the ingress of sodium ions (Na⁺).

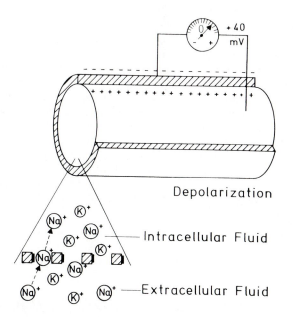

Depolarization

Intracellular Fluid

Extracellular Fluid

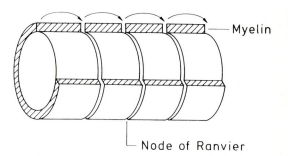

Myelin

Node of Ranvier

Figure 27–5. Diagram of an unmyelinated nerve fiber during depolarization. Note, in comparison with Figure 16–4, that the "gates" are now open, allowing sodium ions to pass into the cell. The electric potential is momentarily 40 mV, the outside of the cell now being negative with respect to the inside.

Figure 27–6. Diagram of depolarization in a myelinated nerve fiber, showing propagation of the electrical impulse from node to node. Voltage changes similar to those described for unmyelinated nerve fibers occur.

MECHANISM OF LOCAL ANESTHETIC ACTION

Almost all of the commercially available local anesthetics are prepared as the hydrochloride (acid) salt of a basic amine. In this form the cation, which is positively charged, is in dissociation equilibrium with the uncharged local anesthetic base:

$$pH = pK_a - \log [BH^+]/[B]$$

Here pH is the hydrogen ion concentration, pK_a is a dissociation constant, $[BH^+]$ is the concentration of positively charged cation, and $[B]$ is the concentration of uncharged base.

The pK_a is a physical constant of any specific local anesthetic, but it is the pH of the solution (or surrounding tissues) that determines the relative concentrations of free base and cation present.

If the pH of the solution or environment decreases, which means the hydrogen ion concentration has increased (more acidic), the equilibrium in the relative concentrations of cation and base shifts so that more local anesthetic will exist in the cationic form. The converse would be true if the pH of the solution were to increase, in which case the equilibrium shifts so that more local anesthetic will occur as the base. This expression is another way of using the principle embodied in the Henderson–Hasselbalch equation:

$$pK_a = pH + \log \frac{(cation)}{(base)}$$

The present theory of local anesthetic action proposes that it is the cationic moiety that is ultimately responsible for producing neural blockade; however, for a local anesthetic to reach its site of action, the base must be present in sufficient concentration to facilitate its passage across (charged) membranes.

The events outlined in Figure 27–7 illustrate the passage of the local anesthetic from its site of deposition outside a nerve into the axon, where its site of action is believed to be. In fact, the description of local anesthetic dissociation is the basis for adding carbon dioxide to local anesthetic solutions to increase the concentration of cation as a result of the lower pH generated by the carbon dioxide inside the nerve membrane.[1] The actual site (receptor) where local anesthetics produce their block is probably at the internal end of the sodium channel. It is believed that displacement of calcium ions from their lipoprotein receptors by local anesthetic cations ultimately blocks the sodium channel, decreasing sodium permeability and thereby inhibiting membrane depolarization. In practice, the local anesthetic moves by diffusion along a concentration gradient from its site of deposition through the tissues and into the nerve. This diffusion continuously decreases the amount of local anesthetic present by dilution and absorption through lymphatic and vascular channels.

Because of an affinity for protein and lipid structures, much of the local anesthetic is also lost to the nerve by binding and dissolution in these structures. One means of achieving a higher concentration of local anesthetic to block the nerve is to add a vasoconstrictor, such as epinephrine, which will decrease its rate of absorption into vascular channels. The size of the fiber also determines the quality of neural blockade. In a mixed nerve, fibers are classified as A, B, and C fibers, representing the different modalities subserved by the nerve. These are of different sizes and in microscopic cross section appear to occur in a random distribution, although in reality there is a certain order. Fibers that subserve proximal structures are situated concentrically on the outer aspect, or mantle, of the nerve, and those fibers that subserve more distal structures occupy the core of the nerve. Attention has been drawn to this order by de Jong. Its practical application is that during the onset of neural blockade, proximal structures will be blocked first and then, as the local anesthetic diffuses into the center of the nerve bundle, those last to be blocked will be the innermost or core fibers.

Because the small C fibers appear to be more easily blocked than large fibers, one might expect that it would be possible to block modalities served by these fibers by means of a given concentration of local anesthetic, thus sparing the function of thicker A fibers; this does indeed occur clinically and is responsible for what is referred to as a "differential block." Recent experimental evidence, however, does not

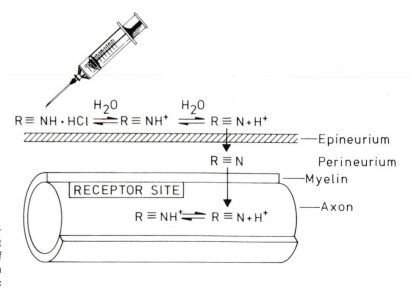

Figure 27–7. Sequence of chemical changes after deposition of the local anesthetic outside of a nerve. It can be seen that the uncharged basic form (R≡N) of the molecule gains access to the inside of the axon where the lower pH causes it to revert to the cationic form.

TABLE 27–1. RELATIONSHIP OF ANESTHETIC POTENCY TO IN VIVO $C_M{}^a$ OF DIFFERENT AGENTS

Drug	Potency	C_M	
		Rat Sciatic Nerve	Cat Sciatic Nerve
Procaine	1	1.000	4.0
Mepivacaine	2	0.500	2.0
Prilocaine	3	0.500	2.0
Chloroprocaine	4	1.000	2.0
Lidocaine	4	0.500	2.0
Tetracaine	16	0.125	0.5
Bupivacaine	16	0.125	0.5
Etidocaine	16	0.125	0.5

^{a} C_M = minimum anesthetic concentration to produce 50% block.
Reprinted, with permission, from Covino BG, Vassallo HG. Local anesthetics: Mechanisms of action and clinical use. New York: Grune & Stratton; 1976.

support this view; in fact, what appears to be a greater sensitivity to local anesthetic action by the small C fibers is in reality an artifact, caused by diffusion barriers, and is not a function of fiber size.[2,3] Therefore, to overcome these diffusion barriers, particularly when muscle relaxation is required in the region for which a nerve block is given, the concentration of the solution must be great enough to block the A fibers responsible for motor activity. A useful concept when considering local anesthetic action has been defined by de Jong as the minimum blocking concentration (C_M). This can be considered analogous to the minimum alveolar concentration (MAC) of a volatile anesthetic that is necessary to provide surgical anesthesia and implies that it is that concentration that will block all elements in a nerve.

One more factor that has a bearing on the effects of local anesthetic block is the frequency with which neural impulses travel along nerve fibers. For example, an isolated axon is much more sensitive to a local anesthetic when the frequency of neural traffic is increased than when fewer impulses are being transmitted. To look at it another way, a weaker local anesthetic solution may produce only partial blockade in a given axon under the influence of a low-frequency stimulus, but the same axon will become completely blocked when subjected to higher frequencies of stimulation. This effect is called *frequency-dependent conduction block* and is shared by all the clinically used local anes-

thetics, particularly those agents like bupivacaine and etidocaine that are highly lipid soluble.[4]

Duration and recovery from nerve block are, again, dependent on the kinetics of local anesthetic action, which are regulated by laws of diffusion (along concentration gradients), and an affinity for lipoprotein structures, which assists in removing local anesthetic and is discussed in more detail later. It is sufficient to say here that during recovery the diffusion gradient is reversed. The outer concentric layer of the nerve loses its local anesthetic to the extracellular fluid first and the core of the nerve somewhat later. The clinical implication of this sequence is that in blocks of the limbs, the proximal region tends to lose its anesthesia before the more distal regions, one of the reasons for early onset of tourniquet pain.

LOCAL ANESTHETIC POTENCY

A standard method of determining the C_M of local anesthetics is the 50 percent reduction of the action potential spike height in a sheathed frog sciatic nerve within 5 minutes, when the nerve is stimulated at a frequency of 30 impulses per second, in a solution of pH 7.2 to 7.4. Under such conditions, the potency of the commonly used anesthetics can be classified as shown in Table 27–1. From this table it can be seen that there is a strong correlation between lipid solubility and potency: procaine (the least lipid soluble) is given a relative potency of 1 and etidocaine (the most lipid soluble) a relative potency of 16. This means that local anesthetics with a high potency will produce their effects at lower concentrations than will agents of intermediate or low potency. It also means that in a mixed nerve, agents of high potency are more likely to block all neural components, that is, A, B, and C fibers, unless only dilute solutions are used. Latency of onset of local anesthesia and duration of neural block are the two most important characteristics clinically. In a manner similar to that used to establish C_M, latency is determined by the concentration of a local anesthetic that will depress the action potential in the frog sciatic nerve by 50 percent in 10 minutes. Latency has no relation to potency but is particularly dependent on the site of injection; there is also a correlation with the pK_a and its lipid solubility concentration, and therefore local anesthetic gradient is also important. Doubling the anesthetic concentration reduces the latency by roughly one third. Etidocaine, which is highly soluble and has the lowest

TABLE 27–2. IN VITRO PHYSICAL AND BLOCK CHARACTERISTICS OF DIFFERENT AGENTS

Drug	Potency	Lipid Solubility	Latency	Duration
Procaine	1	0.6	1.0	1.00
Mepivacaine	2	1.0	1.0	1.50
Prilocaine	3	0.8	1.0	1.50
Chloroprocaine	4	—	0.8	0.75
Lidocaine	4	2.9	0.8	1.50
Tetracaine	16	80.0	2.0	8.00
Bupivacaine	16	28.0	0.6	8.00
Etidocaine	16	141.0	0.4	8.00

Reprinted, with permission, from Covino BG, Vassallo HG. Local anesthetics: Mechanisms of action and clinical use. New York: Grune & Stratton; 1976.

pK$_a$ of all the clinically used local anesthetics, also has the shortest latency (Table 27–2). The duration of neural block is also related to lipid and protein affinity. Most agents can be separated into three groups: those of short, those of intermediate, and those of long duration. The local anesthetics in the latter group not only have the greatest affinity for lipids but are also highly bound to tissue and plasma proteins. Although these in vitro models are important for the establishment of standard pharmacologic criteria, there will invariably be some differences between data obtained from in vitro and in vivo animal studies and data obtained from patients. Most discrepancies, when they do occur, can result from such factors as species differences, different tissue sites, vascularity of the tissues, and vascular tone in the respective tissues. Quite apart from these factors is the intrinsic pharmacologic activity of the different local anesthetics on blood vessels and the effects of vasoconstrictors when added to local anesthetic solutions.

Apart from potency, the most useful clinical criterion is knowledge of the onset (latency) and duration that can be expected from a given local anesthetic.

CLINICAL PHARMACOLOGY AND LOCAL ANESTHETICS

The clinical features of local anesthetics, as well as those factors that govern their uptake, distribution, and metabolism, are now considered.

Uptake and Distribution

Factors governing the uptake of local anesthetic by neural structures have already been discussed. The following discussion focuses on what happens to the portion of a dose of local anesthetic that does not reach the nerve and also the portion that has reached its target, performed its block, and then left the nerve. Four factors primarily affect the absorption of local anesthetics:

1. Site of injection (vascularity and type of immediate tissue, i.e., predominantly fat, muscle, connective)
2. Pharmacology of the particular drug
3. Dose of drug
4. Addition of vasoconstrictor

For example, the highest blood levels of any local anesthetic are obtained after multiple intercostal blocks. The lowest levels are obtained after subcutaneous infiltration, given

that equal volumes and concentrations of local anesthetic are used in each instance. The reasons for the differences are many; not the least important are the greater surface area, greater vascularity, and lower proportion of adipose tissue in the case of intercostal blockade.

The pharmacologic differences between the different amide local anesthetics have been well studied; however, because of the rapid hydrolysis (metabolism) by pseudocholinesterase in body tissues, similar studies for the majority of the ester local anesthetics are lacking. With epidural anesthesia as a model, the amide local anesthetics have been classified according to the blood concentrations obtained after equipotent doses, and, as can be seen in Table 27–3, etidocaine achieved the lowest blood concentrations and mepivacaine the highest. A possible explanation for these differences is the greater rate of tissue redistribution of etidocaine (giving lower blood concentrations). Mepivacaine has less lipid solubility and more vasodilator activity than etidocaine. In the case of prilocaine, which has about the same lipid affinity as mepivacaine, its high clearance (metabolism and excretion) results in low blood concentrations. All the local anesthetics, esters included, except cocaine produce vasodilation in the vicinity of the block site, and, as a rule, those agents that produce the greatest degree of vasodilation are the ones that achieve the greatest benefit from added epinephrine. It is for this reason that epinephrine is added to many commercial preparations of local anesthetics. The vasoconstrictor actions are twofold: first, to increase the duration of action, and second, to reduce the potential toxicity from the absorbed local anesthetic. The dose of epinephrine most commonly used is 1:200,000, or 5 µg/mL. Higher concentrations of epinephrine (except perhaps in oral mucous membranes where solutions may be used containing epinephrine in a dose of 1:80,000) may attain durations that are only marginally longer. As already mentioned, little advantage in duration, despite the reduction in blood concentration, results from the addition of a vasoconstrictor to the two long-acting agents, bupivacaine and etidocaine. Probably the high affinity for lipid structures and the greater vasodilator activity of these agents are responsible. It is the local absorption of local anesthetic by protein in the surrounding tissues (as well as in the nerves) that provides a depot and concentration gradient in favor of the nerves, thereby providing a long duration. This effect offsets the high lipid solubility that favors vascular uptake. Also, epinephrine has only a relatively short duration of effect. The process of absorption of a local anesthetic from its site of deposition is mirrored in the blood, producing a pro-

TABLE 27–3. INFLUENCE OF LIPID SOLUBILITY AND VASODILATOR ACTIVITY ON MAXIMUM BLOOD LOCAL ANESTHETIC CONCENTRATION DURING EPIDURAL BLOCK

	Equipotent Dose (mg)		Lipid Solubility	Relative Vasoactivity	Blood Level (µg/mL)
Lidocaine	300		2.9	1.0	1.4
Prilocaine	300		1.0	0.5	0.9
Mepivacaine	300		0.3	0.8	1.5
Bupivacaine	150		28.0	2.5	1.0
Etidocaine	150		141.0	2.5	0.5

Reprinted, with permission, from Covino BG, Vassallo HG. Local anesthetics: Mechanisms of action and clinical use. New York: Grune & Stratton; 1976.

file that rises and falls at rates dependent on the rate of distribution from the vascular compartment to other tissue compartments and the elimination by metabolism and excretion. The circulatory concentration of local anesthetics may be expressed either as whole blood or plasma concentrations, and these values may differ because of different rates of uptake into blood cells. This knowledge is used by pharmacokineticists, who are able to calculate the relative distribution of these drugs to different tissues. Generally speaking, those tissues receiving a higher proportion of the circulation, such as the lungs and kidneys, also contain higher concentrations of local anesthetics than poorly perfused organs. The rate of tissue redistribution is related in part to the protein binding and lipid affinity of each agent. Therefore agents like prilocaine, which is poorly bound in plasma, and etidocaine, which is very fat soluble, will rapidly equilibrate between the blood and tissue compartments. Such drugs tend to have much lower relative toxicities because the peak blood concentration from the same dose is always much lower than those obtained with other agents that are not so rapidly distributed.

Metabolism and Excretion

Local anesthetics are metabolized along one of two pathways, depending on whether they contain an ester or an amide linkage. Procaine, the forerunner of the ester class, chloroprocaine, and tetracaine are all hydrolyzed in the plasma by pseudocholinesterase to *para*-aminobenzoic acid derivatives. The rate of hydrolysis of chloroprocaine in plasma is extremely fast so that it is almost undetectable in blood after neural blockade. Procaine is hydrolyzed 4 times slower and tetracaine 16 times slower; however, the rates of metabolism of all esters are much faster than for any of the amides. Unfortunately, *para*-aminobenzoic acid can form a hapten with antibodies in certain individuals and in such instances is responsible for allergic phenomena.

The metabolism of amide compounds is quite different from and much more complex than that of the esters. For these compounds the liver is the primary site of metabolism. The rate of metabolism does vary slightly from one agent to another, with prilocaine clearly undergoing the most rapid degradation, followed by etidocaine, lidocaine, mepivacaine, and bupivacaine in that order. The metabolites differ with each drug and may themselves have clinically important actions. Normally, these substances would not be expected to have any untoward or toxic effects, but, in renal failure and cardiac failure, these metabolites may accumulate and, added to their parent substances, generate increased potential for toxic side effects.

Liver disease with severe impairment of normal function can be the cause of toxic sequelae from the accumulation of unmetabolized local anesthetics in the circulation. Consideration of the use of regional anesthesia in such patients must take this factor into account, particularly if the regional anesthetic procedure calls for amounts of local anesthetic that are at the upper range of normal doses.

Impairment of metabolism affects the clearance of these drugs from the body. Generally, greater than 90 percent of all local anesthetics are excreted as metabolites of their parent compounds. In humans, the kidney is the primary ex-

cretory organ. As is the case in impaired liver function, severe renal disease directly affects the clearance and ultimate excretion of local anesthetic metabolites.

Renal disease can also contribute to toxic side effects from systemically absorbed local anesthetic agents when the local anesthetic is displaced from plasma protein by uremic products.

LOCAL ANESTHETICS AND THEIR USES

Esters

The agents in this family of compounds discussed here are cocaine, procaine, chloroprocaine, tetracaine, and benzocaine.

Cocaine. Cocaine is the historical prototype of this group and is supplied as a hydrochloride. The pK_a is 8.6, and it is available in 1 to 20 percent solutions. The most common strength, used in otolaryngology, is 5 percent, which, when applied topically to mucous membranes, provides anesthesia for about 60 minutes. Cocaine is sometimes used in conjunction with epinephrine, but as has already been mentioned, this is usually unnecessary because the drug provides its own vasoconstriction by preventing the reuptake of catecholamines released from vasomotor nerve endings.

The maximum safe dose is now considered to be 200 mg. Because of its stimulatory effects on the sympathetic nervous system, toxic side effects on the central nervous and cardiovascular systems can be expected if high blood levels of the agent occur. Therefore, extreme excitement, convulsions, tachycardia, and hypertension will all precede the depressant effects, which can be fatal when the myocardium is affected. Cocaine is metabolized by the liver and in red blood cells. Accumulation of uremic products in the blood can lead to exaggerated drug responses because the products may displace bound drug molecules from plasma proteins. Therefore, there is the potential for toxic side effects of this local anesthetic in patients with renal disease, although such effects have not been demonstrated experimentally.

Procaine (Novocain). Procaine is a derivative of *para*-aminobenzoic acid and is prepared as the hydrochloride with a pK_a of 9.

Concentrations and Uses. It is available in 1, 2, and 5 percent solutions, the first two strengths being roughly equivalent in potency to similar concentrations of lidocaine when used for infiltration anesthesia; however, the latency and duration are inferior compared with lidocaine. The 5 percent solution can be used with D_5W to provide satisfactory spinal anesthesia with a duration of 30 to 45 minutes. Although it is not used very often today, procaine has been supplied as an alternative to the amide agents to provide anesthesia in patients known to be susceptible to malignant hyperthermia. There is, however, no definite proof that amide agents can precipitate this syndrome.

The maximum safe dose is 500 mg for plain solutions and 750 mg when epinephrine is added.

The drug is hydrolyzed primarily by pseudocholinesterase in the blood and by enzymes in the liver before being excreted in the urine.

Chloroprocaine (Nesacaine). Chloroprocaine shares many of the properties of procaine, the big exception being its greater affinity for lipid (approximately seven times more lipid soluble). This property is responsible for its superior anesthetic quality. The pK_a is 8.7. Because it is the most rapidly hydrolyzed local anesthetic, chloroprocaine achieves very low plasma concentrations and is, therefore, the least toxic local anesthetic. Unfortunately, this quality also results in very short durations, the shortest being about 30 minutes seen in epidural anesthesia. Addition of epinephrine will increase the duration by about 100 percent.

Concentration and Uses. Chloroprocaine is available in 1, 2, and 3 percent solutions. The 1 percent solution is used for infiltration anesthesia or peripheral nerve block and is quite useful for outpatient procedures requiring short durations. Durations of action of 45 to 90 minutes can be realized, depending on whether epinephrine 1:200,000 is used.

The most popular use of this drug has been in obstetric conduction anesthesia, either epidural or caudal. The rapid onset time, poor motor block, and low toxicity all contribute to its popularity in this group of patients. A 2 percent solution is generally adequate, although a 3 percent solution will shorten the latency and improve neural blockade. For this reason, the 3 percent solution is commonly used for emergency cesarean section.

The maximum safe dose is 600 mg for plain solutions, and 800 mg for epinephrine-containing solutions. Like procaine, chloroprocaine is hydrolyzed by pseudocholinesterase in the blood and is excreted by the kidney.

Tetracaine (Pontocaine). Tetracaine is also an ester of *para*-aminobenzoic acid. Its pK_a is 8.5, and it is much more lipid soluble than chloroprocaine. It is readily bound to protein. Tetracaine is available as a solution or as crystals, the latter being more stable to heat sterilization.

Concentrations and Uses. Because of its potency, tetracaine is used in very low concentrations for infiltration and peripheral nerve blocks. A 0.1 to 0.2 percent solution is generally adequate for such blocks, but when larger volumes of solutions are required, as would be the case for multiple intercostal blocks, it is advisable to add epinephrine 1:200,000 to reduce the systemic uptake of drug. The latency is long, and complete block may take 45 minutes to develop fully.

Before the introduction of the long-acting agents, bupivacaine and etidocaine, it was common to add lidocaine to reduce latency and also to improve the quality of sensory block. For epidural or caudal anesthesia, a solution of 0.25 percent is required, and for spinal anesthesia, now its most useful application, a 1 percent solution is used. The 1 percent solution (or crystals of tetracaine) is mixed with distilled water or 10 percent dextrose, depending on whether hypobaric or hyperbaric anesthesia is required. These plain solutions achieve excellent anesthesia for 60 to 90 minutes. Addition of epinephrine 0.2 mg (0.2 mL of 1:1000) prolongs the block by about 60 percent. Phenylephrine 5 mg (0.5 ml of 1 percent solution) prolongs the block by 100 to 150 percent.

Unlike the prolonged latency that occurs when tetra-caine is used for peripheral nerve block or epidural block, the onset of anesthesia after subarachnoid administration is rapid, taking only 5 to 10 minutes.

The maximum dose of 100 mg should not be exceeded unless a vasoconstrictor is added, in which case up to 150 mg can be used. Metabolism of tetracaine by pseudocholinesterase, subsequent breakdown by the liver, and excretion are much slower than for the other esters. Therefore, tetracaine is potentially much more toxic than procaine or chloroprocaine.

Benzocaine. Benzocaine is relatively insoluble in water; it has, however, found considerable use as a topical anesthetic. For this reason it is not available in an injectable form, although it has been incorporated with dextran as a 2 percent solution for the provision of anesthesia lasting many hours, such as for pain from fractured ribs.

Uses. Benzocaine is used as a spray or incorporated into ointments and gels for the anesthesia of mucous membranes and the skin.

Amides

Most of the amides, with lidocaine as the parent congener, are anilides. Only one, dibucaine, is a quinoline derivative. The following agents are discussed: lidocaine, prilocaine, mepivacaine, bupivacaine, etidocaine, and dibucaine.

Lidocaine (Xylocaine). Lidocaine is generally dispensed in aqueous solutions as the hydrochloride salt. It has a pK_a of 7.9, is moderately lipid soluble, and has a plasma protein binding of about 67 percent. In some countries, lidocaine is marketed as a carbonated salt that is buffered to a pH of 6.5. This permits a high proportion of the drug to assist as the "lipid-soluble base" that facilitates its penetration through lipid membranes. As the carbon dioxide is given off (prepared under a pressure of 2 atm), the pH rises to 7.5, again improving conditions for transportation of the uncharged base through lipid barriers. The diffusing carbon dioxide rapidly penetrates the membrane, where the pH falls, thus "trapping" the local anesthetic in the active cationic form.

As a consequence of this activity, the latency is shortened and the quality of anesthesia is improved, although there is little effect on duration.

Concentrations and Uses. Lidocaine is available in 0.5, 1, 2, 4, and 5 percent solutions, to which epinephrine may be added as a vasoconstrictor. Because of the large volumes that may be required, only 0.5 percent solutions are used to provide satisfactory infiltration anesthesia. The duration of action of the 0.5 percent solution may be increased from 75 to about 240 minutes with 1:200,000 epinephrine. A 1 percent solution provides about 120 minutes of anesthesia and, with added epinephrine, 400 minutes. Only in dental anesthesia, because of the highly vascular tissue and the small volumes necessary, is a 2 percent solution with epinephrine 1:80,000 used. The duration that can be expected is about 150 minutes.

A 0.5 percent lidocaine solution provides excellent intravenous analgesia in the upper limbs. Higher concentrations are unnecessary and increase the risk of toxicity. Most peripheral nerve blocks and plexus anesthesia require a 1 percent solution, but satisfactory digital nerve block can be provided by a 0.5 percent solution.

The latency is short, about 5 minutes, for individual nerve blocks and about 20 minutes for plexus anesthesia. A duration of 60 minutes can be increased up to 130 percent by the addition of epinephrine. Epidural and caudal anesthesia requires either a 1 or 2 percent solution, depending on whether less or more motor block is required. Addition of epinephrine 1:200,000 reduces the latency, improves motor block, increases duration, and, when large volumes are used, reduces the potential for toxic side effects. Duration of surgical anesthesia is increased from 60 to 100 minutes when epinephrine is added.

Spinal anesthesia of 45 to 60 minutes' duration can be provided by a plain 5 percent solution of lidocaine in 7.5 percent dextrose. The duration is increased up to 50 percent by addition of 0.2 mg of epinephrine. The solution has a specific gravity of 1.035 at body temperature, which causes it to spread rapidly; therefore, the onset of anesthesia is almost immediate.

A 4 percent solution of lidocaine is available for topical anesthesia, and in some countries, a 10 percent spray is available for the same purposes. The maximum recommended dose of lidocaine is 400 mg, or 500 mg when epinephrine is added.

Lidocaine is metabolized by the liver. Less than 4 percent is excreted unmetabolized in the urine.

Prilocaine (Citanest). The pK_a of prilocaine is 7.9; it has a lower lipid solubility than lidocaine and is approximately 55 percent bound to plasma protein. Unlike the other amides, which are tertiary amines, prilocaine is a secondary amine and is a toluidide (i.e., derivative of *ortho*-toluidine or 2-methylaniline) rather than a 2,6-dimethylaniline like the direct descendants of lidocaine.

Concentrations and Uses. Prilocaine is available in 0.5, 1, 2, and 3 percent solutions. All solutions may be incorporated with a vasoconstrictor.

Like lidocaine, 0.5 to 1 percent prilocaine provides satisfactory infiltration anesthesia lasting from 75 to 280 minutes, depending on whether epinephrine is added.

Prilocaine 0.5 percent solution is probably the anesthetic agent of choice for intravenous regional anesthesia because it is the least toxic of the amide local anesthetics and, therefore, the least likely to produce toxic sequelae during sudden deflation of the tourniquet. In peripheral nerve block, 0.5 to 1.5 percent solutions provide conditions similar to those seen with lidocaine; although in plexus anesthesia, prilocaine generally provides durations 50 percent longer. In this respect, prilocaine is more useful than lidocaine when anesthesia of moderate duration is desired for patients in whom epinephrine is contraindicated.

Although not commonly employed for epidural and caudal anesthesia, prilocaine is used in either a 2 or 3 percent solution. There is little difference in the quality of anesthesia compared with lidocaine; although when the 2 percent solution is used without a vasoconstrictor, excellent anesthesia with minimal motor block and low toxicity make this a very suitable agent for outpatient surgery.

The maximum dose of prilocaine is 400 mg, or 600 mg when epinephrine is added. If a dose of 600 mg is exceeded, the development of clinical methemoglobinemia is possible. This is manifested by cyanosis, which can be treated by the administration of methylene blue in a dose of 1 mg/kg. Although methemoglobin has little effect on the oxygen-carrying capacity of hemoglobin, except in the presence of severe anemia below 5000 mg/100 mL, it is aesthetically displeasing and also masks the normal clinical observation of hypoxia in patients. For this reason, prilocaine should probably not be used in obstetrics patients. It should, however, be emphasized that because prilocaine is four times less cardiotoxic and neurotoxic, it is probably the safest short-acting amide local anesthetic available. Prilocaine is partially metabolized in the liver to *o*-toluidine, and a metabolite of this compound is probably responsible for the production of methemoglobinemia. This metabolic reaction cannot occur with the direct descendants of lidocaine. The metabolites are excreted by the kidneys.

Mepivacaine (Carbocaine). This substance has a pK_a of 7.6 and a lipid solubility similar to that of lidocaine; however, it is more plasma protein bound than either of these two agents, having a range of 68 to 84 percent.

Concentrations and Uses. Mepivacaine is equipotent with lidocaine and is, therefore, available in the same range of concentrations with the exception of topical solutions.

The drug has the same indications as lidocaine, except that it is probably not the drug of choice for obstetric patients, as neonatal metabolism may be slower than is the case with lidocaine; in addition the placental transfer of mepivacaine is greater.

The maximum safe dose of mepivacaine is 400 mg, or 500 mg with epinephrine. Most of the animal studies indicate that mepivacaine is slightly more toxic than lidocaine, and epinephrine is not quite as effective either in increasing the duration of block or in lowering the blood concentrations when added to mepivacaine. Like lidocaine, metabolism of mepivacaine takes place in the liver, with most of the drug being eliminated as metabolites by the kidneys.

Bupivacaine (Marcaine). Bupivacaine belongs to the same group of anilides as mepivacaine, having been synthesized at the same time, although prepared commercially some years later. A butyl group replaces the methyl group in the piperidine ring, and it is this alteration of the molecule that is responsible for its greater lipid solubility compared with mepivacaine.

The pK_a is 8.01. Bupivacaine is 88 percent plasma protein bound and highly lipid soluble. This high lipid affinity accounts for its high potency and also its greater toxicity.

Concentrations and Uses. Solutions of 0.25, 0.5, and 0.75 percent are available. No solution is available for topical anesthesia. A 0.125 to 0.25 percent solution with or without epinephrine is satisfactory for infiltration anesthesia. Latency is short and durations of 200 or 400 minutes are achieved with added epinephrine.

For peripheral nerve block, solutions of 0.25 to 0.5 percent, with or without epinephrine, are satisfactory; however, latencies are long, particularly in the case of plexus anesthesia, which may require 30 minutes to achieve complete block. The 0.5 percent solution provides good motor block and the quality of sensory anesthesia is better than that obtained with the 0.25 percent solution. There is extreme variability in the duration of anesthesia, which may range from 400 minutes to 24 hours. Epinephrine has an unreliable effect on the duration but does reduce the uptake of the drug (and hence its toxicity). In epidural and caudal anesthesia, the most commonly used concentrations are 0.5 and 0.75 percent, depending on whether a more profound motor block is desired. No alteration in duration is achieved by the addition of epinephrine, but the ensuing blood concentrations are lower. Obstetrics is a special situation for which motor block is not required, and bupivacaine in concentrations as low as 0.125 percent, or more commonly 0.25 percent, provides very satisfactory analgesia in this group of patients. The only disadvantage of these weaker solutions is the shorter duration that results.

Bupivacaine is now available in the United States as either a 0.5 percent isobaric or hyperbaric solution for spinal anesthesia. It is very similar to tetracaine with respect to duration of action, the main difference being a superior sensory analgesia but poorer motor block. The maximum safe doses are 150 mg for plain solutions and 200 mg with epinephrine.

Bupivacaine is about four to five times more toxic than lidocaine. The liver is responsible for its metabolism, and the metabolites are excreted via the kidneys.

Etidocaine (Duranest). This drug, also developed from lidocaine, has a pK_a of 7.74. Etidocaine has the highest lipid solubility of all clinical local anesthetics and a plasma binding of 94 percent. It is not equipotent with bupivacaine and is less toxic. It does, however, provide similar durations and a more profound motor block than bupivacaine when twice the concentration is used.

Concentrations and Uses. Etidocaine is available in 0.5, 1, and 1.5 percent solutions. It is not available as a topical anesthetic, but its ability to penetrate lipid barriers would make it a very effective agent. The 0.5 percent solution without epinephrine will provide infiltration anesthesia rapidly with durations similar to those seen with bupivacaine.

When etidocaine is used for peripheral nerve block, the onset is much quicker than with bupivacaine and there is little difference in the durations. A 0.5 percent solution, with or without epinephrine, is used and when large volumes are required. It is safer than bupivacaine because of its lower toxicity.

Epidural and caudal anesthesia is provided by 1 to 1.5 percent solutions, depending on the degree of motor block desired. Even a 1 percent solution of etidocaine provides a motor block superior to that provided by 0.5 percent bupivacaine, which is equally potent. In fact, because of this ability to affect motor function while providing only partial analgesia, etidocaine is not satisfactory for obstetric use.

The latency when a 1.5 percent solution is used is extremely short, and complete anesthesia may take place within 20 minutes. Epinephrine has no effect on duration and a marginal effect on blood concentrations, but does intensify motor block. Because of the degree of motor block, etidocaine is well suited for operations requiring profound relaxation. The maximum dose is 300 mg (400 mg with epinephrine).

Etidocaine is metabolized in the liver with less than 1 percent being excreted in the urine unchanged.

Dibucaine (Nupercainal). Dibucaine is a quinoline derivative having an amide link in the intermediate chain. It has a pK_a of 8.5, is very lipid-soluble, and is very potent.

Concentrations and Uses. The most common solution now available is 0.5 percent in 6 percent dextrose, having a specific gravity of 1.025, which is used for hyperbaric spinal anesthesia. A hypobaric solution is also available. The latency is greater than that for tetracaine, 5 to 10 minutes, and it has a duration of 3 hours. If 0.2 mg epinephrine is added, the duration is increased to 4 hours. Durations up to 130 percent longer can be achieved when phenylephrine 5 mg is added. The range of dose used varies between 5 and 15 mg; the maximum dose is 50 mg.

Dibucaine is metabolized in the liver, but little is known of its metabolites.

Ropivacaine. Ropivacaine is a new, long-acting, amide type of local anesthetic with a chemical structure similar to that of bupivacaine, the butyl group being replaced by a propyl group. Unlike bupivacaine, it is prepared as the *S*-isomer rather than as a racemic mixture. The drug is less lipophilic than bupivacaine and most *in vitro* comparisons have found the drug to be slightly less potent. *In vivo* animal studies suggest that central administration of both drugs produces similar patterns of onset and sensory spread, although ropivacaine has a shorter duration of action and is responsible for less motor block.[5] Interestingly, ropivacaine in test solutions of 0.25 and 0.75 percent (compared with solutions of the same concentration of bupivacaine) causes cutaneous vasoconstriction.[6] It has a pK_a of 8.1 and a protein binding greater than 90 percent.

Concentrations and Uses. In clinical trials, ropivacaine provides excellent surgical anesthesia for subclavian perivascular brachial plexus block in a concentration of 0.5 percent. For epidural anesthesia, solutions of 0.5, 0.75, and 1 percent provide sensory analgesia of good quality and a duration in excess of 5 hours. The motor block is not as effective as that with bupivacaine and a score of 3 (Bromage) is obtained with the 1 percent solution. Because of its vasoconstrictive properties, ropivacaine 0.5 percent would appear to be an excellent solution for infiltration analgesia and peripheral nerve block.

Blood levels of the drug are well within the safe range. Cardiovascular changes are compatible with those associated with autonomic blockade during epidural anesthesia, and there is no evidence of cardiac irritability or myocardial depression.[7] Because of the differential block seen with ropivacaine, it promises to be a useful local anesthetic in obstetrics and in pain control.

As with the other amides, ropivacaine is metabolized in the liver.

Vasoconstrictors

Although a number of vasoconstrictors have been synthesized, epinephrine, introduced by Braun, is still the most widely used and most reliable adjunct for this purpose today.[8] Vasoconstrictors are added to local anesthetic solutions to retard the absorption of the local anesthetic, thereby improving its uptake by nerves, increasing the duration of action, and reducing systemic toxicity.

Epinephrine. Although epinephrine has both alpha- and beta-adrenoreceptor effects, it is only for the alpha effects that epinephrine is incorporated with local anesthetic. It is quite rapidly oxidized, and for this reason it is probably better to add it to the local anesthetic solution immediately prior to its use. Commercially prepared epinephrine-containing solutions, usually in a concentration of 1:200,000 (5 µg/mL), have a low pH (3 to 4.5) and contain an antioxidant, sodium metabisulfite. They can be autoclaved once without materially affecting the potency of the vasoconstrictor. The total dose of epinephrine should be kept below 200 µg. Toxic side effects are caused mainly by the beta-adrenergic stimulatory effects (tachycardia, bradycardia, and cardiac arrhythmias), but high doses also result in the stimulation of alpha-adrenergic receptors causing hypertension.

Epinephrine should be avoided in patients with thyrotoxicosis and hypertension.

Phenylephrine. Phenylephrine is the only other vasoconstrictor that has been used with local anesthetics that is presently available in the United States. It is a synthetic drug with predominantly alpha-agonist effects. Phenylephrine is usually used in a concentration of 1:20,000 (20 µg/mL) and has been very popular as an adjunct for spinal anesthesia, where durations are prolonged by 100 to 150 percent. It is not widely used as a vasoconstrictor for other regional anesthetic procedures because of the widespread systemic effects, but it can be used as an alternative to epinephrine in those cases in which epinephrine is contraindicated.

TOXIC EFFECTS OF LOCAL ANESTHETICS

Because of their ability to influence excitable membranes, local anesthetics can be expected to have far-reaching effects on the central nervous and cardiovascular systems should large amounts enter the systemic circulation.[9]

Central Nervous System

When the local anesthetic level in the blood increases, a recognizable series of reactions are seen in the central nervous system (CNS). Among toxic manifestations are excitatory subjective phenomena such as lightheadedness, dizziness, tinnitus, and difficulty in focusing. Objective signs are slurred speech, shivering, muscular twitching, and tremors. As the blood concentration increases, generalized convulsions ensue. These effects are thought to be an initial action on the inhibitory systems in the CNS, which may be more sensitive to local anesthetic action than are the facilitatory systems, which therefore tend to exert their circulatory effects unopposed. If local anesthetic blood concentrations continue to rise, generalized CNS depression occurs and, if allowed to continue unchecked, leads ultimately to respiratory arrest. Local anesthetic toxicity is enhanced by elevated hydrogen ion (pH) and carbon dioxide (P_{CO_2}) concentrations in the patient. A number of mechanisms may be in-

volved. These include the increased cardiac output associated with a respiratory or metabolic acidosis; the resulting increased cerebral blood flow and vasodilation, which delivers a high local anesthetic dose to the brain; and finally the reduction in intraneural pH, which causes more local anesthetic to exist in the cationic, or active, form. Convulsive activity can be terminated by the administration of an ultrashort-acting barbiturate such as thiopental in a dose of at least 4 mg/kg or diazepam in a dose of 0.1 mg/kg. DeJong has suggested that diazepam be given prophylactically, although other data contradict this suggestion.[10] Excitatory effects can result from local anesthetic overdose. It is not generally realized that all local anesthetics have anticonvulsive activity; however, the doses associated with these effects are much lower than those that cause seizure activity.

Cardiovascular System

Local anesthetics are described as having biphasic effects on cardiac and vascular muscle. This means that at low concentrations stimulatory effects are seen, and at high concentrations depressant effects are manifested. Since the introduction of procaine and, later, lidocaine, these cardiac and vascular actions have been studied extensively. In fact, the margin of safety from cardiovascular toxicity with local anesthetics is very large. Blood concentrations of short-acting local anesthetics must be some ten times greater than those necessary to cause toxic effects on the CNS; those of the long-acting agents, four times greater. Lidocaine, of course, is used extensively as an antiarrhythmic agent and induces its activity at concentrations well below those that cause toxic effects. High blood concentrations of local anesthetic, however, result in depression of both the myocardium and the vascular tissue.

As the local anesthetic concentration in the blood rises, a predictable series of changes are seen in the heart. There are a prolongation of conduction time in most regions of the heart, an increased P-R interval, increased QRS duration, bradycardia, and finally cardiac arrest in asystole. These electrophysiologic changes are identical to the effects that have already been described in relation to the action of local anesthetics on nerve membranes.

On vascular tissue, both in vitro and in vivo studies have demonstrated similar effects, with vasoconstriction occurring at low local anesthetic concentrations and vasodilation with increasing concentrations. The effect that predominates at a given local anesthetic concentration, however, depends on such factors as the background vascular tone and the particular vascular bed concerned. For example, intraarterial administration of mepivacaine to human volunteers caused a decrease in forearm blood flow, but when the concentration was increased, the resistance fell and flows increased. As already discussed, the only local anesthetic that consistently causes vasoconstriction is cocaine; therefore, the toxic vascular effect that can be expected with this agent is profound, widespread vasoconstriction causing hypertension.

High doses of all other local anesthetics cause cardiovascular collapse secondary to cardiac depression and vasodilation.[11] The vascular bed that seems to react differentially is the pulmonary vasculature, which responds with vasoconstriction to high concentrations of most local anesthetics.

Indirect Effects of Local Anesthetics

Because of the interference with the sympathetic nervous outflow, major conduction anesthesia, which includes spinal and epidural anesthesia, is responsible for profound physiologic changes. The degree of disturbance is dependent on a number of factors. These include hypovolemia from whatever cause, the concurrent administration of CNS depressant drugs, the presence or absence of a vasoconstrictor (in the case of epidural anesthesia), and the physiologic status of the patient.

Basically, an increasing tendency toward hypotension can be expected to develop because of vasodilation in the blocked areas and a decrease in venous return caused by pooling in the capacitance system of the skin and muscles. Many of these changes are compensated by vasoconstriction in the unblocked parts of the body. When an increasing number of segments are blocked (above T-5), an increasing inability to make compensatory adjustments to cope with the loss of vasomotor control can be expected. The speed with which hypotension occurs during spinal anesthesia is much faster than is the case during epidural anesthesia; although in most surgical patients with blocks extending to T-5 (which is adequate for most abdominal operations), the ultimate level to which the blood pressure falls in either case is about 15 percent of the control pressure. Therefore, use of either of these two techniques in the presence of uncorrected hypovolemia is contraindicated. When epinephrine-containing solutions are used for epidural anesthesia, there may be an increased tendency for hypotension to develop, even in normovolemic subjects, because of the widespread beta-adrenergic effects that oppose any compensatory vasoconstriction in the unblocked areas, for example, upper limbs and torso.[12] Additional depressant effects on the cardiovascular system must also be expected when CNS depressant drugs, such as those that have been administered for premedication or sedation, are used in conjunction with the conduction anesthetic. These drugs may increase the tendency for hypotension to develop and must be taken into consideration to maintain homeostasis at the desired level.

Finally, although spinal or epidural anesthesia may be selected over general anesthesia for the debilitated patient, it should be remembered that any concurrent circulatory disturbances in such patients also require close observation because of the additional potential for development of hypotension associated with such anesthetic techniques.

The only other toxic effects attributable to local anesthetics are allergy, which can, as has been mentioned, attend the use of the ester local anesthetics, and histotoxic effects, when local anesthetics are repeatedly applied to striated muscle. These histotoxic effects, however, are not permanent and regeneration is usually complete within 2 weeks of the last application of the particular local anesthetic. Recently, the histotoxic effects that have been attributed to the accidental injection of chloroprocaine into the subarachnoid space, causing partial and permanent neurologic lesions, have been shown to have resulted from the antioxidant used to preserve these solutions. Chloroprocaine has been remanufactured with a greatly reduced concentration (from 0.2 to 0.07 percent) of the antioxidant, sodium bisulfite. In vivo and in vitro experiments appear to have reestablished the safety of using this drug as it is now formulated.

REFERENCES

1. Bromage PR, Burfoot ME, Crowell DE, Truant AT. Quality of epidural blockade. III. Carbonated local anesthetic solutions. *Br J Anaesth.* 1967;39:197.
2. Gissen AJ, Covino BG, Gregus J. Differential sensitivities of mammalian nerve fibers to local anesthetic agents. *Anesthesiology.* 1980;53:467.
3. Sprotte G. Thermographic investigations into the physiologic basis of regional anesthesia. In: *Anaesthesiology and intensive care medicine.* Berlin: Springer-Verlag; 1985:159.
4. Courtney KR. Mechanism of frequency-dependent inhibition of sodium currents in frog myelinated nerve by lidocaine derivative GEA 968. *J Pharmacol Exp Ther.* 1977;195:225–236.
5. Arthur GR, Feldman HS, Covino BG. 1988 Comparative pharmacokinetics of bupivacaine and ropivacaine, a new amide local anesthetic. *Anesth Analg.* 1988;67:1053–1058.
6. Steinkamp SL, Katz JA, Sehlhorst CS, et al. Pharmacodynamic effects of ropivacaine after epidural administration in the Rhesus monkey. *Region Anesth.* 1989;14(suppl):5.
7. KerKamp HEM, Gielen MJM, Edstrom HH. Comparison of 0.75% ropivacaine with epinephrine and 0.75% bupivacaine in lumbar epidural anesthesia. *Region Anesth.* 1990;15:204–207.
8. Braun H. Uber den Einfluss Der Vitalitat der Gewebe auf die ortichen und allgemeinen Gifwirkungen localanaesthesirender Mittel und uber die Bedeutung des Adrenalins fur die local Anaesthesie. *Arch Klin Chir.* 1903;69:541.
9. Scott DB, Cousins MJ. Clinical pharmacology of local anesthetic agents. In: Bridenbaugh PO, Cousins MJ, eds. *Neural blockage.* Philadelphia: JB Lippincott; 1980:86–121.
10. deJong RH. *Physiology and pharmacology of local anesthesia.* 2nd ed. Springfield, IL: Charles C Thomas; 1977.
11. Reiz S, Nath S. Cardiotoxicity of local anesthetic agents. *Br J Anaesth.* 1986;58:736–746.
12. Bonica JJ, Akamatsu TJ, et al. Circulatory effects of peridural block. II. Effects of epinephrine. *Anesthesiology.* 1971;34:514.

Pharmacology of Neuromuscular Blockade and Antagonism

Gary D. Zarr

The group of drugs referred to as muscle relaxants block neuromuscular transmission, resulting in muscle paralysis. Muscle relaxants with no central muscle-relaxant capabilities, such as diazepam, are discussed in this chapter. Skeletal muscle relaxants have no sedative, analgesic, or amnestic properties. Their primary contribution to the anesthetic process is to provide a quiet, relaxed surgical field. The degree of neuromuscular blockade can be assessed with a peripheral nerve stimulator. The pharmacology of the drugs in the two classes of muscle relaxants, depolarizing and nondepolarizing, is presented, as is the pharmacology of antagonism of neuromuscular blockade.

HISTORY AND FUTURE OF MUSCLE RELAXANTS

The history of muscle relaxants can be divided into two phases: (1) early investigational research and (2) initial medical and anesthetic uses of muscle relaxants. The early history of muscle relaxants is actually the history of curare, the first muscle relaxant to be studied. The use of curare as arrow poison by various South American Indian tribes is well known. Work by Brody in 1811 demonstrated that death in curare-treated animals could be prevented with the use of artificial ventilation. Additional investigation by Claude Bernard demonstrated that the site of action of curare was the neuromuscular junction. His work showed that a muscle paralyzed by curare could still contract if stimulated directly. Lack of the equipment and expertise necessary to perform oral endotracheal intubation delayed the safe introduction of curare into clinical use. Initial clinical uses by Chisholm in the American Civil War in 1862 and Lawen in 1912 were attempts to reduce the dose of ether necessary to produce muscle relaxation. As a spontaneous ventilatory pattern was an essential component of the open-drop ether technique, these early trials were regarded as unsatisfactory.

The successful clinical use of muscle relaxants is noted in the use of curare to control skeletal muscle spasms in pa-

tients with tetanus.[1] Curare was also used as an adjunct in electroconvulsive therapy.[2] The first use of curare in modern clinical anesthesia was reported in 1942.[3] Reports of higher complication rates in surgical patients who received muscle relaxants caused many anesthetists to avoid the use of muscle relaxants.[4] As the halogenated anesthetics were introduced into clinical practice it became apparent that the use of a muscle relaxant would be necessary to achieve adequate relaxation for intraabdominal procedures if potentially toxic concentrations of these agents were to be avoided. With increased clinical experience and the use of anticholinesterase/antimuscarinic combinations to reverse residual muscle relaxation, the incidence of postoperative respiratory complications decreased. The transition from diethyl ether to halogenated anesthetics to opiate and nitrous oxide anesthesia resulted in the continued increasing use of muscle relaxants in clinical practice. Neuromuscular blockade monitoring was introduced into clinical practice in the late 1960s and early 1970s.[5] This has resulted in better titration of muscle relaxant to maintain the desired levels of muscle relaxation. In addition, neuromuscular blockade monitoring can aid in deciding when the muscle relaxant is ready to be reversed, when it is completely reversed, or if reversal is required at all.

Research efforts to develop nondepolarizing muscle relaxants with intermediate duration of action, such as vecuronium and atracurium, have helped to improve patient safety in the use of muscle relaxants as adjuncts to anesthesia. These agents have fewer complications and a shorter duration of action, giving the clinician better control over the depth and duration of muscle relaxation which is useful in reducing the amount of anticholinesterase drug necessary for reversal and reducing the potential for recurarization in the postoperative phase. With the introduction of long-acting nondepolarizing neuromuscular blocking agents such as pipecuronium and doxacurium, along with intermediate-acting drugs such as vecuronium and atracurium, the challenge with respect to improving patient safety relative to muscle relaxant drugs is to find a nondepolarizing agent with rapid onset and short duration, properties associated with succinylcholine. Introduction of such a nondepolarizing agent would provide the anesthetist with a selection of muscle relaxants that have minimal side effects and a wide spectrum of duration of action.

PHYSIOLOGY OF NERVE CONDUCTION

The transduction of an electrical impulse from a nerve to a chemical impulse that stimulates the endplate of a muscle fiber and produces muscular contraction occurs at the neuromuscular junction. Upper motor neurons that have their origin in the cerebral motor cortex synapse with group A fast-conducting somatic efferent lower motor neurons, the cell bodies of which originate in the gray matter of the anterior horns of the spinal cord. Collections of these lower motor neurons form the efferent spinal motor nerves. When a motor nerve approaches a muscle it loses its myelin sheath and branches to multiple nerve fibers. A single nerve fiber and the muscle fibers it supplies constitute a functional motor unit. Muscle function determines how many muscle fibers will be supplied by a single nerve fiber. Muscles that perform fine movements are supplied by nerve fibers that supply relatively few muscle fibers; muscles that are responsible for sustained contraction are supplied by nerve fibers that supply many muscle fibers. This variability in the size of motor units and the potential for recruitment of additional motor units allow for a high degree of control as to the precision and strength of motor movement. The space between the nerve fiber and the muscle fiber it supplies constitutes the neuromuscular junction. The prejunctional nerve fiber axonal ending contains mitochondria, endoplasmic reticulum, and synaptic vesicles all of which are necessary for the synthesis and storage of the neurotransmitter acetylcholine (ACh). The postjunctional surface is separated from the prejunctional surface by a synaptic cleft 20 to 30 nm wide and is continuous with the extracellular fluid space.[6] The postjunctional surface or the motor endplate is a highly specialized region that is invaginated to increase the surface area of the synapse. Nicotinic cholinergic receptors, the receptors for the neurotransmitter acetylcholine, are located on both the presynaptic axonal terminal and the postsynaptic endplate surface. Acetylcholinesterase (true or tissue cholinesterase), the enzyme necessary to hydrolyze ACh and allow for endplate repolarization, is located in the synaptic cleft.

The resting membrane potential of both large nerve and skeletal muscle fibers is about -90 mV, the reference area inside the cell being 90 mV more negative than the extracellular fluid space outside the cell. This negative resting membrane potential is maintained by a combination of selective membrane permeability to sodium and potassium ions and an energy-dependent electrogenic sodium–potassium pump. In the resting state the membrane is much more permeable to potassium than it is to sodium; in fact, resting membrane potential is closest to the Nernst potential for potassium, which is -94 mV. By use of the Goldman equation and the diffusion potentials for sodium and potassium, a resting membrane potential of -86 mV would be predicted. The energy-dependent electrogenic sodium–potassium pump, which pumps more sodium out of the cell than potassium into the cell, contributes an additional -4 mV to the resting potential. Electrophysiologic measurements have confirmed the calculated resting membrane potential in large nerve and muscle fiber cells.[7]

Should a nerve be stimulated, the resting membrane potential of -90 mV becomes less negative because the ion channels open and allow sodium to enter the nerve. If the membrane potential is reduced to about -65 mV, the threshold potential for an action potential is reached. When threshold potential is reached voltage-sensitive ion channels open and allow sodium to rush into the nerve, causing propagation of an action potential along the course of the nerve. As the wave of depolarization moves along the nerve a wave of repolarization follows. The depolarization resulting from sodium entry into the nerve causes the membrane potential to approach 0 mV, which triggers the opening of voltage-sensitive ion channels and the movement of potassium ions out of the neuron, causing repolarization to -90 mV. Ultimately the restoration of potassium ion concentration inside the nerve and sodium ion concentration outside the nerve is due to the electrogenic sodium–potassium ATP-dependent pump. When the action potential wave of depolarization reaches the nerve fiber axonal terminal, it causes voltage-sensitive calcium channels to open and calcium rushes into the axonal ending. The entry of calcium into the axonal terminal is essential for the exocytotic release of ACh, and low calcium levels or high magnesium levels inhibit the release of ACh.[8,9] The released ACh diffuses across the synaptic cleft and binds to the two alpha subunits of the postsynaptic nicotinic cholinergic receptor, as well as the presynaptic cholinergic receptors.[10] The postsynaptic nicotinic cholinergic ACh receptor is composed of five protein subunits that form an ion pore, which opens when the two 40,000-dalton alpha subunits bind the neurotransmitter ACh (Figs. 28–1 and 28–2).[11] For the ion pore of the acetylcholine receptor to open, each of the alpha subunits must bind a molecule of ACh. Binding of a single antagonist molecule or a molecule of alpha toxin from the venom of the krait or cobra snake to either one of the alpha subunits prevents ion channel opening.[12] The ACh-induced opening of this channel results in movement of sodium into the endplate region, depolarization of the region, and generation of an endplate potential (EPP). An EPP is not like a nerve action potential which is governed by the all-or-none phenomenon. In a nerve, if threshold is reached, an action potential is propagated. EPP resulting from ACh activation of multiple receptors can be summed to produce an endplate voltage change from -90 to about -50 mV, which will then result in a propagated action potential in the muscle fiber. As the action potential spreads throughout the muscle it results in the release of calcium from the sarcoplasmic reticulum and a rise in the free calcium concentration within the muscle fiber. It is believed that the rise in calcium within the muscle fiber results in troponin–tropomyosin interaction with actin, which then allows the active sites on actin to interact with myosin and slide together, producing muscle contraction. Muscle contraction is terminated when calcium is pumped back into the sarcoplasmic reticulum of the muscle fiber, where it is stored until another action potential causes it to be released.

Sustained depolarization of the endplate region is prevented by the action of the enzyme acetylcholinesterase (AChE), which rapidly hydrolyzes ACh to acetate and

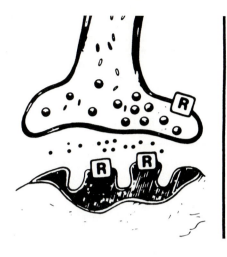

Figure 28–1. Nicotinic cholinergic receptors (R) on postjunctional folds (bottom left) at the motor endplate of skeletal muscle, on motor nerve endings (top left), and in extrajunctional membrane (right) in immature or denervated skeletal muscle. (*Reprinted, with permission, from Katz RL. Muscle relaxants: Basic and clinical aspects.* Seminars in Anesthesia *III(4), December 1984.*)

choline. As AChE rapidly lowers the concentration of ACh present at the receptor, the equilibrium of binding of ACh to the nicotinic receptor alpha subunits reverse. Removal of ACh from the nicotinic receptor allows the channel pore to close and the endplate region to repolarize. Diffusion of ACh away from the synaptic region may play a role in the termination of its effect as well; however, the fact that the endplate region is repolarized over a time course of milliseconds would seem to indicate that the rapid action of AChE is the primary mechanism for the termination of the effects of ACh at the synapse.

ACETYLCHOLINE SYNTHESIS, STORAGE, AND RELEASE

Synthesis of ACh, a quaternary ammonium ester, takes place within cholinergic nerve terminals. ACh is synthesized from acetyl-coenzyme A, derived from glucose metabolism and choline. Choline is present in the extracellular fluid surrounding the nerve terminal. The supply of choline is derived from dietary intake as well as from the enzymatic breakdown of ACh. It has been estimated that as much as 50 percent of the choline used in the synthesis of ACh is de-

rived from the breakdown of this transmitter.[13] Uptake of choline into cholinergic nerve terminals is an active process. It is of pharmacologic interest that hemicholinium can block the uptake of choline and block nerve transmission[14]; however, the nonspecific blockage of choline uptake in all cholinergic nerves demonstrates the lack of any clinical use for hemicholinium.

In the nerve terminal, choline combines with the acetyl group from acetyl-coenzyme A under the influence of choline-O-acetyltransferase to yield ACh and free coenzyme A (Fig. 28–3). After its synthesis in the nerve terminal cytosol, ACh is stored in vesicles. Estimates of the number of ACh molecules in each vesicle range from 1000 to 10,000, and this number is known as the quantal content of the vesicle.[15] Under physiologic conditions the production of ACh is able to keep pace with release as a result of action potentials generated in motor nerves; however, if a motor nerve is stimulated with a tetanic impulse of 200 Hz for 5 seconds, the rate of ACh release is diminished.[16] This fact explains why newer clinical blockade monitors have a limit of 50 to 100 Hz for tetanic stimulation.

It has been proposed that when an action potential in a nerve reaches the nerve terminal, adenylate cyclase is acti-

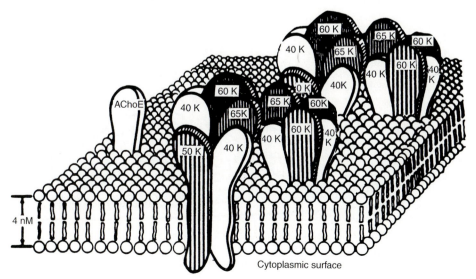

Figure 28–2. Sketch of postjunctional nicotinic acetylcholine receptors with an acetylcholinesterase (AChE) molecule nearby. (*Reprinted, with permission, from Katz RL. Muscle relaxants: Basic and clinical aspects.* Seminars in Anesthesia *III(4), December 1984.*)

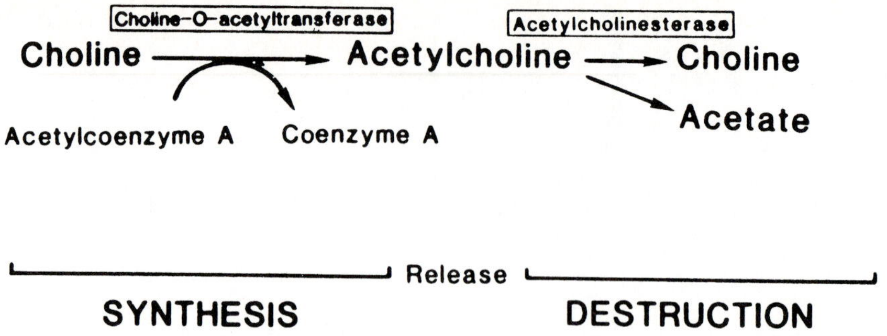

$$\boxed{\text{Choline-O-acetyltransferase}}\qquad\qquad\boxed{\text{Acetylcholinesterase}}$$

Choline ⟶ **Acetylcholine** ⟶ **Choline**

⟶ **Acetate**

Acetylcoenzyme A   **Coenzyme A**

⊢———————————————————⊣ Release ⊢————————————————⊣

SYNTHESIS   **DESTRUCTION**

Figure 28–3. Schematic representation of the synthesis and destruction of acetylcholine within the neuromuscular junction. (*Reprinted, with permission, from Katz RL. Muscle relaxants: Basic and clinical aspects. Seminars in Anesthesia III(4), December 1984.*)

vated causing the conversion of ATP to cyclic AMP (cAMP), which allows calcium channels to open and calcium to enter the nerve terminal. Entry of calcium into the nerve terminal facilitates the fusion of ACh-containing vesicles with the nerve terminal membrane, resulting in the exocytotic release of ACh into the synaptic cleft (Fig. 28–4).[17] The number of vesicles or quanta released into the synaptic cleft by a single nerve terminal has been estimated to be in the range 200 to 400.[18] The importance of cAMP generation and calcium entry into the nerve terminal to allow ACh release has been demonstrated by numerous experimental and clinical observations. Aminophylline has been shown to facilitate the formation of cAMP and promote neuromuscular transmission. Calcium channel blocking drugs such as verapamil and aminoglycoside antibiotics inhibit calcium entry which inhibits neurotransmitter release and decreases neuromuscular transmission. Botulinum toxin and tetanus toxin alter calcium entry into the neuron terminal and inhibit ACh release. Magnesium, a divalent cation, can enter the nerve terminal and replace or decrease the amount of calcium that enters, thereby reducing the release of ACh. Magnesium therapy, such as may be used in obstetrics for preeclamptic and eclamptic patients, has been shown to cause muscular weakness in high doses. In addition, magnesium therapy in obstetric patients has been demonstrated to potentiate both depolarizing and nondepolarizing muscle relaxants.[19]

Neuromuscular Margin of Safety

It should be apparent to the reader that under normal conditions the safety margin to maintain neuromuscular function is high, given the fact that a single action potential at a nerve terminal results in the release of hundreds of vesicles, each with quantal content of thousands of molecules of ACh, which are able to bind with an excess quantity of postsynaptic nicotinic cholinergic receptors to ensure generation of an EPP and muscular contraction. It has been demonstrated that a 0.1-Hz supramaximal stimulus will cause a

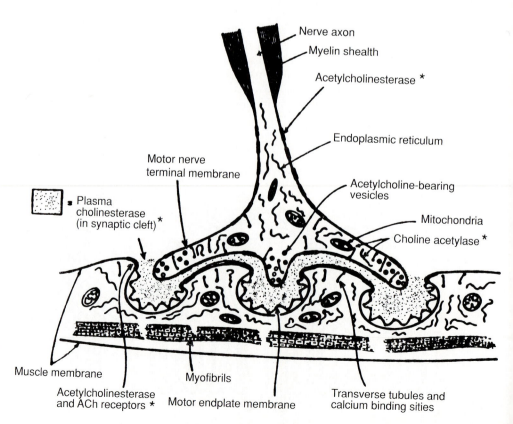

Figure 28–4. Neuromuscular junction and cholinoceptive sites. The acetylcholine-binding (cholinoceptive) sites are indicated by asterisks. (*Reprinted, with permission, from Ali and Savarese.*[20])

Nerve axon
Myelin sheath
Acetylcholinesterase *
Endoplasmic reticulum
Acetylcholine-bearing vesicles
Mitochondria
Choline acetylase *
Motor nerve terminal membrane
Plasma cholinesterase (in synaptic cleft) *
Muscle membrane
Acetylcholinesterase and ACh receptors *
Myofibrils
Motor endplate membrane
Transverse tubules and calcium binding sities

stable twitch response over a long period. For the twitch height response to a 0.1-Hz stimulus to begin to decrease, it has been estimated that 75 percent of the postsynaptic receptors need to be blocked by a nondepolarizing neuromuscular blocking agent before any reduction in motor response occurs.[20] Fade with train-of-four (TOF) stimulation occurs when 70 to 75 percent of receptors are blocked.[21] In addition, fade with tetanic stimulation at 100 Hz occurs when 50 percent of the receptors are blocked at the synapse.[22] The implications of these observations have significant clinical importance. A patient may have normal neuromuscular function, documented by blockade monitoring and motor responses such as sustained head lift for 5 seconds or longer, and still have a large number of nicotinic cholinergic receptors blocked, reducing the margin of safety for neuromuscular transmission. Inability to totally evaluate residual receptor blockade by a competitive nondepolarizing agent would make use of an appropriate reversal agent if there is any question of neuromuscular function a reasonable practice. The anesthetist's decision concerning the adequacy of the paralysis or reversal of paralysis from neuromuscular blocking agents is probably based on evaluation of as few as 25 to 50 percent of the postsynaptic receptors in skeletal muscle depending on the blockade monitoring criteria used. The remaining 50 to 75 percent of the receptors can be likened to the major portion of an iceberg that cannot be seen below the surface of the ocean. In patients receiving neuromuscular blocking agents, loss of muscle strength is not noted until 75 percent of available receptors are occupied by muscle relaxant, and normal function returns when 25 percent of available receptors are available to interact with ACh. Therefore, the status of up to 50 to 75 percent of postsynaptic receptors at the neuromuscular junction is essentially unknown early in the postanesthesia recovery phase.

Although the majority of the ACh is stored in vesicles, action-potential-dependent, all-or-none discharge of ACh vesicle contents to the synaptic cleft ignores the possibility of other forms of storage and release of ACh. Evidence for nonvesicle, non-action-potential-dependent release of ACh has been demonstrated.[23] In addition, non-calcium-dependent vesicle release of quantal amounts of ACh has been shown to occur.[24] These alternate forms of ACh storage and release do not generate sufficient EPPs to produce muscle contraction. These alternate forms of release are associated with the generation of miniature endplate potentials (MEPPs) and sub-MEPPs. The generation of MEPPs may serve a physiologic function to maintain a normal number of receptors in the synaptic region. It has been well documented in numerous experiments that loss of ACh release by denervation injuries or disease states results in extrajunctional overgrowth of nicotinic cholinergic receptors.[25] When denervated muscle is exposed to a nicotinic cholinergic agonist or a depolarizing muscle relaxant like succinylcholine there is exaggerated ion channel opening of extrajunctional receptors with resulting hyperkalemia. Tonic leakage of nonvesicle ACh or isolated vesicle quantal amounts of ACh from the presynaptic nerve terminal may play a role in the maintenance of normal densities and the types of cholinergic receptors present in the synaptic region.

Presynaptic Effects of Acetylcholine

Postsynaptic effects of the binding of released ACh to the nicotinic cholinergic receptor in the endplate region of the muscle have been well understood for some time. The possibility that ACh released from the motor nerve terminal exerts presynaptic effects that result in a positive feedback mechanism to increase mobilization and release of ACh is an action that has been recognized more recently. This presynaptic action of ACh at presynaptic nicotinic cholinergic receptors is supported by data from experiments using cholinergic agonists and depolarizing muscle relaxants as well as nondepolarizing muscle relaxants. Depolarizing muscle relaxants have been shown to increase the mobilization of ACh in motor nerve terminals, a fact that may further explain the fasciculations commonly seen after depolarizing muscle relaxant administration. The fade seen with tetanic and TOF nerve stimulation after administration of a nondepolarizing muscle relaxant is thought to be associated with decreased mobilization of ACh in the nerve terminal as a result of presynaptic receptor blockade.[26] The nondepolarizing muscle relaxant competitively blocking the presynaptic ACh receptor prevents the binding of ACh and prevents activation of the positive feedback loop to maintain adequate mobilization of ACh for release.

MONITORING NEUROMUSCULAR FUNCTION

Nonelectronic Assessment of Neuromuscular Function

Early intraoperative assessment of satisfactory neuromuscular blockade required visual evaluation of reduced muscle tone. If the surgery was an intraabdominal procedure, a relaxed abdominal wall and absence of extrusion of abdominal contents were accepted as evidence of satisfactory neuromuscular blockade. This technique for intraoperative assessment of muscle relaxation provided little quantitative knowledge as to how close to or how far beyond the ideal level of neuromuscular blockade one was. Evaluation of adequate reversal of neuromuscular blockade used clinical evaluation of ability to sustain head lift, adequate vital capacity, negative inspiratory force, hand grasp, or ability to keep the arms extended. These valuable criteria for adequate reversal of neuromuscular blockade are still used today; however, use of these reversal criteria in the presence of postoperative pain, an uncooperative patient, or a patient with residual effects of sedatives or narcotics makes evaluation of possible residual neuromuscular blockade difficult. Poor performance on clinical evaluations that require voluntary skeletal muscle movement may have several causes that are not associated with residual muscle paralysis secondary to neuromuscular blocking agents.

Electronic Assessment of Neuromuscular Function

The need to have a reliable mechanism to evaluate residual muscle paralysis that does not require a cooperative patient led to the use of an electrical impulse to stimulate an action potential in a motor nerve and measure the evoked response of the muscle supplied by the nerve.[5] Early quantitative evaluation of neuromuscular blockade with electrical stimulation of motor nerves employed three types of electronic stimulation. Single twitch or single stimulus at intervals of 0.1 to 1.0 Hz (1 stimulus per 10 seconds to 1 stimulus per second, respectively), tetanic stimulation at a frequency of 30 to 200 Hz (30 to 200 stimuli per second), and posttetanic potentiation. Utilization of single twitch at a frequency of 0.1 Hz was discovered to be of the greatest clinical relevance[27]; however, there are problems with the use of single-twitch stimuli even at 0.1 Hz. For single-twitch stimuli to be of value a control height prior to neuromuscular blocking agent administration must be established to be able to estimate the percentage reduction in control height after administration of neuromuscular blocking agent. In addition, it has been demonstrated that when muscle response to single-twitch stimuli and sustained contraction in response to 50-Hz tetanic stimuli have returned to control height, there may be significant fade to the fourth stimulus of the more sensitive TOF test.[28] In current routine clinical practice, single-twitch stimuli are useful for monitoring the degree of neuromuscular blockade during succinylcholine drip administration.

The appropriate stimulus setting to be used for tetanic stimulation of a nerve during blockade monitoring has varied with the author over time. Gissen and Katz in 1969 recommended the use of high-frequency tetanic stimulation at 100 to 200 Hz to test for fade in muscle contraction that would be associated with residual nondepolarizing blockade.[5] In 1975 Riker demonstrated that high-frequency tetanic stimulation at 200 Hz for 5 seconds or longer could produce fade in normal muscle in the absence of neuromuscular blocking agents.[16] In 1954, Merton showed that the maximal voluntary muscle contraction was equal to the contraction response to tetanus at 50 Hz.[29] In view of these findings tetanic stimulation for 5 seconds at 50 Hz seems to be the most physiologically relevant and clinically useful frequency. Sustained response to tetanic stimulation has been considered partial evidence for absence of neuromuscular blockade; however, as mentioned earlier, despite sustained tetanic contraction without fade, significant fade to the fourth stimulus in the more sensitive TOF test has been demonstrated. Monitoring tetanic stimulation has been useful during continuous infusion of succinylcholine. After establishment of a baseline response to 50-Hz tetanic stimulation, repeat evaluation of the tetanic response should show a dose-dependent suppression of tetanic contraction without fade. The appearance of fade to tetanic contraction during succinylcholine administration is accepted as evidence of conversion from phase I block to phase II block. In addition, tetanic stimulation can be used to differentiate between depolarizing and nondepolarizing neuromuscular blockade, the latter being associated with fade in the tetanic contraction. Evaluation of neuromuscular blockade with tetanic stimulation is not well accepted by conscious patients as it is painful.

Posttetanic twitch stimulation involves administration of a single-twitch stimulus 5 to 10 seconds after a tetanic stimulus at the same intensity at which the single-twitch stimuli were given prior to tetanic stimulation. In the presence of a nondepolarizing neuromuscular block or residual nondepolarizing block, posttetanic potentiation or posttetanic facilitation (posttetanic single twitch greater than pretetanic twitch response) will be seen. The increased single-twitch response is due to increased acetylcholine mobilization for release during the tetanic stimulus. Monitoring for the presence of posttetanic potentiation during continuous succinylcholine administration has been valuable in the detection of conversion from a phase I depolarizing block to a phase II block, as posttetanic potentiation is not present during a normal depolarizing phase I block.

TOF monitoring of neuromuscular blockade, which involves administration of four single-twitch stimuli at a frequency of 2 Hz (1 stimulus per 0.5 second), has numerous advantages over the previously discussed types of nerve stimulation. TOF monitoring can provide a quantitative assessment of the degree of nondepolarizing neuromuscular blockade present without the need for establishing a baseline control.[21] As described earlier, TOF monitoring is the most sensitive monitor of neuromuscular function, and is much less painful than tetanic stimulation.[28] The ratio of the amplitude of the fourth twitch (T_4) to the amplitude of the first twitch (T_1) has been used to determine the degree of nondepolarizing neuromuscular blockade. A ratio of T_4 to T_1 of 0.5 to 0.7 generally indicates satisfactory return of muscle function after administration of nondepolarizing neuromuscular blocking agents.[30] Although the electromyographic or mechanomyographic equipment necessary to establish $T_4 : T_1$ ratios is valuable in a research or teaching environment it is expensive and time consuming in daily clinical practice. A simpler clinical evaluation of the degree of nondepolarizing neuromuscular paralysis using TOF involves observing the number of responses to TOF stimulation that are abolished and correlating this number with a percentage of paralysis. As shown in Figure 28–5 when all four responses are present without fade no neuromuscular blockade exists; when the fourth response in TOF is abolished, 75 percent neuromuscular block exists; 80 percent neuromuscular block is present with loss of the third response; 90 percent neuromuscular block is present with loss of the second response; and 100 percent neuromuscular block is present when first response is abolished.[31] Adequate muscle relaxation for laryngoscopy and abdominal procedures is generally noted with 90 to 95 percent neuromuscular blockade as measured by TOF monitoring. When TOF is used to evaluate neuromuscular blockade during single-dose or continuous infusion of succinylcholine, a dose-dependent reduction in all four responses should be noted during a normal phase I depolarizing block. Fade in response from the first to the fourth response or abolition of some of the responses in the TOF is evidence of early onset of phase II block. Figures 28–6 and 28–7 illustrate depolarizing block TOF monitoring and Figure 28–8 illustrates TOF monitoring in the presence of nondepolarizing neuromuscular blocking agents.

Stimulus Strength of Blockade Monitor

When any form of electrically evoked potential blockade monitoring is used it is assumed that the intensity of all stimuli is supramaximal. The use of supramaximal stimuli ensures adequate nerve depolarization and muscle response. To ensure supramaximal stimulation using gel sur-

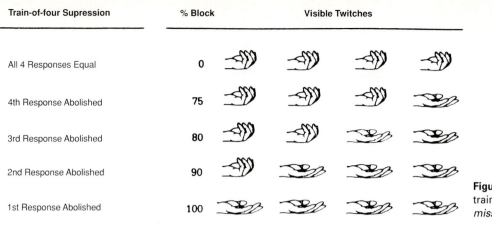

Train-of-four Supression	% Block	Visible Twitches
All 4 Responses Equal	0	
4th Response Abolished	75	
3rd Response Abolished	80	
2nd Response Abolished	90	
1st Response Abolished	100	

Figure 28–5. Interpretation of the train-of-four. (*Reprinted, with permission, from Jones.*[31])

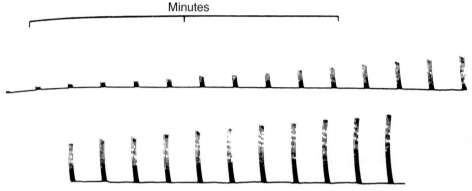

Figure 28–6. Spontaneous recovery of thumb adduction in response to T_4 stimulation at 2 Hz, repeated once every 10 seconds. This recovery followed the administration of succinylcholine 1.0 mg/kg, resulting in complete ablation of the twitches for 8 minutes in a patient anesthetized with thiopental–N_2O–O_2–narcotic. Note that the four responses recovered equally without fade at any degree of block. (*Reprinted, with permission, from Katz RL. Muscle relaxants: Basic and clinical aspects. Seminars in Anesthesia III(4), December 1984.*)

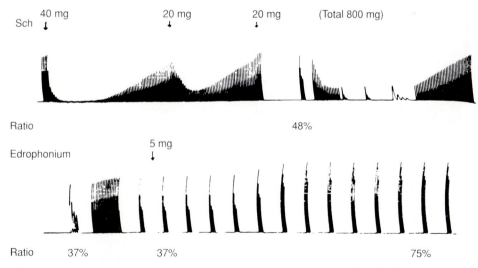

Figure 28–7. The patient whose tracing is depicted here (and also in Fig. 28–6) received a succinylcholine infusion of 10.0 mg/kg over the 2 hours after recovery from the initial dose of succinylcholine. In the upper panel, the response to T_4 after three increments of succinylcholine following discontinuation of the infusion is shown. Note the development of fade which is more evident during the recovery from each dose (recorder speed of 10 mm/min). The lower panel is a continuation of the tracing from the upper panel, showing a T_4 with a ratio of 0.37. Two minutes later, the T_4 ratio persisted at 0.37 despite the continued recovery of the four responses. At the arrow, edrophonium 5.0 mg was injected intravenously, resulting in progressive recovery of the T_4 responses, and the ratio increased from 0.37 to 0.75 in 2 minutes. (*Reprinted, with permission, from Katz RL. Muscle relaxants: Basic and clinical aspects. Seminars in Anesthesia III(4), December 1984.*)

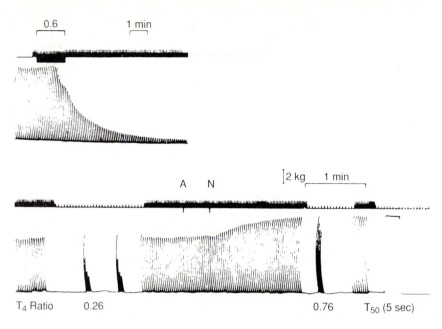

Figure 28–8. The upper panel shows evoked thumb adduction to ulnar nerve stimulation at 0.15 Hz before and after *d*-tubocurarine 0.6 mg/kg. The lower panel shows that the single twitch recovered spontaneously to 75 percent of control height and a train-of-four (T_4) ratio of only 0.26, 150 minutes after the injection of curare. Atropine and neostigmine were administered at A and N, respectively. The single twitch recovered to control height in 4 minutes, and 1 minute later the T_4 ratio increased to 0.76. At T_{50} for 5 seconds, tetanus at 50 Hz was fully sustained. (*Reprinted, with permission, from Katz RL. Muscle relaxants: Basic and clinical aspects.* Seminars in Anesthesia *III(4), December 1984.*)

face electrodes over the ulnar nerve, it is recommended that maximal twitch in the thumb be observed and the current necessary to produce this twitch be multiplied by 2.75 and the resulting current setting used. In adults, however, it is recommended that currents less than 20 mA never be used and, in most cases, currents greater than 20 mA be required to ensure supramaximal stimulation.[32]

Anatomic Sites for Blockade Monitor Stimulation

Sites for nerve stimulation during evoked potential blockade monitoring commonly include the ulnar nerve at the wrist or elbow and the facial nerve. Alternative nerve sites for stimulation have included the radial nerve at the wrist and the peroneal nerve at the ankle. To stimulate the facial nerve the leads should be placed near the tragus of the ear and not over the orbital rima, thereby avoiding the possibility of direct stimulation of the orbicularis oculi muscle which would lead to inaccurate assessment of the lack of neuromuscular blockade.[33] In the presence of 100 percent neuromuscular blockade direct electrical stimulation of muscle will result in muscle depolarization and contraction.

CHARACTERISTICS OF NONDEPOLARIZING, DEPOLARIZING, AND PHASE II NEUROMUSCULAR BLOCK

Nondepolarizing Block

Nondepolarizing neuromuscular blockade can also be referred to as a competitive block. The nondepolarizing muscle relaxants, of which curare is the prototype, are ACh antagonists. They competitively bind to the two alpha subunits of the ACh receptor, blocking the effects of ACh and preventing depolarization and neuromuscular transmission. Binding of nondepolarizing muscle relaxants is reversible and, when enough of the nondepolarizing agent is excreted or "pharmacologically reversed," ACh can successfully compete for the ACh receptor and neurotransmis-

sion can be restored. The peripheral nerve stimulation measurements and clinical observations associated with a nondepolarizing neuromuscular blocking agent can be summarized:

1. Fade with TOF and tetanic nerve stimulation
2. Posttetanic facilitation or potentiation
3. Dose-dependent reduction in single-twitch height
4. Reduction of dose requirement by prior administration of depolarizing agent
5. Reversibility by administration of anticholinesterase agents
6. No fasciculations of muscle

Depolarizing Block

Depolarizing neuromuscular blockade results when drugs with agonistic properties similar to those of ACh are used. Succinylcholine and decamethonium are two drugs that are depolarizing muscle relaxants. Of these two drugs succinylcholine continues to be used clinically; decamethonium is only of historic interest. Depolarizing neuromuscular blocking agents like ACh are able to depolarize the motor endplate and generate an EPP. The true cholinesterase present at the synapse is not able to metabolize the depolarizing neuromuscular blocking agents. As long as drug levels maintain an effective concentration at the synapse repolarization of the endplate region at the synapse will not occur, thereby blocking neuromuscular transmission. The termination of this depolarizing blockade by succinylcholine is dependent primarily on plasmacholinesterase or pseudocholinesterase hydrolysis of succinylcholine to succinylmonocholine in the plasma. The rapid hydrolysis of succinylcholine in plasma rapidly lowers the effective concentration in plasma, resulting in the presence of lower effective concentrations at the synapse. Termination of depolarizing blockade by decamethonium depends primarily on renal excretion as plasma cholinesterase is unable to hydrolyze decamethonium. Peripheral nerve stimulator and clinical findings associated with depolarizing blockade or phase I block would include the following:

1. There is a dose-dependent reduction in single-twitch, TOF, and tetanic stimulation response without fade in any of the tests.
2. There is no evidence of posttetanic potentiation.
3. Fasciculations in skeletal muscle commonly noted.
4. Anticholinesterase drugs given during depolarizing phase I block either show no effect on the peripheral nerve stimulator or intensify the degree of neuromuscular block.

Phase II Block

Phase II block has been reported to occur in individuals who have received succinylcholine. In the past other names were used for phase II block, including desensitization block, dual block, and open channel block. Conversion from a normal depolarizing succinylcholine phase I block to a nondepolarizing type phase II block has been reported to occur after excessive single doses or continuous infusions of succinylcholine for long periods in normal individuals. In patients with atypical pseudocholinesterase, inhibition of pseudocholinesterase (organophosphate exposure), or decreased levels of pseudocholinesterase as a result of disease processes, prolonged paralysis followed by phase II block has been reported to occur with 1 mg/kg intubation doses of succinylcholine. It has been established that phase II block occurs at lower doses of succinylcholine, 4 to 5 mg/kg, if halothane is used, whereas doses of 7 to 8 mg/kg may be required in N_2O/O_2 narcotic anesthesia techniques.[34] Why phase II block occurs is not well defined. The most accepted theory is that the prolonged exposure of the ACh receptor to depolarizing agents such as succinylcholine results in a conformational change of the receptor and the inability to normally depolarize and repolarize in response to cholinergic-type agonists.[35] The pre- and postjunctional ACh receptor conformational change or "desensitization" results in a block with the following peripheral nerve stimulator and clinical observations:

1. Fade with TOF and tetanic nerve stimulation
2. Posttetanic facilitation or potentiation
3. Reduction in single-twitch height
4. Reversal by administration of anticholinesterase agents

The capability to reverse a succinylcholine phase II block has been demonstrated[36]; however, because of the predictability of the quality or safety margin associated with reversal of a phase II block, the conservative clinician may choose to support ventilation and let the passage of time reverse the phase II block.

PHARMACOLOGY AND STRUCTURE–ACTIVITY RELATIONSHIPS OF NEUROMUSCULAR BLOCKING AGENTS

All neuromuscular blocking agents have at least one and in most cases two quaternary nitrogen groups on each mole-

cule (positively charged at physiologic pH) that interact with or bind to a negatively charged region on the two 40,000-dalton alpha subunits on the ACh receptors. The charged quaternary nitrogen moiety of the muscle relaxants results in poor absorption from the gastrointestinal tract, and poor transfer across the placenta and blood–brain barrier. The depolarizing neuromuscular blocking agents are long slender molecules that have structural similarities to the neurotransmitter ACh (Fig. 28–9). In fact, succinylcholine is a dimer of two acetylcholine molecules, and decamethonium is composed of two quaternary ammonium nitrogen groups separated by ten carbon atoms. The structural similarity of succinylcholine and decamethonium to ACh is the reason these compounds have depolarizing agonistic properties at the ACh receptor. The primary action of succinylcholine and decamethonium is to bind to nicotinic ACh receptors in skeletal muscle, producing a depolarizing neuromuscular blockade. Many of the complications associated with the administration of depolarizing muscle relaxants are associated with their capability to bind to muscarinic and nicotinic cholinergic receptors at sites not related to skeletal muscle. Some of the significant sites include nicotinic ACh receptors in the autonomic ganglia, and muscarinic parasympathetic ACh receptors in the heart, gastrointestinal tract, bladder, and bronchi. In contrast to the depolarizing muscle relaxants the nondepolarizing muscle relaxants have a large rigid bulky structure with at least one and in most cases two quaternary nitrogen groups that can bind to the ACh receptor and prevent the binding of ACh to its receptor in a competitive reversible fashion. Other than a quaternary nitrogen group the nondepolarizing muscle relaxants have little resemblance to ACh (Fig. 28–10). The nondepolarizing muscle relaxants have no agonistic properties of their own and in sufficient concentration by mass action will be able to compete for the ACh receptor binding site, preventing depolarization of the endplate region by ACh. The primarily monoquaternary structure of *d*-tubocurarine is thought to be associated with its potential

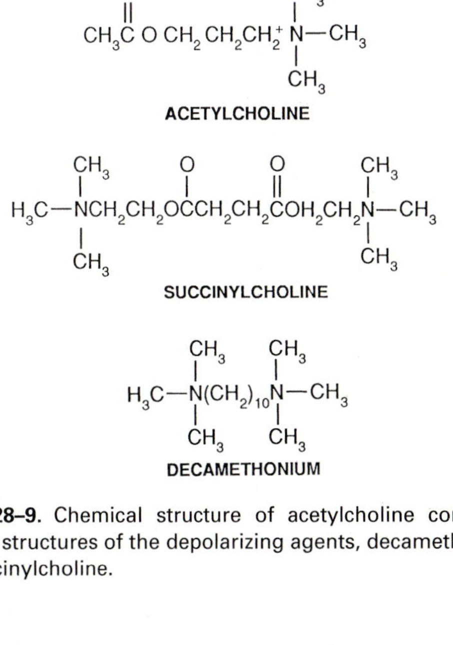

Figure 28–9. Chemical structure of acetylcholine contrasted with the structures of the depolarizing agents, decamethonium, and succinylcholine.

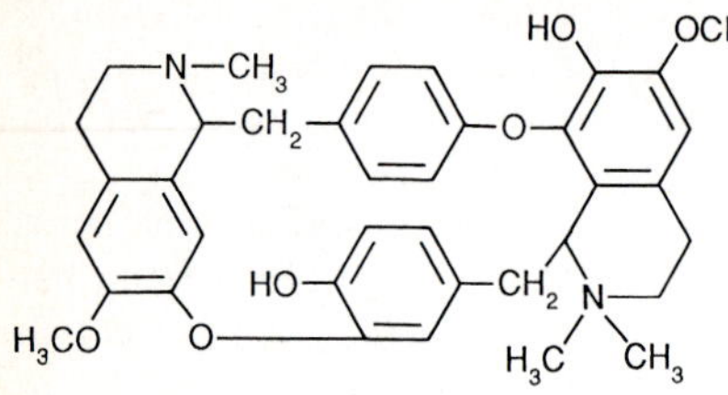

D-TUBOCURARINE

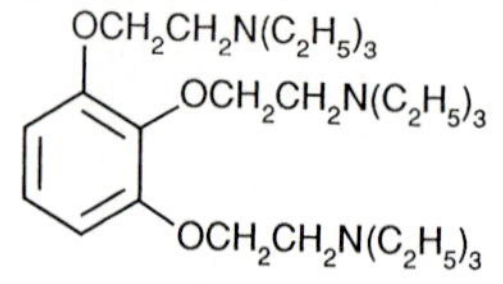

GALLAMINE

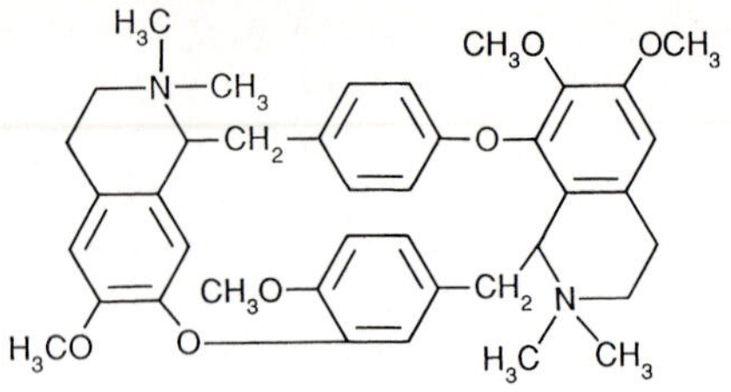

METOCURINE

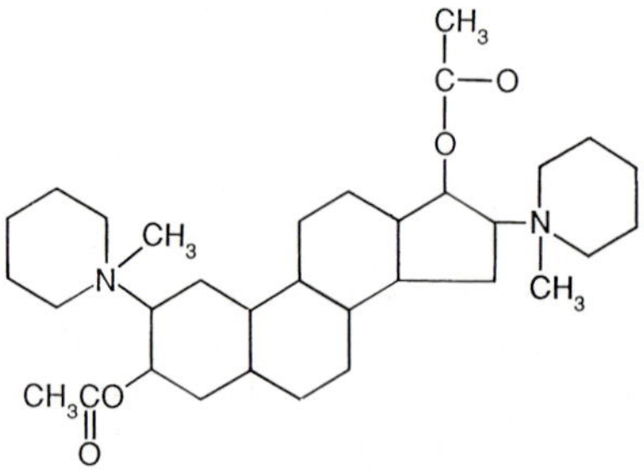

PANCURONIUM

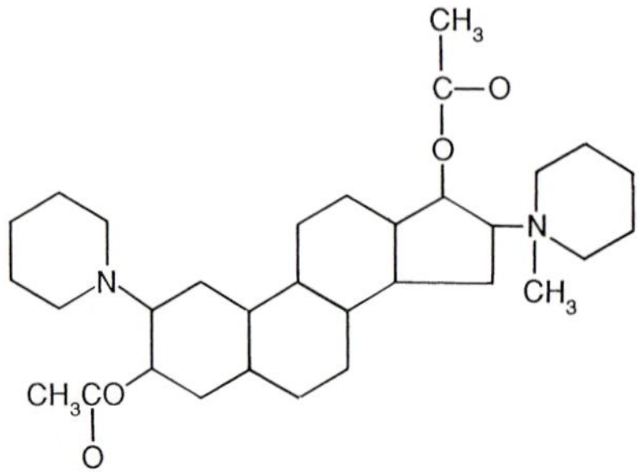

VECURONIUM

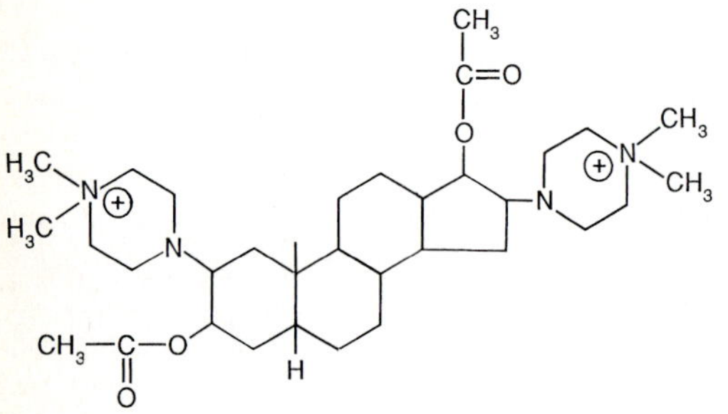

PIPECURONIUM

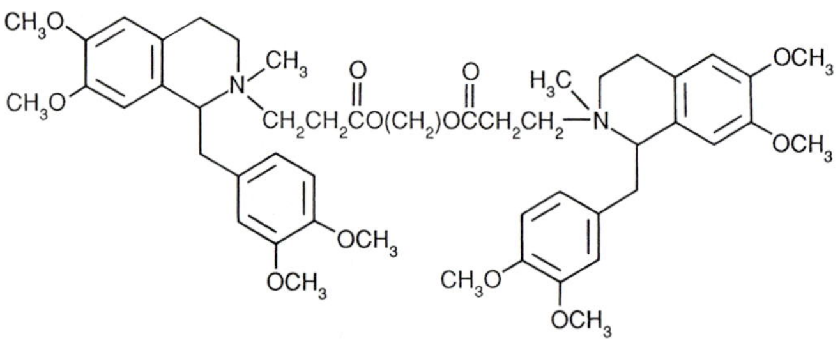

ATRACURIUM

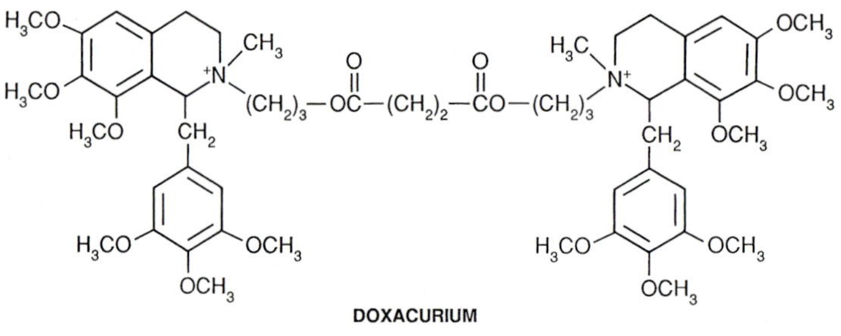

DOXACURIUM

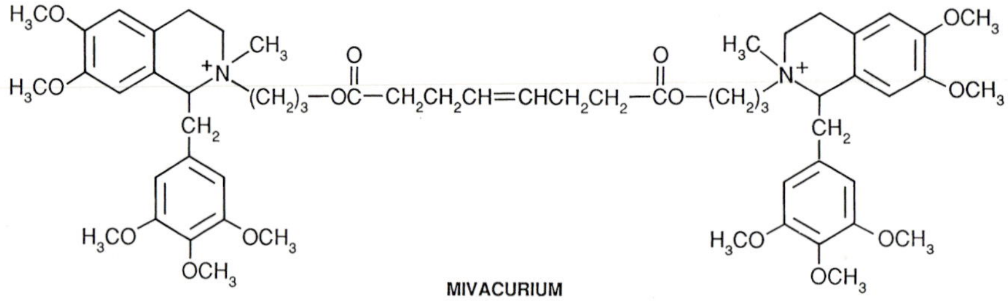

MIVACURIUM

Figure 28–10. Chemical structures of the nondepolarizing neuromuscular blocking agents available in clinical practice.

for autonomic ganglionic blockade and histamine-releasing properties. The additional methylation of d-tubocurarine results in the bisquaternary compound dimethyltubocurarine which is associated with less autonomic ganglionic blockade and histamine-releasing properties. The triquaternary structure of gallamine is thought to be associated with its capability for strong blockade of muscarinic cholinergic receptors, whereas the muscarinic blocking properties of pancuronium are limited primarily to the muscarinic ACh receptors in the heart and autonomic nervous system. The minor modification of removing one methyl group from the steroid structure of pancuronium results in the production of vecuronium, a nondepolarizing muscle relaxant devoid of cardiovascular side effects and having a shorter duration than pancuronium. If there are fewer than eight CH_2 groups between the quaternary nitrogen groups significant autonomic ganglionic blocking will increase and the potency to block nicotinic ACh receptors in skeletal muscle will be decreased. Hexamethonium, a bisquaternary compound with six methylene groups between the quaternary nitrogen groups, is associated with significant autonomic ganglionic blocking properties, whereas decamethonium, a compound with ten methylene groups between the quaternary nitrogen groups, shows significant neuromuscular blocking properties with minimal autonomic ganglionic blocking properties.[37] This finding demonstrated significant differences in the binding affinities for ligands and presumably differences in structure between nicotinic ACh receptors in skeletal muscle and autonomic ganglia.

DEPOLARIZING MUSCLE RELAXANTS

Types of Depolarizing Drugs

Two drugs, decamethonium and succinylcholine, are depolarizing muscle relaxants that have been used clinically. Decamethonium is not in common clinical use today; it has most of the side effects of succinylcholine and its usual duration of action after a single bolus dose is about 20 to 30 minutes. Decamethonium is not broken down by pseudocholinesterase and its action is terminated primarily by renal excretion of unchanged drug. The introduction of intermediate-duration-of-action nondepolarizing muscle relaxants such as vecuronium and atracurium has negated any rational reason for the clinical use of decamethonium. The remaining discussion of depolarizing muscle relaxants is limited to the pharmacology and clinical use of succinylcholine.

Succinylcholine

History. Hunt and de Taveau became aware of the cardiovascular effects of succinylcholine while studying a variety of ACh congeners. Evidently their experiments were performed on curarized animals and the neuromuscular blocking effects of succinylcholine were not noted by these investigators.[38] The neuromuscular blocking effects of succinylcholine were not noted until 1949.[39] By 1951, Bruke et al had introduced succinylcholine into clinical use in Europe, and by 1952 Foldes et al introduced succinylcholine into clinical use in the United States.[40]

Drug Action. Succinylcholine was rapidly accepted into clinical practice because of its ability to produce satisfactory paralysis within 1 minute for intubations or short surgical procedures. The effective dose required for paralysis ranges from 0.3 to 1.1 mg/kg; most clinicians choose a dose of 0.5 to 1 mg/kg which produces satisfactory intubation conditions in 30 to 60 seconds, maximal paralysis for 3 to 5 minutes, and full spontaneous recovery within 10 minutes in normal patients. Succinylcholine infusions at the rate of 0.5 to 5 mg/min monitored by a peripheral nerve stimulator can be used to maintain paralysis for extended periods. The possibility of developing a phase II block with increasing doses of succinylcholine over extended periods has resulted in the recommendation to avoid the use of succinylcholine infusions longer than 1 hour. The introduction of vecuronium and atracurium and the continued trend to avoid the use of depolarizing agents have resulted in a decline in the use of succinylcholine for extended surgical procedures; however, succinylcholine bolus and continuous infusion are useful for short procedures requiring muscle relaxation, such as cesarean sections, closed reductions of fractures, and endoscopy procedures. If a succinylcholine infusion is to be used, addition of methylene blue to color the infusion provides an additional safety factor to avoid confusion with other infusions.

Physical and Chemical Properties. Succinylcholine is a dimer of two ACh molecules bonded together resulting in a bisquaternary compound that has two positively charged regions to interact with the 40,000-dalton alpha subunits of the ACh receptor. Succinylcholine powder is a white crystalline substance that is stable over a wide range of conditions in its unreconstituted state. The water solubility of succinylcholine is high and it easily goes into solution with most common intravenous solutions. Once succinylcholine has been placed in solution it is best to keep the solution refrigerated to avoid hydrolysis and loss of potency. Infusions of succinylcholine should be used only for 24 hours after mixture to avoid the potential for bacterial contamination.

Pharmacokinetics and Pharmacodynamics. Succinylcholine is able to bind to the ACh receptor and produce persistent depolarization of the skeletal muscle endplate region, as the true AChE present at the synapse and in red blood cells cannot hydrolyze succinylcholine. Unlike true AChE, pseudocholinesterase or plasma cholinesterase is synthesized in the liver and high concentrations are present in the plasma but not at the synaptic region. The rapid termination of succinylcholine's effect is due to the ability of pseudocholinesterase to rapidly hydrolyze succinylcholine in the plasma to succinylmonocholine and choline, relatively inactive metabolites of succinylcholine. The elimination half-life for succinylcholine is 1 to 2 minutes. The short half-life of succinylcholine indicates that only a small portion of the total dose administered reaches the synaptic region and that within five half-lives (5 to 10 minutes) breakdown of succinylcholine to succinylmono choline and choline is nearly 100 percent complete. Pseudocholinesterase also is responsible for the slower hydrolysis of succinylmonocholine to succinic acid and choline which is usually complete after 3 hours. The termination of succinylcholine's effect is due to its rapid hydrolysis in the plasma, allowing residual succinylcholine to diffuse out of the synapse to the extracellular fluid, which then allows repolarization of the endplate.

If there are abnormally low levels of pseudocholinesterase the reduction of the pseudocholinesterase activity will be directly related to the increased duration of paralysis.[41] In individuals with atypical pseudocholinesterase, succinylcholine hydrolysis is reduced and the renal excretion of this polar drug becomes a significant factor in the termination of succinylcholine's effect. When the capability for succinylcholine hydrolysis is significantly altered the prolongation of paralysis requires sedation and positive-pressure ventilation until complete spontaneous reversal of paralysis occurs. The use of a peripheral nerve stimulator to document sustained presence of a depolarizing block and its duration enables the clinician to rationally decide when it is safe to extubate the patient. Whenever succinylcholine is administered a peripheral nerve stimulator should be used to demonstrate complete reversal of succinylcholine before additional succinylcholine or a nondepolarizing muscle relaxant is given.

Pseudocholinesterase. Problems with pseudocholinesterase enzyme are either qualitative (the ability to metabolize succinylcholine) or quantitative (the amount of enzyme available to metabolize succinylcholine). Some of the earliest complications associated with succinylcholine administration were related to reductions in the quality or the quantity of pseudocholinesterase present to metabolize succinylcholine, resulting in unexpected prolongation of paralysis after apparently normal doses of the drug. Liver dysfunction, pregnancy, and starvation have been shown to reduce the amount of pseudocholinesterase produced. Owing to the ability of pseudocholinesterase to metabolize succinylcholine rapidly, severe disease or drug inhibition is necessary before a prolongation of succinylcholine paralysis is noted. Foldes et al demonstrated that liver disease must be severe before there is an increase in the duration of paralysis from succinylcholine.[42] Term pregnancy has been shown to produce a 40 percent reduction in pseudocholinesterase activity without a significant increase in the duration of paralysis after succinylcholine.[43] The remaining 60 percent functional enzyme capability and the increase in the volume of distribution of succinylcholine are sufficient to prevent any increase in duration of paralysis. AChE-inhibiting agents that are used in insecticides or the organophosphate AChE-inhibiting agents present in military nerve toxins such as Saran and Soman would inhibit both true and pseudocholinesterase and potentiate the effects of endogenous ACh and exogenous succinylcholine. In addition, the AChE-inhibiting drugs used to treat glaucoma (ecothiopate) and myasthenia gravis (mestanon) and the chemotherapeutic agents nitrogen mustard and cyclophosphamide have been associated with reduction of pseudocholinesterase activity and increased duration of paralysis after succinylcholine administration.

In 1957 Kalow and Genest were able to demonstrate three phenotypes of pseudocholinesterase as expressed in an in vitro assay using the amide local anesthetic dibucaine.[44] Normal or typical pseudocholinesterase will hydrolyze succinylcholine and benzoylcholine. When typical pseudocholinesterase is exposed to benzoylcholine in the presence of dibucaine the hydrolysis of benzoylcholine is inhibited to 80 percent of normal. Therefore, the "dibucaine number" is an expression of the percentage pseudocholinesterase inhibition of benzoylcholine hydrolysis in the presence of dibucaine. Individuals with normal or typical pseudocholinesterase show 80 percent dibucaine inhibition, constitute 96.25 percent of the population (Canadian population data), and react normally to succinylcholine. Individuals who are heterozygotes (one normal and one abnormal allele for pseudocholinesterase) have dibucaine numbers of 70 to 30 percent inhibition, constitute 3.7 percent of the population, and may show a modest prolongation of paralysis after normal doses of succinylcholine. Individuals who are homozygotes for atypical pseudocholinesterase (two abnormal alleles for pseudocholinesterase) have dibucaine numbers showing less than 30 percent inhibition, constitute 0.05 percent of the population, and may require 2 to 4 hours or longer to recover from a single 1 mg/kg dose of succinylcholine.

In about 20 percent of the homozygous atypical pseudocholinesterase individuals a third type of allele is thought to exist and has been referred to as the *silent allele*. A genotype consisting of one atypical allele and one silent allele results in the phenotype of an atypical homozygote. A genotype of two silent alleles results in the phenotypical expression of an individual with no pseudocholinesterase activity at all, and would therefore have a dibucaine number of 0 percent inhibition as there is no enzyme to inhibit. An individual who is a homozygote for the silent allele would demonstrate severe sensitivity to succinylcholine as the only mechanism for termination would be renal excretion.

A fourth allele is thought to exist based on the observation that rare forms of serum cholinesterase are not resistant to inhibition by dibucaine but are resistant to inhibition by fluoride. If an individual is heterogeneous or a homozygote for the "fluoride-resistant" allele there will be some degree of increased sensitivity to the paralytic effects of succinylcholine.

A fifth isoenzyme of pseudocholinesterase has been identified. The existence of this fifth isoenzyme for pseudocholinesterase would suggest the existence of a fifth allele governing the production of pseudocholinesterase. It is of interest that unlike the other forms of atypical pseudocholinesterase that show increased sensitivity to succinylcholine, this fifth isoenzyme of pseudocholinesterase is associated with a shorter-than-normal duration of paralysis and presumably an increased rate of hydrolysis of succinylcholine.[45]

If a patient is known or suspected of having a form of atypical pseudocholinesterase it would be reasonable to choose a nondepolarizing muscle relaxant that would have a predictable duration of action. In many cases it would be acceptable to use the priming principle with a nondepolarizing agent in conjunction with ventilation through cricoid pressure to achieve intubating conditions in a slightly longer time than would be noted with succinylcholine. In a patient with atypical pseudocholinesterase the short duration of action of succinylcholine could not be relied on even if the dose were significantly reduced.

Adverse Effects of Succinylcholine

Hyperkalemia. In normal patients succinylcholine will produce an increase in serum potassium of about 0.5 to 1.0 mEq/L.[46] Severe hyperkalemic episodes after succinylcholine administration to burn patients were initially reported by Lowenstein in 1966.[47] Since this report was published, the conditions associated with hyperkalemia that result in ventricular fibrillation and cardiovascular collapse after succinylcholine have expanded to include massive trauma, severe intraabdominal infections, denervation with muscle atrophy, upper motor neuron lesions, tetanus, muscular dystrophy, and multiple sclerosis. The mechanism for hyperkalemia in massive trauma is thought to be related to muscle membrane dysfunction and inability to move potassium back to the intracellular space after depolarization by succinylcholine. The mechanism for hyperkalemia in patients with upper motor neuron disease or denervation injuries is better understood. The loss of presynaptic neurotransmitter release results in the excessive growth of extrajunctional cholinergic receptors on the muscle surface and, when succinylcholine binds to these extrajunctional receptors and depolarizes the muscle, a large amount of intracellular potassium is released to the extracellular space. The length of time after injury during which the patient is at risk for a hyperkalemic response to succinylcholine administration varies. In burn patients, serum potassium may begin to rise within days of the burn and peak 3 weeks after burn injury. The burn patient remains at risk for hyperkalemia after succinylcholine administration until all burns are healed. Patients with upper motor neuron denervation injuries are at risk for 6 to 12 months after the initial injury if disease does not continue to progress. Succinylcholine has not been associated with hyperkalemia when given less than 24 hours after a burn injury or within the first 1 to 2 hours of injury in trauma patients. It is reasonable to avoid the use of succinylcholine more than 24 hours after initial burn injury or 1 to 2 hours after a traumatic injury until all wounds or burns are healed or infection has been cleared. In the case of denervation injuries and upper motor neuron injuries it may be safest to avoid succinylcholine for 6 to 12 months after neurologic loss has stabilized.

In the case of a patient with a potassium of 5.5 or greater the slight increase in potassium of 1 to 0.5 mEq seen in all patients who are given succinylcholine may be sufficient to cause the patient to experience an acute onset of arrhythmias. In chronic renal failure patients with potassium elevations who are dialysis dependent and present for emergency surgery, the use of succinylcholine may be contraindicated. Pretreatment or defasciculation with a nondepolarizing neuromuscular blocking agent (10 percent of a normal paralyzing dose) has been shown to attenuate the hyperkalemic response; however, defasciculation has not been shown to reliably provide full protection from the occurrence of hyperkalemia.

Cardiac Dysrhythmias.

The development of dysrhythmias without associated hyperkalemia is associated with the ability of succinylcholine to stimulate cholinergic receptors at autonomic ganglia in both the sympathetic and the parasympathetic nervous systems, as well as muscarinic receptors for ACh in parasympathetic effector organs such as the conduction system of the heart. Supraventricular dysrhythmias most commonly reported after the use of succinylcholine include sinus bradycardia, junctional rhythms, and, more rarely, sinus arrest. Sinus bradycardia after an initial dose of succinylcholine is more common in nonatropinized children who normally have a higher resting sympathetic tone. When the sympathetic nervous system is very active, as it is in many children additional equal stimulation of both limbs of the autonomic nervous system results in what appears to be a greater effect in the parasympathetic nervous system, as there is greater potential for change in activity in the branch of the autonomic nervous system that was less active (the parasympathetic nervous system). As noted earlier, this parasympathetic nervous system activation is due to succinylcholine stimulation of the autonomic nervous system at nicotinic cholinergic receptors at the autonomic ganglia as well as cholinergic muscarinic receptors in the cardiac conduction system. Stoelting has noted that gallamine 0.3 mg/kg is more effective than atropine 0.006 mg/kg in preventing bradycardia after the initial dose of succinylcholine.[48]

Junctional bradycardia is most commonly reported in adults who have received a second dose of succinylcholine 5 minutes after the initial dose. The occurrence of this dysrhythmia is most likely due to greater stimulation of muscarinic receptors in the sinus node than in the atrioventricular node, causing the atrioventricular node to become the predominant pacemaker. The interval of 5 minutes between doses suggests that hydrolysis of succinylcholine and generation of succinylmonocholine play a role in potentiation of the bradycardiac effects of succinylcholine. Mathias et al demonstrated that the incidence of junctional bradycardia increases after a second dose of succinylcholine, but can be prevented by prior administration of *d*-tubocurarine.[49]

Increases in heart rate and blood pressure have also been reported after succinylcholine administration. The magnitude of the heart rate increase would be potentiated by a preexisting high parasympathetic nervous system tone (an effect opposite to that seen with high sympathetic tone in children). In addition, the prior administration of small doses of atropine will further increase the heart rate, as the effects of succinylcholine on the parasympathetic system will be blocked by atropine at the muscarinic receptors, leaving the effects of succinylcholine on the sympathetic ganglia unopposed.[50] The increased blood pressure is due to succinylcholine stimulation of nicotinic cholinergic receptors at the autonomic ganglia, resulting in an increase in release of norepinephrine and epinephrine from the adrenal medulla. The potential for increased blood pressure and heart rate can be significant in patients who have coronary insufficiency, cerebral aneurysms, or other vascular conditions in which sudden changes in blood pressure could be damaging.

Intragastric Pressure Increases.

Succinylcholine is often the muscle relaxant of choice in intubation of a patient who presents with a full stomach. It is ironic that the drug that can establish intubation conditions the fastest can place the patient at increased risk for regurgitation and aspiration. There are conflicting reports in the literature as to succinylcholine's effects on intragastric pressure. Miller and Way have suggested that the fasciculations associated with succinylcholine can significantly increase intragastric pressure to produce regurgitation of gastric contents.[51] Salem et al found that succinylcholine did not significantly alter intragastric pressure in infants and children.[52] Miller and Way suggested that *d*-tubocurarine 3 mg, gallamine 20 mg, or lidocaine 6 mg/kg prevents succinylcholine-mediated increases in intragastric pressure.[51] A study by Smith et al demonstrated that the difference between the intragastric pressure and the pressure in the high-pressure zone of the lower esophageal sphincter was the critical element that prevented gastric regurgitation.[53] As long as the pressure in the high-pressure zone of the lower esophageal sphincter is higher than the intragastric pressure, regurgitation does not take place. In addition, Smith et al found that during succinylcholine administration increases in intragastric pressure are always associated with increases in high-pressure-zone esophageal sphincter pressures, eliminating the increased risk of regurgitation associated with succinylcholine administration.[53] Marchand demonstrated that intragastric pressures greater than 28 cm H_2O result in incompetence of the cardioesophageal junction in cadavers[54]; however, the assumption that regurgitation will never occur at intragastric pressures below 28 cm H_2O is not accurate. An intragastric pressure of 15 cm H_2O is sufficient to produce gastroesophageal incompetence in patients who have increased intraabdominal contents (pregnancy, bowel obstruction, obesity, ascites, hiatal hernia), conditions that alter the normal oblique angle of entry of the esophagus into the stomach.

In current practice if succinylcholine is to be used for a patient at risk for vomiting or regurgitation and aspiration, it would be reasonable to pretreat the patient with a nondepolarizing relaxant. In addition, if time and patient condition permit, pharmacologic pretreatment with metoclopramide, an H_2-receptor blocker (ranitidine), and a nonparticulate antacid can be beneficial. Finally, whenever the induction agent and succinylcholine are administered, Sellick's maneuver is maintained until the airway is secured. Should arterial desaturation become evident during a rapid sequence induction on a patient with a full stomach, mask ventilation with Sellick's maneuver in place is more acceptable than the effects of persistent hypoxemia. If the patient's condition permits, light sedation and awake intubation can overcome many of the concerns of regurgitation in the patient with a "full stomach."

Intraocular Pressure Increases. The patient with an open eye injury poses a dilemma in patient management to the anesthetist. In most cases, patients with open eye injuries present emergently and have a full stomach. Succinylcholine muscle relaxation will allow the most rapid intubation and control of the airway; however, it is well known that succinylcholine produces an increase in intraocular pressure that peaks within 2 to 4 minutes and lasts 5 to 10 minutes.[55] The increase in intraocular pressure in response to succinylcholine is presumed to result from its ability to produce contracture or fasciculations of extraocular and orbital muscles.[56] It was suggested that a small dose or defasciculatory dose of a nondepolarizing muscle relaxant (3 to 6 mg of *d*-tubocurarine) would reduce or prevent succinyl-

choline-induced increases in intraocular pressure. Cook has since demonstrated that no pretreatment regimen can consistently reduce increases in succinylcholine-induced intraocular pressure.[57] The recommendation that succinylcholine not be given to patients with open eye injuries remains clinically valid. Techniques in common practice for intubation of patients with open eye injuries generally involve a priming dose followed by an intubation dose of a nondepolarizing muscle relaxant and mask ventilation with Sellick's maneuver until intubation conditions exist. One case that could possibly justify the use of succinylcholine in a patient with an open eye injury would be the patient who has a difficult-to-visualize airway. In this case defasciculation prior to administration of succinylcholine and the possibility of a slight rise in intraocular pressure may be more tolerable than the inability to intubate a patient who will be paralyzed for an extended period.

Intracranial Pressure Increases. Succinylcholine 1 mg/kg has been shown to increase intracranial pressure in animals and more importantly in humans. Minton et al demonstrated that in anesthetized patients with brain tumors succinylcholine produced an average intracranial pressure increase of 4.9 mm Hg and, in some patients, maximal increases of 9 mm Hg.[58] The rise in intracranial pressure can be prevented by defasciculation with a nondepolarizing muscle relaxant.[59] In cases where immediate control of the airway is not necessary, induction of an adequate depth of anesthesia, maintenance of ventilation and hypocarbia, and slower production of muscle paralysis with nondepolarizing non-histamine-releasing muscle relaxants will avoid increases in intracranial pressure. If there exists a need to establish intubation conditions rapidly, succinylcholine can be safely used if the patient is defasciculated, the anesthetic depth is adequate, and controlled ventilation with hypocarbia is ensured.

Myoglobulinemia and Myoglobulinuria. Myoglobulinemia has been reported after succinylcholine administration in pediatric patients.[60] Significant elevations of plasma creatine phosphokinase (CPK) have also been demonstrated after the administration of succinylcholine. These findings would indicate some degree of muscle damage in children who receive succinylcholine; however, the occurrence of actual myoglobulinuria in conjunction with the myoglobulinemia is rare. The mechanism responsible for myoglobulinemia after succinylcholine administration in children is poorly understood and rarely seen in normal adult patients. There is no correlation between the occurrence of fasciculations, the use of defasciculatory doses of nondepolarizing muscle relaxants, or the total dose of succinylcholine administered and the degree of myoglobulinemia seen in children.[61] Based on the long history of clinical use of succinylcholine in normal children, it would appear that myoglobulinemia after succinylcholine administration is an interesting biochemical finding with minimal clinical significance.

Myalgia. Muscle pain in the shoulders, back, neck, abdomen, chest, and extremities has been reported after succinylcholine administration. The incidence is highest in young adults undergoing minor surgical procedures that are associated with minimal postoperative pain and allow for early ambulation. The onset of pain is usually noted less than one day after succinylcholine administration and generally lasts a couple of days. The pain is described as that usually associated with extended physical exertion. Initially the myalgia after succinylcholine was thought to be caused by fasciculation of skeletal muscle, which is most likely due to presynaptic ACh receptor depolarization by succinylcholine.[16] Drugs with the strongest presynaptic ACh receptor blocking capability, such as *d*-tubocurarine, have been found to be the most reliable defasciculatory agents. Defasciculatory doses of nondepolarizing muscle relaxants clearly reduce the incidence of fasciculations as well as the incidence and severity of postoperative myalgia[62]; however, Manchikanti et al showed little correlation between the incidence of fasciculation and postoperative myalgia.[63] Other pharmacologic agents that have been used to prevent fasciculations or reduce myalgias include lidocaine,[64] fentanyl,[65] calcium gluconate,[66] and diazepam.[67] The incidence of succinylcholine-induced myalgia in the absence of fasciculations leaves the exact mechanism of action for this problem open to question.

Abnormal Muscle Responses. Rare conditions exist in which succinylcholine produces muscle contraction rather than relaxation. Patients with myotonia congenita or myotonia dystrophica who are given succinylcholine develop jaw rigidity as well as generalized body rigidity, which can make intubation and ventilation difficult. The rigidity observed in patients with myotonias given succinylcholine is rarely related to the malignant hyperthermia syndrome and symptoms of a hypermetabolic state are not noted.

The syndrome of malignant hyperthermia was first described by Denborough and Lovell in 1960.[68] A wide variety of stimuli can precipitate the onset of malignant hyperthermia in genetically sensitive individuals; in fact, in genetically sensitive pigs, the stress of transport to market was sufficient to trigger fatal episodes of malignant hyperthermia. Rare reports of hyperthermia and death associated with ether anesthesia had been reported in the early 1900s prior to Denborough and Lovell's report. Halogenated anesthetics (most commonly halothane) by themselves can trigger sustained muscle contraction and a malignant hyperthermic episode; however, halogenated anesthetics in conjunction with succinylcholine constitute an especially potent pharmaceutical trigger of this hypermetabolic state. Any muscular rigidity that occurs in association with unexplained tachycardia after succinylcholine administration must be evaluated as a potential case of malignant hyperthermia until proven otherwise. For a detailed discussion of malignant hyperthermia the reader is referred to the review by Gronert.[69]

Allergic Responses and Histamine Release. Succinylcholine has a low potential for producing clinically significant histamine release and is stated to have 1/100th of the histamine-releasing potential of *d*-tubocurarine. The possibility of anaphylaxis exists for nearly every pharmacologic compound introduced into clinical practice. Rare true anaphylaxis related to succinylcholine administration has been reported with signs and symptoms of tachycardia, hypotension, bronchospasm, and pharyngeal and facial edema. As with any anaphylactic reaction maintenance of effective circulation and oxygenation are paramount in patient survival.

Use in Pregnancy. Succinylcholine has been safely used in obstetric patients for years without adverse effects on the fetus. The quaternary ammonium structure of succinylcholine results in a substance that is highly charged and poorly transferred across the placental barrier in normal clinical doses. Succinylcholine has not been shown to reduce the rate or force of uterine contraction.

Summary of Depolarizing Relaxants

Succinylcholine has enjoyed a unique role in clinical anesthesia. Its primary advantages are its rapid onset and short duration of action. Despite its many potential complications and drug interactions it will remain in clinical use until a nondepolarizing muscle relaxant with rapid onset and a duration of action profile similar to that of succinylcholine is introduced. The recent introduction of mivacurium (BW B1090U) represents the beginning of the rewards of research and development directed at isolation of nondepolarizing muscle relaxants that may one day replace succinylcholine.[70]

LONG-ACTING NONDEPOLARIZING MUSCLE RELAXANTS

Common Factors of Nondepolarizing Relaxants

The mechanism of action of all nondepolarizing muscle relaxants is their ability to function as competitive antagonists at the ACh receptor. These agents have no cholinergic agonist activity and, by binding to the ACh receptor, block the action of ACh. Inhibition of neuromuscular transmission and development of EPPs is dependent on the presence of a greater concentration of nondepolarizing muscle relaxant than of ACh at the synapse to effectively compete for ACh binding sites at alpha subunits of the ACh receptor. The competitive reversible binding of the nondepolarizing relaxants to the ACh receptor is the basis for reversal of paralysis. When the concentration of nondepolarizing agent decreases or the concentration of ACh is increased by an anticholinesterase drug, binding of ACh to the ACh receptor is favored and neuromuscular transmission is restored. Activation and channel opening of the ACh receptor require occupation of both alpha subunits, whereas competitive blockade of the ACh receptor channel can be accomplished by occupation of only one alpha subunit of the ACh receptor.

The nondepolarizing agents available for clinical use include *d*-tubocurarine, metocurine, gallamine, pancuronium, pipecuronium, and doxacurium which all have moderately long durations of action. Nondepolarizing agents with intermediate durations of action include atracurium and vecuronium. Mivacurium is a new short-acting nondepolarizing relaxant with a duration roughly half as long as that of atracurium or vecuronium.

d-Tubocurarine

History and Pharmacologic Action. *d*-Tubocurarine (Fig. 28–10) was the first muscle relaxant used clinically and is often the prototype muscle relaxant with which all new nondepolarizing muscle relaxants are compared, with respect to potency, side-effect profile, and duration of action. Therefore, an understanding of the pharmacology of *d*-tubocurarine is essential to the understanding of other nondepolarizing agents. The history and clinical pharmacology of *d*-tubocurarine have been discussed previously. All nondepolarizing neuromuscular blocking agents produce paralysis by competing with ACh for binding to nicotinic cholinergic receptors at the motor endplate. Neuromuscular blocking agents are highly ionized at physiologic pH and cross the lipid barriers of cell membranes poorly. Measurable amounts of *d*-tubocurarine have been detected in cerebrospinal fluid.[71] No alteration in cognitive function or analgesic properties has been shown to be associated with any nondepolarizing muscle relaxant in clinical use. The characteristics of nondepolarizing neuromuscular blockade can be summarized as (1) dose-dependent reduction in single-twitch height, (2) fade with TOF and tetanic stimulation, (3) posttetanic potentiation, (4) absence of fasciculations, (5) reversibility with anti-AChE agents, and (6) augmentation of nondepolarizing agent effect by prior administration of a depolarizing agent. Paralysis of skeletal muscle is first noted in the small muscle groups of the eyes, which explains the frequency of diplopia after defasciculatory doses of nondepolarizing agents. As the plasma concentration of nondepolarizing agents increases larger muscle groups are paralyzed, with the diaphragm being the most resistant to paralysis by nondepolarizing muscle relaxants.

Physical and Chemical Properties. *d*-Tubocurarine (Fig. 28–10) is a monoquaternary compound with one stable quaternary ammonium group.[72] The monoquaternary structure is thought to be related to its potential histamine-releasing and autonomic ganglia blocking properties. Methylation of the tertiary amine group of *d*-tubocurarine to yield dimethyltubocurarine or metocurine (Fig. 28–10) results in a muscle relaxant with three times less autonomic ganglia blocking and histamine-releasing ability than the parent compound.[73] *d*-Tubocurarine, unlike succinylcholine, is not subject to hydrolysis and has a stable shelf life in solution without refrigeration.

Pharmacokinetics and Pharmacodynamics. The ED95 for *d*-tubocurarine is 0.51 mg/kg; the bolus loading dose for intubation is 0.6 mg/kg and has a duration of action of 60 to 90 minutes. Subsequent maintenance doses under N_2O-O_2- narcotic anesthesia are approximately 0.1 mg/kg or one-fifth the original dose because of continued receptor occupation by the initial loading dose. The recommended maintenance dose during concurrent halogenated agent anesthesia is 0.05 mg/kg because of the potentiation of nondepolarizing muscle relaxants by all halogenated anesthetics. Halothane at 1.25 MAC (minimum alveolar concentration) reduces the requirement of *d*-tubocurarine by 50 percent when compared with an equipotent dose required to produce a similar degree of muscle relaxation during N_2O-O_2-opiate anesthesia. Isoflurane and enflurane under similar conditions will reduce the dose of *d*-tubocurarine by 70 percent.[20] It should be noted that maximal potentiation of nondepolarizing muscle relaxants will be achieved once a stable minimum alveolar concentration is reached; during the initial induction or during emergence, when inspired concentrations of inhaled anesthetic are low, the magnitude of potentiation will be decreased.

d-Tubocurarine is not highly bound to plasma proteins (40 to 50 percent). Cohen et al demonstrated that in dogs *d*-tubocurarine is not highly metabolized; 75 percent of the dose administered is recovered unchanged in the urine, and 10 to 15 percent of the dose is recovered in the bile within the first 24 hours of administration.[74] This group also demonstrated that in nephrectomized animals, hepatic elimination of *d*-tubocurarine is increased three- to fourfold. Elderly patients require doses similar to those given younger patients to achieve effective plasma concentrations for paralysis; however, the half-life for terminal elimination in elderly patients is longer than that seen in younger patients.[75] Presumably the reduction in glomerular filtration is primarily responsible for the increased time required for terminal elimination of *d*-tubocurarine and the resulting increased duration of action in the elderly.

Cardiovascular Effects. It is well known that rapid administration of intubating doses of *d*-tubocurarine is associated with significant hemodynamic changes. Rapid administration of *d*-tubocurarine 0.4 mg/kg is associated with 20 percent or larger reductions in mean arterial pressure (MAP); this dose was also associated with reductions in systemic vascular resistance (SVR), cardiac output (CO), central venous pressure (CVP), stroke volume (SV), and increases in heart rate (HR).[76] The hemodynamic changes associated with *d*-tubocurarine are due primarily to its histamine-releasing properties and, to a lesser extent, the potential for blockade of nicotinic cholinergic receptors in autonomic ganglia. *d*-Tubocurarine reductions in MAP are associated with a parallel dose-dependent increase in plasma histamine concentrations.[77] The extent of MAP reduction with *d*-tubocurarine use is related to total dose administered and depth of anesthesia.[78] The magnitude of histamine release and the reduction in MAP are also related to the rate of *d*-tubocurarine administration. Administration of an intubating dose of *d*-tubocurarine over 90 seconds rather than a single rapid bolus reduces the magnitude of MAP reduction.[79] The rate of histamine release and reduction in MAP can be further reduced by slow administration of paralyzing dose of *d*-tubocurarine over a period of 5 to 10 minutes. In view of the relationship between plasma histamine increases and hemodynamic changes associated with *d*-tubocurarine, it appears that autonomic ganglionic blockade is minimal in clinically relevant dosages. In the past the hypotensive effects of *d*-tubocurarine have been exploited when controlled hypotension was part of the anesthetic plan. With the current availability of hypotensive agents that are more predictable and titratable, this practice has decreased. The hemodynamic effects of *d*-tubocurarine are of greatest concern in patients with compromised cardiovascular systems or in individuals who are extremely sensitive to the effects of histamine.

Use in Pregnancy. *d*-Tubocurarine is a quaternary ammonium compound and, because of its highly ionized nature, crosses the placental barrier poorly. No reports of significant fetal blood levels or effects on the fetus have been reported. Current clinical use in obstetrics is generally limited to defasciculatory doses prior to succinylcholine administration, which further limits the potential for fetal effects. The duration of action of succinylcholine is generally too long for many obstetric procedures.

Metocurine

History and Pharmacologic Action. Metocurine is a synthetic derivative of *d*-tubocurarine that has three additional methyl groups added to its structure which was first described by King in 1935. It is a long-acting nondepolarizing muscle relaxant with the same mechanism of action as the parent compound, which was introduced into clinical practice in 1950.

Physical and Chemical Properties. Addition of an additional methyl group to *d*-tubocurarine results in the production of metocurine which then has two stable quaternary nitrogen groups. This structural modification results in a muscle relaxant that is twice as potent as *d*-tubocurarine but is markedly reduced in histamine-releasing and autonomic ganglia blocking properties.

Pharmacokinetics and Pharmacodynamics. An ED95 of metocurine of 0.28 mg/kg will produce a 95 percent reduction in twitch height in 3 to 5 minutes and a duration of 60 to 90 minutes. Like *d*-tubocurarine metocurine is potentiated by halogenated anesthetics, and it is recommended that the normal incremental dose of 0.07 mg/kg be reduced to 0.04 mg/kg in the presence of halogenated anesthetics. The recommended intubation dose is 0.4 mg/kg. Metocurine does not undergo significant metabolism and termination occurs primarily through excretion in the unchanged form in the urine.[80] Atracurium provides a reasonable alternative to metocurine in renal failure as its elimination is not dependent on renal function.

Cardiovascular Effects. Metocurine is not associated with any of the vagal blocking properties of pancuronium or gallamine. Large bolus doses of metocurine 0.4 mg/kg, given rapidly, are associated with slight increases in heart rate and a 7 percent reduction in MAP.[81] As with *d*-tubocurarine, the hypotensive effect is thought to result primarily from histamine release[81] and can be eliminated when the dose is administered more slowly.[82] Combinations of pancuronium 0.025 mg/kg and metocurine 0.1 mg/kg have been recommended to exploit the synergistic combinations of these two nondepolarizing muscle relaxants. Synergistic combinations of metocurine and pancuronium potentiate neuromuscular blockade and significantly reduce the increase in heart rate seen with pancuronium alone.[83] The sympathomimetic and vagolytic properties of intubating doses of pancuronium increase the potential for myocardial ischemia, which can be reduced by administration of metocurine–pancuronium combinations.[84] Introduction of agents such as doxacurium, pipecuronium, vecuronium, and atracurium has resulted in

a decreased need for metocurine or metocurine–pancuronium combinations in many practice settings. With time, metocurine will likely be of historic pharmacologic interest only.

Pancuronium Bromide

History and Pharmacologic Action. Pancuronium bromide (hereafter referred to as pancuronium) is a bisquaternary ammonium steroid without steroid activity that was synthesized in 1964 and introduced into clinical practice in 1977 by Baird and Reed (Fig. 28–10). It is considered to be a long-acting nondepolarizing relaxant and is not associated with significant histamine release or autonomic ganglionic blockade, which was a major advantage when it was introduced. Pancuronium is a highly ionized compound and lacks the structural modifications that would allow it to cross lipid barriers to bind to intracellular steroid receptors or produce receptor–steroid complexes that would translocate to the nucleus. Pancuronium is the precursor of the more modern steroid nondepolarizing muscle relaxants vecuronium and pipecuronium. Pancuronium has the ability to inhibit plasma cholinesterase which can prolong the action of succinylcholine. When pancuronium is used for defasciculation the normal nondepolarizing muscle relaxant inhibition of succinylcholine will be offset by decreased pseudocholinesterase breakdown of succinylcholine, which will result in higher effective succinylcholine concentrations. Defasciculation with nondepolarizing agents other than pancuronium increases the dose of succinylcholine needed for effective blockade.

Pharmacokinetics and Pharmacodynamics. The ED95 required for 95 percent suppression of twitch height, 0.07 mg/kg, produces satisfactory muscle relaxation for 60 to 90 minutes. Maintenance doses of pancuronium are 0.015 mg/kg without halogenated agents and 0.007 mg/kg with halogenated agents. Initial doses of 0.03 to 0.04 mg/kg after recovery from succinylcholine for intubation have provided adequate muscle relaxation for abdominal surgery. Attempts to shorten the time to onset of paralysis with pancuronium by increasing the dose from 1 ED95 to 2 ED95 given as a single rapid bolus have been successful. The duration of time necessary to satisfactorily blockade is shortened from 4.2 to 1.8 minutes, with an increase in the intensity of blockade; the time to 5 percent spontaneous recovery of twitch height increases from 43 to 129 minutes.[85] Should this increased duration of blockade be undesirable when attempting to avoid succinylcholine for intubation, vecuronium can be substituted for pancuronium. At the low dose of 0.02 mg/kg, pancuronium is approximately five times as potent as *d*-tubocurarine; at a higher dose of 0.08 mg/kg, pancuronium is approximately eight times more potent than *d*-tubocurarine.

The primary mechanism for elimination of pancuronium, as with other highly ionized compounds, is renal elimination of unchanged drug. The liver has limited ability to deacetylate pancuronium to less active metabolites that can be excreted in the bile. When anephric patients are given pancuronium, the half-life for elimination is increased to five times the normal half-life and prolonged paralysis is noted.[86]

Cardiovascular Effects. The classic hemodynamic effect of pancuronium is a dose-dependent 10 to 15 percent increase in heart rate, cardiac output, and mean arterial pressure.[76] The hemodynamic effects of pancuronium are due primarily to increases in heart rate, as little change in systemic vascular resistance is noted.[87] Pancuronium's ability to increase heart rate is due principally to its ability to block muscarinic ACh receptors (M_2 subtype) in the sinoatrial node. Heart rate increases associated with pancuronium can be blocked by prior administration of atropine which blocks muscarinic ACh receptors.

The clinical significance of the sympathomimetic effects of pancuronium in the autonomic nervous system is difficult to determine because of the potential for species variation differences in some studies. The drug interactions between pancuronium and other sympathomimetic drugs may, however, be explained by the potential for activation of the sympathetic nervous system that exists with pancuronium administration. Experimental evidence indicates that vagal cholinergic nerve terminals synapse with the sympathetic nerve terminals and decrease the release of norepinephrine.[88] Pancuronium and gallamine may block the muscarinic receptors (M_2 subtype) on the sympathetic nerve terminals and thus the inhibition of vagal cholinergic nerve terminal transmitter release, resulting in increased release of norepinephrine.[89] Additionally, pancuronium and gallamine have the ability to increase the release of norepinephrine in a noncholinergic muscarinic receptor blocking mechanism. In addition to increasing the release of norepinephrine from nerve terminals it has been proposed that pancuronium inhibits the reuptake of norepinephrine into postganglionic sympathetic neurons.[90–92]

A final mechanism for the expression of sympathomimetic effects of pancuronium at the autonomic ganglionic level is related to the drug's ability to block muscarinic receptors (M_2 subtype) for ACh on dopaminergic interneurons that synapse with postganglionic norepinephrine neurons. Normally the release and binding of ACh to muscarinic receptors on dopamine interneurons increase the release of dopamine, an inhibitor transmitter, which hyperpolarizes the postganglionic norepinephrine neuron, decreasing the release of norepinephrine.[93] The ability of pancuronium and gallamine to block muscarinic receptors on dopaminergic interneurons inhibits this negative effect on norepinephrine release; the net effect is an increase in the release of norepinephrine from postganglionic sympathetic neurons.[94]

The hemodynamic effects of pancuronium are probably of greatest concern in patients with compromised cardiovascular systems caused by coronary artery disease or in patients on tricyclic antidepressants. Patients with coronary artery disease are dependent on slow heart rates to decrease myocardial oxygen demand and to increase myocardial oxygen supply during the diastolic interval. Many patients with coronary artery disease are treated with calcium channel blocking agents and beta-adrenergic receptor blocking compounds to maintain slow heart rates. The greatest increases in heart rate with pancuronium have been reported in patients that had low resting heart rates. Increases in heart rate can be especially detrimental in this population of patients because of the increases in myocardial oxygen consumption and corresponding decreases in oxygen supply.[84] Dogs pretreated with imipramine, a first-generation tricyclic antidepressant, and given pancuronium during halothane anesthesia experience a high incidence of severe premature ventricular contractions that rapidly progress to ventricular tachycardia and ventricular fibrillation.[95] This finding has resulted in the obvious recommendation to avoid the triad of pancuronium, halothane, and tricyclic antidepressants.

Gallamine

History and Pharmacologic Action. Gallamine is a synthetic triquaternary ammonium compound (Fig. 28–10) with nondepolarizing muscle relaxant properties and one-sixth to one-seventh the potency of *d*-tubocurarine. It was first prepared by the Frenchman Bovet in 1947, and first used in clinical anesthesia in France by Huguenard and Boue in 1948. Gallamine has two outstanding pharmacologic features, its ability to reliably increase heart rate by its potent vagal blocking properties and its near-total dependence on renal function for elimination.

Pharmacokinetics and Pharmacodynamics. Gallamine 2 mg/kg produces good intubating conditions equivalent to those obtained with 0.4 to 0.5 mg/kg *d*-tubocurarine, and the duration of neuromuscular blockade is equal to or greater than that of *d*-tubocurarine. The duration of action is prolonged; thus, gallamine is best avoided in renal disease as it is almost totally eliminated unchanged by the kidney.[96] In the event of renal failure the liver is a poor alternative organ for excretion, as minimal amounts of gallamine are excreted in bile by the liver and the only other mechanism of elimination is dialysis.

Cardiovascular Effects. Gallamine causes dose-dependent increases in heart rate; an average increase of 30 to 40 percent may be noted within 1 to 2 minutes of drug administration, which is maximized at a dose of 1 mg/kg.[97] Like pancuronium, gallamine is associated primarily with blockade of muscarinic ACh receptors (M_2 subtype) in the sinoatrial node. Heart rate increases of nearly 100 percent have been noted when the resting heart rate was low prior to administration of gallamine.[99] The potent vagal blocking properties of gallamine are comparable to those of intravenous atropine administration when defasciculatory doses as small as 20 mg are given prior to succinylcholine administration.[98] The vagolytic effects of gallamine administration persist even after the neuromuscular blocking effect wears off.[99] Heart rate increases with gallamine 0.5 to 2 mg/kg result in mean arterial pressure increases of 10 to 20 torr and cardiac output increases of 25 to 50 percent.[97]

The primary hemodynamic effects of gallamine are most likely due to the vagolytic block and resulting increase in heart rate; however, experimental evidence shows that gallamine has the potential to exert sympathomimetic effects at the autonomic ganglia and at postganglionic nerve endings. As seen with pancuronium gallamine can increase the release of norepinephrine from postganglionic adrenergic nerve terminals,[88,89] can prevent dopaminergic interneuron hyperpolarization of postganglionic adrenergic neurons,[93,94] and can increase norepinephrine release by a mechanism not related to muscarinic receptor blockade.[90] If the patient's compromised cardiovascular status causes concern over the use of pancuronium, then gallamine certainly is a neuromuscular blocking agent to be eliminated from the anesthetic plan.

Doxacurium Chloride

Chemical Properties, Pharmacokinetics, and Pharmacodynamics.
Doxacurium is a competitive nondepolarizing muscle relaxant with a bisquaternary structure (Fig. 28–10) that is compatible with commonly used intravenous solutions and requires no refrigeration. A dose of 0.025 mg/kg (1 ED95) has a volume of distribution of 0.15 L/kg, indicating that the drug is poorly lipid soluble and not widely distributed in body tissues. It is associated with low plasma protein binding, approximately 30 percent, and is 2.5 to 3 times more potent than pancuronium. Duration of action is dose dependent; doses of 0.025 mg/kg (1 ED95), 0.05 mg/kg (2 ED95), and 0.075 mg/kg (3 ED95) are associated with mean clinically effective blockade times to 25 percent recovery of 60, 100, and 160 minutes, respectively. Satisfactory intubation conditions in 90 percent of patients are achieved in 5 minutes after a dose of 0.05 mg/kg; increasing the dose to 0.08 mg/kg decreases the time to satisfactory intubation conditions by only 1 minute.[100] Doxacurium is not associated with significant drug accumulation after repeated doses and plasma clearance remains stable over a wide range of dosages in normal patients.[101] Incremental doses after 25 percent recovery of blockade are usually one-fifth the initial dose (0.005 mg/kg after a bolus of 1 ED95 or 0.01 mg/kg after a bolus of 2 ED95) and produce additional clinical relaxation for 30 to 45 minutes. As with other nondepolarizing relaxants, doxacurium is potentiated by inhalation anesthetics up to approximately 25 percent.

Cardiovascular Effects.
Doxacurium is a nondepolarizing muscle relaxant with a duration of action similar to that of pancuronium and a cardiovascular profile similar to that of vecuronium. With up to 0.075 mg/kg (3 ED95), no significant changes in mean arterial pressure are noted.[102] A slight reduction in heart rate was observed; however, it was not as great as the reductions noted with comparable doses of vecuronium. After a high dose of doxacurium no increase in plasma histamine levels was noted.[101] Doxacurium is an agent with a high margin of safety and provides a reasonable alternative when a muscle relaxant with a duration longer than that of atracurium or vecuronium is desired and the vagolytic effects of pancuronium are not desired.

Metabolism.
Doxacurium is not metabolized in the body. It is excreted unchanged in the urine and the bile. It is reasonable to expect that there will be an increased duration of action if renal or hepatic failure is evident. In addition, a higher degree of variability of response will be noted in elderly patients because of their varying degrees of reduced renal and hepatic function.

Reversal.
As with all other long-acting nondepolarizing muscle relaxants it is not recommended that reversal be attempted until some signs of spontaneous reversal are evi-

dent on blockade monitoring. Prostigmine is recommended for reversal; edrophonium has not been recommended for reversal of doxacurium muscle relaxation.[103]

Pipecuronium Bromide

History and Chemical Properties.
Pipecuronium bromide (hereafter referred to as pipecuronium) was extensively studied in 1980 by Ka'rpa'ti and Bir'o,[104] and initial clinical use in 1980 was reported by Boros et al.[105] Pipecuronium was introduced into common clinical practice in the United States in 1991.

Pipecuronium is a competitive nondepolarizing neuromuscular blocking agent that is structurally similar to the other steroid-based muscle relaxants vecuronium and pancuronium. Both pipecuronium and pancuronium have bisquaternary ammonium structures, but pipecuronium has piperazine rings attached to the steroid nucleus whereas pancuronium has piperidine rings (Fig. 28–10). The structural modifications of pipecuronium result in a muscle relaxant that lacks cholinergic muscarinic receptor blocking properties in the sinoatrial node and has remarkable hemodynamic stability. It is supplied as a sterile lyophilized white crystalline cake that requires reconstitution prior to intravenous use. The potency of pipecuronium compared with pancuronium is 1:1.5, or stated another way, pipecuronium is approximately 30 percent more potent than pancuronium.[106]

Pharmacokinetics and Pharmacodynamics.
Estimates of the ED95 range from a high of 0.05 mg/kg,[106,107] to a low of 0.035 mg/kg for pipecuronium during intravenous balanced anesthesia.[108,109] The rate of onset of blockade with pipecuronium does not seem to be dose dependent; 90 percent suppression of T_1 twitch height in TOF testing was noted 2.6, 2.0, and 2.1 minutes after doses of 0.07, 0.085, and 0.1 mg/kg, respectively.[110] Good intubation conditions are generally achieved within 2 to 3 minutes of administration of pipecuronium 0.07 mg/kg and maximum paralysis is achieved 5 minutes after administration. Mean time to 25 percent recovery of initial twitch height is dose dependent, occurring 69.9, 98.3, and 94.6 minutes after doses of 0.07, 0.085, and 0.1 mg/kg, respectively under nitrous oxide–narcotic anesthesia.[108] The durations of action for pipecuronium 0.07 mg/kg and pancuronium 0.1 mg/kg were similarly prolonged by halothane anesthesia in normal patients, with mean duration to 25 percent recovery of initial twitch height at 98 and 117 minutes, respectively.[109]

Data from Caldwell et al confirm potentiation of pipecuronium (0.07 mg/kg) by concurrent halothane administration with times to recovery to 25 percent of initial twitch height of 98 minutes in normal patients and 103 minutes in patients with end-stage renal disease.[110] The similar mean recovery times for pipecuronium in normal patients and those with end-stage renal disease may seem confusing on the surface as pipecuronium is heavily dependent on renal elimination. It has been demonstrated that up to 56 percent of the administered dose is recovered in the urine within 24 hours and 25 percent of the recovered drug is the metabolite, 3-desacetyl pipecuronium.[111] Further evaluation of the data from Caldwell et al, however, demonstrates a greater degree of variability of recovery in normal patients and patients with end-stage renal disease, 55 to 198 and 30 to 267 minutes, respectively. Additionally, the mean clearance and half-life for elimination (normal versus renal failure) were 2.4 mL/kg/min^{-1} versus 1.6 mL/kg/min^{-1} and 118 minutes versus 247 minutes, respectively.[110] Increased variability in time to 25 percent recovery of twitch height, decreased clearance, and increased time for terminal elimination of pipecuronium indicate a high possibility for increased duration of action of pipecuronium in patients with renal disease.

If succinylcholine is used prior to pipecuronium it is recommended that the initial dose of pipecuronium be reduced to 0.05 mg/kg to avoid excessive increases in duration of action.

Cardiovascular Effects. In numerous studies pipecuronium in doses as high as 0.15 mg/kg has not been associated with any significant hemodynamic changes.[106,108,112] Pipecuronium has not been associated with any significant histamine release or autonomic ganglia blocking properties. This remarkable cardiovascular stability has allowed the bradycardic effects of high-dose narcotic to be more evident in some cases. Pipecuronium is a reasonable choice when a muscle relaxant with cardiovascular stability is desired for procedures that last 90 minutes or longer.

Use in Pregnancy. Currently studies on placental transfer and fetal accumulation of pipecuronium are not available. Should experience with other highly ionized bisquaternary ammonium compounds hold true for pipecuronium, significant placental transfer to produce effects in the fetus would not be expected. The duration of action of pipecuronium is longer than many obstetric procedures and in most cases would be a poor choice for use even if studies showed it was safe to use in pregnancy.

Reversal. Patients with spontaneous mean recovery of T_1 to 28.7 percent and a $T_4 : T_1$ ratio of 9.2 percent demonstrated adequate reversal with T_1 greater than 90 percent and $T_4 : T_1$ ratios greater than 75 percent within 10 minutes of administration of 2.5 mg neostigmine with the appropriate antimuscarinic agent. Those with a spontaneous mean recovery of T_1 to 13.2 percent showed a mean T_1 recovery of 67.9 percent and a $T_4 : T_1$ ratio of 51.4 percent 10 minutes after reversal with 2.5 mg neostigmine and required additional time for adequate reversal or additional neostigmine administration.[110]

Edrophonium 0.5 mg/kg, given to patients with spontaneous recovery of 25 percent TOF, produced adequate reversal of pipecuronium (> 70 percent recovery of TOF) within 10 minutes in patients who received pipecuronium with nitrous oxide–oxygen–narcotic anesthesia. In patients who received isoflurane 10 minutes after the initial 0.5 mg/kg dose of edrophonium, an additional 0.25 mg/kg dose of edrophonium was required to achieve marginally acceptable reversal at slightly greater than 70 percent recovery of TOF.[107] Edrophonium has been judged as a less than safe agonist for pipecuronium, which has been a similar finding for most of the other long-acting nondepolarizing agents in the dose range 0.5 to 0.75 mg/kg.

INTERMEDIATE-DURATION NONDEPOLARIZING MUSCLE RELAXANTS

Vecuronium

Chemical Properties. Vecuronium, a competitive nondepolarizing muscle relaxant, is a structural analog of pancuronium in which the methyl group from the A ring of the steroid nucleus has been removed (Fig. 28–10). This minor structural modification results in major clinical differences between vecuronium and pancuronium. Vecuronium has not been associated with muscarinic receptor blocking properties in clinically relevant doses. The absence of muscarinic receptor blocking capability results in loss of the vagolytic effects and potential sympathomimetic effects associated with pancuronium. The monoquaternary structure of vecuronium is still ionized and hydrophilic but the loss of one quaternary nitrogen results in a slight increase in lipid solubility and a greater dependence on hepatic function for elimination. When equipotent doses are compared vecuronium duration of action of clinically effective muscle relaxation is approximately 30 percent that of pancuronium. Because of its lack of stability in solution vecuronium is supplied as a lipophilized cake that is reconstituted with sterile water prior to use.

Pharmacokinetics and Pharmacodynamics. If given at 1 ED95 (0.05 mg/kg) vecuronium has an onset time of 4 minutes.[113] Attempts to increase the time of onset with vecuronium have employed the priming principle, the administration of larger doses (3 to 5 ED95), or both. The time of onset is dose dependent, with vecuronium in doses of 3 and 5 ED95, onset times are 2.8 and 1.1 minutes, respectively. Recovery from vecuronium is also dose dependent; at 5 ED95 83 minutes is required for recovery of the second twitch in TOF monitoring.[114] Incremental doses of 0.01 to 0.02 mg/kg given when the initial twitch returns to 10 percent of control or when the fourth twitch in TOF monitoring becomes prominent will maintain satisfactory abdominal muscle relaxation.

Use of the priming principle with vecuronium is an attempt to increase the time of onset and to reverse residual paralysis earlier than is allowed with vecuronium at 5 ED95. One technique of priming involves giving one-tenth the calculated 2 ED95 dose of vecuronium (0.01 mg/kg) and, after 4 minutes, giving the full calculated 2 ED95 dose of vecuronium (0.1 mg/kg).[115] By use of vecuronium and the priming principle, time to intubation can be reduced to under 1.5 minutes. After 2 ED95 bolus doses of vecuronium can be successfully reversed within 20 to 30 minutes. When recovery from the initial bolus dose of vecuronium begins, muscle relaxation can be maintained with an infusion of vecuronium at a mean steady-state rate of 1.2 μg/kg/min^{-1}. Mean recovery time to 25 percent of initial twitch height when this infusion rate is stopped is 12.7 minutes.[116]

Vecuronium is normally highly dependent on hepatic function for excretion.[117] When high-dose vecuronium (0.2 mg/kg) is administered to patients with cirrhosis of the liver a decreased plasma clearance and an increased elimination half-life are observed.[118] When similar doses of vecuronium are administered to patients with cholestasis undergoing biliary surgery an increased duration of action is noted.[119] When lower doses of vecuronium (0.1 mg/kg) are given to patients with cirrhosis of the liver the elimination half-life is the same as that of normal patients.[120] These lower doses of vecuronium given to patients with cirrhosis are most likely cleared by compensatory renal excretion. Under normal conditions about 30 percent of an administered dose of vecuronium is excreted in the urine as unchanged drug or drug metabolites in the first 24 hours.[121] In patients with end-stage renal disease compensatory hepatic excretion of vecuronium occurs and no significant increase in duration of action is noted, so vecuronium can be safely used in patients with renal failure.[121]

Cumulative effects of vecuronium are clinically insignificant. Incremental doses given at consistent points of twitch recovery produce the same duration and intensity of neuromuscular blockade each time they are given.[122] The differences in potentiation by halogenated agents and the effects of concentration changes are less pronounced with vecuronium than with the parent compound pancuronium. Potentiation of vecuronium muscle relaxation under steady-state isoflurane and enflurane is only 20 to 30 percent higher than noted with halothane.[123]

Cardiovascular Effects. Vecuronium has not been associated with any significant hemodynamic changes or histamine-releasing or autonomic ganglia blocking properties. Doses 20 times greater than those required for neuromuscular blocking produced no cardiovascular changes in dogs or cats.[124] In humans anesthetized with halothane doses of 0.28 mg/kg (12 ED90) no changes in heart rate or arterial blood pressure were noted.[125] As has been noted with pipecuronium and doxacurium, vecuronium will allow the bradycardic effects of narcotic agents to be noticed to a greater degree.

Use in Pregnancy. Vecuronium has been safely used in patients undergoing cesarean section without harmful effects to the fetus. If succinylcholine is contraindicated for reasons other than pseudocholinesterase abnormalities, mivacurium may be a more reasonable choice than vecuronium or atracurium.

Atracurium Besylate

History. Atracurium besylate (hereafter referred to as atracurium) (Fig. 28–10) was first synthesized by Stenlake and colleagues who concentrated on producing a muscle relaxant that would be able to use the Hofmann elimination pathway for spontaneous breakdown of quaternary ammonium compounds at physiologic temperature and pH.[126] This was not an easy process, as chemical breakdown of quaternary ammonium compounds usually occurs at the boiling point of water in strong alkaline solutions. Initial pharmacologic studies were conducted by Hughes and Chapple,[127] and atracurium was first used clinically in 1979.[128]

Chemical Properties. Atracurium is a bisquaternary ester, competitive nondepolarizing neuromuscular blocking agent. A unique feature of atracurium is that under normal physiologic conditions, renal or hepatic function is not required for its metabolism. The normal elimination half-life of atracurium is unchanged by renal[129] or hepatic[120] failure. Chemical breakdown and elimination of atracurium take place by the Hofmann elimination process, which involves removal of a beta hydrogen and disruption of an alpha C—N bond; and by ester hydrolysis in plasma by nonspecific esterases, not pseudocholinesterase (Fig. 28–11). To minimize the Hofmann elimination process under storage atracurium is buffered to a pH of 3.25 to 3.65 and maintained under refrigeration at 5C. Under refrigeration loss of potency of atracurium is limited to approximately 6 percent per year, or approximately 5 percent per month if not refrigerated.

Hofmann elimination breakdown of atracurium yields a monoacrylate and laudanosine, a tertiary amine that can enter the brain. Ester hydrolysis of atracurium yields a quaternary acid and a quaternary alcohol, both of which can be further metabolized by the Hofmann elimination to yield laudanosine. Studies have indicated that laudanosine can cause seizures in dogs,[130] and evidence of arousal on electroencephalography has been noted after administration of atracurium 1 to 2.5 mg/kg to dogs.[131] Transient reductions in blood pressure of 14 percent were noted after 1 mg/kg laudanosine was given to dogs under halothane anes-

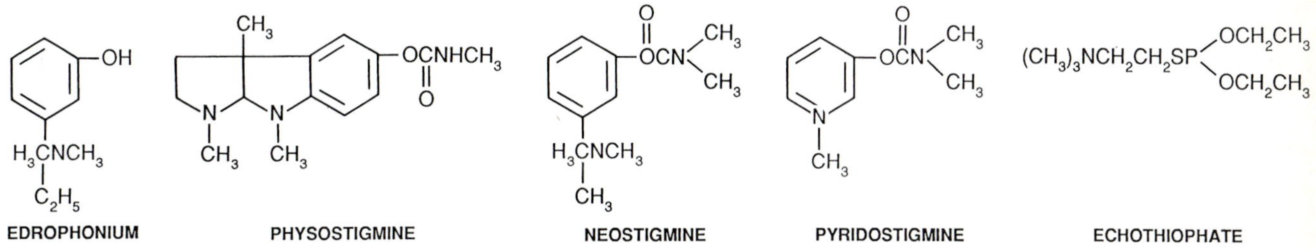

EDROPHONIUM   PHYSOSTIGMINE   NEOSTIGMINE   PYRIDOSTIGMINE   ECHOTHIOPHATE

Figure 28–11. Chemical structures for neostigmine, physostigmine, pyridostigmine, edrophonium, and echothiopate. The methyl carbamate moiety is essential for the pharmacologic activity of physostigmine, a tertiary amine. Neostigmine is a quaternary ammonium derivative with a dimethyl carbamate side chain. Edrophonium is a hydroxy analog of neostigmine lacking the carbamate group. Incorporation of a quaternary nitrogen into the ring yields pyridostigmine. Echothiopate is an organophosphate anticholinesterase used topically in the treatment of glaucoma (see Chapter 35).

thesia[132]; however, the atracurium or laudanosine doses given to laboratory animals in the above studies are far greater than ever administered or could be generated by clinically relevant doses. Similar neurologic side effects or cardiovascular findings have not been noted in acute care patients receiving atracurium infusions for 38 to 219 hours, which is longer than even the slowest surgical teams usually operate.[133]

Pharmacokinetics and Pharmacodynamics. The average ED95 dose of atracurium, 0.20 mg/kg, produces its maximal effect in approximately 4 minutes, and spontaneous recovery of 95 percent of twitch height occurs in 44 minutes.[134] Equipotent 1 ED95 bolus doses of both vecuronium and atracurium can generally be reversed within 20 minutes. A dose of 0.5 mg/kg produces a more rapid onset to maximal block (2.5 minutes) and a recovery to 10 percent of T_1 height within 40 minutes,[135] a point that allows for easy reversal of atracurium with neostigmine or edrophonium. Time to spontaneous 90 percent recovery of twitch height was 66 minutes.[135] Attempts to speed onset and use atracurium rather than succinylcholine for intubation have been based on the priming principle and a bolus dose of 2.5 ED95 (0.5 mg/kg), which is the maximal dose that has not been associated with significant histamine release. In one priming technique, 0.06 to 0.08 mg/kg is given and, after 3 minutes, the remaining 0.5 mg/kg is given.[136]

After signs of recovery from the initial bolus of atracurium are evident (10 percent recovery of T_1 height) adequate muscle relaxation can be maintained with a mean steady-state atracurium infusion of 7.9 µg/kg/min^{-1}.[118] With this infusion rate 25 percent T_1 recovery can be expected within 12.5 minutes after the atracurium infusion is discontinued.[116]

Both atracurium and vecuronium have been associated with slight evidence of a cumulative effect,[124] with the effect of atracurium being even less noticeable than that of vecuronium; neither drug has been associated with significant clinical cumulative effects. If succinylcholine is used for intubation, reduction of the initial atracurium dose to 0.3 mg/kg may be desirable. Incremental doses of atracurium to maintain satisfactory muscle relaxation range from 0.05 to 0.1 mg/kg every 15 to 30 minutes.

Halogenated agent potentiation of the intermediate-acting muscle relaxants is not as agent or dose sensitive as is potentiation by the long-acting muscle relaxants. With steady-state concentrations of isoflurane and enflurane approximately 30 percent potentiation of atracurium is noted; 20 percent potentiation is noted with halothane.

Cardiovascular Effects. There is less potential for cardiovascular changes with atracurium than with *d*-tubocurarine or metocurine. When cardiovascular effects are noted they are transient and associated with histamine release. Atracurium given in rapid bolus doses up to 2 ED95 (0.4 mg/kg) are not associated with changes in heart rate or blood pressure.[134] When 3 ED95 atracurium was given, heart rate increased 8.3 percent and mean arterial pressure decreased 21.5 percent; these changes were evident in 60 to 90 seconds and disappeared within 5 minutes.[136] Cardiovascular changes and histamine release with atracurium are

related to total dose and rate of administration. A dose of 0.8 mg/kg given over 5 seconds produced a 25 percent reduction in blood pressure, slower injection of the same dose over 75 seconds or antihistamine pretreatment result in significant reduction of blood pressure and histamine changes.[137]

Use in Pregnancy. Atracurium has been safely used in obstetric anesthesia, with the fetal umbilical venous blood levels of atracurium below the sensitivity of the assay.[138]

SHORT-ACTING NONDEPOLARIZING MUSCLE RELAXANTS

Mivacurium Chloride

Chemical Properties. Mivacurium chloride (hereafter referred to as mivacurium) is a synthetic bisbenzylisoquinolinium diester that is structurally related to atracurium (Fig. 28–10). It is a competitive nondepolarizing neuromuscular blocking agent that is hydrolyzed by plasma cholinesterase but not true cholinesterase. Mivacurium is not subject to spontaneous hydrolysis in the absence of pseudocholinesterase.

Pharmacokinetics and Pharmacodynamics. ED95 dose varied with the investigator, all of whom used nitrous oxide–narcotic anesthesia. The ED95 ranged from a low of 0.058 mg/kg[139], to 0.067 mg/kg[140], to 0.075 mg/kg[134] and a high of 0.08 mg/kg.[141] The most commonly accepted mean ED95 was 0.075 mg/kg in nitrous oxide–narcotic anesthesia. The potency and duration of mivacurium are increased by halogenated anesthetics and under stable enflurane anesthesia the ED95 was reduced to 0.052 mg/kg.[140] During nitrous oxide–narcotic anesthesia the mean time to complete block was not dose dependent at 0.15, 0.20, or 0.25 mg/kg and was 2.5, 2.4, and 2.7 minutes, respectively. Mean time to 10 percent recovery of twitch height is dose dependent with 15.6, 18.0, and 20.6 minutes, respectively being required from the lowest dose to the highest dose.[134] When a patient has demonstrated 10 percent recovery of twitch height mivacurium is easily reversed. Even if reversal is not attempted mean time to 95 percent recovery of twitch height occurs in 26.9 minutes.[116]

In a study by Ali et al, patients were intubated with approximately 1.5 to 3 ED95 of mivacurium, maintained under enflurane anesthesia, and allowed to recover to a twitch height of 18.2 percent.[116] A mivacurium infusion was started at the rate of 8.4 µg/kg/min^{-1} for the first 15 minutes and then reduced to 6.6 µg/kg/min^{-1} to maintain 90 to 99 percent twitch suppression. At the end of infusions as long as 2 hours, no cumulative effects were noted and mean time for recovery of $T_4 : T_1$ greater than 70 percent was 17 minutes without reversal. When edrophonium or neostigmine was given at the time the infusion was terminated, recovery of $T_4 : T_1$ was greater than 70 percent within 8.2 minutes of edrophonium 0.75 mg/kg and within 11.2 minutes of neostigmine 0.04 mg/kg. Essentially rates of recovery from comparable levels of twitch suppression with either single-bolus or steady-state infusion are similar. When infusions of mivacurium are used in nitrous oxide–narcotic anesthesia, the mean rate of infusion necessary to maintain 95 percent suppression of twitch height is 8.3 μg/kg/min^{-1},[116] which is greater than the 6.6 μg/kg/min^{-1} rate used during enflurane anesthesia.[142] Equipotent doses of mivacurium have approximately half the duration of vecuronium or atracurium.

In vitro studies have shown that mivacurium is metabolized in a first-order process by pseudocholinesterase and not true cholinesterase with a half-life for elimination of 5.3 minutes; the half-life for elimination of succinylcholine by pseudocholinesterase is 2.3 minutes. The rate of hydrolysis of mivacurium by pseudocholinesterase is 70 percent as fast as that of succinylcholine.[143] Chemical inhibition and qualitative or quantitative abnormalities of pseudocholinesterase prolong the action of mivacurium.

Attempts to speed the onset of paralysis using 4 ED95 (0.30 mg/kg) along with a priming technique produced excellent intubation conditions within 60 seconds.[144] Rapid injection of large doses of mivacurium has been associated with transient histamine release and hypotension.

Cardiovascular Effects. Mivacurium in a dose of 0.10 mg/kg or less given intravenously over 10 to 15 seconds is not associated with facial flushing, significant hemodynamic changes, or histamine release. At 0.25 mg/kg there is a high incidence of facial flushing associated with increases in plasma histamine and a transient mean reduction in arterial pressure from baseline of 13 percent. The incidence of facial flushing, hemodynamic changes, and histamine levels associated with mivacurium 0.10 mg/kg given over 10 to 15 seconds is equivalent to that associated with 0.25 mg/kg given over 60 seconds.[141]

Mivacurium is a nondepolarizing agent that is not associated with many of the potential complications of succinylcholine. Its relatively rapid rate of onset and short duration of action should allow for its use in many situations where succinylcholine would have been the drug of choice in the past.

DRUG INTERACTIONS WITH NONDEPOLARIZING MUSCLE RELAXANTS

Potent Inhalation Anesthetics

The most common drug interaction with nondepolarizing muscle relaxants is the well-documented ability of potent inhalation anesthetics to potentiate all nondepolarizing muscle relaxants to varying degrees. In current clinical practice isoflurane is slightly more potent than enflurane, and both agents are more potent than halothane.[20] The mechanism of potentiation is probably due to a combination of central nervous system effects and effects in the postsynaptic surface or in the muscle. Discussion of inhalation agent effects on specific nondepolarizing agents has been included in the presentation of each agent.

Antibiotics

The aminoglycoside antibiotics have both pre- and postjunctional effects that potentiate nondepolarizing muscle relaxants. Aminoglycosides are thought to have an effect similar to magnesium which decreases calcium availability and

ACh release.[145] Calcium's ability to only partially reverse the effects of the aminoglycoside demonstrates the existence of both pre- and postjunctional effects of these agents. Polypeptide antibiotics (polymyxin) have potent neuromuscular blocking properties on their own that are thought to be related to a local anesthetic-like action.

Local Anesthetics

The fast sodium channel blocking capability of local anesthetics can depress all electrically excitable tissues in a dose-dependent fashion. This action results in decreased transmission of action potentials, the release of neurotransmitter, stabilizing effects on postjunctional membranes, and excitability of muscle cells. Nondepolarizing neuromuscular blockade can be potentiated by all local anesthetics.[146]

Anticonvulsants

Phenytoin therapy has been reported to increase the dose of pancuronium, vecuronium, and metocurine necessary to produce satisfactory muscle relaxation.[147] Carbamazepine has also been reported to produce increased dose requirements for pancuronium.[148]

Diuretics

Furosemide in low doses (< 10 μg/kg) potentiates nondepolarizing agents, whereas high doses (1 to 4 mg/kg) antagonize nondepolarizing agents.[149,150] It is thought that low-dose furosemide inhibits a protein kinase, which decreases cAMP and transmitter release, whereas high doses inhibit phosphodiesterase, which increases cAMP and transmitter release. The mechanism of action for potentiation of muscle relaxants by high-dose furosemide is similar to that reported for aminophylline. Mannitol, a substance that is filtered by the glomerulus and not reabsorbed by the renal tubule, has no direct effect on nondepolarizing relaxants because it does not affect glomerular filtration rates and muscle relaxant excretion.[151] Although biphasic effects of furosemide on muscle relaxants have been reported, measurable effects in routine clinical practice may be difficult to observe.

Ionic Effects

Acute changes in potassium concentration will alter transmembrane potential. For chronic changes in potassium concentration, there is sufficient time for intracellular and extracellular concentrations of potassium to equilibrate, leading to no net change in transmembrane potential. Acute hypokalemia produces increased transmembrane potential, making it more difficult to depolarize a neuron and thereby reducing transmitter release and potentiation of nondepolarizing muscle relaxants. Acute increases in extracellular potassium decrease transmembrane potential, making it easier to depolarize a neuron and thereby increasing transmitter release and reducing the effectiveness of nondepolarizing muscle relaxants.

Increased serum concentrations of magnesium reduce neurotransmitter release presynaptically and reduce the sensitivity of the postjunctional membrane to the neurotransmitter. Magnesium has been shown to potentiate the effects of nondepolarizing muscle relaxants.[19]

The effects of lithium are controversial. In a single case report lithium was found to potentiate muscle relaxation from pancuronium administration.[152] Other evidence indicates that lithium has a negligible effect on degree of muscle relaxation produced with pancuronium or d-tubocurarine.[153]

AGE AND NONDEPOLARIZING MUSCLE RELAXANTS

Geriatric Patients

Prolonged duration of action with long-acting nondepolarizing muscle relaxants in elderly patients is usually related to decreased renal or hepatic clearance. Decreased elimination and prolonged duration of action have been demonstrated for the long-acting nondepolarizing muscle relaxants.[75] The dose–response curves for elderly and young patients receiving long-acting nondepolarizing muscle relaxants are similar.[75] These findings suggest that both the elderly and the young require comparable doses of long-acting nondepolarizing muscle relaxants to achieve a given degree of paralysis, with effective paralysis lasting longer in the elderly than in the young. Newer intermediate or short-acting nondepolarizing muscle relaxants such as atracurium and mivacurium may provide the advantage of more predictable duration of action in the elderly.

Pediatric Patients

Remarkable differences in the pharmacokinetic data for d-tubocurarine exist between neonates and adults with respect to volume of distribution (0.74 and 0.31 L/kg), elimination half-life (174 and 89 minutes), and ED50 plasma concentration (0.18 and 0.53 $\mu g/mL^{-1}$, respectively). The rate of clearance is similar for neonates and adults, 3.7 and 3.0 $mL/kg/min^{-1}$, respectively.[154] It is clear that neonates and infants are more sensitive to the effects of d-tubocurarine; however, the larger volume of distribution in neonates and children than adults may offset the increased sensitivity to d-tubocurarine, and in similar doses may be necessary to produce a given degree of neuromuscular blockade in both neonates and adults.[154] Because of the potential for greater variability in response in pediatric patients, long-acting nondepolarizing agents are often given in increments of one-half the adult ED95 and with blockade monitoring titrating the dose to the desired effect.

REVERSAL OF NONDEPOLARIZING MUSCLE RELAXANTS

Pharmacologic Principles and Practical Considerations

The primary goal of pharmacologic reversal of muscle relaxants is to increase the concentration of ACh present at the myoneural junction. Increasing the concentration of ACh molecules relative to residual nondepolarizing muscle relaxant molecules can prevent the binding of muscle relaxant molecules to ACh receptors by simple mass action competition, which would allow reversal of residual paralysis. Anticholinesterase drugs are used to inhibit AChE, the resulting inhibition of ACh hydrolysis allows the buildup of ACh necessary to overcome the action of residual muscle relaxant molecules at the myoneural junction. Timely muscle relaxant administration is required so that the residual concentration of muscle relaxant present at the synapse is low enough to allow the anticholinesterase-induced ACh to effectively compete for viable ACh receptor binding sites. Measurement of peripheral nerve stimulation should show some evidence of spontaneous recovery from nondepolarizing muscle relaxant paralysis before reversal is attempted; mechanical ventilation should be continued until some evidence of spontaneous recovery is present. None of the recommended doses of anticholinesterase agents are intended to successfully reverse a 100 percent block. Anticholinesterase compounds currently in clinical use are not selective and inhibit both pseudocholinesterase and true cholinesterase. Nonselective inhibition of true cholinesterase allows the accumulation of ACh at all cholinergic synaptic regions, both nicotinic and muscarinic. Although accumulation of ACh at nicotinic cholinergic receptors of the myoneural junction is desirable in this process, the accumulation of ACh at nicotinic cholinergic receptors of autonomic ganglia and muscarinic receptors in the autonomic nervous system is accepted as a necessary side effect of the reversal process. To avoid the symptoms of a cholinergic crisis, which would be similar to the symptoms seen with exposure to military nerve agents or organophosphate insecticides (i.e., bradycardia, bronchoconstriction, salivation, urination, lacrimation, and defecation), an antimuscarinic agent such as atropine or glycopyrrolate is administered prior to or with the anticholinesterase compound. Antimuscarinic agents are effective in blocking the effects of ACh at muscarinic receptors on the effector organs of the parasympathetic nervous system but have not been effective at blocking the effects of ACh at nicotinic cholinergic receptors in the autonomic ganglia.

Available Anticholinesterase Compounds

Drugs that inhibit AChE are chemically related to the naturally occurring compound eserine or physostigmine, an alkaloid derived from the calibar bean that was used by African tribes in witchcraft trials. To someone with a thorough understanding of the autonomic nervous system, the mental image of an individual forced to consume extracts of the calibar bean would be quite repulsive and was probably a significant emotional event for members of the tribes who witnessed this type of ordeal. Physostigmine (Fig. 28–11) is a tertiary amine, and as such crosses the blood–brain barrier to produce predictable central nervous system effects. For this reason it is not used to reverse residual effects of muscle relaxants but has been used in anesthesia as an analeptic to reverse the effects of central anticholinergic syndrome. The synthetic anticholinesterase agents neostigmine, pyridostigmine, and edrophonium (Fig. 28–11) are quaternary ammonium compounds that cross the blood–brain barrier poorly. They are associated with minimal central nervous system effects and are useful agents for reversal of residual muscle relaxant effects.

The organophosphate cholinesterase inhibitor echothiophate (Fig. 28–11) is used in medicine; other organophosphate inhibitors of AChE are used either as military nerve agents (Taubun, Saran, Soman, VX) or insecticides (Malathion, Parathion). Useful anticholinesterase compounds in anesthesia produce reversible inhibition of AChE. Organophosphate inhibitors of AChE result in covalent binding of organic phosphate to the esteratic site of the enzyme (Fig. 28–12) that requires hours to regenerate active enzyme or inhibition that may require days or weeks to be overcome by synthesis of new AChE enzyme. Untreated high-dose exposure to potent organophosphate toxins is potentially lethal, as physiologically the living organism cannot survive the toxic effects long enough to regenerate or synthesize active AChE enzyme.

Anticholinesterase Mechanism of Action

AChE enzyme can exist in five different states: (1) normally active without substrate present, (2) acetylated, (3) sterically inhibited, (4) carbamylated, and (5) phosphorylated. The enzyme acetylcholinesterase has two active sites, an anionic (negative) site and the esteratic site, which contains the amino acids serine and histidine, which can interact to donate a pair of electrons to break ester bonds. Under normal conditions the cationic (positive) quaternary ammonium portion of ACh is attracted to the anionic region of AChE while the esteratic site interacts with the ester bond between choline and acetate. The electrons transferred from the serine residue allow choline to split off, leaving acetylated AChE enzyme which cannot be enzymatically active until reactivated. Within microseconds hydrolysis splits off acetate from the acetylated enzyme, leaving regenerated or active AChE enzyme and free acetate (Fig. 28–13).

Edrophonium lacks a carbamate group and inhibits AChE by electrostatic interaction with the anionic site and hydrogen bonding at the esteratic site of AChE. The com-

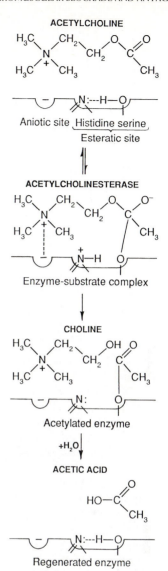

Figure 28–13. Diagram of the interaction between acetylcholine and acetylcholinesterase at the anionic and esteratic sites. Subsequent hydrolysis to choline and acetate is accompanied by regeneration of the active enzyme.

petitive reversible steric obstruction of AChE enzyme that edrophonium produces prevents interaction between AChE and substrate ACh. This action results in accumulation of ACh as long as effective concentrations of edrophonium are present at the synapse (Fig. 28–14).

The anticholinesterase agents neostigmine, pyridostigmine, and prostigmine are carbamate-containing compounds. These carbamate ester cholinesterase inhibitors are competitive substrates for the AChE enzyme, and drug that binds to the AChE is metabolized by the esteratic site. Neostigmine and pyridostigmine interact with the anionic and esteratic sites of AChE in the same manner as does ACh. When the esteratic site breaks the ester bond of carbamate-containing anticholinesterase agents, the carbamate portion of the molecule covalently binds to the esteratic site, resulting in a carbamylated AChE enzyme that will not be able to break down ACh until the carbamate group is re-

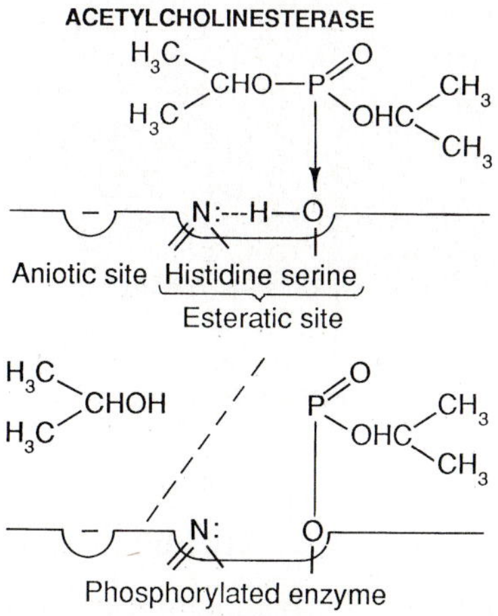

Figure 28–12. Organophosphate anticholinesterase drugs produce irreversible inhibition of acetylcholinesterase by forming a phosphorylated complex at the esteratic site of the enzyme which does not undergo hydrolysis. Therefore, spontaneous regeneration of acetylcholine requires a long period (several hours) if it occurs at all. These factors account for its potency.

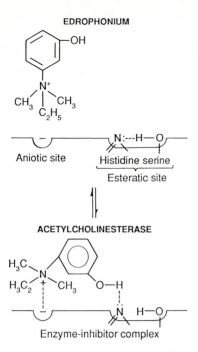

Figure 28–14. Stages in binding of edrophonium and neostigmine to acetylcholinesterase.

moved from the enzyme (Fig. 28–15). Unlike acetylated AChE enzyme carbamylated enzyme is much more resistant to regeneration by hydrolysis and has a half-life for regeneration that is measured in minutes rather than microseconds for acetylated enzyme regeneration. Competitive inhibition of AChE with anticholinesterase agents is what many practitioners commonly think of when considering muscle relaxant reversal. The action of cholinesterase-inhibiting agents is more complex than simple inhibition of AChE enzyme. Anticholinesterase drugs can generate antidromic action potentials and repetitive firing of motor nerve endings.[155] Anticholinesterase agents are also capable of directly depolarizing motor nerve terminals and cholinergic receptors on the postsynaptic surface. These actions increase mobilization and release of ACh to the synapse at the myoneural junction and aid in competing for available binding sites on the alpha subunits of the receptor to prevent binding of the depolarizing muscle relaxant. Anticholinesterase reversal of muscle relaxants is a combination of AChE enzyme inhibition and the direct pre- and postsynaptic effects of these agents.

The elimination of anticholinesterase agents is dependent on renal and hepatic function. Nondepolarizing muscle relaxants other than atracurium and mivacurium are also dependent on renal function for elimination. If anticholinesterase agents are used to reverse nondepolarizing muscle relaxants in patients with decreased renal function the excretion of anticholinesterase drug will be decreased as much as or more than that of the muscle relaxant.[156,157] This should make recurarization unlikely; the only concern left is that a long-acting antimuscarinic agent will prevent the reappearance of muscarinic side effects. The entire question of recurarization in patients with renal disease can be eliminated by choosing a muscle relaxant that is not dependent on renal function for elimination.

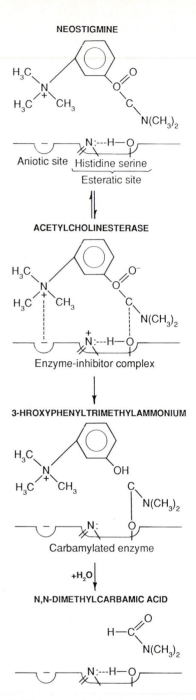

Figure 28–15. Diagram of the interaction between anticholinesterase, neostigmine, and acetylcholinesterase. Because of the stability of the bond of the carbamylated enzyme, the enzyme is functionally inhibited.

Clinical Use of Specific Anticholinesterase Agents

Edrophonium. At 0.5 mg/kg edrophonium will produce an antagonism of residual nondepolarizing muscle relaxant paralysis that is equivalent in magnitude and duration to that seen with 0.043 mg/kg neostigmine.[158] Because of edrophonium's rapid onset and lower potential to produce muscarinic side effects, it has been recommended that atropine 7 μg/kg be given with edrophonium 0.5 mg/kg.[158] If reversal with edrophonium is inadequate after the initial 0.5 mg/kg dose an additional 0.25 mg/kg atropine can be given. In cases where twitch height has returned to only 10 percent of control 1.0 mg/kg edrophonium may be required to produce a rate of reversal equal to that of neostigmine.[159] Edrophonium is probably best suited for cases where TOF monitoring demonstrates the presence of two to three twitches with fade or where intermediate-acting (vecuronium and atracurium) or short-acting (mivacurium) muscle relaxants have been used. The need for pharmacologic reversal when all monitoring criteria demonstrate complete reversal after the use of short- or intermediate-acting muscle relaxants may be an area where edrophonium could be helpful. Edrophonium has the ability to reverse the subclinical effects of muscle relaxants, increase the margin of safety for neuromuscular transmission, and reduce the potential for recurarization to the lowest point possible with minimal muscarinic side effects. Clinicians who, if only for litiginous reasons, believe pharmacologic reversal of subclinical effects of nondepolarizing muscle relaxants is necessary may find edrophonium to be a reasonable choice. Peak neuromuscular blocking antagonism occurs in less than 5 minutes with edrophonium, whereas peak effects of neostigmine require 7 to 10 minutes.[158] It is difficult for this author to envision a surgical team efficient enough to justify the use of edrophonium on the basis that it takes 2 to 5 minutes less to produce maximal reversal and thus makes a significant difference in the patient's overall anesthetic time. Edrophonium has not been recommended for reversal with the new long-acting muscle relaxants pipecuronium or doxacurium either because of inadequate reversal or because of the decreased safety margin of reversal and the potential for recurarization.

Neostigmine

Neostigmine is an anticholinesterase drug that is suitable for reversal of all nondepolarizing muscle relaxants at any depth of residual paralysis as long as some evidence of spontaneous reversal is demonstrated by blockade monitoring. The usual dose of neostigmine is 35 to 45 μg/kg given with either 15 μg/kg atropine or 7.5 μg/kg glycopyrrolate. This dose may be repeated once if satisfactory reversal is not evident after the initial dose. Maximal inhibition of AChE is achieved with neostigmine 70 to 80 μg/kg. Should this dose produce incomplete reversal, positive-pressure ventilation to support respiration should be continued until neuromuscular blockade dissipates with the passage of time.

Glycopyrrolate's onset and duration of antimuscarinic action is better matched to the onset and duration of the anticholinesterase action of neostigmine or pyridostigmine. Simultaneous administration of glycopyrrolate with neostigmine or pyridostigmine produces reversal of residual paralysis with minimal change in heart rate.[160] Glycopyrrolate is a tertiary amine and does not cross the blood–brain barrier to the degree atropine does to produce central nervous system depression. Patients who receive glycopyrrolate with neostigmine for reversal show more rapid arousal than patients who receive atropine neostigmine reversal.[161]

Pyridostigmine

When compared with neostigmine and edrophonium, pyridostigmine is the anticholinesterase agent with the slowest time to maximal reversal (12 to 15 minutes) and the longest duration of action.[158] The average dose is 150 to 200 μg/kg given with either atropine 15 μg/kg or glycopyrrolate 7.5 μg/kg. As with neostigmine, this dose may be repeated once if the first dose does not produce adequate reversal. If the second dose fails to produce complete reversal of residual paralysis, positive-pressure ventilation should be used to support ventilation until time dissipates the effects of the muscle relaxant. During this time patient comfort must be ensured by providing analgesia and sedation if needed. When compared with neostigmine, pyridostigmine has been associated with a lower incidence of arrhythmias in the elderly.

SUMMARY

Successful use of muscle relaxants requires adherence to three principles: acquisition of knowledge, vigilant monitoring, and titration of dose to desired effect. Comprehensive knowledge of the pharmacology of all muscle relaxants allows the practitioner to choose the muscle relaxant best suited to the surgical procedure as well as the general medical condition of the patient. Frequent assessment of neuromuscular junction status with peripheral nerve stimulation monitors will allow rational decisions about the extent and nature of paralysis present and the need for additional muscle relaxant doses. Based on the results of vigilant monitoring, the size and timing of additional muscle relaxant doses can be titrated to produce adequate paralysis during the procedure and to allow for some degree of spontaneous recovery prior to time for reversal at the end of the anesthetic. With adherence to these principles rapid reversal of residual paralysis is possible, the margin of safety for neuromuscular conduction after reversal is high, and the incidence of recurarization is zero or low.

REFERENCES

1. West R. Curare in man. *Proc R Soc Med*. 1932;25:1107–1116.
2. Bennett AE. Preventing traumatic complications in convulsive shock therapy by curare. *JAMA*. 1940;114:322–324.
3. Griffith HR, Johnson GE. The use of curare in general anesthesia. *Anesthesiology*. 1942;3:418–420.
4. Beecher HK, Todd DP. A study of deaths with anesthesia and surgery. *Ann Surg*. 1940;140:2–34.
5. Gissen AJ, Katz RL. Twitch, tetanus and post-tetanic potentiation as indices of nerve-muscle block in man. *Anesthesiology*. 1969;30:491–497.
6. Drachman DA. Myasthenia gravis. *N Engl J Med*. 1978;298:136–142.
7. Guyton AC. *Textbook of medical physiology*. 8th ed. Philadelphia: WB Saunders; 1991.
8. Katz B. *Nerve, muscle and synapse*. New York: McGraw-Hill; 1966.
9. Hubbard JI, Jones SF, Landau EM. On the mechanism by which calcium and magnesium affect the release of transmitter by nerve impulses. *J Physiol*. 1968;196:75–86.
10. Taylor P. Are neuromuscular blocking agents more efficacious in pairs? *Anesthesiology*. 1985;63:1–3.

11. Guy HR. A structural model of the acetylcholine receptor channel based on partition energy and helix packing calculations. *Biophys J.* 1984;45:249–262.

12. Taylor P, Brown RD, Johnson DA. The linkage between ligand occupation and response of the nicotinic acetylcholine receptor. In: Kleinzeller A, Martin BD, eds. *Current topics in membranes and transport.* New York: Academic Press; 1983;18:407–444.

13. Plotter LT. Synthesis and release of ^{14}C acetylcholine in isolated rat diaphragm muscle. *J Physiol.* 1970;206:145–166.

14. Elmqvist D, Quastel DMJ. Presynaptic action of hemicholinium at the neuromuscular junction. *J Physiol.* 1965;177:463–482.

15. Del Castillo J, Katz B. Quantal components of the end-plate potential. *J Physiol.* 1954;124:560–573.

16. Riker WF. Prejunctional effects of neuromuscular and facilitory drugs. In: Katz RL, ed. *Muscle relaxants.* Amsterdam: Excerpta Medica; 1975:59–102.

17. Standaert FG, Dretchen KL. Cyclic nucleotides in neuromuscular transmission. *Anesth Analg.* 1981;60:91–99.

18. Hubbard JI, Wilson DF. Neuromuscular transmission in a mammalian preparation in the absence of blocking drugs and the effect of *d*-tubocurarine. *J Physiol.* 1973;228:307–325.

19. Ghoneim MM, Long JP. The interaction between magnesium and other neuromuscular blocking agents. *Anesthesiology.* 1970;32:23–27.

20. Ali HH, Saverese JJ. Monitoring of neuromuscular function. *Anesthesiology.* 1976;45:216–249.

21. Waud BE, Waud DR. The relation between the response to "train-of-four" stimulation and receptor occlusion during competitive neuromuscular blockade. *Anesthesiology.* 1972;37:413–416.

22. Waud BE, Waud DR. The relation between tetanic fade and receptor occlusion in the presence of competitive neuromuscular block. *Anesthesiology.* 1971;35:456–464.

23. Katz B, Miledi R. Transmitter leakage from motor nerve endings. *Proc R Soc Lond.* 1977;196:59–72.

24. Thesleff S, Molg'o J. A new type of transmitter release at the neuromuscular junction. *Neuroscience.* 1983;9:1–8.

25. Carter JG, Sokoll MD. Effect of spinal cord transection on neuromuscular function in the rat. *Anesthesiology.* 1981;55:542–546.

26. Bowman WC, Marshall IG, Gibb AJ. Is there feedback control of transmitter release at the neuromuscular junction? *Semin Anesth.* 1984;3:275–283.

27. Ali HH, Savarese JJ. Stimulus frequency and the dose response to *d*-tubocurarine in man. *Anesthesiology.* 1980;52:35–39.

28. Ali HH, Savarese JJ, Lebowitz PW, et al. Twitch, tetanus, and train-of-four as indices of recovery from nondepolarizing neuromuscular blockade. *Anesthesiology.* 1981;54:294–297.

29. Merton PA. Voluntary strength and fatigue. *J Physiol.* 1954;123:553–564.

30. Jones RM, Pearce AC, Williams JP. Recovery characteristics following antagonism of atracurium with neostigmine or edrophonium. *Br J Anaesth.* 1984;56:453–457.

31. Jones RJ. Use of the peripheral nerve stimulator. *AANA J.* 1980;48:152–154.

32. Kopman AF, Lawson D. Miliamperage requirements for supramaximal stimulation of the ulnar nerve with surface electrodes. *Anesthesiology.* 1984;61:83–85.

33. Moore G, Williams JR. Monitoring of neuromuscular function of the facial nerve: A noninvasive technique. *AANA J.* 1984;52:171–172.

34. Futter ME. Prolonged suxamethonium infusion during nitrous oxide anesthesia supplemented by halothane or fentanyl. *Br J Anaesth.* 1983;55:947–953.

35. Bowman WC. Prejunctional and postjunctional cholinoreceptors at the neuromuscular junction. *Anesth Analg.* 1980;59:935–943.

36. Donati F, Bevan DR. Antagonism of phase II succinylcholine block by neostigmine. *Anesth Analg.* 1985;64:773–776.

37. Paton WDM, Zaimis EJ. The methonium compounds. *Pharmacol Rev.* 1954;4:219–253.

38. Hunt R, de Taveau MR. On the physiologic action of certain choline derivatives and new methods for detecting choline. *Br Med J.* 1906;2:1178–1791.

39. Dorkins HR. Suxamethonium—The development of a modern drug from 1906 to the present day. *Med Hist.* 1982;26:145–168.

40. Foldes FF, McNall PG, Borrengo-Hinojosa JM. Succinylcholine: A new approach to muscular relaxation in anesthesiology. *N Engl J Med.* 1952;247:596–600.

41. Viby-Mogensen J. Correlation of succinylcholine duration of action with plasma cholinesterase activity in subjects with genotypically normal enzyme. *Anesthesiology.* 1980;53:517–520.

42. Foldes FF, Rendell-Baker L, Birch JH. Causes and prevention of prolonged apnea with succinylcholine. *Anesth Analg.* 1956;35:609–613.

43. Leighton BL, Cheek TG, Gross JB, et al. Succinylcholine pharmacodynamics in peripartum patients. *Anesthesiology.* 1986;64:202–205.

44. Kalow W, Genest K. A method for the detection of atypical forms of human serum cholinesterase. Determination of dibucaine numbers. *Can J Biochem.* 1957;35:339–353.

45. Sugimori T. Shortened action of succinylcholine in individuals with cholinesterase C5 isozyme. *Can Anesth Soc J.* 1986;33:321–327.

46. Lowenstein E. Succinylcholine administration in the burned patient. *Anesthesiology.* 1966;27:494–496.

47. Mazze RI, Escue HM, Houston JB. Hyperkalemia and cardiovascular collapse following administration of succinylcholine to the traumatized patient. *Anesthesiology.* 1969;31:540–547.

48. Stoelting RK. Comparison of gallamine and atropine as pretreatment before anesthesia induction and succinylcholine administration. *Anesth Analg.* 1977;56:493–495.

49. Mathias JA, Evans-Prosser CDG, Churchill-Davidson HC. The role of nondepolarizing drugs in the prevention of suxamethonium bradycardia. *Br J Anaesth.* 1970;42:609–613.

50. Perez HR. Cardiac arrhythmias after succinylcholine. *Anesth Analg.* 1970;49:33–38.

51. Miller RD, Way WL. Inhibition of succinylcholine-induced increased intragastric pressure by non-depolarizing muscle relaxant and lidocaine. *Anesthesiology.* 1971;34:185–188.

52. Salem MR, Wong AY, Lin YH. The effect of suxamethonium on the intragastric pressure in infants and children. *Br J Anaesth.* 1972;44:166–170.

53. Smith G, Dalling R, Williams TIR. Gastro-esophageal pressure gradient changes produced by suxamethonium. *Br J Anaesth.* 1978;50:1137–1143.

54. Marchand P. A study of the forces productive of gastro-esophageal regurgitation and herniation through the diaphragmatic hiatus. *Thorax.* 1957;12:189–202.

55. Pandey K, Badola RP, Kumar S. Time course of intraocular hypertension produced by suxamethonium. *Br J Anaesth.* 1972;44:191–196.

56. Katz RL, Eakins KE. Mode of action of succinylcholine on intraocular pressure. *J Pharmacol Exp Ther.* 1968;162:1–9.

57. Cook JH. The effect of suxamethonium on intraocular pressure. *Anaesthesia.* 1981;36:359–365.

58. Minton MD, Grosslight K, Stirt JA, Bedford RF. Increases in intracranial pressure from succinylcholine: Prevention by prior nondepolarizing blockade. *Anesthesiology.* 1986;65:165–169.

59. Stirt JA, Grosslight K, Bedford RF. "Defasciculation" with metocurine prevents succinylcholine-induced increases in intracranial pressure. *Anesthesiology.* 1987;67:50–53.

60. Ryan JF, Kagan LJ, Hyman AL. Myoglobinemia after a single dose of succinylcholine. *N Engl J Med.* 1971;285:824–825.

61. Harrington JF, Ford DJ, Striker TW. Myoglobinemia and myoglobinuria after succinylcholine in children. *Anesthesiology.* 1983;59:A439.

62. Stoelting RK, Peterson C. Adverse effects of increased succinylcholine dose following *d*-tubocurarine pretreatment. *Anesth Analg.* 1975;54:282–288.

63. Manchikanti L, Grow JB, Colliver JA, et al. Atracurium pretreatment for succinylcholine-induced fasciculations and postoperative myalgia. *Anesth Analg.* 1985;64:1010–1014.

64. Chatterji S, Thind S, Daga S, et al. Lignocaine pretreatment for suxamethonium. A clinicobiochemical study. *Anaesthesia.* 1983;38:867–870.

65. Lindgren L, Saarnivaara L. Effects of competitive myoneural blockade and fentanyl on muscle fasciculations caused by suxamethonium in children. *Br J Anaesth.* 1983;55:747–750.

66. Shrivastava O, Chatterji S, Kachhawa S, et al. Calcium gluconate pretreatment for prevention of succinylcholine myalgia. *Anesth Analg.* 1983;62:59–62.

67. Davies AO. Oral diazepam premedication reduces the incidence of post-succinylcholine muscle pains. *Can Anaesth Soc J.* 1983;30:603–606.

68. Denborough MA, Forster JFA, Maplestone PA, et al. Anesthetic deaths in a family. *Br J Anaesth.* 1962;34:395–396.

69. Gronert GA. Malignant hyperthermia. *Anesthesiology.* 1980;53:395–425.

70. Goldhill DR, Whitehead RS, Emmott AP, et al. Neuromuscular and clinical effects of mivacurium chloride in healthy adult patients during nitrous oxide–enflurane anesthesia. *Br J Anaesth.* 1991;67:289–295.

71. Matteo RS, Pua EK, Khambatta HJ, Spector S. Cerebrospinal fluid levels of *d*-tubocurarine in man. *Anesthesiology.* 1977;46:396–399.

72. Everett AJ, Cowe LA, Wilkonson S. Revision of the structures of (+)-tubocurarine chloride and (+)-chondrocurine. *Chem Commun.* 1970:1020–1021.

73. Hughes R, Chapple DJ. Cardiovascular and neuromuscular effects of dimethyltubocurarine in anaesthetized cats and rhesus monkeys. *Br J Anaesth.* 1976;48:847–852.

74. Cohen EN, Corbascio A, Fleischli G. The distribution and fate of *d*-tubocurarine. *J Pharmacol Exp Ther.* 1965;147:120–129.

75. Matteo RS, Backus WW, Dudley DM, et al. Pharmacokinetics and pharmacodynamics of *d*-tubocurarine and metocurarine in the elderly. *Anesth Analg.* 1985;64:23–29.

76. Stoelting RK. The hemodynamic effects of pancuronium and *d*-tubocurarine in anesthetized patients. *Anesthesiology.* 1972;36:612–615.

77. Moss J, Rosow CE, Savarese JJ, Philbin DM, Kniffen KJ. Role of histamine in the hypotensive action of *d*-tubocurarine in humans. *Anesthesiology.* 1981;55:19–25.

78. Munger WL, Miller RD, Stevens WC. The dependence of *d*-tubocurarine-induced hypotension on alveolar concentration of halothane, dose of *d*-tubocurarine, and nitrous oxide. *Anesthesiology.* 1974;40:442–448.

79. Stoelting RK, McCammon RL, Hilgenberg JC. Changes in blood pressure with varying rates of administration of *d*-tubocurarine. *Anesth Analg.* 1980;59:697–699.

80. Brotherton WP, Matteo RS. Pharmacokinetics and pharmacodynamics of metocurine in humans with and without renal failure. *Anesthesiology.* 1981;55:272–276.

81. Savarese JJ, Ali HH, Antonio RP. The clinical pharmacology of metocurine: Dimethyltubocurarine revisited. *Anesthesiology.* 1977;47:277–284.

82. Hughes R, Ingram G, Payne JP. Studies on di-methyltubocurarine in anesthetized man. *Br J Anaesth.* 1976;48:969–974.

83. Lebowitz PW, Ramsey FM, Savarese JJ, et al. Potential of neuromuscular block in man produced by combination of pancuronium and metocurine or pancuronium and *d*-tubocurarine. *Anesth Analg.* 1980;59:604–609.

84. Thompson IR, Putnins CL. Adverse effects of pancuronium during high-dose fentanyl anesthesia for coronary artery bypass grafting. *Anesthesiology.* 1985;62:708–713.

85. Lebowitz PW, Ramsey FM, Savarese JJ. Combination of pancuronium and metocurine: Neuromuscular and hemodynamic advantages over pancuronium alone. *Anesth Analg.* 1981;60:12–16.

86. McLeod K, Watson MJ, Rawlins MD. Pharmacokinetics of pancuronium in patients with normal and impaired renal function. *Br J Anaesth.* 1976;48:341–345.

87. Scott RPF, Savarese JJ. The cardiovascular and autonomic effects of neuromuscular blocking agents. *Semin Anesth.* 1985;3:319–334.

88. Loffelholz K, Muscholl E. Inhibition of parasympathetic nerve stimulation of the release of adrenergic transmitter. *Naunyn Schmiedeberg's Arch Pharmacol.* 1970;267:181.

89. Vercruysse P, Bossuyt P, Hanegreefs G, et al. Gallamine and pancuronium inhibit prejunctional and post-junctional muscarinic receptors in canine saphenous veins. *J Pharmacol Exp Ther.* 1979;209:225–230.

90. Brown BR, Crout JR. The sympathomimetic effect of gallamine on the heart. *J Pharmacol Exp Ther.* 1970;172:266–273.

91. Ivankovich AD, Miletich DJ, Albrecht RF, Zahed B. The effect of pancuronium on myocardial contraction and catecholamine metabolism. *J Pharm Pharmacol.* 1975;27:837–841.

92. Salt PJ, Barnes PK, Conway CM. Inhibition of neuronal uptake of noradrenaline in the isolated perfused rat heart by pancuronium and its homologues ORG 6368, ORG 7268, and ORG NC45. *Br J Anaesth.* 1980;52:313–317.

93. Greengard P, Kebabian JW. Role of cyclic AMP in synaptic transmission in the mammalian peripheral nervous system. *Fed Proc.* 1974;33:1059–1067.

94. Gardier RW, Tsevdos EJ, Jackson DB, et al. Distinct muscarinic mediation of suspected dopaminergic activity in sympathetic ganglia. *Fed Proc.* 1978;37:2422–2428.

95. Edwards RP, Miller RD, Roizen MF. Cardiac responses to imipramine and pancuronium during anaesthesia with halothane and enflurane. *Anesthesiology.* 1979;50:421–425.

96. Agoston S, Vermeer GA, Kersten UW, et al. A primary investigation of the renal and hepatic excretion of gallamine triethoiodide in man. *Br J Anaesth.* 1978;50:345–351.

97. Stoelting RK. Hemodynamic effects of gallamine during halothane–nitrous oxide anesthesia. *Anesthesiology.* 1973;39:645–647.

98. Stoelting RK. Comparison of gallamine and atropine as pretreatment before anesthetic induction and succinylcholine administration. *Anesth Analg.* 1977;56:493–495.

99. Longnecker DE, Stoelting RK, Morrow AG. Cardiac and peripheral vascular effects of gallamine in man. *Anesth Analg.* 1973;52:931–935.

100. Scott RPF, Norman J. Doxacurium chloride: A preliminary clinical trial. *Br J Anaesth.* 1989;62:373–377.

101. Basta SJ, Savarese JJ, Ali HH. Clinical pharmacology of doxacurium chloride: A new long-acting nondepolarizing muscle relaxant. *Anesthesiology.* 1988;69:478–486.

102. Emmott RS, Bracey BJ, Goldhill DR, et al. Cardiovascular effects of doxacurium, pancuronium and vecuronium in anaesthetized patients presenting for coronary artery bypass surgery. *Br J Anaesth.* 1990;65:480–486.

103. Scott RPF, Norman J. Doxacurium chloride: A preliminary clinical trial. *Br J Anaesth.* 1989;62:373–377.

104. Ka'rpa'ti E, Bir'o K. Pharmacological study of a new competitive neuromuscular blocking steroid, pipecuronium bromide. *Arzneim Forsch Drug Res.* 1980;30:346–354.

105. Boros M, Szenohradszky J, Marosi GY, Toth I. Comparative clinical study of pipecuronium bromide and pancuronium bromide. *Arzneim Forsch Drug Res.* 1980;30:389–393.

106. Tassonyi E, Neidhart P, Pittet JF, et al. Cardiovascular effects of pipecuronium and pancuronium in patients undergoing coronary artery bypass grafting. *Anesthesiology.* 1988;69:793–796.

107. Wierda JMKH, Richardson FJ, Agoston S. Dose–response relation and time course of action of pipecuronium bromide in humans anesthetized with nitrous oxide and isoflurane, halothane, or droperidol and fentanyl. *Anesth Analg.* 1989;68:208–213.

108. Larijani GE, Bartkowski RR, Azad SS, et al. Clinical pharmacology of pipecuronium bromide. *Anesth Analg.* 1989;68:734–739.

109. Caldwell JE, Castagnoli KP, Canfell PC, et al. Pipecuronium and pancuronium: Comparison of pharmacokinetics and duration of action. *Br J Anaesth.* 1988;61:693–697.

110. Caldwell JE, Canfell PC, Castagroli KP, et al. The influence of renal failure on the pharmacokinetics and the duration of action of pipecuronium bromide in patients anesthetized with halothane and nitrous oxide. *Anesthesiology.* 1989;70:7–12.

111. Wierda JMKH, Karliczek GF, Vandenbrom RHG, et al. Pharmacokinetics and cardiovascular dynamics of pipecuronium bromide during coronary artery surgery. *Can J Anaesth.* 1990;37:183–191.

112. Foldes FF, Nagashima H, Nguyen HD, et al. Neuromuscular and cardiovascular effects of pipecuronium. *Can J Anaesth.* 1990;37:549–555.

113. Krieg N, Crul JF, Booij LHDJ. Relative potency of ORG NC45, pancuronium, alcuronium, and tubocurarine in man. *Br J Anaesth.* 1980;52:783–787.

114. Lennon RL, Olson RA, Gronert GA. Atracurium or vecuronium for rapid sequence endotracheal intubation. *Anesthesiology.* 1986;64:510–513.

115. Taboada JA, Rupp SM, Miller RD. Refining the priming principle for vecuronium during rapid-sequence induction of anesthesia. *Anesthesiology.* 1986;64:242–247.

116. Ali HH, Savarese JJ, Enbree PB, et al. Clinical pharmacology of mivacurium chloride (BW B1090U) infusion: Comparison with vecuronium and atracurium. *Br J Anaesth.* 1988;61:541–546.

117. Bencini AF, Houwertjes MC, Agoston S. Effects of hepatic uptake of vecuronium bromide and its putative metabolites on their neuromuscular blocking actions in the cat. *Br J Anaesth.* 1985;57:789–795.

118. Lebrault C, Berger JI, D'Hollander AA, et al. Pharmacokinetics and pharmacodynamics of vecuronium (ORG NC45) in patients with cirrhosis. *Anesthesiology.* 1985;62:601–605.

119. Lebrault C, Duvaldestin P, Henzel D, et al. Pharmacokinetics and pharmacodynamics of vecuronium in patients with cholestasis. *Br J Anaesth.* 1986;58:983–987.

120. Bell CF, Hunter JM, Jones RS, et al. Use of atracurium and vecuronium in patients with esophageal varices. *Br J Anaesth.* 1985;57:160–168.

121. Bencini AF, Scaf AHJ, Sohn YJ, et al. Disposition and urinary excretion of vecuronium bromide in anesthetized patients with normal renal function or renal failure. *Anesth Analg.* 1986;65:245–251.

122. Fahey MR, Morris RB, Miller RD, et al. Clinical pharmacology of ORG NC45 (Norcuron™): A new nondepolarizing muscle relaxant. *Anesthesiology.* 1981;55:6–11.

123. Rupp SM, Miller RD, Gencarelli PJ. Vecuronium-induced neuromuscular blockade during enflurane, halothane and isoflurane in humans. *Anesthesiology.* 1984;60:102–105.

124. Marshall RJ, McGrath JC, Miller RD, et al. Comparison of the cardiovascular actions of ORG NC45 with those produced by other non-depolarizing neuromuscular blocking agents in experimental animals. *Br J Anaesth.* 1980;52(suppl):21S–32S.

125. Morris RB, Cahalan MK, Miller RD, et al. The cardiovascular effects of vecuronium (ORG NC45) and pancuronium in patients undergoing coronary artery bypass grafting. *Anesthesiology.* 1983;58:438–440.

126. Stenlake JB, Waigh RD, Urwin J, et al. Atracurium: Conception and inception. *Br J Anaesth.* 1983;55(suppl):3S–10S.

127. Hughes R, Chapple DJ. The pharmacology of atracurium: A new competitive neuromuscular blocking agent. *Br J Anaesth.* 1981;53:31–44.

128. Hunt TM, Hughes R, Payne JP. Preliminary studies with atracurium in anesthetized man. *Br J Anaesth.* 1980;52:238P–239P.

129. deBros FM, Lai A, Scott R, et al. Pharmacokinetics and pharmacodynamics of atracurium during isoflurane anesthesia in normal and anephric patients. *Anesth Analg.* 1986;65:743–746.

130. Chapple DJ, Miller AA, Ward JB, et al. Cardiovascular and neurologic loss effects of laudanosine. *Br J Anaesth.* 1987;59:218–225.

131. Lanier WL, Milde JH, Michenfelder JD. The cerebral effects of pancuronium and atracurium in halothane-anesthetized dogs. *Anesthesiology.* 1985;63:589–597.

132. Hennis PJ, Fahe MR, Canfell PC, et al. Pharmacology of laudanosine in dogs. *Anesthesiology.* 1986;65:56–60.

133. Yate PM, Flynn PJ, Arnold RW, et al. Clinical experience and plasma laudanosine concentrations during infusion of atracurium in the intensive therapy unit. *Br J Anaesth.* 1987;59:211–217.

134. Basta SJ, Ali HH, Savarese JJ, et al. Clinical pharmacology of atracurium besylate (BW33A): A new non-depolarizing muscle relaxant. *Anesth Analg.* 1982;61:723–729.

135. Caldwell JE, Heier T, Kitts JB, et al. Comparison of the neuromuscular block induced by mivacurium, suxamethonium or atracurium during nitrous oxide–fentanyl anesthesia. *Br J Anaesth.* 1989;63:393–399.

136. Naguib M, Abdulatif M, Gyasi HK, et al. The pattern of train-of-four fade after atracurium: Influence of different priming doses. *Anesth Analg.* 1987;66:427–430.

137. Scott RP, Savarese JJ, Basta SJ, et al. Clinical pharmacology of atracurium given in high dose. *Br J Anaesth.* 1986;58:834–838.

138. Frank M, Flynn PJ, Hughes R. Atracurium in obstetric anaesthesia. *Br J Anaesth.* 1983;55:113S–114S.

139. Brandom BW, Woelfel SK, Cook DR, et al. Comparison of mivacurium and suxamethonium administered by bolus and infusion. *Br J Anaesth.* 1989;62:488–493.

140. Caldwell JE, Kitts JB, Heier T, et al. The dose–response relationship of mivacurium chloride in humans during nitrous oxide–fentanyl or nitrous oxide enflurane anesthesia. *Anesthesiology.* 1989;70:31–35.

141. Savarese JJ, Ali HH, Basta SJ, et al. The cardiovascular effects of mivacurium chloride (BW1090U) in patients receiving nitrous oxide–opiate–barbiturate anesthesia. *Anesthesiology.* 1989;70:386–394.

142. Goldhill DR, Whitehead JP, Emmott RS, et al. Neuromuscular and clinical effects of mivacurium chloride in healthy adult patients during nitrous oxide–enflurane anesthesia. *Br J Anaesth.* 1991;67:289–295.

143. Cook DR, Stiller RL, Weakly JN, et al. In vitro metabolism of mivacurium chloride (BW B1090U) and succinylcholine. *Anesth Analg.* 1989;69:452–456.

144. Savarese JJ, Ali HH, Basta SJ, Embree PB, et al. Sixty-second tracheal intubation with BN B1090U after fentanyl thiopental induction. *Anesthesiology.* 1987;67:A351.

145. Sokoll MD, Gergis SD. Antibiotics and neuromuscular function. *Anesthesiology.* 1981;55:148–155.

146. Matuso S, Rao DBS, Chaundry I, et al. Interaction of muscle relaxants and local anesthetics at the neuromuscular junction. *Anesth Analg.* 1978;57:580–587.

147. Plotkin CN, Ornstein E. Resistance to pancuronium: Adult respiratory distress syndrome or phenytoin. *Anesth Analg.* 1986;65:820–821.

148. Roth S, Ebrahim ZY. Resistance to pancuronium in patients receiving carbamazepine. *Anesthesiology.* 1987;66:691–693.

149. Scappaticci KA, Ham JA, Sohn YJ, et al. Effects of furosemide on the neuromuscular junction. *Anesthesiology*. 1982;57:381–388.

150. Azar I, Cottrell, Gupta B, et al. Furosemide facilitates recovery of evoked twitch response after pancuronium. *Anesth Analg*. 1980;59:55–57.

151. Matteo RS, Nishitateno K, Pua E, et al. Pharmacokinetics of *d*-tubocurarine in man: Effect of an osmotic diuretic on urinary excretion. *Anesthesiology*. 1980;52:335–338.

152. Borden H, Clarke MT, Katz H. The use of pancuronium in patients receiving lithium carbonate. *Can Anaesth Soc J*. 1974; 21:79–82.

153. Waud BE, Farrell L, Waud DR. Lithium and neuromuscular transmission. *Anesth Analg*. 1982;61:399–402.

154. Fisher DM, O'Keefe C, Stanski DR, et al. Pharmacokinetics and pharmacodynamics of *d*-tubocurarine in infants, children, and adults. *Anesthesiology*. 1982;57:203–208.

155. Donati F, Ferguson A, Bevan DR. Twitch depression and train-of-four ratio after antagonism of pancuronium with edrophonium, neostigmine, or pyridostigmine. *Anesth Analg*. 1983; 62:314–316.

156. Cronnely R, Stanski DR, Miller RD. Renal function and the pharmacokinetics of neostigmine in anesthetized man. *Anesthesiology*. 1979;51:222–226.

157. Cronnely R, Stanski DR, Miller RD, et al. Pyridostigmine kinetics with and without renal function. *Clin Pharmacol Ther*. 1980;28:78–81.

158. Cronnely R, Morris RB, Miller RD. Edrophonium: Duration of action and atropine requirement in humans during halothane anesthesia. *Anesthesiology*. 1982;57:261–266.

159. Rupp SM, McChristian JW, Miller RD, et al. Neostigmine and edrophonium antagonism of varying neuromuscular blockade induced by atracurium, pancuronium, or vecuronium. *Anesthesiology*. 1986;64:711–717.

160. Salem MG, Richardson JC, Meadows GA, et al. Comparison between glycopyrrolate and atropine in mixture with neostigmine for reversal of neuromuscular blockade. *Br J Anaesth*. 1985;57:184–187.

161. Sheref SE. Pattern of CNS recovery following reversal of neuromuscular blockade: Comparison of atropine and glycopyrrolate. *Br J Anaesth*. 1985;57:188–191.

Pharmacology of Cardiovascular Drugs

J. L. Reeves-Viets and
D. E. Supkis, Jr.

A variety of pharmacologic agents are available for cardiovascular management during anesthesia. The availability of agents with precise sites of action has increased the sophistication with which the practitioner can induce or manage hemodynamic alterations when indicated. This array of agents, however, offers the opportunity for confusion in management as well. This chapter addresses the common agents used during anesthetic and perioperative management, according to the classification of the agent, and their clinical applications.

The majority of agents employed for hemodynamic control during anesthesia operate by modulating the effects of the autonomic nervous system. This mechanism of action gives the practitioner the ability to augment or reduce autonomic tone by the use of selective agonists or antagonists. For the purposes of this review, the drugs are broken down into several categories: sympathetic agonists, which include the inotropes and vasopressors; sympathetic antagonists, which include the alpha and beta blockers; direct-acting vasodilators; antihypertensives; calcium channel blockers; and antiarrhythmics.

SYMPATHETIC AGONISTS

The sympathetic agonists operate through two mechanisms, following the routes of sympathetic innervation and control. The intrinsic route operates from sympathetic fibers, which terminate in the systemic and pulmonary vasculature and in the heart at several sites, including the sinoatrial (SA) node, the atrioventricular (AV) node, and the Purkinje fibers responsible for transmission of the impulses to the ventricles.[1] The primary neurotransmitter for the intrinsic route is norepinephrine, released at the site of the myoneural junction.[2] In contrast, the hormonal or humoral route operates through release of catecholamines from the adrenal medulla, with actions similar to those of the intrinsic route.[3] The primary neurotransmitter for the humoral

route is epinephrine,[1,3–6] carried through the vascular tree after release from the adrenal medulla in response to stress.

Both sympathetic routes operate by enhancing the inotropic state of the ventricles, enhancing the rate of intrinsic depolarization in pacemaker cells, and enhancing the development of arrhythmias. The effects on the peripheral vasculature increase with increasing dose. Stimulation of the humoral route, which induces the release of low concentrations of epinephrine, produces beta-mediated peripheral dilation, whereas the release of norepinephrine or higher concentrations of epinephrine results in an overriding alpha-mediated peripheral vasoconstriction. The development of an overriding alpha tone does not, however, eliminate the beta-induced increases in inotropy, rate, and arrhythmogenicity.

Sympathetic agonists may operate in several fashions. Direct stimulation of the sympathetic terminals may produce the corresponding beta or alpha effects, as is the case with direct-acting catecholamines. Alternately, indirect pathways may enhance the release of the sympathetic neurotransmitter or delay neurotransmitter breakdown and reuptake.[7,8] The sympathetic agonists can be divided into three major groups: (1) catecholamines, which directly produce the classic graduated effects with increasing dosage; (2) inodilators, which indirectly produce increases in inotropy without increases in systemic vascular resistance at higher doses; and (3) vasoconstrictors, which directly mimic the vascular effects of norepinephrine or high-dose epinephrine. Although there is overlap between these groups, general patterns can be defined that direct their clinical application. Commonly employed agents, along with their doses and prominent clinical effects, are listed in Table 29–1.

Catecholamines

The catecholamines include four direct-acting agents: epinephrine, norepinephrine, dopamine, and isoproterenol. Except when used as emergency drugs, these agents are all generally employed as titratable continuous infusions. The first three are native sympathetic neurotransmitters; isoproterenol is a synthetic molecule. These agents all produce in-

TABLE 29–1. COMMONLY USED SYMPATHETIC AGONISTS

Drug	Dosage (µg/kg/min)	Effect	Indications/Benefits	Disadvantage
Epinephrine				
	0.0–0.4	Beta	Low CO,[a] CHF, failure to wean from bypass, bradycardia	Atrial tachycardia
	0.04–0.1	Mixed beta/alpha	Low CO with low SVR Low arterial pressure with low SVR	Arrhythmias (PACs, PVCs) As above
	> 0.1	Alpha effects predominate	Profound hypotension low SVR, anaphylaxis	Induction of arrhythmias, vasoconstriction: reduced peripheral perfusion and metabolic acidosis
Isuprel				
	(All doses) 0–0.2	Beta agonist	Bradycardia, CHF, low CO, pulmonary HTN, failure to wean from bypass	Profound peripheral dilation and systemic hypotension
Norepinephrine				
	(All doses) 0–0.2	Alpha agonist	Profound hypotension from low SVR, failure to wean from bypass	Induction of arrhythmias, vasoconstriction: reduced peripheral perfusion and metabolic acidosis
Dopamine				
	0–3	Dopaminergic	Renal dilation, oliguria (renal)	
	0–5	Beta	Low CO, CHF, failure to wean from bypass	Atrial tachycardias, mild increase in PA pressure
	5–15	Mixed beta/alpha	Low CO with low SVR, low arterial pressure with low SVR	As above
	> 15	Alpha effects predominate	Profound hypotension, low SVR, failure to wean from bypass	Peripheral vasoconstriction: reduced peripheral perfusion and metabolic acidosis, tachycardia
Dobutamine				
	0–15	Beta	Reduces PA pressure: failure to wean from bypass, CHF, low CO	Systemic hypotension in higher doses
	> 15	Alpha effects demonstrated		
Amrinone				
	(All doses) 0–40	Beta	Reduces PA pressure: failure to wean from bypass, CHF, low CO	Systemic hypotension in higher doses

[a] CO, cardiac output; CHF, congestive heart failure; SVR, systemic vascular resistance; PACs, premature atrial contractions; PVCs, premature ventricular contractions; HTN, hypertension; PA, pulmonary artery.

creases in inotropic state, in the rate of spontaneous depolarization in pacemaker cells, and in arrhythmogenicity. Their effects on the systemic vasculature vary according to the specific drug. Among these agents, epinephrine and dopamine demonstrate the classic graduated response to increasing doses. Isoproterenol produces beta agonism, which increases inotropic state and heart rate without producing alpha-agonist systemic vasoconstriction. Norepinephrine produces primarily alpha-agonist increases in systemic vasomotor tone, with less effect on inotropic state and heart rate. An additional agent, ephedrine, produces its effects through an increase in the release of native catecholamines, and operates as a weak neurotransmitter itself. It is generally used for bolus administration rather than as a continuous infusion.

Epinephrine produces the classic graduated response with increasing dosage. Clinical effects are rapid, usually occurring within 2 minutes, and lasting 5 to 15 minutes after administration, depending on the dose employed. In low doses (below 0.04 µg/kg/min), it produces increased inotropy, increased rate of spontaneous depolarization in the pacemaker cells, and increased arrhythmogenicity. As the dose is increased to the midrange (0.04 to 0.15 µg/kg/min), a gradual increase in systemic vascular resistance is noted, with increased blood pressure. At high doses (over 0.15 µg/kg/min), the alpha effects of increased vasomotor tone predominate, whereas beta-induced increases in inotropy eventually plateau.[9] The arrhythmogenic effects of epinephrine increase with increasing dosage, as does the increase in the rate of spontaneous depolarization of the pacemaker cells. Hence, with increasing dosages, tachycardia and tachyarrhythmias become a prominent feature.[2]

Norepinephrine has similar onset and duration, and operates through the intrinsic pathway similar to epinephrine in low doses, producing an increase in inotropic state and arrhythmogenicity.[10] In contrast to epinephrine, its hormonal effect produces a direct increase in peripheral vasomotor tone, which is a prominent effect at all rates of administration. It is generally used in titratable form with doses up to 0.1 µg/kg/min. In response to increased systemic pressure, slowing of the heart rate may occur as a reflex rather than a direct effect. Because the peripheral constrictor effects outweigh inotropic benefit, norepinephrine is seldom used in the clinical setting as an inotrope. Its use is generally restricted to that of a vasoconstrictor in patients demonstrating high cardiac output with unsatisfactory systemic pressures.

Isoproterenol was the first synthetic sympathetic agonist developed for clinical use in a continuous infusion. It has a rapid onset within 2 minutes and slightly shorter duration of action than epinephrine, which may be related to the dose employed. It is generally titrated according to clinical response at rates up to 0.2 µg/kg/min. At all clinical doses, isoproterenol produces a pure beta-mediated increase in inotropic state,[2,11] which is otherwise similar to that of the other catecholamines. Drawbacks to the use of isoproterenol include enhancement of arrhythmias and the development of frequent tachycardias.[2] Additionally, isoproterenol is devoid of any demonstrable alpha effect on the peripheral and pulmonary vasculature.[12,13] Hence, the effects on systemic pressure are unpredictable. When beta-induced inotropic benefits outweigh the reduction in systemic vascular resistance, blood pressure may be increased. When the beta-induced reduction in systemic vascular resistance predominates, systemic pressures may decline with its use. For these reasons, isoproterenol has found progressively less application in the management of the adult patient.[2] It is currently commonly used for maintaining heart rate in patients with SA node dysfunction (sick sinus syndrome, refractory bradycardia with secondary hypotension) and in patients with cardiac transplant, or in managing pediatric patients in whom the systemic pressure is not maintained in the adult range.[9]

Dopamine is probably the most commonly employed catecholamine, and maintains a physiologic profile slightly different from those of the other agents. It has a slightly slower onset than epinephrine, at 2 to 5 minutes for clinical effect, and a duration up to 10 minutes on termination of infusion. Dopamine is itself a native sympathetic neurotransmitter and a precursor in the formation of both norepinephrine and epinephrine.[14] Dopamine is a weaker inotropic agent than epinephrine, requiring severalfold the dosage to produce similar effects. Part of the effects demonstrated by dopamine are indirect, being mediated by an augmented release of norepinephrine at the intrinsic terminals.[15] Hence, it demonstrates its greatest effect in the intact heart and has less potency in the denervated organ. Further, long-term usage may demonstrate a reduction in the benefit of dopamine, as native neurotransmitter stores are depleted and replaced by dopamine. As a neurotransmitter, it demonstrates a physiologic profile similar to that of epinephrine.[16] At low doses (< 5 µg/kg/min), it produces an increase in inotropy and in the rate of spontaneous depolarization of the pacemaker cells, with only minimal increases in arrhythmogenicity. With progressive increases in dosage

to the midrange (5 to 15 µg/kg/min), it produces a gradual increase in systemic vascular resistance. At high doses (> 15 to 20 µg/kg/min), the alpha-induced peripheral vasoconstriction predominates. Dopamine has been reported to be less arrhythmogenic than either epinephrine or isuprel when used at equipotent inotropic doses.[9] In addition to its inotropic effects, dopamine demonstrates intrinsic renal and mesenteric vasodilator effects at low doses, mediated through specific dopaminergic receptors in the renal and mesenteric vasculature.[17,18] This may produce increases in renal blood flow and augment urinary output when the drug is used at low to intermediate doses. At high doses, the renal dilatory effect is overridden by the alpha-induced peripheral vasoconstriction.

Ephedrine produces both direct and indirect effects.[2] It stimulates the release of endogenous stores of the native catecholamines,[12] producing an augmented alpha and beta response on administration. Ephedrine usually demonstrates an initial clinical effect within 2 to 5 minutes and demonstrates clinical effects for up to 15 minutes after a bolus administration. It is also taken up in the sympathetic nerve terminal, where it functions as a weak neurotransmitter in its own right.[9] Patients receiving repeated doses or continuous administration may demonstrate tachyphylaxis as ephedrine is taken up in nerve terminals and produces its weak direct effect. It is generally used only in bolus doses of 2.5 to 10 mg for short-term hemodynamic support in the treatment of bradycardia and hypotension that follows mild myocardial depression in response to anesthetic agents.

Inodilators

Two drugs are included in the class of agents termed inodilators: dobutamine and amrinone. These agents produce only mild beta agonism directly, and their mechanism of action is dependent on indirect effects as well, including inhibition of the phosphodiesterase enzyme system (PDE-III)[19] that is responsible for breakdown of endogenous catecholamines. Thus, both agents produce increases in inotropic state without the increase in systemic vasomotor tone that accompanies administration of the native catecholamines. Both agents reportedly produce less frequent and less severe tachycardia, and are less arrhythmogenic, than native catecholamines. Additionally, they produce reductions in pulmonary vascular resistance that may prove beneficial in management of patients with pulmonary hypertension. Finally, inhibition of PDE-III provides a mechanism of action independent of direct beta agonism, making these agents useful in management of patients with ventricular dysfunction who have been treated with beta-blocking agents.

Dobutamine provides direct, mild beta agonism and possesses an indirect mechanism of action that may represent either norepinephrine accumulation or inhibition of PDE-III.[20] It produces an increase in inotropic state with generally only mild increases in heart rate. Dobutamine is slower in onset than the catecholamines, requiring 5 to 7 minutes to demonstrate clinical effects, and duration of action is similarly extended to 10 to 12 minutes. Although there was initially less frequent tachycardia and less arrhythmogenicity reported with the use of dobutamine than with the native catecholamines, mild increases in heart rate may be noted.[21,22] Dobutamine is a relatively mild inotrope, requiring severalfold the dosage of epinephrine to produce similar increases in inotropic state. Reductions in systemic vasomotor tone and ventricular afterload augment the effects of increased inotropic state in the failing ventricle. The reduction in pulmonary vascular resistance may be proportionately greater than the increase in cardiac output, which results in a decrease in pulmonary artery pressure.[23,24] Dobutamine is devoid of the renal effects seen with dopamine. When high doses (over 15 to 20 µg/kg/min) are employed, a mild increase in systemic vascular resistance may be demonstrated, although profound systemic vasoconstriction is not noted with its use.[21,22]

Amrinone is likewise a mild direct beta agonist, the physiologic effects of which have yet to be fully elucidated. The effects are felt to be mediated primarily through inhibition of PDE-III.[19] Amrinone has an onset and duration of action similar to those of dobutamine. It produces increases in inotropic state with minimal increases in heart rate and no increase or a reduction in systemic vascular resistance. As amrinone acts primarily through enzyme inhibition, it is a comparatively weak inotrope, requiring relatively high doses (up to 40 µg/kg/min) to produce inotropic increases similar to those produced with epinephrine. Amrinone is an effective pulmonary vasodilator, decreasing pulmonary vascular resistance proportionately with the increase in cardiac output. As amrinone is available in oral form, it is frequently used for prolonged management of the patient with congestive heart failure, for management of patients in coronary care units, and for medical management of patients prior to cardiac transplantation.

Vasoconstrictors

The vasoconstrictors used in current clinical practice employ direct stimulation of the alpha receptors to produce an increase in systemic and pulmonary vasomotor tone. The result is increased systemic vascular resistance and an increase in the corresponding arterial pressure when cardiac output is held constant. As a result of the increase in systemic arterial pressure, slowing of the heart rate may occur with their use through a reflex rather than a direct effect. Only two agents are commonly used in infusion form: norepinephrine and phenylephrine. A third agent, methoxamine, is generally used in bolus form rather than as a continuous infusion.

Norepinephrine has been previously discussed as a sympathetic agonist. It possesses direct sympathetic activity and is the primary neurotransmitter in the intrinsic sympathetic terminals in the myocardium. In infusion form at all doses up to 0.1 µg/kg/min, this effect is overshadowed by its role in the humoral route in which norepinephrine produces alpha-mediated increases in vasomotor tone. The overriding systemic alpha agonism makes it more suitable as a vasoconstrictor than an inotrope. Hence, it is most commonly used for maintenance of systemic vascular resistance in the management of patients with high cardiac output and low systemic blood pressure.

Phenylephrine is a less potent vasoconstrictor, producing effects similar to those of norepinephrine when used at approximately tenfold dosage. It has a rapid onset within 1 to 2 minutes and a duration of action of 5 to 10 minutes after termination of the infusion.[11] Phenylephrine is also practically devoid of beta effects except at high doses,[25–28] producing alpha-mediated systemic vasoconstriction that increases with doses up to 1 µg/kg/min. As with norepinephrine, it finds primary application in the management of patients with high cardiac output and low systemic arterial pressure. Phenylephrine provides effective, titratable increases in vasomotor tone and permits maintenance of normal systemic vascular resistance in most patients with pharmacologically induced reduction in sympathetic vasomotor tone.

Methoxamine is a direct-acting alpha stimulant[29] that produces prompt, sustained peripheral vasoconstriction. It is usually used in a single bolus dose of 2 mg and demonstrates an increase in systemic pressure within 2 minutes of administration.[30] It has a sustained duration of action, lasting 15 minutes to 1 hour after a single dose.[11,28,31] Methoxamine appears to be totally devoid of any beta effects,[32,33] and does not stimulate tachycardias or arrhythmias.[34] Reflex bradycardia may follow its administration as a result of the increase in systemic arterial pressure. Because of its extended duration of action, methoxamine is not employed as a continuous infusion.

Clinical Applications of Sympathetic Agonists

When employed in a physiologically sound fashion, the use of inotropes and vasoconstrictors permits the practitioner to maintain both cardiac output and systemic blood pressure within a desired range. When the required preload is maintained, inotropic agents may be used to support the contractile state, the second determinant of stroke volume, and, therefore, cardiac output. When cardiac output is maintained, the use of vasoconstrictors permits adjustment of the systemic vascular resistance, which is the second determinant of systemic blood pressure. Appreciation of basic physiologic principles and the pharmacologic actions of each of the agents will identify their individual applications.

The use of catecholamines generally produces an increase in the inotropic state, along with mild to moderate increases in heart rate and progressive increases in vasomotor tone. These effects in combination permit the maintenance of both cardiac output and systemic arterial pressure. Ephedrine is frequently used to elicit both alpha and beta effects in the treatment of relatively mild myocardial depression. It proves effective short-term cardiovascular support when prolonged myocardial depression is not expected. Additionally, its enhancement of sympathetic tone may also make ephedrine useful in accelerating SA node automaticity in the patient with SA node depression and secondary AV nodal electrical mechanism. This may prove beneficial in the management of patients having myocardial revascularization who fail to reestablish normal sinus mechanism on rewarming from the cold ischemia of cardioplegia.

Among the catecholamines used in continuous infusion, only isoproterenol is a pure beta agonist, permitting the practitioner to increase heart rate and provide inotropic support without increasing the systemic vascular resistance. It is primarily used in the management of patients with profound, hemodynamically significant bradycardia or in patients requiring inotropic support without increases in systemic vascular resistance. Isoproterenol may in fact produce profound beta-induced reductions in systemic vascular resistance at higher doses, and its lack of alpha activity makes it unsuitable as a sole agent in the management of patients requiring both inotropic support and maintenance of systemic vascular resistance. When isoproterenol is employed for maintenance of heart rate in patients with reduced systemic vascular resistance, it may prove necessary to employ a second agent as a direct vasoconstrictor to maintain systemic vasomotor tone. Combined therapy with isoproterenol and phenylephrine or norepinephrine may permit maintenance of heart rate and inotropic state, while permitting the practitioner to directly augment systemic vascular resistance and therefore systemic pressures.

Although combined therapy with pure alpha and beta agonists is possible, it is more common practice to employ those catecholamines that produce the classic graduated response. Epinephrine and dopamine are frequently used in the management of patients with poor cardiac output based on myocardial depression alone. In those patients, the use of epinephrine is supported for its direct action and by its role as the natural sympathetic neurotransmitter in the humoral sympathetic route. In contrast, dopamine is an effective sympathetic agonist with the additional benefit of renal vasodilation and improved renal blood flow. It proves popular for both its direct cardiac effects and its systemic, noncardiac action; however, because dopamine is a relatively less potent inotropic agent and part of its effect is indirect, it is less effective in maintaining the necessary alpha-mediated increase in systemic vascular resistance in patients with profound cardiovascular depression. Therefore, dopamine is frequently used in patients with comparatively mild myocardial depression and finds most application in weaning patients from cardiopulmonary bypass or in treatment of the comparatively mild myocardial depression that may occur in the patient with compromised ventricular function in response to the use of anesthetic agents that possess myocardial depressant effects. Epinephrine is more frequently used in patients with severe myocardial depression that has proven refractory to therapy with less potent agents such as dopamine and in patients requiring both inotropic support and maintenance of systemic vascular resistance.

The role of the noncatecholamine sympathetic agonists is rapidly developing. Both dobutamine and amrinone are indirect-acting agents, dependent on inhibition of PDE-III for their effects and producing only weak direct sympathetic stimulation. These agents offer several advantages over the direct-acting sympathetic agonists. Both inodilators are effective pulmonary vascular dilators, producing reductions in pulmonary vascular resistance that correspond to or exceed the increase in cardiac output. These agents may produce reductions in pulmonary artery pressure and prove valuable in the management of patients with acute increases in pulmonary pressure, unloading the right ventricle and maintaining cardiac output without increased risk of right ventricular failure. Additionally, both agents provide inotropic support to the failing left ventricle without increasing systemic vascular resistance, which may prove undesirable in the patient with left ventricular failure, and are popular in

the management of patients with chronic failure and high systemic vascular resistance whose cardiac function would be expected to deteriorate with further increases in afterload. Additionally, both inodilators operate through indirect action, which bypasses direct stimulation of the sympathetic axis, and are effective in treatment of ventricular failure in patients who are treated with beta antagonists chronically. They find application in acute management of the depressed ventricle as a primary inotropic agent or as a supplemental agent in the management of patients who have demonstrated an inadequate response to direct-acting catecholamines. In this fashion, dobutamine and amrinone are frequently employed in weaning patients from cardiopulmonary bypass who have failed to wean with only the use of direct-acting catecholamines and in managing patients with ventricular failure after cross-clamping of the aorta in whom inotropic support is required without the concomitant increase in systemic vascular resistance.

The vasoconstrictors provide a means of supporting systemic arterial pressure in those patients who maintain adequate cardiac output but demonstrate systemic hypotension secondary to reductions in systemic vascular resistance. They also find application in the management of patients requiring higher-than-normal systemic vascular resistance to maintain coronary perfusion, as in those patients with left ventricular outflow obstruction from critical aortic stenosis. In the patient with ventricular failure, they find little application because the increase in systemic resistance produces an increase in left ventricular afterload. Finally, vasoconstrictors may be used to effectively "autotransfuse" the patient with reduced vascular volume by augmenting vasomotor tone in the venous capacitance vessels. This permits the practitioner to maintain preload, cardiac output, and systemic perfusion pressures while gradually increasing vascular volume. The vasoconstrictors may be useful in the volume-depleted patient on chronic diuretic therapy or in the patient with acute hemorrhage requiring emergency intervention. Because massive vasoconstriction reduces total systemic perfusion, these agents may cause hypoperfusion of selected organs with high doses, and produce metabolic acidosis. Therefore they are not recommended for chronic therapy except for those patients with demonstrated low systemic vascular resistance, such as the septic patient, and attention should be given to indices of systemic organ perfusion when they are employed.

SYMPATHETIC ANTAGONISTS

The sympathetic antagonists directly antagonize the systemic and cardiac effects of the agonist agents. They operate through the sympathetic route to reduce the inotropic state, slow heart rate, and reduce arrhythmogenicity through antagonism of beta-mediated effects, or to produce systemic dilation through antagonism of alpha-mediated vasomotor tone. In contrast to the agonist agents, most antagonists have very specific alpha- or beta-antagonist effects. Only one agent, labetalol, that combines both alpha and beta antagonism is currently available for clinical use. The majority of sympathetic antagonists have a far longer duration of action than their corresponding agonist agents and are not available for use as a continuous infusion. At present only one beta antagonist, esmolol, has sufficiently short duration of action to be considered practical for use in continuous infusion.

Beta Antagonists

Two beta antagonists are currently available that readily lend themselves to use in anesthetic practice: propranolol and esmolol. Both of these agents are effective in antagonizing the beta-mediated sympathetic effects. Therefore, they provide safe and effective means of slowing the heart, reducing arrhythmogenicity, and depressing the hyperdynamic ventricle. They are used most commonly in the treatment of acute intraoperative hypertension and tachycardia, and they can be used to achieve similar goals. Esmolol has a very quick onset and is an extremely short-acting agent. This makes esmolol titratable and of use in acute management; it has too short a duration of action to provide long-term suppression of sympathetic stimulation. Propranolol, in contrast, has a slower onset combined with a prolonged duration of action. This makes it nontitratable for short-term management and, therefore, more suitable for long-term suppression. This combination of agents permits the practitioner to achieve short-term acute control of sympathetic overdrive, with the option of converting to long-acting activity when indicated.

Propranolol is a pure beta antagonist with a comparatively longer duration. It finds clinical application primarily in three roles: reduction of heart rate in the tachycardic patient, treatment of hypertension, and as an adjunct in treatment of malignant ventricular dysrhythmias refractory to standard therapy. The purpose for which propranolol is used generally determines the dose employed. For treatment of acute tachycardia, propranolol may be used in intravenous doses beginning at 0.1 to 0.25 mg and titrated to effect. Control of acute-onset tachycardias is generally achieved with a total dose of 1 to 2 mg, although a total dose of up to 5 mg may be employed in younger patients. In the management of sinus or atrial tachycardias, it generally provides suppression of heart rate within 5 to 15 minutes of administration. It has an extended duration of action, lasting 8 to 12 hours after administration.[2,35] As a myocardial depressant, it finds application in the management of hypertension. For the management of hypertension, larger doses are required, and it is employed usually in incremental doses of 0.25 to 0.5 mg. In patients who are on chronic beta-blocker therapy, larger initial doses may be employed. Control of ventricular hypertension is generally achieved with a total dose of 2 to 5 mg. When used for the control of hypertension, propranolol generally demonstrates its clinical effect within 15 to 30 minutes, with duration of action remaining 8 to 12 hours. Because of its extended duration of action, however, it is not readily titratable, which makes it undesirable for short-term use.

Esmolol is a rapid-acting, pure beta antagonist with rapid onset (approximately 2 minutes) and short duration of action (approximately 10 to 20 minutes),[36] which makes it titratable. This is particularly beneficial in the short-term management of sinus or atrial tachycardias or for use as an adjunct to standard antiarrhythmic therapy for patients with refractory ventricular dysrhythmias. It may prove ben-

eficial in the short-term management of the hyperdynamic ventricle,[37] and its short duration of action permits rapid recovery from overdosage or quick return to baseline when used to treat overdose of sympathetic agonists. When used for the treatment of tachycardia, graduated boluses of 10 mg permit the practitioner to titrate the effect of esmolol without producing severe reductions in heart rate or resultant bradycardia. Esmolol can be used in a continuous infusion. When so employed, it is recommended that a loading dose up to 500 µg/kg be used, then titrated to effect starting at the rate of 50 to 100 µg/kg/min.[2] At rates of administration up to 200 µg/kg/min, esmolol proves effective in controlling tachycardias; doses over 200 µg/kg/min have not been shown to offer any additional benefit. When used in infusion form, its rapid onset and rapid recovery permit adjustment of the effect of the drug without prolonged cardiac depression after termination of the infusion.

Alpha Antagonists

At present, only two agents are available for direct antagonism of alpha-mediated sympathetic effects: phentolamine and phenoxybenzamine. Both of these agents produce rapid reductions in alpha-mediated vasomotor tone and are effective in reducing systemic blood pressure; however, neither has an ultrashort duration of action, which makes them less popular for control of systemic vascular resistance than the direct-acting vasodilators. For that reason, they find less application in broad practice. Both agents directly antagonize alpha-mediated systemic vasoconstriction.

Phentolamine is a rapid-acting agent with an onset of 1 to 2 minutes when used in doses of 2.5 to 5.0 mg intravenously.[2] It has a half-life of about 19 minutes.[38] Because it proves less titratable than the direct-acting vasodilators[39] and has a longer duration of action, it finds little application in general practice, although it may still be useful in the management of acute hypertensive crises in patients with autonomic hyperreflexia following spinal cord injury and in the acute management of paroxysmal hypertension in patients with pheochromocytoma.[2]

Phenoxybenzamine is another direct alpha antagonist available only in oral form. As such, it has a slower onset of action than phentolamine and a half-life of 24 hours. It has little clinical application during anesthesia, but it may be found as a preoperative treatment for patients with pheochromocytoma.[2]

Combined Antagonists

Labetalol is the only combined alpha and beta antagonist currently available. It provides effective, readily titratable control of sympathetic tone with an approximate 1:7 ratio of alpha : beta blockade when used intravenously.[40–42] Labetalol proves effective for management of patients with transient hypertension and tachycardia, particularly during emergence from anesthesia.[43] Labetalol has a rapid onset of action, usually producing reductions in blood pressure within 5 minutes of intravenous administration. It is generally administered in doses beginning at 0.25 mg/kg and titrated in doubled doses at intervals of 5 to 10 minutes to achieve the desired endpoint.[2] When used during the course of anesthesia, it is recommended that the drug dose be halved, which corresponds to an initial dose of 10 mg in the standard (70-kg) adult. It has a clinical duration of action of 16 to 18 hours. Labetalol may be administered in a continuous infusion, starting at a recommended dose of 2 mg/min²; however, because of its prolonged duration of action, it lacks the tight controllability of direct-acting vasodilators and the rapidly metabolized beta blocker esmolol.

Clinical Applications of Sympathetic Antagonists

The use of sympathetic antagonists during anesthesia is directed primarily to management of the hyperdynamic heart. Both beta antagonists are valuable in the management of tachyarrhythmias and may be useful in the management of acute-onset ventricular dysrhythmias that are unresponsive to or poorly controlled by standard antiarrhythmic therapy. Propranolol is frequently employed in the management of patients with primary hypertension, both intraoperatively and as a chronic medication. The availability of the rapidly metabolized, short-acting beta blocker esmolol has extended the usefulness of these agents for the short-term management of hemodynamically significant tachycardias. When it proves necessary to convert to long-term suppression, it is possible to titrate esmolol dosage down while administering a longer-acting beta antagonist such as propranolol. This permits the practitioner to achieve both immediate suppression without delay and long-term suppression without interruption. This method may be particularly useful in reducing arterial shear forces that may be increased during induced hypotension with direct-acting vasodilators such as nitroprusside. Thus, the combination of direct-acting vasodilators with short-acting beta blockers may prove useful in the management of aortic aneurysms suspected of dissection. Further, the rapid titratability of esmolol makes it useful when treatment of catecholamine overdosage is required.

Because their beta-antagonistic effects may precipitate exacerbation of the underlying pulmonary dysfunction, it is recommended that beta blockers be used only with caution in patients with bronchospastic disease.[44,45] Propranolol has been demonstrated to produce exacerbations of pulmonary disease; esmolol appears to have less effect.[46,47] Similarly, beta antagonists are not recommended for treatment of patients with primary ventricular failure, as their use may exacerbate the underlying ventricular dysfunction.[48] Additionally, their use may produce marked reductions in blood sugar in the diabetic patient whose blood glucose should be carefully monitored when it is required.[49,50] Because of their synergistic effects, beta antagonists should be used cautiously in patients receiving calcium channel blockers or digoxin.[51] Profound bradycardia can ensue with the administration of beta antagonists in standard doses when given to patients receiving these agents.

Alpha antagonists find comparatively less application in anesthetic practice. They may be used in the management of patients with acute hypertension resulting from autonomic hyperreflexia following spinal cord injury or in the management of patients with uncontrolled pheochromocytoma. In the latter, it is recommended that alpha blockade be achieved before beta blockade, to prevent development of heart failure when a depressed ventricle operates against excessive afterload. The availability of a variety of shorter-duration, rapidly titratable, direct-acting vasodilators such as nitroprusside has generally made control of systemic hypertension easier to achieve and maintain than the use of alpha antagonists permits. Their application in anesthetic practice has therefore declined.

The combined alpha and beta antagonist labetalol provides rapid and effective control of hypertension and tachycardia, which is particularly effective in the management of postoperative hypertension. This is particularly valuable in the management of patients undergoing systemic vascular procedures, such as carotid endarterectomy, in whom wide swings in pressure might otherwise be expected and in whom severe hypertension is to be avoided. Labetalol may also prove very effective as an adjunct in long-term control of postoperative hypertension in the general surgical population for periods of up to 16 hours postoperatively.[52]

DIRECT-ACTING VASODILATORS

At present, only three direct-acting vasodilators have broad clinical applications in the practice of anesthesia: nitroprusside, trimethaphan, and nitroglycerin. Both nitroprusside and nitroglycerin produce direct relaxation of the smooth muscle in the vessels, although nitroprusside is more effective in low doses on the arterial tree and nitroglycerin is more effective in low doses on the venous capacitance vessels. Trimethaphan has the additional effect of ganglionic blockade, which prevents increases in heart rate. The vasodilators are used primarily in the control of preload and afterload in anesthetic management, although nitroglycerin is also used in the management of cardiac ischemia.

Nitroprusside

Nitroprusside is an extremely rapid-acting, short-lasting direct vasodilator. It has an onset of 1 to 2 minutes when administered in continuous infusion, and the clinical effects last less than 5 minutes. It produces direct relaxation of the smooth muscle in the vessel wall and does not invoke alpha antagonism for its action.[53–55] It operates primarily on the medium and small arteries and arterioles in low doses (< 1.5 μg/kg/min), and it demonstrates progressively greater arterial dilation and dilation of the venous capacitance vessels when used in higher doses (up to 5 μg/kg/min).[2] It is not recommended that nitroprusside be used as a sole agent at doses in excess of 5 to 10 μg/kg/min or for prolonged maintenance because of the risk of cyanide toxicity.[2,55]

Trimethaphan

Trimethaphan provides both direct-acting vasodilation and an accompanying autonomic ganglionic blockade.[1,2,56–58] It does cause the release of histamine, although this does not appear to have significant impact on the production of hypotension.[1,59] It is generally delivered as a continuous infusion with a starting dose of 1 to 2 mg/min and titrated to control blood pressure in the desired range. It has a somewhat slower onset than nitroprusside, reaching clinical effect usually within 5 to 7 minutes, and the ganglionic blockade demonstrates an extended duration of action; however, systemic arterial pressure generally returns to the low normal range within about 10 minutes of discontinuation of the infusion because of metabolism by plasma pseudocholinesterases.[60]

Nitroglycerin

Nitroglycerin is a rapid-acting, short-lasting direct vasodilator that affects primarily the venous capacitance vessels in low doses.[2,61,62] It has a slightly slower onset than does nitroprusside (2 to 3 minutes) and a longer duration of action (5 to 10 minutes). At low doses (< 1.5 µg/kg/min) it is an effective venodilator, reducing preload and pulmonary artery pressures.[62] When used in higher doses (up to 5 µg/kg/min), it produces a progressive decrease in systemic resistance as well.[63] When used in the recommended range, nitroglycerin has not been shown to have any toxicity.[61] Nitroglycerin has also been shown to dilute the medium-sized coronary arteries, making it a mainstay in the treatment of myocardial ischemia.

Clinical Applications of Direct-Acting Vasodilators

All the direct-acting dilators are useful in the management of patients with systemic hypertension or in the induction of deliberate hypotension, although nitroprusside is sometimes preferred for its more specific arterial action. Nitroglycerin may be used effectively in high doses for the control of mild to moderate hypertension, and it proves to be effective in managing mild to moderate degrees of pulmonary hypertension as well. Trimethaphan proves useful in the management of hypertension and is sometimes preferred because its ganglionic blockade prevents the development of the tachycardia that frequently accompanies rapid reductions in systemic arterial pressure. In the management of hypertension, nitroprusside is usually begun at doses of 0.5 to 2 µg/kg/min and titrated to effect. Control of hypertension secondary to increased systemic vascular resistance is usually possible with doses less than 5 µg/kg/min. When doses greater than 5 to 10 µg/kg/min are required for management of primary hypertension in the patient not undergoing aortic cross-clamping, the risk of toxicity from cyanide is increased. When used for control of hypertension in patients undergoing surgical cross-clamping of the aorta, doses in excess of 10 µg/kg/min may be required briefly during the interval of cross-clamping. When used in that clinical setting, higher doses are not demonstrated to have any serious risk of toxicity. Nitroglycerin is generally used as a primary venodilator or to control pulmonary hypertension. In that capacity, it is useful in the management of excessive preload in patients with congestive heart failure or in the treatment of patients with volume overload in conjunction with diuresis. Nitroglycerin may also be used singly or in combination with nitroprusside in the management of patients undergoing aortic cross-clamping. When placement of the cross-clamp is low (e.g., infrarenal aneurysms or patients with Leriche occlusion of the distal aorta), nitroglycerin alone may prove effective in controlling hypertension. In the management of patients undergoing procedures involving cross-clamping of the

thoracic aorta, nitroglycerin does not prove as effective in controlling hypertension during cross-clamping as nitroprusside. It may, however, be used as an adjunct vasodilator to reduce preload and to unload the ventricle faced with excessive afterload.

Although trimethaphan has proven to be an effective arterial dilator, its ganglionic blockade lasts longer than the peripheral dilatory effect. That extended recovery time limits its use in patients susceptible to the hypotensive effects of ganglionic blockade. Because of the ganglionic blockade, it does prove effective in the management of hypertension and reduction of shear forces in patients with aortic dissection, and it may be employed in that setting as an alternative to combined therapy with vasodilators and beta blockade. As it produces histamine release, it may produce an exacerbation of symptoms in patients with bronchospastic disease, and it should be used with caution in that population.

ANTIHYPERTENSIVE AGENTS

The antihypertensive agents are a mixed group of agents with variable sites of action that are generally administered in bolus form for maintenance of blood pressure exclusively. In contrast to beta antagonists, the actions of the antihypertensive agents may center on centrally mediated control of hypertension, on peripheral vasomotor tone, or both. In contrast to the direct-acting vasodilators used in continuous infusion form, these agents have an extended duration of action, lasting several hours after a single bolus administration. A comprehensive listing of a variety of agents is provided in Table 29–2. Three drugs in this class find application during anesthetic management: hydralazine, methyldopa, and diazoxide.

Hydralazine

Hydralazine appears to produce an antihypertensive effect by direct peripheral vasodilation, possibly through the release of endothelial factors[64,65] which reduce systemic vascular resistance without producing myocardial depression.[2] In the patient with ventricular dysfunction, this may augment stroke volume and produce an increase in cardiac output. Hydralazine is generally administered in divided doses of 10 to 20 mg up to a total dose of 0.5 mg/kg.[2] The reduction in blood pressure is generally noted within 10 minutes of administration, although peak reductions may not be noted for as long as 1 hour after administration. Tachycardia is a frequent accompaniment of the reduction in blood pressure after administration of hydralazine, and it may represent baroreceptor reflex or the release of endogenous catecholamines.[2,66] Hydralazine appears to have a clinical half-life of 3 to 7 hours, though it may last up to 12 hours. No mechanism is known for the discrepancy in duration of action.[60]

Methyldopa

Methyldopa appears to operate on the central axis by competing for metabolism with natural transmitter to yield α-methylnorepinephrine or α-methylepinephrine,[67–69] which

TABLE 29–2. ANTIHYPERTENSIVE AGENTS EMPLOYED DURING ANESTHESIA

Drug	Dose[a]	Latency	Duration	Side Effects
Diuretics				
Furosemide	20–40 mg IV	5–10 min	4 h	Hypokalemia, hypovolemia
Sympatholytics				
α-Methyldopa	250–500 mg SIV	20 min	24 h	Sedation, hepatitis, hemolytic anemia
Clonidine	0.2 mg in 10 mL NS per rectum	20 min	12–24 h	Sedation, dry mouth, withdrawal syndrome
Vasodilators				
Hydralazine	5–10 mg IV	15–20 min	4–6 h	Lupuslike syndrome, drug fever, rash
	10–40 mg IM	20–40 min		
Nifedipine	10 mg SIV	5–10 min	7 h	Headache, fluid retention
Verapamil	5 mg IV	2–5 min	4–6 h	Heart block, myocardial failure
Diazoxide	300 mg SIV	3–5 min	5–12 h	Decreased cerebral blood flow, hyperuricemia
Sodium nitroprusside	0.25–0.5 µg/kg/min	1–2 min	2–5 min	Cyanide toxicity, increased cerebral blood flow
Nitroglycerin		2–5 min	3–5 min	Headache, fluid retention

Doses shown are for a 70-kg adult. IV, intravenous push; SIV, slow intravenous infusion; IM, intramuscular; SL, sublingual; NS, normal saline.
Reprinted, with permission, from Barash PG, Cullen BF, Stoelting RK, eds. Clinical anesthesia. *Philadelphia: JB Lippincott; 1989.*

operates as a weak false neurotransmitter producing central inhibitory alpha tone. Methyldopa may also produce a reduction in plasma renin activity. Because of its central action, the effects of methyldopa are slow in onset and may require up to 6 to 8 hours.[70] It has a clinical duration of action of 10 to 16 hours after a single administration. The usual dose of methyldopa is 250 to 500 mg administered slowly. Because it has slow onset, it is usually used only as maintenance in those patients receiving chronic therapy.

Diazoxide

Diazoxide operates directly on the smooth muscle in the systemic arterial tree, producing a prompt reduction in systemic vascular resistance and arterial blood pressure.[2,71] The reduction in resistance may result in an increase in cardiac output, particularly in the patient with underlying left ventricular failure. Diazoxide is avidly and tightly protein bound, which makes it necessary to administer the drug intravenously as a rapid bolus to prevent complete binding of the administered dose.[2] Because of its protein binding, it is useful only for short-term control of hypertension. Diazoxide may be administered as a single rapid bolus of 150 to 300 mg or as a series of smaller divided boluses of 1 to 3 mg/kg at intervals greater than 5 minutes.[72,73] It has a rapid clinical effect, producing reductions in blood pressure within 5 to 10 minutes and peak effects within less than 30 minutes. The clinical duration of action is generally less than 12 hours.[2]

Clinical Applications of Antihypertensive Agents

The antihypertensive agents are generally used in management of patients who are on chronic antihypertensive therapy or in the control of comparatively mild degrees of hypertension. Their relatively slow onset compared with the direct-acting continuous-infusion vasodilators makes them less titratable, and their extended duration of action makes them less controllable.

Hydralazine finds application in the treatment of patients with acute hypertension that is not related to light anesthesia. It is an effective vasodilator for the patient expected to require treatment for hypertension for several hours following anesthesia when preoperative medications cannot be reinitiated during that interval. Likewise, it proves effective in reducing blood pressure in patients requiring sustained control of systemic arterial pressure for a prolonged interval in whom wide swings in arterial blood pressures are not expected to accompany the surgical procedure or anesthetic management. It is synergistic when administered with the titratable, continuous-infusion agents, the rate of administration of which should be reduced to half the baseline when hydralazine is added to prevent severe hypotension from the summated effects. Because the development of clinically significant tachycardias may accompany hydralazine-induced reductions in blood pressure, it is frequent practice to administer beta blockers concomitantly to reduce myocardial oxygen demand. This may prove critical in the patient with symptomatic myocardial ischemia.

Diazoxide has a pattern of use similar to that of hydralazine. It finds application only for short-term maintenance during the perioperative period, and it is not recommended for use for more than 10 days. It is generally employed only for the acute perioperative period. Patients receiving diazoxide may demonstrate increases in blood glucose levels, and diabetic patients should be monitored closely when it is administered.

In contrast to the other antihypertensive agents, methyldopa demonstrates a comparatively long onset and finds little application in the short-term management of intraoperative hypertension. Its primary use in anesthesia is as a maintenance drug for those patients receiving methyldopa as a chronic medication in the treatment of hypertension. The use of methyldopa may produce a positive Coombs test in patients,[60] leading to difficulty in establishing an accurate crossmatch for compatible homologous blood. In general, when only the direct Coombs test is positive, a crossmatch can be completed. When both direct and indirect Coombs tests are positive, crossmatching for compatible blood may be complex.

The advent of the rapid-onset, continuous-infusion agents has reduced the use of antihypertensive agents in the practice of anesthesia because of the greater controllability of the former agents. The use of classic antihypertensive agents, however, should not be ignored. They may be employed to establish and maintain prolonged reductions in blood pressure when desired. These agents are effective in producing a mild sustained reduction in systemic vascular resistance that can then be augmented by the use of reduced doses of the titratable agents when brief periods of profound hypotension are required, or to reduce the requirement for direct-acting, titratable vasodilators when sustained reductions in systemic vascular resistance and systemic pressure are required in the perioperative period.

CALCIUM CHANNEL BLOCKERS

Only two calcium channel blockers are currently in common anesthetic use: verapamil and nifedipine. These represent two different actions in the group of drugs and have different applications. Calcium channel blockers have been grouped into two forms based on their blocking of the slow or fast calcium channels[74,75]; however, it is likely that both forms block the slow calcium channel with the differentiating feature being the rate of recovery.[76-78] Calcium channel blockers may be used in the control of tachycardias as in the treatment of supraventricular tachycardias, or in the control of vasomotor tone, as in the control of pulmonary artery hypertension or coronary spasm.

Verapamil

Verapamil was originally described as a slow channel blocker that slows the rate of recovery.[79,80] It provides effective treatment of supraventricular tachycardia.[81] It effectively blocks the reuptake of calcium and prolongs the rate of spontaneous depolarization in pacemaker cells. It also appears to possess some alpha-blocking activity, which produces reductions in peripheral vasomotor tone, operating at the level of the resistance vessels.[82,83] Verapamil demonstrates only mild myocardial depressant effect in the normal heart; however, when administered to the patient with ventricular dysfunction, the depressant effect may become clinically significant.[84] When administered in doses of 2.5 to 5 mg intravenously, it generally provides control of tachycardias, which is hemodynamically significant within 3 to 5 minutes.[85] Total doses of up to 10 mg may be required in young patients; elderly patients usually respond satisfactorily to a total dose of 5 mg. Verapamil has an initial redistribution half-life of about 4 hours and an elimination half-life of 2 to 5 hours, which may be extended in patients receiving chronic therapy.[61,86,87]

Nifedipine

Nifedipine is a calcium channel blocker that demonstrates little effect on the rate of recovery of the slow calcium channels. It has little benefit in the control of tachycardias.

Nifedipine produces effective systemic and pulmonary artery dilation when administered in sublingual form.[88] It also produces effective coronary artery dilation in the patient suffering coronary artery spasm or Prinzmetal's variant angina[89,90] and is the treatment of choice for that condition. In addition, nifedipine appears to be effective in dilating internal mammary artery grafts that develop vasospasm, and it may be used for this purpose during myocardial revascularization. The usual dose of nifedipine is 0.1 to 0.25 mg/kg, which may be given sublingually, corresponding to 10 to 20 mg in the typical (70-kg) adult.[75,89] It has an onset of less than 5 minutes and a half-life of 1 to 2 hours.[2] At present, nifedipine is available only in the sublingual or oral form; however, current work is under way to prepare an intravenous form that will facilitate its use in clinical anesthesia.

Clinical Applications of Calcium Channel Blockers

Verapamil may be used during the course of anesthesia as an adjunct in the management of paroxysmal tachycardias. It proves effective when used as a sole agent for the control of tachycardias, although with rapid administration marked decreases in systemic blood pressure may be seen because of its alpha-blocking effects and myocardial depression in response to calcium channel blockade. When declines in blood pressure are precipitous, as in the patient with impaired ventricular function, administration of calcium chloride titrated in increments of 100 to 250 mg may block myocardial depression and peripheral dilation without antagonizing the antiarrhythmic effects of the drug. Verapamil demonstrates no significant effect on coronary vasospasm, but it is not shown to be effective in controlling primary coronary spasm. It should be used with caution in conjunction with either beta-blocking agents or digoxin as the effects of these agents may be additive or synergistic and severe bradycardias may occur, although it has also been used effectively in the treatment of digoxin-induced ventricular arrhythmias.[91]

Nifedipine finds application preoperatively in the management of coronary vasospasm. It also finds use in the patient with coronary artery spasm during surgery or in the treatment of spasm of the internal mammary artery used as a coronary graft. As with verapamil, it should be used with caution in patients with primary ventricular dysfunction as it may demonstrate myocardial depressant effects that can be antagonized with calcium in incremental boluses. It should also be used with caution in patients receiving beta blockers as it may prove additive or synergistic. Because of its more potent pulmonary dilation, nifedipine may prove effective in the management of patients with acute pulmonary hypertension in response to stresses, such as aortic crossclamping or acute left ventricular dysfunction.

ANTIARRHYTHMIC AGENTS

The antiarrhythmic agents represent a broad class of drugs with a variety of actions. Their primary use is to control ventricular or supraventricular arrhythmias during the course of anesthesia. There is considerable overlap among antiarrhythmic agents, and a number of previously discussed agents are employed as antiarrhythmics. Sympathetic antagonists, particularly the beta blockers, are used to control supraventricular tachycardias, and may find application in the control of ventricular dysrhythmias that fail to respond to the usual antiarrhythmic therapy, as previously outlined. Calcium channel blockers, particularly verapamil, may be used in the treatment of supraventricular tachycardias, as previously discussed. A comprehensive listing of antiarrhythmics is provided in Table 29–3. Six agents typically find application in anesthesia: the local anesthetics lidocaine and procainamide, bretylium, phenytoin, quinidine, and digoxin.

Local Anesthetics

The local anesthetics are used primarily to treat or control ventricular dysrhythmias. Two agents are typically employed during anesthetic management: lidocaine and procainamide. Both appear to operate at the site of the Na–K channel, producing a slowing in the rate of spontaneous depolarization and extending the refractory period in the conductive tissue. Hence, their action as antiarrhythmic agents parallels their action as anesthetic agents.

Lidocaine appears to specifically extend the phase 4 period of depolarization in the myocardial conductive tissue, thereby decreasing the rate of automaticity without producing significant changes in membrane function when used in the recommended therapeutic range.[92] When administered in the usual dose of 1 mg/kg, it generally produces a quelling of ventricular excitability within 1 to 2 minutes. Lidocaine has a short clinical duration, with a bolus dose demonstrating activity for no more than 10 to 15 minutes. Therefore, it is generally continued as a prolonged infusion at a rate of 1 to 4 mg/min for long-term control of ventricular dysrhythmias. The appearance of continued ventricular ectopy may be treated with smaller boluses of 0.5 mg/kg and an increase in the rate of administration of the continuous infusion.

Procainamide has a mechanism of action similar to that of lidocaine, but it also appears to produce electrophysiologic changes in the atria and AV node.[92] It appears to be a more potent suppressant of ventricular ectopy but is also a more potent myocardial depressant and produces peripheral vasodilation through ganglionic blockade.[92] For these reasons, procainamide is seldom used unless therapy with lidocaine alone has proven insufficient. Procainamide generally demonstrates a clinical effect within 2 minutes and lasts 10 to 15 minutes after a single bolus. When administered as a bolus, it should be given slowly because of its myocardial depressant effect. It is recommended that no more than 50 to 100 mg be given in any bolus; a total of no more than 500 mg is recommended in divided boluses to control ventricular ectopy, although persistent ectopy may require a total loading dose of up to 1 g.[93] When administered as a continuous infusion, procainamide should be maintained at the rate of 1 to 2 mg/min.

Bretylium

Bretylium appears to operate by accumulating in the sympathetic intrinsic nerve terminal and blocking the release of

norepinephrine.[92] It does not therefore alter the depolarization of normal conductive tissue, but it does appear to restore the normal depolarization pattern in cells injured by ischemia or other events.[94] It may additionally increase the duration of the action potential in conductive tissue. The administration of bretylium is associated with an early phase of increased catecholamine release, which may produce a brief interval of aggravated ectopy, increased inotropy, and increased systemic vascular resistance.[92,95] This is followed by a second phase of suppression of sympathetic activity that produces the antiarrhythmic effects.[92] Therefore, bretylium is generally used only as an antiarrhythmic when other therapies such as the local anesthetics have failed to adequately control ventricular ectopy. The standard dose of bretylium is a 5 mg/kg bolus administered over several minutes. When ventricular ectopy persists, an additional bolus may be required, for a total of 10 mg/kg.[92] The clinical effects are slow to appear, and peak effects in suppression of ventricular ectopy are not noted for up to 6 hours after administration,[95] so that bretylium may be administered as intermittent slow boluses or it may be maintained as a continuous infusion of 1 to 2 mg/min.

Quinidine

Quinidine is generally administered orally for the treatment of arrhythmias resulting from states of enhanced atrial or ventricular automaticity, while providing enhancement of the rate of transmission of impulses across the AV node.[92] It appears to reduce atrial and ventricular automaticity by extending phase 4 of depolarization and to extend the duration of the refractory period by slowing the rate of depolarization and repolarization and reducing the amplitude of the action potential generated.[96] The action on the AV node appears to be mediated by a direct anticholinergic effect that blocks vagal tone,[97] which may also account for its mild myocardial depressant effect. Because it is usually administered orally, quinidine finds little direct application in anesthesia and is most frequently used in chronic maintenance therapy. It has been demonstrated to induce ventricular dysrhythmias and produce Torsade de pointes in the presence of decreased serum potassium concentrations.[98]

Phenytoin

Phenytoin is most commonly used as an anticonvulsant. Its ability to promote the efflux of sodium from the cell, resulting in a stabilization of the membrane potential,[99] makes it useful in the management of atrial dysrhythmias also. Because it continues to depress ventricular automaticity, it may not be recommended in patients with second- or third-degree heart block.[92] The standard dose of phenytoin is a 50-mg bolus administered through a fast-flowing intravenous line, as it will precipitate if not given proximally. It has a clinical effect within 5 minutes, and the duration of action appears to be up to 12 hours. Phenytoin may increase conduction across the AV node, enhancing the transmission of rapid atrial rates transiently.[92]

TABLE 29–3. PHARMACOLOGY OF ANTIARRHYTHMIC AGENTS

Class	Drug	Commonly Used Dosage	Elimination Half-Life	Therapeutic Plasma Level (μg mL^{-1})	Side Effects
IA	Quinidine	Oral: 200–600 mg q 6–8 h IV: 6–10 mg kg^{-1} over 30 min followed by 2–3 mg min^{-1}	6 h	2–6	Quinidine syncope, conduction disturbances, nausea, vomiting, diarrhea, thrombocytopenia, hypotension
	Procainamide	Oral: 250–1000 mg q 4 h (q 6 for sustained-release form) IV: 10–20 mg kg^{-1} over 20–40 min followed by 2–6 mg min^{-1}	2–4 h	4–12 (8–15, N-acetyl procainamide)	Conduction disturbances, nausea, diarrhea, fever, lupus syndrome, hypotension
	Disopyramide	Oral: 150–300 mg q 6–8 h IV: 2 mg kg^{-1} over 3–5 min	6–8 h	5–7	Cardiac depression, conduction disturbances, anticholinergic symptoms
IB	Lidocaine	IV: 1–2 mg kg^{-1} bolus followed by 20–40 μg kg^{-1} min^{-1}	1–2 h	2–5	Drowsiness, hallucination, seizures, paranoid ideation
	Tocainide	Oral: 400–600 mg q 8 h	13–15 h	4–10	Tremor, dizziness, ataxia, paresthesia, rash, hepatitis, nausea, vomiting
	Mexiletine	Oral: 150–300 mg q 6–8 h	10–20 h	0.75–2.0	Tremor, convulsion, dizziness, photosensitivity, dermatitis, hypotension, nausea, vomiting
	Phenytoin	Oral: 200–400 mg once daily IV: 50–100 mg every 5 min to maximum 1 g	24 h	10–18	Hypotension, vertigo, lethargy, dysarthria, gingivitis, macrocytic anemia, lupus, pulmonary infiltrates
	Moricizine (ethmozine)	Oral: 75–200 mg q 8 h	4–10 h		Dizziness, headache, pruritus
IC	Encainide	Oral: 25–75 mg q 6–8 h IV: 0.5–1 mg kg^{-1} over 15 min	3–4 h	0.01–0.02	Conduction disturbances, blurred vision, nystagmus, dizziness, ataxia, vertigo, paresthesia, nausea, proarrhythmic
	Flecainide	Oral: 100–200 mg q 12 h IV: 2 mg kg^{-1} over 10 min	18–20 h	0.2–1.0	Blurred vision, headache, lightheadedness, ataxia, proarrhythmic
	Lorcainide	Oral: 100–200 mg q 12 h IV: 1–2 mg kg^{-1} over 30 min	7–13 h (norlorcainide, 24 h)	0.05–0.3 0.08–0.3	Sleep disturbances, nightmares, tremor, hyponatremia, nausea, diarrhea
Unclassified					
	Propafenone	Oral: 100–300 mg q 8 h IV: 2 mg kg^{-1} over 15 min	4–8 h	0.5–2.0	Dizziness, metallic taste, conduction disturbances, nausea
II	Propranolol (β_1/β_2)[a]	Oral: 20–80 mg q 6 h IV: 0.5–1 mg q 2 min to maximum 6–10 mg	3–6 h	0.05–0.1	Depression, fatigue, atrioventricular block, bradycardia, myocardial depression
	Acebutolol (β_1/β_2)	Oral: 600–1200 mg once daily	24 h		As above
	Atenolol (β_1)	Oral: 50–200 mg once daily	24 h		As above
	Nadolol (β_1/β_2)	Oral: 40–240 mg	24 h		As above
	Timolol (β_1/β_2)	Oral: 20–60 mg	15 h		As above
III	Amiodarone	Oral: 800–1600 mg d^{-1} for 2 wk, then 200–600 mg d^{-1} maintenance IV: 5–10 mg kg^{-1} bolus over 5–15 min, then 800–1600 mg d^{-1} as a continuous infusion or in divided doses	13–60 d		Corneal deposit, gastrointestinal disturbances, altered thyroid function, interstitial pulmonary disease, peripheral neuropathy, bradycardia, conduction block, hepatic dysfunction

TABLE 29–3. PHARMACOLOGY OF ANTIARRHYTHMIC AGENTS (continued)

Class	Drug	Commonly Used Dosage	Elimination Half-Life	Therapeutic Plasma Level (μg mL^{-1})	Side Effects
Unclassified					
	Bretylium	IV: 5–10 mg kg^{-1} bolus over 10–30 min, then 1–4 mg min^{-1}	6–8 h	0.8–2.0	Transient hypertension, sinus tachycardia, postural hypotension, proarrhythmic
IV	Verapamil	Oral: 80–160 mg q 6–8 h IV: 5–10 mg bolus, repeated after 10 min to a maximum of 20 mg Continuous infusion: 1–5 μg kg^{-1} min^{-1}	4–8 h	0.1	Cardiac depression, hypotension, atrioventricular block, asystole, edema, headache, constipation
	Diltiazem	Oral: 60–90 mg q 6 h	3–5 h		Edema, postural hypotension
Other Agents					
	Digoxin	Oral: 1–1.5 mg in divided doses over 24 h for digitalization, 0.125–0.25 mg once daily for maintenance IV: 0.75–1 mg in divided doses over 24 h for digitalization	1.5 d	1–2	Anorexia, nausea, vomiting, diarrhea, malaise, fatigue, confusion, headache, colored vision, arrhythmias, aggravation of heart failure

[a] β_1/β_2, noncardioselective beta blockers; β_1, cardioselective beta blockers.
Reprinted, with permission, from Barash PG, Cullen BF, Stoelting RK, eds. Clinical anesthesia. *Philadelphia: JB Lippincott; 1989. Platia EV.* Management of cardiac arrhythmias. *Philadelphia: JB Lippincott.*

Digoxin

Digoxin is the only cardiac glycoside currently used in intravenous form for the control of atrial dysrhythmias. Digoxin produces alterations in both sympathetic outflow and vagal tone.[100–103] The latter produces a slowing of SA automaticity and conduction of impulses at the AV node, and it is the basis for the use of digoxin in controlling the ventricular response rate in patients with atrial fibrillation. Digoxin may also be used as an inotropic agent in the patient with congestive failure, in whom it increases sympathetic tone and reduces systemic vascular resistance.[101] The effects of digoxin administration on the ventricular response rate may be seen within 5 to 30 minutes of administration of a 0.25-mg bolus intravenously. Repeated doses may be necessary to establish a therapeutic response in the patient who has not been previously digitalized. Peak effects may not be seen for up to 4 to 6 hours.[104] In the patient receiving digoxin preoperatively, supplemental doses of 0.125 to 0.25 mg may be sufficient. It has a clinical half-life of up to 2 days, which is variable depending on the patient's condition.[104] Because of the sympathetic axis stimulation, digoxin may also predispose the patient to ventricular ectopy.

Clinical Applications of Antiarrhythmic Agents

The use of antiarrhythmic agents is necessarily determined by the appearance of atrial or ventricular ectopy. The management of ventricular ectopy or fibrillation is generally predicated on the use of the local anesthetics. Of those, lidocaine is generally preferred because it appears to produce less myocardial depression than procainamide and has fewer drug reactions. The management of refractory ventricular ectopy or fibrillation may incorporate the use of beta antagonists, such as propranolol, to suppress sympathetic tone and augment the effects of the local anesthetics.

Alternately, the use of bretylium permits the practitioner to quell ventricular ectopy without suppressing the normal mechanism for depolarization in the conductive tissue in the myocardium. Bretylium, however, does have an associated interval of sympathetic discharge, during which the patient may demonstrate hyperdynamism and increased irritability. It is not generally used unless previous efforts at therapy have failed and ventricular fibrillation persists despite the use of local anesthetics and countershock.

The use of quinidine permits control of atrial and ventricular dysrhythmias effectively, although its myocardial depressant effects may reduce ventricular function in the impaired ventricle. It should be used with caution in patients with atrial flutter, as it does enhance transmission across the AV node and may predispose to rapid ventricular response rates in that situation. It should also be used cautiously in the presence of incomplete AV block. Administration of quinidine has been shown to increase the serum digoxin level in patients receiving both agents, and it should be used with caution in that patient population.

The use of phenytoin permits the practitioner to control atrial arrhythmias, although the availability of the calcium channel blockers and the beta antagonists has decreased its utilization. For the management of atrial tachycardias, verapamil and beta antagonists offer more rapid control of rate and are preferred. Phenytoin does block the effects of digoxin at the level of the AV node, making it an effective treatment for digoxin-induced bradycardia or dysrhythmias.[105,106] Phenytoin does cause an increase in blood glucose levels; therefore, diabetic patients should be monitored closely when it is employed.

The use of digoxin for both treatment of congestive heart failure and control of ventricular response rates in the patient with atrial fibrillation or flutter is long established. In the patient with new-onset atrial fibrillation, digoxin may quell atrial irritability and reestablish a sinus mechanism. For this reason, some practitioners use digoxin prophylactically in patients undergoing pneumonectomy in whom there is a high incidence of new-onset atrial fibrillation in response to the increased pulmonary artery pressures. In the patient with long-standing atrial fibrillation, digoxin produces a reduction in AV node transmission of the electrical impulse that tracks with the plasma level, permitting the practitioner to control ventricular response rate effectively. Caution should be used in the treatment of atrial flutter with digoxin as there is a narrow threshold at which the corresponding AV block must be maintained. Conversion of a 3 : 1 or 4 : 1 block permits the maintenance of a ventricular rate of 100 to 75 beats per minute, whereas increases in the dose of digoxin may easily convert the 4 : 1 to a greater ratio resulting in significant bradycardia. For that reason, the availability of continuous monitoring is paramount, and treatment of bradycardia with either pacing or the use of phenytoin may be indicated. Digoxin may predipose to ventricular dysrhythmias, particularly in the presence of associated electrolyte disturbances. As these ventricular dysrhythmias are generally difficult to convert, it is important to follow the electrolyte profile in patients receiving digoxin, paying particular attention to the serum potassium level.

SUMMARY

Increases in the availability of intravenous agents suitable to application in anesthetic practice have improved the sophistication and precision with which practitioners can manage the cardiovascular and hemodynamic profile of their patients; however, the effective use of these agents requires an appreciation of their basic pharmacologic and physiologic effects. By applying principles of cardiovascular physiology and integrating the pharmacologic effects of the variety of agents available, complex cases can be more effectively and safely managed than previously possible. The benefits in terms of availability of care and safety mandate critical review and application of the agents currently available.

REFERENCES

1. Merin RG. Autonomic nervous system pharmacology. In: Miller RD, ed. *Anesthesia.* 3rd ed. New York: Churchill Livingstone; 1990.
2. Durrett LR, Lawson NW. Autonomic nervous system physiology and pharmacology. In: Barash PG, Cullen BF, Stoelting RK, eds. *Clinical anesthesia.* Philadelphia: JB Lippincott; 1989.
3. Guyton AC. The autonomic nervous system: The adrenal medulla. In: Guyton AC, ed. *Textbook of medical physiology.* Philadelphia: WB Saunders; 1986.
4. Lake CR, Chernow B, Feuerstein G, et al. The sympathetic nervous system in man: Its evaluation and the measurement of plasma NE. In: Ziegler MG, Lake CR, eds. *Norepinephrine.* Baltimore: Williams & Wilkins; 1984.
5. Bexton RS, Milne JR, Cory-Pearce R, et al. Effect of beta blockade on exercise response after cardiac transplantation. *Br Heart J.* 1983;49:584.
6. Thomas J, Fouad FM, Tarazi RC, et al. Evaluation of plasma catecholamines in humans: Correlation of resting levels with cardiac responses to beta-blocking and sympatholytic drugs. *Hypertension.* 1983;5:858.
7. Zaimis E. Vasopressor drugs and catecholamines. *Anesthesiology.* 1968;29:732.
8. Smith NT, Corbascia AN. The use and misuse of pressor agents. *Anesthesiology.* 1970;8:58.
9. Waller JL. Inotropes and vasopressors. In: Kaplan JA, ed. *Cardiac anesthesia.* vol. 2: *Cardiovascular pharmacology.* New York: Grune & Stratton; 1983.
10. Makabali C, Weil MH, Henning RJ. Dobutamine and other sympathomimetic drugs for the treatment of low cardiac output failure. *Semin Anesth.* 1982;1:63.
11. Weiner N. Norepinephrine, epinephrine and the sympathomimetic amines. In: Gilman AG, Goodman LS, Rall TW, Murad F, eds. *Goodman and Gilman's the pharmacologic basis of therapeutics.* 7th ed. New York: Macmillan; 1985.
12. Zaritsky AL, Chernow B. Catecholamines, sympathomimetics. In: Ziegler MG, Lake CR, eds. *Frontiers of clinical neuroscience.* vol. 2: *Norepinephrine.* Baltimore: Williams & Wilkins; 1984.
13. Chernow B, Rainey TG, Lake CR. Catecholamines in critical care medicine. In: Ziegler MG, Lake CR, eds. *Frontiers of clinical neuroscience.* vol. 2: *Norepinephrine.* Baltimore: Williams & Wilkins; 1984.
14. Axelrod J, Weinshilboum R. Catecholamines. *N Engl J Med.* 1972;287:237.
15. Goldberg LI, Hsieh Y-Y, Resnekov L. Newer catecholamines for treatment of heart failure and shock: An update on dopamine and a first look at dobutamine. *Prog Cardiovasc Dis.* 1977; 19:327.
16. Rajfer SI, Goldberg LI. Sympathetic amines in the treatment of shock. In: Shoemaker WC, Thompson WL, Holbrook RP, eds. *Textbook of critical care.* Philadelphia: WB Saunders; 1984.
17. Hilberman M, Maseda J, Stinson EB, et al. The diuretic properties of dopamine in patients following open heart operations. *Anesthesiology.* 1984;61:489.
18. Goldberg LI. The dopamine vascular receptor: New areas for biochemical pharmacologists. *Biochem Pharmacol.* 1975;24:651.
19. Rutman HI, LeJemtel TH, Sonnenblick EH. Newer cardiotonic agents: Implications for patients with heart failure and ischemic heart disease. *J Cardiothorac Anesth.* 1987;1:59.
20. Hug CC, Kaplan JA. Pharmacology—Cardiac drugs. In: Kaplan JA, ed. *Cardiac anesthesia.* New York: Grune & Stratton; 1979.
21. Kopin IJ. Catecholamine metabolism and the biochemical assessment of sympathetic activity. *Clin Endocrinol Metab.* 1977;6:525.
22. Leier CV, Unverferth DV. Dobutamine. *Ann Intern Med.* 1983;99:490.
23. Pank JR, Tinker JH. Cardioactive drugs and their monitorable effects. *Semin Anesth.* 1983;11:268.
24. Furman WR, Summer WR, Kennedy TP, et al. Comparison of the effects of dobutamine, dopamine and isoproterenol on hypoxic pulmonary vasoconstriction in the pig. *Crit Care Med.* 1982;10:371.
25. Schmid PG, Eckstein JW, Abboud FM. Comparison of the effects of several sympathomimetic amines on resistance and ca-

pacitance vessels in the forearm of man. *Circulation*. 1966;34:209.

26. Rude RE. Pharmacologic support in cardiogenic shock. *Adv Shock Res*. 1983;10:35.

27. Benfey BG. Cardiac adrenoreceptors at low temperature and the adrenoreceptor interconversion hypothesis. *Br J Pharmacol*. 1977;61:167.

28. Shibata S, Seriguchi DG, Iwadare S, et al. The regional and species differences on the activation of myocardial alpha-adrenoreceptors by phenylephrine and methoxamine. *Gen Pharmacol*. 1980;11:173.

29. Garcia-Sainz JAG, Molina RV, Corvera S, Bahena JH, Tsujimoto G, Hoffman BB. Differential effects of adrenergic agonists and phorbol esters on the alpha-adrenoreceptors of hepatocytes and aorta. *Eur J Pharmacol*. 1985;112:393–397.

30. Nathanson MH, Miller H. Clinical observations on a new epinephrine-like compound, methoxamine. *Am J Med Sci*. 1952;223:270–279.

31. Goldberg LI, Bloodwell RD, Braunwald E, et al. The direct effects of norepinephrine, epinephrine and methoxamine on myocardial contractile force in man. *Circulation*. 1960;22:1125–1132.

32. King BD, Dripps RD. The use of methoxamine for maintenance of the circulation during spinal anesthesia. *Surg Gynecol Obstet*. 1950;90:659–665.

33. Aviado DM, Wnuck AL. Mechanisms for cardiac slowing by methoxamine. *J Pharmacol Exp Ther*. 1957;119:99–106.

34. Lahti RE, Brill IC, McCawley EL. The effect of methoxamine hydrochloride (Vasoxyl) on cardiac rhythm. *J Pharmacol Exp Ther*. 1955;115:268–274.

35. Hoffman BB, Lefkowitz RJ. Adrenergic receptor antagonists. In: Gilman AG, Rall TW, Nies AS, Taylor P, eds. *Goodman and Gilman's the pharmacologic basis of therapeutics*. 8th ed. New York: Pergamon Press; 1990.

36. Gorcynski R. Basic pharmacology of esmolol. *Am J Cardiol*. 1985;56:3F.

37. Gray RJ, Bateman TM, Czer LSC, et al. Esmolol: A new ultrashort-acting beta-adrenergic blocking agent for rapid control of heart rate in postoperative supraventricular tachyarrhythmias. *J Am Coll Cardiol*. 1985;5:1451.

38. Stoelting RK. *Pharmacology and physiology in anesthetic practice*. 2nd ed. Philadelphia: JB Lippincott; 1991;295–296.

39. Weiner N. Drugs that inhibit adrenergic nerves and block adrenergic receptors. In: Gilman AG, Goodman LS, Rall TW, eds. *Goodman and Gilman's the pharmacologic basis of therapeutics*. 8th ed. New York: Macmillan; 1985.

40. Blakeley AG, Summers RJ. The effects of labetalol (AH5158) on adrenergic transmission in the cat spleen. *Br J Pharmacol*. 1977;59:643–650.

41. Drew GM, Hilditch A, Levy GP. Effect of labetalol on the uptake of [³H]-(−)-noradrenaline into the isolated vas deferens of the rat. *Br J Pharmacol*. 1978;63:471–474.

42. Gold EH, Chang W, Cohen M, et al. Synthesis and comparison of some cardiovascular properties of the stereoisomers of labetalol. *J Med Chem*. 1982;25:1363–1370.

43. deBruihn NP, Reves JG, Croughwell N, et al. Pharmacokinetics of esmolol in anesthetized patients receiving chronic beta blockade therapy. *Anesthesiology*. 1987;66:323.

44. Tattersfield AE, Harrison RN. Effect of beta blocker therapy on airway function. *Drugs*. 1983;25(suppl 2):227.

45. Chang LCT. Use of practolol in asthmatics: A plea for caution. *Lancet*. 1971;2:321.

46. Stech J, Sheppard D, Byrd R, et al. Pulmonary effects of esmolol. *Clin Res*. 1985;33:472A.

47. McDevitt DB. Clinical significance of cardioselectivity. State of the art. *Drugs*. 1983;25:211.

48. Cohn JN. Hemodynamic effects of beta blockers. *Drugs*. 1983;25(suppl 2):100.

49. Hansten PD. Beta blocking agents and antidiabetic drugs. *Drug Intell Clin Pharmacol*. 1980;14:46.

50. Rizza RA, Cryer PE, Hammond MW, et al. Adrenergic mechanisms of catecholamine action on glucose homeostasis in man. *Metabolism*. 1980;29:1155.

51. Lewis JG. Adverse reactions to calcium antagonists. *Drugs*. 1983;25:196.

52. Malsch E, Katonah J, Gratz I, Scott A. The effectiveness of labetalol in treating postoperative hypertension. *Nurse Anesth*. 1991;2:65–71.

53. Stoelting RK. Peripheral vasodilators. In: Stoelting RK, ed. *Pharmacology and physiology in anesthetic practice*. 2nd ed. Philadelphia: JB Lippincott; 1987.

54. Cohn JN, Burke LP. Nitroprusside. *Ann Intern Med*. 1979;91:752.

55. Tinker JH, Michenfelder JD. Sodium nitroprusside: Pharmacology, toxicology and therapeutics. *Anesthesiology*. 1976;45:340.

56. Hareioka T, Hatano Y, Mori K, Toda N. Trimethaphan is a direct arterial vasodilator and an alpha-adrenoreceptor antagonist. *Anesth Analg*. 1984;63:290–296.

57. Wang HH, Liu LMP, Katz RL. A comparison of the cardiovascular effects of sodium nitroprusside and trimethaphan. *Anesthesiology*. 1977;46:40–48.

58. Knight PR, Lane GA, Hensinger RN, Bolles RS, Bjoraker DJ. Catecholamine and renin–angiotensin response during hypotensive anesthesia induced by sodium nitroprusside or trimethaphan camsylate. *Anesthesiology*. 1983;59:248–253.

59. Fahmy NR, Soter NA. Effects of trimethaphan on arterial blood histamine and systemic hemodynamics in humans. *Anesthesiology*. 1985;62:562–566.

60. Gerber JG, Nies AS. Antihypertensive agents and the drug therapy of hypertension. In: Gilman AG, Rall TW, Nies AS, Taylor P, eds. *Goodman and Gilman's the pharmacologic basis of therapeutics*. 8th ed. New York: Pergamon Press; 1990.

61. Murad F. Drugs used for the treatment of angina: Organic nitrates, calcium-channel blockers and beta-adrenergic antagonists. In: Gilman AG, Rall TW, Nies AS, Taylor P, eds. *Goodman and Gilman's the pharmacologic basis of therapeutics*. 8th ed. New York: Pergamon Press; 1990.

62. Ferrer MI, Bradley SE, Wheeler HO, et al. Some effects of nitroglycerin upon the splanchnic, pulmonary and systemic circulations. *Circulation*. 1966;33:357–373.

63. Fremes SE, Weisel RD, Mickle D, et al. A comparison of nitroglycerine and nitroprusside. I. Treatment of postoperative hypertension. *Ann Thorac Surg*. 1985;39:53.

64. Spokas EG, Folco G, Quilley J, Chander P, McGiff JC. Endothelial mechanism in the vascular action of hydralazine. *Hypertension*. 1983;5(suppl 1):I107–I111.

65. Kruszyna H, Kruszyna R, Smith RP, Wilcox DE. Red blood cells generate nitric oxide from directly acting, nitrogenous vasodilators. *Toxicol Appl Pharmacol*. 1987;91:429–438.

66. Azuma J, Sawamura A, Harada H, Awata N, Kishimoto S, Sperelakis N. Mechanism of direct cardiostimulating actions of hydralazine. *Eur J Pharmacol*. 1987;135:137–144.

67. Beart PM, Rowe PR, Louis WJ. Alpha methyladrenaline is a central metabolite of alpha methyldopa. *J Pharm Pharmacol*. 1980;35:519.

68. Bobik A, Jennings G, Jackman G, Oddie C, Korner P. Evidence for a predominantly central hypotensive effect of alpha-methyldopa in humans. *Hypertension*. 1986;8:16–23.

69. Reid JL. Alpha-adrenergic receptors and blood pressure control. *Am J Cardiol*. 1986;57:6E–12E.

70. Wright JM, Orozco-Gonzalez M, Polak G, Dollery CT. Duration of effect of single daily dose methyldopa therapy. *Br J Pharmacol*. 1982;13:847–854.

71. Standen NB, Quayle JM, Davies NW, Brayden JE, Huang Y, Nelson MT. Hyperpolarizing vasodilators activate ATP-sensitive K⁺ channels in arterial smooth muscle. *Science*. 1989:245:177–180.

72. Wilson DJ, Viet DG. Control of severe hypertension with pulse doses of diazoxide. *Clin Pharmacol Ther.* 1978;23:135–140.

73. Garrett BN, Kaplan NM. Efficacy of slow infusion of diazoxide in the treatment of severe hypertension without organ hypoperfusion. *Am Heart J.* 1982;103:390–394.

74. Gagnon RM, Morissette M, Priesant S, et al. Hemodynamic and coronary effects of intravenous labetalol in coronary artery disease. *Am J Cardiol.* 1982;49:1267.

75. Stoelting RK. Calcium entry blockers. In: Stoelting RK, ed. *Pharmacology and physiology in anesthetic practice.* 2nd ed. Philadelphia: JB Lippincott; 1987.

76. Coraboeuf E. Ionic basis of electrical activity in cardiac tissues. *Am J Physiol.* 1978;234:H101–H116.

77. Henry PD. Mechanisms of action of calcium antagonists in cardiac and smooth muscle. In: Stone PH, Antman EM, eds. *Calcium channel blocking agents in the treatment of cardiovascular disorders.* Mount Kisco, NY: Futura; 1983.

78. Ehara T, Kaufmann R. The voltage- and time-dependent effects of (–)-verapamil on the slow inward current in isolated cat ventricular myocardium. *J Pharmacol Exp Ther.* 1978;207:49–55.

79. Antman EM, Stone PH, Muller JE, et al. Calcium channel blocking agents in the treatment of cardiovascular disorders. Part I. Basic and clinical electrophysiologic effects. *Ann Intern Med.* 1980;93:875.

80. Atlee JA. Drugs used for treatment of cardiac dysrhythmias. In: Atlee JA, ed. *Perioperative cardiac dysrhythmias.* Chicago: Year Book Medical; 1985.

81. Haft JI, Habbab MA. Treatment of atrial arrhythmias—Effectiveness of verapamil when preceded by calcium infusion. *Arch Intern Med.* 1986;146:1085.

82. Robinson BF, Dobbs RJ, Kelsey CR. Effects of nifedipine on resistance vessels, arteries and veins in man. *Br J Clin Pharmacol.* 1980;10:433–438.

83. Tosone SR, Reves JG, Kissin I, et al. Hemodynamic responses to nifedipine in dogs anesthetized with halothane. *Anesth Analg.* 1983;62:903.

84. Chew CYC, Hecht HS, Collett JT, McAllister RG, Singh BN. Influence of severity of ventricular dysfunction on hemodynamic responses to intravenously administered verapamil in ischemic heart disease. *Am J Cardiol.* 1981;47:917–922.

85. Klein HO, Kaplinsky E. Digitalis and verapamil in atrial fibrillation and flutter. Is verapamil now the preferred agent? *Drugs.* 1986;31:185.

86. Singh BN, Ellrodt G, Peter CT. Verapamil: A review of its pharmacological properties and therapeutic use. *Drugs.* 1978;15:169–197.

87. Raemsch KD, Sommer J. Pharmacokinetics and metabolism of nifedipine. *Hypertension.* 1983;5(suppl II):II18–II24.

88. Ono H, Hashimoto K. In vitro tissue effects of calcium flux inhibition. In: Stone PH, Antman EM, eds. *Calcium channel blocking agents in the treatment of cardiovascular disorders.* Mount Kisco, NY: Futura; 1983.

89. Reves JG, Kissin I, Lell WA, et al. Calcium entry blockers: Uses and implications for anesthesiologists. *Anesthesiology.* 1982;57:504.

90. Reves JG. The relative hemodynamic effects of calcium entry blockers: Uses and implications for anesthesiologists. *Anesthesiology.* 1982;61:3.

91. Rosen MR, Danil P Jr. Effects of tetrodotoxin, lidocaine, verapamil and AHR-2666 on ouabain-induced delayed after depolarizations in canine Purkinje fibers. *Circ Res.* 1980;46:117–124.

92. Bigger JT, Hoffman BF. Antiarrhythmic drugs. In: Gilman AG, Rall TW, Nies AS, Taylor P, eds. *Goodman and Gilman's the pharmacologic basis of therapeutics.* 8th ed. New York: Pergamon Press; 1990.

93. Giardina EGV, Heissenbuttel RH, Bigger JT. Intermittent intravenous procainamide to treat ventricular arrhythmias. *Ann Intern Med.* 1973;78:183.

94. Cardinal R, Sasyniuk BI. Electrophysiological effects of bretylium tosylate on subendocardial Purkinje fibers from infarcted canine hearts. *J Pharmacol Exp Ther.* 1978;204:159.

95. Heissenbuttel RH, Bigger JT. Bretylium tosylate: A newly available antiarrhythmic drug for ventricular arrhythmias. *Ann Intern Med.* 1979;91:229.

96. Aps C, Clement AJ. The cardiovascular system. In: Churchill-Davidson HC, ed. *A practice of anesthesia.* 5th ed. Chicago: Year Book Medical; 1984.

97. Treatment of cardiac arrhythmias. *Med Lett Drugs Ther.* 1989;31:35.

98. Roden DM, Hoffman BF. Action potential prolongation and induction of abnormal automaticity by low quinidine concentrations in canine Purkinje fibers. Relationship to potassium and cycle length. *Circ Res.* 1985;56:857–867.

99. Barnhart ER, ed. *Physicians desk reference.* 44th ed. Oradell, NJ: Medical Economics Co.; 1990:1601–1603.

100. Gillis RA, Onset JA. The role of the nervous system in the cardiovascular effects of digitalis. *Pharmacol Rev.* 1980;31:19.

101. Ferguson DW, Berg WJ, Sanders JS, Roach PJ, Kempf JS, Kienzle MG. Sympathoinhibitory responses to digitalis glycosides in heart failure patients. Direct evidence from sympathetic neural recordings. *Circulation.* 1989;80:65–77.

102. Gillis RA, Quest JA. The role of the central nervous system in the cardiovascular effects of digitalis. *Pharmacol Rev.* 1980;31:19–97.

103. Vasalle M. Cardiac glycosides: Regulation of force and rhythm. In: Nathan RD, ed. *Cardiac muscle: The regulation of excitation and contraction.* New York: Academic Press; 1986.

104. Hoffman BF, Bigger JT. Digitalis and allied cardiac glycosides. In: Gilman AG, Rall TW, Nies AS, Taylor P, eds. *Goodman and Gilman's the pharmacologic basis of therapeutics.* 8th ed. New York: Pergamon Press; 1990.

105. Peon J, Ferrier GR, Moe GK. The relationship of excitability to conduction velocity in canine Purkinje tissue. *Circ Res.* 1978;43:125–135.

106. Rosen MR, Danil P Jr, Alonso MB, Pippenger CE. Effects of therapeutic concentrations of diphenylhydantoin on transmembrane potentials of normal and depressed Purkinje fibers. *J Pharmacol Exp Ther.* 1976;197:594–604.

PART V

Anesthesia and Subspecialties

Anesthesia for General and Genitourinary Surgery

John Aker

The development of general surgery has a long and illustrious tradition. Surgical procedures that are commonly executed today required years of technical development and scientific validation. Undoubtedly the advancement of general surgery would have been delayed without the introduction of general anesthesia, which allowed surgical endeavors to be completed painlessly and without time constraints. The demonstration of successful inhalation anesthesia by Crawford Long and William T. G. Morton empowered surgeons to develop surgical treatments for a wide variety of disorders. The understanding that disease was localized to specific organ systems and remedied by surgical treatment led to the development of the surgical subspecialties.

Complementing a discussion of anesthetic administration for general and genitourinary surgical procedures, it is the author's intent to examine some of the representative general and genitourinary surgical procedures, providing a brief description of required monitoring and anesthetic equipment (if unique to the procedure), a brief explanation of the surgical procedure, and complications that may confront the anesthetist during anesthetic administration. Consideration of the preoperative evaluation for general and genitourinary surgical procedures is confined to problems that are unique to patient pathology or the intended surgical procedure. Although a number of factors influence the selection of a suitable anesthetic technique (see evaluation, Chapter 11), knowledge of the intended surgical procedure complements the anesthetist's preoperative evaluation and facilitates the development of a deliberate plan of care.

GENERAL SURGICAL PROCEDURES

Thyroidectomy

Prior to the development of antithyroid drugs, subtotal thyroidectomy was the fundamental treatment for goiter. Today, thyroid surgical procedures are reserved for the treatment of multinodular goiter and malignant disease.[1]

Although a discussion of thyroid hormone function is beyond the scope of this chapter, the anesthetist should appreciate the physiologic responses and the clinical signs and symptoms that accompany the overproduction or underproduction of thyroid hormones (Table 30–1).

Anesthetic management for thyroid surgery presents many challenges to the anesthetist. Preoperative preparation should include a consultation by an endocrinologist. It is imperative that the patient be rendered euthyroid prior to surgical intervention. This can be accomplished in the hyperthyroid patient with a variety of antithyroid drugs including Lugol's iodine and propylthiouracil. Propranolol may also be administered to control the adrenergic excess that develops from increased circulating levels of thyroxine. Preoperative preparation of the hypothyroid patient will likely require thyroid supplementation to establish a euthyroid state. Whether the patient is hyperthyroid or hypothyroid, a period of 2 to 6 weeks may be required to situate the patient in a euthyroid state.

A careful preoperative evaluation is crucial to the development of any anesthetic plan. The preoperative physical exam for the patient with an enlarged thyroid should include an attentive examination of the airway. The presence of a goiter may produce varying degrees of airway obstruction as a result of tracheal compression from the enlarged gland. Patients with large goiters may have tracheal deviation and may benefit from a preoperative radiographic appraisal of the airway. The presence of tracheal deviation may require an awake laryngoscopy and intubation, a fiberoptic approach to endotracheal intubation to secure the airway prior to the induction of general anesthesia, or both. The selection of a smaller endotracheal tube may be required as the cross-sectional diameter of the trachea may be decreased as a result of the thyroid enlargement.

The positioning requirements for thyroid surgery ensure anatomic access for the surgeon and facilitate exposure and dissection of the gland. Requisite to positioning for thyroid surgery is the necessity to appreciate potential problems that are inherent in this position. The operating table is manipulated into a "lawn-chair" position, with the table flexed at the knees and the head elevated, placing the pa-

TABLE 30–1. CLINICAL SIGNS AND SYMPTOMS OF THYROID DYSFUNCTION

Condition	Symptoms		
	Cardiovascular	Metabolic	Miscellaneous
Hyperthyroidism	Tachycardia Increased cardiac output Tachydysrythmias	Increased appetite Weight loss Fatigue Heat intolerance	Exophthalmus Dermopathy Emotional liability
Hypothyroidism	Bradycardia Decreased cardiac output Peripheral vasoconstriction	Decreased appetite Decreased sweating Lethargy Cold intolerance	Cool dry skin

tient in a semisitting position. The arms are placed at the sides and secured after proper protection of the ulnar nerve with suitable padding. A small blanket, towel, or intravenous fluid container is placed under the thoracic spine which facilitates neck extension and dorsal displacement of the shoulders, providing acceptable exposure of the anterior neck (Fig. 30–1). A small towel is placed under the occiput to support the head in the midline. After patient positioning, it is imperative that the anesthetist auscultate the chest for the presence of bilateral equal breath sounds. Alterations in head position influence the position of the endotracheal tube within the trachea.[2] Neck extension produces a cephalad displacement of the endotracheal tube, and may result in an unexpected extubation of the trachea.[2] A simple expression to recall the displacement of the endotracheal tube with manipulation of the neck is "the tube follows the chin."

Although the "thyroid position" provides the required surgical access, the position involuntarily endangers the facial structures (particularly the eyes) from the application of

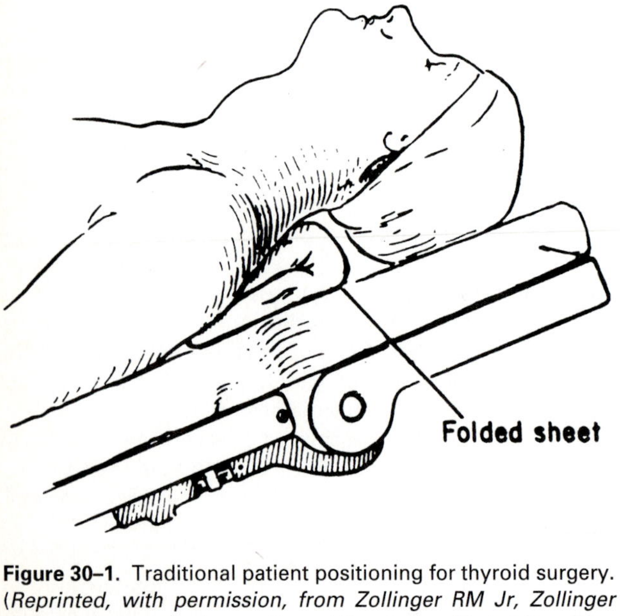

Figure 30–1. Traditional patient positioning for thyroid surgery. (*Reprinted, with permission, from Zollinger RM Jr, Zollinger RM.* Atlas of surgical operations. *6th ed. New York: Macmillan; 1988:Plate CLXXVI.*)

surgical drapes and the unintended pressure from encroachment by the surgeon and surgical assistants. The eyes should be protected with a suitable lubricant and taped closed to prevent corneal abrasion. This eye care may be difficult in the patient with exophthalmos, as the eyelids may not approximate when closed, necessitating the placement of sutures to approximate the eyelids.

Anesthesia is ideally induced with a short-acting barbiturate (thiopental). Thiopental has been demonstrated to exhibit antithyroid activity through a decrease in serum thyroxine levels.[3] Endotracheal intubation is facilitated with a muscle relaxant which is chosen contingent on the preoperative evaluation of the airway and the intended method for securing the airway. Enflurane or isoflurane are acceptable agents for the maintenance of anesthesia. Halothane should be avoided in patients exhibiting a hyperthyroid state as increased serum triiodothyronine (T_3) levels have been shown in an animal model to influence the development of centrilobar hepatic necrosis irrespective of the presence of hypoxia.[4] A balanced anesthetic technique is acceptable; however, the anesthetist must consult the surgeon with respect to the continued use of neuromuscular blocking drugs after endotracheal intubation. The surgeon may desire to preserve neuromuscular function to facilitate identification of important anatomic structures during dissection. Independent of the technique selected, a satisfactory depth of anesthesia is required to prevent patient movement (bucking on the endotracheal tube) during surgical dissection adjacent to the trachea.

Meticulous dissection is carried out within the vicinity of the carotid sinus. The sudden occurrence of bradycardia and hypotension may result from stimulation of the carotid sinus. Surgical dissection should cease and intravenous increments of atropine or glycopyrrolate may be required to restore normal sinus rhythm and normotensive blood pressure. The infiltration of the carotid sinus with 1 percent lidocaine will prevent further hemodynamic insult.

Complications that attend thyroid surgery are associated with the use of a semisitting position and the potential for injury to vascular and neurologic structures surrounding the thyroid. Intraoperative blood loss is influenced by the vascularity of the thyroid and the surgeon's technical skill, but generally averages 300 mL.[5] Venous air embolism, although rare, may occur as the "thyroid position" places the surgical site above the level of the heart. Hematoma formation in the postoperative period may produce acute

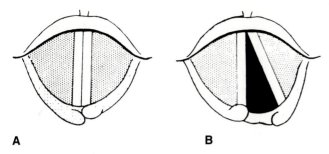

Figure 30–2. Stretching of the left recurrent laryngeal nerve producing an abductor palsy of the left vocal cord. **A.** The right vocal cord meets the left in the midline during phonation, but lies anterior to the left vocal cord. **B.** The uninjured right vocal cord abducts normally during inspiration. (*Reprinted, with permission, from Linton.*[6(p14)])

swelling in the neck and airway obstruction necessitating immediate endotracheal intubation and surgical exploration.

Surgical excision of the thyroid requires meticulous dissection to avoid unintentional injury to the recurrent laryngeal nerve. Injury to the recurrent laryngeal nerve may consist of a "stretch" or "bruising" resulting from traction on the nerve. Transection of the nerve is also a potentiality.

Figures 30–2, 30–3, and 30–4 illustrate the physical findings that accompany left recurrent laryngeal nerve injury.[6] The recurrent laryngeal nerve provides motor innervation to the vocal cord. *Add*uctor fibers are contained within the core (center); the *Abd*uctor fibers are carried by mantle (peripheral) layer of the nerve.[6] Stretching of the nerve produces injury to the abductor fibers and an abductor palsy. With inspiration, the left vocal cord remains in the midline position unable to abduct, whereas the uninjured right vocal cord abducts during inspiration permitting inspiration (Fig. 30–2). Figure 30–3 illustrates vocal cord function after transection of the left recurrent laryngeal nerve which produces both an abductor/adductor palsy. With the loss of function of both adductor and abductor fibers, the vocal cord situates in an abducted position. With phonation, the right vocal cord crosses the midline to meet the injured left vocal cord. The uninjured cord abducts normally during inspiration. Figure 30–4 illustrates vocal cord function after

bilateral injury to the recurrent laryngeal nerve. With a bilateral stretch and injury to the abductor fibers the vocal cords remain near the midline unable to abduct, creating airway obstruction (see Fig. 30–4A). With the transsection of both nerves (abductor/adductor palsy), the vocal cords remain stationary in an abducted position, allowing airway exchange (see Fig. 30–4B). It is therefore understandable that patients with bilateral injury to the abductor fibers of the recurrent laryngeal nerve experience airway obstruction after endotracheal extubation as adduction is unopposed and the vocal cords are closed at the midline, preventing air exchange. This necessitates immediate reintubation to maintain the patient's airway.

If the surgical team is suspicious that unilateral or bilateral injury of the recurrent laryngeal nerve may have occurred, evaluation of vocal cord function may be advisable at the completion of the surgical procedure immediately after extubation. This visualization is best accomplished within the operating theater prior to transport to the recovery room. With the resumption of respiration and after the intravenous administration of lidocaine, the endotracheal tube is removed under direct vision and vocal cord abductor and adductor function is evaluated. As previously discussed, unilateral injury will likely be tolerated, whereas bilateral injury may result in complete airway obstruction necessitating immediate reintubation and ventilation.

Cholecystectomy

Cholecystectomy is the third most frequently performed general surgical procedure; 500,000 are performed annually.[7,8] Cholecystectomy was performed first by Langenbuch of Berlin in 1882 and later by Ohage in the United States in 1886.[9(p1128)] The original surgical technique (incisional removal of the gallbladder) developed by these pioneers has prevailed with minimal modification until recently. As a result of the explosive technologic developments in optics and video imaging, laparascopic cholecystectomy is rapidly replacing this traditional technique.

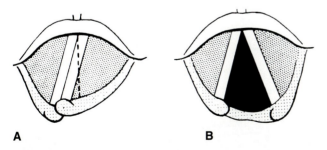

Figure 30–3. Transection of the left recurrent laryngeal nerve produces an abductor and adductor palsy. **A.** During phonation the right vocal cord shifts past the midline to meet the injured left vocal cord. **B.** During inspiration, the right vocal cord abducts normally, as the left vocal cord remains in its injured position. (*Reprinted, with permission, from Linton.*[6(p14)])

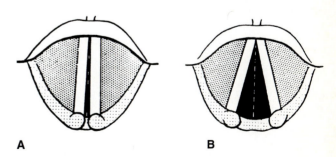

Figure 30–4. A. Bilateral trauma or complete transection of the recurrent laryngeal nerves produces a partial palsy. The vocal cords remain in the midline during inspiration as the adductor fibers are unopposed, producing airway obstruction. This is life threatening as the patient shows signs of respiratory obstruction. **B.** Bilateral stretch of the recurrent laryngeal nerves results in a total palsy where the vocal cords lie in abduction and are unable to adduct. (*Reprinted, with permission, from Linton.*[6(p14)])

Cholecystectomy is the definitive treatment for the acute or chronic inflammation of the gallbladder (cholecystitis). Calculi are often present within the gallbladder. These may advance through the cystic duct into the common bile duct, producing biliary stasis (cholestasis) and jaundice. Patients with cholecystitis experience a variety of symptoms including epigastric and right upper quadrant abdominal pain, nausea and vomiting (60 to 70 percent), and jaundice (10 percent).[9(p1128)] Other acute abdominal pathology as well as ischemic coronary artery disease may produce analogous clinical findings. During the preoperative evaluation, attention should be directed to the cardiovascular system, as cardiovascular complications are largely responsible for the morbidity following cholecystectomy. Laboratory findings that accompany cholecystitis include elevations in the white blood count, serum amylase, and bilirubin. A prothrombin time should be obtained in the patient with biliary obstruction, as there is a decrease in the production of vitamin K-dependent coagulation factors secondary to the decrease in vitamin K absorption in the intestine.

Traditional Cholecystectomy. Traditional cholecystectomy involves the removal of the gallbladder through an upper abdominal incision. The duration of the procedure cannot be stated with certainty, although it can usually be completed by an experienced surgeon in approximately 1 hour. The surgical exploration of the common bile duct and removal of impacted stones require additional operative time. Blood loss averages 200 mL for cholecystectomy and approaches 500 mL with common duct exploration.[5]

General endotracheal anesthesia is the preferred anesthetic technique although both spinal and epidural techniques have been used successfully. A regional technique requires a sensory block to the T-4 dermatome and produces physiologic alterations that can be avoided with the administration of general anesthesia.

After the application of the standard monitoring devices and prior to the induction of general anesthesia, the patient is positioned on the operating table with the arms secured at the sides. After acceptable positioning, a "scout" radiograph of the right upper quadrant is obtained in preparation for the intraoperative cholangiogram which may be obtained for the examination of the common bile duct (Fig. 30–5).

Anesthesia is induced with a short-acting induction agent with or without the concomitant administration of an opioid. The anesthetist should recall that bolus doses of several opioids (including meperidine, fentanyl, and morphine) increase the tone in the sphincter of Oddi, producing pain as a result of an increase in biliary pressure.[10] Endotracheal intubation is facilitated with the administration of either succinylcholine or an intermediate-acting nondepolarizing muscle relaxant. The administration of intravenous lidocaine (1.5 mg/kg) 3 minutes prior to intubation attenuates the expected increase in sympathetic tone that accompanies laryngoscopy and intubation.[11] Patients experiencing episodes of acute cholecystitis with peritonitis may likely have paralytic ileus and delayed gastric emptying, necessitating the use of a rapid-sequence induction.[9(p1139)] After the induction of anesthesia, the surgeon may request the insertion of a nasogastric tube to decompress the stomach.

Anesthesia is maintained with a combination of nitrous oxide in oxygen, narcotic, and muscle relaxant. An air–oxygen combination can be used in place of nitrous oxide. A potent inhalation agent (enflurane or isoflurane) may be administered in addition to, or substituted for, the opioid. Halothane is avoided in patients with intrinsic liver disease or those undergoing hepatic or biliary surgery.

Surgical access of the gallbladder is obtained through either a midline, paramedian, or subcostal incision of the anterior abdominal wall (Fig. 30–6). Skeletal muscle relaxation is required for the duration of the procedure; muscle relaxation facilitates entry into the abdominal cavity as well as closure of the peritoneum and abdominal musculature. Muscle relaxation is monitored with a neuromuscular function monitor and maintained with an intermittent bolus or constant infusion of a nondepolarizing muscle relaxant. An 80 percent block (disappearance of last two twitches of train-of-four) provides adequate muscle relaxation.

As previously mentioned, the surgeon may elect to visually evaluate the common bile duct for the presence of "stones." Cholangiography is accomplished by the injection of radiocontrast material into the duct with the simultaneous exposure of radiographic film placed under the patient. Although thousands of radiologic procedures are enhanced with radiocontrast media, it has been estimated that adverse systemic reactions occur in approximately 4 percent of patients.[12,13] The anesthetist should be aware that patients with an allergic history have an increased risk of adverse reaction to radiocontrast media on the order of 1.5 to 10 times that of

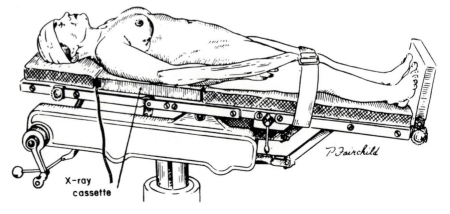

Figure 30–5. Positioning for traditional cholecystectomy. The radiographic plate positioned under the patient will be exposed during cholangiography. (*Reprinted, with permission, from Zollinger RM Jr, Zollinger RM. Atlas of surgical operations. 6th ed. New York: Macmillan; 1988:Plate XXVII.*)

X-ray cassette

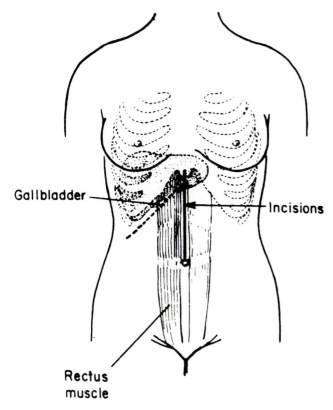

Figure 30–6. Incision sites for surgical access for traditional cholecystectomy. (*Reprinted, with permission, from Zollinger RM Jr, Zollinger RM.* Atlas of surgical operations. *6th ed. New York: Macmillan; 1988:Plate XXVII.*)

the nonallergic patient.[14,15] During general anesthesia, allergic reactions may manifest through the cutaneous, respiratory, or cardiovascular system. Characteristic signs and symptoms of anaphylaxis elicited during general anesthesia are depicted in Table 30–2. The reader is referred to the excellent review by Levy for a discussion of the treatment strategies for allergic reactions.[12]

At the conclusion of the surgical procedure, neuromuscular blockade is reversed with a suitable combination of anticholinergic and anticholinesterase. The author prefers to titrate the "reversal" mixture after closure of the anterior rectus muscle fascia. Spontaneous ventilation resumes and ventilation is assisted during closure of the subcutaneous tissue and skin. The use of either isoflurane or enflurane is discontinued with the commencement of skin closure. A 50 to 70 percent combination of nitrous oxide and oxygen is continued until the surgical dressing is applied; 100 percent oxygen is administered in preparation for endotracheal extubation.

Laparoscopy Cholecystectomy. The use of laparoscopy for the diagnosis and treatment of general surgical conditions is gaining wide popularity. Procedures amenable to laparoscopy include appendectomy, adhesiolysis, and cholecystectomy.[16–18] The application of laparoscopy for cholecystectomy is riding a wave of popularity since the first independent development of the surgical procedure by Reddick and Olsen[19] and Dubois et al.[19] It has been esti-

TABLE 30–2. RECOGNITION OF ANAPHYLAXIS IN INTUBATED PATIENTS

System	Signs
Respiratory	Cyanosis
	Wheezing
	Increased peak airway pressure
	Acute pulmonary edema
Cardiovascular	Tachycardia
	Dysrhythmias
	Hypotension
	Pulmonary hypertension
	Decreased systemic vascular resistance
	Cardiovascular collapse
Cutaneous	Urticaria
	Flushing
	Perioral edema
	Periorbital edema

Reprinted, with permission, from Levy.[12(p19)]

mated that approximately 20,000 procedures are being performed yearly since the advent of this surgical technique.[20]

The indications for laparoscopic cholecystectomy parallel those of traditional cholecystectomy. Surgical contraindications are listed in Table 30–3. Operative time is longer than for traditional cholecystectomy but decreases as the surgeon becomes proficient with the surgical technique. It should also be noted that presence of an upper abdominal scar and acute cholecystitis are less constraining contraindications as surgical proficiency develops. Laparoscopy cholecystectomy offers several advantages over traditional cholecystectomy, as postoperative recovery time is decreased, providing for a rapid return to activities of daily living and employment, patients experience less postoperative pain, there is less postoperative respiratory embarrassment, and the surgical incisions are aesthetically acceptable to the patient.

Preoperative preparation of the patient for general anesthesia, as well as the immediate preinduction preparation (positioning and acquisition of a "scout" radiograph), is managed as previously discussed. A great deal of technical support equipment is required for the procedure which limits the anesthesia workspace (Figure 30–7). General anesthesia is induced and endotracheal intubation is facilitated with a depolarizing or nondepolarizing muscle relaxant. After the airway is secured by means of an endotracheal tube, the stomach should be decompressed with an orogastric tube (rather than nasal tube as this is removed at

TABLE 30–3. CONTRAINDICATIONS TO LAPAROSCOPIC CHOLECYSTECTOMY

Absolute Contraindications	Relative Contraindications
Inability to tolerate general anesthesia	Coagulopathy
	Upper abdominal scar
Required concomitant upper abdominal operation	Acute cholecystitis
	Choledocholithiasis

Reprinted, with permission, from Schirmer et al.[20(p666)]

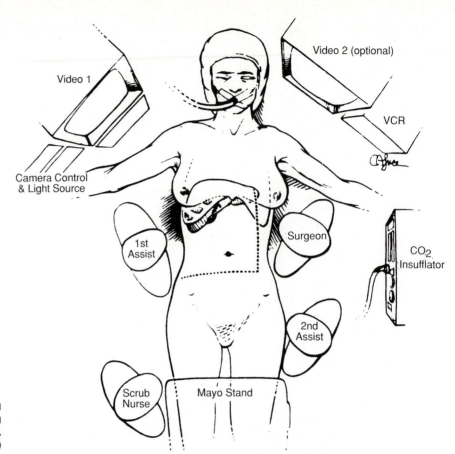

Figure 30–7. Positioning of the operating room personnel and equipment during laparoscopy cholecystectomy. (*Reprinted, with permission, from Schirmer et al.*[20(p666)])

the conclusion of the surgical procedure), and a Foley catheter inserted. Bladder and gastric decompression lessens the chance of injury during establishment of the pneumoperitoneum.

Pneumoperitoneum is established with the introduction of carbon dioxide into the abdomen by means of a Verres needle inserted through an umbilical incision or by means of a surgical incision and the placement of an operating trocar. Manual ventilation should be temporarily halted during the insertion of the Verres needle or trocar to limit the risk of injury to abdominal contents. The insufflation of carbon dioxide into the peritoneal cavity produces increased abdominal pressure and distension, a decrease in diaphragmatic excursion, and decreased tidal volumes with excessively insufflated volumes of carbon dioxide. Carbon dioxide retention may follow.[21] Unlike gynecologic laparoscopy where severe degrees of Trendelenburg position may be required, the laparoscopy cholecystectomy patient is typically placed in a reverse Trendelenburg position to encourage a caudad displacement of the omentum, providing exposure of the gallbladder. This positioning may lessen the respiratory embarrassment that accompanies pneumoperitoneum.

Carbon dioxide is passively absorbed from the abdomen; however, carbon dioxide retention is typically not problematic in patients without cardiopulmonary disease and can be prevented with hyperventilation of the patient.[21] Wittgen and colleagues found that patients with preoperative cardiopulmonary disease may experience significant in-

creases in arterial carbon dioxide and decreases in pH during CO_2 insufflation during laparoscopy cholecystectomy.[22] In addition, increases of end-tidal carbon dioxide did not parallel the increases in arterial carbon dioxide.[22] Hence, the patient with preoperative cardiopulmonary dysfunction may require serial arterial blood gas monitoring during prolonged periods of insufflation.

Cardiovascular embarrassment (hypotension and dysrhythmia) may occur with excessively insufflated volumes of carbon dioxide as intraabdominal pressure compromises venous return to the heart. Treatment consists of cessation of insufflation and temporary deflation of the abdomen.

Figure 30–8 illustrates the location of the operative trocars. A cautery spatula electrode and microdissection scissors are introduced through the operative trocar for surgical dissection of the gallbladder, and surgical clips are placed prior to division of the cystic duct and the arterial supply to the gallbladder. As in the traditional cholecystectomy, an operative cholangiography may be performed. Cholangiography will increase the operative time by approximately 20 minutes. After dissection from the liver bed, the gallbladder is extracted through the umbilical trocar. The operative site is then irrigated, hemostasis is ensured, and the surgical incisions are closed after removal of the remaining pneumoperitoneum. The residual muscle relaxant is reversed during closure of the trocar sites, the orogastric tube is removed, spontaneous ventilation is reestablished, and the patient is extubated.

It should be noted that unforeseen complications that

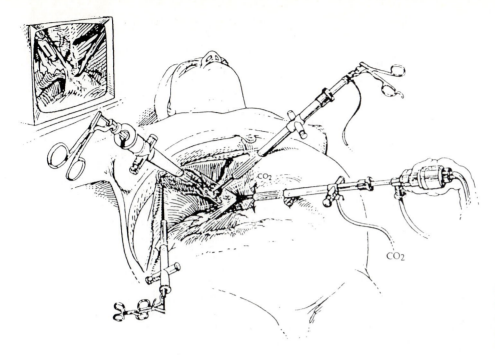

Figure 30–8. Introduction of four operative trocars for laparoscopy cholecystectomy. (*Reprinted, with permission, from Schirmer et al.*[20(p667)])

arise during laparoscopy cholecystectomy (difficulty defining anatomy, uncontrolled bleeding, bile duct injury, bile leak) may necessitate a conversion to the traditional procedure.

Surgical Procedures on the Breast

The surgical treatment of breast pathology accounts for a large proportion of outpatient as well as inpatient general surgical procedures. Breast biopsy, lumpectomy (removal of benign or malignant breast tissue), simple mastectomy, and modified radical mastectomy with axillary dissection are the most frequently scheduled procedures.

Breast cancer is the leading cause of death in women between the ages of 40 and 44.[23] A sensitive approach to the patient scheduled for surgery of the breast is beneficial as this individual is understandably fearful of the potential diagnosis of malignancy, as well as the pain and potential disfigurement that may follow the procedure. Indeed, these fears may be responsible for a delay in surgical treatment.

A number of considerations must be acknowledged when selecting an appropriate anesthetic technique, including the anticipated surgical procedure, the patient's willingness to accept the anesthetic technique, and the surgeon's personal surgical preferences. The patient may elect a general anesthetic because of the fear of diagnosis and the fear of the accompanying pain of the procedure.

Excisional breast biopsy is usually facilitated with the radiographic placement of a penetrating wire (needle localization), or the injection of a dye (methylene blue) into the affected area of breast tissue. This procedure assists the surgical identification and removal of the questionable tissue. The aforementioned procedure is scheduled in the radiology department, a few hours prior to the scheduled surgical procedure.

The infiltration of a local anesthetic is acceptable for su-

perficial breast biopsies (without the excision of deep breast tissue) although the substantial removal of breast tissue will likely require supplementary intravenous analgesia, general anesthesia, or both. General anesthesia allows the surgeon to obtain hemostasis and the ability to ensure an acceptable cosmetic result as the breast contour may be altered with the removal of breast tissue. Breast biopsy is generally less than 1 hour in duration and blood loss is typically less than 100 mL.

Segmental breast resection, simple mastectomy, and modified radical mastectomy are generally accomplished with general endotracheal anesthesia. After endotracheal intubation, the additional administration of muscle relaxant is discouraged; muscle relaxation during the procedure is not essential, and neuromuscular function is important in the preservation of the axillary nerves and the long thoracic nerve during surgical dissection. Blood loss during simple mastectomy approaches 200 mL, with losses approaching 800 mL during modified radical mastectomy.[5] Humidification of inspired gases and the maintenance of an acceptable operating room temperature will abet decreases in core temperature that are likely to result from surgical exposure.

Hernia

Hernia is defined as the protrusion of abdominal contents through the fascial and muscular layers of the abdomen. Hernia occurs as a consequence of a congenital defect (indirect inguinal hernia and umbilical hernia) or an acquired defect (direct and incisional hernia) of the abdominal wall. Incisional hernia typically develops in vertical rather than transverse abdominal incisions. Mortality from hernia is a genuine concern as the associated intestinal obstruction that may ensue has been shown to be one of the leading causes of death.[24]

Herniorrhaphy is performed in the newborn, child,

adult, and geriatric patient. The choice of anesthesia is dictated not only by the patient's age and physical status but also with respect to the location of the hernia. Herniorrhaphy is generally an elective surgical procedure as the majority of patients are young, healthy, and physically active. The procedure can be safely undertaken on an outpatient basis. When the patient presents with trapped abdominal contents, however, herniorrhaphy is an emergent situation.

Elective herniorrhaphy in the adult and geriatric patient can be performed with local anesthesia, local anesthesia with conscious intravenous sedation, or regional or general anesthesia techniques. Preparation for conscious sedation begins with attentive patient positioning. The patient should be placed in the flexed "lawn-chair" position with a pillow under the knees. It is exhausting for the patient to lie on an uncushioned, completely flat operating table, and the patient will likely become uncomfortable despite the intravenous administration of sedative-analgesic drugs. Carefully titrated doses of a benzodiazepine and a short-acting opioid will provide anxiolysis and supplemental analgesia. Monitoring requirements for general anesthesia are also germane for the patient during local/conscious sedation. The patient should receive supplemental oxygen by either face mask or nasal cannula as the sedative-hypnotic combination may produce respiratory depression. With a local/conscious sedation technique, the surgeon is solely responsible for administration of anesthesia (the infiltration of local anesthetic at the operative site). If the patient is uncooperative because of incisional pain, the anesthetist should encourage the surgeon to infiltrate the operative site with additional local anesthetic, rather than administer additional doses of sedative-analgesic agents. The judicious administration of sedative-hypnotic agents will produce a patient who is comfortable, without respiratory depression, and who will respond verbally to the anesthetist when stimulated. Precipitation of respiratory depression and unresponsiveness occur with excessive administration of these agents. A surgeon's request that the patient be sedated to the point of unresponsiveness dictates that the patient be managed with a general anesthetic.

General anesthesia can be managed by mask or endotracheal tube. Assuming that herniorrhaphy is undertaken in the outpatient setting, the anesthetist should choose agents that provide a rapid return of consciousness and a shortened time in the postanesthesia recovery room to attain street fitness. After repair, the infiltration of bupivacaine into the surgical site will provide postoperative analgesia.[25]

Umbilical and incisional herniorrhaphy and procedures that involve manipulation of abdominal contents (sliding hernia) require muscle relaxation to facilitate repair and, therefore, are not amenable to a local anesthesia or local/conscious intravenous sedation technique. Use of a potent inhalational agent or an opioid–nitrous oxide technique with an intermediate-duration nondepolarizing muscle relaxant provides optimal operating conditions. Prior to endotracheal extubation, residual muscle relaxation is reversed, and intravenous lidocaine (1.5 mg/kg) is administered to minimize "bucking" and straining which may disrupt the surgical repair.

Spinal and epidural techniques are acceptable alternatives to general anesthesia, as they provide analgesia and muscle relaxation. The surgeon may evaluate the surgical repair during regional anesthesia by having the patient perform a Valsalva maneuver; however, some practitioners are reticent about the use of spinal anesthesia for the outpatient because of the fear of postdural puncture headache.[26]

Patients who present emergently for herniorrhaphy have either incarcerated (contents of hernia sac cannot be returned to abdomen) or strangulated (blood supply is compromised by compression) bowel. The potential for regurgitation and aspiration is a genuine concern because of intestinal obstruction. If general anesthesia is chosen, a rapid-sequence induction with endotracheal intubation is the prudent approach. The selected induction agents must be administered cautiously as the entrapped bowel may contain translocated fluid and protein which may create a relative hypovolemia. This relative hypovolemia may become clinically evident after the administration of vasodilating induction agents.

After emergent surgical repair, endotracheal extubation should not be attempted until the patient has demonstrated the return of protective airway reflexes and the residual neuromuscular block has been successfully reversed.

Abdominal Surgical Procedures

A number of abdominal procedures may be performed by the general surgeon. Table 30–4 lists representative upper and lower abdominal surgical procedures. Surgical access to the abdominal cavity is obtained through a midline or transverse abdominal incision, division of the abdominal musculature, and incision of the peritoneum.

Recall that the sensory innervation of the peritoneum and abdominal contents is by way of the sympathetic and parasympathetic nervous system. The sensory supply to the pelvic structures (bladder, uterus, rectum) originates from the sacral distribution (S-2, S-3, and S-4) of the parasympathetic nervous system; the remainder of the abdominal contents is innervated by the sympathetic system.

Several preoperative conditions (history of gastroesophageal reflux, potential for delayed gastric emptying, presence of intestinal obstruction, fluid and electrolyte imbalance, preoperative antibiotic therapy, to list a few) influ-

TABLE 30–4. INTRAABDOMINAL SURGICAL PROCEDURES

Abdominal Region	Procedures
Upper	Gastrectomy
	Vagotomy
	Pancreatic resection
	Splenectomy
Lower	Hysterectomy
	Colon resection
	Small bowel resection
	Appendectomy

ence the selection of specific anesthetic techniques for abdominal surgery.

GENITOURINARY SURGICAL PROCEDURES

Genitourinary surgery is performed either through a surgical incision or with the use of a lighted-lens instrument introduced through the urethra. The subsequent discussion provides an overview of common genitourologic surgical procedures as well as rationale for the selection of specific anesthetic agents or techniques.

Cystoscopy

The examination of the urinary bladder is achieved in a *closed* procedure with the insertion through the urethra of a rigid lighted-lens instrument (endoscope). Cystoscopy allows visual evaluation of the urethra and bladder. Radiographic evaluation of the upper urinary system (ureters, renal pelvis) at the time of cystoscopy can also be accomplished with the retrograde injection of contrast medium. A nonelectrolyte irrigating solution is infused through the cystoscope to distend the bladder and improve operator visualization.

Cystoscopic procedures are generally less than 1 hour in duration and are traditionally performed in the lithotomy position; however, cystoscopy may be performed in the supine position with a flexible cystoscope.

There are a number of suitable anesthetic techniques for cystoscopy including local anesthesia with or without conscious sedation and general or regional anesthesia techniques. Local anesthesia is presumably not appropriate for the pediatric patient but may be selected for the cooperative adult or poor-risk patient. Anesthesia is achieved with the instillation of 2 percent topical lidocaine jelly through the urethra into the bladder. After a suitable period (approximately 5 minutes) urethral instrumentation can be undertaken. The use of carefully titrated doses of midazolam and a short-acting opioid (fentanyl or alfentanil) provides anxiolysis and supplemental analgesia. During "local" cystoscopy, patients experience discomfort from bladder distension as a result of the continuous infusion of irrigating solution into the bladder. This discomfort can be easily and quickly relieved by the surgeon with the intermittent drainage of the bladder during the procedure.

The selection of a regional technique (spinal or epidural) requires a sensory block to T-10 as the sensory fibers of the bladder accompany the sympathetic and parasympathetic distribution from T-11 to L-2.[27(p52)] General anesthesia is initiated with a short-acting intravenous induction agent and maintained with oxygen, nitrous oxide, and an inhalation anesthetic by mask. A short-acting opioid may be substituted for, or administered in addition to, the inhalation agent. A muscle relaxant is not essential for cystoscopy (see discussion below) but may be administered to facilitate endotracheal intubation. The decision to place an endotracheal tube is at the discretion of the anesthetist.

Patients with spinal cord injury are prone to urinary tract infections and hypercalcemia as a result of recumbency. These patients are frequent visitors to the operating room for diagnostic cystoscopy or the manipulation of ureteral calculi.[28] Quadriplegics or paraplegics who require cystoscopic examinations and stone manipulation are at risk for autonomic hyperreflexia if the spinal cord injury is at or above T-5. Approximately 66 to 85 percent of these patients may experience the symptoms of autonomic hyperreflexia.[29] Autonomic hyperreflexia is exhibited as a response to noxious stimuli (i.e., bladder catheterization or irrigation) below the level of the spinal cord lesion. Clinical manifestations include paroxysmal hypertension, bradycardia, ventricular dysrhythmia, and heart block.[30] The development of severe hypertension occurs in patients when the spinal cord injury is above the splanchnic outflow (between T-4 and T-6). Patients with spinal cord injury between T-5 and T-10 experience less severe increases in blood pressure.[31] General, spinal, and epidural anesthesia are all suitable in the prevention of autonomic hyperreflexia, although the administration of regional anesthesia in these patients may be technically difficult.[32] Figure 30–9 lists the sequence of events associated with the clinical presentation of autonomic hyperreflexia.

In addition to its diagnostic benefit, cystoscopy is frequently employed for the treatment of urethral or bladder wall tumors. Specially designed biopsy forceps or an electrically energized wire loop may be introduced through the cystoscope to excise tissue and arrest subsequent bleeding. Electrical resection of urethral and bladder wall tumors dictates the use of a nonelectrolyte bladder irrigation solution to facilitate dispersion of electrical current. Unlike cystoscopy, the electrosurgical resection of bladder wall tumors requires an immobile patient. Bladder perforation may follow unexpected patient movement (bucking on the endotracheal tube) during tumor resection.[33] Unexpected patient movement can also be precipitated during resection by inadvertent electrical stimulation of the obturator nerve by the endoscopist. Although infrequent, stimulation of the obturator nerve may occur during resection of lateral bladder wall tumors, provoking sudden leg adduction. On stimulation, the endoscopist should be prepared to quickly terminate the resection to avoid perforation. The selection of a regional technique or general anesthesia with the administration of a nondepolarizing muscle relaxant will serve to secure an immobile surgical field; however, the use of muscle relaxants during general anesthesia should not be relied on to produce immobilization in insufficiently anesthetized patients.

With perforation, the conscious patient may complain of periumbilical, inguinal, or suprapubic pain.[33] The urologist may also note the failure of return of bladder irrigation. Additional signs and symptoms include pallor, sweating, abdominal rigidity, nausea with or without vomiting, and hypotension.[33]

Perforation during general anesthesia is more difficult to diagnose. Again, the urologist may note the failure of return of bladder irrigation. A reflexive movement of the limbs has been reported in unconscious patients at the time of perforation.[33,34] Hemodynamic changes may assist in the diagnosis, but these are dependent on the size and location of the perforation, as well as the amount of irrigating fluid that extravasates. Small perforations with little extravasa-

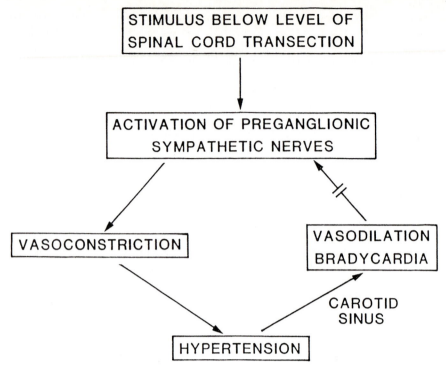

Figure 30–9. Sequence of events leading to the clinical manifestation of autonomic hyperreflexia. (*Reprinted, with permission, from Stoelting RK, Dierdorf SF, McCammon RL, eds.* Anesthesia and co-existing disease. *2nd ed. New York: Churchill Livingstone; 1988:326.*)

tion will produce minimal changes in hemodynamics, whereas the extravasation of large amounts of fluid is associated with a gradual increase in blood pressure preceding the onset of severe hypotension and tachycardia.[35] Holtgrewe and Valk examined factors that influenced morbidity and mortality in 2015 cases of transurethral resection of the prostate and found the incidence of bladder perforation to be 1.1 percent (25 patients).[36] Four deaths and five major complications occurred in 12 patients when suprapubic cystotomy was delayed beyond 2 hours after perforation, emphasizing the importance of prompt diagnosis.[36]

Ureteral Endoscopy

Ureteral endoscopy provides for the evaluation of pathology in the ureter with the use of either a rigid or a flexible urethroscope introduced through the urethra. Ureteral endoscopy and instrumentation is employed for the injection of radiocontrast medium for visualization of the upper urinary drainage system, the placement of ureteral stints, and the manipulation and removal of ureteral calculi. Ureteral calculi are removed with the use of a special catheter that encloses a flexible wire basket. The catheter is directed into the ureter; beyond the calculus, the basket is opened and, on withdrawal of the catheter, the calculus is captured and removed.

The urologist may use fluoroscopy or inject radiocontrast material (or both) and obtain serial radiographs for visualization of the ureters and renal pelvis during urethroscopy. Again, the anesthetist should recall that patients with an allergic history have an increased risk of adverse reaction to radiocontrast medium on the order of 1.5 to 10 times that of the nonallergic patient.[9(p1139),12] Allergic reactions are, however, infrequent with the retrograde injection of contrast medium into the urinary system, as there is inconsequential systemic absorption.

During the course of endoscopy, the surgeon may request the intravenous administration of a diagnostic dye. Indigo carmine dye (0.8 percent) is administered in a 5-mL volume to color the urine and aid the identification of the ureteral orifice. Indigo carmine may increase systemic vascular resistance and consequently arterial blood pressure via its alpha-sympathomimetic stimulating effects. A 1 percent solution of methylene blue may be substituted for indigo carmine. The intravenous administration of methylene blue has been associated with the occurrence of hypotension.

The intravenous administration of these diagnostic dyes is associated with an abrupt decrease in SpO_2 as determined by pulse oximetry.[37] These two dyes absorb light in the region of 660-nm wavelength of light emitted by the pulse oximeter. The decrease in SpO_2 after intravenous administration lasts approximately 30 to 45 seconds, with recovery to baseline readings within 3 minutes in young healthy subjects.[37] The duration of decreased SpO_2 may be more prolonged in the elderly, the debilitated, or patients with decreased cardiac outputs.[37] Scheller and colleagues found that the largest decreases in SpO_2 from baseline occurred after the administration of methylene blue and that the smallest change occurred after the administration of indigo carmine.[37] In the event of sudden decreases in SpO_2 after the intravenous administration of diagnostic dyes, the prudent anesthetist should confirm that the patient is being adequately ventilated with inspection of capnography and auscultation of the chest to confirm the presence of bilateral breath sounds.

Anesthesia for urethroscopy and instrumentation is longer in duration than cystoscopy (1 to 1.5 hours). Unexpected patient movement during urethroscopy or manipulation of ureteral calculi may precipitate ureteral injury and laceration (see previous discussion under Cystoscopy). Urethroscopy may be safely conducted with either general or regional anesthesia. Conscious sedation (monitored anesthesia care) is occasionally chosen for poor-risk patients, although these patients may be quite uncomfortable with instrumentation and dilation of the ureter. Pain originating from ureteral manipulation is transmitted along visceral afferent nerve fibers that accompany the sympathetic and parasympathetic distribution from T-11 to L-2.[27(p52)] To effectively abolish the pain associated with ureteral instrumentation would therefore require general anesthesia or a regional technique (spinal or epidural) which provides a sensory block to T-10.[27(p26)] General anesthesia is induced and maintained as previously discussed.

Transurethral Resection of the Prostate

Transurethral resection of the prostate (TURP) is one of the most common genitourinary procedures; 350,000 were performed in 1985.[38] Greater than 90 percent of male patients with bladder neck obstruction as a result of a benign or malignant processes are treated with TURP.[39]

The prostate is anatomically subdivided into five lobes (one anterior, two lateral, one median, one posterior) and surrounds the prostatic urethra at the base of the bladder. Under the influence of testosterone, the periurethral glands and the lateral and medial lobes of the prostate hypertrophy and compress the prostate tissue, producing bladder neck obstruction. Patients with bladder neck obstruction may experience hematuria, large residual urine volumes, acute urinary retention, and recurrent urinary tract infections.[40] Patients with these symptoms are candidates for TURP.[40]

Men in the fifth, sixth, and seventh decades of life usually present for TURP. These patients may have extensive preexisting medical problems. The American Urological Association Cooperative Study found that 77 percent of patients presenting for TURP suffer from significant medical problems.[40] The most frequent medical problems encountered were pulmonary (14.5 percent), gastrointestinal (13.2 percent), cardiovascular (history of myocardial infarction [12.5 percent] or arrhythmias [12.4 percent]), and renal (9.8 percent) insufficiency.[40] Today patients scheduled for TURP are routinely admitted on the day of surgery, necessitating a thorough medical workup prior to admission. The medical evaluation should critically examine the patient's cardiovascular, pulmonary, and renal function prior to admission.

Transurethral resection of the prostate is performed in the dorsal lithotomy position through a modified cystoscope. The medial and lateral lobes of the prostate are resected with an electrically energized wire loop. The electrical current is also used to coagulate areas of bleeding. As in cystoscopy, irrigating fluid is infused into the bladder to improve visualization and flush the resected prostatic tissue from the bladder.

There are a number of potential problems that the anesthetist may encounter during the intraoperative and immediate postoperative period. The most common complications include (1) the intravascular absorption of irrigating fluid through opened prostatic venous sinuses with the development of transurethral resection (TUR) syndrome,

(2) the potential for substantial blood loss, and (3) bladder perforation during resection. The reader is referred to the previous discussion concerning bladder perforation.

Absorption of Irrigating Fluid. Intravascular and extravascular absorption of irrigating fluid may ensue during TURP. The opening of prostatic venous sinuses during resection provides a route for the intravascular absorption of irrigating fluid when the irrigating fluid pressure exceeds venous pressure. A number of factors influence the amount of irrigating solution that is absorbed; (1) the hydrostatic pressure of the irrigating solution (determined by the height of the solution above the bladder), (2) the type of irrigating fluid employed, (3) the number of venous sinuses exposed during resection, (4) the duration of the resection, and (5) the experience of the surgeon.[41]

The height of the irrigation solution above the bladder determines the pressure of the fluid in the prostatic fossa and the amount of fluid absorbed. Irrigating fluid absorption increases twofold when the height of the fluid is increased from 60 to 70 cm.[42] The amount of fluid absorbed is also influenced by the resection time. Hagstrom and colleagues have estimated that between 10 and 30 mL of irrigating fluid is absorbed per minute of resection time.[43] Oester and Madsen using a double-isotope technique found that approximately 1 L of irrigating fluid was absorbed during the course of resection.[44] Irrigating fluid absorption probably occurs throughout the period of resection; however, Hahn and colleagues have established that irrigating fluid absorption was greatest 30 minutes subsequent to the beginning of the resection.[45] The amount of fluid absorbed during TURP is difficult to predict as a result of the many factors that influence irrigating fluid absorption. The American Urological Association Cooperative Study found that the incidence of TUR syndrome was increased if the prostate gland was larger than 45 g or resection time was longer than 90 minutes.[40] To limit fluid absorption, resection time should be limited to 90 minutes, the height of the fluid should not be greater than 60 cm above the bladder, and the surgeon should avoid resection near the venous sinuses lying deep within the prostate capsule.[40,41]

Complications arising from the absorption of irrigating solution depend on the type of fluid used as well as the rate of absorption. A variety of irrigating fluids have been used during TURP. Distilled water was initially employed because of its accessibility and the superior visibility afforded to the endoscopist. Creevy and Webb illustrated the hazards of using distilled water, reporting a fatal hemolytic reaction after TURP.[46] The intravascular absorption of distilled water (a hypotonic solution) produced dilutional hyponatremia and hemolysis of red blood cells favoring the development of anemia and death.

Table 30–5 lists the desirable characteristics of the ideal irrigating fluid for TURP. As previously discussed, a nonelectrolyte solution must be used to facilitate dispersion of electric current. Nonelectrolyte solutions have been manufactured with the addition of solutes to distilled water to increase the osmolarity of the solution. Glucose, glycine, urea, mannitol, sorbitol, and the combination of sorbitol and mannitol (Cytal) have all been successfully used during TURP. Although these fluids are not isotonic, they are non-

TABLE 30–5. CHARACTERISTICS OF THE IDEAL IRRIGATING FLUID FOR TRANSURETHRAL RESECTION OF THE PROSTATE

Optically inert
Isotonic
Nonhemolytic
Nonelectrolytic
No toxic metabolic products
Rapidly excreted

Reprinted, with permission, from Jenson V. Can J Anaesth. 1991;38:91.

hemolytic. Currently the most popular irrigating fluid is 1.5 percent glycine.

Transurethral Resection Syndrome. The TUR syndrome is a consequence of the absorption of irrigating fluid during TURP and is exhibited by alterations in cardiovascular and central nervous system functioning. Table 30–6 lists the clinical presentation of the TUR syndrome. Intravascular absorption of irrigating fluid may precipitate the development of this syndrome intraoperatively. Oester and Madsen have estimated that only 29 percent of absorbed irrigating solution enters the circulation, with the rest accumulating in the interstitial spaces.[44] With extravascular absorption into the retroperitoneal and periprostatic spaces, the TUR syndrome may not manifest until the first postoperative day.[45]

The intravascular absorption of irrigating fluid increases intravascular volume and dilutes plasma proteins, decreasing plasma oncotic pressure. Circulatory overload increases myocardial oxygen requirements which may be detrimental to the patient with coronary artery disease. The decrease in plasma oncotic pressure encourages the relocation of fluid from the intravascular to the interstitial compartment.[47] The clinical presentation of TUR syndrome is a consequence of this relocation of intravascular fluid.

TURP should be postponed in patients with a preoperative serum sodium of 120 to 130 mEq/L. Dilutional hyponatremia follows the absorption of large amounts of electrolyte-free irrigating fluids. The movement of 100 mL of fluid into the interstitial compartment produces a 10- to 15-

mEq decrease in intravascular sodium concentration.[48] The onset of central nervous system (CNS) symptoms is dependent on the speed with which the serum sodium decreases.

Table 30–7 enumerates the signs and symptoms that accompany acute decreases in serum sodium. Recall that extracellular sodium is required for cellular excitability and plays a formidable role in the initiation of cellular action potentials. Acute decreases in serum sodium concentration may disturb myocardial and cerebral function. The absorption of a large quantity of irrigating fluid will acutely decrease the serum sodium concentration. A decrease in serum sodium to 120 mEq/L results in the clinical presentation of CNS symptoms and is indicative of a severe reaction. The patient will likely exhibit central nervous symptoms clinically recognized as restlessness, confusion, and hypotension. Further decreases in serum sodium concentration are accompanied by changes in the electrocardiogram (widened QRS and ST segment elevation) and progressive CNS depression. A decrease in serum sodium to 100 mEq/L is associated with seizures, coma, and respiratory and cardiac arrest.

The absorption of large amounts of glycine irrigation fluid and the increase in serum glycine levels may contribute to the CNS effects of the TUR syndrome. Gecelter and Gascoigne found that serum glycine concentrations increased to ten times normal plasma levels despite normal serum sodium levels.[49] Glycine, a nonessential amino acid, functions as an inhibitory neurotransmitter whose distribution parallels that of γ-aminobutyric acid (GABA) in the brainstem and spinal cord.[50] Increased concentrations of glycine within the CNS may produce various degrees of CNS depression including transient blindness, nausea and vomiting, confusion, and coma.[51,52] Ovassapian and colleagues measured a serum glycine concentration of 1029 mg/L (normal plasma glycine level 13 to 17 mg/L) which was associated with transient blindness.[51] The patient's vision returned approximately 12 hours later, with the serum glycine level decreasing to 143 mg/L. Ammonia, the metabolic by-product of glycine, may contribute to the CNS depression and has been implicated as contributing to delayed awakening after general anesthesia.[53]

The TUR syndrome appears to be a consequence of the absorption of irrigating fluid which produces circulatory overload, hyposmolarity, and hyponatremia. The development and clinical presentation of the syndrome are dependent on the type of irrigating fluid employed, as well as the amount and the rate of absorption. Increased serum glycine levels may also be a consequence of the use of glycine irrigating fluid. Ammonia, the metabolic by-product of glycine, as well as glycine may contribute to the development of this clinical condition.

The anesthetist must accurately recognize the onset of TUR syndrome and institute corrective measures. Intraoperative changes in mental status are easily recognized in lightly sedated patients during regional anesthesia. As previously discussed, a sensory blockade to T-10 provides a quiet surgical field and sufficient sensory blockade for TURP. The selection of a regional technique would allow the observation of cardiovascular and CNS changes during the intraoperative period. Marx and Orkin describe a clinical triad of subjective signs for the identification of ir-

TABLE 30–6. CLINICAL PRESENTATION OF TRANSURETHRAL RESECTION SYNDROME

	Symptoms	
Onset	**Cardiovascular/ Respiratory**	**Central Nervous System**
Early	Angina	Anxiety/apprehension
	Bradycardia	
	Hypertension	Disorientation
	Increased central venous pressure	Visual disturbances
		Nausea/vomiting
Late	Electrocardiographic changes	Stupor
		Seizures
	Pulmonary edema	Coma

Reprinted, with permission, from Aasheim.[47]

TABLE 30–7. CLINICAL PRESENTATION OF HYPONATREMIA

Serum Concentration (mEq/L)	Electrocardiographic Changes	Central Nervous System Symptoms
120	Widened QRS (?)	Restlessness Confusion
115	Widened QRS ST elevation	Nausea Stupor
100	Ventricular tachycardia Ventricular fibrillation	Seizure Coma

Reprinted, with permission, from Jenson V. Can J Anaesth. 1991;38:92.

rigating fluid absorption.[35] These signs include (1) a rise in systolic and diastolic blood pressure, with an increase in pulse pressure (the difference between systolic and diastolic pressure); (2) a decrease in pulse rate; and (3) the presentation of CNS symptoms such as restlessness, confusion, headache, nausea and vomiting, with progression to a stuporous state. Hypoxia and cyanosis may also accompany these changes.[35] During general anesthesia, the anesthetist would observe the hemodynamic changes that accompany fluid overload (increases in systolic and diastolic pressure

and increasing pulse pressure); however, the subjective CNS symptoms would not be possible to evaluate.

Figure 30–10 illustrates the steps for the initiation of treatment for the TUR syndrome. A delay in the identification and treatment may result in progression of the syndrome, creating further complications such as pulmonary edema, cardiovascular collapse, and death. Fluid overload should be initially treated with the administration of a loop diuretic (Lasix) followed in the postoperative course with fluid restriction. The surgeon should be notified and the operative procedure promptly concluded. Increased concentrations of oxygen should be administered by nasal cannula or mask. Endotracheal intubation and positive-pressure ventilation may be required for the patient who develops pulmonary edema. Oxygenation and ventilation can be assessed with arterial blood gas analysis. A serum sodium level should be determined. The acute treatment of hyponatremia may be initiated with the intravenous administration of hypertonic saline. Hypertonic saline (3 or 5 percent) is slowly infused until the serum sodium concentration returns to 120 mEq/L. The use of hypertonic saline solutions for the acute correction of hyponatremia is not without clinical complications. Rapid correction of hyponatremia with hypertonic saline solutions has been associated with cerebral demyelinating lesions.[54]

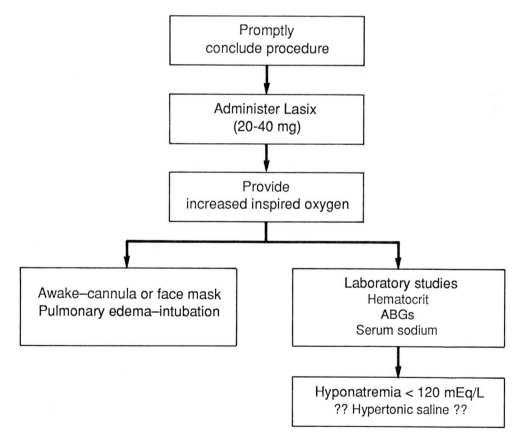

Figure 30–10. Flow diagram illustrating the initiating treatment for transurethral resection (TUR) syndrome. ABGs, arterial blood gases.

Blood Loss. The visual determination of blood loss in this procedure is inexact as the anesthetist frequently underestimates or overestimates the actual loss.[54,55] The irrigating fluid is drained from the bladder into a receptacle inserted into the floor or may be drained into a "kick bucket." This collection of irrigating fluid makes it impossible to visually determine the blood loss. The reliance on hemodynamic changes (tachycardia, hypotension) as an evaluation of blood loss is unreliable as the intravascular absorption of irrigating fluid may mask these signs. Serial determinations of hematocrit during the intraoperative period may also be inaccurate as a result of intravascular absorption.

Levin and his colleagues have found that blood loss is correlated with the size of the prostate and the duration of resection.[56] The blood loss during TURP has been estimated to be 15 mL per gram of prostate tissue.[56] Mebust and his colleagues contend that blood loss is typically 500 mL per 25 g of prostate.[57]

Blood loss can be excessive. With the intravascular absorption of irrigating fluid, a dilutional thrombocytopenia may develop. With prostatic resection, tissue thromboplastin may be released into the circulation, leading to the development of a coagulopathy (see Fig. 30–10).[58] The released tissue thromboplastin stimulates the conversion of plasminogen to plasmin, leading to the breakdown of fibrin, producing a diffuse disseminated coagulopathy.

Extracorporeal Shock Wave Lithotripsy

Extracorporeal shock wave lithotripsy (ESWL) has evolved as the predominant method for the treatment of urolithiasis. Approximately 85 percent of patients with urinary tract stones are treated with ESWL.[59] There are two prevalent types of lithotripsy machines being used in the United States. The first-generation lithotripter, the Dornier HM3, necessitates the immersion of the patient in a water bath after the induction of anesthesia. The second-generation lithotripters (Siemens Lithostar and the Dornier HM4) eliminate the use of a water bath.

Immersion Extracorporeal Shock Wave Lithotripsy. Immersion ESWL necessitates the placement of the patient in a lawn-chair position in a hydraulic gantry which is subsequently lowered into a water bath. An underwater spark plug with a current of 18,000 to 24,000 V produces a high-voltage discharge within a brass ellipsoid at the base of the water bath (Fig. 30–11). The shock wave is triggered by the patient's electrocardiogram and fires 20 milliseconds after the R-wave to avoid the development of shock wave-generated arrhythmias. Subsequently to this discharge, a shock wave is generated as a result of the explosive evaporation of water. A single shock wave with a force of approximately 15,000 pounds per square inch is generated with each high-voltage discharge. With the use of dual-axis fluoroscopy and hydraulic alignment of the gantry, the urologist precisely positions the patient, orientating the urinary stone within the focal point of the generated shock wave. The typical ESWL treatment consists of approximately 1000 to 2000 repetitive shocks. The imposing mechanical stresses disintegrate the stone into fine fragments which may be passed in the urine.

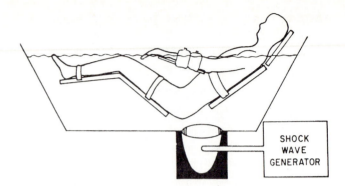

Figure 30–11. For extracorporeal shock wave lithotripsy, the patient is positioned on a gantry (movable frame) and lowered into the water bath until immersed. The arms are supported by arm floats. (*Reprinted, with permission, from Liu WS, Wong KC. Anesthesia for genitourinary surgery. In: Barash PG, Cullen BF, Stoelting RK, eds.* Clinical anesthesia. *Philadelphia: JB Lippincott; 1989:1113.*)

Table 30–8 lists the contraindications for the use of ESWL. Patients over 52 in. in height and under 295 lb (135 kg) are suitable candidates. The presence of a transvenous pacemaker is a relative contraindication. Although patients with ventricular inhibited pacemakers have been successfully treated, some of the new programmable pacemakers may be damaged if the shock wave is directed toward the pacemaker generator.

A general or regional anesthetic technique is required when the energy levels meet or exceed 18,000 V. Although the shock wave energy is directed at the urinary stone, the generated energy is partially released at the entry and exit sites (the patient's flank and anterior chest wall). Patients experience varying degrees of discomfort (described as a burning or bruising sensation) with each shock wave. The patient must also remain motionless to maintain the orientation of the urinary stone within the focal point of the shock wave.

The second-generation lithotripters have eliminated the use of a water bath. Shock waves are generated within an enclosed water container surrounded by a plastic membrane that is placed against the patient. The shock wave is triggered by the patient's respiration or by the R-wave of the electrocardiogram (ECG). Anesthesia requirements are minimal with these lithotripters. Intravenous sedation with the administration of small doses of a benzodiazepine and narcotic produces a comfortable and cooperative patient. The application of a transcutaneous electrical nerve stimula-

TABLE 30–8. CONTRAINDICATIONS TO EXTRACORPOREAL SHOCK WAVE LITHOTRIPSY

Contraindication	Examples
Abnormal laboratory findings	Coagulopathies
Implanted devices	Lumbar orthopedic implants Transvenous pacemaker
Altered physiology	Obesity (>135 kg) Abdominal aortic aneurysm

tion (TENS) unit without the use of intravenous sedation has been demonstrated to provide comfort for over 90 percent of patients requiring fewer than 3000 shock waves for stone destruction.[60]

Physiologic Changes with Immersion. Immersion produces tangible alterations of the cardiovascular, respiratory, renal, and gastrointestinal systems (Table 30–9). These alterations appear to be sustained for the duration of immersion. For every 1 ft of immersion, an external pressure of 22.4 mm Hg is produced. The hydrostatic pressure compresses the peripheral veins of the lower extremities and abdomen, producing an increase in venous return and preload. Central venous pressure and blood volume increase with an accompanying increase in cardiac output and blood pressure and a reflexive decrease in heart rate.[61] The increase in blood pressure with immersion usually offsets the modest drop that follows the induction of general anesthesia or the sympathetic block produced with regional anesthesia. The patient with borderline cardiac reserve (i.e., congestive heart failure) may not tolerate this sudden increase in central blood volume. Immersion of patients with borderline cardiac reserve should be instituted slowly with vigilant cardiovascular monitoring.

Hydrostatic pressure compresses the thorax, producing a 30 to 36 percent decrease in the functional residual capacity (decreased expiratory reserve volume) as well as an 8 to 22 percent decrease in vital capacity.[62] Airway resistance is also noted to increase.[62]

Body temperature may also be altered during ESWL. Neglect of the water bath temperature may result in the development of hypothermia or hyperthermia. The water bath should be maintained at 37C to avoid shivering. Shivering precipitated by hypothermia may produce excessive patient movement, redirecting the focus of the shock wave, and create a poor ECG signal which would interfere with the triggering of the shock wave. Hypothermia can be prevented with the maintenance of an adequate room temperature and the prompt drying and covering of the patient after removal from the water bath.

Anesthetic Management. The immersion of the patient in the water bath complicates the anesthetic management, as the patient is remote from the anesthesia machine and mon-

itoring devices. Water immersion may loosen tape that secures the intravenous line and digital pulse oximetry, and dislodge ECG pads from contact with the skin. After the introduction of an intravenous infusion in the hand, a latex glove may be applied over the hand, and the cuff of the glove secured with additional surgical adhesive drape. Additional invasive monitoring catheters can also be protected with application of adhesive surgical drape. Immersion jeopardizes the function of a digital pulse oximetry probe. Placement of the patient's hand on the side of the water tank will prevent water contact. The application of a nasal pulse oximetry probe will ensure uninterrupted function. It is imperative that a faultless ECG signal be obtained to ensure proper triggering of the shock waves. ECG electrodes should be placed high on each shoulder, with the third electrode placed high in the left midaxillary line. The electrodes can be covered with a 2×2 gauze pad followed by the application of a clear surgical adhesive drape to ensure a watertight seal. The Velcro closure on the noninvasive blood pressure cuff may be ineffectual after immersion. The cuff may be supported with a light wrap of adhesive tape around the cuff. Protected positioning of the patient in the gantry is mandatory. Great detail should be paid to positioning, and this should be properly reflected on the anesthetic record (see Chapter 13).

The patient is strapped in a lawn-chair position in the gantry with the arms placed above the head prior to immersion in the water bath. The patient cart should follow the movement of the gantry as the patient is moved toward the water bath. After immersion, the arms may be placed on the sides of the water tub or allowed to float.

Both general and regional anesthesia have been successfully employed for ESWL. The induction of general anesthesia is facilitated with a short-acting intravenous induction agent with the patient on the transport cart prior to transfer to the hydraulic gantry. Endotracheal intubation is mandatory to ensure a secure airway during transport to and from the water bath. Anesthesia may be maintained with either an inhalation or narcotic-relaxant technique. Treatment duration is dependent on the patient's intrinsic heart rate. The use of vagotonic narcotics may prolong the procedure. The Dornier HM3 can sense an intrinsic heart rate as fast as 120 beats per minute. To hasten the procedure, heart rate can be pharmacologically manipulated with the intravenous administration of atropine or glycopyrrolate. This should be cautiously executed in the patient with ischemic coronary artery disease.

Considerable attention has been directed to the mode of ventilation employed during general anesthesia for ESWL, as diaphragmatic excursion may move the stone out of the focal point of the generated shock wave. Minimizing stone movement may increase the success rate of stone destruction. High-frequency jet ventilation (HFJV) and high-frequency positive-pressure ventilation (HFPPV) have been advocated to minimize stone movement; however, there appears to be no difference in the treatment outcome after the use of either technique.[63] A satisfactory alternative to HFPPV and HFJV is the use of small tidal volumes (300 mL) delivered with a conventional volume ventilator, with the adjustment of the respiratory rate to achieve a normal end-tidal carbon dioxide.[63]

TABLE 30–9. PHYSIOLOGICAL CHANGES ACCOMPANYING IMMERSION DURING EXTRACORPOREAL SHOCK WAVE LITHOTRIPSY

System	Physiological Alteration
Cardiovascular	Increased preload
	Increased cardiac output
	Increased blood pressure
Respiratory	Decreased functional residual capacity (30–36%)
	Decreased vital capacity (20%)
Temperature	Hyperthermia
	Hypothermia
Gastrointestinal	Increased gastric reflux

Both spinal and continuous epidural regional techniques have been successfully used; however, a continuous epidural technique is advantageous as the duration of the procedure is unpredictable. A sensory blockade between T-4 and T-6 provides satisfactory anesthesia. Preservative-free saline rather than air should be used for the "loss of resistance" technique when identifying the epidural space, as the presence of epidural air may decrease the shock wave energy. Likewise, the presence of air in Microfoam tape that may be used to secure the epidural catheter may decrease the successful destruction of the stone.[64] After advancement into the epidural space, the insertion site and catheter can be covered with a surgical adhesive drape to establish a watertight seal.

The judicious titration of midazolam and a short-acting narcotic (fentanyl or alfentanil) will provide anxiolysis and supplemental analgesia. As previously discussed, immersion produces restrictive changes in respiratory mechanics, requiring vigilant monitoring during the administration of sedatives. The generation of shock waves produces a great deal of noise which is particularly disturbing to the patient. The sound that accompanies shock wave generation can be suppressed with the application of protective headphones. The patient is instructed to remain motionless during the treatment. A predetermined patient gesture such as the movement of a hand can alert the anesthetist and allow the cessation of shock wave delivery if a problem arises.

REFERENCES

1. Harrison TS. The thyroid gland. Historical aspects and anatomy. In: Sabiston D, ed. *Textbook of surgery.* Philadelphia: WB Saunders; 1986:579.

2. Conrardy PA, Goodman LR, Lainge F, Singer MM. Alteration of endotracheal tube position: Flexion and extension of the neck. *Crit Care Med.* 1976;4:8–12.

3. Wase AW, Fostyer WC. Thiopental and thyroid metabolism. *Proc Soc Exp Biol Med.* 1956;91:89–91.

4. Wood M, Berman ML, Harbison RD, Hoyle P, Phython JM, Wood AJJ. Halothane-induced hepatic necrosis in triiodothyronine-pretreated rats. *Anesthesiology.* 1980;52:470–476.

5. Collins VJ. Monitoring in anesthesia. In: Collins VJ, ed. *Principles of anesthesiology.* Philadelphia: Lea & Febiger; 1980:83.

6. Linton RAF. Structure and function of the respiratory tract. In: Churchill Davidson HC, ed. *A practice of anesthesia.* Chicago: Year Book Medical; 1984;14–15.

7. McKernan JB. Laparoscopic cholecystectomy. *Am Surg.* 1991;57:311.

8. Nahrwold, DL. Chronic cholecystitis and cholelithiasis. In: Sabiston DC Jr, ed. *Textbook of surgery.* Philadelphia: WB Saunders; 1986:1147.

9. Nahrwold DL. The biliary system. In: Sabiston DC Jr, ed. *Textbook of surgery.* Philadelphia: WB Saunders; 1986.

10. Radney PA, Duncalf D, Novakovic M, Lesser ML. Common bile duct pressure changes after fentanyl, morphine, meperidine, butorphanol, and naloxone. *Anesth Analg.* 1984;63:441–444.

11. Tam S, Chung F, Campbell M. Intravenous lidocaine: Optimal time of injection before endotracheal intubation. *Anesth Analg.* 1987;66:1036–1038.

12. Levy JH. *Anaphylactic reactions in anesthesia and intensive care.* Boston: Butterworths; 1986.

13. Shehadi WH, Toniolo G. Adverse reactions to contrast media. *Radiology.* 1980;136:299–302.

14. Ansell G, Tweedie MCK, West CR, Evans P, Cough L. The current status of reactions to intravascular contrast media. *Invest Radiol.* 1980;15:532–539.

15. Greenberger P, Patterson R, Kelly J, Stevenson DD, Simon R, Liberman P. Administration of radiographic contrast media in high risk patients. *Invest Radiol.* 1980;15:540–543.

16. McKernan JB, Saye WB. Laparoscopic laser appendectomy with argon laser. *South Med J.* 1990;83:84.

17. Semm K. Endoscopic appendectomy. *Endoscopy.* 1983;15:59–64.

18. Reddick EJ, Olsen DO. Laparoscopy laser cholecystectomy: A comparison with mini-lap cholecystectomy. *Surg Endosc.* 1989;3:131–133.

19. DuBois F, Icard P, Berthelot G, Levard H. Coelioscopic cholecystectomy. Preliminary report of 36 cases. *Ann Surg.* 1990;211:60–62.

20. Schirmer BD, Edge SB, Dix J, Hysner MJ, Hanks JB, Jones RS. Laparoscopy cholecystectomy: Treatment of choice for symptomatic cholelithiasis. *Ann Surg.* 1991;213:665.

21. Motew M, Iavanovich AD, Bieniarz J, Albrecht RF, Zabed B, Scommenga A. Cardiovascular effects and acid base and blood gas during laparoscopy. *Am J Obstet Gynecol.* 1973;155:1002–1012.

22. Wittgen CM, Andrus CH, Fitzgerald SD, Baudendistel LJ, Dahms TE, Kaminski DL. Analysis of the hemodynamic and ventilatory effects of laparoscopic cholecystectomy. *Arch Surg.* 1991;1265:997–1001.

23. Wilson RE. The breast. In: Sabiston DC Jr, ed. *Textbook of surgery.* Philadelphia: WB Saunders; 1986:541.

24. Gaster J. *Hernia: One day repair.* Darien, CT: Hafner; 1970.

25. Ryan JA Jr, Adye BA, Jolly PC, et al. Outpatient inguinal herniorrhaphy with both regional and local anesthesia. *Am J Surg.* 1984;148:313–316.

26. Flaatten H. Spinal anesthesia for outpatient surgery. *Anaesthesia.* 1985;40:1108–1111.

27. Tanagho EA. Anatomy and surgical approach to the urogenital tract. In: Walsh PC, Gitts RF, Perlmutter AD, Stamey TA, eds. *Campbell's urology.* Philadelphia: WB Saunders; 1986.

28. Chaussy C, Schmiedt E, Jochiam O, et al. First clinical experience with extracorporeal induced destruction of kidney stones by shock waves. *J Urol.* 1982;127:417.

29. Bors E. The challenge of quadriplegia. *Bull LA Neurol Soc.* 1956;21:105.

30. Bendo AA, Griffin JP, Cottrell JE. Anesthetic and surgical management of acute and chronic spinal cord injury. In: Cottrell JE, Turndorf H, eds. *Anesthesia and neurosurgery.* St. Louis, MO: CV Mosby; 1986:399–401.

31. Guttman L, Whitteridge D. Effects of bladder distension on autonomic mechanisms after spinal cord injury. *Brain.* 1947;70:361.

32. Lambert DH, Deane RS, Mazuzan JE. Anesthesia and control of blood pressure in patients with spinal cord injury. *Anesth Analg.* 1982;61:344.

33. Kenyon HR. Perforation in transurethral operations: Technique for immediate diagnosis and management of extravasation. *JAMA.* 1950;142:798.

34. Simpson RA. Rupture of the bladder during transurethral resection of the prostate and possibility of aid by anesthesiologist in its diagnosis. *Urol Cutan Rev.* 1946;50:628.

35. Marx GF, Orkin LR. Complications associated with transurethral surgery. 1962;23:6;809–810.

36. Holtgrewe HL, Valk WL. Factors influencing the mortality and morbidity of transurethral prostatectomy: A study of 2015 cases. *J Urol.* 1962;87:450.

37. Scheller MS, Unger RJ, Kelner MJ. Effects of intravenously administered dyes on pulse oximetry readings. *Anesthesiology.* 1986;65:550–552.

38. Holtgrewe HL, Mebust WK, Dowd JB, et al. Transurethral prostatectomy: Practice aspects of the dominant operation in American urology. *J Urol.* 1989;141:248–253.

39. Mebust WK. Transurethral prostatectomy. *Urol Clin North Am.* 1990;17:577.

40. Mebust WK, Holtgrewe HL, Cockett ATK, et al. Transurethral prostatectomy immediate and postoperative complications: A cooperative study of 13 participating institutions evaluating 3,885 patients. *J Urol.* 1989;141:243–247.

41. Fillman EM, Hanson OL, Gilbert LO. Radioisotopic study of effects of irrigating fluid in transurethral prostatectomy. *JAMA.* 1959;171:1488.

42. Madsen PO, Naber KG. The importance of the pressure in the prostatic fossa and absorption of irrigating fluid during transurethral resection of the prostate. *J Urol.* 1973;109:446–452.

43. Hagstrom RS, Dennise SA, Rowland HS, et al. Studies on fluid absorption during transurethral prostate resection. *J Urol.* 1955;73:852.

44. Oester A, Madsen PO. Determination of absorption of irrigating fluid during transurethral resection of the prostate by means of radioisotopes. *J Urol.* 1969;102:714–719.

45. Hahn R, Berlin T, Lewenhaupt A. Irrigating fluid absorption and blood loss during transurethral resection of the prostate studied with regular interval monitoring (RIM). *Scand J Urol Nephrol.* 1988;22:23–30.

46. Creevy CD, Webb EA. A fatal hemolytic reaction following transurethral resection of the prostate gland: A discussion of its prevention and treatment. *Surgery.* 1947;21:56–66.

47. Aasheim GM. Hyponatremia during transurethral surgery. *Can Anaesth Soc J.* 1973;20:247.

48. Desmond J. Serum osmolality and plasma electrolytes in patients who develop dilutional hyponatremia during transurethral resection. *Can Anaesth Soc J.* 1970;17:25.

49. Gecelter LG, Gascoigne H. Safety and efficacy of a 1.5 percent glycine solution as an irrigation medium in prostatic surgery. *S Afr Med J.* 1984;65:693–694.

50. Richter JJ. Current theories about the mechanisms of benzodiazepines and neuroleptic drugs. *Anesthesiology.* 1981;54:67.

51. Ovassapian A, Joshi CW, Brunner EA. Visual disturbance: An unusual symptom of transurethral prostate resection reaction. *Anesthesiology.* 1982;57:332.

52. Creel DJ, Wang JML, Wong KC. Transient blindness associated with transurethral resection of the prostate. *Arch Ophthalmol.* 1987;105:1537.

53. Roesch RP, Stoelting RK, Lingman JE, Kahnoski RJ, Backes DJ, Gephardt SA. Ammonia toxicity resulting from glycine absorption during a transurethral resection of the prostate. *Anesthesiology.* 1983;58:577–579.

54. Clough D, Higgins P. Discrepancies in estimating blood loss. *Am J Nurs.* 1981;2:331–333.

55. Lucas WJ, Tyler EP. Errors in estimating blood loss. *Anesthesiology.* 1989(September suppl):A99.

56. Levin K, Nyren O, Pompeius R. Blood loss, tissue weight, and operating time in transurethral prostatectomy. *Scand J Urol Nephrol.* 1981;15:197.

57. Mebust WK, Foret JD, Valk WL. Transurethral surgery. In: Harrison JH, Gittes RF, Perlmutter AD, Walsh PC, Stamey TA, eds. *Campbell's urology.* 4th ed. Philadelphia: WB Saunders; 1979:2367.

58. Freidman NJ, Hoag MS, Robinson AJ, Aggeler PM. Hemorrhagic syndrome following transurethral prostate resection for benign adenoma. *Arch Intern Med.* 1969;124:341–349.

59. Clayman RV, McClennan BL, Garvin TJ, Denstedt JD, Andriole GL. Lithostar: An electromagnetic acoustic shock wave unit for extracorporeal lithotripsy. *J Endourol.* 1989;3:307.

60. Fernandez J, Clayman RV, Gray D, et al. Transcutaneous electric nerve stimulator: An approach to anesthesia-free shock wave lithotripsy with the Lithostar unit. In: Lingeman JE, Newman DM, eds. *Shock wave lithotripsy: State of the art.* New York: Plenum Press; 1988.

61. Behnia R, Shanks CA, Ovassapian A, Wilson LA. Hemodynamic responses associated with lithotripsy. *Anesth Analg.* 1987;66:354.

62. Duvall J, Griffith D. Epidural anesthesia for extracorporeal shock wave lithotripsy. *Anesth Analg.* 1985;64(5):80–87.

63. Zetlin GL, Roth RA. Effect of three anesthetic techniques on the success of extracorporeal shock wave lithotripsy in nephrolithiasis. *Anesthesiology.* 1988;68:272–276.

64. Pandit SK, Powell RB, Crider B, McLaren ID, Rutter T. Epidural fentanyl is not effective for analgesia for extracorporeal lithotripsy (ESWL). *Anesthesiology.* 1988;68:176.

Obstetric Anesthesia and Analgesia

*Charles H. Moore,
Norman H. Blass, and
Jonathan H. Skerman*

Obstetric anesthesia has developed into a recognized specialty within the field of anesthesia. Historically, nurse anesthetists have played an integral role in the care of the parturient. To continue to provide optimal care to the mother and fetus, nurse anesthetists must be cognizant of the basic principles and advances in this evolving anesthesia specialty.

PHYSIOLOGIC CHANGES DURING PREGNANCY

Pregnancy produces profound physiologic changes in all major organ systems.[1] The cardiovascular system shows alterations as early as 5 to 8 weeks of gestation. Cardiac output starts to increase in early pregnancy, reaches its zenith at approximately 30 to 34 weeks of gestation, and then declines toward term. There had been some dispute about the rate of decline in maternal cardiac output as term approaches. It is now known that many factors modify cardiac output, including age of the mother, maternal position (especially near term), pain of uterine contractions, bearing down efforts of Valsalva maneuvers, type of delivery, and type of anesthesia/analgesia.[2]

The cardiovascular system imposes significant demands on the pregnant mother, but these demands are usually well tolerated during gestation; however, the parturient with heart disease or reduced cardiac reserve may not be able to meet the increased requirement during pregnancy or labor.[3] During pregnancy, red blood cell volume, total blood volume, and total plasma volume all increase. As the increase in total blood volume is greater than that in red cell volume, physiologic anemia ensues. The total blood volume is usually 40 percent above the nonpregnant state but is ordinarily well tolerated by the gravida.[4]

There is a slight fall in both systolic and diastolic pressure during the midtrimester of pregnancy, but a return to the nonpregnant or early trimester level usually occurs in the last trimester. The white blood cell count also increases during pregnancy. The reason for this is not obvious, but the increase may be estrogen induced. In the attempt to evaluate leukocytosis as an indicator of infection, the shift to the left of the white blood cell count is more important than the actual rise in the blood count itself.[5]

Pregnancy produces a hypercoagulable state in the parturient. It is known that there is a change in the coagulation mechanism, with an increase in fibrinogen, prothrombin, and factors VII, VIII, IX, and X and augmentation of the fibrolytic inhibitors. There is a decrease in the concentrations of factors XI and XIII; however, a triggering mechanism is needed to begin the coagulation mechanism.[1]

Respiratory System

The enlarging uterus produces a mechanical change in the configuration of the abdomen and a concomitant rise in the diaphragm of approximately 4 cm. There is an increase in the transverse and anteroposterior diameter of the thoracic cage plus an outward and upward movement of the rib cage. This produces alterations in the lung volume during pregnancy. These alterations in lung volume usually occur at approximately 4 to 5 months of gestation, so that at term the expiratory reserve capacity is reduced 20 to 25 percent from the nonpregnant state; however, respiratory capacity increases so there is compensation. Minute alveolar ventilation is increased. This is produced by a mild increase in the respiratory rate and a greater increase in the depth of the ventilatory tidal volume. Hyperventilation occurs producing a mild respiratory alkalosis. A decrease in the functional residual capacity at term is a constant finding. This decrease is exaggerated by the supine or Trendelenburg position, which is usually assumed by the patient on the delivery or operating table. (This accentuation does not occur in the sitting position.)

The decrease in functional residual capacity and the increased alveolar ventilation facilitate washout of anesthetic gases, producing rapid induction of general anesthesia, especially with the more volatile inhalation agents. The reduced functional residual capacity and the low $Paco_2$ in the pregnant patient can lead to a rather precipitous decline in Pao_2 during periods of apnea. Denitrogenation prior to the induction of general anesthesia and before intubation is thus essential to minimize the risk of hypoxemia.

Maternal PaO_2 is increased because of the increased alveolar ventilation. Nevertheless, airway closure occurs at normal tidal volume range in many parturients approaching term. This is particularly prevalent in the supine position and may lead to ventilation–perfusion abnormalities and reduced PaO_2. Hyperventilation and mechanical positive-pressure ventilation may reduce uterine blood flow and fetal oxygenation. Similarly, the distraught hyperventilation of uncontrolled labor patients may be detrimental to the fetus, and it is not unusual to see maternal carbon dioxide levels as low as 20 to 25 mm Hg and pH levels as high as 7.65.[5]

Central Nervous System

The dosage of local anesthetics used in conduction anesthesia during pregnancy should be less than that used for nonpregnant patients. Epidural veins are swollen, leading to a diminution in the size of the epidural and subarachnoid spaces; this is the cause of the reduced amount of local anesthetic required.

There is an increase in cerebrospinal fluid pressure, which may be the reason for the high dermatome level of spread of local anesthetics during pregnancy. There is a reduction in minimal alveolar concentration (MAC) during pregnancy. The cause is not known, but it may be related to the sedative effects of progesterone.[6]

Gastrointestinal Tract

As the pregnancy progresses, the enlarging uterus pushes the intestines and the stomach cephalad. This contributes to the increase in the risk of regurgitation and pulmonary aspiration. There is a rise in intragastric pressure, particularly when the patient is in the lithotomy or modified lithotomy position, and there is a decrease in gastroesophageal sphincter tone. The motility of the stomach is reduced, and there is an increase in gastric contents as well as a reduction in gastric pH. During labor, anxiety and pain also tend to reduce the motility of the stomach, delaying emptying time even further and increasing gastric acidity and volume.

The administration of an antacid to women in labor has been shown to increase gastric pH, although pulmonary aspiration of particulate matter is still possible. Clear antacids such as 0.3 M sodium bicitrate have become the accepted standard. Several measures are recommended to minimize the risk of maternal aspiration:

1. Avoid general anesthesia if possible.
2. Administer prophylactic antacid.
3. Employ rapid-sequence induction of anesthesia when indicated, using intubation with cricoid pressure and a cuffed endotracheal tube.
4. Avoid positive-pressure ventilation prior to intubation and inflation of the endotracheal tube cuff.[7]

Although results of many liver function tests are altered during pregnancy, the appropriate dose of drugs such as succinylcholine is safe to use.

Renal, Endocrine, and Metabolic Changes

Progesterone contributes to the dilation of the smooth muscle of the kidney, pelvis, and ureters starting as early as the third month of gestation. As the pregnant uterus enlarges, the growing uterus encroaches on the ureters, producing a mechanical cause of kidney dilation.

There is a gradual increase in renal blood flow and glomerular filtration, leading to a lowering of blood urea nitrogen (BUN) and creatinine. A patient whose creatinine and BUN are in the normal range for nonpregnant females may be abnormal when pregnant. The anesthetist must be aware of this prior to the administration of potentially nephrotoxic drugs. As tubular reabsorption of increased amounts of glucose filtered by the glomerulus is relatively fixed, glycosuria during pregnancy is not uncommon.

Pregnancy induces increased activity of the endocrine system. The pituitary gland enlarges during pregnancy, producing more adrenotropic and thyrotropic hormones along with prolactin.

The elevated basal metabolic rate during pregnancy has been attributed to pregnancy per se, but studies have shown that this apparent hypermetabolic state is produced by the needs of the fetus for increased oxygen.

There is an increase in thyroxine-binding globulin produced by the excess amount of estrogen in the pregnant state, and there is an increase in the size of the thyroid gland over the nonpregnant state. During pregnancy, results of thyroid function tests must be interpreted carefully.

The adrenal gland produces more aldosterone, and the parathyroid glands show enlargement. The pancreas is stimulated to increase insulin production, in response to the diabetogenic action of pregnancy.

Maternal metabolism and oxygen consumption increase steadily throughout gestation, and metabolism of protein, fat, and carbohydrate is altered.[8]

MATERNAL AND FETAL PHARMACOLOGY

Most drugs administered to a pregnant woman readily cross the placenta, although a few of large molecular size do not. Although it is true that more consideration is given to drugs administered to the mother during labor and delivery, a number of studies have shown that there is a tendency for pregnant women to take medications throughout pregnancy. The number of drugs taken by any patient during pregnancy averages from 5 to 10: 80 percent of these are taken without a physician's knowledge or supervision.

The drugs most frequently used during labor and delivery are analgesics, sedatives, tranquilizers, and local and general anesthetics. It is axiomatic that almost all medication can be found in the fetus within minutes of administration to the mother.[9]

For years it was believed that the placenta was a barrier to the passage of drugs from mother to baby. It is now known that nonionized, fat-soluble, low-molecular-weight drugs are transferred rapidly.

Most muscle relaxants in the usual dosage pass poorly from the mother to fetus, but in doses of high magnitude they readily cross the placenta. Anesthetic gases, narcotics, and barbiturates pass readily. Nitrous oxide approaches 80 percent of the maternal level in about 10 minutes. Pregnancy-induced hypertension (toxemia) and other maternal diseases may interfere with this so-called placental barrier and may allow even more rapid and complete transfer.

Fetal brain concentration of medication can be reduced by giving an intravenous dose at the time of a uterine contraction so that less drug will go to the fetus because of the placental vasoconstriction. Fetal liver metabolism and the dilution of drugs in the fetal circulation prior to their reaching the fetal brain also contribute to a lessening of the anesthetic effect.

Whether any drug that is given to the mother has an adverse effect on the fetus or the mother can be determined only by direct observation. Ideally, maternally administered analgesics should provide maternal pain relief without any adverse effects on the newborn. We have not achieved this goal, but research efforts of this nature are ongoing. It behooves us, however, to use the minimum amount of anesthetic agents and other drugs to produce any desired effect.

FETAL MONITORING

The rational use of anesthesia for labor and delivery requires careful surveillance and monitoring of the mother, the uteroplacental unit, and the fetus. Changes in physiology of the obstetric patient may affect the fetus. These changes can increase during the progress of parturition and may be further aggravated by the administration of anesthesia.[10]

The electronic fetal heart rate monitor, developed in the United States by Hon and in Europe by Hammacher, has an advantage over intermittent auscultation of the patient in that it provides a continuous beat-to-beat record of the fetal heart rate and a record of uterine activity. Electronic intrapartum fetal heart rate monitoring is now considered mandatory for high-risk pregnancies, but its value for the low-risk parturient is still undetermined. Electronic monitoring accompanied by an evaluation of the fetal acid–base status has given the obstetrician and anesthetist a more comprehensive understanding of the changes in homeostasis that occur in the fetus and possible alterations associated with anesthetic administration.

Antepartum fetal assessment and the evaluation of antepartum fetal well-being using various modalities have been done for years by the obstetrician. Surveillance of the fetus prior to contemplated delivery is ordinarily not in the province of the anesthesiologist or anesthetist; however, knowledge of fetal monitoring during labor and in preparation for delivery is essential.

The various modalities available for intrapartum determination of the fetal status are discussed next.[11]

Phonocardiography

Fetal heart rate signals are obtained through an abdominal microphone but are generally unsatisfactory during labor.

Ultrasound (Abdominal Doppler)

In ultrasound, a transducer directs a low-energy ultrasonic beam toward the fetal heart. A small part of the original signal is reflected back to the transducer. Problems have been encountered in the use of Doppler ultrasound technique to measure beat-to-beat variability, which is one of the earliest and most reliable signs of fetal distress.

Electrocardiography

There are two modes of electronic monitoring: (1) an external mode in which external transducers placed on the maternal abdominal wall are used to determine both fetal heart rate and uterine activity; (2) an internal mode in which a spiral electrode is used to assist in obtaining the fetal electrocardiogram and an intrauterine catheter (or transverse cervical catheter) is used to assess intrauterine pressure.

The technique for obtaining the fetal heart rate by use of the abdominal electrocardiogram (ECG) is associated with problems related to maternal muscle noise and overlapping maternal ECG complexes. Beat-to-beat variability is also difficult to assess by this method. Therefore, this technique is not entirely satisfactory. Attachment of a transcervical bipolar electrode to the fetal presenting part (scalp or buttocks) gives an accurate fetal heart rate, and the beat-to-beat variability can be reliably determined. This direct fetal heart rate determination requires that the fetal membranes be ruptured and that the cervix be dilated at least 1 cm. A complication associated with this technique is a fetal scalp infection rate of approximately 5 percent. Serious scalp difficulties may be seen in approximately 1 of 800 to 1 of 1000 newborn infants.

For years, nurses and physicians have carefully auscultated fetal heart sounds 30 seconds after the end of the uterine contraction to assess fetal well-being during labor. The fetal heart rate frequently was counted for 15 seconds and then multiplied by 4. This was thought to be a reliable indicator of fetal well-being. It has been determined in a well-documented collaborative study that the auscultatory method is of dubious value. Benson and his colleagues[14] demonstrated that there was no correlation between the fetal heart rate as determined with the fetoscope and neonatal condition, except in the most extreme circumstances.

Fetal bradycardia as determined by auscultation is a late finding of fetal distress. By definition, a fetal heart rate above 160 is considered to be tachycardia and a rate below 100 is bradycardia. Some authorities express the opinion that a rate between 100 and 120 should be termed *moderate bradycardia*.

Fetal Heart Rate Patterns

When the fetus is stimulated, as with loud sounds or by uterine contractions, the fetal heart rate often changes. These periodic changes may be either decelerations or accelerations. Accelerations are considered to be a sign of an aroused fetus and are generally indicative of an intact internal fetal milieu; on the other hand, decelerations may reflect a poor fetal status.

Periodic Decelerations

The three major forms of fetal heart rate decelerations are (1) early, (2) late, and (3) variable.

Early Decelerations (Type I). Decelerations are usually greater than 15 beats per minute, begin at the onset of a uterine contraction, and return gradually to baseline after the contraction subsides. Early decelerations are generally due to pressure on the fetal skull causing an increase in intracranial pressure or a decrease in cerebral blood flow. This activates the vagus nerve, producing a decrease in the fetal heart rate. Recovery occurs as the pressure is relieved.

Head compression may occur from uterine contractions, vaginal examinations, fundal pressure, or occasionally from the placement of an internal electronic fetal monitor. Characteristically, early decelerations have a uniform shape and mirror the contraction phase. They begin early in the contraction phase, before the peak of the contraction. The low point of the deceleration occurs at the peak of the contraction. The return to baseline occurs by the end of the contraction. The fetal heart rate rarely drops below 100 beats per minute and the depth of the deceleration keeps pace with the intensity of the contraction. These decelerations are usually associated with normal baseline variability and are repetitive with each contraction. Early decelerations are almost always of little clinical significance.

Late Decelerations (Type II). There is a lag between the onset of the uterine contraction and the deceleration, or between the end of the uterine contraction and the return of the fetal heart to its baseline (Fig. 31–1). The deceleration is uniform and the fetal heart rate seldom drops below 100 beats per minute. Return of the fetal heart rate to baseline after a contraction most often occurs 15 to 20 seconds after the contraction has ceased. Late decelerations are considered ominous, particularly when they occur with more than

50 percent of contractions, and are associated with the loss of beat-to-beat variability. The smoother the late deceleration and the slower the recovery, the more ominous is the pattern. The etiology is thought to be fetal myocardial hypoxia resulting from uteroplacental insufficiency. Characteristically, uterine hyperactivity or maternal hypotension decreases the intervillous space blood during contractions. This hypoxia and myocardial depression activate a vagal response, producing bradycardia. When accompanied by placental dysfunction, there is anaerobic metabolism and the development of lactic acidosis, which then contributes to the deceleration.

Uteroplacental insufficiency may result from the following:

1. Hyperstimulation of the uterus from oxytocin administration
2. Maternal hypotension
3. Toxemia
4. Postmaturity
5. Infection
6. Small-for-gestational-age babies
7. Maternal diabetes
8. Bleeding disorders
9. Maternal cardiac disease

Variable Decelerations (Type III). Variable decelerations generally indicate that the fetus is responding to stress. The

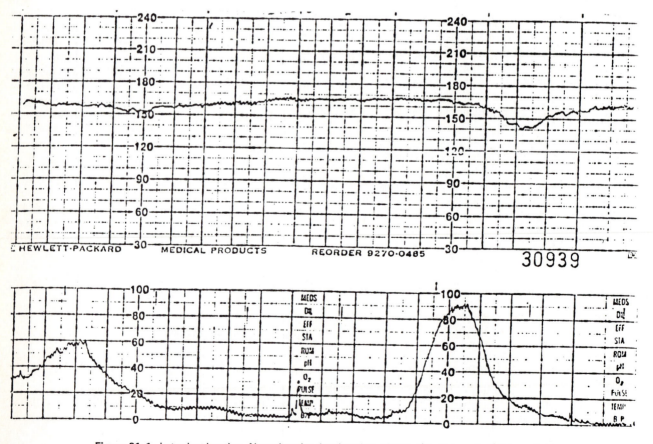

Figure 31–1. Late deceleration. Note that the deceleration occurs after the peak of the contraction.

tracing lacks constancy in its configuration and its time relationship to a uterine contraction. It is the most common variety of deceleration. It is often preceded or followed by a brief period of acceleration. Variable decelerations are thought to be caused by umbilical cord compression and its consequent cardiovascular reflexes. Administration of oxygen to the mother is without effect; this is not the case with a late deceleration. Fetal acidosis may develop if the compression becomes severe, prolonged, or repetitive. Variable decelerations that last more than a minute or manifest a decrease in heart rate to less than 60 beats per minute are indicative of acute distress and can indicate impending death in utero. The pathophysiology of this condition is a transitory umbilical cord compression, and accelerations may occur first. The ensuing hemodynamic changes lead to activation of chemoreceptors and baroreceptors that stimulate the vagus nerve, thus producing the deceleration. The etiology is usually umbilical cord compression resulting from maternal position, cord around a fetal part, short cord, knot in the cord, or prolapsed cord. The fetal heart rate usually is below 100 beats per minute and is frequently associated with average baseline variability (Fig. 31–2). It is not necessarily repetitive.

Short-Term Variability (Beat-to-Beat Variability)

The normal fetal heart rate can be described as having a variance of 6 to 10 beats as seen on an electrocardiographic

tracing (Fig. 31–3). This is due to the interaction of the sympathetic and parasympathetic divisions of the central nervous system. This beat-to-beat variability of the fetal heart rate, as demonstrated by the fluctuation from the baseline, is an indication of normal neurologic control of the heart rate and a measure of fetal reserve. Increased variability usually is produced by fetal stimulation. This may be caused by uterine contractions, fetal activity, and maternal activity. Decreased variability as seen in Figure 31–4 may be brought about by prematurity; the administration of drugs (narcotics, tranquilizers, anesthetics); hypoxia and acidosis; the physiologic state of fetal sleep; and the suppression of cardiac control mechanisms by heart block in the fetus.

The relationship between reduced fetal heart rate variability and hypoxia was noted by Hon and has been successfully demonstrated in an animal model.[11] Normal variability as seen on fetal heart rate tracings can predict a satisfactory neonatal outcome. Clinical studies have demonstrated better acid–base balance and viability in those fetuses with normal variability during labor, regardless of the specific fetal heart rate pattern. There is a greater likelihood of normal neurologic function at 1 year of age in those infants who displayed normal variability in labor when compared with infants displaying reduced variability. Shiffrin showed a significant correlation between normal variability and good Apgar scores.[12] Cetrulo et al[13] found a loss of baseline variability to be a consistent feature of fetal heart rate patterns preceding fetal death. Reduced beat-to-beat vari-

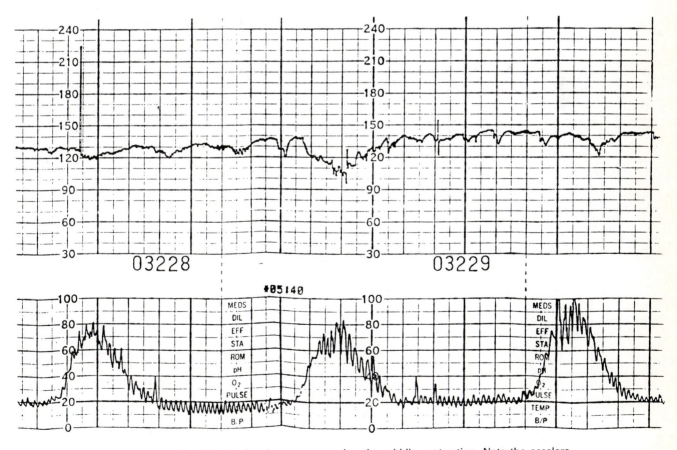

Figure 31–2. Variable deceleration accompanying the middle contraction. Note the acceleration that precedes the deceleration.

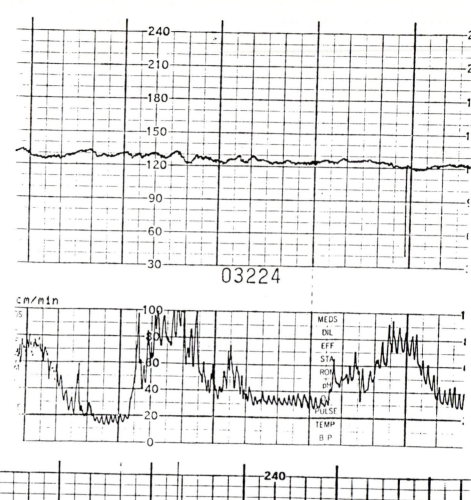

Figure 31–3. Normal heart rate with good beat-to-beat variability.

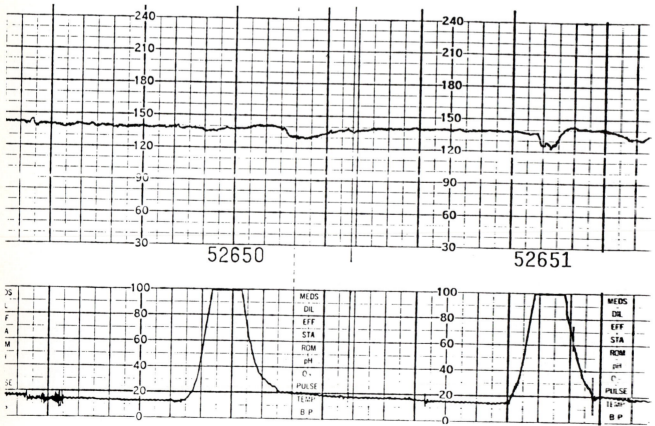

Figure 31–4. Poor beat-to-beat variability with variable decelerations.

ability does not always mean that the fetus is hypoxic because several factors can reduce fetal heart rate variability without reducing fetal oxygen tension: fetal sleep; immaturity; fetal tachycardia; congenital anomalies; drugs such as alphaprodine, secobarbital, and morphine.

Parasympatholytic agents and local anesthetics have been related to diminished variability. Magnesium sulfate has been reported to decrease variability; however, it should be noted that it may actually increase the fetal heart rate because as a uterine relaxant it can increase uterine blood flow.[12]

Prolonged Deceleration

The term *prolonged deceleration* may be applied to a deceleration of the fetal heart rate of more than 30 beats per minute that persists for more than 2 minutes. It may be caused by hypoxia or may be purely reflex in nature. Even in those cases where the deceleration is reflex in nature, hypoxemia may occur because with severe bradycardia fetal cardiac output is reduced. Prolonged decelerations are frequently observed with compression of the umbilical cord and with other hypoxic patterns such as loss of beat-to-beat variability, baseline shifts in fetal heart rate, and late decelerations.

Many factors trigger this reflex or result in sufficient hypoxemia to elicit prolonged decelerations. Hypotension from regional anesthesia, excessive uterine activity, maternal hemorrhage, and supine hypotension can cause fetal bradycardia. Paracervical block in particular has been shown to produce this condition. Management of this pattern requires a coordinated effort in several areas. It occurs frequently in advanced second stage. Delivery can often be accomplished easily by the use of outlet forceps; however, if the patient is not deliverable more conservative action is indicated and preparations should be made for delivery by cesarean section. Fetal monitoring should be continued even into the delivery room to ascertain if the pattern will spontaneously resolve, thereby averting an operative delivery. Concomitant efforts should be directed to correcting the etiology of the uterine hypertonus, decreased uterine blood flow, or cord compression. Changing maternal position, checking for cord prolapse, and correcting any maternal hypotension should be done quickly.

When the maternal condition is satisfactory, most instances of prolonged bradycardia resolve before fetal acidosis occurs and progression to vaginal delivery may be allowed.[13] If the fetal ECG shows improvement in the fetal heart rate, a fetal scalp blood sample can be obtained to help clarify the condition of the fetus. If the intrauterine environment can be improved to allow fetal recovery, the fetus will correct its hypoxia and acidosis more quickly in utero than it will if delivered in a hypoxic state. If no trend toward recovery is observed, delivery should be accomplished as soon as possible by an assisted vaginal delivery or cesarean section.[14] General anesthesia probably is the technique of choice for cesarean section of such a compromised fetus.

Baseline Shifts

As defined previously, fetal heart rate normally ranges between 120 and 160 beats per minute. A rate exceeding this range is considered tachycardia, and a rate below, bradycardia. Fetal tachycardia is commonly seen with chorioamnionitis in which the variability may be reduced and acidosis is also present. Fetal movement, maternal anxiety, and beta-adrenergic stimulation cause fetal tachycardia, but in these situations variability is normal and acidosis is generally absent.

Treatment for Abnormal Fetal Heart Rate Changes

The mother should be turned onto her side preferably to the left initially, which may relieve compression of the umbilical cord and relieves any compression of the aorta and inferior vena cava by the occluding pregnant uterus. Aortocaval compression occurs more frequently when the gravida is supine and if she has had major conduction anesthesia. It should be mandatory that gravidas in labor lie on their side or with a left uterine displacement, rather than supine. The occurrence of this compression syndrome is noncompensated in about 10 percent of patients, even those who have not been administered anesthesia.

If the mother is receiving oxytocin, this should be discontinued immediately to prevent fetal hypoxia caused by the decreased uterine perfusion produced by the drug. Oxygen should be administered to the mother because maternal hyperoxia may alter the uteroplacental insufficiency as manifested by late decelerations.

Correctable causes of abnormal fetal heart rate patterns (such as hypotension) should be treated with fluids and ephedrine should be administered as necessary. Fetal scalp biochemical monitoring should be used in these situations.

Biochemical Monitoring

Fetal scalp sampling was introduced initially as an independent means of fetal surveillance during labor. Most authorities now agree that a combination of heart rate monitoring and fetal scalp sampling is the preferred method of fetal evaluation during labor. Fetal scalp sampling is used when abnormal heart rate patterns occur that cannot be readily abolished or the significance of which cannot be determined. The technique consists of analyzing blood drawn from the fetal scalp for determination of pH, PO_2, PCO_2, and base excess.[15] This scalp sampling may be accomplished with the patient in the lithotomy or Sim's position, on either the labor bed or the delivery table. The cervix must be dilated at least 2 to 3 cm and the presenting part must be in the pelvis. The membranes must be ruptured before the procedure becomes technically feasible. Today most centers determine only the scalp blood pH and the method is generally reserved for situations in which the fetal heart rate pattern is ominous or confusing.

The reliability of capillary blood in assessing fetal acid–base status has been firmly established. Numerous studies have shown that a fetal capillary blood pH of 7.25 or greater can be classified as normal, a pH of 7.20 to 7.24 is preacidotic, and a pH of 7.20 is defined as the lowest limit of normal.[16] Furthermore, a good correlation has been found between the pH of capillary blood and the fetal condition as based on Apgar score. It should be recognized, however, that a single measurement of blood pH may be misleading.

Therefore, if the fetal pH is reported at 7.18, it is recommended that the mother be delivered as expeditiously as possible. When the pH equals or exceeds 7.25, labor is observed and samplings are repeated intermittently. Scalp sampling should be repeated immediately if the fetal heart rate pattern becomes more ominous. If, however, the scalp pH is between 7.18 and 7.25, sampling should be repeated every 15 to 20 minutes until delivery.

Normal fetal pH values are found in approximately 10 percent of infants who are delivered in a depressed condition as reflected by the Apgar score. Some causes for these so-called false normal values follow[17]:

1. Newborn depression from analgesic drugs or anesthesia administered to the mother
2. Infection
3. Maternal hyperventilation
4. Airway obstruction in the newborn infant
5. Prematurity
6. Congenital anomalies
7. Asphyxia occurring between the time of sampling and delivery

Evaluation and Management of Fetal Distress as Determined by Electronic and Biochemical Measurement

Reassuring signs to both obstetrician and anesthesia personnel would be a normal baseline rate, normal baseline variability, and lack of variable or late decelerations.[18] Warning signs would be decreasing variability, increasing baseline rate, variable decelerations with abnormal baseline variability, and meconium staining of amniotic fluid. Ominous signs would be no baseline variability, late decelerations, severe variable decelerations, and bradycardia. With the onset of warning and ominous signs, the position of the patient should be corrected. Uterine activity should be decreased by stopping any oxytocin infusion. If not already being given, oxygen should be administered to the mother at the rate of 6 to 7 L/min with a tight face mask. Preparation should be made for operative delivery.

If the ominous fetal heart rate pattern persists 10 minutes after the initiation of these restorative maneuvers, immediate termination of labor should be considered by the most expeditious means: either vaginal delivery or cesarean section.

ANESTHESIA FOR VAGINAL DELIVERY

Most women experience a great deal of discomfort during labor and delivery. The pain of the first stage of labor is the pain resulting from dilation and effacement of the cervix as well as uterine ischemia because of uterine contractions. This pain is primarily visceral in nature and is transmitted by spinal nerves entering the spinal cord at T-10, T-11, and T-12. In the second stage of labor, there is the addition of somatic pain resulting from the stretching of the vagina and the tearing of the perineum. These impulses are carried via the pudendal nerves entering S-2 to S-4. The degree of discomfort that a parturient may experience cannot be accurately predicted. Ideally, analgesia for labor and delivery should alleviate the pain of labor for the mother and not interfere with the mechanics or progress of labor. There should be no undue risk to the mother or to the fetus. Early bonding between the mother and baby should be possible, and adequate working conditions for the obstetrician should not be ignored.

Obstetric analgesia may be provided by such techniques as acupuncture, hypnosis, and natural childbirth,[19] all of which may play a satisfactory role but are beyond the scope of this chapter. There are many satisfactory books on these subjects.

Analgesia for labor and delivery can be provided by systemic medications such as narcotics, sedatives, tranquilizers, and inhalation analgesia; local anesthetics and regional anesthesia are also used.[20] It is important to remember that all systemic medications used for analgesia or to relieve anxiety rapidly cross the placenta.

Tranquilizers, hypnotics, and amnestics may all be given to the mother to alleviate anxiety, but they assist little in the relief of pain. Use of these drugs with concomitant narcotics may cause the patient to become disoriented and uncontrollable during painful contractions. Most of these drugs are additive in their depressant effects on both the mother and newborn.

Systemic narcotics are frequently used to lessen the pain of the first stage of labor. Analgesic doses of narcotics cause equal maternal and neonatal depression. The primary difference in the narcotics used is the duration of action in the mother. Thus longer-acting narcotics such as meperidine are indicated early in labor, whereas fentanyl is more appropriate toward the end of labor.[9]

Naloxone is a specific narcotic antagonist with no narcotic action of its own. It is effective in both the mother and newborn. Rarely should it be given to the mother before delivery unless another form of analgesia is begun, because it will rapidly antagonize any narcotic analgesia at a time when it is most needed. The neonatal dose of naloxone is 0.1 to 0.2 mg intramuscularly or intravenously. Its duration of action is only about 1 hour, and renarcotization may follow its use. The use of naloxone in patients who are chronic narcotic users or in their newborn children may produce rapid symptoms of narcotic withdrawal. Recent evidence has shown that naloxone may cause problems in patients with cardiovascular disease and probably should be used most cautiously in parturients with compromised cardiac status. Doses of meperidine as low as 50 mg have been associated with decreased Apgar scores at birth and depressed neurobehavioral function. Depression in the newborn may be minimal if delivery occurs within the first hour of intramuscular injection; however, drugs given by the intravenous route may still be associated with newborn depression when delivery rapidly follows drug administration.

Opioid agonist–antagonists such as butorphanol and nalbuphine have the advantage of lower incidence of nausea and vomiting and dysphoria as well as a "ceiling effect" on depression of ventilation. Butorphanol has the disadvantage of producing a high level of maternal sedation, whereas nalbuphine may produce an abstinence syndrome in mothers dependent on morphinelike drugs. Recommended analgesic doses of these agents are 1 to 2 mg IM or IV for butorphanol and 10 mg IV or IM for nalbuphine.

Intermittent Inhalational Analgesia

Intermittent inhalation analgesia involves the administration of synesthetic concentrations of inhalation agents to the mother. Self-administration of volatile inhalational agents during labor and delivery by means of a Duke or Cyprane inhaler, once a popular analgesic technique, has been surpassed by more modern modalities. Nitrous oxide (30 to 40 percent in oxygen with or without a small added concentration of isofluorane) can give satisfactory analgesia for delivery. The use of enflurane in concentrations of 0.5 to 0.8 percent with oxygen has also been effective as an analgesic agent for delivery; however, caution must be exercised in administering enflurane or isofluorane because of the ease of rapid deepening to general anesthesia. When inhalation analgesia is combined with a pudendal block or local infiltration of the perineum, adequate analgesia for episiotomy and outlet forceps delivery can be obtained.[20]

The administration of nitrous oxide with contractions may not be satisfactory because the peak effect of concentration is not reached until 50 seconds after inhalation has begun. Better relief of pain is obtained with continuous administration of 50 percent nitrous oxide and oxygen starting in the delivery room before delivery and continuing through expulsion of the placenta and postpartum examination of the vagina and cervix.

Inhalation analgesia causes little neonatal depression, even when used for long periods. Uterine activity is not depressed, and when inhalation agents are properly administered, the mother remains awake. She maintains the urge to push and can protect her own airways, which minimizes the threat of pulmonary aspiration of stomach contents; however, the depths of analgesia can be rapidly altered and anesthesia may ensue. It is therefore essential that inhalation analgesia be constantly supervised. The mother should be able to answer questions and remain cooperative.

Low-dose ketamine in the range 0.25 to 0.3 mg/kg of maternal body weight provides effective analgesia for vaginal delivery with little or no neonatal depression. There is a minimal amount of hallucinatory response and very little increase in salivation. Ketamine produces profound analgesia and amnesia and as such takes away the mother's ability to relate to her newborn and thus could decrease bonding. As far as the fetus is concerned, there is no hypotonia and apparently no thermoregulatory inhibition, nor is there any decrease in the Apgar score. This particular type of analgesia is most satisfactory in those patients who do not want to view the birth because they are giving the baby up for adoption or because there is a fetal demise and they do not want to be aware of the delivery. In a normal vaginal delivery, low-dose ketamine probably does not contribute much because of the amnesia it produces and today may even be contraindicated by this fact alone.[9]

General anesthesia is rarely required for normal vaginal delivery. It abolishes the bearing down reflex and is associated with neonatal depression correlating with the depth of the anesthesia and the elapsed time until delivery.

General anesthesia, when administered, removes from the mother the awareness of her newborn and definitely increases the risk of pulmonary aspiration. The parturient is particularly prone to aspiration because her stomach usually is not empty even if she has not eaten for a long period, and the enlarged uterus together with the lithotomy position causes a marked rise in intragastric pressure.

When general anesthesia is necessary, it is mandatory to intubate the trachea with a cuffed endotracheal tube. It may be placed either as an awake intubation or immediately after rapid-sequence induction with correct cricoid pressure (Sellick's maneuver) applied from the time of induction to the time of intubation. General anesthesia for the parturient without intubation is totally unacceptable anesthetic practice.

General anesthesia is indicated when acute fetal distress occurs and prompt vaginal delivery is possible. It may be used in a patient who becomes uncontrollable during delivery or when regional anesthesia is contraindicated or refused and operative obstetrics is required. General anesthesia is often indicated when depression of uterine activity is required. Such uterine relaxation may be necessary to abolish a tetanic uterine contraction or to allow internal uterine manipulation, as in the extraction of a second twin. For uterine relaxation, halothane and probably enflurane and isoflurane may be used because they cause rapid relaxation of the uterus, but accompanying this relaxation of the uterus, there is always the danger of hemorrhage. After the baby has been delivered, the halothane, enflurane, or isoflurane should be discontinued. If it is necessary to maintain general anesthesia, a nitrous oxide–oxygen–narcotic technique is the anesthetic technique of choice.[21]

Regional Anesthesia

Conduction anesthesia is suitable for vaginal delivery, and there are distinct advantages associated with the use of regional anesthesia for both mother and fetus. Maternal airway reflexes usually remain intact provided severe hypotension or reactions to local anesthetics are avoided. The mother remains awake and can react to her newborn early in the postpartum period. There is a decrease in the need for narcotics or sedatives, and regional anesthesia usually eliminates the need for general anesthesia and its potentially depressant effect on the neonate. When properly administered, regional anesthesia is associated with minimal or no neonatal depression.

There is some evidence that nontoxic doses of some local anesthetics, particularly mepivacaine when used in a continuous lumbar epidural block, may be associated with a prolonged half-life in the neonate. Chloroprocaine and bupivacaine do not seem to cause this problem.[22]

Repeated doses of an amide type of local anesthetic may be associated with increased blood levels of the drug in the mother and fetus, probably associated with their prolonged elimination, extended half-life, and high protein binding capabilities. This is not a problem with the ester-type local anesthetics such as procaine and chloroprocaine because of their short half-lives and rapid metabolism in the bloodstream.

Chloroprocaine has been implicated in creating neurotoxic reactions when injected into the subarachnoid space. Recent research has shown that chloroprocaine itself is probably not the causative factor, but rather the high concentration of the antioxidant sodium metabisulfite is the noxious agent. In addition, preservative-containing local anesthetics should not be used for major conduction block anesthesia because of their potential cytotoxic effects. The paraben derivatives are the most common preservatives used and have also been associated with allergic reactions. Chloroprocaine is now available in a methylparaben-free solution, and ethyldiaminotetraacetate (EDTA) has been substituted for sodium metabisulfite.[23–25]

Bupivacaine in high concentrations (0.5 and 0.75 percent) injected intravascularly as large boluses has been blamed for a large number of cardiovascular arrests in parturients who were unable to be resuscitated. Action by the Food and Drug Administration subsequently led to the banning of the use of 0.75 percent bupivacaine in all obstetric suites. These controversies further emphasize the need for vigilance when administering epidural blocks, through either a needle or a catheter. Negative aspiration of blood or spinal fluid should always be used with an appropriate test dose volume of suitable local anesthetic. This test, in and of itself, is not always conclusive of appropriate needle catheter placement. Fractionated intermittent doses of the agent of choice are absolutely essential, along with continuous observation and communication with the patient.[26]

When regional anesthesia is used, maternal monitoring is required in both the labor room and the delivery room. A reliable, large-bore intravenous line must be in place. It is mandatory that the airway be kept patent, and someone must always be available to treat any untoward reaction, whether caused by a high level of anesthetic block, hypotension, or intravascular or accidental intrathecal injection.

Paracervical block is produced by infiltration submucosally of a local anesthetic into the fornix of the vagina lateral to the cervix. It provides relatively rapid relief of pain and is associated with minimal maternal side effects, but it gives no perineal relief, even though the block does not interfere with the second stage of labor.

Unfortunately, paracervical block may cause fetal bradycardia and can lead to fetal acidosis and sometimes even fetal demise. These effects are thought to be secondary to rapid placental passage of the drug, decreased uterine blood flow caused by absorption in the uterine arteries, as well as the direct uterine vasoconstrictive effect created by the local anesthetic. These effects are minimized by using small amounts of less toxic anesthetics and by injecting carefully into the parametrium.

Paracervical block is best avoided when the fetus is at risk. Studies have shown that after paracervical blocks parturients have had decreased baseline variability in real heart rate, and some also have variable decelerations. Bilateral lumbar sympathetic blocks at the L-2 level eliminate uterine pain alone. Because the block is rather difficult to perform and is somewhat painful during its administration, it is rarely used in obstetrics today.

Pudendal nerve block alleviates most of the vaginal and perineal pain associated with delivery. It provides no uterine pain relief and does not provide analgesia for uterine manipulation. Pudendal block does, however, provide adequate analgesia for an episiotomy repair. Supplemented with inhalation analgesia, it may provide sufficient analgesia for outlet forceps delivery or low forceps rotation. As pudendal block does not produce complete pelvic analgesia, the bearing down reflex usually is not abolished.

If local anesthetic toxicity is avoided, pudendal block has a minimal depressant effect on the mother and newborn and is not associated with maternal hypotension. It is a safe and effective block and is usually administered in the delivery room shortly before delivery by the obstetrician.

Subarachnoid block is one of the more versatile types of regional anesthesia available for use in obstetrics. Various names are given to this anesthetic technique, such as saddle block, subarachnoid block, or spinal anesthesia, but all are essentially the same technique. A saddle block, giving alleviation of pain from S-1 to S-5, is no longer deemed a satisfactory method for delivery, as a true spinal anesthetic with a T-10 sensory level block alleviates all pain of labor and delivery and allows uterine manipulation. Use of 40 to 50 mg of lidocaine (5 percent in dextrose 7.5 percent) provides a satisfactory block for most operative vaginal procedures. For a longer-duration block, approximately 4 mg of tetracaine (1 percent in dextrose 10 percent) or 5 to 7 mg of hyperbaric bupivacaine (0.75 percent in 8.5 percent dextrose) gives a satisfactory dermatome level and a block lasting approximately 1.5 to 2 hours.

The major drawbacks of subarachnoid analgesia may include a marked degree of maternal hypotension[27] (particularly if adequate rapid prehydration of intravenous fluids is not infused prior to initiation), "total spinal" abolishment of the urge to bear down, possible prolongation of the second stage of labor, and postdural puncture headache. Severe and sudden hypotension leading to maternal cardiovascular collapse is a leading cause of maternal mortality. Prophylaxis includes left uterine displacement along with preblock hydration of an intravenous balanced salt solution. Treatment consists of the above plus a primary acting central vasopressor such as ephedrine (10 to 20 mg) intravenously and a high FiO_2.

Vasoconstrictors such as methoxamine and phenylephrine correct hypotension, but they cause a further decrease in uterine blood flow and compromise the fetus because they are alpha-adrenergic agents.

Total spinal block may lead to apnea and probably loss of consciousness and cardiovascular collapse. It may be prevented by limiting the dose of local anesthetic to two-thirds or even one-half that used in a nonpregnant woman and not injecting the medication during a contraction. Treatment consists of correction of the hypotension and protection of the upper airway with an endotracheal tube and ventilation (i.e., intermittent positive-pressure ventilation with 100 percent oxygen). Even though subarachnoid analgesia abolishes the bearing down reflex, the mother can be coached to push, and forceps delivery is easily performed. Postdural puncture headache occurs very commonly in the parturient, probably because of the increased pressure of cerebrospinal fluid and the venous engorgement discussed earlier. Prophylaxis includes the use of a small-gauge spinal needle (25, 26, or 27 gauge), adequate postpartum hydration, and use of a tight abdominal binder when a parturient assumes the upright position. Treatment consists of all of the above plus bed rest in the supine position (the prone position is even more efficacious), hydration, and appropriate analgesics. If severe headache persists, an epidural blood patch may be indicated. Maintaining the supine position after postdural puncture does not prevent headaches.

Lumbar epidural analgesia is becoming more popular than ever for vaginal delivery.[28] The use of a continuous catheter technique, specifically localized for segmental anesthesia and with a T-10 to L-1 sensory block, is efficacious. This allows a mother to have a relatively pain-free labor and still maintain her motor ability. She can easily push for the vaginal delivery. When the baby is to be delivered, anesthesia of the vagina and perineum (S2-4) can be achieved. This allows for all necessary obstetric maneuvers.

Segmental lumbar epidural anesthesia has mostly replaced caudal anesthesia. The perineal analgesia that caudal anesthesia provides is out of logical sequence, requires more local anesthetic, is less reliable, and technically may be more difficult to perform. Lumbar epidural anesthesia can be extended cephalad and caudad to provide satisfactory levels for cesarean section. If the dose is not accidentally placed in the subarachnoid space, postspinal cephalalgia is almost always avoided. Continuous epidural analgesia frequently eliminates the necessity for depressant drugs that are used during labor and delivery. The mother is awake, mostly pain free, and cooperative.

Today many obstetric anesthesiologists are using continuous-infusion pumps to maintain continuous local anesthetic infusions of lower-concentration solutions of the customarily used local anesthetics. The technique is very effective, even at the extremely low concentrations used in maintaining adequate analgesia for the pain of labor and contractions. A "top-up" dose prior to delivery provides superb anesthesia for either forceps delivery or episiotomy repair. An important advantage is that the low concentrations seem to cause no change in the labor pattern or curve. There is no prolongation of labor, and even if, as often occurs with a primigravida, there should be acute pain in the early stages of an extended labor, the possibility of accumulation leading to toxic levels is minimized. The facilitated ease of maintenance does not mean that the patient needs any less observation or monitoring, but safety is certainly enhanced. Furthermore, low-dose continuous infusion eliminates the magnitude of changes that occur as analgesia wanes.

An exciting recent development has been the use of epidural opioids in labor,[29,30] usually in conjunction with extremely low-concentration local anesthetic solutions (see Table 31-1 for dosing recommendations). Epidural opiates provide pain relief without producing hypotension or motor blockage and seem to be more effective in relieving visceral pain (first stage of labor) than somatic pain (second stage). The more lipid-soluble agents such as fentanyl, alfentanil, and sufentanil are minimally associated with maternal or fetal respiratory depression; however, the hydrophilic opiate morphine has been implicated in producing significant respiratory depression as late as 12 to 16 hours after its administration.

Although epidurally administered opiates are more effective when used in conjunction with low concentrations of local anesthetics, they can be used as the sole agent. When given alone they may provide complete analgesia in early labor and can be used in situations where the prevention of hypotension is mandatory, such as in a laboring cardiac patient. Epidural opiates such as fentanyl, sufentanil, and alfentanil are also highly effective in reducing the "perineal discomfort" seen during the middle of the first stage of labor. Epidurally administered opiates can also result in bothersome side effects such as pruritus and urinary retention; the frequency of these problems may be dose related. Many different protocols are being tried with varying dosages of morphine, fentanyl, sufentanil, alfentanil, and butorphanol to investigate the quality of analgesia, effects on the progress of labor, and effects on the fetus. The results of these investigations should improve the use of these agents.

Postoperative pain relief after surgery has similarly been shown to be extraordinarily effective with epidural administration of narcotics without the need for parenteral medications.[31] Vigilance is essential, however, and close monitoring of these patients is mandatory because of the variable side effects that may occur in a small percentage of patients.[32]

Hypotension after epidural anesthesia is usually slower in onset than after a subarachnoid block; however, its sever-

TABLE 31-1. DOSING RECOMMENDATIONS FOR COMMON LOCAL ANESTHETICS AND NARCOTIC–LOCAL ANESTHETIC COMBINATIONS

	Drug		
	Bupivacaine	*Bupivacaine-Fentanyl*	*Lidocaine*
Loading dose			
Local anesthetic	0.25–0.5%	0.125–0.25%	1–1.5%
Narcotic	None	50–75 μg	50–75 μg
Volume	5–10 mL	8–12 mL	8–12 mL
Continuous infusion			
Local anesthetic	0.25%	0.125–0.25%	Switch to bupivacaine
Narcotic	None	1.5–2 μg/mL	
Volume	8–12 mL/h	8–12 mL	
Intermittent bolus			
Local anesthetic	Same as loading dose 2–3 h	Same as loading dose 2–3 h	Same as loading dose 1.5–2 h
Duration			

ity can be just as marked. Prevention and treatment are the same as in subarachnoid injection of local anesthetic, and hypotension may be avoided by giving a test dose of 3 to 4 mL of local anesthetic, waiting 2 to 3 minutes, and then checking the dermatome level before giving the remainder of the local anesthetic in fractionated or incremental doses. Epidural anesthesia requires five to ten times the amount of local anesthetic to produce the same level of anesthesia as spinal anesthesia. Unrecognized subarachnoid injection usually results in a very high or total block.

Epidural analgesia of the perineum does decrease the urge to bear down and may result in an increased tendency for forceps delivery. There may also be an increase in the incidence of persistent posterior presentations.

A disadvantage of lumbar epidural anesthesia as compared with subarachnoid anesthesia is that a larger dose of anesthetic agent is required, resulting in higher local anesthetic blood levels in the mother and fetus.

The parturient in labor deserves as good, if not better, anesthetic care than a patient for surgery, particularly because the anticipated life expectancy of both mother and fetus totals more than 120 years. Failure to provide this care during labor, delivery, and the postpartum period can lead to tragedy such as the death of a young mother or the birth of a stillborn or brain-damaged child.

ANESTHESIA FOR CESAREAN SECTION

The type of anesthesia for cesarean section should be determined by the reason for the surgery, any underlying medical problems, and the presence of complicating anatomic abnormalities. There are guidelines on which to base the choice of regional or general anesthesia. If the patient has had an uneventful labor and the fetus has shown no signs of depression of heart rate patterns, then the choice between epidural, spinal, or general anesthesia is essentially a decision agreed on by the patient, obstetrician, and anesthetist.[33] An example of this type of situation would be a young mother with cephalopelvic disproportion after a trial of labor without progress. If the fetus has shown signs of hypoxia and has had deleterious changes in fetal heart rate patterns, late decelerations, prolonged tachycardia, or loss of beat-to-beat variability, then general anesthesia may be preferable to either spinal or epidural anesthesia.[33] General anesthesia maintains uterine perfusion more uniformly than regional anesthesia, with less chance of hypotension. In the face of an emergency procedure and a possibly mildly dehydrated acidotic mother with a hypoxic fetus, maternal hypotension is probably an unjustified risk to the fetus.

For cesarean section for a prolapsed cord or for the patient with potential hemorrhage, such as in placenta previa, general anesthesia is again preferable. One of the most important factors in this choice is the longer time required for regional anesthesia to be induced and to take effect. This is often noxious to the fetus. The second consideration is the sympathetic blockade produced by regional anesthesia in the face of possible hemorrhage.

In the extremely obese patient (weight greater than 250 lb or 100 kg), general anesthesia may be preferable because of the decrease in vital capacity and other respiratory parameters associated with the supine position and the decrease in functional residual capacity associated with the supine position, pregnancy, and obesity. This judgment will be tempered somewhat by the obstetrician doing the operative procedure and the time required to empty the uterus. Prior to giving a general anesthetic to an extremely obese patient, the anesthetist must be certain that he or she will be able to intubate the patient without undue difficulty. If this cannot be accomplished, an awake intubation definitely should be considered.

Conduction Anesthesia for Cesarean Section (Spinal or Epidural)

It is important to preload the patient with between 1500 and 2000 mL of intravenous fluids (non-glucose-containing crystalloid) prior to initiating the block, but this does not pertain to the patient who is cardiac compromised.[34] The obese patient may require an even greater prehydration volume (25 to 30 mL/kg).[35] The block should be instituted with the patient in either the right lateral decubitus position or the sitting position. After the block is given and the patient has been placed supine, the operating table should be tilted approximately 10 degrees to the left and a wedge should be placed under the patient's right hip.[36] The blood pressure should be checked every 30 seconds until stable and thereafter at a minimum of every 5 minutes. Oxygen saturation should be continuously monitored by means of pulse oximetry, and supplemental oxygen may be administered by nasal cannula or face mask. A dull safety pin should be used to determine the dermatomal level of anesthesia.

If the systolic blood pressure begins to fall from its preanesthetic level, it is advisable that the uterus be displaced further to the left and an intravenous fluid bolus of crystalloid be given. Ephedrine in increments of 10 to 12 mg should be given intravenously. No longer does one wait until the systolic blood pressure drops below 100 mm Hg (or 20 percent less than the preanesthetic block level) before instituting ephedrine as a vasopressor. If the patient is toxemic and is running a diastolic blood pressure in the range 100 to 120 mm Hg, the limit of the drop in blood pressure should not be below 90 to 100 mm Hg (diastolic).

It is important to realize that the dose of local anesthetic necessary to achieve a T4–5 level is approximately two-thirds to one-half the dose normally used in a nonpregnant patient. The compression of the subarachnoid space by engorged epidural veins, the pressure of the uterus on the pelvic veins, and the hypertrophy of the vertebral veins all lead to diminution of the epidural space. This produces the alteration in dosages of local anesthetic solutions required for cesarean section.

Epidural anesthesia is being used more often for cesarean section, particularly after being administered for pain relief during labor and then extended for cesarean section. The dosage required is again usually two-thirds that for the normal nonpregnant woman, and the blood pressure must be taken every 5 minutes for the first 15 to 20 minutes after injection. The dermatomal level that should be achieved is T3–4.[37,38]

General Anesthesia for Cesarean Section

General anesthesia for cesarean section requires the same preliminary maneuvers as for conduction anesthesia; however, capnography and pulse oximetry should be considered mandatory monitoring modalities. A large-bore intravenous line should be adequately secured, and the patient, after being placed on the operating table, should be denitrogenated for 4 to 5 minutes because of the increased oxygen demands of pregnancy along with the increased risk of hypoxia. If immediate delivery is necessary and 4 to 5 minutes is not available to denitrogenate, four or five deep breaths of 100 percent oxygen can be substituted. While the patient is lying on the operating table, the table should be tilted 10 degrees to the left and a wedge placed under her right hip.

There is considerable controversy about precurarization 3 minutes prior to the administration of succinylcholine used to facilitate intubation in the rapid-sequence induction. One school of thought claims the use of a nondepolarizing muscle relaxant prior to succinylcholine helps prevent an increase in intragastric pressure and the fasciculations produced by succinylcholine. The other school of thought says that a parturient rarely complains of muscle soreness from excessive fasciculations and that the increased time delay to the onset of action of the succinylcholine is too heavy a price to pay in an already compromised situation. Precurarization should not be used.

After the patient is completely prepared and draped, thiopental sodium (Pentothal) in the amount of 3 to 4 mg/kg is given as a bolus intravenously (up to a maximum of 250 mg, 300 mg in the obese); this is followed by succinylcholine in the range 80 to 100 mg. With the sodium pentothal, cricoid pressure should be instituted. The reservoir bag should not be squeezed. The face mask should be kept on the patient's face. Once the endotracheal tube is passed into the trachea and the cuff has been inflated slightly beyond the vocal cords, the operation can begin. To maintain muscle relaxation throughout the procedure, a succinylcholine drip or an intermediate-duration nondepolarizing muscle relaxant may be used (atracurium, vecuronium).[39]

It is accepted practice today for halogenated inhalational agents such as halothane (0.5 percent), isoflurane (0.75 percent), and enflurane (1.0 percent) to be used prior to abdominal delivery of a fetus to provide supplemental anesthesia and to help in prevention of the mother's recall if skin incision to delivery time should be extended. At these concentrations, uterine bleeding is not magnified and can be counteracted by pitocin administration after delivery of the fetus. After clamping and cutting of the cord, the halogenated agents most often are discontinued and a narcotic agent such as fentanyl and an amnestic such as midazolam are then used to deepen the anesthesia.

If general anesthesia has to be used in an emergency situation when the mother or fetus may already be severely compromised and after the rapid-sequence induction already described, 100 percent oxygen only with the addition of one of the above agents in low concentrations may contribute toward a better outcome (so long as delivery is rapid). The high FiO_2 delivered without nitrous oxide would seem to cause less depression to either mother or fetus, with the extremely low concentration of the halogenated agent preventing maternal recall.

Endotracheal intubation is mandatory when general anesthesia is chosen for cesarean section; however, it must be anticipated that the anesthetist may be unable to intubate the trachea. It is therefore necessary to have a plan to fall back on to protect the patient from developing hypoxia. Cricoid pressure must be maintained. The patient should be turned head down with her face toward the side, and an airway should be inserted. Oxygenation should be established by face mask while maintaining the cricoid pressure. The patient should be ventilated with 100 percent oxygen, the nitrous oxide turned off, and the anesthetic allowed to wear off. Local or regional anesthesia should be carried out as a safer alternative, or an awake oral intubation or fiberoptic technique should be considered. If the operation is an emergency and there is no time to consider another form of anesthetic technique, the patient should be ventilated using nitrous oxide–oxygen and anesthesia maintained with an agent such as isoflurane or enflurane to establish surgical anesthesia with spontaneous ventilation, after the succinylcholine has worn off. If a nondepolarizing muscle relaxant has been used, ventilation has to be continued by the anesthetist. The operation should be allowed to proceed via the face mask, but cricoid pressure must be maintained. If intubation and mask ventilation are unsuccessful an emergency cricothyroidotomy should be performed to accomplish transtracheal ventilation.

ACUTE POSTOPERATIVE PAIN RELIEF

Patient-controlled analgesia (PCA) and epidural and subdural opioids are newly emerging alternatives to traditional forms of postoperative pain relief methods. Intravenous PCA devices consist of a microprocessor-controlled pump triggered by the patient (pressing a button). When triggered, a preset amount (incremental dose) of narcotic is delivered into the patient's intravenous line. A timer in the pump prevents administration of an additional bolus until a specified period has occurred. This technique has the advantage of allowing for consistent titration of analgesic drugs, which can be tailored to the patient's needs.

Spinal and epidural analgesia for cesarean delivery has enhanced the use of intraspinal narcotics for postoperative pain control. Duramorph (morphine without preservatives), in a dose of 5 mg epidurally or 0.5 mg subarachnoid (one time), can provide 18 to 24 hours of satisfactory pain relief. Pruritus, nausea, vomiting, urinary retention, and respiratory depression are the most common complications associated with this technique. Side effects seem to be related, at least in part, to dosage. Factors that may increase the risk of respiratory depression include advanced age or opioid sensitivity, highly water soluble narcotics (morphine), concomitant administration of systemic opioids, and intrathecal versus epidural administration.[31]

ANESTHESIA FOR ABNORMAL OBSTETRICS

Abnormal obstetrics may be defined as situations in which conditions unfavorable to the mother or the fetus already exist or are predicted and anticipated. Women with pregnancy-induced hypertension (toxemia), antepartum or postpartum hemorrhage, preterm labor, or abnormal presentation all fall within this category. A myriad of medical conditions may influence the management of the pregnant patient. Such conditions include diabetes mellitus, congenital and acquired heart disease, preexisting renal disease, and chronic hypertension.

Pregnancy-Induced Hypertension (Preeclampsia, Eclampsia)

It is important for the anesthetist to understand the physiologic factors that alter the condition of the toxemic patient: renal and hepatic involvement, hypovolemia, anemia, and electrolyte imbalance. Classically, the patient presents with hypertension, peripheral edema, and albuminuria. If blood pressure is elevated above 140/90 or increased 30 torr above baseline, edema is generalized and not restricted to the ankles or feet, and more than 0.3 g protein is excreted in a 24-hour period, the diagnosis of mild preeclampsia is made. Preeclampsia becomes severe when the blood pressure is elevated above 160/110 or proteinuria is in excess of 5 g in a 24-hour period. The presence of oliguria, pulmonary edema, visual disturbances, epigastric pain, or cerebral disturbances also supports the diagnosis of severe preeclampsia. Pathophysiologically, there is generalized arterial spasm and general vasoconstriction, with swelling of the renal glomeruli and epithelial cells, leading to reduction of the capillary lumen and a subsequent decrease in glomerular filtration rate and renal blood flow. There is vascular hyperactivity with an increased pressor response to angiotensin, probably from the shift of sodium into the arterial wall. In approximately 7 to 8 percent of the patients, there is a decrease in platelets, fibrinogen, and prothrombin, leading to a potentially disseminated intravascular coagulopathy.

The central nervous system becomes edematous, irritable, and sensitive to all depressant drugs. Uterine blood flow is diminished. Hypovolemia is a common occurrence despite the presence of peripheral edema. It is noteworthy that blood pressure may be very sensitive to autonomic blockage from epidural anesthesia. There also is frequent uterine irritability, which may lead to a marked response to small doses of oxytocin (Pitocin).

Treatment prior to the termination of pregnancy is bed rest with the patient on her side, a low-salt diet, and some sedation. If the patient requires an antihypertensive drug, a direct vasodilator such as hydralazine usually is effective. Magnesium sulfate is given for control of central nervous system irritability, and the dosage is determined by serum magnesium levels and tendon reflexes.

If vaginal delivery is planned, the patient should labor on her side, and if the diagnosis is severe pregnancy-induced hypertension, pulmonary artery catheterization may be indicated as the hypovolemia that is present can be quite marked. Coagulation studies should be performed, and the patient should receive magnesium sulfate as indicated. Crystalloid solutions are quite useful in combating the severe vasoconstriction that exists. Serial hematocrits may be useful in determining whether the treatment is improving the patient's condition.

Recent work has verified that there are often gross fluid shifts in these parturients with pregnancy-induced hypertension. Effective and judicious use of volume expanders, such as albumin or human plasma protein (Plasmanate), along with continuous monitoring of pulmonary artery pressure and pulmonary capillary wedge pressure, may assist in shifting the extravascular fluids back to the intravascular compartment, raising the central venous pressure to nearly normal levels without compromising the already altered blood pressures. Epidural anesthesia, well administered, without epinephrine, provides satisfactory analgesia for labor if the above criteria are met. Epidural anesthesia will help to eliminate the stressful, painful contractions and can be used to correct the blood pressure elevation. It is necessary that the hemodynamic parameters be at a known level and that the coagulation profile and platelet count be stable prior to initiating the block. A pudendal block may also be a suitable adjunct for vaginal delivery.

For cesarean section, epidural anesthesia is excellent if there are no blood volume problems, bleeding, or convulsions. Spinal anesthesia is never the anesthetic technique of choice when severe preeclampsia is present and is contraindicated because of the probability of a rather severe drop in blood pressure that would be detrimental to the fetus. General anesthesia is preferred to spinal anesthesia. If general anesthesia is used, endotracheal intubation and denitrogenation are mandatory.

If a parturient with severe pregnancy-induced hypertension requires emergent delivery via general anesthesia, protection against increasing the already hypertensive state with laryngoscopy and intubation procedures will often necessitate an infusion of a potent antihypertensive agent such as nitroglycerin for protection, despite the fact that hydralazine and magnesium sulfate may have already been given.

Labetalol in doses of 0.5 to 1 mg/kg may also be useful in preventing the hypertensive response to laryngoscopy and intubation. Labetalol may also have the advantage of improving uterine perfusion.

During laryngoscopy, the blood pressure will increase but will usually not exceed pretreatment levels. By preventing marked exacerbations of hypertension, intracranial hemorrhage and pulmonary edema may be avoided. If circumstances allow, it would probably be better if such a severely affected parturient could be managed and treated at a tertiary care facility or a high-risk obstetric center where every resource is immediately available.

When preeclampsia is accompanied by grand mal convulsions not related to other neurologic conditions it becomes eclampsia. The first priority in managing the eclamptic patient is controlling convulsions. Thiopental 50 to 100 mg or diazepam 2.5 to 5 mg is usually effective in terminating convulsions. Further therapy includes the administration of magnesium sulfate. Oxygen should be administered to the mother and, on occasion, tracheal intubation is necessary to prevent pulmonary aspiration and ensure adequate ventilation. It is generally recommended that the mother be stabilized before delivery of the fetus be attempted. Once the convulsions are controlled the management of the eclamptic patient is similar to that of the severe preeclamptic patient.

HELLP syndrome, a variant of severe preeclampsia, is evidenced by hemolysis, elevated liver enzymes, and low platelets.[40] It is a multisystem disorder that usually requires general anesthesia for cesarean section. Because of the clotting dysfunction, regional anesthesia is rarely used.

Acute Intrapartum Hemorrhage

Hemorrhage is the most common cause of obstetric shock, but the blood pressure may not decrease nor the pulse rate increase until a liter or more of blood has been lost. Placenta previa and abruptio placentae are the most common causes of external hemorrhage.

Placenta previa, which may be total, partial, or marginal, occurs in approximately 0.4 percent of pregnancies and has a greater incidence in the multipara. It is painless and is frequently accompanied by malpresentation and prematurity. The diagnosis of placenta previa is determined by the patient's history of painless vaginal bleeding, the use of ultrasonography, and the "double setup." In the double setup, the patient undergoes pelvic examination in the operating room while being prepared for a stat cesarean section, as the vaginal examination may cause uncontrollable bleeding. General anesthesia and crossmatched blood should be immediately available prior to this procedure.

Abruptio placentae, which is often associated with toxemia, may present with mild to moderate bleeding or with a stormy onset, severe pain, and continuous heavy bleeding. There is significant risk of fetal death and maternal shock. Extensive infarction of the placenta with the release of thromboplastin and activation of the clotting mechanism can lead to a defect in clotting, hypofibrinogenemia, and disseminated intravascular coagulopathy.

The anesthetic management of patients with hemorrhage reflects the effects and manifestations of hypovolemia and loss of oxygen-carrying capacity. This usually precludes the use of spinal or epidural anesthesia. For vaginal delivery of a patient with partial placenta previa or partial abruptio placentae, pudendal block, nitrous oxide, and oxygen with the use of low-dose ketamine can be recommended. High FiO$_2$ should be used. When cesarean section is indicated, general anesthesia with endotracheal intubation is the anesthetic of choice. Ketamine and oxygen are an excellent general anesthetic combination. If there is a need to decrease uterine tone, as in abruption, lower doses of thiopental sodium plus lower doses of ketamine should be considered.

MEDICAL CONDITIONS ASSOCIATED WITH OBSTETRICS

Diabetes Mellitus

The current thoughts about the management of the insulin-dependent pregnant patient include strict control of maternal hyperglycemia and the maintenance of maternal blood glucose concentration between 80 and 120 mg/100 mL.

Problems encountered in the diabetic patient during pregnancy include an increased tendency to ketoacidosis in the last half of pregnancy, alterations in insulin dosage, and the diabetogenic nature of pregnancy itself. There is an increased risk of preeclampsia and hydramnios.

As far as the fetus is concerned, macrosomia and death in utero are relatively common if the diabetic parturient is not carefully supervised throughout her pregnancy. Placental pathology with premature aging of the placenta is not uncommon and may lead to hypoxia in utero.

Anesthesia care includes intelligent fluid therapy during labor and delivery. If cesarean section is indicated, an insulin technique that is time tested consists of half the usual A.M. dose of insulin and an intravenous infusion of 5 percent dextrose just prior to the delivery; however, hypoglycemia has been a problem in infants because of the release of insulin produced by stimulation of the infant pancreas. A newer insulin technique that seems to be an improvement is the microinsulin technique used by endocrinologists. This maintains strict maternal blood glucose control and has just about eliminated hypoglycemia in the neonate.

It is now advocated by neonatologists and understood by anesthesia personnel that the mother should not receive a bolus of dextrose prior to receiving an epidural anesthetic for cesarean section. It is again important to avoid aortocaval compression by careful positioning of the parturient. If cesarean section is necessary, it has been shown that both epidural and general anesthesia are satisfactory. Spinal anesthesia may increase the acidosis that is encountered in the fetus. It is noteworthy that once the baby is delivered, the mother may be diabetic for several days.[41-44]

Heart Disease

The incidence of heart disease in pregnant women is relatively small but is a major nonobstetric cause of death. Patients who have left-to-right shunts usually tolerate labor and delivery without any major problems unless a drop in blood pressure causes a reversal in the shunt. Patients with right-to-left shunt have a higher incidence of fetal wastage. Myocardial infarction is rare in pregnant women but does occur and can lead to fatalities.[3,45]

In rheumatic heart disease, the valvular lesions can cause decreased cardiac response to the demands of pregnancy and labor. Mitral stenosis is the most common lesion associated with rheumatic heart disease, and it produces increased pulmonary blood volume and decreased cardiac output throughout pregnancy. It is important to minimize increases in the central blood volume and avoid marked increases in pulmonary artery pressure.

When a patient with rheumatic heart disease enters the hospital in labor, her clinical status, as represented by the classification of either the New York Heart Association or the American Heart Association, should be ascertained. If the patient is in category 1 or 2 (almost no limitation of activity and no evidence of congestive heart failure), she should be treated with caution, but the usual standards of care are sufficient. On the other hand, patients who have marked symptoms probably should be monitored with an arterial line and a pulmonary artery catheter.

Anesthesia for vaginal delivery in a patient with rheumatic heart disease would be best carried out with segmental epidural anesthesia to lessen the stress of labor and to relieve the anxiety of labor with its effects on the heart. Ephedrine should be avoided and, if possible, so should excess fluids. If general anesthesia is necessary, drugs that produce tachycardia such as pancuronium, meperidine, and ketamine should be avoided.

The pregnant patient with congenital heart disease presents the problem of reversal of a left-to-right shunt. The systolic pressure must be maintained, and the stress and the strain of delivery should not be allowed to create further impositions on the heart. Continuous segmental lumbar epidural anesthesia and spinal anesthesia for delivery are both useful.

Pulmonary Disease

In patients with pulmonary disease such as bronchial asthma, the anesthetic management that should be used is regional anesthesia. Reactive airways are prone to bronchospasm under rapid-sequence induction of general anesthesia with endotracheal intubation. For patients with nonasthmatic chronic obstructive pulmonary disease, regional anesthesia is satisfactory. If there is reduced total lung volume and reduced vital capacity, general anesthesia may be more effective and safer for cesarean section.

ANESTHESIA FOR PRETERM LABOR AND DELIVERY

Preterm delivery is one of the leading causes of perinatal mortality in the United States and occurs in about 1 in 12 births. Preterm labor is described as labor occurring between the 20th and 37th weeks of gestation.[46] Many factors have been associated with preterm labor including: exposure to diethylstilbestrol (DES), low socioeconomic status, smoking, drug use (cocaine), infection, multiple gestation, cervical incompetence, surgery, and acute or chronic systemic disease.[47,48] Not all preterm births result from preterm labor, however. Elective preterm delivery may be considered for the treatment of severe pregnancy-induced hypertension or when hemolytic disorders such as Rh sensitization compromise the mother or fetus.[49]

The initial obstetric management of preterm labor includes bed rest, hydration, and fetal surveillance. If these measures prove ineffective, tocolytic therapy may be implemented. Terbutaline, a beta-adrenergic agonist that increases levels of cyclic AMP, and magnesium sulfate, which decreases intracellular calcium, are the mainstay of tocolytic therapy in the United States today. Terbutaline is a relatively specific beta-2 receptor agonist (e.g., uterine smooth muscle); however, some beta-1 receptor stimulation does occur. Side effects of beta-adrenergic tocolytics include pulmonary edema, myocardial ischemia, hypotension, cardiac arrhythmias, metabolic acidosis, hypokalemia, hyperglycemia, and a reduced hematocrit.

Fluid administration in patients receiving beta-adrenergic agonists should be approached with caution as they are vulnerable to fluid overload.[50] This is a particularly important consideration when determining the hydration needs prior to the placement of an epidural or spinal block. Because of the potential for serious complications it is generally recommended that the beta-adrenergic agonist ritodrine, which is administered intravenously and has a distribution half-life of 32 ± 21 minutes, be discontinued 1 hour prior to the initiation of anesthesia.[49]

Magnesium sulfate, which has long been used as an anticonvulsant in the treatment of preeclampsia, is also proving to be useful as both a primary tocolytic agent and an adjunct to other tocolytic agents. The site of action of magnesium sulfate is the calcium-binding sites of smooth muscle and the neuromuscular junction; here it decreases

the sensitivity of the endplate to acetylcholine.[51] Because of the effect on acetylcholine, patients who are receiving magnesium tocolysis may be more sensitive to both depolarizing and nondepolarizing muscle relaxants. Magnesium tocolysis is also associated with some of the same side effects seen with the use of beta-adrenergic agents (pulmonary edema and chest tightness); however, these complications occur less frequently with magnesium therapy.

Because of their effect on smooth muscle, calcium-entry blocking agents such as nifedipine, verapamil, and diltiazem are being studied to determine their effectiveness in treating preterm labor. Reports of adverse effects, such as decreased uterine blood flow and fetal acidosis in animals, have, however, tempered enthusiasm toward these drugs. Prostaglandin synthetase inhibitors, which inhibit cyclooxygenase, and cause a decrease in uterine contractions, are also under investigation as tocolytic agents. These drugs have the advantage of producing minimal maternal side effects with the exception of transient platelet function abnormality; however, uncertainty regarding the effect of in utero fetal exposure to these agents may curtail their use.

If tocolysis fails and anesthesia services are required, it must be remembered that the preterm fetus is different from the term fetus. Management of the preterm fetus for labor and vaginal or cesarean delivery presents many challenges to the anesthetist. The preterm fetus is thought to be more susceptible to the effects of depressant drugs; this is believed to be the result of a lower protein binding capability, an immature blood–brain barrier, and a decreased ability to metabolize and excrete drugs. The preterm infant is also less capable of tolerating the stress of labor and delivery and is vulnerable to asphyxia. A poorly developed calvaria and friable intracranial vessels increase the risk of intracranial hemorrhage and brain injury, especially during a poorly controlled delivery.

The ideal management for delivery of the preterm infant is unknown. Regional anesthesia offers several advantages. The need for depressant drugs is reduced or eliminated and excellent conditions for delivery are maintained. Epidural analgesia can decrease the mother's urge to bear down and help facilitate a controlled vaginal delivery. The use of forceps and episiotomy, both of which may enhance protection of the fetal head, are better tolerated during epidural analgesia. In addition, there may be an increased incidence of retained placenta associated with prematurity; therefore, a functioning epidural catheter may make manual extraction of the placenta easier and safer.

MATERNAL COMPLICATIONS OF OBSTETRIC ANESTHESIA

It would be impossible to list all the potential complications that may follow obstetric anesthesia. This discussion is limited to acute complications that may develop intrapartum or postpartum and that the anesthetist may be called on to recognize or treat immediately.

Hypotension

Hypotension as a consequence of obstetric anesthesia usually is a sequela of conduction anesthesia techniques (i.e., spinal or epidural anesthesia). The development of hypotension may be defined as blood pressure falling 20 percent below the initial baseline blood pressure or systolic pressure decreasing below 100 mm Hg.

Prevention is preferable to treatment. The patient should not be allowed to labor on her back because of the consequences of aortocaval compression,[52] which can lead to supine hypotensive syndrome. A mild to moderate drop in blood pressure can usually be corrected by placing the patient in a slight head-down lateral position and giving a rapid infusion of fluids, preferably crystalloid. Oxygen tends to reduce nausea and vomiting associated with the hypotension and may aid in transplacental oxygenation of the fetus. Ephedrine given in small incremental doses of 10 to 12 mg at the initial onset of the hypotension usually eliminates the syndrome rather rapidly and helps prevent hypoxia of the fetus. Approximately 1 out of 10 or 12 pregnant women in the last trimester of pregnancy, when placed in the supine position, sustains these significant reductions in blood pressure.[53] There is definite obstruction of the vena cava and the aorta by the gravid uterus when the patient lies supine. The majority of parturients compensate for this by shunting blood from the lower extremities through the azygos veins and the paravertebral circulation into the superior vena cava and then into the right atrium. There is an accompanying increase in sympathetic tone and peripheral vascular resistance; however, approximately 30 percent of women who have conduction anesthesia (spinal or epidural) have significant hypotension, as the sympathetic blockade produced by the conduction anesthetic tends to eliminate the compensatory mechanisms of the body. Treatment consists of placing the patient on her left side, placing a wedge under her right hip, infusing fluids, and administering oxygen. If she is to be transported to the delivery or operating room, she should always be placed in the lateral position, not on her back.

Postdural Puncture Headache

Although not considered dangerous, the postdural puncture headache (often called a postspinal headache) is one of the most annoying and bothersome complications of anesthesia. Postdural puncture headache occurs twice as frequently in the postpartum patient as in a nonpregnant woman of equivalent age. Apparently, the incidence of headache is related to the size of the needle. The 26- or 27-gauge needle has helped to reduce the incidence and severity of these headaches. Presumably leakage of CSF via the puncture site and a subsequent drop in CSF pressure is the cause of the headache. The headache is generally located in the frontal or occipital areas and is relieved when the patient lies flat. It is aggravated in an upright position. Conservative therapy in the manner described may very often eliminate the problem. An abdominal binder should be placed over the site of puncture because it may help to increase the tone and peripheral vascular resistance. Rapid infusion of 250 mL/h of crystalloid solution over a period of 8 hours with a Foley catheter in place, with the patient being kept supine or flat (denied bathroom privileges), very often relieves the problem. Appropriate analgesics should be used, and if severe headache persists, an epidural blood patch usually provides immediate relief.

If there is an accidental dural puncture during lumbar epidural anesthesia, the epidural catheter should be placed either one lumbar space above or one lumbar space below the area of the dural puncture. This should be followed by a small bolus of normal saline (3 to 4 mL), which is placed into the epidural space through the needle at the site of puncture prior to withdrawal of the needle. The catheter is kept in place after the delivery. Continuous infusion of sterile saline at 8 to 10 mL/h for approximately 24 hours can successfully prevent a postdural puncture headache in about 70 percent of patients who incur an unintentional dural puncture. This technique, although effective, is somewhat cumbersome and can be restricting to the patient. As an alternative to the infusion of saline epidurally, a prophylactic epidural blood patch via the in situ epidural catheter has been shown to be an effective means of preventing a postdural puncture headache (80 percent).[54] A volume of no less than 15 to 20 mL of autologous blood should be injected through the epidural catheter after delivery.

Pulmonary Aspiration

Anesthesia complications are a leading cause of maternal mortality. Approximately 30 to 40 percent of the patients who die from anesthesia during labor or delivery die from pulmonary aspiration.[55] Several predisposing factors make pulmonary aspiration a great risk in the parturient.

1. General anesthesia may be required with great urgency, for example, in the event of a prolapsed cord, fetal distress, or acute hemorrhage.
2. The patient may have had a meal just prior to admission or even after the onset of labor. Pregnant patients have delayed gastric emptying time, with retention of food and solids, particularly after the onset of labor. Sedation, anxiety, and pain also delay gastric emptying.
3. Hiatal hernia has been demonstrated radiographically to exist in 20 percent of all women in the last trimester of pregnancy.
4. Increased intraabdominal pressure produced by the pregnant uterus is aggravated by the lithotomy position; the fasciculations from succinylcholine may also predispose to regurgitation and vomiting.

Pathophysiologically, particulate matter may cause difficulty, and acid aspiration, particularly if the pH is below 2.5, causes a chemical burn. If the pH is less than 1.2, actual necrosis occurs. Mortality may be high even if the pH is less than 1.75.

When the aspiration syndrome occurs, there is intense bronchospasm and an increase in lower airway resistance. There is a rapid fall in arterial blood pressure and an initial rise in pulmonary artery blood pressure followed by a return to normal. This is then followed by a fall in the pulmonary artery pressure. Acute pulmonary edema ensues, with a large loss of plasma into the lungs. The resultant decrease in plasma volume allows a consequent hemoconcentration to occur. There is a progressive fall in the PaO_2 and pH and a moderate rise in the $PaCO_2$. Right-sided aspiration is favored by the bronchial configuration. If the patient is in Trendelenburg position, the apical segment of the upper lobe and the apical segment of the lower lobe are more frequently involved. Infection is an infrequent but serious complication; however, most patients are afebrile and the chest usually clears in 7 to 10 days, if the patient survives.

When the patient aspirates solid material, there is massive collapse of the lung independent of the pH, with airway obstruction and atelectasis. There is no free fluid in the pleural or pericardial cavities, but there is a rise in the $PaCO_2$ despite less exudation or fluid loss.

The clinical picture of aspiration may occur during induction, maintenance of anesthesia, or recovery from anesthesia. Trivial amounts of acid cause severe illness. The syndrome itself may occur immediately after the aspiration or may be delayed several hours. The patient becomes restless, dyspneic, tachypneic, and cyanotic; her blood pressure falls rapidly; and she progresses into shock. Generalized bronchospasm, rales, and rhonchi with sanguineous secretions of frothy sputum from the frank pulmonary edema are noted. Chest x-rays show mottled densities, as in pulmonary edema or bronchopneumonia.

The clinical picture of a patient who has aspirated solid particles depends on the size of these particles. Acute bronchospasm and often massive atelectasis of a lobe or the entire lung may occur. Cyanosis, tachycardia, dyspnea, and mediastinal shift can develop.

Prevention is preferable to actual treatment. Although it is not guaranteed that local or regional anesthesia will circumvent pulmonary aspiration, it does lower the incidence. It is important to ensure that patients do not eat during labor. Use of a nasogastric tube or induction of vomiting for patients in labor is very controversial. Antacids definitely cause a rise in the pH of gastric contents and help alleviate the potential for acid aspiration. Antacids do not eliminate pulmonary aspiration. It has been suggested that there is a danger of aspirating particulate-matter antacids and producing particulate-matter aspiration. Therefore, the use of a nonparticulate antacid such as sodium bicitra (Bicitra) is recommended. If general anesthesia is to be used, it is essential that the patient be intubated with a cuffed endotracheal tube, and cricoid pressure be applied and maintained from the moment induction is begun. Awake intubation should not be ignored or neglected in the case of a patient with a difficult airway.

Recent research studies using H_2 blockers such as cimetidine and ranitidine in conjunction with the gastric emptying drug, metoclopramide, have been producing interesting but controversial results. Metoclopramide,[56] for example, is ineffective if narcotics were previously administered and may produce extrapyramidal effects and neurologic reactions. The intravenous administration of H_2 blockers may be contraindicated, as they can produce biliary dysfunction. The oral route and intramuscular route (the night before and the morning of), if elective cesarean section is to be performed, appear to be beneficial in all respects. It should be emphasized that these are useful adjuncts to our armamentarium and that they should not be considered a substitute for prevention and vigilance.

The management of the actual aspiration, if it should occur, consists of clearing the airway immediately with the head down in a lateral position, the right side being preferred. The pH of the vomitus should be tested, the patient oxygenated, and the airway secured with endotracheal intu-

bation prior to suction. If solid material is aspirated, immediate bronchoscopy may be required. Artificial ventilation with 100 percent oxygen, positive end-expiratory pressure, and chest therapy may be necessary. If there is hypovolemia, cardiovascular support based on central venous pressure, arterial blood gases, and the wetness of the lungs should be considered. The use of steroids is controversial, but there is no evidence that steroids help the patient. Antibiotics probably should not be used unless infection supervenes.

Total or High Spinal Anesthesia

High spinal or total spinal anesthesia can occur after an accidental injection of an epidural dose into the subarachnoid space or a miscalculation in the injection of local anesthetic into the subarachnoid space. Epidural anesthesia predisposes to a massive total spinal, as the dose of local anesthetics used in epidural anesthesia is 5 to 20 times that used in spinal anesthesia.

Patients with a high spinal characteristically suffer from difficulty in breathing, tingling in the fingers of the hand, difficulty in coughing, nausea, and possibly vomiting. If the dermatome level reaches T1–2 or even T-3, bradycardia may ensue.

Total spinal anesthesia leads to vascular hypotension, cessation of respiration, and unconsciousness. Treatment of a massive subarachnoid injection consists of administration of fluids to support the circulation, immediate intubation with an endotracheal tube, and ventilation with 100 percent oxygen. Blood pressure, circulation, and respiration should be maintained until the effects of the block are terminated. A vasopressor may be necessary.

Intravenous Injection of Local Anesthetics

A toxic level of local anesthesia may follow from accidental injection of a local anesthetic into a vein or may be the end result of an accumulation of local anesthetic after prolonged administration. An anesthetist usually encounters the former. This occurs when local anesthetic has been injected into a vein instead of into the epidural space. It may occur via the epidural needle or the epidural catheter. The engorged nature of the veins and the fact that there are numerous veins in the epidural space predispose to this situation. There are no valves in the veins of the epidural space, and the local anesthetic therefore easily reaches the brain and the heart, producing the symptoms of toxicity. Patients may complain of sleepiness, ringing in the ears (tinnitus), circumoral numbness, or a funny taste in the mouth. Grand mal seizures may rapidly follow. There may be bradycardia and cardiovascular collapse. The drop in blood pressure is due to both the lowering of cardiac output and peripheral vasodilation. Prevention is preferable to treatment and consists of making sure the epidural catheter is placed in the midline, not in the lateral portion of the epidural space. Careful aspiration of the catheter before injection of any local anesthetic and the use of a test dose help to prevent problems and do decrease their incidence, although they do not guarantee safety. Treatment consists of turning the mother to a lateral position, giving 100 percent oxygen, and performing tracheal intubation immediately if indicated. Utilization of a barbiturate such as thiopental (50 mg) or intravenous diazepam aids in terminating convulsions. Succinylcholine will control the outward manifestations of the convulsions, but if an electroencephalogram still reveals convulsive activity, this is not the treatment of choice. Maintenance of circulation and cardiovascular stability by vasopressors or fluids may be necessary. With a convulsion, there is a tremendous increase in oxygen demand and oxygenation is mandatory.

EVALUATION AND RESUSCITATION OF THE NEWBORN

A newborn's first breath usually occurs 20 to 30 seconds after the appearance of its nose. The stimulus for initiation of this first breath is unknown, but within 90 seconds rhythmic respirations usually occur under the control of the medullary centers.

It is best if someone other than the obstetrician is available to resuscitate a compromised infant. The baby should have its mouth and nose cleared of secretions, as 80 percent of infants are obligatory nasal breathers. The baby should be kept dry to reduce heat loss and then placed in an infrared warming device. The Apgar score is the sum of scores on five variables—heart rate, respiratory effort, muscle tone, reflex irritability, and color—each rated from 0 to 2, and should be evaluated at 1 and 5 minutes.[57] If the 1-minute Apgar score is between 5 and 7, the baby should be stimulated, kept dry, and ventilated with oxygen by bag and mask. If the Apgar score is 0 to 2, the trachea should be intubated, the lungs ventilated with oxygen, and cardiac resuscitation initiated. Acute neonatal asphyxia may manifest first with an accelerated heart rate and then an abrupt decrease. Proper resuscitation can bring a rise in heart rate followed in several minutes by spontaneous breathing. An infant heart rate of less than 100 is an indication for active, vigorous resuscitation.[58]

When ventilating a newborn, the adequacy of ventilation is determined by equal expansion of the chest, an increase in the heart rate to normal, improvement of color, and equal bilateral strong breath sounds in the axilla. The ventilatory pressure should be maintained between 25 and 30 cm H_2O, but if the lungs remain stiff, higher pressures may be necessary. If meconium is present, an endotracheal tube should be used as a suction catheter. Laryngoscopy should be performed to see if there is meconium present at or below the vocal cords, and if so, the newborn should be suctioned. If meconium is not present, visualization alone is sufficient.

Cardiac massage should be performed if the heart rate is less than 60 beats per minute. This is done by compressing the sternum two-thirds the distance to the vertebral column at a rate of 120 times a minute with the thumbs placed at the junction of the middle third of the body. Cardiac massage and ventilation should be maintained until the heart rate is above 100 beats per minute.

If pH determination shows evidence of metabolic acidosis, 2 to 3 mL of sodium bicarbonate should be administered into the umbilical vein and the ventilation continued. If the pH remains below 7.10 despite ventilation, the anesthetist should try to correct one fourth of the metabolic component with the initial sodium bicarbonate.

It is important to maintain volume, as 60 percent of asphyxiates in utero are volume depleted and the correction of acidosis may reveal unrecognized hypovolemia. To detect hypovolemia, the anesthetist checks arterial pressure, capillary filling, skin color, and pulse. Treatment consists of giving blood, 10 mL/kg; albumin, 25 percent, 1 g/kg; crystalloid solution, 10 mL/kg; or plasma, 10 mL/kg. The blood pressure is evaluated regularly.

Recognizing those infants who need special observation or therapy and placing them in intensive care nurseries will definitely reduce perinatal mortality, particularly among premature infants.

REFERENCES

1. Cohen SE. Why is the pregnant patient different? *Semin Anesth.* 1982;1(2):73–82.
2. Cheek TG, Gutsche BB. Maternal physiologic alterations during pregnancy. In: Shnider SM, Levinson G, eds. *Anesthesia for obstetrics.* 2nd ed. Baltimore: Williams & Wilkins; 1987:3–13.
3. Joyce TH III, Palacios QT. Cardiac disease. In: James FM, Wheeler AS, Dewan DM, eds. *Obstetric anesthesia—The complicated patient.* 2nd ed. Philadelphia: FA Davis; 1988:159–180.
4. Bonica JJ. Maternal physiologic alterations of pregnancy. In: Bonica JJ, ed. *Obstetric analgesia and anesthesia.* Amsterdam: World Federation of Societies of Anaesthesiologists; 1980:1–56.
5. Cohen SE. Why is the pregnant patient different? 1982 ASA Annual Refresher Course Lectures. 1982;119:1–7.
6. Blass NH. Regional anesthesia in the morbidly obese parturient. *Region Anaesth.* 1979;4(10):20–22.
7. Gibbs CP, Banner TC. Effectiveness of Bicitra as a preoperative antacid. *Anesthesiology.* 1984;61:97–99.
8. Cohen SE, Brose WG. Endocrine disease. In: James FM, Wheeler AS, Dewan DM, eds. *Obstetric anesthesia—The complicated patient.* 2nd ed. Philadelphia: FA Davis; 1988:243–266.
9. Conklin KA, Murad SHN. Pharmacology of drugs in obstetric anesthesia. *Semin Anesth.* 1982;1(2):83–100.
10. Fiedler MF. AANA Journal Course: Advanced scientific concepts: Update for nurse anesthetists—An introduction to fetal heart rate monitoring. *AANA J.* 57(8):1989:257–264.
11. Hon EH. The clinical evaluation of fetal heart rate. In: Hon EH, ed. *An atlas of fetal heart rate patterns.* New Haven, CT: Harty Press; 1968:25–31.
12. Schifrin BS, Dame L. Fetal heart rate patterns: Prediction of Apgar score. *JAMA.* 1972;219:1322–1325.
13. Cetrulo CL, Schifrin BS. Fetal heart rate patterns preceding death in utero. *Obstet Gynecol.* 1976;48:521–527.
14. Benson RC, Schubeck F, Deutschberger J. Fetal heart rate as a predictor of fetal distress. *Obstet Gynecol.* 1968;32:259–266.
15. Parer JT. The current role of intrapartum fetal blood sampling. *Clin Obstet Gynecol.* 1980;23:565–582.
16. Quilligan EJ. Monitoring the fetus using acid–base studies. *Clin Obstet Gynecol.* 1979;6:309.
17. Chan WH, Paul RH, Toews J. Intrapartum fetal monitoring: Maternal and fetal morbidity and perinatal mortality. *Obstet Gynecol.* 1973;41:7–13.
18. Quilligan EJ, Paul RH. Fetal monitoring: Is it worth it? *Obstet & Gynecol.* 1975;45:96–100.
19. LeBoyer F. Natural childbirth. In: LeBoyer F, ed. *Birth without violence.* New York: Knopf; 1975:1–114.
20. Schaer HM. History of pain relief in obstetrics. In: Marx GF, Bassel GM, eds. *Obstetric analgesia and anesthesia.* Amsterdam: Elsevier/North-Holland; 1980:12–16.

21. Crawford JS, Burton OM, Davies P. Anaesthesia for section: Further refinements of a technique. *Br J Anaesth.* 1973;45:726–731.

22. Covino BG. Pharmacology of local anaesthetic agents. *Br J Anaesth.* 1986;58:701–716.

23. Gissen AJ, Datta S, Lambert D. The chloroprocaine controversy. Is chloroprocaine neurotoxic? *Region Anesth.* 1984;9(4):135–145.

24. Moore DC, Spierdijk J, Van Kleef JD, et al. Chloroprocaine neurotoxicity: Four additional cases. *Anesth Analg.* 1982;61:155–159.

25. Reisner LS, Hochman BN, Plumer MH. Persistent neurologic deficit and adhesive arachnoiditis following intrathecal chloroprocaine. *Anesth Analg.* 1980;59:452–454.

26. Albright GA. Cardiac arrest following regional anesthesia with etidocaine or bupivacaine. *Anesthesiology.* 1979;51:285–287.

27. James FM III, Greiss FC, Kemp RD. An evaluation of vasopressor therapy for maternal hypotension during spinal anesthesia. *Anesthesiology.* 1970;33:25.

28. Redick LF. Epidural analgesia. *Clin Perinatol.* 1982;9(1):63–76.

29. Abboud TK, Shnider SM, Dailey PA, et al. Intrathecal administration of hyperbaric morphine for the relief of pain in labour. *Br J Anaesth.* 1984;56:1351–1360.

30. Hughes SC, Rosen MA, Shnider SM, et al. Maternal and neonatal effects of epidural morphine for labor and delivery. *Anesth Analg.* 1984;63:319–324.

31. Kotelko DM, Dailey PA, Shnider SM, et al. Epidural morphine analgesia after cesarean delivery. *Obstet Gynecol.* 1984;63: 409–413.

32. Rawal N, Wattwil M. Respiratory depression after epidural morphine: An experimental and clinical study. *Anesth Analg.* 1984;63:8–14.

33. Datta S, Alper MH. Anesthesia for cesarean section. *Anesthesiology.* 1980;53:142.

34. Ramanathan S, Masih A, Rock L, et al. Maternal and fetal effects of prophylactic hydration with crystalloids or colloids before epidural anesthesia. *Anesth Analg.* 1983;62:673–678.

35. Blass NH. Anesthesia for the morbidly obese. In: Katz J, Benumof J, Kadis LB, eds. *Anesthesia and uncommon diseases: Pathophysiology and clinical correlations.* 2nd ed. Philadelphia: WB Saunders; 1981:450–462.

36. Eckstein KL, Marx GF. Aortocaval compression and uterine displacement. *Anesthesiology.* 1974;40:92–96.

37. Datta S, Corke BC, Alper MH, et al. Epidural anesthesia for cesarean section: A comparison of bupivacaine, chloroprocaine and etidocaine. *Anesthesiology.* 1980;52:48–51.

38. James FM III, Crawford JS, Hopkinson R, et al. A comparison of general anesthesia and lumbar epidural analgesia for elective cesarean section. *Anesth Analg.* 1977;56:228.

39. Gibbs CP. Anesthesia for the high risk parturient. *IARS Rev Course Lectures.* 1984;58(7):49–61.

40. Weinstein L. Syndrome of hemolysis, elevated liver enzymes and low platelet count: A consequence of severe hypertension in pregnancy. *Am J Obstet Gynecol.* 1982;142:159–167.

41. Datta S, Brown WU Jr. Acid–base status in diabetic mothers and their infants following general or spinal anesthesia for cesarean section. *Anesthesiology.* 1977;47:272.

42. Datta S, Kitzmiller JL. Anesthetic and obstetric management of diabetic and pregnant women. *Clin Perinatol.* 1982;9(1):154–166.

43. Datta S. The Diabetic Parturient. In: James FM, Wheeler AS, Dewan DM, eds. *Obstetric anesthesia—The complicated patient.* 2nd ed. Philadelphia: FA Davis; 1988:401–410.

44. Kitzmiller JL, Cloherty JP, Younger D, et al. Diabetic pregnancy and perinatal morbidity. *Am J Obstet Gynecol.* 1978;131:560–580.

45. Metcalfe J, Ueland K. Maternal cardiovascular adjustments to pregnancy. *Prog Cardiovasc Dis.* 1974;16:363–374.

46. Rush RW, Keirse MJNC, Howat P, et al. Contribution of preterm delivery to perinatal mortality. *Br Med J.* 1976;2: 965–968.

47. Frederick J, Anderson AM. Factors associated with spontaneous preterm birth. *Br J Obstet Gynaecol.* 1976;83:342–350.

48. MacGregor S, Keith LG, Chasnoff IJ, et al. Cocaine use during pregnancy: Adverse perinatal outcome. *Am J Obstet Gynecol.* 1987;157:686–690.

49. Chestnut DH. Anesthesia for preterm labor and delivery. In: Hood DD, ed. *Problems in anesthesia: Anesthesia in obstetrics and gynecology.* 1989;3(1):32–44.

50. Eggleston MK. Management of preterm labor and delivery. *Clin Obstet Gynecol.* 1986;29:230–239.

51. Gambling D, Birmingham CL, Jenkins C. Magnesium and the anaesthetist. *Can J Anaesth.* 1988;35:644–654.

52. Holmes F. The supine hypotensive syndrome: Its importance to the anaesthetist. *Anaesthesia.* 1960;15:298–306.

53. Howard BK, Goodson JH, Mengert WF. Supine hypotensive syndrome of late pregnancy. *Obstet Gynecol.* 1953;1:371–377.

54. Colonna-Romano P, Shapiro BE. Prophylactic epidural blood patch in obstetrics. *Anesthesiology.* 1988;69(3A):A665.

55. Roberts RB, Shirley MD. Reducing the risk of acid aspiration during cesarean section. *Anesth Analg.* 1974;53:859–868.

56. Cohen SE, Jasson J, Talafre L, et al. Does metoclopramide decrease the volume of gastric contents in patients undergoing cesarean section? *Anesthesiology.* 1984;61:604–607.

57. Apgar V. A proposal for a new method of evaluation of a newborn infant. *Anesth Analg.* 1953;32:260–267.

58. Ostheimer GW. Newborn resuscitation. *Semin Anesth.* 1982;1(2): 168–176.

Pediatric Anesthesia

Timothy D. Saye

The conduct of pediatric anesthesia requires increased vigilance as the margin of safety for managing complications is much less than with the average adult. Increased technology in monitoring has greatly enhanced our ability to safely anesthetize the pediatric patient, but a thorough understanding of pediatric anatomy, physiology, and pathophysiology is essential to providing appropriate anesthesia tailored to individual patient requirements.

HISTORICAL PERSPECTIVES

Elective pediatric surgery preceded the advent of surgical anesthesia. Surgical correction of club foot, strabismus, and cleft lip and palate was performed without anesthesia. On July 3, 1842, Crawford W. Long anesthetized an 8-year-old boy with ether dropped onto a towel for the amputation of a toe. Long reported that "the operation was performed without the boy evincing the least sign of pain."[1] This was the second patient to be anesthetized with ether by Long. He failed to publish his report of ether anesthesia until 1849, three years after William Morton, a New England dentist, performed the first public demonstration of ether anesthesia at the Bullfinch ampitheatre of the Massachusetts General Hospital. After Morton's public demonstration in 1846, others began using ether for surgical anesthesia.

When news of ether anesthesia reached England in December 1846, John Snow, an established physician and physiologist, took an interest in an anesthesia practice. He undertook detailed clinical and pharmacologic studies of ether, chloroform, and other anesthetics. Snow published several books. In the last, *On Chloroform and Other Anesthetics*, he makes a keen pharmacokinetic observation pertaining to anesthesia for infants: "The effects of chloroform are more quickly produced and also subside more quickly in children than in adults, owing no doubt to the quicker breathing and circulation."[2(p49)] Snow continues with a description of how he delivered chloroform anesthetics to as many as 186 infants under 1 year old, some as young as 8 days old. Furthermore, he states that there had been no ill effects of chloroform when administered to children.[2(pp258–259)] As more cases were performed it was recognized that children were also susceptible to the hepatic and cardiovascular complications of chloroform. In fact, the first recorded anesthetic death was a healthy 15-year-old girl undergoing toenail excision under chloroform anesthesia in 1848.

Occurring simultaneously with the development of anesthesia was the initiation of formalized nursing training schools and the integration of nurses into every aspect of hospital function. Through the tireless efforts of nurses, aseptic surgical technique became a reality, surgical mortality decreased, and the numbers of operations soared. Nurses also played a vital role in postoperative care of surgical patients.

The first American text offering advice on pediatric anesthetic techniques was James T. Gwathmey's *Anesthesia*, published in 1914. He suggested inducing children in the presence of their mother, with a gentle manner of both voice and movement. He also added the essence of bitter orange to the mask to disguise the anesthetic odor.[3]

The concept of the "steal" induction was advocated by Arthur Guedel in 1921. He would begin with the mask concealed in his hand above the face of the sleeping child, then would slowly lower it to cover the face and increase the inspired concentration of anesthetic.[4]

In the early years of the 20th century, there arose a great deal of interest in regional anesthesia. One Minneapolis surgeon, Robert Emmett Farr, performed a variety of abdominal and extremity surgeries on children with the use of regional anesthesia. In the 1923 text *Practical Local Anesthesia*, he explained his dependence on the support of the anesthetist by giving her a special title, the "psychoanesthetist," whose job it was to comfort and divert the attention of the younger patients during the procedure.[5]

As the number and complexity of pediatric surgical procedures increased, there developed a need for specific pediatric equipment and specialty training. In the years following World War II, pediatric anesthetists have endeavored to advance the frontiers of knowledge regarding the uniqueness of the pediatric patient when undergoing anesthesia and surgery. They have been instrumental in the development of specific equipment designed for the pediatric patient and have been committed to the communication of their knowledge and skills to others in the field.

GENERAL APPROACH TO THE PEDIATRIC PATIENT

It is important for the anesthetist to recognize that the infant or child who is having a surgical procedure is not the only member of the family who is experiencing stress related to the operation. In fact, with infants less than 6 months of age, the parents certainly suffer far more trauma associated with separation from their child than does the infant. This stress on the parents can be worsened by feelings of guilt about the condition of the child. If the child has a congenital defect or has suffered an accident, the parents may unfairly blame themselves. The preoperative period is one in which the anesthetist can express empathy with and compassion for the parents. This helps build a bond between the anesthetist and the parents that will endure throughout the perioperative period.

The reasons for stress to the child during the surgical period include (1) separation from the parents, (2) painful procedures, (3) strange surroundings, (4) frightening procedures, and (5) survival. One of the principal ways the physician may help the parents and child cope with the stress is through honest communication. With younger children, the communication is directed at the parents; with older children it is directed toward the patient. Procedures and plans for induction should be explained fully, with particular attention regarding painful parts of the perioperative period. These should be addressed honestly, but with understanding and concern for the patient's feelings.

Age, or cognitive awareness, is probably the most important factor in determining the child's response to the stress of the surgical experience. Therefore age is an important determinant of the type or need for premedication. Young children are most concerned with separation from their parents. With the development of memory comes the fear of pain. Older children fear the unknown, whereas teenagers fear loss of control and dignity.

Steward has divided the ages into useful groups on the basis of cognitive development and response to stressful situations.[6] Birth to 6 months of age is the period of maximum stress for the parents and of least stress for the infant, who is not old enough to understand what is happening. There is no need for sedative premedication. The only premedication needed is an anticholinergic (atropine 0.01 mg/kg IV or 0.02 mg/kg PO or IM; or glycopyrrolate 0.01 mg/kg IV or IM or 0.05 mg/kg PO) to diminish secretions and control vagal-induced bradycardia. Six months to four years is an age when separation anxiety is at its maximum. The child is able to remember painful experiences, but not able to understand that they may be necessary or that they will end. Sedative premedication by whatever route chosen is especially helpful in reducing stress to the child, parents, and anesthetist. It should be emphasized that parents are the best premedication available, and they should be allowed to remain with the child as long as possible. Four to six years has been called the "almost" age because the child can almost understand the surgical experience and can usually tolerate separation from their parents. At this age, the child becomes the focus of communication and should be given choices within reason as to premedication, induction options, and other factors. All issues and questions should be discussed fully with the patient. Six years to adolescence has been termed the *golden age,* for these patients are able to understand what is going to happen and make well-informed decisions regarding premedication, induction techniques, and postoperative pain control options. Adolescents and teenagers have significant concerns of dignity and privacy related to their developing sexuality, and it is imperative that their modesty be respected by all members of the operating room team.

Regardless of how much skill and knowledge is exercised by the anesthetist in the operating room, what the parents and patient remember is the quality of care, understanding, and concern expressed in the preoperative and postoperative visits.

PHYSIOLOGIC AND ANATOMIC DIFFERENCES BETWEEN PEDIATRIC AND ADULT PATIENTS

Patients identified as pediatric can encompass a wide range of ages, weights, and levels of maturation. The difference in physiology and anatomy between adults and pediatric patients is exaggerated in younger patients and reaches a zenith with the premature patient. To safely manage the anesthesia for the newborn, a thorough knowledge of the physiology of the neonate is needed. This includes the abrupt transition of the fetus to the newborn state and the subsequent maturation of the neonatal systems. The newborn period is said to be the first 24 hours of life, the neonatal period being the first month of life. All of the newborn's systems exhibit dramatic changes but the circulatory, respiratory, renal, and metabolic systems are of the most interest to the anesthetist.

Circulatory System

The circulatory system of the fetus has a parallel configuration, where the majority of blood that enters the fetus through the umbilical vein is shunted from the right atrium and pulmonary artery across the foramen ovale and ductus arteriosus respectively, bypassing the lungs and flowing into the left atrium and descending aorta. This circulatory pattern is maintained by high pulmonary pressures and low systemic pressures. At birth, as the alveoli are filled with air, there is a sharp decrease in pulmonary vascular resistance and, therefore, an increase in pulmonary blood flow. Left atrial pressure increases as systemic vascular pressure increases, and the foramen ovale is functionally closed. A series circuit is established in which the majority of the cardiac output passes through the pulmonary vasculature.

The oxygen content of the blood is increased at birth, and this inhibits the synthesis of prostaglandins which results in closure of the ductus arteriosus. The muscular wall of the ductus is very sensitive to the dilating effects of prostaglandins and the constricting effects of increased Pa_{O_2}.[7] The premature infant has less muscle in the wall of the ductus and therefore is less sensitive to the changes in prostaglandins and Pa_{O_2}, which partially accounts for the higher incidence of patent ductus arteriosus in premature patients.

The pulmonary circulation remains very sensitive to changes in PaO_2 and pH during the neonatal period. Any pathophysiologic process that results in hypoxia, acidosis, or hypothermia can cause an increase in pulmonary vascular resistance and reopening of the ductus arteriosus and foramen ovale. This would result in a persistent fetal circulation and systemic hypoxia.

Having completed the transition from fetal to adult circulation, the neonate is left with an immature cardiovascular system. The myocardium contains less contractile tissue than does the adult heart. This results in a decreased ability to develop large degrees of muscle contraction.[8] Furthermore, the decreased amount of contractile tissue reduces the compliance of the ventricle, limiting the ability of the neonate to increase stroke volume. The neonate therefore relies on increasing heart rate to increase cardiac output in times of stress; however, this may be limited by a relatively greater vagal input to the heart in neonates than in adults. Neonates are considered highly vagotonic. Bradycardia during anesthesia can result from hypoxia, vagal stimulation, or volatile anesthetics. Furthermore, the arterial baroresponse, that reflex response to hypotension resulting in an increase in heart rate, has been found to be reduced to a larger degree in the newborn rabbit given small amounts of inhalation anesthetic than in adult rabbits.[9] If the same is true in humans, the neonate has a very limited ability to increase cardiac output. Any heart rate in the neonate below 120 beats per minute should be considered bradycardia; and any rate below 100 beats per minute should be treated with atropine, with cardiac compressions considered depending on the patient's hemodynamic status (Table 32–1).

The neonate has a higher percentage of fetal hemoglobin than does the adult. Fetal hemoglobin has a greater affinity for oxygen than does adult hemoglobin, which results in a decreased release of oxygen to the peripheral tissues. The oxygen hemoglobin dissociation curve is shifted to the left. This effect is offset by the increased concentration of hemoglobin in the neonate. By 4 to 6 months of age, the relative concentration of fetal hemoglobin begins to resemble that of an adult. Because of the decreased cardiac reserve of the neonate and the increased affinity of fetal hemoglobin for oxygen, the hematocrit of the neonate generally should be maintained at 40 percent or higher.

Respiratory System

In several respects the neonate is at a disadvantage in terms of respiratory function. The anatomy of the head and neck influences the airway management of the neonate (Fig. 32–1). Neonates are obligate nose breathers and the nares are narrow and easily obstructed by secretions and nasogastric tubes. The occiput of the neonate is relatively larger than that of the adult, so that when the neonate is lying supine on a flat surface, the head is flexed forward and the airway may become obstructed. A pad placed beneath the neck and shoulders will allow the head to be tilted back, improving airway patency and facilitating laryngoscopy and intubation. The tongue is relatively large, which can cause obstruction and interfere with laryngoscopy. The glottic opening, which is at the level of the fifth cervical vertebra in the adult, is between C-3 and C-4 in the neonate. This makes the glottis appear more anterior during laryngoscopy. The most narrow portion of the airway in an adult is the glottic opening. In the newborn, however, this is at the cricoid ring. Therefore, an endotracheal tube may pass easily through the vocal cords but not be able to be advanced further. A smaller tube should then be used. The epiglottis in the neonate is stiffer and relatively larger than that in the older child. Also, the vocal cords in the neonate slant more anteriorly than in the adult. The cumulative effect of all these anatomic differences between adult and neonate is that the neonate's airway is more dependent on proper positioning for patency and the intubation of the neonate is a more difficult and skill-dependent procedure.

The mechanism of breathing also undergoes a maturation process. The ribs of the newborn are relatively horizontal. They assume a more vertical angle as the infant grows. This change of angle improves the contracting mechanism of the intercostal muscles. Furthermore, the ribs and cartilage of the neonate are more pliable than those of older infants and may not support large negative intrapleural pressures.

The neonate's muscles also undergo a maturation process. There are two types of muscles in the body, type I and type II. Type I muscles are slow-twitch, high oxidative fibers that maintain prolonged muscle activity. Type II muscle fibers are fast-twitch, low oxidative fibers that can maintain short contractions only. The premature infant has a very low concentration of type I muscle fibers. In the diaphragm, type I muscles achieve maturity at 8 months of life, whereas the intercostal muscle type I fibers achieve maturation at 2 months of life. This obviously predisposes the 3- to 4-month-old infant to fatigue in the face of respiratory obstruction, chronic illness, and disease.

The closing volumes of infants are higher than those of adults. The closing volume is the volume of gas in the lungs below which the alveoli will collapse on expiration. There is an overlap between the closing volume and the normal tidal volume in the neonate. This allows atelectasis and hypoxia to develop more easily.

TABLE 32–1. CARDIOVASCULAR DATA

	Heart Rate	Blood Pressure (mm Hg)	Blood Volume (mL/kg)	Hemoglobin (g/100 mL)
Neonate (0–4 wk)	120	60/40	80	16–18
Infant (4 wk–6 mo)	110	90/60	75	10–11
Child (6 mo–6 y)	100	100/70	70	12–14
Adult	80	120/70	60–65	12–14

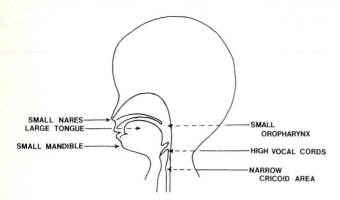

SMALL NARES
LARGE TONGUE

SMALL MANDIBLE

SMALL OROPHARYNX

HIGH VOCAL CORDS

NARROW CRICOID AREA

Figure 32–1. The pediatric airway.

The neonate also has a paradoxical response to hypoxia. In the adult, hypoxia causes tachypnea, whereas in the neonate, the respiratory rate can decrease or even apnea may result. The principal differences between the respiratory values and lung volumes of the neonate and those of an adult are respiratory rate and oxygen consumption (Table 32–2). Tidal volume, dead space, and functional residual capacity are all approximately equivalent when expressed in cc/kg. The O_2 consumption is 6 to 8 cc/kg/min for the neonate as compared with 3 cc/kg/min for the adult. As the tidal volumes are the same, the respiratory rate must be faster, resulting in a higher alveolar ventilation. This in turn results in a faster induction of inhalation anesthesia and a faster emergence. Moreover, this implies a relatively low O_2 reserve when the airway is obstructed for any reason, resulting in hypoxia and bradycardia.

Renal System

During fetal life the kidney forms urine which contributes to the formation of amniotic fluid, which is important in the development of the lung and acts as a shock absorber for the fetus. The renal blood flow and glomerular filtration rate are low because (1) the systemic arterial pressure is low, (2) renal vascular resistance is high, (3) glomerular capillaries have a very low permeability, and (4) the glomeruli are of small size and diameter. The first two conditions change at birth, thereby increasing the renal blood flow and glomerular filtration rate markedly.

TABLE 32–2. LUNG VOLUMES

	Adult	Child	Neonate
VA (mL/kg/min)	60	80	100–150
Frequency (per min)	10	20	40
TLC^a (mL/kg)	80	70	60
FRC (mL/kg)	34	32	30
RV (mL/kg)	17	19	20
Vt (mL/kg)	7	7	6

^{a} TLC, total lung capacity; FRC, functional residual capacity; RV, residual volume.

Glomerulogenesis is completed at the 34th week of gestation. The renin–angiotensin–aldosterone system is intact in the newborn. There is an increase in aldosterone secretion in the newborn above that of the adult, which is thought to be due to the need for sodium salts in the bone and the lack of a mature renal feedback mechanism.

The distal tubule cannot efficiently reabsorb all of the sodium from the filtrate, despite the increased aldosterone secretion. The neonate is therefore referred to as an "obligate sodium loser" and should receive sodium in all intravenous solutions. Moreover, in the first 24 to 48 hours of life, the neonate has a limited ability to both concentrate and dilute the urine; however, during the first 3 or 4 days, with the increase in glomerular filtration rate, the neonate is able to dilute and concentrate the urine appropriately. Renal function approximates 70 to 80 percent of normal values at the end of 1 month of life.

Metabolic System

The infant maintains a precarious balance between endogenous energy stores and the high energy demand associated with the infant's high metabolic rate. Prolonged NPO (nothing by mouth) states and the stress of surgery and disease may disturb this balance and lead to hypoglycemia. On the other hand, the injudicious use of glucose-containing solutions may lead to hyperglycemia and the establishment of a hyperosmotic state. This in turn may cause an osmotic diuresis.

Endogenous energy stores are not developed until the last trimester. The 28-week-old fetus has practically no fat stores; the 34-week-old fetus contains 7 to 8 percent of body weight as fat with 9 g of glycogen; and the full-term newborn has 16 percent of body weight as fat with 34 g of glycogen. The normal rate of glucose metabolism is approximately 6 to 8 mg/kg/min. The hepatic and muscle glycogen stores are rapidly depleted in the first few hours of life. Therefore an exogenous source of glucose should be provided to the infant in the perioperative period. Although many authors have studied the perioperative glucose requirements of infants,[10–12] there is no consensus on a regimen of glucose administration; however, infusion of a solution containing 5 percent dextrose at maintenance rates seems to provide adequate substrate to meet metabolic demands. It must be remembered that in times of great stress to the infant, this regimen might prove inadequate, and therefore blood glucose concentrations should be followed periodically during the perioperative period, and the administration of dextrose modified accordingly.

PHARMACOLOGIC DIFFERENCES

There are significant differences in the pharmacodynamics and pharmacokinetics of the inhalation and intravenous anesthetic agents between infants and adults. These differences underscore the importance of titrating dosages to the patient's responses and monitoring for these responses appropriately.

There are developmental differences in body tissue composition. The preterm neonate has a high total body water (TBW) content approaching 85 percent of body weight.

This decreases to 78 percent at term and 60 percent at 1 year of age. Most intravenous agents tend to distribute throughout the TBW before reaching their target receptor sites. Therefore, the amount of TBW influences the final drug concentration, and in general the larger the TBW the higher the required dose to achieve the same target organ concentration or effect.

There are also age-related differences in drug metabolism. Most drugs are metabolized by either degradative pathways (e.g., oxidation reduction or hydrolysis) or synthetic reactions, also called conjugation reactions. The concentration and activity of the synthetic reactions are more profoundly affected by age, improving at 3 months and peaking at 2 to 3 years. The half-lives of barbiturates and benzodiazepines are markedly prolonged in the infant. The pharmacokinetics of narcotics may yield acceptable plasma levels after injection, but they may have a prolonged depressant effect on respiratory drive.

Infants have a different response to neuromuscular blocking agents than do adults. On a weight basis, infants require more succinylcholine than do adults to produce apnea[13,14]; however, when the dose is based on surface area, there is no age difference in the response.[15] A more pronounced respiratory depression following *d*-tubocurarine injection has been seen in the neonate when compared with the adult. Electromyographic studies demonstrate equivalent levels of neuromuscular blockade. The infant simply appears to be more sensitive to weakening of the respiratory musculature.

There are important differences in the pharmacodynamics and pharmacokinetics of inhalation anesthetics between pediatric and adult patients. To understand these differences it is necessary to review the factors that determine the uptake and distribution of inhaled agents. These factors determine the rate at which the anesthetic partial pressure in the alveolus approaches the inspired anesthetic partial pressure. Inspired concentration, alveolar ventilation, and functional residual capacity determine the rate of delivery of the inspired anesthetic to the lung. The cardiac output, solubility of the agent, and the alveolar-to-venous partial pressure gradient determine the rate of uptake of the anesthetic from the lungs.[16] It has been reported that the alveolar partial pressures of halothane,[17] isoflurane, and enflurane[18] rise more rapidly, approaching the inspired partial pressure of the agent, in children than in adults. There are four differences between neonates and adults that contribute to this more rapid rise.

The first of these is the difference in the ratio of alveolar ventilation to functional residual capacity. This is a measure of the rate of "wash-in" of the anesthetic into the alveoli. This ratio is 5 : 1 in the neonate compared with 1.5 : 1 in adults. The difference is secondary to a much greater alveolar ventilation in neonates, as the functional residual capacity remains constant on a weight basis as the person grows.

The second difference is attributed to the higher proportion of the cardiac output distributed to the vessel-rich group (VRG) in the neonate. The VRG is composed of the brain, heart, kidneys, and splanchnic and endocrine organs. In adults, an increase in cardiac output slows the rate of rise of alveolar to inspired anesthetic partial pressure. In con-

trast, the increased cardiac output in the neonate speeds the rate of induction of inhaled agents, because the cardiac output is preferentially distributed to the VRG. This occurs because the VRG constitutes 18 percent of the body weight of the neonate as opposed to only 6 percent in adults. Therefore the anesthetic partial pressure in the VRG, which includes the brain, equilibrates more rapidly with the alveolar partial pressure.

The third difference between neonates and adults that contributes to the more rapid rise in alveolar partial pressure is the lower blood/gas solubility of inhaled anesthetics in the neonate. The less soluble an anesthetic is in blood or tissue, the greater the amount of the anesthetic that remains in the alveolus and, therefore, the more rapid rise of the alveolar to inspired anesthetic partial pressure. The cortical partial pressure is a reflection of the alveolar partial pressure. The solubilities of halothane, isoflurane, enflurane, and methoxyflurane in blood are 18 percent less in neonates than in adults.[19] The solubility in preterm neonates of isoflurane, halothane, and sevoflurane is similar to that in full-term infants; that is, solubility is independent of gestational age.[20]

The fourth difference between neonates and adults is the lower tissue/blood solubility of inhaled anesthetics in neonates. The less soluble an agent is in tissues, the less anesthetic is removed from the blood to achieve a partial pressure that is equal to alveolar pressure. Therefore, the partial pressure of the anesthetic in the blood returning to the lungs increases and the alveolar-to-venous partial pressure gradient decreases. It follows that less anesthetic is then removed from the alveolus and a more rapid rise of alveolar to inspired anesthetic partial pressure occurs. The solubilities of halothane, isoflurane, enflurane, and methoxyflurane in the VRG of neonates are approximately 50 percent less than in adults.[21] The lower tissue solubility may be the result of the greater water content and lower protein and lipid concentrations in neonatal tissues.

The pharmacokinetics of inhaled anesthetics during the first 15 to 20 minutes of exposure depends on the solubility of the agent in the VRG. For the next 20 to 200 minutes, primarily the uptake of the anesthetic by the muscle tissues determines the pharmacokinetics of that agent. The solubility of anesthetic agents in skeletal muscle varies directly with age, being lower in neonates than in adults.[21]

The net effect of all these differences between neonates and adults is that the alveolar partial pressure of inhalation anesthetics rises more rapidly to equal the inspired concentration of the anesthetics in the neonate. This can contribute to a more rapid inhalation induction of anesthesia in neonates than in adults.

There are also age-related differences in the minimum alveolar concentration (MAC) of inhaled anesthetic agents. The MAC of halothane in neonates (0.87 ± 0.03 percent) is 25 percent less than it is in older infants 1 to 6 months of age (1.20 ± 0.06 percent).[22] The MAC of isoflurane in neonates is 15 percent less than in infants 1 to 6 months of age.[23] MAC also varies with gestational age. The MAC of isoflurane in preterm neonates less than 32 weeks of gestational age (1.28 ± 0.17 percent) is 10 percent less than it is in neonates 32 to 37 weeks of gestational age (1.41 ± 0.18 percent), which is 12 percent less than in full-term neonates (1.60 ± 0.03 percent).[24]

ANESTHETIC MANAGEMENT OF INFANTS AND CHILDREN

A thorough knowledge of the physiologic, pharmacologic, and anatomic differences between pediatric and adult patients allows the anesthetist to approach the anesthetic management of infants and children in a rational and safe manner. There are, however, additional differences with regard to preoperative evaluation, equipment needs, induction, maintenance, emergence from anesthesia, and recovery room care that the pediatric anesthetist must be cognizant of.

Preoperative Evaluation

The preoperative evaluation starts with a thorough history. In younger children and in all patients with congenital abnormalities, this must include a history of the pregnancy, delivery, and newborn period. Details regarding extended hospital stays postdelivery, intensive care unit management, and oxygen and mechanical ventilatory requirements are critical. Information regarding other persons in the family with congenital abnormalities or a history of sudden infant death syndrome is helpful. Of course these questions are in addition to a routine preoperative history, including the patient's and family's previous anesthetic experiences. A common problem that the pediatric anesthetist encounters is the child with a cold. This condition must be approached in a careful manner giving consideration to all parties involved. The patient or parents should be questioned regarding the presence of symptoms such as rhinorrhea, coughing (productive or nonproductive), nasal and sinus congestion, laryngitis, changes in activity level and appetite, presence of fever, and disruption of sleep patterns. It should be determined if there are other children at home or in school who are ill, as this can help to confirm a diagnosis and indicate the time course of the illness. On physical examination, special attention should be paid to auscultation of the lungs and examination of the ears and oropharynx. A white blood cell count with a lymphocyte differential is helpful; a left shift may indicate an infective process.

The parents' judgment as to the severity of the illness or its time course can be very accurate, and should sometimes be trusted over a brief examination of the patient. The child with a florid upper respiratory infection (URI) is at increased risk of laryngospasm, bronchospasm, stridor, breath holding, and hypoxia during anesthesia. The incidence of postoperative complications including oxygen requirements and need for mechanical ventilation is also increased. Therefore, the child appearing for elective surgery with an URI must be carefully examined; a history questioning the presence of the above symptoms must be taken, the surgeons and parents must be consulted, and if the child is deemed to be at increased risk for anesthesia, the surgery should be postponed until the URI resolves. With lower respiratory infections, the surgery should be delayed 4 to 6 weeks so that the respiratory tract can return to normal levels of reactivity and the infective process can completely clear.[25]

Volume status should be evaluated, especially in patients with surgical conditions predisposing to dehydration, for example, gastroschisis. Length of NPO period, time of last void, history of diarrhea or vomiting, skin turgor, tenseness of fontanelles, and physical appearance can all aid in this determination (Table 32–3). Laboratory values of blood urea nitrogen, creatinine, hematocrit, and urine specific gravity can also be useful, as can a comparison of current weight and previous weights. The following formula can be used to calculate the percentage fluid deficit:

$$\text{Percentage fluid deficit} = \frac{\text{usual weight} - \text{current weight}}{\text{usual weight}}$$

Proper volume repletion should be completed prior to induction of anesthesia.

The airway must figure prominently in any preoperative examination of a child. A cleft lip or palate, oropharyngeal masses, presence of teeth, and size and position of tongue should all be clarified preoperatively. The presence of congenital anomalies affecting the airway, like the Pierre Robin, Goldenhar, and Treacher Collins syndromes, should be determined. Parents should be questioned as to what position the child prefers to sleep at night, the presence of snoring, or apneic spells during sleep. On physical examination, the anesthetist should pay special attention to the limits of opening of the mouth and extension and flexion of the neck, ensuring that the trachea is midline and evaluating the potential displacement area. This area is the space between the middle of the inside of the mentum of the mandible and the hyoid bone, where the tongue can be displaced to visualize the cords. It should be at least 1.5 cm in newborns and 3 cm in adults.[26]

The preoperative evaluation also includes examination of the heart for murmurs and of the abdomen for distension or masses, palpation of peripheral pulses, and examination of extremities and the neck for venous access.

The medical record should be consulted if the patient has had surgery before to examine the anesthetic record. Much information can be learned from the response of the patient in the past to anesthetics and from the written report on airway management by the anesthetist.

Finally, all appropriate laboratory work should be complete and the results reviewed prior to the induction of anesthesia. Any consultations that are required based on the above history and physical should be sought.

Preoperative Preparation

As discussed previously, the need for sedative preoperative medication varies with age. The need is most acute at ages 6 months to 3 years. Today, there exist a variety of medica-

TABLE 32–3. DEHYDRATION CRITERIA

Physical Sign	Dehydration (%)
Dry mouth and mucous membranes, infrequent voiding	5
Sunken eyes or fontanelle, lethargy, poor capillary filling	10
Tenting of the skin, anuria, hypotension	15

tions as well as routes by which they may be administered. Oral pentobarbital sodium (Nembutal) may be given on the ward prior to transport of the patient to the operating room holding area. The anesthetist may choose rectal brevital; oral, rectal, or intravenous midazolam; intramuscular or intravenous ketamine; or intranasal narcotics. The principle guiding all these premedications must be the careful titration of dose according to weight and physical condition of the patient and close observation of the child by the anesthetist after administration. In some cases, for example, the child with a difficult airway, severe asthma, or congenital cyanotic heart disease, it may be injudicious to administer any sedative premedication. A possible exception would be the child with tetralogy of Fallot prone to "tet" spells, in whom adequate preoperative sedation can prevent an acute decompensation. Other premedications that may be appropriate are H_2 antagonists, metoclopramide, and anticholinergics. It is often useful to have a syringe with ketamine and glycopyrrolate ready to administer intramuscularly if a premedication or inhalation induction is inadequate or not proceeding smoothly.

Although there has been considerable debate recently as to the length of the NPO period required for an empty stomach, the vast majority of pediatric anesthetists recommend a 4-hour fast for neonates and infants up to 2 years of age. From 2 to 6 years, a 6-hour fast is recommended, and above 6 years of age, an 8-hour NPO period. This does not, however, guarantee an empty stomach, especially in children with swallowing difficulties, malrotation of the bowel, or small bowel obstruction. These special circumstances deserve individual attention.

The idiom "proper preparation prevents poor performance" is nowhere as true as with pediatric anesthesia. It is incumbent on the anesthetist to have a wide selection of age-appropriate equipment like endotracheal tubes laryngoscope blades, angiocaths, masks, and blood pressure cuffs in the operating room prior to induction (Fig. 32–2). The monitors, drugs, and airway equipment must be arranged in such a way as to be readily available to the anesthetist. Once the infant is brought into the room the anesthetist

must be able to focus all attention on the patient (Fig. 32–3). This requires extensive preparation.

Straight laryngoscope blades are usually more helpful with infants, the Wis-Hippel 1.5 being an ideal blade for neonates and small infants. Miller blades should be available as well. Small laryngoscope handles are more appropriate with infants. A good face mask fit is imperative during inhalation inductions; a larger mask should be chosen if the choice is between one that is too large and one that is too small. Flavored scents can be added to the mask to cover the smell of the anesthetic gases. A choice of endotracheal tube (ETT) sizes should be available, one age-appropriate size and one size smaller and one size larger. A useful equation for determining appropriate ETT size (internal diameter) is (16 + age of patient)/4. Uncuffed tubes are appropriate for children less than 10 years of age. Intravenous lines should be prepared in advance; a Buretrol setup is appropriate for children less than 6 years old or in special circumstances like renal failure or congenital heart failure.

The patient should be monitored with the basic monitors; electrocardiogram (ECG), noninvasive blood pressure monitor, temperature monitor, precordial or esophageal stethoscope, O_2 supply analyzer, O_2 saturation monitor, $ETCO_2$ analyzer, and inspiratory pressure monitor. Additional invasive monitors like arterial lines and a Foley catheter should be considered in special cases. With neonates and infants, the ambient room temperature should be elevated to prevent the rapid surface cooling of the infant. Also, warming lights should be used in these cases.

Induction of Anesthesia

On entry into the operating room, an oxygen saturation probe, ECG, and blood pressure cuff should be attached to the patient. Then depending on the patient's age, inhalation or intravenous induction should proceed. If the patient has been given a premedication, the inhalation induction merely completes the induction process. Halothane is most frequently used as it is the least noxious of the inhalation

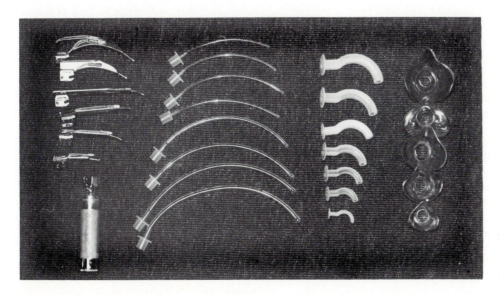

Figure 32–2. Pediatric airway equipment. From left to right, laryngoscope blades—Nos. 0, 1, 2 Miller, No. 1.5 Wis-Hipple, Nos. 2, 3 Macintosh; uncuffed endotracheal tubes—2.5 to 6.0 mm by half sizes; oral airways—40 to 100 mm; Rendell–Baker–Soucek masks, Nos. 00, 0, 1, 2, 3.

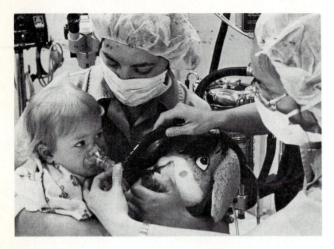

Figure 32–3. A child undergoing induction. Note that the child's security object is with her, that she is in a sitting position, and that eye contact is maintained between the child and the anesthetist.

agents, and, therefore, there is less breath holding and laryngospasm on induction. The inspired concentration should be increased slowly, 0.2 percent for each three breaths, and preceded by nitrous oxide if the patient's oxygen saturation tolerates it. If the child should begin to cough and hold his or her breath, the induction must cease, and the patient must be given 100 percent oxygen. The anesthetist then waits for the child to resume a normal respiratory pattern and begins again. Laryngospasm can be treated first with positive-pressure ventilation and, if that fails, intramuscular or intravenous succinylcholine and atropine. In addition, if the child becomes very uncooperative during the inhalation induction, an intramuscular injection of ketamine (3 to 5 mg/kg) and glycopyrrolate can sometimes be the kindest maneuver for everyone involved.

When the induction has continued to such a point that the patient is unresponsive to tactile stimuli, an intravenous line should be established. This can be done on the hands or feet, but the external jugular should provide a suitable alternative if the attempts at veins in the extremities fail. In older children in whom an intravenous line is established prior to induction, the sequence of drugs is similar to that in adults, except that an anticholinergic should usually be administered prior to succinylcholine.

Once intravenous access is ensured, the patient is intubated. This can be done with a muscle relaxant or with deep halothane anesthesia. If the latter is chosen, the heart tones can be used as an indicator of the depth of anesthesia. Halothane is a negative inotropic agent, and as the tissue partial pressure increases, the contractility of the heart decreases, and the heart sounds lose their sharp snap, and begin to sound muffled. This is then the time to intubate the patient.

Because of the large occiput of the infant in relation to body size, a small roll placed under the shoulders can help place the patient in a "sniffing" position for intubation. The trachea is intubated under direct visualization with laryngoscopy, and the endotracheal tube should be placed midway between the vocal cords and the carina. This can be

ensured by placing the tube into the right mainstem bronchus and withdrawing it 1 cm after breath sounds become bilaterally equal. Or the tube can be placed into the trachea until the double line on the Sheridan ETT lies at the cords. Bilateral breath sounds should confirm the proper position.

Maintenance of Anesthesia

General anesthesia can be maintained with inhalation agents, intravenous agents, or a combination. Except in very ill children, inhalation agents are preferred because of the unpredictable respiratory depressant effects of narcotics; however, narcotics have been used safely in all age groups. Once again, the overriding principle is to administer only what is needed and observe for side effects. Muscle relaxation can be maintained with any of a variety of agents; however, pancuronium with its vagolytic effect, increasing heart rate, is a distinct advantage in the heart rate-dependent neonate. Of course, a nerve stimulator should guide neuromuscular blockade therapy. The agents should be completely reversed prior to emergence from anesthesia.

Fluids and Blood Replacement

In the pediatric population, fluids and blood status must be monitored very carefully. Even small losses may be substantial in the smallest of patients. Although many systems for estimating and replacing fluid and blood losses have been proposed, the anesthetist should use these as guidelines only and tailor her or his clinical actions to the individual patient's requirements. These requirements can vary dramatically with changes in temperature, metabolic state, and type of surgical procedure. The most widely used fluid replacement regimen is based on caloric expenditures. In this system, the maintenance requirements are 4 cc/kg/h for the first 10 kg of weight, 2 cc/kg/h for the second 10 kg, and 1 cc/kg/h for the remaining weight above 20 kg. These estimates must be corrected for different clinical conditions. For example, in a hypermetabolic state, the estimates are increased 20 to 75 percent. As temperature varies, there is a 10 percent change with each degree centigrade. Infants placed under radiant warmers have much increased fluid requirements.

In addition to maintenance fluids which consist of 5 percent dextrose with lactated Ringer's or Plasmalyte for neonates and lactated Ringers or Plasmalyte for older infants and children, patients undergoing surgery need additional replacement fluids to compensate for losses in third-space edema and increased insensible losses. These losses result from surgical trauma and the removal of the skin as a barrier to evaporation. For replacement, 2 to 10 cc/kg/h of an isotonic solution is given depending on the severity of the surgery.

Infants require a higher hematocrit because of the increased concentration of fetal hemoglobin and their limited cardiac reserve. For this reason, blood loss must be followed closely and blood administered appropriately. A method has been proposed for calculating estimated blood volume and the need for transfusion of red cells:

Estimated blood volume (EBV)

$$= 90 \text{ mL/kg} \quad \text{in} \quad \text{neonates}$$

$$80 \text{ mL/kg} \quad \text{in} \quad \text{infants up to 1 year}$$

$$70 \text{ mL/kg} \quad \text{in} \quad \text{patients older than 1 year}$$

Estimated red cell mass (ERCM)

$$= EBV \times \frac{Hct}{100}$$

Acceptable red cell loss (ARCL)

$$= ERCM - ERCM_{25}$$

Acceptable blood loss in mL (ABL)

$$= ARCL \times 3$$

$ERCM_{25}$ is ERCM at a hematocrit of 25 percent. This term should be modified according to the patient's age and clinical condition.

Transfusion of 10 cc/kg packed red blood cells raises the hematocrit by 4 percent. Hypocalcemia can result secondary to binding of calcium by citrate, which is contained in blood products. The mainstay of modern transfusion therapy is the use of blood components instead of whole blood to treat specific clinical needs, as this conserves blood resources and is safer. Red blood cells should be used for increasing oxygen-carrying capacity alone, not for volume expansion as this can be accomplished in a safer manner using crystalloid. The major risks of transfusion therapy are infection and alloimmunization. The infective agents are non-A, non-B hepatitis, human immunodeficiency virus, hepatitis B, cytomegalovirus, and malaria. Hemolytic transfusion reactions are caused principally by ABO incompatibility as a result of errors in blood labeling and patient identification.

Emergence

Time to emergence from anesthesia can vary with the age of the patient, the agents used during the case, and, in very short procedures, the residual effects of the sedative premedication. Smooth and timely awakening from anesthesia is a result of planning both before and during the case. For very short cases, a decreased dose of a sedative premedication might be chosen or no premedication may be given. The avoidance of "fixed" intravenous agents during the case in very young patients may facilitate a smooth emergence. Using a muscle relaxant of appropriate duration ensures the ability to reverse the agent at the end of the case. Preventing infants from getting cold during the procedure can avoid a lengthy warming period prior to extubation.

The timing of extubation is critical in all patients. In neonates and infants, who cannot respond to verbal commands to open eyes or move extremities, other objective criteria must be sought (Table 32–4). One should wait for a regular respiratory pattern, with adequate tidal volumes, swallowing, and movement. Grimacing and furrowing of the brow to noxious stimuli (e.g., suctioning of the oropharynx) indicate the patient is awakening. And finally, when the patient reaches for the endotracheal tube or opens his or her eyes, extubation can be performed. The ETT should be removed under positive pressure so that oropharyngeal se-

TABLE 32–4. EXTUBATION CRITERIA

Good respiratory effort
Good cough and gag
Good muscle strength
Eye opening

cretions are not aspirated. Immediately after extubation, the lungs should be auscultated and breath sounds, wheezing, or obstruction listened for. If laryngospasm should occur, it can be treated first with positive pressure by mask and then with intramuscular succinylcholine with atropine. If there is any question as to the patient's ability to remain well oxygenated en route to the recovery room, portable oxygen should be administered by face mask.

Recovery Room Care

The modern recovery room is merely an extension of the operating room, and the patient should be given the same level of care and attention there as in the operating room. This care is delivered by the recovery room nurse under the direction of an anesthetist. On admission to the recovery room, initial vital signs and a cursory examination of the child should be performed with particular attention paid to respiratory effort, color, state of consciousness, and muscular strength. The anesthetist should provide the nurse with a detailed history of the patient and the operative course and should alert the nurse to any potential postoperative problems. A review of the lines placed, fluids given, blood lost, and surgical procedure is mandatory.

Frequent postoperative problems in the pediatric population include hypoxia secondary to airway obstruction or apneic spells (Table 32–5), hypovolemia from inadequate fluid replacement in the operating room, continued blood loss or third spacing, and delayed awakening secondary to administration of central nervous system depressants or inadequate ventilation preventing removal of inhalation agents. When alerted by the recovery room nurse to one of these problems, the anesthetist must examine the patient, make a decision as to the cause, and outline effective treatment. The surgeon should be notified if the treatment is of such a nature as to alter the patient's postoperative course significantly.

Patient-controlled analgesia (PCA) has found increasing acceptance with anesthetists and surgeons for pediatric patients. The dosages are of course on a weight basis, with similar lockout intervals as for adults. PCA has been successful in children age 6 and older. Regional techniques for

TABLE 32–5. SIGNS OF AIRWAY OBSTRUCTION

Cyanosis
Grunting
Retractions
Nasal flaring
Tachycardia

intraoperative and postoperative analgesia are being used more frequently for pediatric patients. For some time, "one-shot" caudal blocks have been placed, usually with 0.25 percent bupivacaine 0.5 to 1 cc/kg, for urologic or lower abdominal procedures. Recently, epidural and intrathecal routes have been used for both intraoperative anesthesia and postoperative analgesia. Brachial plexus blocks have also been widely used in some centers to provide anesthesia during upper extremity surgery. The discovery of peripheral opiate receptors has stimulated research into more regional use of opioids in postoperative pain control.

SPECIAL CONSIDERATIONS FOR THE PREMATURE PATIENT

The introduction of mechanical ventilation and intensive care for premature infants has decreased mortality significantly but has not affected morbidity.[27,28] Chronic lung disease, damaged central nervous system, malnutrition, and necrotizing enterocolitis are as difficult to treat today as hyaline membrane disease was 20 years ago.[29] Disease secondary to treatment has become increasingly important in these patients' morbidity. Also, because of the excellent care these patients receive, they appear for surgical treatment in greater numbers, in more critical condition, and with multi-organ system dysfunction.

The respiratory tract is especially vulnerable to injury because of the immature condition of the lungs at birth and the frequent need for mechanical ventilation. The more common upper respiratory tract pathology consists of subglottic stenosis and tracheomalacia. Alveolar proliferation only begins after birth and then continues for the first 8 years of life. Surfactant is not produced in sufficient quantities until 34 to 35 weeks.[30] Furthermore, the extremely compliant chest wall of the premature infant causes inward rather than outward movement of the sternum during forced inspiration, making respirations more difficult. Chronic lung disease can result from pneumonia, meconium aspiration, pulmonary edema, gastroesophageal reflux with recurrent aspiration, and persistent pulmonary hypertension. Prolonged mechanical ventilation can cause pulmonary damage from disruption of ciliary activity, oxygen toxicity, and formation of hyaline membranes.

The cardiovascular system of the premature infant is less able to compensate for the stresses placed on it by disease processes. This is due to the decreased sympathetic innervation, decreased amount of contractile tissue, and elevated pulmonary resistance seen in these patients. The ductus arteriosus and foramen ovale provide conduits for right-to-left cardiac shunting, worsening hypoxia and increasing the likelihood of paradoxical air emboli. These patients lose heat rapidly because of a lack of subcutaneous tissue, lack of brown fat, and high body surface area-to-weight ratio. Theoretically, all infants less than 44 weeks of conceptual age are susceptible to retinopathy of prematurity; however, most cases occur in infants under 30 weeks of age. Therefore, extremes of PaO_2 and $PaCO_2$ should be avoided in this age group for prolonged surgical periods. There is an increased incidence of postoperative apnea in patients who are born premature. This has been observed in patients who are less than 54 weeks of conceptual age. It is

therefore recommended that any infant with a history of prematurity who is less than 60 weeks of conceptual age[31] or who has received narcotic anesthetics should be on an apnea monitor postoperatively, and may need to be ventilated postoperatively.

CONCLUSION

The practice of pediatric anesthesia has a magnificent history filled with individuals dedicated to the care of children, the nurturing of the parent–child relationship, and the conveyance of these skills to others. When equipped with a thorough knowledge of the uniqueness of the pediatric patient's anatomy, physiology, and response to anesthetics, and consideration of the special emotional needs of the family undergoing a surgical experience, the anesthetist can embark on a challenging but exceedingly rewarding course of endeavor.

REFERENCES

1. Long CW. An account of the first use of sulphuric ether by inhalation as an anaesthetic in surgical operations. *South Med Surg J*. 1849;5:705–713.
2. Snow J. *On chloroform and other anesthetics*. London: Churchill; 1858.
3. Gwathmey JT. *Anesthesia*. New York: Appleton; 1914:322–327.
4. Guedel AE. Unpublished personal papers. Guedel Anesthesia Center, San Francisco.
5. Farr RE. *Practical local anesthesia*. Philadelphia: Lea & Febiger; 1923:492.
6. Steward OJ. Some aspects of paediatric anesthesia. In: Hunter AR, ed. *Monographe in Anaesthesiology*. Amsterdam: Excerpta Medica; 1982.
7. Clyman R. Ontogeny of the ductus arteriosus response to prostaglandins and inhibitors of their synthesis. *Semin Perinatol*. 1980;4:115.
8. Friedman WF. The intrinsic physiologic properties of the developing heart. *Prog Cardiovasc Dis*. 1972;56:188.
9. Wear R. The effect of halothane on the baroresponse of adult and baby rabbits. *Anesthesiology*. 1982;56:188.
10. Welborn LG, McGill WA, Hannallah RS, Nesselson CL, Ruttiman UE, Hicks FM. Perioperative blood glucose concentrations in pediatric outpatients. *Anesthesiology*. 1986;65(5):543–547.
11. Srinivasan G, Jain R, Pildes RS, Kannan CR. Glucose homeostasis during anesthesia and surgery in infants. *J Pediatr Surg*. 1986;21(8):718–721.
12. Anand KJ, Brown MJ, Bloom SR, Aynsley-Green A. Studies on the hormonal regulation of fuel metabolism in the human newborn infant undergoing anaesthesia and surgery. *Horm Res*. 1985;22(1/2):115–182.
13. Cook DR, Fischer CG. Neuromuscular blocking effects of succinylcholine in infants and children. *Anesthesiology*. 1975;142:662.
14. Cook DR, Fischer CG. Characteristics of succinylcholine neuromuscular blockade in infants. *Anesth Analg*. 1978;57:63.
15. Walts LF, Dillon JB. The response of newborns to succinylcholine and *d*-tubocurarine. *Anesthesiology*. 1969;31:35.
16. Eger EL II. *Anesthetic uptake and action*. Baltimore: Williams & Wilkins; 1974.
17. Salanitre E, Rackow H. The pulmonary exchange of nitrous oxide and halothane in infants and children. *Anesthesiology*. 1969; 30:388–394.

18. Gallagher TM, Black GW. Uptake of volatile anesthetics in children. *Anaesthesia*. 1985;40:1073–1077.

19. Lerman J, Willis MM, Gregory GA, Eger EI II. Age and the solubility of volatile anesthetics in blood. *Anesthesiology*. 1984;61: 139–143.

20. Malviya S, Lerman J. The blood/gas solubilities of sevoflurane, isoflurane, halothane and serum constituent concentrations in neonates and adults. *Anesthesiology*. 1990;72:793–796.

21. Lerman J, Schmitt BI, Willis MM, Gregory GA, Eger EI II. Effect of age on the solubility of volatile anesthetics in human tissues. *Anesthesiology*. 1986;65:63–67.

22. Lerman J, Robinson S, Willis MM, Gregory GA. Anesthetic requirements for halothane in young children 0–1 month old and 1–6 months of age. *Anesthesiology*. 1983;59:421–424.

23. Cameron CB, Robinson S, Gregory GA. The minimum anesthetic concentration of isoflurane in children. *Anesth Analg*. 1984;63:418–420.

24. LeDez KM, Lerman J. The minimum alveolar concentration (MAC) of isoflurane in preterm neonates. *Anesthesiology*. 1987;76:301–307.

25. Empey W, Laitinen LA, Jacobs L, et al. Mechanics of bronchial hyperreactivity in normal subjects after upper respiratory tract infection. *Am Rev Respir Dis*. 1976;113:131.

26. Berry FA. Anesthesia for the child with a difficult airway. In: Berry FA, ed. *Anesthetic management of difficult and routine pediatric patients*. New York: Churchill Livingstone; 1986:149.

27. Cohen RS, Stevenson DK, Malachowski N, et al. Favorable results of neonatal intensive care for very low birth weight infants. *Pediatrics*. 1982;69:613.

28. Horwood SP, Boyle MH, Torrance GW, et al. Mortality and morbidity of 500 to 1499 gram birth weight infants live-born to residents of a defined geographic region before and after neonatal intensive care. *Pediatrics*. 1982;69:613.

29. Finholt DA. The anesthetic management of the premature nursery graduate. In: Berry FA, ed. *Anesthetic management of difficult and routine pediatric patients*. New York: Churchill Livingstone; 1986:315.

30. Farrell PM, Hamosh M. The biochemistry of fetal lung development. *Clin Perinatol*. 1978;5:197.

31. Kurth CD, Spitzer AR, Broemle AM, Downes JJ. Post-operative apnea in preterm infants. *Anesthesiology*. 1987;66:483–488.

Geriatric Anesthesia

Wynne R. Waugaman and
Benjamin M. Rigor

Aging is a complex of phenomena, partly exogenous and partly endogenous, in which physiologic and pathologic processes are often inextricably mixed. Since World War II, our society has undergone profound changes, including rapid growth and greater sophistication in the delivery and technology of medicine. As a result, we are presented daily with large numbers of patients who have lived longer and survived the physiologic effects of age and disease only to require extensive surgery.

As the aged population increases, so will the incidence of Alzheimer's disease. The impact of this age factor is significant as demographic trends illustrate that the population susceptible to Alzheimer's disease is increasing rapidly. The risk for developing Alzheimer's disease in those who survive to 80 years of age is 20 percent.

The risk of surgery for many elderly patients is complicated by chronic disease processes. The reported incidences of the most prevalent diseases among the aged are 78 percent for osteoarthritis, 40 percent for hypertension, 40 percent for heart disease, and 4 percent for diabetes mellitus.

When adequately prepared, elderly people can tolerate many types of operations as well as young people; however, in the case of extensive major operations, the mortality rate for the aged may be four to eight times higher than that for young patients. Patients over 70 years of age have an overall elective surgery mortality under 5 percent compared with nearly 10 percent for emergency surgery, with variations depending on anatomic site and development of complications. At least 2 percent of this mortality can be attributed to anesthesia. It has been reported that more than 100,000 patients over the age of 65 die postoperatively each year.

The success of anesthesia and surgery with these patients in part depends on the nurse anesthetist's knowledge of physiologic alterations caused by the aging process and of the possible effects of anesthetics and adjuvant and supportive drugs on the aged.

Although age alone does not preclude surgery, it is apparent that the anesthetic management of the aged is influenced by the frequency and severity of degenerative diseases and chronic illnesses.

AGING AND MORTALITY

There is no consensus as to the true definition of old age but most authors and experts consider age 65 and above as elderly and the true scope of geriatric medicine. It has been known that chronologic age has no direct relationship with physiologic age and aging can be characterized as a process where there are well-documented changes in the chemical composition of the body, a broad spectrum of progressive deteriorative changes, reduced ability to respond adaptably to environmental changes, an increased vulnerability to many diseases, and an increase in mortality. At present, people older than 65 years of age constitute approximately 11 percent (23 million) of the population; they will constitute 13 percent by the year 2000 and 17 percent or 52 million by the year 2030. Five million Americans reach the age of 65 every day and, in 1980, 32,194 Americans were at least 100 years of age or older. The average human life span in the United States was 47 in the year 1900 and 73 years in 1981 and will be 82.4 by 2010 because of improved nutrition, sanitation, health care, alterations in life-styles, advancements in medical technology and drug therapy despite the increased incidence of AIDS and "life-style" diseases, for example, chemical dependency and motor vehicular accident deaths. As birth rate decreases, the percentage of geriatric people increases. The biologic limit to the human life span now appears to be around 100 years of age. A person reaching the age of 85 has only 1 in 10,000 chances of reaching the age of 110. The population of Americans 65 and over is a large and diverse group; however, there is a considerable heterogeneity in the manner in which these people mature, and the elderly population is in itself aging. There is also a trend toward higher mortality rates for males compared with females for all age groups. It seems that the elderly of the new era or the coming decades will be better educated and therefore more demanding and sophisticated health care consumers.[1] Eighty percent of Americans over 65 years of age have at least one chronic disease and many more have more than one. The most common coexisting conditions in the elderly are congestive heart failure, depression, dementia, chronic renal failure, angina pectoris, osteoarthritis, gait disorders, urinary incontinence, vascular insufficiency, constipation, diabetes, sensory and perceptual deficits, sleep disorders, adverse drug reactions, and anemia. Over 80 percent of all health care resources in the United States are devoted to chronic medical conditions.

HEALTH CARE EXPENDITURES FOR THE ELDERLY

Older persons are more likely to have health problems and physical infirmity. The per capita health care cost for persons 65 and older is approximately three times that of the younger person. Whereas older persons represent 11 percent of the total population, they account for 29 percent ($41.3 billion) of the total personal health care costs. Of these costs, one third is paid by private source and two thirds by Medicare, Medicaid, and other state and federal programs (Fig. 33–1). More than half of older Americans have some chronic medical conditions and 18 percent have limited ability to work or care for themselves. Older people make 40 to 50 percent more outpatient physician visits and are 2.5 times more likely to be admitted to a hospital where they spend 70 percent more time per admission than younger patients. Thus, per capita, the elderly accumulate three times more hospital bed days than do the young, and they constitute over 90 percent of our long-term care patients. These long-term care patients now occupy more beds than all general hospital beds in the United States combined at an annual cost exceeding $15 billion per year. In 1988 alone, the financial risk of an average older adult for long-term care in a nursing home setting was an average of $22,000. The realistic assumption about the current and future cost of health care and personal economic resources of adults are that no more than 30 to 40 percent of adults will be able to insure long-term care adequately. The other 60 to 70 percent will depend on public provision for care.[2]

Twelve percent of the elderly had self-pay expenses of more than $500 per year. Those who did average $5000 accounted for nearly 50 percent of all self-pay expenditures. The 5.9 percent of Medicare patients who die each year account for nearly 30 percent of the total program expenditure because of the increase in service volume, intensity of newer technologies, and reimbursement structure of Medicare.

The implications are plain and simple. Aging is here to stay and aging has many of the characteristics of a long-term growth industry. The aged are growing older; retirement as currently patterned may no longer be anticipated. The aged are less homogeneous as a group than the middle-aged, young adults, and children. Statistically the variability among physiologic and psychologic determinants increases with age: the aged become less alike when compared with other age groups. Aging is a process of change that enhances individual differences in abilities, interests, and background. The aged have the greatest experience in living. Many have good health, emotional resources, creativity, and a sense of survival that is enviable, and most of the mythology of incapacity is at times unwarranted.

The success of anesthesia and surgery with these patients in part depends on the nurse anesthetist's knowledge of physiologic alterations caused by the aging process and of the possible effects of anesthetics and adjuvant and supportive drugs on the aged. Although age alone does not preclude surgery, it is apparent that the anesthetic management of the aged is influenced by the frequency and severity of degenerative diseases and chronic illnesses.

ANESTHETIC IMPLICATIONS OF PHYSIOLOGIC ALTERATIONS IN THE AGED

The geriatric patient differs little from the young patient, even when the physiologic aspects of aging are considered, because, in general, neither group tolerates prolonged anesthesia or extensive surgery. It can, however, be said that the margin of safety and capacity for compensation are reduced appreciably at the extreme ages of life. The influ-

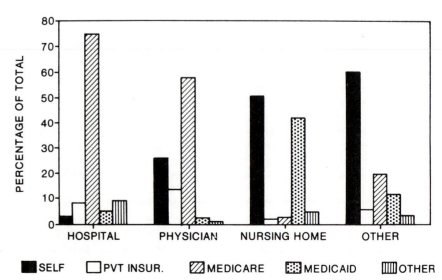

Figure 33–1. Source of payment for health care services for persons 65 and older. (*Reprinted, with permission, from Pawlson.*[2(p161)])

ence of age on the risks of anesthesia and surgery is determined by the type of associated disease and dysfunction; however, separating the effects of aging from those of degenerative disease processes is often difficult.

The aging process is not only a function of chronologic age. Organs and organ systems do not regress at the same rate and speed; thus patients must be assessed individually. Organ function declines 1 percent per year of the functional capacity present at age 30 (Fig. 33–2). These physiologic changes of aging often interfere with the uptake, distribution, biotransformation, and elimination of anesthetics. The significant physiologic alterations from the aging process and their implications in anesthetic management are discussed in the following sections.

General and Constitutional Changes

The elderly undergo a decrease in body fat and adipose tissue, which decreases their ability to retain body heat and, in turn, exposes them to hypothermia in the cool environment of the operating room.

Accurate determination of weight and weight changes is profoundly significant. Acute, sudden loss is usually due to loss of body water. Chronic loss is due to depletion of body stores of protein and fat. As a person ages, his or her body water naturally decreases; however, nutritional deficiencies may also occur in the elderly and are associated with a reduction in intracellular water and in total potassium. Hypovolemia, a natural consequence of this decrease in total body water, renders these persons vulnerable to hypotension during induction of anesthesia with potent intravenous agents such as sodium thiopental. Patients who are sedentary, bedridden, or immobilized for long periods are usually hypovolemic and have more difficulty compensating for changes in circulatory physiology caused by altering their posture or position. Their lowered basal metabolic rate (hypothyroid-like state) reduces tolerance to increasing con-

centrations of premedications, anesthetic agents, postoperative sedatives, hypnotics, and analgesics.

Senile atrophy with collagen loss and decreased elasticity of tissue makes the skin more sensitive to trauma from tape and monitoring electrodes. When the patient is placed on the operating table, close attention must be paid to bony prominences and other areas sensitive to pressure. Arm boards should be padded properly and the patient's arms positioned comfortably. Care must be taken when a warming blanket is used because burns may occur more frequently in the elderly, particularly in those with peripheral vascular disease.

The airway of the geriatric patient presents several problems. There is a progressive decrease in reactivity of protective airway reflexes, such as coughing and swallowing, associated with age. The aged are often edentulous or have a few loose teeth remaining. These factors make an anesthetic mask fit tenuous and increase the likelihood of regurgitation of stomach contents with aspiration of vomitus into the lungs. Cervical osteoarthritis and laryngeal changes that accompany rheumatoid arthritis, as well as irregular dentition, often increase the difficulty of inserting an endotracheal tube into the trachea to maintain a proper airway and adequately ventilate the lungs.

Cardiovascular System

Arteriosclerotic vascular changes and reduced myocardial reserve decrease cardiac output and stroke volume, prolong circulation time, and decrease perfusion of the vital organs such as the brain, heart, liver, and kidneys. Heart rate also decreases during the aging process. When anesthesia is induced, these cardiac and vascular changes can cause disastrous consequences, such as hypotension, myocardial ischemia or infarction, cerebral vascular accidents, and renal failure from decreased renal artery perfusion.

Coronary artery disease is prevalent in younger patients as well as geriatric patients; however, coronary obstructive lesions are seen more frequently in the elderly. It is important to remember that the patient with coronary disease is unable to significantly increase coronary flow. Therefore, preventive measures should be directed against increasing myocardial oxygen demand.

Rapid intravenous induction of potent short-acting barbiturates such as sodium thiopental or methohexital can provoke cardiovascular collapse as a result of poor compensatory hemodynamic response and inadequate cardiac function and blood volume.

A prolonged circulation time has profound implications for the intravenous agents. One can anticipate an induction time period of up to twice as long as would be expected in a younger individual. This prolonged circulation time not only prolongs the onset of action of succinylcholine but also decreases the tendency to fasciculate and increases the time during which pseudocholinesterase can act.

The age-related decrease in cardiac index provides a faster induction with volatile inhalation agents because of a more rapid rise in alveolar concentration. Hypotension may therefore appear sooner, especially in the patient who is hypovolemic.

Bradycardia in the aged is probably best treated with

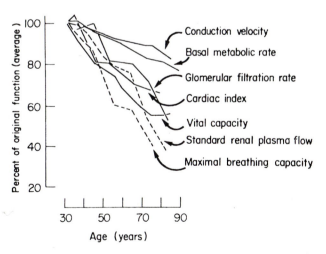

Figure 33–2. Changes in physiologic function with age in humans expressed as percentages of mean values at age 30. (*Reprinted, with permission, from Miller RD. Anesthesia for the elderly. In: Miller RD, ed.* Anesthesia. *2nd ed. New York: Churchill Livingstone; 1986:1801–1819.*)

glycopyrrolate, as it does not cross the blood–brain barrier. This drug appears to be more desirable in the elderly than atropine.

The aging myocardium becomes thicker during both systole and diastole. There is a decrease in size and number of individual muscle fibers and an increase in fibrous and adipose tissue. Afterload increases with age. The elastic and muscular tissue in the arterial walls is replaced by fibrous tissue and calcium.

Peripheral vascular resistance increases with age to a greater degree than the decrease in cardiac output, so the blood pressure increases. The most notable increase is generally in the systolic pressure. Hypertension in the elderly may be considered to be above 160 systolic and 90 diastolic. These numbers may be acceptably increased as age increases.

The baroreceptor reflex is diminished during the aging process. There is less tachycardia to warn of hypovolemia and less increase in vascular tone to maintain perfusion pressure.

Respiratory System

Significant respiratory changes that occur with aging include decreased breathing capacity, stiffening and rigidity of air passages as a result of fibrosis, distension of peripheral air sacs, reduction of forced expiratory volume and forced vital capacity, decrease in diffusion properties, and an increase in closing volume. The consequences of these respiratory changes, especially in patients with chronic obstructive airway problems such as emphysema, predispose the elderly to infection and collapse of airways in the early postoperative period. Changes in pulmonary dynamics also decrease or prolong uptake and distribution of less soluble inhalation anesthetics.

After 65 the closing volume becomes greater than the functional residual capacity. There is airway closure with each breath and relatively decreased ventilation–perfusion, resulting in shunting and a decrease in the PaO_2. An 80-year-old patient may have normal lungs but have a PaO_2 of 75 torr. This level may be adequate to maintain the oxygen saturation of the blood, but a smaller margin of error exists for periods of hypoxia such as those created by airway obstruction and momentary apnea. This decrease in arterial oxygen tension as a result of age can be predicted by the equation $PaO_2 = 109 \text{ torr} - 0.43 \times \text{age (in years)}$. Other similar equations exist for the computation of expected PaO_2.

There is an increased risk of pulmonary embolism in the aged during the perioperative period, especially for operations conducted in the head-up position or for those involving prolonged immobility and bed rest. Miniheparinization, antiembolism stockings, and early ambulation may be helpful in reducing the incidence of pulmonary embolism.

Central and Peripheral Nervous Systems

The decreased requirement for both inhalation and intravenous anesthetics is related not only to circulatory and constitutional changes but also to decreased neuronal density. Decreased sensitivity to local anesthetic drugs was shown by Bromage[3] to be caused by changes such as alter-

ations in vascular supply (arteriosclerosis), abnormal neural structures, and differences in the permeability coefficient of the drugs. The peripheral nerve changes that occur with aging are diminution in size and in number of motor units.

Brain weight and number of neurons decrease with increased age. This causes the patient to become more sensitive to sedative and hypnotic drugs in terms of a more pronounced initial response and a prolonged recovery. There is also greater sensitivity to the toxic effects of anticholinergic agents such as atropine; doses that are normal for a young adult (0.4 to 0.8 mg) often cause psychosis in the elderly person.

Autoregulation of cerebral blood flow maintains flow independent of pressure until a critical mean pressure is reached; below this pressure a direct pressure–flow relationship is observed. This critical pressure may be raised in the elderly and in arteriosclerotic individuals. The anesthetist must be alert to avoid even a mild degree of hypotension in these patients.

Reduction in the dopaminergic receptors and postreceptor alterations (cell membrane, ion transport systems, etc.) occur during the aging process. Animal studies have shown that a reduction in total dietary intake of up to 40 percent causes no change in the number of dopaminergic receptors in the aged versus the young adult. Therefore, one may predict that obesity further contributes to reduction in these receptors.

Hepatorenal System

The decrease in liver enzymes such as plasma pseudocholinesterase reduces the detoxification and elimination of ester-type local anesthetics such as procaine and tetracaine, muscle relaxants such as succinylcholine, and ganglionic blocking agents such as trimethaphan. Therefore, reduced dosages of these drugs are required. Poor or sluggish biotransformation and detoxification prolong and magnify the effects of anesthetics and other adjuvant or supportive drugs.

Changes in renal function as a result of aging influence other body physiology. Degenerative changes in renal circulation begin early. In fact, renal perfusion decreases by 1.5 percent per year, which means that there is a 40 to 50 percent decrease from ages 25 to 65. Reduction in plasma albumin and synthesis increases the levels of active drugs that are unbound to plasma proteins such as barbiturates, local anesthetics, and certain muscle relaxants. Glomerular filtration rate abruptly decreases after the age of 60, and effective renal plasma flow decreases 10 percent per decade. Creatinine clearance is the most sensitive indicator of renal function in the elderly. These hepatorenal changes not only reduce drug elimination but also raise, prolong, or sustain drug levels in blood and tissue.

Other Physiologic Changes Pertinent to Anesthesia

The aged patient has decreased capacity for thermal regulation, as shown by tests for regional cooling, and homeostatic reaction to external temperature. Prolonged and extensive surgery with massive blood loss and exposed body cavities and organs induces hypothermia, which antagonizes the effect of nondepolarizing muscle relaxants such as *d*-tubocurarine and pancuronium bromide.

Although procedures preparing the large bowel for surgery have many attributes from the standpoint of reducing bowel flora, they have the disadvantage of disturbing the fluid and electrolyte balance. Cleansing enemas and cathartics cause significant losses of fluids containing quantities of sodium and potassium. There is also a loss of bicarbonate and chloride. The frequently diminished renal function in the elderly may not permit prompt compensation for these abrupt body fluid and electrolyte shifts. Not only is adequate fluid needed, but additional sodium bicarbonate or sodium lactate is required to correct the hyperchloremic acidosis that may be caused by bowel preparation.

Because of a decrease in lean body mass, in the presence of drugs that are distributed primarily to this compartment, such as diazepam, the plasma levels are increased with a calculated dose and the half-life is increased.

Stress accentuates biologic differences between individuals, and there tends to be a wider variation among the elderly with regard to their responses to stress. The organic and physiologic alterations from aging decrease the rate of compensatory responses and recovery from the stress of anesthesia and surgery. This may be compounded by a decrease in adrenocortical secretions, also associated with the aging process.

APPLIED GERIATRIC CLINICAL PHARMACOLOGY

Although 11 percent of the American population is age 65 or older, this age group spends about $3 billion per year for prescription and nonprescription drugs, which represents 20 to 25 percent of the total national expenditure and is predicted to increase to 35 to 45 percent over the next four decades.

Approximately one quarter of all drugs prescribed are consumed by elderly individuals and an estimated 85 percent of elderly ambulatory patients and 95 percent of institutionalized patients receive drugs. About 25 percent of all drug reactions occur in the elderly, and of the medications prescribed for the elderly, 25 percent may not be needed or are known to be ineffective! The average number of drug categories used by patients varies directly with increasing age, that is, 1.64 under 70 years of age and 2.64 over 84 years of age. The rate of failure of elderly to comply with physician's treatment plan may be as high as 50 percent. Three fourths of this noncompliance consists of either omitting necessary medications or taking inappropriate drugs. Fifteen percent of these patients suffered from visual handicaps of significant magnitude to cause problems in reading labels and following instructions accurately. Adverse reactions varied from 10.2 to 24 percent in a variety of elderly patients. The complexity of these problems relative to multiple drug intake, problems with possible overuse or noncompliance, and gastrointestinal, hepatic, renal, and other significant factors affecting drug absorption, distribution, biotransformation, and rate of excretion presents a challenge to the practitioner of anesthesiology. Therefore, every professional must be adept and familiar with the pharmacokinetics and pharmacodynamics of drugs used by the elderly including their interactions with anesthetics and other adjuvant drugs used in our daily armamentarium.

Pharmacokinetics is the study of the time course of absorption, distribution, metabolism, and excretion of drugs and their metabolites from the body and the relationship of drug deposition to the intensity and duration of therapeutic effect, or in short what the body does to the drug. Pharmacodynamics refers to the physiologic or psychologic response of the body to a drug or combination of drugs, or what the drug does to the body.

The most commonly used drugs are cardiovascular agents and drugs for hypertension, analgesics and antiarthritic preparations, sedatives and tranquilizers, and gastrointestinal preparations such as laxatives and antacids. About 40 percent of these medications are over-the-counter drugs, and for all inpatients, the number of drugs prescribed increases linearly with age and the length of stay in the hospital or in a nursing or convalescent home.

The ability of the drug to produce side effects depends on the amount that reaches specific receptors. In the absorption of the drug, the amount administered is very important. In geriatric patients, drugs taken orally can be absorbed slowly or may not be absorbed at all. There are sufficient studies showing that tablets taken orally can appear in the feces of elderly patients unchanged. These are related to the changes in the gastrointestinal mucosa, a marked reduction in blood supply, alteration in gastric emptying and intestinal motility, and reduction in gastric acidity. Most drugs absorbed by passive facilitation and not involving an active transport process are probably not limited, in contrast with nutrients such as sugar, amino acids, calcium, iron, thiamine, and others that are absorbed by an active transport mechanism. Drugs that are administered parenterally, either intramuscularly or intravenously, behave differently, because with the former there is slower or erratic absorption as a result of poor and slow peripheral and tissue perfusion, and with the latter, the practitioner must be aware that the slow circulation time and reduced cardiac output together with reduced receptor sensitivity cause a protracted and prolonged onset of effect, for example, sedation with barbiturates during intravenous induction. Systemic availability is a function of the fraction of the drug absorbed, and of that absorbed, the fraction that is metabolized by the intestine and hepatic enzymes. The amount of drug metabolized during the "first pass" of the absorption phase in the liver decreases with age, increasing the total amount of drug reaching the systemic circulation and necessitating dosage reduction for the elderly. In the practice of anesthesiology, it is prudent and safe to reduce the dose of drug to one-third to one-half the adult dose and to titrate to effect after sufficient observation and monitoring for tangible effects.

There is a 10 to 15 percent reduction in total body water between ages 20 and 80 years, as well as a reduction in the plasma volume and extracellular fluid. There is a gradual decline in the lean body mass and a proportionate increase in body fat, which is about 18 percent in men and 12 percent in women. These changes in body composition affect the volumes of distribution of drugs as they distribute into the total body water and body fat. The volumes of distribution for some of the lipophilic drugs such as diazepam, chlordiazepoxide, and pentothal will be larger; those of the water-soluble drugs such as cimetidine and digoxin decline with age. The serum albumin concentration can be reduced as much as 15 to 20 percent with an increase in the globulin fraction and an increase in the concentration of α_1-acid glycoprotein (AGP) which tend to increase with age. Acidic drugs such as diphenylhydantoin and warfarin are bound to plasma albumin, whereas weak bases such as lidocaine and propranolol are bound primarily to AGP. With the decline in albumin and the increase in AGP concentration, there is a reduction in the binding of weakly acidic drugs and an increase in the binding of weak bases. There is a resultant shift in the free drug concentration and an increase in the availability of free drug for metabolism or receptor binding sites. Caution should be exercised when using multiple drug therapy, as displacement from receptors and binding sites by other drugs that are competing for the same receptors may liberate other drugs the pharmacologic effects of which can be toxic and fatal to geriatric patients.

There is also a reduction in the activity of the microsomal mixed function oxidase system and microsomal enzyme induction. There is a reduction in hepatic mass and regional blood flow to the liver of up to 40 to 45 percent. This is shown by the benzodiazepine class of sedative-hypnotic and analgesic agents. Clearance of midazolam (Fig. 33–3) and of chlordiazepoxide and its metabolite desmethyldiazepam is reduced in older patients, especially among men. Many of the other drugs in this class have long elimination half-lives up to 220 hours, and because of this tendency for accumulation and excessive sedation, doses of these drugs should be reduced in elderly patients. The rates of elimination of drugs metabolized by nonmicrosomal enzymes, such as lorazepam, do not seem to be affected by these changes in the liver.

The clearance and excretion of these drugs are heavily influenced by the changes in the kidneys, which include a reduction in or diminished renal function, both glomerular and tubular. There is a decline in the capacity to concentrate during water deprivation and renal sodium conservation with an increased sensitivity to hyperosmolarity. It is essential that plasma levels of potentially toxic drugs that accumulate in the body such as digoxin and the newer-generation aminoglycoside antibiotics be measured. Many of the muscle relaxants that are eliminated primarily by renal excretion, such as vancuronium, gallamine, and cimetidine, showed a reduction in excretion with age.

Based on our knowledge of pharmacokinetics and the recommendation for the reduction of dosages and frequency of administration of potent medications for elderly patients, it should be emphasized that older people are more sensitive to the effects of analgesics and sedatives such as the benzodiazepines but not to the effects of cardiovascular drugs such as propranolol, verapamil, and calcium blockers.

The basic principle in prescribing and providing preanesthesia medications for geriatric patients include the evaluation of the need for drug therapy, obtaining a complete history of habits and drug usage, good working knowledge of the pharmacokinetics and pharmacodynamics of the drugs used, reduction in the dose, and titration of the drug dosage based on the patient's response. As much as possible, the patient should be encouraged to comply with therapeutic regimen which is simple, easy to understand, practical, and cost effective and has a high margin of safety. The patient's medications should be continuously reviewed and drugs that are not necessary should be discontinued to avoid complex drug interactions and drug reactions.

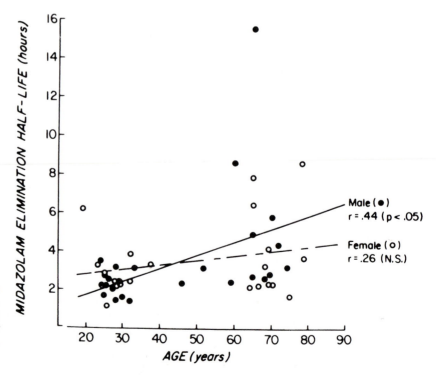

Figure 33–3. Relation of age to midazolam elimination half-life in men and women. (*Reprinted, with permission, from Reves JG, Fragen RJ, Vinik HR, et al. Midazolam: Pharmacology and uses.* Anesthesiology. *1985;62:316.*)

PREOPERATIVE EVALUATION AND PERIOPERATIVE ANESTHETIC CARE

All geriatric patients scheduled for elective surgery must have a preoperative visit from the anesthesiologist or anesthetist. Increased fear resulting from a previous unpleasant anesthesia experience may be alleviated by a pleasant preoperative experience. These fears and anxieties can provoke sympathetic nervous system responses and cardiac dysrhythmia during induction of anesthesia. Tactful and sympathetic visits allay apprehension, as well as give lasting, genuine reassurance.

After a review of the patient's chart and results of standard laboratory examinations, a physical examination is conducted with emphasis on the airway and airway problems, endocrine and metabolic signs of disease, and stability of the hemodynamic components. The patient should be assessed with a simple tilt test. A positive result implies either hypovolemia or an unstable sympathetic nervous system.

Standard laboratory examinations must include a complete blood count, liver and renal function profile, electrolytes, chest x-ray, and electrocardiogram. Other examinations such as arterial blood gases, pulmonary function tests, blood coagulation profile, and highly specialized studies such as blood volume and urinary steroids should be ordered on an individual basis where indicated.

Elderly patients may take multiple drugs; therefore, a careful history of drug intake will reduce the incidence of undesirable drug interactions (Table 33–1). Prolonged intake of steroids in patients with arthritis or allergies indicates the possibility of adrenal insufficiency, necessitating

an adjustment in this medication to compensate for the stress of anesthesia and surgery. Many medications, particularly the antihypertensive agents, should be continued up to the time of surgery. One drug that requires preoperative withdrawal and substitution of another drug on an elective basis is clonidine. This drug may cause profound rebound hypertension if withdrawn suddenly. Clonidine should be withdrawn 2 to 3 weeks prior to elective surgery and substitution therapy made.

One of the most useful elements of the history is the patient's exercise tolerance. This gives the anesthetist an indication of cardiopulmonary reserve.

When assessing the anesthetic and operative risks, potential airway problems should be noted, as described earlier. Individuals with chronic obstructive pulmonary disease or a smoking habit may require respiratory aerosol therapy, bronchial dilators, chest physical therapy, and antibiotic therapy for existing infections, for an appropriate length of time preoperatively. Correction or control of other associated medical problems such as diabetes, hypertension, angina, and congestive heart failure is mandatory. Elective surgery should be postponed if the medical conditions cannot be controlled or stabilized in time.

Surgical priorities and criteria for operability should include proper assessment of operative risk, assessment and treatment of functional abnormalities and other associated diseases, as well as the fine-tuning necessary to optimize conditions for anesthesia and the surgical procedure. It has been shown that surgical mortality rates increase linearly with American Society of Anesthesiologists (ASA) physical status classification (I–V), which can be used to critique op-

TABLE 33–1. DRUGS AND ADVERSE EFFECTS AFTER CHRONIC INTAKE WITH POSSIBLE DRUG–DRUG INTERACTIONS IN THE AGED

Drug	Effect/Interaction
Digitalis	Hypokalemia; arrhythmias
Diuretics	Hypokalemia; arrhythmias
Alcohol dependence	Hepatic disease; chronic intake—decreased response to anesthetics
Sedatives, tranquilizers, barbiturates	Liver enzyme induction; need reduced dose of anesthetics following intake
Tricyclic antidepressants	Interface with myocardial conduction; arrhythmias after relaxant reversal; discontinuation 48–72 h preop probably advantageous
Echothiophate eyedrops	Pseudocholinesterase inhibition—avoid or decrease succinylcholine
Monoamine oxidase inhibitors	Discontinue 10–14 d prior to surgery; hypotensive response with most anesthetics; hypertensive crisis with meperidine
Lithium carbonate	Atrial arrhythmias; muscle relaxant interaction
Antibiotics (streptomycin, gentamycin, neomycin)	Muscle relaxant interaction (prolonged response)
Quinidine	Muscle relaxant interaction
Aspirin	Bleeding and ulceration of gastrointestinal tract
Propranolol hydrochloride	Bradycardia and hypotension with potent halogenated anesthetic agents
Calcium channel blockers	Interaction with beta blockers can lead to cardiac decompensation; interaction with halogenated anesthetics at minimum alveolar concentration may enhance drug effects

erative mortality. Patients can also be classified on the basis of functional cardiorespiratory status derived from physiologic parameters obtained by peripheral, arterial, and central Swan-Ganz catheterization as shown by Del Guercio and Cohn.[4] The proper management of elderly surgical patients requires an understanding of the normal decline in physiologic reserves and the common pathologic conditions associated with the aging process. Assessment of cardiac risk factors (Table 33–2), improvement of pulmonary function including exercise tolerance, and prevention of pulmonary, cardiac, renal, and other vital organ failure are tantamount to obtaining the proper optimal conditions for the administration of anesthesia and performance of the surgical procedure.

There is consensus that factors associated with increased risks in surgery among elderly patients include age of 75 or older; emergency procedures; anatomic site, for example, chest and upper abdomen; length of surgical procedure greater than 2 hours; and poor exercise tolerance or low level of activity prior to procedure. Other significant factors to be considered are the skill of the surgeon and the adequacy of the anesthesia care and management plan. The most common reasons for preoperative medical consultations include chronic medical problems (56 percent); specific signs and symptoms, for example, angina and fever (18 percent); ECG and other laboratory anomalies (15 percent); acute illness or recent change in condition (6 percent); and specific management and therapeutic issues, for example, antibiotic prophylaxis, steroid coverage, and bleeding and coagulation problems (5 percent).[5]

All possible complications, risks, and alternatives must be explained to the patient and family. The type of anes-thetic management planned and the reason for the choice should be discussed with the patient, stressing that the patient's safety and welfare are the foremost considerations in this selection.

Specific medical problems that are to be controlled and corrected prior to elective surgery include hypertension, congestive heart failure, cardiac dysrhythmias, preexisting pulmonary conditions, fluid and electrolyte imbalance, endocrine and metabolic disorders, bleeding and coagulation abnormalities, neuropsychiatric disorders, and possible drug interactions or drug reactions. The most significant preoperative medical problems encountered during the preoperative period are shown in Table 33–3 and the mortality rates for these conditions are shown in Table 33–4. There is no question that involvement of more than one organ system with organic diseases increases morbidity and mortality from a surgical procedure. The mortality rate is 29 percent for patients with multiple-organ disease aged 95 and older compared with 4.7 percent among healthy patients of similar age.[6]

For certain patients with specific problems, useful and meaningful laboratory data such as blood volume, electrolytes, renal and hepatic function, chest x-rays, ECG, arterial blood gases, and pulmonary function must be assessed thoroughly. The adequacy of blood volume and compensatory autonomic nervous system reflexes can be assessed by blood volume determinations using dye dilution studies. To assess forced expiratory volume and forced vital capacity, simplified pulmonary function tests can be done with a portable respirometer.

Invasive monitoring techniques such as right-sided heart catheterization, balloon-flotation catheterization

---

TABLE 33–2. COMPUTATION OF THE CARDIAC RISK INDEX

Criterion	Multivariate	"Points"
History		
Age > 70 y	0.191	5
MI[a] in previous 6 mo	0.384	10
Physical examination		
S3 gallop or JVD	0.451	11
Important VAS	0.119	3
Electrocardiogram		
Rhythm other than sinus or PACs	0.283	7
>5 PVCs/min documented at any time before operation	0.278	7
General status		
$Po_2 < 60$ or $Pco_2 > 50$ mm Hg	0.132	3
K < 3.0 or $HCO_3 < 20$ mEq/L		
BUN > 50 or Cr > 3.0 mg/dL		
Abnormal SGOT		
Signs of chronic liver disease or patient bedridden from noncardiac causes		
Operations		
Intraperitoneal, intrathoracic, or aortic operation	0.123	3
Emergency operation	0.167	4
Total possible		53 points

[a] MI, myocardial infarction; JVD, jugular vein distension; VAS, valvular aortic stenosis, PACs, premature atrial contractions; ECG, electrocardiogram; PVCs, premature ventricular contractions; Po_2, partial pressure of oxygen; Pco_2, partial pressure of carbon dioxide; K, potassium; HCO_3, bicarbonate; BUN, blood urea nitrogen; Cr, creatinine; SGOT, serum glutamic–oxalacetic transaminase.
Reprinted, with permission, from Goldman L. Multifactorial index of cardiac risk in non-cardiac surgical patients. N Engl J Med. 1977;297:848.

TABLE 33–3. PREANESTHETIC COMPLICATIONS[a]

Complication	Number of Patients	Percent
Hypertension	466	46.6
Arteriosclerotic cardiovascular disease	269	26.9
Myocardial infarction	185	18.5
Cardiomegaly	136	13.6
Congestive heart failure	75	7.5
Angina	64	6.4
Cardiovascular accident	58	5.8
Chronic obstructive pulmonary disease	140	14.0
Pulmonary (other)	135	13.5
Diabetes	92	9.2
Renal dysfunction	314	31.4
Liver dysfunction	85	8.5

[a] Preexisting complications by history or examination.
Reprinted, with permission, from Stephen CR. The risk of anesthesia and surgery in the geriatric patient. In: Krechel SE, ed. Anesthesia and the geriatric patient. *New York: Grune & Stratton; 1984:231.*

(Swan-Ganz), and arterial catheterization for sampling may be indicated to assess the physiologic status of the patient for severe or extensive surgery. This invasive preoperative assessment may disclose serious physiologic abnormalities that require a delay in surgery or even cancellation of the procedure.

When gross physiologic decompensation is absent, the elderly patient may tolerate and demand effective premedication. Premedication should be prescribed to suit individual situations, but generally consists of a narcotic, a tranquilizer or hypnotic, an anticholinergic, or a combination of these. Doses should be reduced from a "normal adult dose" to one suitable for an aged patient. Ideally, the patient should be premedicated 1 hour before transport to the operating room so that the medication can achieve maximum effectiveness. Some controversy exists over the need for a narcotic as part of the preoperative medication routine in a patient who is not in pain. The consequences of producing respiratory depression in these patients must be considered.

MANAGEMENT OF PREOPERATIVE MEDICAL PROBLEMS

Uncontrolled hypertension is a risk for end-organ failures, for example, stroke, myocardial infarction, and renal failure, aside from the inherent hypovolemic state of the patient. In general, patients with uncontrolled hypertension have more hemodynamic instability during the perioperative period especially with intubation, conditions causing fluid shifts such as third-space fluid losses, and the emergence period where there is catecholamine release as a result of pain, stress, hypoxia, and hypercarbia. Elective procedures on patients with diastolic pressures higher than 100 mm Hg should be postponed or rescheduled and the patient's compliance to their antihypertensive medication should be monitored for adequate and proper control of blood pressure prior to surgery. Recent advances in the pharmacotherapy of hypertension have revolutionized and made blood pressure control easier by adjusting doses of drugs used on

TABLE 33–4. MORTALITY BY SELECTED PREOPERATIVE CONDITION

Condition	Number of Deaths	Number of Operations	Mortality Rate (%)
Cardiac failure	186	1,175	15.8
Impaired renal function	84	779	10.8
Vomiting	154	1,529	10.1
Previous general anesthetic	219	3,014	7.3
Angina, arteriosclerosis, or ischemic heart disease	544	7,776	7.0
Impairment of general health by surgical diagnosis	631	10,681	5.9
Diabetes	82	1,462	5.7
Chronic lower respiratory tract infection	408	8,060	5.1
Obesity	116	5,434	2.1
No preoperative condition	206	43,483	0.5

Reprinted, with permission, from Farrow SC, Fowkes FGR, Lunn JN, et al. Epidemiology in anaesthesia. II. Factors affecting mortality in hospital. Br J Anaesth. 1982;54:811.

a monotherapy mode and preferably once a day to increase patient compliance, such as angiotensin converting enzyme inhibitor (ACE), beta and calcium channel blockers, and the newer generation of antihypertensive medications.[7] In a patient with labile hypertension, intraoperative direct arterial line blood pressure monitoring is mandatory with properly prepared and mixed vasopressors and depressor agents to obtain optimal control of blood pressure and prevent extremes (i.e., profound hypotension, which can precipitate myocardial infarction, or massive hypertension which can result in stroke and other cardiac disastrous events such as cardiac arrest).

The classic signs of congestive heart failure in elderly patients include jugular venous distension, dyspnea on exertion, hepatomegaly, dependent pedal edema, and S_3 gallop. Depending on the etiology, aggressive treatment with diuretics, inotropes, and vasodilators, close monitoring of hemodynamic parameters with Swan-Ganz pulmonary artery catheters, and intraoperative transesophageal echocardiography monitoring of filling pressures, wall motion, and ejection fraction are warranted.[8]

There is a greater incidence of ventricular dysrhythmias and conduction abnormalities among elderly patients, probably as a normal progression of the diseases of the heart, but also from a previous myocardial infarction affecting the conduction system. Patients with complete heart block and sick sinus syndrome require preoperative pacemaker placement. Among patients with demand pacemakers undergoing transurethral resection of the prostate, a fixed-rate pacemaker is recommended to decrease the possibility of electrical cautery interference and other extraneous sources of electricity in the operating room. Blood levels of antiarrhythmic agents must be monitored for adequacy of dosage and optimal effect. Conditions that increase arrhythmia perioperatively include anxiety and stress, exogenous catecholamines, adverse hemodynamic extremes, hypoxia, and hypercarbia; these should be prevented and properly monitored.

Changes in the respiratory reserve as a normal part of aging are also magnified in the elderly patient, especially those with many years of smoking or history of primary pulmonary lung diseases. The surgical morbidity and mortality resulting from a respiratory complication can be as high as 40 percent. Anesthetic risk increases because of the obtunded protective airway reflexes, such as coughing, gagging, and swallowing, and the altered level of consciousness, which increases the probability of aspiration pneumonitis. The decrease in functional cilia of the tracheobronchial tree hampers the clearance of tracheal secretions which is already aggravated by dry and nonhumidified anesthetic gases. Bedridden and sedentary patients are also more susceptible to venous stasis and pulmonary embolism. High-risk patients should be identified not only by a thorough workup and medical history but also by pulmonary function tests and evaluation of exercise tolerance. Patients who require pulmonary function tests include those scheduled for thoracic and upper abdominal surgery, those with a prolonged history of heavy smoking and other primary pulmonary diseases, and those patients 70 years of age and older.[9] Patients with a maximum breathing capacity less than 50 percent of the predicted value, a forced expira-

tory volume in 1 second (FEV_1) less than 2 L, and a P_{CO_2} greater than 45 mm Hg are very high pulmonary surgical risks. It is recommended that these patients decrease or stop smoking, submit sputum culture for proper antibiotic therapy, and undergo bronchodilator, aerosol, and humidification therapy, postural drainage, and chest physiotherapy.[10] Enteral or parenteral nutrition improves integrity of respiratory muscles. It is important to overemphasize the continuation of a rigorous pulmonary regimen after the postoperative period, including well-supervised incentive spirometry, reduction of narcotic and depressant drugs with the use of selected regional anesthesia techniques and epidural opiates, use of effective breathing exercises to prevent splinting during deep breathing, effective coughing, and early ambulation.

The mortality for acute operative–postoperative renal failure is between 40 and 80 percent in elderly patients. With an awareness of the renal changes in the elderly and the effects of anesthesia and surgery, the goal is to decrease the risk of postoperative renal failure. Factors that compromise renal blood flow during the perioperative period include the decrease in cardiac output caused by halogenated inhalation anesthetics, positive-pressure ventilation, hypovolemia from surgical losses, and retraction and pressure on renal blood vessels by surgical instruments. The patient should be hydrated to ensure a good urinary output of 0.5 to 1 mL/kg/h. As much as possible, the use of potentially nephrotoxic drugs such as aminoglycosides must be avoided. Any patient with terminal renal failure or disease should be dialyzed to treat the hypovolemia, hyperkalemia, metabolic acidosis, or uremic encephalopathy.[11] Fluid and electrolyte problems resulting from surgical procedures include water or irrigation fluid absorption during transurethral resection of the prostate, profound hypovolemia and massive fluid replacement in major trauma, vasopressin deficiency in pituitary surgery, and gastrointestinal obstruction with continuous vomiting and suction for the decompression of dilated bowels, and any other massive extracellular fluid shifts and translocations.

Many elderly patients with adult- or maturity-onset diabetes (non-insulin-dependent, non-ketoacidosis-prone, type II, or stable diabetes) for many years present as a challenge to anesthesia because of complications associated with the progress of the disease, such as ketoacidosis, neuropathies, atherosclerosis, microangiopathy, increased incidence of infection, and delayed wound healing. Ketoacidosis is diagnosed in patients with metabolic acidosis and hyperglycemia (more than 300 mg dL^{-1}). Glycosuria and osmotic diuresis accentuate hyperosmolality and loss of electrolytes, resulting in hypovolemia that can lead to circulatory collapse. Patients with severe autonomic neuropathy manifest orthostatic hypotension, resting tachycardia, and reduction of beat-to-beat variability with deep breathing signifying autonomic instability that are resistant to vasopressors, inotropes, and anticholinergic agents, and there is an inherent sensitivity to respiratory depressant drugs. There is a higher incidence of silent myocardial infarction and unexplained cardiorespiratory arrest that is resistant to aggressive cardiopulmonary efforts and a greater tendency to aspiration as a result of gastroparesis.[12] The perioperative anesthesia care includes frequent monitoring of blood sugar and of ketone bodies in the blood and urine. There is no evidence that tight or close control of blood glucose concentration is beneficial over other methods as long as the blood glucose concentration is maintained between 100 to 250 mg percent, titrating it properly with additional glucose or regular insulin as often as necessary or as needed. The presence of ketone bodies is a good reason for postponement of elective surgery. In the presence of peripheral neuropathy, conduction or regional anesthesia should be used with caution because of a predisposition to nerve injury; this also emphasizes the importance of proper positioning and padding of bony prominences and external nerve distributions to prevent traction, pressure, and ischemia. It is prudent to decrease the dose of local anesthetics, and caution must be exercised in the use of epinephrine and other vasoactive drugs with local anesthetics in patients with diabetes complicated by atherosclerosis. Patients suffering from nonketonic hyperglycemic coma require immediate correction of hypovolemia and hyperosmolarity with intravenous balanced electrolyte solution, potassium supplementation, and small doses of intravenous regular insulin.

The prevalence of hypothyroidism in hospitalized elderly patients is reported to be 9.4 percent and as high as 13.2 percent.[13] The anesthetic implications of hypothyroidism include a marked sensitivity to depressant drugs, for example, drugs for premedication, agents for induction, and medications for pain relief postoperatively; a hypodynamic cardiovascular system with reduced cardiac output, heart rate, and stroke volume; a slower drug metabolism and detoxification, for example, for hypnotics, sedatives, and opiates; unresponsive baroreceptor reflexes; decreased intravascular volume; impaired ventilatory response to arterial hypoxemia, elevated partial pressure of carbon dioxide (PCO_2), or both; delayed gastric emptying time; impaired clearance of free water resulting in hyponatremia; hypothermia; anemia; hypoglycemia; and primary adrenal insufficiency.[14] There is a reduced requirement for premedication, anesthetic agents, and muscle relaxants because of the previously mentioned effects of the aging process and the fragile general constitution of the patient who is very susceptible to congestive heart failure and hypothermia. Appropriate monitoring modalities are recommended. Conservative use of adjuvant drugs such as vasopressors, inotropes, and other sympathetic amines; maintenance of normal body temperature; optimal ventilatory support; and conservative use of opiate analgesics are essential during the postoperative period.

Bleeding and coagulation problems among elderly patients result from excessive use of aspirin and nonsteroidal anti-inflammatory drugs (NSAIDs) for degenerative osteoarthritis, vitamin deficiency from poor nutrition and use of broad-spectrum antibiotics, liver disease associated with chronic alcoholism, indiscriminate use of coumadin, and, recently, use of dipyridamole for coronary, cerebral, and other vascular occlusive diseases. Patients with liver disease have complex hemostatic abnormalities and platelet dysfunction. Alcohol or ethanol may interfere with arachidonate metabolism in the platelets. There is now good evidence that aspirin increases operative blood loss in heparinized patients undergoing open heart surgery.[15]

ANESTHETIC MANAGEMENT

No shortcut anesthesia regimen can be used for the aged because their physiologic condition and the associated risks leave a very narrow margin of safety. The monitoring and surveillance of the aged must minimally include blood pressure, pulse, respiration, and temperature. In addition to the standard noninvasive monitoring modes mentioned, monitoring of end-tidal carbon dioxide concentration and oxygen saturation is particularly useful in assisting the anesthetist to maintain homeostasis intraoperatively. Invasive monitoring techniques such as measurement of central or peripheral arterial pressure, central venous pressure, and pulmonary artery pressure (Swan-Ganz) by catheterization are generally reserved for extensive surgery, where massive blood loss and fluid shifts are anticipated, and for patients with moderate-to-severe cardiopulmonary disease. Insertion of a urinary catheter for the monitoring of urinary output is helpful but may be contraindicated for patients with histories of multiple genitourinary infections or prostatic obstruction.

Temperature must be carefully monitored intraoperatively. Body temperature may decrease rapidly in the cool operating room environment. Preventive measures to maintain body heat include warming or use of a hyperthermia blanket, warmed intravenous and irrigation fluids, a heated nebulizer, and reduction in total gas flows.

It is mandatory that the correction of abnormal physiologic parameters be confirmed, including blood volume in patients with chronic or acute hemorrhage, blood pressure stability and control in hypertensive patients taking diuretics and antihypertensive agents, and blood glucose levels in brittle diabetics prone to diabetic ketoacidosis. After prolonged diuretic therapy, the serum potassium level must be measured because electrolyte imbalance can cause fatal arrhythmias during anesthesia. Blood sugar determination by the glucose oxidase method (Dextrostix) is essential for patients who receive their maintenance insulin dose on the day of surgery and may be indicated for other insulin-dependent diabetics as well as for adult-onset diabetics prone to hypoglycemia.

The criteria for operability must take into account the possibility of partial-to-complete restoration of function, diminution of disability, alleviation of pain, and prolongation of life. Choice of anesthesia is based on the patient's condition, the type of surgery, and the skills of the anesthesia care team and surgeon. The ideal anesthetic is one that can be controlled with very little effect on the already altered physiology. The anesthetic technique should be reversible so that, if complications arise, it can be discontinued abruptly and all vital functions may recover quickly.

General Anesthesia

General anesthesia includes intravenous and inhalation agents. In comparison to regional anesthesia, general anesthesia with insertion of an endotracheal tube has the advantages of better control of the airway and fast and smooth induction of anesthesia with unlimited duration, but it carries the hazard of aspiration of vomitus into the lungs, especially in patients with full stomachs.

Intravenous induction agents should be administered slowly in incremental doses so that the drug effect can develop completely and physiologic changes can be analyzed. Hypovolemia is common in the aged and, coupled with the reduced ability of the circulatory system to compensate for this, tends to make the induction of anesthesia with drugs such as thiopental potentially hazardous by producing poorly controlled swings in blood pressure and pulse. Hypertension and cardiac arrhythmias may occur if laryngoscopy is performed under light anesthesia. This is particularly dangerous in a patient with coronary insufficiency. Rapid, efficient laryngoscopy after intratracheal or intravenous treatment with lidocaine may help control the occurrence of arrhythmias during this procedure.

For many years, a balanced anesthetic technique—nitrous oxide, narcotic, tranquilizer, and muscle relaxant—was considered the safest for the aged patient; however, this technique has been reexamined and has been shown to cause myocardial or respiratory depression, or both (depending on which narcotic had been used). There is renewed interest in inhalation agents for anesthetic management of the aged, particularly since the introduction of isoflurane. It has been illustrated that, with age, the minimum alveolar concentration (MAC) of inhaled agents progressively decreases (Fig. 33–4). Other investigators have made similar findings with different anesthetic agents when comparing MACs of inhalation agents with age. That is, age decreases the requirements for anesthesia with an inhalation agent.

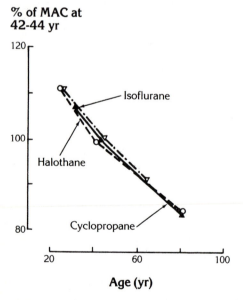

Figure 33–4. Anesthetic requirement (minimum alveolar concentration [MAC]) decreases with age. MAC values for nine groups of patients with mean ages ranging from 25 to 81 years are expressed as percentages of MACs at 42 to 44 years for each agent. The parallelism of the slopes indicates similar responses. (*Reprinted, with permission, from Munson ES, Hoffman JC, Eger EI II. Use of cyclopropane to test generality of anesthetic requirement in the elderly. Anesth Analg. 1984;63:998–1000.*)

Some of the effects of halogenated anesthetic agents on organs and organ systems include cerebral vasodilation with an increase in cerebral blood flow, early obtundation of laryngeal and pharyngeal reflexes, respiratory depression, and depression of myocardial and vascular smooth muscles, which causes a decrease in systemic blood pressure, cardiac contractile force, cardiac output, total peripheral resistance, and whole-body oxygen consumption. The anesthetist should be aware of the incompatibility of halothane with exogenous and endogenous catecholamines, such as epinephrine, because depending on the dose of exogenous catecholamines or blood level of endogenous catecholamines, cardiac arrhythmias may result. Enflurane (and isoflurane), however, can be used in anesthetic management when a limited amount of exogenous epinephrine may be required to control capillary oozing. The ability of halogenated anesthetic agents to produce hepatorenal toxicity is related to the amount of biotransformation and the final or intermediate products of detoxification. This is possibly not a direct effect but an indirect or autoimmune mechanism.

Inhalation agents have been associated with a higher incidence of intraoperative hypotension and arrhythmias than intravenous agents. The intravenous or balanced anesthesia technique gives a smoother intraoperative course but, reportedly, greater postoperative morbidity and mortality.

Regional Anesthesia

Regional block or conduction anesthesia is ideal for surgery on the extremities and for many types of surgery below the level of the umbilicus. Because the aged may have degenerative and vascular changes, their local anesthetic requirement is low, and incorporating drugs such as epinephrine to prolong nerve blocks is not recommended.

The obvious advantages of regional anesthetics are a conscious patient and probably a better, faster recovery with less likelihood of aspiration and other postoperative pulmonary complications.

The disadvantages of spinal or epidural anesthesia are that the sympathetic blockade can result in profound hypotension or cardiovascular collapse and there may be technical difficulty with inserting the spinal needle into a patient with spinal arthritis or calcified ligaments. Also, some patients tend to refuse this anesthetic technique in spite of its relative safety compared with general anesthesia. Many cling to unscientific traditional beliefs and fears that spinal anesthesia can cause paralysis, even though this complication is rare in this day and age.

SPECIAL ANESTHETIC CONSIDERATIONS

Geriatric Ambulatory Surgery

In many hospitals in the United States today, more than 60 percent of surgical procedures can be done in outpatient or ambulatory surgery centers. The benefits for outpatient surgery include better psychologic and emotional support from less distraction of daily routines, decreased morbidity and mortality (0.01 to 0.02 deaths per 10,000 procedures), less exposure to hospital-acquired or nosocomial infections, improved utilization of inpatient hospital beds, and cost effectiveness. These outweigh the disadvantages such as lack of immediate availability or care should a sudden complication arise. Patient selection is extremely important because of the known physiologic changes of aging and their effects on organ systems, drug action, elimination, and the perioperative and postoperative conduct of anesthesia and surgery. There is always the proverbial argument as to whether elderly patients can be operated on an outpatient basis if no responsible adult or guardian will take care of the postoperative needs and requirements, for example, medications, feeding, wound care, and complications. There is no argument that adequate and proper postoperative home care is mandatory for the optimal care of these patients. Many hospital-based ambulatory surgery centers now use the 23-hour postoperative admit unit to handle the previously mentioned scenario and there is usually no additional charge to the patient or the insurance carrier. The type, anatomic location, and duration of the surgical procedure are also extremely important. Most elderly patients should not require extensive or prolonged medical and nursing postoperative care, which may increase health care costs. In a series of 1553 patients, Meridy reported that age did not affect the duration of recovery from anesthesia and the complication rate.[16] The selection of anesthesia depends on the surgical procedure, the patient's state of health and psychologic and emotional adequacy, and the skill and experience of the surgeon and the anesthesia care team. Local and regional anesthesia when adequate and effective provides patients with a better sense of control and psychologic gratification, and there is evidence to show that there are fewer complications and a more expedient and pleasant recovery. In a series of 2951 patients over 60 years of age, the postoperative admission rate was 0.8 percent, which is only 0.2 percent higher than that for all patients.[17] The overall ambulatory anesthesia care of these patients must be considerate, sympathetic, understanding, and relaxed; these attitudes are true virtues in addition to the safe conduct of anesthesia and surgery. There are special patients requiring special handling and dedication contributing to the total quality care in ambulatory surgery centers.

Alzheimer's Disease

Alzheimer's disease, or senile dementia of the Alzheimer type (SDAT), is a complex degenerative process involving selective neuronal pathways. To date, no risk factors have been identified directly with the development of Alzheimer's disease although a familial tendency seems to exist. Advanced chronologic age itself appears to be the only factor directly related to the development of this disorder.

Because people are living longer, more elderly people may be faced with the prospect of elective or emergency surgery. Therefore, the number of patients with Alzheimer's disease undergoing surgery will continue to increase. Significant cognitive impairment is a cardinal sign of the disease and may not be a function of the aging process. Other symptoms of Alzheimer's disease are variable, but the patient may present a good state of physical health or have a health status compromised by other concurrent chronic disease processes. The overall physical condition of the Alzheimer patient should be a primary factor when considering outpatient, ambulatory, or inpatient surgery.

Cognitive impairment in the patient with Alzheimer's disease may include memory loss and reduced ability to concentrate. These factors make it difficult to take an accurate history from the patient. A close family member or guardian should be queried regarding the patient's past and current medical and surgical history including drug therapy. Patients with Alzheimer's disease may be taking a cadre of medications to modify behavioral changes such as aggressiveness, anxiety, depression, agitation, insomnia, and paranoia that may have resulted from the disease process. These patients are extremely sensitive to the effects of all medications and generally require reduced dosages to achieve the desired effect. The Alzheimer patient should be observed carefully for any side effects from medications, both those taken preoperatively and those taken for concurrent chronic disease processes.

Any directions that the patient will be expected to follow should be written down for the patient clearly and concisely. The written word is very helpful to reinforce any preoperative and postoperative instructions for the patient with Alzheimer's disease.

In all discussions with the patient regarding the upcoming surgery, the day and time of surgery should be mentioned. This assists the patient to remain oriented to time and place. If the patient will be moved to a new unit or require special care postoperatively, the patient and family should be apprised of this preoperatively if feasible. The family should be involved as much as possible in the plans for postoperative care. In some cases, private-duty nurses or family members may plan to stay with the patient postoperatively. If the quality of care the patient requires can be provided in this manner, this may be optimal for the patient with Alzheimer's disease. Because of the difficulty with orientation to time and place exhibited by these patients, the routines of specialty care units may add to their cognitive difficulties. The continuity of care provided by supportive family members and nurses familiar to the patient reinforces the patient's orientation to time and place. The charge nurse of the patient care unit should make every effort to assign a small number of nurses to care for the patient with Alzheimer's disease. The consistency of caregivers provides stability for the patient during the hospital stay.[18]

Patients with Alzheimer's disease requiring emergency surgery need special preoperative consideration. Explanations to the family and patient and an accurate accounting of the patient's history, particularly of drug therapy, are crucial. The number of individuals making a preoperative assessment of the patient should be kept to a minimum to reduce the degree of confusion associated with many new faces.

The same physical preparation should be made for Alzheimer's patients as for other elderly patients. A patient in the late stages of Alzheimer's disease may exhibit agitation and combative behavior. Restraint of the patient may be necessary to prevent accidental or self-inflicted injury.

Preoperative medication administered to these patients should be minimal as the patient may exhibit an exaggerated or untoward response to the medication which will make communication with and cooperation by the patient more difficult. Patients with Alzheimer's disease may be very sensitive to the depressant effects of hypnotics and narcotics as they generally are taking tranquilizers of some type. If a narcotic or sedative is administered preoperatively, the patient should be carefully monitored and observed for signs of respiratory depression. Administration of these drugs further depresses airway reflexes which increases the risk of passive regurgitation and aspiration of gastric contents. Vital signs must be monitored as these patients also may be sensitive to cardiovascular side effects such as hypotension from any narcotic or sedative preoperative medications administered.

Because the cholinergic system of these individuals has been shown to be impaired, anticholinergics such as atropine and scopolamine should be avoided. The use of these drugs could lead to an exacerbation of behavioral symptoms. The use of preoperative medication should be reserved for those instances when the patient requires analgesia or treatment of agitation. Patient rapport and understanding often serve as the most effective form of "preoperative medication."

Most patients with Alzheimer's disease will have their surgery performed under general anesthesia. Because of their difficulty with mentation and lack of understanding or cooperation, these patients generally are not good candidates for regional or local anesthesia, except in the very early stages of the disease process when cognitive abilities are well maintained.

Delayed recovery from anesthesia is not uncommon in these patients. Therefore, prolonged observation of the patient will be required in the postanesthesia care unit as well as in the patient care unit. Every effort should be made intraoperatively and postoperatively to keep the patient normothermic. Hypothermia can delay recovery from anesthesia. Confusion in the postoperative phase has been attributed to low body temperature and inadequate hydration.

Preserving optimum body temperature and maintaining adequate hydration help reduce the incidence of confusion postoperatively in patients with Alzheimer's disease. Outpatients should be apprised preoperatively by the surgeon or anesthetist of the prospect of hospital admission overnight after surgery should recovery be delayed. Some patients have shown temporary improvement in their cognitive abilities in response to administration of the anticholinesterase physostigmine. The long-term effects of the use of physostigmine as part of the treatment regimen in Alzheimer's disease are still under investigation.

POSTOPERATIVE EVALUATION AND MANAGEMENT

Postoperative management includes proper monitoring of all vital signs and parameters, including fluid intake and output, adequacy of ventilation, and cardiac stability.

Among the most frequent postoperative complications are those that are pulmonary in nature. Prevention of these problems begins as soon as the operative procedure is completed. Tracheobronchial suctioning before removal of the endotracheal tube and oropharyngeal suctioning are basic methods for ensuring that ventilatory exchange is maintained in the immediate postoperative period. Often it is safer to leave the endotracheal tube in place after the operation until the patient reacts to its presence rather than to remove the endotracheal tube before the patient is conscious, is breathing adequately, and has regained control of all reflexes.

Despite preventive measures, tenacious sputum and atelectasis of the lung still may cause difficulties postoperatively. Forceful coughing must be encouraged and tracheal suctioning must be resorted to if coughing is ineffectual. Oxygen should be administered routinely through a high-flow mask; patients with chronic obstructive pulmonary disease who retain carbon dioxide should be provided with a Venturi-type mask for the delivery of low concentrations of oxygen.

If the patient exhibits delirium in the recovery room, hypoxemia should be suspected. If arterial blood gases are normal, 1 to 2 mg of physostigmine may be used to reverse the effect of anticholinergic toxicity if symptoms displayed are related to administration of anticholinergic drugs.

Hypothermia must be prevented in the early postoperative period. Shivering in response to hypothermia increases tissue oxygen demand by as much as 400 to 500 percent. This can initiate a cycle of increased minute volume and cardiac output. Unless cardiopulmonary compensation occurs, anaerobic cellular metabolism will ensue, leading to severe metabolic acidosis. Postoperative hypothermia is more prolonged in the patient who has had regional anesthesia than in one who has had general anesthesia.

Narcotics may be used with caution in older patients. The usual dosage may produce profound respiratory depression. For the majority of patients, a reduced analgesic dose will control pain and allay restlessness without having an adverse effect on respiratory or circulatory function.

The metabolic response to surgery in elderly patients is similar to what is seen in younger patients, but certain important aspects particularly influence postoperative management and are especially important when cardiac or renal function is impaired. In the postoperative period, increased output of antidiuretic hormone by the posterior pituitary enhances reabsorption of water by the renal tubules and produces increased water retention. More adrenal hormones, principally aldosterone, are secreted and result in sodium retention. Basic fluid requirements, therefore, are limited to not more than 1000 mL (1 L) to cover insensible water losses and not more than 1500 mL to provide sufficient water for urine formation to excrete nitrogenous waste products. Not more than 500 mL of this should be isotonic sodium (normal saline solution). As soon as urinary output is ensured, potassium should be added to infused fluids, 40 to 60 mEq daily, to provide for potassium loss. Extrarenal losses of fluid, such as by gastric drainage, should be replaced by volume with appropriate solutions in addition to the quantities outlined.

After an operation, daily weighing is a valuable aid in determining hydration. Patients should be weighed at the same time each morning after voiding. After major surgery, weight loss should be anticipated. If weight loss does not occur by the third day, overhydration should be suspected and administration of fluids curtailed. Overzealous administration of fluids is a common cause of cardiac decompensation in the aged during the postoperative period.

Early ambulation and mobilization should be encouraged to prevent clot formation in the lower extremities and pelvic vessels. Pulmonary embolism is a complication that frequently occurs in the aged, particularly if there is no ambulation early in the postoperative period or if patients are not encouraged to wear antiembolism stockings. The goal for these patients is early rehabilitation and return to community activities and functions.

SUMMARY

The field of anesthesia for the aged or geriatric patient is very broad. This chapter has presented only a brief summary of the major points, issues, and physiologic alterations resulting from the aging process that influence anesthetic management.

Information gained through studying our expanding life spans, coupled with increased technology and research in gerontology, will enhance our skill in anesthetic management of the aged.

REFERENCES

1. Moritz DJ, Ostfeld AM. The epidemiology and demography of aging. In: Hazzard WR, Andres R, Bierman EL, Blass JP, eds. *Principles of geriatric medicine and gerontology.* New York: McGraw-Hill; 1990:146–156.
2. Pawlson LG. Health care implications of an aging population. In: Hazzard WR, Andres R, Bierman EL, Blass JP, eds. *Principles of geriatric medicine and gerontology.* New York: McGraw-Hill Information Services Co., Health Professions Division; 1990: 157–166.
3. Bromage P. *Epidural analgesia.* Philadelphia: WB Saunders; 1978.
4. DelGuercio LRM, Cohn JD. Monitoring operative risk in the elderly. *JAMA.* 1980;243:1350–1355.
5. Charlson ME, Cohen RP, Sears CL. General medical consultation: Lessons from a clinical service. *Am J Med.* 1983;75:121–128.
6. Denny JH, Denson JS. Risk of surgery in patients over 90. *Geriatrics.* 1972;27:115.
7. Goldman L, Caldera DL. Risk of general anesthesia in elective operation in the hypertensive patient. *Anesthesiology.* 1979;50: 285–292.
8. Cahlan MK, Litt L, Botvinick EH, et al. Advances in noninvasive cardiovascular imaging: Implications for the anesthesiologist. *Anesthesiology.* 1987;66:356–372.
9. Tisi GM. Preoperative evaluation of pulmonary function: Validity, indications, and benefits. *Am Rev Respir Dis.* 1979; 119:293–310.
10. Tine M, Cassara EL. Preoperative pulmonary evaluation and therapy for surgery patients. *JAMA.* 1970;211:787–790.
11. Pompei P. Preoperative assessment and perioperative care. In: Cassel CK, et al, eds. *Geriatric medicine.* 2nd ed. New York: Springer-Verlag; 1990.
12. Page MM, Watkins PJ. Cardiorespiratory arrest in diabetic autoimmune neuropathy. *Lancet.* 1978;1:14–16.
13. Livingstone EH, Hershman JM, Sawin CT, et al. Prevalence of thyroid disease and abnormal thyroid tests in older hospitalized and ambulatory persons. *J Am Geriatr Soc.* 1987;35:109–114.
14. Murkin JM. Anesthesia and hypothyroidism: A review of thyroxin, physiology, pharmacology, and anesthetic implications. *Anesth Analg.* 1982;61:371–383.
15. Goldman S, Copeland J, Moritz T, et al. Improvement in early saphenous vein graft patency after coronary artery bypass surgery with antiplatelet therapy: Results of a Veterans Administration Cooperative Study. *Circulation.* 1988;77:1324.
16. Meridy HW. Criteria for selection of ambulatory patients and guidelines for anesthesia management. A retrospective study of 1,553 cases. *Anesth Analg.* 1982;61:921.
17. Lichtider MD, Wetchler BV, Philip BK. The adult and geriatric patient. In: Wetchler BV, ed. *Anesthesia for ambulatory surgery.* Philadelphia: JB Lippincott; 1985:216.
18. Waugaman WR. Preoperative and postoperative considerations for patients with Alzheimer's disease. *Geriatr Nurs.* 1988;9: 227–230.

Outpatient Anesthesia

Gerald David Allen

The emphasis on outpatient surgical procedures has had significant impact on the practice of anesthesia, especially in the last decade. The move to outpatient facilities has resulted largely from attempts by the federal government and others to contain health care costs, especially those incurred with traditional hospital stays which are usually longer, more labor intensive, and more expensive. Outpatient anesthesia may be performed in a hospital-based satellite, a special area of a hospital operating suite, a separate outpatient surgical unit, or a free-standing outpatient surgical clinic. Surgical procedures performed in the outpatient area have demonstrated an enviable safety record. In 1978, the Free-Standing Ambulatory Surgical Association recorded only 1 death in 283,658 cases, with a hospitalization rate of 0.007 percent.[1] Morbidity and mortality rates from outpatient anesthesia provided in oral surgeons' offices in California, revealed only 1 death in 673,000 general anesthetics.[2] It should be noted that these statistics were from facilities that were either state or federally approved, inspected, or certified. Unfortunately, many general anesthetics are still provided in less well maintained or staffed outpatient facilities. Many states have yet to enact or enforce universal standards devised to protect the public by providing a quality of care equal to that provided by traditional inpatient settings. Consequently, it behooves the CRNA to determine the appropriateness of providing care in outpatient facilities that lack peer review mechanisms, adequate facilities and equipment, or licensed personnel. The recent upsurge in outpatient anesthesia does not indicate an innovation in patient care as the concept of a free-standing outpatient clinic was developed in 1919 by Waters and described in "The Downtown Anesthetic Clinic."

MEDICAL ECONOMICS OF OUTPATIENT SURGERY

Current data reveal that nearly 40 percent of surgery can be performed on an outpatient basis and enthusiastic pursuit of this concept will promote further expansion of outpatient anesthesia in the future. In the past 5 years alone, outpatient anesthesia has increased from 11 to 29 percent and some policymakers project that this may reach 80 percent by the end of the century. The financial necessity of outpatient anesthesia is a further imperative for selection of this mode of patient care. Analysis of hospital costs show that it is possible to save 40 to 50 percent of the expenses of a surgical procedure by having the surgery performed on an outpatient basis, and consequently, a commitment to outpatient anesthesia has now been afforded by all insurance carriers. In fact, a major concern of anesthesia providers has been to secure agreements from carriers to admit patients prior to the day of surgery in those cases where a medical necessity exists, which requires a more extensive workup than is traditionally provided to patients in the inpatient area of the hospital.

Organizational Concerns

The proper organization and administration of an outpatient anesthesia facility or department are critical determinants of success in the provision of quality patient care. Ideally, all such facilities should be recognized by the Joint Commission on Accreditation of Hospital Organizations (JCAHO) or other state certifying or accreditation bodies. Many of these agencies publish standards of practice and patient care standards, as well as standards relating to facility equipment and services, that must be met to receive recognition. In addition, all facilities should have a quality assessment program not only to satisfy accreditation requirements, but also to ensure ongoing high-quality care. Therefore, the anesthetist must have significant input into developing the guidelines for the administration of outpatient anesthesia.

The hospital outpatient facility should be in a separate location from the routine hospital inpatient surgical units. The importance of a separate waiting area from the discharge area must be emphasized, and a circular pattern of patient flow provides the smoothest form of organization. The recovery room should be provided with a changing area, and again the separation of waiting and recovery areas must be emphasized. A free-standing ambulatory anesthesia clinic should have firm and defined arrangements for the admission of patients for whom hospital admission is considered essential. These arrangements should be organized and implemented prior to the development of a problem. The provision of suitable parking areas and collection points is essential.[3]

Patient Acceptance

Patient acceptance of outpatient anesthesia is evident from available data. Between 93 and 96 percent of patients react favorably to the concept of outpatient anesthesia and between 87 and 91 percent of patients indicated they would repeat the experience.[4] Frequently, patient rejection of outpatient anesthesia experience is related to sociologic problems of handling the difficult child or prolonged nausea and vomiting. Many patients, particularly those who suffered nausea and vomiting, attribute their unfortunate experience to the outpatient anesthetic. As noted in Table 34–1, the incidence of nausea and vomiting remains the most significant factor leading to an unplanned hospital admission. The experiences of the SurgiCenter in Phoenix indicate that the most common age group for acceptance of outpatient anesthesia is between 15 and 45 years of age. Only 3.5 percent of their patients are over 65.[5]

PREOPERATIVE PREPARATION

Patient Selection

Perhaps the most significant factor in determining the overall success of outpatient anesthesia relates to proper patient selection. Not every patient is suited for the outpatient experience, usually because of medical reasons that relate to the degree of surgical or anesthesia risk or invasiveness or length of surgery or preexisting disease. Patients must also agree with the concept of outpatient anesthesia and consider it to be the most ideal situation for them. Social factors are of considerable importance. A lack of adequate home care for the patient in the immediate postoperative period would mitigate against an outpatient procedure. It has been suggested that the outpatient should reside within 1 hour's distance from the operative facility. This is usually considered driving time and not, as has been interpreted by some,

TABLE 34–1. COMPLICATIONS[a]

Nausea and vomiting	12–25%
Headache	13–50%
Sore throat	25–40%
Muscle pain	12–25%
Temporomandibular joint pain	4%
Drowsiness	30%

[a] The common complications of outpatient anesthesia are not particularly related to the outpatient setting. Women are more likely to suffer complications, and the greater the length of operation (20 minutes) the more frequent the complication.

flying time. Arrangements can frequently be made for the patient to remain at an adjacent motel for 24 hours after the procedure if required, and even this can still be a more economical and more comfortable experience than admission to a hospital.

The extremes of age do pose some problems. For instance, full-term infants can be accepted for outpatient surgery at 2 weeks, but any suspicion that apnea may develop postoperatively calls for overnight admission. The significance of the outpatient setting for the geriatric patient should be based on physiologic, not chronologic, age. In selecting patients for outpatient anesthesia, it is usually preferred that they be American Society of Anesthesiologists (ASA) physical status 1 or 2. If patients have another complicating disease, it must be controlled and present no immediate or obvious threat to the perioperative course. There are exceptions to this rule, however, as many physical status ASA 3 patients are operated on in outpatient clinics. In fact, the outpatient anesthesia area can provide unique benefits to more medically compromised patients. For instance, patients with leukemia or cystic fibrosis or those on immunosuppressant drugs would benefit from situations where they can avoid contact with hospital bacteria, such as would be provided in the outpatient area.

Surgical Considerations

The desire of the surgeon to operate in an outpatient facility must be considered. Most surgeons like the outpatient area as case turnover times are significantly reduced and greater flexibility is afforded in the types of surgical procedures undertaken. In addition, surgeons perceive that their patients like the convenience of same-day admission and increased cost savings. Factors relating to the type of surgery should also be considered, especially as they relate to operative time and the probability of complications. Outpatient operations should be of a superficial nature, with a preferable duration of 5 to 90 minutes. This should not be considered an absolute duration as some dental and plastics procedures may extend to 6 hours; however, the surgical trauma in such cases is usually minimal. The critical surgical factor that precludes use of an outpatient anesthetic facility is the potential for postoperative bleeding. Any suggestion that this might occur would indicate a day-stay facility with overnight admission rather than an outpatient center. The potential range of operations performed in the outpatient area covers the spectrum of surgery and final determinations may be based on patient condition, availability of hospital support services, adequacy of professional staffing, and duration and invasiveness of the planned operation. Complications, if they arise, are usually related to those commonly found in the general surgical population or to surgical technique (Table 34–2).

The anesthetist should appreciate the fact that there are no absolute indications and relatively few contraindications to outpatient procedures. The suitability of each should be determined individually and in accordance with available resources, patient condition, and patient safety concerns. Such decisions can be illustrated in the following examples. The patient undergoing thoracentesis may have extremely

TABLE 34–2. MAJOR MORBIDITY[a]

Hypotension
Arrhythmia
Hemorrhage
Hypoventilation
Extended surgery

[a] The major problems that occur in outpatient anesthesia are usually surgical problems. Hypoventilation will not occur with alert anesthetists, and arrhythmias are not necessarily related to outpatient anesthesia.

severe postoperative pain which may preclude adequate analgesic control under medical supervision postoperatively. The breast cyst, if malignant, may require instant radical mastectomy, a much more time consuming procedure. The skin graft may require extensive postoperative care for immobility, whereas for the most common of all outpatient procedures, the dilation and curettage, bleeding may present a problem. It has also been suggested that a herniorrhaphy is unsuitable for an outpatient setting, as it requires the patient to lie immobile in bed, whereas a vasectomy, if done on an outpatient basis, can pose problems with postoperative hemorrhage. The immobility required after some orthopedic operations could mitigate against outpatient anesthesia. Many procedures involving the ear, nose, and throat have a tendency to result in high blood losses. Pain associated with an anal fissure or hemorrhoidectomy may be a contraindication to outpatient care, and operations on the eye muscles have a high incidence of postoperative nausea and vomiting, requiring inpatient care. Although all these types of surgeries may be performed on outpatients, postoperative care and complications must be carefully considered.

Patient Instruction and Chart Documentation

Once the patient and surgeon have determined that an outpatient surgical procedure is appropriate, written instructions governing the pre- and postoperative period should be provided by the surgeon or anesthesia provider. The anesthetist should determine that this document contains requisite anesthesia-related information that must be followed for the surgery to commence and safety standards to be maintained. These instructions should include the following information: patients will be discharged only to a responsible adult and arrangements should be made for postoperative care by a competent individual; patients should be instructed to abide strictly by NPO (nothing by mouth) orders; any change in the patient's physical condition preoperatively, such as development of acute respiratory infection, should be reported to the anesthesia provider immediately. Instructions for preoperative care should include a warning to avoid consumption of alcohol the night before the procedure; patients should be informed not to undertake any heavy physical or important decision-making activities for 24 hours postoperatively, as judgment may be impaired; and finally, patients should be informed of relevant physical signs and symptoms that may indicate impending complications, such as severe pain, excessive bleeding, and elevated temperature.

In every case, a qualified anesthesia provider should conduct a thorough history and physical. If an outpatient anesthesia screening clinic is used, documentation can be obtained at that time. A standard anesthesia history form is of value, as screening can be performed rapidly and pertinent points reviewed. A preoperative note should be written to include the anesthetic plan, informed consent, patient ASA classification and any other noteworthy data relative to the patient's physical condition that must be addressed in the course of the anesthetic. A copy of the patient's history and preoperative instructions should be signed by the patient or guardian and retained in the chart.

Physical Evaluation

In a properly organized outpatient facility, the patient's history can be reviewed and the physical examination conducted adequately the day of surgery, provided the instructions given at the initial examination have been followed. This is possible via preoperative screening clinics or phone interviews that reveal the necessity for the patient to be evaluated in advance of the surgery by anesthesia personnel subsequent to complex medical problems. The history should include at a minimum the following: past surgical procedures/anesthetic complications in self or family, recent/acute illnesses, medications taken within the last 3 months, allergies, any current medical problems currently being treated by a physician, diagnosed lung disease, shortness of breath, coughing, wheezing, current upper respiratory infection, diagnosed cardiovascular disease, ankle swelling, chest pain, peripheral numbness. Recent studies of abbreviated physical examinations that were inclusive of cyanosis, clubbing, dyspnea, and head and neck abnormalities were sufficient to successfully evaluate 96 percent of the patients presenting for anesthesia. This is not to suggest that a private physician should not perform a complete physical examination, but standard screenings performed by the anesthetist and surgeon are usually sufficient to provide for an adequate physical evaluation of the patient prior to anesthesia. Screening tests for asymptomatic patients have recently been reevaluated. Typical screening tests are indicated in Table 34–3. The cost effectiveness of routine laboratory tests in asymptomatic patients prior to anesthesia indicated that the only truly cost-effective laboratory test was an examination of the hemoglobin and urine.

Premedication

Premedication is best avoided in outpatient anesthesia. It has been found that the use of opiates in premedications will delay recovery; however, those patients receiving sedative medications did not experience delayed recovery. In the patient who may be mobile soon after the operative procedure, premedications may induce nausea and vomiting. In addition, the unnecessary injection of standard intramuscular premedication adds to the discomfort of the patient. If, as some authorities promote, an anticholinergic drug is given, oral forms of atropine should be used, as they are equally effective. In this regard, oral cimetidine 300 mg has been shown to effectively reduce gastric fluid pH and vol-

TABLE 34–3. SCREENING TESTS FOR ASYMPTOMATIC PATIENTS[a]

< 40 y	
Men	None
Women	Hemoglobin or hematocrit
40–60 y	
Men	BUN[b], glucose, ECG
Women	Hemoglobin or hematocrit, BUN, glucose, ECG
> 60 y	
Men	BUN, glucose, ECG, hemoglobin or hematocrit, chest x-ray
Women	Hemoglobin or hematocrit, BUN, glucose, ECG, chest x-ray

[a] Additional tests may be indicated for existing conditions.
[b] BUN, blood urea nitrogen; ECG, electrocardiogram.

ume in outpatients and might be a useful premedication.[6,7] Studies of secobarbital and propiomazine resulted in recovery within 90 minutes of their intravenous administration. If secobarbital was administered orally, recovery was delayed an additional 45 minutes, giving further support for the avoidance of premedication. As the majority of patients receive intravenous induction of anesthesia, preoperative sedation, if indicated, is administered immediately prior to induction of anesthesia by the intravenous route rather than by painful and unpredictable intramuscular routes. This technique is usually followed also for those patients undergoing regional blocks.

Diazepam produces good amnesia and sedation, but there have been reports of delayed effects from the metabolites up to 48 hours postoperatively. Lorazepam is a very good amnesic if given 45 minutes before the procedure but, in moderate dosage, produces little sedation. Midazolam has proven to be the most satisfactory benzodiazepine for intravenous premedication, as recovery and absence of delayed effects are evident.[8] Intravenous pentobarbital has a well-established record of producing good sedation. If a narcotic is to be administered prior to the procedure, pentobarbital decreases the incidence of nausea with intravenous narcotics. The sedative technique consisting of pentobarbital, meperidine, and scopolamine (Jorgensen technique) provides good supplemental sedation for regional anesthesia in anxious patients. This technique does delay recovery, and selection of sedation for outpatient premedication should be made with the knowledge that recovery may be delayed. Hypnosis is an excellent adjunct for outpatient anesthesia, and even a short amount of time spent inducing a hypnotic state in patients benefits smooth induction. A technique for rapid hypnotic induction has been introduced by Barber.[9] Specifics relative to a broader range of preoperative medications can be found in Chapter 14.

Pediatric Factors

An overly anxious parent, or one with inadequate home facilities, is not a candidate to care for a child after a surgical procedure. This is unfortunate as there are many positive factors to encourage the use of outpatient anesthesia in pediatric practice. The anxiety exhibited by the pediatric patient is reduced, and separation is less traumatic if it is for a short time, a situation usually accommodated well in outpatient facilities. Nosocomial infections are greatly reduced in the outpatient population. For instance, the outpatient generally contacts only 9 people during their stay, but an inpatient comes in contact with an average of 27 people while in the hospital. A 17 percent infection rate in a hospital surgical practice was reduced 50 to 70 percent by using outpatient surgery. These reductions in infections are among indications for performing outpatient anesthesia on pediatric patients, especially those of higher ASA classifications (above 3).

Pediatric procedures should be scheduled early in the morning to abbreviate the time during which the patient has no food intake and remains NPO. Studies have revealed that outpatient scheduling may actually enhance serum blood sugars in pediatric patients by decreasing NPO time. One study noted that the plasma glucose levels in children under 5 years of age were 46 mg/100 mL for inpatients and 88.5 mg/100 mL for outpatients. This could be attributed to a less restrictive fluid intake or possibly to the increased activity of the patient prior to outpatient treatment. In addition, postoperative admission rates for complications in pediatric outpatient anesthetic practice have ranged from 0.1 to 2 percent, a most acceptable level.

The only relative consistent contraindications to outpatient procedures in the pediatric population are infants with a history of acute respiratory distress syndrome requiring ventilatory support or a history of bronchopulmonary dysplasia and preterm infants younger than 44 weeks of postconceptual age. All groups tend to develop some element of postoperative pulmonary dysfunction. Most notable are studies that indicate that premature infants may be prone to postoperative apnea up to 12 hours after emergence. It has also been suggested that pediatric patients with siblings who died of sudden infant death syndrome (SIDS) be treated in an inpatient facility.

In premedication and induction of the pediatric patient, much has been made of the use of a solution of rectal methohexital 20 mg/kg or thiopental paste 40 mg/kg. Experience with these drugs varies. Delayed recovery is a major problem with this form of *induction* of anesthesia. Unnecessary injections in children remain a determining factor in selecting premedication in children. Both oral sodium citrate 0.4 ml/kg and cimetidine syrup 10 mg/kg 1 hour before induction have proven to be effective in increasing gastric pH.

Geriatric Factors

Although considered in greater detail in Chapter 33, some salient factors relating to outpatient anesthesia in the elderly should be emphasized. The consideration of age is important as it relates to the lack of activity associated with diseases accompanying increasing age, even more so than physiologic and pharmacologic changes affecting drug disposition. It should be remembered that age alone is not considered a contraindication for outpatient surgery in the geriatric patient. There have been no studies that indicate that the recovery rates for the general geriatric population are increased in this setting or that complication rates are higher, given that patients meet all preoperative screening criteria. In fact, the outpatient setting may provide these patients with the ability to decrease the total time away from their home environment, which will decrease any potential for confusion or inability to cope effectively with a new environment.

Especially significant to anesthetic practice are the pulmonary changes as well as the 20 to 30 percent decrease in cardiac output that occur by age 65. PaO_2 decreases progressively as ventilation–perfusion abnormalities develop as a result of the increase in closing volumes beyond functional residual capacity. The ventilatory response to hypoxemia and hypercapnia is diminished and metabolism may be depressed. These physiologic changes in the elderly require particular care during intravenous anesthesia and monitored anesthesia care, as apnea has been noted to occur with as little as 2.5 mg of diazepam. Renal function is decreased in the elderly, such that drugs dependent on renal function for elimination exhibit decreased plasma clearance. Pharmacodynamic changes in drug profiles are due to alterations at the receptor level and to altered responsiveness of the homeostatic mechanisms that would normally counteract drug effects.

INTRAOPERATIVE TECHNIQUES

Timing of admission of patients to the surgical outpatient clinic is important and early arrival times and long waiting periods until surgery should be avoided. A major advantage of having a separate outpatient surgical unit lies in the fact that surgical scheduling is not dependent on the scheduling problems often encountered in the hospital setting. There are definite physiologic changes that relate to the duration of wait prior to anesthesia; however, interpretations of their significance may vary. For instance, protracted waits may exacerbate patient anxiety and increases in circulating catecholamines, which may result in arrhythmias during induction or requirements for increased drug dosage levels. Peripheral vascular tone must also be preserved prior to the introduction of agents that cause vasodilation. Consequently, long periods during which patients are NPO may result in situations where the patient becomes less responsive to normal mechanisms of homeostasis.

Conscious Sedation

For many outpatients, conscious sedation is the anesthetic technique of choice. It provides sedation and patient comfort while allowing the surgery to proceed under local anesthesia. The anesthetist is charged with the responsibility of titrating various drugs to the level at which the patient is comfortable yet retains spontaneous, unassisted ventilation and airway reflex patency and can respond appropriately to verbal command. Monitoring standards are the same as those that apply to general anesthesia. The technique of conscious sedation has also been found to be useful as an adjunct to regional anesthesia to afford the patient an advanced degree of comfort and reduction in stress. The technique is also beneficial in that it may obviate a full general anesthesia and the risks and longer recovery attendant to it.

The success of a sedation technique hinges on the patient's understanding of what he or she will experience dur-

ing the procedure. Therefore, proper patient selection and teaching is important. It is incumbent on the CRNA to provide a clear explanation of what may occur during the procedure, such as "feelings of pressure from the surgical intervention, maintenance of consciousness, ability to talk and swallow and breathe freely without impairment." The CRNA should keep in constant verbal contact with the patient to assure him or her that the procedure is going well and also to assess more clearly the patient's level of consciousness, airway patency, and level of comfort. This can be accomplished by requiring the patient to follow simple commands such as taking a deep breath or squeezing the anesthetist's hand.

A fine line exists between the analgesia provided via conscious sedation techniques and the anesthesia that may result from inadvertent overdose. Such situations may essentially leave the patient with an unprotected airway in situations where such is indicated. Therefore, constant vigilance is required to maintain an optimal balance between analgesia, sedation, consciousness, and maintenance of normal homeostatic mechanisms. In addition, other risks are attendant to this technique that are not unique to the outpatient setting, but rather are potentially characteristic of any surgical procedure. These may include allergic or idiosyncratic drug responses, hypertension/hypotension, and especially airway problems including frank obstruction, bronchospasm, and potential aspiration. It is usually considered appropriate for the patient to receive low-flow air/oxygen via mask while the procedure is being conducted. As for all surgical procedures, full monitoring equipment, including pulse oximetry, should be used as induction of general anesthesia may be unexpectedly required.

Drugs used for conscious sedation include a wide range of short-acting narcotics and sedative drugs, as well as some inhalation agents such as nitrous oxide. Inhalation sedation with 20 to 40 percent nitrous oxide in oxygen produces minimum cardiorespiratory change, with almost instant recovery of all the patient's faculties at the conclusion of a procedure. Studies have shown complete return of full faculties after breathing room air for 15 minutes. Twenty-five percent nitrous oxide in oxygen will produce analgesia equivalent to that provided by 10 mg of morphine. A personal practice with the majority of regional anesthetics is to supplement the block with nitrous oxide–oxygen sedation if the patient desires transient amnesia. Low-dose continuous intravenous administration of methohexital and propofol have been found useful. The administration of alfentanil as a continuous infusion or in bolus doses provides short-lived supplementary anesthesia with minimal sedation. Drug selection and dosages should be titrated only to effect, keeping in mind that all ministrations of the technique should be directed toward minimizing delay of recovery.

Alternate techniques of sedation may include small doses of diazepam, midazolam, or pentobarbital or the use of incremental doses or continuous infusion of thiopental or methohexital during short periods of increased surgical stress or discomfort. These short-acting intravenous anesthetics produce greater depression than the sedatives but are frequently used to supplement regional anesthetics.

Regional Anesthesia

Regional anesthesia is frequently considered to be the most suitable form of outpatient anesthesia, as the extent of anesthesia is restricted to the surgical site. These techniques are often supplemented by some degree of sedation for patient comfort and relaxation. The extent to which regional techniques are used in the outpatient setting are usually dependent on the skill of the practitioner and time factors required to administer and "set" the block without delaying the surgical schedule. Often, regional anesthetics are avoided because of their protracted recovery time; however, this characteristic can afford the patient significant analgesia during the postoperative phase. Decisions to use a regional block should be made on the basis of several factors including the extent to which this technique is most suitable for the patient, considering surgical requirements and patient acceptance of the technique. It is also paramount that the patient be properly schooled in the proper care of the affected extremity postoperatively as normal protective mechanisms of pain and pressure are obtunded for a time.

Early ambulation, usually a desirable feature of outpatient anesthesia, may become problematic when some regional techniques are used in an outpatient setting. Subarachnoid blocks would seem generally to be contraindicated in outpatient use primarily because of the potential for postspinal headache. It should be noted, however, that some studies report that with proper technique, patient hydration, selection of 25- or 26-gauge needles, and proper bevel position, this risk is significantly attenuated. Early ambulation after a subarachnoid block is one of the most frequent causes of headache and should thus be avoided in an outpatient setting or delayed for several hours.

The incidence of pneumothorax after a supraclavicular block or stellate ganglion block on an outpatient basis is much greater if the patient is extremely active after these blocks. Perforation of the apex of the lung does not result in a pneumothorax unless vigorous breathing turns the puncture into a tear. It is usually considered advantageous to reserve the supraclavicular nerve block for inpatient procedures. The stellate ganglion block is commonly employed in pain clinic patients on a recurring basis, but these patients are usually less active; however, warnings with regard to the extent of exercise after the use of such a block must be given.

Other techniques of regional anesthesia advocated are pudendal, perianal, axillary, and trigeminal blocks, all of which are suitably performed in an outpatient setting. The intravenous regional (Bier) block is a most suitable form of outpatient anesthesia and easy to administer. Major blocks such as the four-quadrant or sciatic–femoral block may be used for outpatient procedures particularly in the pain clinic, as may intercostal nerve blocks. Again, if precautions are not taken with the intercostal nerve block, pneumothorax may result. Lumbar and splanchnic nerve blocks can be performed in the correct setting for diagnostic and therapeutic purposes. Lumbar epidural blocks have been proven to be advantageous for anesthesia involving the pelvic and abdominal areas as well as lower extremity surgery. A particular advantage of most of these techniques is that postoperative nausea and vomiting are significantly reduced.

Provided follow-up is adequate, the patient can be discharged the same day.

Antiseptics that would stain clothing should be avoided and patients should be instructed not to wear expensive or cumbersome clothing. In selection of an agent, consideration should be given to the avoidance of including epinephrine in the solution as the block may be prolonged. Chloroprocaine and Xylocaine appear to be the most popular agents for most blocks because of their short duration of action and wide margins of safety. Agents such as bupivacaine and tetracaine are usually avoided because of their prolonged durations.

General Anesthesia

For selected cases, general anesthesia may be preferable. As with any agent or technique to be used in the outpatient setting, the drugs should be selected to avoid delay of emergence and prolong recovery. Because of the need to "tailor" the anesthetic to the patient and the procedure, the balanced anesthesia technique has gained widespread popularity in the outpatient setting. This technique provides minimal physiologic (primarily cardiorespiratory) change and early recovery. Judicious combinations of sedatives, analgesics, and muscle relaxants with or without nitrous oxide may be used. Low concentrations of isoflurane or other inhalation agents can also be employed in the technique as a substitute for narcotics and, to some degree, amnestic agents. Narcotic premedication should be restricted to that minimal dose producing euphoria. Further, studies have demonstrated that narcotics produce little reduction in the minimum anesthetic concentration of inhalation agents and also may delay recovery.

Various induction agents can be considered appropriate to the outpatient area. Intravenous induction of anesthesia with 1 mg/kg methohexital or 3 mg/kg thiopental is the most satisfactory form of outpatient anesthetic induction. Methohexital allows for earlier recovery, although it produces more dramatic cardiovascular changes, such as a fall in peripheral resistance with compensatory increases in heart rate (Table 34–4). Intravenous etomidate 0.4 mg/kg is also available for induction of anesthesia, but it has the disadvantage of frequently causing venous thrombosis, pain on injection, and myoclonus. Ketamine in doses of 5 to 7 mg/kg appears to be particularly suitable for intramuscular induction in children, but has been found to pose

TABLE 34–4. CHANGE IN CARDIAC RATE[a]

Atropine	30%
Hydroxyzine, methohexital	14%
Thiopental	25%
Diazepam	31%
Methohexital	45%
Ketamine	82%

[a] Studies in outpatients show changes in rate subsequent to administration of various medications indicated. The changes in cardiac rate may be considered arrhythmias. With methohexital and ketamine, particularly in the elderly with a fixed cardiac output, the rate alone could cause problems.

other problems, especially relative to recovery. Recovery may be prolonged, but this can be taken into account in the scheduling of the patient if ketamine is considered the most desirable agent. Intravenous ketamine doses are usually limited to 1.0 mg/kg. All of these intravenous induction agents can be used as supplements to nitrous oxide–oxygen for maintenance of anesthesia and recovery is usually rapid. Propofol 1.5 to 2.5 mg/kg is a useful agent for induction of anesthesia in the outpatient, as a single dose has a duration of action of only 3 to 5 minutes. Pain on injection is a problem, but the principal disadvantage is cardiovascular depression. It should be used with caution in the elderly. As with thiopental, sensitivity to propofol does not change with age, nor does the initial volume of distribution decrease with age.

The use of inhalation induction with nitrous oxide–oxygen in combination with halothane, enflurane, or isoflurane is a satisfactory technique in outpatients. Induction with nitrous oxide–oxygen–halothane lasts only a few minutes and, for the majority of patients, is a pleasant experience. Certainly in children, it is a frequent technique of induction prior to the insertion of an intravenous cannula. Halothane is preferred to isoflurane, as it is not as pungent. Even though the physical characteristics of enflurane and isoflurane indicate more rapid induction, this has not been confirmed by clinical experience, especially in children.[10]

Maintenance of anesthesia is preferable with nitrous oxide–oxygen and enflurane, isoflurane, or halothane. Ventricular arrhythmias are common with halothane in the unmedicated patient, but are worsened with addition of atropine (Table 34–5). Arrhythmias are frequently ventricular in nature. The use of short-acting narcotics, such as fentanyl, with nitrous oxide–oxygen has been suggested for maintenance. Although fentanyl or alfentanil decreases the amount of thiopental needed for general anesthesia, the incidence of apnea is greater than if thiopental alone is used as a supplement for nitrous oxide–oxygen.[11] Longer-acting narcotics are used less frequently and reversal at the conclusion of the procedure with drugs such as naloxone 0.1 mg may be required. If reversal is contemplated, it should be appreciated that repeated doses of the reversal may be required as the half-life of naloxone is shorter than that of most narcotics. Vomiting is also a frequent concomitant of overdose with naloxone, and there is usually total reversal of the analgesia produced if the dose is not carefully titrated.

Propofol is used for induction and maintenance by continuous infusion (10 mg/kg/h) or intermittent injection. Recovery from the neurologic effects of general anesthesia by this technique is more rapid than by any other combination of drugs. Some difference in recovery time is noted between narcotic and inhalation cases. Recovery from a volatile agent, although significantly more rapid in the period 0.5 to 1 hour postoperatively, was found to equal recovery time from narcotics after 1 hour.

The use of an endotracheal tube is dependent on the surgery rather than the anesthetic, as it will frequently require the administration of a muscle relaxant, an added complication for the anesthetic. The use of an endotracheal tube is advisable if intraoperative regurgitation is considered a potential problem. It should be noted that postoperative regurgitation and aspiration in the recovery room are more frequent when an endotracheal tube has been used. If a muscle relaxant is required throughout a procedure, as in tubal ligation, then endotracheal intubation is essential. Ventilation without a tube may inflate the stomach, resulting in postoperative nausea and vomiting. A good guideline for duration, in this respect, is that up to 2 hours of placement of an endotracheal tube results in microscopic damage of the trachea, whereas 6 hours produces macroscopic damage to the tracheal wall.

If the requirement for an endotracheal tube is dependent on limited access to the head, a useful alternative is the laryngeal mask. It will not prevent aspiration, and this is not an alternative if regurgitation is predicted. Artificial ventilation can be performed adequately without inflation of the stomach.[12] Still, the use of a mask is preferable in those cases where there are no strict indications for intubation.

Muscle relaxants are frequently employed in outpatient surgical practice. The use of intravenous drip succinylcholine is still considered by many to be a satisfactory means of providing relaxation in balanced anesthesia. There are potential problems in using succinylcholine, although these are usually manifested only after prolonged administration; however, the incidence of abnormal pseudocholinesterase is considered to be 1 in 3000, and the chances of prolonged apnea are considerable. If nondepolarizing relaxants are used in outpatient anesthesia, as for example in laparoscopy, the more recently introduced agents atracurium and vecuronium are preferable.[13]

The concept of a minor anesthetic, that is, an anesthetic used for a procedure taking less than 1 hour, is well substantiated in outpatient anesthesia.[14] For instance in 1969, outpatient tonsillectomy had a zero mortality in 40,000 patients, when these patients were not subject to endotracheal intubation and the procedure was brief. As a general rule, the shorter the operation, the fewer physiologic effects. However, a short general anesthetic can cause acute changes in renal hemodynamics related to a decrease in the mean arterial pressure. The changes are rapidly reversed and appear to be related to the effect on the afferent arteriolar circulation. General anesthesia lasting more than 60 minutes appears to cause afferent arteriolar vasoconstriction, with subsequent changes in the filtration factor (Fig. 34–1).

Monitoring

The use of a precordial stethoscope, temperature probe, blood pressure monitor, pulse oximeter, and capnography are considered essential to all outpatient cases. The CRNA should remember that the standards of care or of perioperative monitoring should not differ between inpatient or outpatient sites.

TABLE 34–5. VENTRICULAR ARRHYTHMIA[a]

N₂O–halothane	25%
+ Thiopental	10%
+ Thiopental and atropine	20%
+ Propranolol	0%

[a] Ventricular arrhythmias are related to catecholamine release in light anesthesia and are worsened by the addition of atropine.

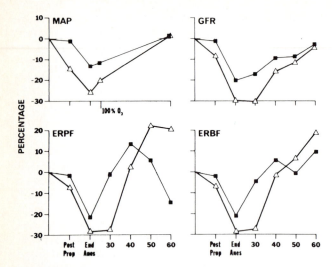

Figure 34–1. Renal effects relative to mean arterial blood pressure after administration of a brief outpatient anesthetic. In brief anesthesia, the renal changes parallel effects in mean arterial blood pressure. (*Reprinted, with permission, from Everett GB, Allen GD, et al. Renal hemodynamic effect of general anesthesia in outpatients.* Anesth Analg. *1973;52:470.*)

POSTOPERATIVE PATIENT CARE

The recovery room must be staffed by competent nurses who will be alert to the problems of aspiration, vomiting, and delayed recovery. Blood pressure and other vital signs should be routinely checked until full recovery. The duration of stay will be dependent on the surgical procedure and the duration of the anesthetic.[14] The use of specific drug antagonists, such as naloxone and flumazenil, can hasten recovery. These drugs have demonstrated that rapid reversal of narcotics and benzodiazepines is possible, although they must be employed with caution to ensure that the time course of their activity parallels the action of the agonist.[15]

In many instances, if an endotracheal tube has been placed, particularly in children, the patient should be monitored in the recovery room for 2 hours. If analgesia is required, then short-acting narcotics such as fentanyl are indicated, and the patient should be detained until the respiratory depression of the analgesic has dissipated. If intravenous morphine is given, vomiting may become a problem; thus parenteral narcotics should be avoided, if possible. Other potential analgesics are aspirin rectal suppositories. If oral medication can be taken, then aspirin and codeine combinations are the most efficacious.

DISCHARGE CRITERIA

Discharge criteria are important, and are commonly referred to as an assessment for "street fitness"; however, controversy continues to exist over which criteria constitutes this definition. Definitions have been further clouded as patient performance on street fitness assessments vary, depending on the type of anesthetic administered. Such an assessment is critical to the proper care of patients, as they are released to home care without strict supervision and con-

sequently must rely on their own innate abilities to function in a safe and lucid manner. One can appreciate this need, as it has been demonstrated that intravenous barbiturates, such as thiopental, produce electroencephalographic changes up to 24 hours postoperatively (Table 34–6), and active metabolites of diazepam have been found in plasma more than 48 hours after administration.

Many psychomotor tests are available to assess street fitness, including the simple face–hand test (Fig. 34–2). These tests in isolation are not necessarily sole indicators of patient fitness and should be used in combination with other vital signs and general physiologic condition.[16] Most of the tests used today are patterned after examinations in common use to assess drug and alcohol effect on driving performance. These involve skills of observation, judgment, motor performance, and possibly complete psychomotor testing. The simple alcoholic evaluation tests are the finger–nose test, the Romberg test, and "walking the line," all of which can be readily performed in an evaluation for street fitness. More advanced testing involving the use of a car simulation, use of body sway indicators, and measurements of ocular balance are generally more difficult to administer and have not as yet found general acceptance in busy clinical practices.

Some evaluation or score is of value in the assessment of recovery from outpatient anesthesia, both to quantify recovery and to legally document the standard of care. Although not considered an absolute indication for release, it is a repeatable measure of recovery. Complete recovery is often considered to occur at least 48 hours after introduction of the agent. The metabolism of halothane and enflurane produces metabolites that are present for some considerable time postoperatively and account for the hangover noted by some patients. In reviewing the postoperative morbidity of outpatients, changes up to and in excess of 5 days after the operation were noted in a few patients. Nonetheless, the essential feature of the assessment in recovery is the ability of the patient to be discharged from the recovery room *in the care of a responsible adult.*

Perhaps a more pragmatic approach is provided by the following criteria which in most cases allow the patient to be dismissed to a responsible adult.

1. Vital signs remain stable for 1 hour.
2. Patient has not experienced nausea and vomiting for 30 minutes after the last episode.

TABLE 34–6. RECOVERY[a]

	Thiopental	Methohexital
Verbal command	8.5 min	4.5 min
Wakening	30 min	20 min
Face–hand test	40 min	30 min
Driving reactor	21 min	14 min
Electroencephalogram	24 h	24 h

[a] The duration of recovery with thiopental and methohexital single doses is related to various assessments of recovery. The electroencephalogram may not return to normal for 24 hours.

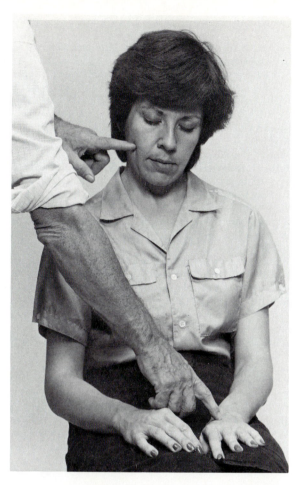

Figure 34–2. The face–hand test is useful to assess recovery from anesthesia or sedation. Because of facial dominance, extinction occurs in the sedated patient when the cheek and contralateral dorsum of hand are touched simultaneously. The patient notices only touching of the cheek until recovery is complete.

3. Patient is appropriately oriented to time and place with little or no dizziness after sitting in chair for 15 minutes.
4. Patient is able to urinate.
5. Pain relief does not require intravenous agents.
6. Bleeding and oozing are attenuated and there is no increase in pain, which would indicate problems.

For those patients who have undergone regional anesthesia, written instructions should be given to the patient regarding wound, cast, or prosthesis care; indications of problems such as high fever and emergent nausea and vomiting; dietary instructions; and directions for activity and pain medications for the first 24 hours. Patients who have had a spinal anesthetic should be encouraged to rest quietly for 24 hours, maintain bathroom privileges, and watch for headache or other unrelieved pain. Ability to urinate indicates that the sympathetic block has abated sufficiently for dismissal. Walking should be undertaken to normal levels until general proprioceptic orientation is

achieved and normal sensation to the affected area of block is restored. The CRNA or anesthesiologist should always conduct or confirm that a dismissal evaluation has been made and document on the chart that the patient has met an acceptable set of evaluative criteria.

COMPLICATIONS

The patient, in spite of the numerous advantages of outpatient care, is predisposed to a variety of postoperative complications, some of which are listed in Table 34–1. It behooves the anesthetist to avoid, if possible, problems such as nausea and vomiting, the headache associated with halothane outpatient anesthesia, and the additional special problems of pediatric patients. Nausea and vomiting remain the most predominant justification for hospital admission from the outpatient surgery recovery room. These complications may exist in as many as 20 to 30 percent of all patients presenting for outpatient surgery. The etiologies are numerous and may include a predisposition for motion sickness, use of intraoperative narcotics, quick motion such as standing or sitting, unrelieved surgical pain, and the anatomic site of surgery. Low-dose droperidol has been found to be most efficacious in reducing the incidence of both nausea and vomiting postoperatively. The adult dose of 0.625 mg is effective and does not delay discharge when given within 30 minutes of emergence of anesthesia.[17] Prophylactic use of droperidol in conjunction with metoclopramide 10 to 20 mg IV has been found to decrease the incidence of nausea further. Droperidol has also been found to be effective in the pediatric population even after ocular surgery, where nausea and vomiting may be especially severe and protracted because of extraocular muscle manipulation. Admission to the hospital is relatively rare but must be available. Major morbidity has been attributed to hypotension, arrhythmia, hemorrhage, hypoventilation, and extended surgery. Although complications occur, they are generally unrelated to the outpatient setting. Other complications relate to the amount of sedation the patient receives and the ability to concentrate on tasks. In some individuals, the response to sedation may necessitate a delay in returning to work. This individual response should be noted in discussions with the patient prior to the procedure.

Temporomandibular joint pain is probably related to anterior dislocation of the jaw in an attempt to maintain an airway. In one study, convulsions were noted in a few outpatients. No mention was made of the agent, nor if pyrexia was a feature. Compliance with instructions is variable in outpatients. Written instructions and verbal communication with an individual responsible for the patient regarding instructions are essential. The ambulatory surgery unit should contact patients for follow-up by phone within 24 hours of the surgery.

CONCLUSION

Anesthesia for the outpatient is similar to that for the inpatient: the object is to achieve minimal yet effective anesthesia that produces few if any complications that would prolong the recovery phase. There is an emphasis on early recovery and minimal cardiorespiratory and other physiologic disturbances. The equipment for the administration of anesthesia and monitoring should be identical to that available for the inpatient, and there should be no compromise in the care or preoperative evaluation of the outpatient. Outpatient anesthesia has proven to be a relatively uncomplicated and more economical means of providing patient care without the disruption or separation from the home environment for both adult and child. A major benefit is the avoidance of nosocomial infections. Emphasis on the brevity of the operation results in less trauma to the patient than would occur in the main operating suite.

Patient acceptance is generally good in both pediatric and adult populations. A frequent cause for rejecting the opportunity to repeat the outpatient experience is that of the stress of patient care for the parent or guardian. All patients should be warned that there may be a delay in returning to work. The delay varies from 5.4 percent of patients being unable to work the day after anesthesia to 9 percent requiring more than 5 days away from work.

REFERENCES

1. Natof HE. Complications associated with ambulatory surgery. *JAMA.* 1980;244:1116–1118.
2. Lytle JJ, Stamper EP. The 1988 Anesthesia Survey of the Southern California Society of Oral and Maxillofacial Surgeons. *J Oral Maxillofac Surg.* 1989;47:834–842.
3. *Accreditation handbook for ambulatory health care.* Chicago: Joint Commission on Accreditation of Hospitals; 1987–1988.
4. Nathanson BN. Ambulatory abortion, experience with 26,000 cases (July 1, 1970 to August 1, 1971). *N Engl J Med.* 1972;286:403–407.
5. Ford JL, Reed WA. The surgicenter—An innovation in the delivery and cost of medical care. *Ariz Med.* 1969;26:801–804.
6. Manchikanti L, Roush JR. Effect of pre-anesthetic glycopyrrolate and cimetidine on gastric fluid pH and volume in outpatients. *Anesth Analg.* 1984;63:40.
7. Ong BY, Palahuniuk RJ, Cumming M. Gastric volume and pH in outpatients. *Can Anaesth Soc J.* 1978;25:36–39.
8. Raybould D, Bradshaw EG. Premedication for day care surgery. *Anaesthesia.* 1987;42:591–595.
9. Barber J. Rapid induction analgesia procedure. In: Allen GD, ed. *Dental anesthesia and analgesia.* 3rd ed. Baltimore: Williams & Wilkins; 1984:41.
10. Fisher DM, Robinson S, Brecht CM, et al. Comparison of enflurane, halothane, and isoflurane for diagnostic and therapeutic procedures in children with malignancies. *Anesthesiology.* 1985;63:647–650.
11. White PF, Coe V, Shafer A. Comparison of alfentanil with fentanyl for outpatient anesthesia. *Anesthesiology.* 1986;64:99–107.
12. Griffin RM, Hatcher IS. Aspiration and the laryngeal mask airway. *Anaesthesia.* 1990;45:1039–1040.
13. Fragen RJ, Shanks CA. Neuromuscular recovery after laparoscopy. *Anesth Analg.* 1984;63:51.
14. Allen GD. Minor anesthesia. *J Oral Surg.* 1973;31:330–335.
15. Philip PK, Simpson TH, Hauch MA, et al. Flumazenil reverses sedation after midazolam-induced general anesthesia in ambulatory surgery patients. *Anesth Analg.* 1990;71:371–376.
16. Doenicke A, Jugler J, Laub M. Evaluation of recovery and "street fitness" by EEG and psychodiagnostic tests after anesthesia. *Can Anaesth Soc J.* 1967;14:567–583.
17. Valanne J, Kortilla K. Effect of a small dose of droperidol on nausea, vomiting and recovery after outpatient enflurane anesthesia. *Acta Anaesthesiol Scand.* 1985;29:359–362.

Anesthesia for Ophthalmic Surgery

Wynne R. Waugaman,
Lesa J. Hirschman, and
Don R. Hirschman

Over the last decade ophthalmic surgery has made tremendous advances because of increased technology. As a result, our anesthetic management of these patients has greatly improved. The utilization of regional anesthesia for a majority of these procedures has contributed to successful outcomes. Most ophthalmic surgical patients are outpatients and the anesthetic techniques selected must be conducted with minimal side effects to afford a timely discharge from the hospital, physician's office, or ambulatory surgical unit. The vast majority of patients presenting for ophthalmic surgery are either geriatric or pediatric, and all require careful assessment and anesthetic management. This chapter reviews pertinent anatomy, physiology, and pathophysiology of the eye. In addition, the anesthetic management for a variety of ophthalmic techniques and procedures is presented. This chapter focuses on regional anesthesia and the unique aspects of general anesthesia for ophthalmic surgery.

OCULAR ANATOMY AND PHYSIOLOGY

The bony orbit houses the eyeball and its associated structures. The outer periosteal layer of the dura covers the orbit whose walls comprise the frontal, zygomatic, greater wing of the sphenoid, palatine, lacrimal, maxilla, and ethmoid bones. This protective structure also contains the nerves, blood vessels, and muscles necessary for proper functioning of the eye.[1] The orbit contains nine canals and fissures. The most important of these are the optic foramen, the superior and inferior orbital fissures, and the supraorbital and infraorbital foramina.

The infraorbital foramen is located approximately 4 mm below the orbital rim in the maxilla. This foramen contains the infraorbital nerve, artery, and vein. The lacrimal fossa which houses the lacrimal gland is located in the superior temporal orbit. At the junction of the medial one third and temporal two thirds of the superior orbital rim, the anesthetist can palpate the supraorbital notch con-taining the supraorbital nerve, artery, and vein. These anatomic structures—the supraorbital notch, the infraorbital foramen, and the lacrimal fossa—can be palpated and serve as the major landmarks for the administration of ocular regional anesthesia.[2]

The normal globe of the eye is approximately 24 mm in diameter (anteroposterior).[1] The three layers of the eyeball are the fibrous outside layer comprising the cornea and sclera; the middle layer which is vascular in nature and made up of the iris, ciliary body, and choroid; and the inner neural layer containing the retina. Intraocular contents include the crystalline lens and the aqueous and vitreous humors[1] (Fig. 35–1).

Six extraocular muscles control the movements of the globe. Four rectus muscles (superior, medial, inferior, and lateral) originate from a common tendon ring which encircles the optic foramen.[1] The other two muscles controlling globe movement are the superior and inferior oblique muscles. The levator muscle of the upper lid is also located in the orbit. The motor innervation of these striated ocular muscles is by cranial nerves III (oculomotor), IV (trochlear), and VI (abducens). Sensory supply to the eye is from the ophthalmic division of cranial nerve V (trigeminal).[1]

Intraocular Pressure

One of the primary physiologic functions of the eye is the formation and drainage of aqueous humor and the effects on intraocular pressure (IOP). Two thirds of the aqueous humor is formed in the posterior chamber by the ciliary body and one third is formed by passive filtration from the vessels on the anterior surface of the iris.[2] Aqueous humor from the posterior chamber flows into the anterior chamber, where it mixes with aqueous formed by the iris through the pupillary aperture. From the peripheral segment of the anterior chamber, it leaves the eye through the trabecular network, the canal of Schlemm, and the episcleral venous system, enters the general venous system, and eventually flows to the superior vena cava and the right atrium.[2]

Normal IOP ranges from 10 to 22 mm Hg. A pressure above 25 mm Hg is considered pathologic. Many factors

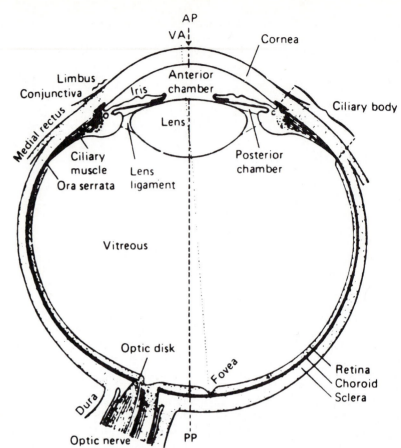

Figure 35–1. Anatomy of the eye. AP, anterior pole; PP, posterior pole; VA, visual axis. (*Reprinted, with permission, from Warwick R.* Eugene Wolff's anatomy of the eye and orbit. *7th ed. Philadelphia: WB Saunders; 1977.*)

such as obstruction of venous return, patient position, systemic blood pressure, intracranial pressure, coughing, straining, depolarizing muscle relaxants, external pressure (e.g., from an anesthetic mask), and endotracheal intubation can influence IOP by producing mild, transient rises in pressure. Control of IOP is essential as any sustained marked rise in IOP during anesthesia could produce permanent visual loss.

Oculocardiac Reflex

The oculocardiac reflex was first described in 1908. This term is used to designate a variety of cardiac arrhythmias that may result from manipulation of the eye. Traction of the extraocular muscles, especially the medial rectus, pressure on the globe, and traction on the conjunctiva and orbital structures stimulate the afferent component. Afferent impulses originate in the long and short ciliary nerves and subsequently traverse the ciliary ganglion, the ophthalmic division of the trigeminal nerve, and the trigeminal ganglion to terminate in the main sensory nucleus of the trigeminal nerve near the fourth ventricle. The efferent limb is vagal and stimulation most often manifests in a 10 to 50 percent decrease in heart rate.[3]

Cardiac standstill, atrioventricular block, ventricular bigeminy, idioventricular rhythm, and junctional rhythm can also occur. These arrhythmias occur frequently during ophthalmic surgery, particularly in surgery on the muscles of the eye. In addition, this reflex can be elicited by ocular trauma, retrobulbar block,[3] or pressure on tissue left in the orbital apex after enucleation.[4] A variety of methods to obliterate this reflex have been recommended. Retrobulbar block is controversial because it can cause as well as protect against the oculocardiac reflex. This block also has the potential to produce hemorrhage and optic nerve injury. Preoperative atropine sulfate administered intramuscularly does not provide effective protection against this reflex. Intravenous administration of atropine as surgery commences or within 30 minutes prior to surgery may reduce the incidence of this reflex and the severity of bradycardia; however, atropine administration also appears to cause or contribute to more serious arrhythmias.

If prophylactic measures do not provide effective protection against the elicitation of the oculocardiac reflex, what is the best course of action? The patient must be continuously monitored with a precordial or esophageal stethoscope and an electrocardiogram (ECG). At the first indication of dysrhythmia or bradycardia, the surgeon is asked to release all pressure or traction from the eye. The rhythm usually returns to normal within seconds. If bradycardia persists, atropine sulfate may be administered intravenously only after ocular stimulation by the surgeon has stopped. Once a regular rhythm has been reestablished, the surgeon may be advised to continue surgery. The oculocardiac reflex fatigues rapidly at the level of the cardioinhibitory center.

It is important to remember that hypoxia or hypercarbia can be the underlying cause of the elicitation of the oculocardiac reflex as it can for any arrhythmia. Therefore, an assessment of the patient's ventilatory status should be made concurrently with cardiac evaluation. Monitoring cardiac rhythm, assessing ventilation, and rapidly responding to the initial appearance of the oculocardiac reflex lessen the chance of a life-threatening arrhythmia.

OCULAR PATHOPHYSIOLOGY

Glaucoma

Glaucoma results in impairment of capillary blood flow to the optic nerve, eventually leading to loss of optic nerve tissue and function, producing blindness. Glaucoma is characterized by an elevated IOP. Open-angle (chronic simple) and closed-angle (acute) glaucoma are the two anatomic types of glaucoma. Open-angle glaucoma is thought to result from impaired aqueous filtration and drainage. The treatment includes eyedrops such as epinephrine, timolol maleate, and similar agents to produce miosis and trabecular stretching.[2] Closed-angle glaucoma results from obstruction of aqueous outflow. This pathology can result from chronic conditions and trauma to the lens producing anterior dislocation and blockage of the anterior chamber. Primary congenital glaucoma is classified according to age: infantile and juvenile. Early diagnosis is essential in the successful management of infantile glaucoma. This form of glaucoma is frequently associated with outflow obstruction of aqueous humor. Juvenile glaucoma is often associated with a family history of open-angle glaucoma. Juvenile glaucoma is treated with the same regimen as primary open-angle glaucoma.[2]

Atropine sulfate may be safely administered preoperatively to prevent parasympathetic reflexes and decrease oral secretions in the patient presenting with glaucoma. Atropine sulfate premedication appears to have no effect on IOP in either open-angle or closed-angle glaucoma. When 0.4 mg of atropine is given to a 70-kg person, approximately 0.0001 mg is absorbed by the eye.[5] Scopolamine appears to produce a greater mydriatic effect than atropine and, therefore, is not recommended in patients with diagnosed or suspected closed-angle glaucoma.[6]

Diabetes Mellitus

Since the introduction of exogenous insulin for the treatment of diabetes mellitus, the length and often the quality of life of the diabetic patient have greatly improved. Because diabetics are living longer, anesthesia providers are often faced with managing this multisystem disease for elective surgeries.

The ophthalmic complications of diabetes are well known. Laser photocoagulation and vitrectomy surgery have maintained visual function in many patients who would have otherwise become blind. For these patients whose ocular signs and symptoms can be treated reasonably effectively, the application of the treatment may be complicated by other organ system disease. The primary ocular pathology of diabetes is ischemia of the tissues of the eye. Diabetic retinopathy is the leading cause of blindness. This retinopathy is not usually seen until 10 years after the diagnosis of diabetes has been made. It progresses from the early phases of microaneurysm formation, intraretinal hemorrhage, and retinal edema to the proliferative phases of

neovascularization of the retina and optic nerve.[7] The proliferative phases are complicated by vitreous hemorrhage and traction detachment. Vitrectomy alone and in combination with scleral buckling, photocoagulation, lensectomy, and gas–fluid exchange has been applied to treat these later phases of retinopathy.

Neovascular glaucoma is very difficult to treat and control. Initially, drugs such as timolol maleate and diuretics are employed. If medical therapy fails, surgical intervention may be indicated to control the disease process. As ophthalmic surgery is generally elective, there is usually ample time to have the patient's diabetes controlled medically to provide optimal anesthetizing conditions. Unfortunately, the functions of other organ systems are deteriorating concurrently, increasing the surgical and anesthetic risk for these patients.

Cataracts

A cataract is an opacity of the lens and may be congenital or acquired. A number of metabolic diseases may predispose patients to the development of cataracts. Cataracts occur more frequently and at an earlier age in diabetics than in nondiabetics. Histopathologically, cataracts occurring in the diabetic are identical to those in the nondiabetic. Proper control of IOP is essential for intraocular surgeries, particularly traditional intracapsular cataract extraction. This traditional technique has been replaced by phacoemulsification and extracapsular extraction of the lens followed by an intraocular lens implant. With the latest advances in cataract surgery, IOP is less of a factor; however, when necessary, reduction of IOP must be accomplished prior to opening of the eye. When the IOP is reduced, the plane of the iris becomes concave or more posterior and the anterior chamber is deepened. This facilitates safe lens extraction. A number of devices and methods have been used to reduce IOP and produce a "soft eye," for example, the Honan balloon.[8] It is important for the nurse anesthetist to appreciate when reduction in IOP is necessary and when production of a "soft eye" may be problematic. Cataract surgery is one of the most common elective ophthalmic procedures performed. Currently, cataract extraction is most often accomplished under regional anesthesia with monitored anesthesia care (referred to as orbital epidural anesthesia); however, some circumstances may require general anesthesia for this procedure.

PHARMACOLOGY OF OPHTHALMIC DRUGS AND ANESTHETIC IMPLICATIONS

Anesthetic agents can alter the patient's ocular physiology. Ophthalmic medications can alter the response to anesthesia. Although not all inclusive, the drugs encountered most often during the interface of ophthalmic surgery and anesthesia are discussed in this section (Table 35–1).

Topical and Intraocular Agents

Acetylcholine. Acetylcholine may be used intraocularly after lens extraction to produce a rapid miosis. Parasympathetic side effects, including bradycardia, bronchial secretions and bronchospasm, hypotension, and salivation, have

TABLE 35–1. ANESTHETIC IMPLICATIONS OF OPHTHALMIC DRUGS

Drug	Concentration (%)	Amount per Drop (mg)	Potential Problems	Indications
Acetylcholine	1	0.5	Bradycardia, hypotension, increased salivation and bronchial secretions, bronchospasm	Miosis
Atropine	1	0.2–0.5	Flushing, thirst, tachycardia Agitation	Mydriasis Cycloplegia
Cocaine	1–10	0.5–5	Hypertension, dysrhythmias, agitation, hyperthermia, cardiorespiratory arrest contraindicated in patients taking sympathomimetics	Vasoconstriction
Cyclopentolate	0.5–1 2	0.25–0.5 1	Usually well tolerated CNS[a] toxicity: dysarthria, disorientation, convulsions	Mydriasis, cycloplegia Mydriasis, cycloplegia
Echothiophate	0.03–0.25	0.01–0.1	Prolonged action of succiny-choline, procaine, cocaine, chloroprocaine, and so forth	Antiglaucoma
Epinephrine	0.25–2	0.1–1	Nervousness, hypertension, dysrhythmias, headache, faintness (usually with 2% solution)	Antiglaucoma
Phenylephrine	2.5–10	1.2–5	Usually well tolerated Hypertension, headache, tremulousness, cerebral hemorrhage, myocardial ischemia and infarction	Mydriasis Vasoconstriction Decongestion
Scopolamine	0.5	0.25	CNS excitation and disorientation	Mydriasis Cycloplegia
Timolol	0.25–0.5	0.1–0.25	Systemic, nonselective beta blockade	Antiglaucoma
SF_6, C_3F_6, C_4F_8	Not applicable	Not applicable	In the presence of N_2O, may compromise retinal blood flow	Retinal reattachment
Fluorescein	10 or 25	Not applicable	Nausea, vomiting, extravasation, pruritus, headache, urticaria, allergic reactions, hypertension, myocardial infarction (rare), pulmonary edema (rare), anaphylactic shock (rare)	Diagnostic

[a] CNS, central nervous system.

Reprinted, with permission, from McGoldrick KE. Anesthesia for ophthalmic and otolaryngologic surgery. *Phildelphia: WB Saunders; 1992:228.*

been noted after intraocular administration. These side effects can be reversed by intravenous administration of atropine.

Atropine Sulfate. Ophthalmic atropine solution is available in a 1 percent solution and is used to produce mydriasis and cycloplegia. Systemic absorption generally occurs through the conjunctiva or the nasal mucosa after drainage through the nasolacrimal duct.[9] Applying light finger pressure on the sac medially for 1 minute after instillation of the eyedrop or tilting the patient's head to the side of the operative eye will help to reduce the systemic absorption of any eyedrop. Geriatric and pediatric patients are more likely to

exhibit systemic reactions to atropine including tachycardia, dry skin, increased body temperature, flushing, and, occasionally, agitation. The effects of atropine may persist up to 10 days, are not readily reversed by eserine and miotics, and could precipitate an attack of closed-angle glaucoma.

Cocaine. Cocaine was introduced into ocular use as a local anesthetic by Koller in 1884. The vasoconstriction that follows cocaine application may produce corneal injury. This drug has limited use in ophthalmic surgery, but is used to saturate nasal packing during dacryocystorhinostomy because of its vasoconstrictive properties. Numerous cardiovascular side effects such as tachycardia, hypertension, and premature ventricular contractions have been noted following the use of this sympathomimetic amine. Several other topical local anesthetics are indicated for ophthalmic procedures including tetracaine (0.5 percent solution) and proparacaine (0.5 percent solution). These drugs are both esters chemically.

Cyclopentolate. Cyclopentolate is a short-acting mydriatic agent, with maximum mydriasis occurring in 30 minutes and maximum cycloplegia in approximately 45 minutes. The duration of action is 30 minutes. This drug has been reported to have undesirable central nervous system side effects including convulsions and psychosis.[10,11] Side effects are more often noted when concentrations greater than 1 percent are used.

Echothiophate Iodide. The long-acting anticholinesterase echothiophate iodide produces parasympathetic miosis and has been used to treat glaucoma. Because it inhibits pseudocholinesterase, patients receiving this drug must be observed carefully during any anesthesia procedure that includes the administration of drugs metabolized by plasma cholinesterase such as succinylcholine, chloroprocaine, procaine, and cocaine. A decrease in pseudocholinesterase activity has been reported for 4 weeks following echothiophate therapy.[12] When succinylcholine is used for muscle relaxation, caution must be exercised to avoid an inadvertent overdose resulting in prolonged apnea. A peripheral nerve stimulator is imperative and the succinylcholine must be given in small incremental doses. Administration of intermediate-acting nondepolarizing muscle relaxants such as vecuronium and atracurium rather than succinylcholine is recommended.

Epinephrine. Topical epinephrine in a 2 percent solution has been used to decrease aqueous secretion, enhance aqueous outflow, and reduce IOP in patients presenting with open-angle glaucoma.[9] As one drop of a 2 percent solution contains between 0.5 and 1 mg of epinephrine (the maximum safe dose for an adult), the anesthetist should observe for systemic sympathetic side effects such as hypertension, tachycardia, pallor, and cardiac arrhythmias. The tendency of cardiac arrhythmias to occur after administration of systemic doses of epinephrine during general anesthesia with volatile agents such as halothane is well known; however, epinephrine has been used successfully with few side effects in doses up to 68 µg/kg administered in the anterior chamber during cataract surgery involving phacoemulsification and aspiration.[13] This may be attributed to the facts that there is very little systemic drug absorption from the globe of the eye and topically administered epinephrine is rapidly captured by the adrenergic receptors of the iris.

Phenylephrine Hydrochloride. Phenylephrine produces pupillary dilation and capillary decongestion without cycloplegia. Systemic side effects are rare after topical application, but constant surveillance of the blood pressure is mandatory. Side effects including severe hypertension, headache, reflex bradycardia, and even subarachnoid hemorrhage have been reported after instillation of more concentrated (10 percent) solutions.[14] Children and the elderly

seem to be especially susceptible to these hypertensive side effects. Therefore, the 2.5 percent solution is recommended for pediatric and geriatric patients.

Pilocarpine Hydrochloride. By mimicking the action of acetylcholine at the junction of parasympathetic nerve endings in the smooth muscle cells of ocular structures, pilocarpine hydrochloride causes the iris, ciliary body, and sphincter muscles to contract. The resulting miosis helps to open the trabecular meshwork in the anterior chamber angle of the eye, enhancing the flow of aqueous humor and reducing IOP. This miotic agent is used clinically in solutions of 0.5 to 1 percent to treat open-angle glaucoma and to overcome mydriasis produced by atropine. When alternated with mydriatics, pilocarpine is employed to break adhesions between the iris and the lens. Chronic use of pilocarpine may result in hypotension, bradycardia, bronchospasm, and increased bronchial secretions and salivation.

Timolol Maleate. Timolol maleate is a beta-adrenergic blocking agent used topically for the treatment of chronic open-angle glaucoma, aphakic glaucoma, and secondary glaucoma. This drug acts to reduce the production of aqueous humor by the ciliary body, thereby reducing IOP. Systemic absorption of timolol does occur and this drug should be used cautiously if at all in patients with bronchospastic disease, heart block, bradycardia, or heart failure, since timolol is 5 to 10 times more potent than propranolol.[15] Caution must be used when reversing neuromuscular blockade with anticholinesterase agents after general anesthesia in patients receiving ophthalmic timolol. A profound bradycardia unresponsive to atropine may occur. Betaxolol hydrochloride, a beta-1-adrenergic blocking agent with a reduced potential to produce systemic side effects, may be a more desirable antiglaucoma drug than timolol maleate.

Systemic Agents

Osmotics. Hypertonic agents such as urea, mannitol, and glycerine, when administered, elevate plasma osmolarity, allowing fluid to leave the intraocular space along an osmotic gradient, which produces a temporary acute reduction in IOP. Mannitol, an osmotic diuretic, is often administered preoperatively and sometimes postoperatively to achieve this desired reduction in IOP. The dose for the reduction of IOP during an acute attack of congestive glaucoma or for ophthalmic surgery is not to exceed 1.5 to 2 g/kg IV over a 30- to 60-minute period.[15] The maximum reduction in IOP occurs in 30 to 90 minutes, with a return to baseline levels in approximately 5 to 6 hours. The subsequent diuresis may result in distension of the bladder, which may cause systemic hypertension under anesthesia and may necessitate placement of a urinary catheter. Administration of mannitol has been associated with an acute intravascular volume overload. Therefore, the anesthesia care team must evaluate the patient's cardiac status preoperatively and assess the patient's ability to tolerate a sudden increase in the circulating blood volume. Mannitol should be administered through a filter and warmed to avoid infusion of crystals.[9]

Intravenous administration of urea will produce results similar to those produced by mannitol, but it is associated with tissue damage if extravasation occurs. Glycerin is effective when administered orally. The onset of action occurs within 10 minutes. The oncotic effect peaks at 30 minutes and lasts 5 to 6 hours. It is rapidly metabolized yielding little diuresis. The adult dose is 1 to 1.5 g/kg and is given as a 50 or 75 percent solution. The ocular hypotensive effect of glycerine is less predictable than that of either mannitol or urea. Glycerine also increases the risk of aspiration because it may trap gastric fluid in the stomach. Isorbid is another oral osmotic agent that is effective in lowering the IOP and it is better tolerated by patients than glycerin. The recommended dose is 1 to 3 g/kg.[15]

Acetazolamide. Acetazolamide is a carbonic anhydrase inhibitor. It is used in acute glaucoma to depress the sodium pump process responsible for the secretion of aqueous humor. IOP is reduced correspondingly. Acetazolamide administered intravenously, usually in two divided doses of 250 mg diluted in 5 mL of sterile water, acts within 5 minutes and exhibits its maximum effect in 20 to 30 minutes.[15] During the initial phase of treatment, acetazolamide produces a marked increase in potassium excretion, attributable to enhanced secretion in the distal nephron. Unfortunately, the cardiac instability and anesthetic implications related to a low plasma potassium are too well known. The patient population most likely to require this agent is middle-aged or older and may be taking other drugs such as digitalis that further enhance the risk of electrolyte depletion. A patient receiving acetazolamide therapy should have plasma electrolyte levels surveyed prior to administration. If the serum potassium level is less than 3.0 mEq/L, elective surgery should be cancelled. As acetazolamide is a sulfonamide, it should not be administered to patients with a history of sulfa allergy. Acetazolamide is also contraindicated in patients with serious hepatorenal disease.

EFFECTS OF ANESTHETIC AGENTS AND ADJUNCT DRUG THERAPY ON INTRAOCULAR PRESSURE

Anesthetic Agents

Volatile inhalation anesthetic agents produce a dose-related decrease in IOP. Nitrous oxide (N_2O) must be used cautiously in any case where this agent could cause undesirable expansion of a space or tissues such as during surgery for repair of retinal detachment. Often the surgeon injects sulfur hexafluoride (SF_6) gas into the vitreous to facilitate reattachment of the retina. Concurrent administration of N_2O could promote a rapid and substantial increase in IOP by diffusing into the area of the injected SF_6 gas bubble, causing expansion of the volume and a marked increase in IOP. This increase in IOP could seriously compromise retinal blood flow. Therefore, it has been recommended that N_2O be terminated 15 minutes prior to gas injection.[16] In addition, should the patient require general anesthesia for any surgical procedure within 10 days of SF_6 injection, N_2O should not be used.[17]

All central nervous system depressants including barbiturates, narcotics, tranquilizers, and hypnotics reduce IOP. This reduction in IOP occurs irrespective of whether the eye is normal or glaucomatous.[9] Contrary to earlier data, ketamine appears to have no significant effect on IOP[18]; however, it is not suitable for a variety of ophthalmic procedures because it can produce nystagmus and blepharospasm. Etomidate administration has generally been associated with a significant decrease in IOP, even though skeletal movement and pain on injection have been reported.[19] Propofol also appears to produce a dose-related decrease in IOP and is particularly useful for a number of ophthalmic procedures because of its short duration of action.

Neuromuscular Blocking Agents

Nondepolarizing muscle relaxants are associated with a decrease or no change in the IOP; however, succinylcholine is well known for its ability to significantly elevate IOP. A number of theories have been postulated to explain this phenomenon. Some clinicians believe that the transient muscle fasciculations that follow succinylcholine administration cause a rise in IOP by producing a sustained contracture of the extraocular muscles, thereby increasing the external pressure on the eye. Others believe that a concurrent rise in systemic blood pressure during induction and intubation may actually be responsible for the increase in IOP. An increase in IOP occurs within the first minute of injection. The average peak increase in IOP is 6 to 8 mm Hg between 1 and 4 minutes after injection, with a return to control measurements by 5 to 7 minutes.[20]

Pretreatment with a small dose of a nondepolarizing muscle relaxant or incremental doses of succinylcholine administered slowly appear to have no effect on controlling the rise in IOP. Lidocaine has been studied for its effects on controlling IOP. Grover et al.[21] found that 1.5 mg/kg lidocaine given 1 minute prior to a thiopental induction prevented an increase in IOP above baseline after both succinylcholine administration and intubation. The use of sublingual nifedipine prior to induction has been studied; 10 mg sublingually 20 minutes prior to induction of anesthesia prevented an increase in IOP.[22] It would appear that agents producing a decrease in systemic blood pressure also reduce IOP.

Adjunct Drugs and Miscellaneous Effects

Ganglionic blocking agents such as trimethaphan produce a dramatic reduction in IOP. This phenomenon could be related to the overall effect of reduction in blood pressure on decreasing the IOP. It is of interest to note that trimethaphan lowers IOP in patients who do not have glaucoma despite the fact that this agent produces mydriasis.[9]

A number of other factors can influence IOP. Respiratory acidosis has been reported to increase both choroidal blood volume and IOP, and respiratory alkalosis appears to decrease volume and IOP.[23] The opposite holds true for metabolic derangements: metabolic acidosis reduces choroidal blood volume and IOP and metabolic alkalosis increases them.

Hypoxia increases IOP by producing dilation of

choroid vessels. Hypothermia reduces IOP because it decreases the production of aqueous humor and induces vasoconstriction.[9]

PREOPERATIVE ASSESSMENT

As the health care industry has become more cost conscious, patients are seldom admitted to the hospital preoperatively prior to surgery. This is particularly true for ophthalmic surgery where only 15 years ago, the majority of these procedures were done on hospital inpatients. Today, a very small percentage of patients presenting for elective ophthalmic surgery are actually hospital inpatients. With this move to the outpatient ambulatory surgical setting and advances in surgical techniques, procedures that once required patients to remain in the hospital 5 days now allow them to leave the hospital or ambulatory surgical center the same day of their surgery.

Many patients are assessed preoperatively by the anesthesia provider several days or weeks preceding the date of surgery. Some patients are interviewed in person at this time. Other patients are interviewed preoperatively by telephone and the actual physical assessment occurs on the day of surgery.

A thorough history and physical examination of the patient are essential for the provision of a safe anesthetic. In addition, appropriate laboratory studies should be performed based on the patient's medical history. A complete review of all drug therapy is important to the anesthetic plan as some systemic drugs may have ocular effects or interact with anesthetic agents. The patient should be informed of all anesthesia risks and benefits and the type of anesthesia planned should be discussed in length. Patients should have ample opportunity to ask questions regarding their impending anesthesia and surgery. The anesthetist should emphasize the importance of preoperative fasting, according to hospital or surgery center guidelines, with instructions to continue chronic cardiorespiratory or other essential drug therapy perioperatively. Continuation of coumadin therapy is controversial and should be negotiated between the surgeon and the patient's primary physician. Aspirin may be discontinued 1–2 weeks preoperatively.

Many patients presenting for ophthalmic surgery are elderly, so detailed explanations in simple terminology should be given clearly and slowly. It is often helpful to provide explanations in the presence of another family member. One of the main purposes of the preoperative interview is to allay fear and apprehension. Elderly patients are likely to have multiorgan chronic illnesses. Therefore, it may be necessary to obtain consultation from a number of specialists such as cardiologists and pulmonologists before scheduling a surgical time. The reader is referred to Chapter 33 for a comprehensive discussion of the anesthetic management of the geriatric patient.

Preoperative sedation is useful to calm the patient prior to surgery and reduce the incidence of anxiety-induced hypertension. Diazepam (5 to 10 mg) may be given orally 1 hour preoperatively with a sip of water. Some anesthetists prefer to premedicate the patient with intravenous medications shortly before the scheduled surgery. Midazolam administered intravenously in 0.5- to 1-mg incremental doses provides excellent sedation and amnesia. Most patients require no more than a total dose of 2 to 4 mg of midazolam. Short-acting narcotics such as fentanyl and alfentanil may be administered cautiously along with midazolam intravenously. Fentanyl is administered in 25–50-μg doses. Alfentanil is generally given in 125–250-μg doses. Intravenous sedation is often administered several minutes prior to the regional anesthetic block.

Patients with a history of hiatal hernia or gastric reflux may require preoperative treatment with H_2-receptor antagonists such as cimetidine. The usual preoperative dose is 300 mg orally, but this drug can be administered intravenously if necessary. Other centrally acting antiemetics may be given either preoperatively or once intravenous access has been established. Metaclopramide can be given orally or intravenously. The usual preoperative dose is 10 to 20 mg. Postoperatively, metoclopramide 0.15 mg/kg can be given should nausea and vomiting occur. Droperidol is the most frequently used antiemetic in anesthesia practice. Preoperatively or early in the anesthetic course, a dose of 0.625 to 1.25 mg may be administered intravenously. Preoperative doses do not usually exceed 2.5 mg. Droperidol can cause excessive drowsiness or hypotension in large doses. Droperidol is not given concomitantly with metoclopramide to awake patients because of the possible extrapyramidal reactions stemming from additive dopamine blockade in the central nervous system. Both drugs are relatively contraindicated in the presence of Parkinson's disease for this same reason. The use of antiemetics is recommended in patients who will be receiving general anesthesia or in those who are undergoing ophthalmic surgical procedures with a high incidence of postoperative nausea and vomiting, such as strabismus surgery. Postoperative retching and vomiting after ophthalmic surgery can be very dangerous as vomiting significantly increases IOP which could lead to permanent eye damage.

ANESTHETIC MANAGEMENT

Anesthetic Techniques

Ophthalmic surgical procedures can be safely managed under general, regional, or local anesthesia. Objectives of ophthalmic anesthesia should include analgesia, prevention of the oculocardiac reflex, avoidance of drug–drug interactions, akinesia of the eye as appropriate, and prevention of an increase in IOP through the avoidance of coughing, bucking, retching, and vomiting. The choice of anesthetic should be tailored to the patient's safety and needs as well as to considerations for optimizing the surgical environment. The anesthetist must be aware of the complications that may arise no matter which anesthetic technique is employed. Trends in anesthetic management of the ophthalmic patient have changed over the last decade or so particularly for cataract surgery. Standard anesthetic protocol for cataract surgery nearly always entailed general anesthesia, whereas current management leans almost exclusively to regional anesthesia. The indications and techniques of both general and regional anesthesia for ophthalmic surgery are discussed in this section.

General Anesthesia. The goal of general anesthesia for ophthalmic surgery is to provide a motionless eye and stable IOP. As was discussed in the section on pharmacology, certain drugs often used as part of general anesthesia such as succinylcholine may increase IOP, whereas other drugs such as barbiturates may actually lower IOP. The primary risk posed by an increased IOP during open eye surgery is expulsion of the intraocular contents. A number of factors or components of general anesthesia can induce increases in IOP. Therefore, every effort should be made to employ agents that reduce or have no effect on the intraocular pressure such as nondepolarizing muscle relaxants, barbiturates, and volatile anesthetic agents. IOP is substantially increased during routine intubation. Laryngoscopy and intubation stimulate the sympathetic nervous system, which releases catecholamines that subsequently increase blood pressure. Rises in systemic blood pressure appear to parallel increases in IOP. Therefore, deep levels of general anesthesia are necessary. This can be achieved through inhalational anesthesia or through a combination of agents such as muscle relaxants, narcotics, sedatives, and reduced concentrations of inhaled gases. Appropriate anesthetic depth should be maintained until the last suture is placed. Ventilation should be controlled either manually or mechanically during the surgical procedure. Adequacy of ventilation must be assessed with an end-tidal carbon dioxide monitor and with mass spectroscopy whenever possible. Oxygen saturation should be monitored with a pulse oximeter. This is particularly important as the anesthetist is usually at the patient's side and does not have access to the head or the ability to observe facial skin color.

The administration of intravenous lidocaine (1.5 to 2 mg/kg) approximately 4 to 5 minutes before extubation has been recommended to reduce the incidence of coughing.[9] Whenever possible, patients should be extubated while anesthetized once adequate ventilatory levels have been ascertained. Any residual effects of a nondepolarizing muscle relaxant must be antagonized with an anticholinesterase prior to extubation. Full return of neuromuscular function should be established with the assistance of a peripheral nerve stimulator. McGoldrick[9] recommends extubating patients while they are in the lateral position with the operative side superior.

As mentioned previously, preventive measures should be taken preoperatively to avoid nausea and vomiting after surgery. If despite these measures postoperative nausea and vomiting should develop, 10 μg/kg droperidol can be administered intravenously. The most prevalent cause of hospital admission after ambulatory ophthalmic surgery, particularly in pediatric patients, is protracted vomiting.[24]

Regional Anesthesia. Many types of ophthalmic procedures can be performed under regional anesthesia. Because the patient will be awake for the procedure, it is essential to assess preoperatively whether the patient has any physical or psychologic problems that would preclude lying relatively flat and still on the operating room table for one or more hours. A thorough explanation of the procedure is often helpful. Good communication skills on the part of the anesthetist are extremely important with these patients as drapes cover their faces and they are unable to see what is happening to them. Speaking in a comforting tone and holding the patient's hand are often more successful than drug therapy in calming the patient during surgery. A warming blanket can be used to maintain body temperature. Head and body position are of crucial importance to the surgeon, anesthesia provider, and patient. For all procedures using the microscope, proper positioning with the iris parallel to the floor and the pupil aligned coaxially with the microscope light is especially important, particularly for cataract surgery. The position of the torso in relation to the head is important for physiological reasons. The patient should be alerted not to move his or her head or cough without first warning the surgeon. Monitoring standards for regional anesthesia are the same as for any general anesthetic. Intravenous induction drugs and intubation equipment should be prepared in case the regional block and supplementation fail or the patient requires intubation for some other reason.

Historically, regional anesthesia was administered by ophthalmologists; however, with the increased utilization of peribulbar blocks and the greater employment of regional anesthetics in outpatient facilities, anesthesia care providers have become both interested and skillful in the administration of a variety of regional anesthetic blocks for ocular surgery. This section is limited to a discussion of retrobulbar and peribulbar anesthesia.

Selection of the Local Anesthetic. Important considerations in the selection of a local anesthetic for either retrobulbar or peribulbar block include onset and duration of action, efficacy, toxicity, and ability to provide postoperative analgesia. The regional anesthetic is generally achieved using a combination of local anesthetics such as lidocaine, mepivacaine, and bupivacaine. Hyaluronidase is a soluble enzyme product that splits molecular bonds, thereby decreasing the viscosity of the cellular cement and promoting diffusion and absorption of the injected local anesthetic.[15] This enzyme is an extremely important additive to ophthalmic blocks in concentrations ranging from 10 to 30 units/mL of local anesthetic. Addition of hyaluronidase to the local anesthetic together with utilization of a pressure-reducing device allow the volume of local anesthetic to disperse and the IOP to return to normal or below-normal levels prior to surgery.

Topical anesthesia generally precedes the regional anesthetic block. Tetracaine, 0.5 percent solution, can be used for topical anesthesia of the eye. Proparacaine hydrochloride, 0.5 percent solution, is also useful. Although both tetracaine and proparacaine are esters, there appears to be no cross-sensitization between proparacaine and other local anesthetic agents.[15] Proparacaine is similar in potency to tetracaine; however, unlike tetracaine, it produces little or no initial irritation. Proparacaine begins to act within 20 seconds and its effects usually last 10 to 15 minutes.

Often sedation is desired prior to administration of the regional block. A combination of a tranquilizer, such as midazolam, and a narcotic, such as alfentanil, is usually sufficient to produce amnesia with respect to the regional block but still allow the patient to cooperate and follow directions. In some cases, administration of a small dose of thiopental or methohexital is necessary prior to administration of the regional block. In the "painless technique" developed by Hustead[25] the use of a sharp 27-gauge, 1¼-in. needle to perform the block is recommended. Some controversy has existed over whether a blunt or sharp needle is superior for the performance of ophthalmic regional anesthesia. Grizzard et al.[26] found that eyes penetrated with blunt needles were more likely to have total loss of vision than those perforated by sharp needles.

Other components of the "painless technique" include dilution of the topical proparacaine hydrochloride 0.5 percent solution with 15 parts balanced salt solution. Warmed drops of this solution are instilled in the cul de sac to produce topical anesthesia without irritation. To prepare the injectable solution for regional ophthalmic anesthesia, 1.5 mL of a solution containing 1 part 2 percent mepivacaine, 2 parts 0.75 percent bupivacaine, and 0.5 unit/mL hyaluronidase should be mixed into a 15-mL vial of balanced salt solution.[25] This solution can also be used for making a skin wheal prior to venipuncture. As the pH of the commercial balanced salt solution may be lowered to extend shelf life, 1 mL of 8.4 percent sodium bicarbonate may be added to balance pH. Hustead uses epinephrine 1: 300,000 as a component of the injectable solution[25]; however, this addition of epinephrine should be based on the patient's needs for any given case.

Retrobulbar Block Technique. Once the patient is adequately prepared and sedated as necessary, the anesthetist may proceed with administration of the regional block. The Gills-Lloyd modification of the retrobulbar block is performed by inserting a 1-in., 30-gauge sharp needle and injecting local anesthetic solution, prepared as previously described, while advancing the needle with the patient looking straight ahead (Fig. 35–2).[27] The conjunctiva is entered at 4 o'clock for the left eye and 8 o'clock for the right eye. While pulling gently downward to evert the eyelid, the anesthetist injects 0.3 to 0.5 mL of the dilute solution subconjunctivally, while advancing the needle 5 to 8 mm at a

170-degree angle downward. The anesthetist then withdraws the needle 3 to 5 mm, redirects it posteriorly at a 135-degree angle, and injects the remainder of the 1 mL of solution at a depth of approximately 0.75 in. (Fig. 35–3). There should be no resistance or motion of the globe. If this occurs, the needle must be withdrawn immediately as motion of the globe can lead to penetration of the muscle or sclera.[28] This injection causes the patient little or no discomfort.

After 1 minute of gentle massage and verbal reassurance of the patient, 5.5 mL of the warmed (approximately body temperature or slightly below) full-strength solution is injected inferotemporally following the same track used to inject the dilute local anesthetic. One milliliter is injected slowly, anterior to the orbital septum for lid anesthesia. A slow injection hurts less and thus reduces the need for sedation which may produce respiratory depression. In addition, the likelihood that the patient will move in response to pain is reduced. Vascular complications are more likely to occur when the patient moves during injection. Prior to administration of the local anesthetic, the patient should be encouraged to vocalize any discomfort rather than move in response to it. It is extremely important to communicate to the patient the necessity of lying still during the injection. Injecting the local anesthetic slowly also allows the anesthetic to be deposited properly within the muscle cone.

After the injection is complete, the patient is observed for immediate symptoms of potential complications. Proptosis, or hardening of the eye; whitening of the cornea from increased IOP; and decreased respirations, pulse, and blood pressure are all symptoms of complications of this technique. In addition, the Honan balloon or pressure-reduction device should be applied at this point. After approximately five minutes, the block can be assessed.

Numerous orbital septa surround the eye interconnecting the muscles and attaching them to the orbit. These structures support the globe and check ocular movements. The annulus of Zinn contains the entrance of the optic artery, vein, and nerve into the orbit. The inferior oblique muscle,

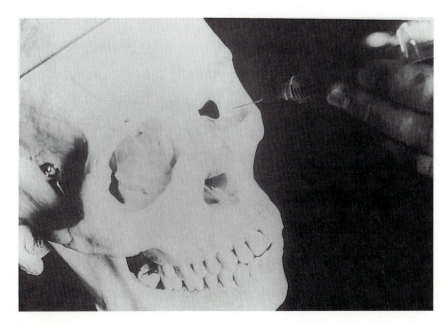

Figure 35–2. Skull with syringe depicting the anatomical position for inferotemporal landmark for the retrobulbar or peribulbar injection. (*Reprinted, with permission, from LB Bloomberg media collection, Bloomberg Eye Center, 1651 W. Main Street, Newark, Ohio 43055*).

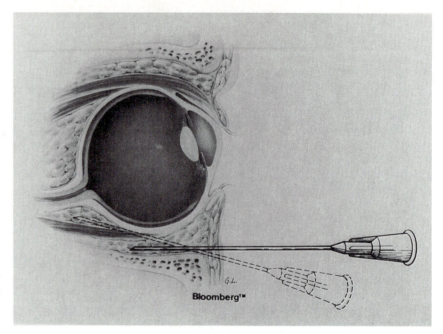

Figure 35–3. The peribulbar (solid line to needle) and the retrobulbar (inferior, dotted line to needle) needle positions for injection. (*Reprinted, with permission, from LB Bloomberg media collection, Bloomberg Eye Center, 1651 W. Main Street, Newark, Ohio 43055*).

being outside this area, may be more difficult to block. Likewise, the trochlear nerve is located outside the muscle cone and a separate injection may be required to block the superior oblique muscle. The 12 o'clock position is preferred to supplement the superior rectus and the superior oblique and often to complete the orbicularis and levator muscle blocks.[29] The needle is inserted transcutaneously, parallel to and outside the muscle cone, to a depth of approximately 1 in. The index finger of the hand not used to inject can depress the eye to ensure appropriate location. Negative aspiration may be difficult due to the needle gauge used. However, negative aspiration must be assessed prior to each injection to reduce the incidence of sequelae from unintended vascular injections. Three to five milliliters of the anesthetic is then injected. Care is taken not to inject on insertion into or withdrawal from the levator palpebrae.

A medial peribulbar supplement may be needed to block the medial rectus and possibly the superior and inferior rectus muscles. A 30-gauge, 1-in. needle is inserted through the caruncle conjunctival area tangential to the globe, proceeding medially and posteriorly until contact is made with the lacrimal bone posterior to the lacrimal sulcus. The needle is then redirected just superficial to the periosteum of the lacrimal bone and parallel to the globe, entering the medial peribulbar space. Directing the needle toward the lacrimal bone helps avoid any penetration of the lacrimal ductwork. After negative aspiration, 1.5 to 2.5 mL of the anesthetic solution is injected.

The original modified retrobulbar block may need to be repeated if the inferior and lateral rectus muscles are fully functional. The volume may be decreased from the first injection using the original mixture. Four percent lidocaine 3 to 4 mL may be used to provide a rapid onset of regional blockade. When supplements of local anesthetic are administered, it is important to use a pressure reduction device, such as the Honan, as any increase in volume injected in or around the eye will increase IOP.

If the aforementioned blocks have not produced satisfactory results, an orbicularis oculi block may be needed. The orbicularis is innervated by the facial nerve. The levator palpebrae superioris muscles are innervated by the oculomotor nerve. Together, these muscles provide for movement of the eyelid, and blockade is necessary to achieve lid akinesia for intraocular surgery. The method of lid akinesia described by van Lint in 1914 requires needle insertion inferotemporal to the lateral canthus (Fig. 35–4).[30] The injection is directed nasally along the lower margin of the orbit. The needle is withdrawn to 1 mm and redirected upward along the superotemporal margin. Injection of the local anesthetic solution must reach deep into the orbicularis where nerve fiber innervation occurs. This technique blocks the terminal branches of the facial nerve to the orbicularis.[31] If this block is performed after the retrobulbar or peribulbar injection, it does not produce much discomfort for the patient.

Traditionally lid akinesia has been achieved through blockade of the facial nerve. The O'Brien technique advocates injection anterior to the tragus of the ear. This block anesthetizes the facial nerve branches near the condyloid of the mandible, resulting in total facial nerve paralysis (see Fig. 35–5).[32] This profound facial nerve paralysis may enhance the patient's anxiety. Other methods have been described to achieve facial nerve paralysis. Atkinson described a technique of blocking the facial nerve without blocking the branches that supply the lip and lower face (Fig. 35–6).[33] The anesthetic is injected midway between the landmarks in the techniques of van Lint and O'Brien with the needle directed toward the pinna of the ear. Some danger is involved in injecting the vessels anterior to the ear when using this technique. A modification of the hand position during injection may help prevent this complication. Nadbath and Rehman described a technique in which the facial nerve is blocked as it exits the skull below the auricular cartilage (Fig. 35–7).[34] This technique is often painful and has very se-

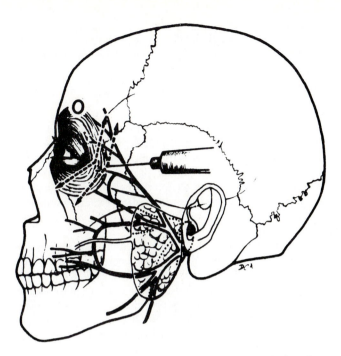

Figure 35–4. Van Lint block. (*Reprinted, with permission, from Zahl K. Blockade of the orbicularis oculi. In: Zahl K, Meltzer MA, eds:* Regional anesthesia for intraocular surgery. Ophthalmol Cli North Am. *1990;3:94.*)

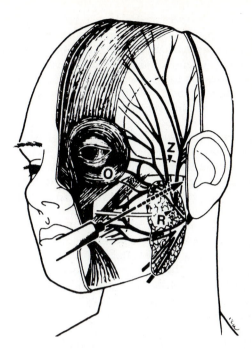

Figure 35–6. Atkinson block. (*Reproduced, with permission, from Zahl K: Blockade of the orbicularis oculi. In: Zahl K, Meltzer MA, eds:* Regional anesthesia for intraocular surgery. Ophthalmol Cli North Am. *1990;3:97.*)

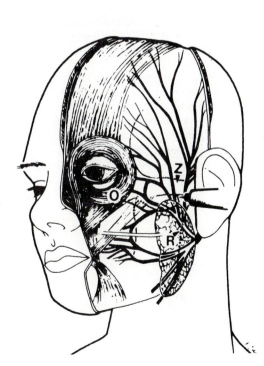

Figure 35–5. O'Brien block. (*Reprinted, with permission, from Zahl K. Blockade of the orbicularis oculi. In: Zahl K, Meltzer MA, eds:* Regional anesthesia for intraocular surgery. Ophthalmol Cli North Am. *1990;3:95.*)

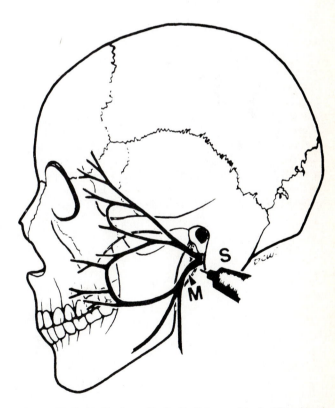

Figure 35–7. Nadbath or Nadbath–Rehman block. (*Reprinted, with permission, from Zahl K. Blockade of the orbicularis oculi. In: Zahl K, Meltzer MA, eds:* Regional anesthesia for intraocular surgery. Ophthalmol Cli North Am. *1990;3:98.*)

rious potential complications including damage to the facial nerve, facial paralysis (including Bell's palsy), and even brain damage when a long needle is used. Infiltration of the facial nerve may cause diffusion to the vagus nerve and intrinsic laryngeal muscles, resulting in stridor, dysphagia, and possible aspiration. Overall, injecting the facial nerve separately is generally avoidable.

Assessment of the Block. Analgesia of the globe generally precedes akinesia of the eye muscles. Akinesia is usually assessed by having the patient follow the anesthetist's or ophthalmologist's finger visually, looking up and down and then side to side. Amaurosis or loss of vision in the blocked eye may or may not occur. It is more likely to occur after instillation of local anesthetic into the muscle cone. Some patients may find this loss of vision very disconcerting, particularly if vision is impaired in the nonoperative eye. As the oculomotor nerve is blocked, the pupil may dilate and the lid may relax as it also supplies motor function to the levator palpebrae muscles and contains parasympathetic fibers to constrict the iris sphincter muscles.

Peribulbar Block Technique. Davis and Mandel described a posterior peribulbar technique wherein the muscle cone is never entered.[35] This technique can include a single or multiple injections. Most commonly, the first injection deposits 4 to 5 mL of local anesthetic at the inferotemporal position after a slightly cephaloposterior angled placement of the needle (Fig. 35–8). During the second injection, 4 to 5 mL of local anesthetic is administered at the superonasal position just below and medial to the supratrochlear notch (Fig. 35–9). McGoldrick uses a 25-gauge, 1.25-in. needle and directs it just beyond the equator of the globe.[9] Local anesthetic agent diffuses into the lid during the placement of this block.

Peribulbar anesthesia, also known as periconal anesthesia, appears to be safe and is associated with a reduced incidence of complications. No life-threatening complications have been reported but globe perforation and peribulbar hemorrhage have occurred.[9] The major disadvantage of this block is its slower onset which necessitates administration 20 to 30 minutes prior to the intended start of surgery. Also, an increased volume of local anesthetic is placed in the orbit which could increase IOP; however, the

avoidance of major complications may outweigh the disadvantages of the technique. Amaurosis rarely occurs with peribulbar block when compared with retrobulbar block.

Special Anesthetic Considerations for Ophthalmic Surgery

There are numerous ophthalmic procedures that can be performed under local anesthesia. Many of these procedures are extraocular, such as ectropian, entropian, and ptosis surgery. The discussion of all of these surgeries is not within the scope of this chapter. Therefore, the types of surgery will be limited to intraocular, retinal eye muscle, and eye trauma.

Intraocular Surgery. Proper management of IOP is essential in successful intraocular surgery. There seems to be little difference in outcome of this type of surgery whether the patient has received a regional or a general anesthetic as long as an increase in IOP is prevented. Because the main concern is reduction or control of IOP, premedication or intraoperative medication to prevent postoperative emesis is essential. The anesthesia provider must also appreciate the potential impact of an increase in IOP caused by the coughing of an awake patient intraoperatively. Lidocaine (1.5 to 2.0 mg/kg) may be administered intravenously to the awake patient to avoid this problem. Intraocular surgery frequently requires pupillary dilation. This is almost always accomplished by continuous infusion of epinephrine (1 : 200,000) in a balanced salt solution. Although drug uptake is usually limited to the iris, the anesthetist must continually monitor for any systemic effects from potential absorption of epinephrine. Vigilance is essential when volatile anesthetic agents such as halothane are employed. The most common intraocular surgical procedures are cataract aspiration or extraction, trabeculectomy, and corneal transplant or penetrating keratoplasty.

Retinal Surgery. Repair of retinal detachment involves procedures that affect intraocular volume and often use some synthetic material to produce scleral buckling or injection of an expandable gas such as SF_6 into the vitreous as previously described. As a reduction in IOP is desirable for retinal surgery, intravenous mannitol or acetazolamide may

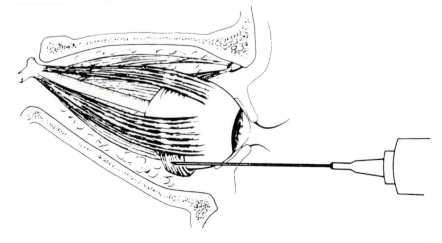

Figure 35–8. Peribulbar block, the inferotemporal injection. (*Reprinted, with permission, from McGoldrick KE. Anesthesia for ophthalmic and otolaryngologic surgery. Philadelphia: WB Saunders; 1992:246.*)

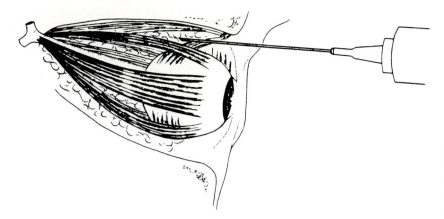

Figure 35–9. Peribulbar block, the supero-nasal injection. (*Reprinted, with permission, from McGoldrick KE. Anesthesia for ophthalmic and otolaryngologic surgery. Philadelphia: WB Saunders; 1992:246.*)

be required preoperatively or intraoperatively. Rotation of the globe with concurrent traction on the extraocular muscles may elicit the oculocardiac reflex intraoperatively. Retinal detachment surgery is often emergency surgery. Therefore, the patient may not present in optimal physical condition. Although either general or regional anesthesia is appropriate for retinal surgery, these procedures are generally long and some patients may find it extremely difficult to lie quietly for the entire procedure.

Strabismus Surgery. Strabismus surgery is the most common pediatric ophthalmic procedure performed in the United States.[9] Eye muscle surgery is conducted increasingly more often on infants aged 6 months to 1 year to improve vision results; however, much older pediatric patients and even adults may present for eye muscle repair. Potential problems associated with strabismus surgery include oculocardiac reflex-induced cardiac arrhythmias, an increased incidence of malignant hyperthermia,[36] succinylcholine-induced tonic contracture of the extraocular muscles,[9] and an increased incidence of postoperative nausea and vomiting.

Anesthetic management should include any special considerations for the pediatric patient (see Chapter 32). Antiemetics should be administered early in the operative course as a high incidence of postoperative nausea and vomiting is associated with this surgery. The recommended antiemetic dose of droperidol for patients undergoing strabismus surgery is 75 µg/kg administered either during induction or intraoperatively.[9] This dose of droperidol used during strabismus surgery has not been associated with delayed hospital discharge. Routine prophylaxis against arrhythmias associated with elicitation of the oculocardiac reflex can be accomplished with preoperative administration of intravenous atropine 0.02 mg/kg or glycopyrrolate 0.1 mg/kg.[9] The oculocardiac reflex, should it appear, is treated according to the guidelines previously discussed in this chapter.

Surgery for Traumatic Eye Injuries. The dilemma in dealing with a patient who has recently eaten and has sustained a penetrating eye injury is a difficult one. There is no ideal anesthetic management for this problem. A sudden increase in IOP caused by intubation of the trachea or succinylcholine administration may lead to extrusion of ocular contents, including prolapse of the iris, lens, and vitreous. Aspiration of gastric contents can produce Mendelson's syndrome, with subsequent cardiopulmonary morbidity

and even death. Striving toward prevention of one complication may increase the risk of occurrence of the other. The possible loss of vision in the affected eye must be weighed against the possible loss of life. An awake intubation would safeguard the lungs and risk the eye. An increased dose of a nondepolarizing muscle relaxant, such as pancuronium, for intubation would preserve the integrity of the eye but might leave the airway vulnerable for minutes before a smooth intubation could be performed. A middle ground must be found between these two extremes.

First, consider that most of the patients presenting with traumatic eye injuries are young and healthy. Some irreversible damage has more than likely already been done to the eye. Avoiding aspiration must be the dominant consideration, and at present, rapid-sequence induction and intubation constitute the most effective method. Although vecuronium 0.2 mg/kg has been used effectively in these situations to lessen the chance of increasing IOP, many clinicians still are concerned about the increased chance for vomiting and aspiration should endotracheal intubation prove to be difficult. Pretreatment with a defasciculating dose of a nondepolarizing muscle relaxant, for example, *d*-tubocurarine, 0.06 mg/kg, and with adequate doses of intravenous lidocaine (1.5 mg/kg) and sublingual nifedipine (10 mg) may afford the best protection against a rise in IOP as well as enable the use of succinylcholine for intubation to ensure the greatest airway protection.

Patients with full stomachs are as likely to vomit during emergence from anesthesia as they are during induction. The endotracheal tube should be left in place with the cuff inflated until the patient is awake and airway reflexes are intact. Intravenous lidocaine may be administered prior to extubation to reduce the incidence of coughing and bucking on the endotracheal tube. Extubation may be performed with the patient in a lateral head-down position or lateral position with operative eye "up" with suction immediately available. Decompression of the stomach prior to extubation may be advisable.

POSTOPERATIVE COMPLICATIONS

Corneal Abrasions

The most common ocular complication following general anesthesia is corneal abrasion caused either by the anesthesia mask, by surgical drapes, or by some injury resulting from failure to close and protect the eyes during surgery.[37] Because general anesthesia decreases tear production, drying of the cornea may occur, making patients vulnerable to the development of corneal abrasions. Eyes should be protected by taping the eyelids closed and by instilling a petroleum-based ointment producing artificial tears. A thorough history should be elicited from the patient regarding any potential allergy to eye ointments or other sensitivities of the eye. Postoperatively, patients present with symptoms of tearing, pain, and sometimes photophobia. Treatment of corneal abrasions includes application of antibiotic ointment and patching of the injured eye. Healing generally occurs within 24 hours.[9]

Complications of Retrobulbar Block

Hemorrhage. Hemorrhage fortunately does not occur frequently. The hemorrhage results from puncture of a vein or artery within the retrobulbar space. The onset with a venous puncture may be slow and self-limiting. With an arterial puncture, however, the eye immediately becomes firm and proptotic, and the cornea may turn white and appear hazy. The eyelid becomes tense, in either the open or the closed position. Subconjunctival hemorrhage may be seen as the blood follows the path of least resistance. Firm manual pressure should be applied on the closed eyelid. The surgeon, if not already present, should be consulted immediately. A lateral canthotomy may need to be done if IOP increases. Administration of intravenous mannitol or acetazolamide may be indicated. Occlusion or spasm of the central retinal artery and vein may follow an elevation of IOP. Therefore, immediate reduction of IOP is essential.

Local Anesthetic Toxicity. If the local anesthetic is injected directly into a vessel, seizure activity, tinnitus, blurred vision, and other symptoms leading to cardiorespiratory arrest may be observed. A grand mal seizure may also result from penetration of the optic nerve sheath. Respiratory arrest is usually seen within 2 to 5 minutes of the injection but can occur as long as 10 minutes after injection. Intubation and ventilatory support are indicated. Cardiovascular support and appropriate drug therapy are needed to combat the resulting hypotension and bradycardia.

Perforation of the Globe. Perforation of the globe may occur after regional anesthesia irrespective of the type or length of needle used. Signs and symptoms of perforation include pain on contact with the globe, globe movement as the needle penetrates, resistance to injection, and immediate dilation and paralysis of the pupil. The cornea becomes edematous as IOP increases. Subconjunctival hemorrhage occurs and finally the globe becomes hypotonic. Myopic patients with an axial length (anteroposterior diameter) greater than 25 mm are at increased risk for perforation of the globe. This perforation usually results in a posterior retinal tear associated with retinal detachment, and vitreous hemorrhage, or both.

Choroidal Hemorrhage

The choroid, which is composed of three layers of blood vessels, extends from the optic nerve posteriorly to where it joins with the ciliary body anteriorly. A choroidal hemorrhage or effusion results in increased IOP and may occur as a result of needle trauma or during surgery. The vortex veins which drain the choroid are near the superior and inferior rectus muscles. Preoperatively, pressure is applied if a hemorrhage is suspected. This complication can occur intraoperatively. Mannitol may be indicated if IOP is greatly increased or the surgeon may perform a vitreous tap. The anesthetist should be alerted to the possibility of a vagal response as a result of increased IOP.

Ptosis

One complication of intraocular surgery is ptosis. The ptosis is generally unilateral. Ptosis may be due to the myotoxicity of the local anesthetic, the pressure reducing device, the bridle suture used to steady the eye during surgery, or the lid retraction device. Ptosis, as a complication, may be a result of the aging process.[38]

Chemical and Thermal Injury

Improper rinsing of anesthetic face masks after cleansing with a disinfectant and spilling of solutions during preparation may result in chemical injury of the eye. Any germicidal skin preparation is also hazardous to the eye. The best treatment for this injury is prevention; however, should a chemical injury occur, the affected eye must be thoroughly rinsed with water or balanced saline solution to remove residual chemicals. As thermal injury of the eyes is possible during laser surgery, the patient's eyes should be protected with moist gauze pads and metal shields.

Hemorrhagic Retinopathy

Hemorrhagic retinopathy may occur in otherwise healthy patients secondary to hemodynamic changes occurring during a particularly difficult emergence from anesthesia or after vomiting. These venous hemorrhages do not usually require treatment and generally resolve in a relatively short period. Visual changes do not occur unless the macula is affected. If hemorrhage is massive, permanent visual damage may occur.[39] Vitrectomy may be indicated in these cases.

Retinal Ischemia

Retinal ischemia, infarction, or both may result from arterial bleeding, ocular trauma, embolism, or injection of a large volume of SF_6 in the presence of N_2O. Ocular trauma can result from a poorly fitting anesthesia face mask. Patients are more vulnerable to this complication during periods of hypotension.[9]

Acute Glaucoma

Acute glaucoma may develop postoperatively not necessarily as a direct result of the anesthetic technique employed. Topical application of some mydriatics such as atropine and scopolamine has been associated with an increased incidence of acute glaucoma as previously described. A thorough preoperative evaluation by the ophthalmologist including a penlight examination to detect a shallow anterior chamber should alert the surgical team to the potential for development of this complication. Postoperatively, patients should be observed for reddened eyes or any complaints of pain or blurring of vision. Immediate therapy for acute closed-angle glaucoma is essential to preserve vision.

SUMMARY

Anesthesia for ophthalmic surgery may be likened to baseball. Many may find baseball boring because they see only the obvious, not the strategy, goals, and nuances of the game. This is often true of anesthetic management during ophthalmic surgery. If the anesthetist knows little about the surgery, and the procedure is not displayed on a video monitor to follow the progress of the surgery, it may all seem very tiresome and boring. If the anesthetist is an active participant and recognizes and accepts the challenge of providing anesthesia for an exceptionally delicate and largely successful surgery, he or she will find it a most rewarding and professionally challenging opportunity.

REFERENCES

1. Feitl ME, Krupin T. Neural blockade for ophthalmologic surgery. In: Cousins MJ, Bridenbaugh PO, eds. *Neural blockade in clinical anesthesia and management of pain.* 2nd ed. Philadelphia: JB Lippincott; 1988:577–592.
2. McGoldrick KE. Anesthesia and the eye. In: Barash PG, Stoelting RK, eds. *Clinical anesthesia.* Philadelphia: JB Lippincott; 1989:1049–1065.
3. Berler DK. Oculocardiac reflex. *Am J Ophthalmol.* 1963;12:954.
4. Kirsch RE, Sumet P, Kugel V, et al. Electrocardiographic changes during ocular surgery and their prevention by retrobulbar injection. *Arch Ophthalmol.* 1957;58:348.
5. Duncalf D, Foldes FF. Effect of anesthetic drugs and muscle relaxants on intraocular pressure. In: Smith RB, ed. *Anesthesia in opthalmology.* Boston: Little, Brown; 1973:21.
6. Garde JF, Aston R, Endler GC, et al. Racial mydriatic response to belladonna preparations. *Anesth Analg.* 1978;57:572.
7. Diseases of the endocrine system. In: Katz J, Benumof J, Kadis LB, eds. *Anesthesia and uncommon diseases: Pathophysiologic and clinical correlation.* 3rd ed. Philadelphia: WB Saunders; 1991.
8. Hunt L. Use of the Honan intraocular pressure reducer. *J Ophthalmic Nurs Tech.* 1988;7:59–61.
9. McGoldrick KE. Anesthetic ramifications of ophthalmic drugs. In: McGoldrick KE, ed. *Anesthesia for ophthalmic and otolaryngologic surgery.* Philadelphia: WB Saunders; 1992:227–234.
10. Kennerdall JS, Wucher FP. Cyclopentolate associated with two cases of grand mal seizure. *Arch Ophthalmol.* 1972;87:634.
11. Blinkhorst RD, Weinstein GW, Baretz RM, et al. Psychotic reaction induced by cyclopentolate: Results of pilot study and a double-blind study. *Am J Ophthalmol.* 1963;55:1243.
12. DeRoeth A, Dettbar WD, Rosenberg P. Effect of phospholine iodide on blood cholinesterase levels. *Am J Ophthalmol.* 1963;59:586.
13. Smith RB, Douglas H, Petruscak J, et al. Safety of intraocular adrenaline with halothane anesthesia. *Br J Anaesth.* 1972;44:1314.
14. Fraunfelder FT, Scafidi AF. Possible adverse effects from topical ocular 10 percent phenylephrine hydrochloride. *Am J Ophthalmol.* 1978;84:447.
15. Gilman AG, Rall TW, Nies AS, Taylor P, eds. *Goodman and Gilman's the pharmacological basis of therapeutics.* 8th ed. New York: Macmillan; 1990.
16. Stinson TW, Donlon JV Jr. Interaction of SF_6 and air with nitrous oxide. *Anesthesiology.* 1979;51:S16.
17. Wolf GL, Capuano C, Hartung J. Nitrous oxide increases intraocular pressure after intravitreal sulfur hexafluoride injection. *Anesthesiology.* 1983;59:547–548.
18. Ausinisch B, Rayburn LR, Munson ES, Levy NS. Ketamine and intraocular pressure in children. *Anesth Analg.* 1976;55:773–775.
19. Thompson MF, Brock-Utne JG, Bean P, et al. Anaesthesia and intraocular pressure: A comparison of total intravenous anaesthesia using etomidate with conventional inhalational anaesthesia. *Anaesthesia.* 1982;37:758.
20. Pandey K, Badola RP, Kumar S. Time course of intraocular hypertension produced by suxamethonium. *Br J Anaesth.* 1972;44:191–195.
21. Grover VK, Lata K, Sharma S, et al. Efficacy of lignocaine in the suppression of the intraocular pressure response to succinylcholine and tracheal intubation. *Anaesthesia.* 1989;44:22–25.
22. Indu B, Batra YK, Puri GD, Singh H. Nifedipine attenuates the intraocular pressure response to intubation following succinylcholine. *Can J Anaesth.* 1989;36:269–272.
23. Duncalf D, Weitzner SW. Ventilation and hypercapnia on intraocular pressure in infants and children. *Anesth Analg.* 1963;43:232–237.
24. Patel RI, Hannallah RS. Anesthetic complications following pediatric ambulatory surgery: A 3 year study. *Anesthesiology.* 1988;69:1009–1012.
25. Hustead AF. *Painless awake eye blocks.* Wichita, KS: Hustead Anesthesiology; 1990. Videotape.
26. Grizzard WS, Kirk NM, Pavan PR, Antworth MV, Hammer ME, Roseman AL. Perforating ocular injuries caused by anesthesia personnel. *Ophthalmology.* 1991;98:1011–1016.
27. Gills JP, Loyd TL. A technique of retrobulbar block with paralysis of orbicularis oculi. *Am Intra-ocular Implant Soc J.* 1983;9:339–340.
28. Pautler SE, Grizzard WS, Thompson LN, et al. Blindness from retrobulbar injection into the optic nerve. *Ophthalmic Surg.* 1986;17:334–337.
29. Kimbrough RL, Stewart RH, Okereke PC. A modified Gills' block and its effectiveness for lid akinesia. *Ophthalmic Surg.* 1987;18:14–17.
30. van Lint A. Paralysie palpebrae temporaire provoquee dans l'operation de la cataracte. *Ann Ocul (Paris).* 1914;151:420–424.
31. Bruce RA, McGoldrick KE, Oppenheimer PM. *Anesthesia for ophthalmology.* Birmingham, AL: Aesculapius; 1982:39.
32. O'Brien CS. Akinesia during cataract extraction. *Arch Ophthalmol.* 1929;1:447–449.
33. Atkinson WS. Akinesia of the orbicularis. *Am J Ophthalmol.* 1953;36:1255–1258.
34. Nadbath RP, Rehman I. Facial nerve block. *Am J Ophthalmol.* 1963;55:143–146.
35. Davis DB, Mandel MR. Posterior peribulbar anesthesia: An alternative to retrobulbar anesthesia. *J Cataract Refractive Surg.* 1986;12:182–184.
36. Beasley H. Hyperthermia associated with ophthalmic surgery. *Am J Ophthalmol.* 1974;77:76.
37. Betra YK, Bali M. Corneal abrasions during general anesthesia. *Anesth Analg.* 1977;56:363.
38. Rainin EA, Carlson BM. Postoperative diplopia and ptosis. *Arch Ophthalmol.* 1985;103:1337–1339.
39. Madsen PH. Traumatic retinal angiopathy. *Ophthalmologica.* 1972;165:453.

Anesthesia for Ear, Nose and Throat, Head and Neck, and Oral and Maxillofacial Surgery

Joel M. Weaver

The anesthetic management of the patient undergoing any otolaryngologic procedure or oral and maxillofacial surgery requires an understanding not only of basic anatomy and physiology but of the anesthetic implications of the presenting pathophysiology. Reliable control of the airway is particularly important in many of these cases as the airway may already be compromised. Once control of the airway is established, the anesthetist may be positioned some distance from the patient's head, making direct access to the airway difficult once the surgical procedure has begun. This chapter discusses the anesthetic selection and management, monitoring, and special patient considerations for a variety of procedures of the head and neck.

PREOPERATIVE EVALUATION

Preoperative evaluation of patients for ear, nose and throat, head and neck, and oral and maxillofacial surgery is performed in the usual manner, with particular emphasis on the airway. Conditions such as nasal polyps, maxillary and mandibular fractures, tumors, trismus, hemorrhage, edema, retrognathia, and previous neck radiation and surgery may cause the anesthetist unusual difficulty in establishing and securing a patent airway. Additionally, because the airway is the common focus of attention of both the anesthetist and the surgeon, cooperation is essential for the safe anesthetic management of the patient.

Patients undergoing head and neck cancer surgery usually have chronic bronchitis, obstructive pulmonary disease, and emphysema. Preoperative evaluation of pulmonary status with arterial blood gas analysis and pulmonary function testing can help the anesthetist decide on appropriate anesthetic techniques and monitoring devices for such patients.

The patient should be examined for ability to open the mouth and for neck mobility. A normal distance between upper and lower incisor teeth is 35 mm for adult women and 40 mm for adult men. Patients with limited opening should be further evaluated and consultation with the surgeon is suggested to determine the etiology. An awake intubation may be necessary if a mechanical problem such as a depressed zygomatic arch fracture limits mandibular opening. Previous radiation therapy to the neck may decrease the mobility of soft tissues and certain anatomic structures, making laryngoscopy and intubation difficult. Likewise a previous cervical spine fusion or neck arthritis may also cause a decrease in neck mobility.

PATIENT POSITIONING

The head is placed in the "sniffing position" prior to induction and intubation. A 1-liter intravenous fluid bag wrapped in a pillowcase or folded sheets placed under the occiput may facilitate this maneuver. Extension at the atlanto-occipital joint and flexion of the cervical spine help to properly align the airway structures. Proper positioning prior to the initiation of surgery is important to avoid strain on the neck, particularly when the head is turned to one side or when a shoulder roll is used to hyperextend the neck for laryngeal or thyroid surgery. Pressure points such as the elbows and heels should be padded, and a pillow should be placed under the knees. For nasal, maxillary, or sinus surgery, placing the patient at a 15- to 20-degree head-up tilt may help decrease bleeding when used in conjunction with other local methods such as topical cocaine or epinephrine. The eyes should be protected not only from dryness during anesthesia, but also from inadvertent damage from the surgeon as he or she operates near them. Lubrication with a bland ointment and taping of the eyelids are recommended in most instances. The surgeon may suture the lids for protection in some facial procedures.

Frequently the anesthetist assumes a position that is remote from the surgical site, where direct access to the airway is difficult or impossible. Problems such as disconnection and kinking of the endotracheal tube must be anticipated and should be immediately recognized by the anesthetist, who continuously monitors breath sounds with an esophageal or precordial stethoscope, observes for proper chest expansion, and monitors end-tidal carbon dioxide concentrations.

MONITORING

The standard monitoring devices used in these types of surgery include blood pressure cuff, temperature probe, electrocardiogram (ECG) monitor, pulse oximeter, end-tidal carbon dioxide monitor, and either a precordial or an esophageal stethoscope. If possible, the patient's hand should be readily available to the anesthetist to permit palpation of the pulse, observation of the nail beds, and arterial blood sampling. Breath-by-breath analysis of end-expiratory carbon dioxide and pulse oximetry provides useful information on ventilatory status, although hypotension or hypothermia may decrease the accuracy of the pulse oximeter. Medically compromised patients or those undergoing exceptionally extensive surgical procedures may benefit from arterial cannulation for direct blood pressure and blood gas monitoring, central venous pressure monitoring, and pulmonary artery catheterization. Urinary catheterization is necessary for procedures longer than 4 hours or when monitoring urinary output is desirable, that is, when major blood loss is expected or during induced hypotensive anesthesia.

CHOICE OF ANESTHETIC

Although there are many variables to consider in choosing a particular anesthetic technique, several generalizations can be made. A rapid, smooth, and reasonably pleasant induction with oxygen–nitrous oxide–halothane is most often used for children. Patients with oral, pharyngeal, or laryngeal carcinomas usually have significant smoking histories, which may indicate the use of potent volatile agents to dilate bronchioles and permit the delivery of high concentrations of oxygen. Limited cardiac reserve in some patients may indicate a nitrous oxide–oxygen–narcotic (fentanyl or sufentanil) anesthetic to maintain adequate cardiac output. Patients without significant cardiorespiratory disease who are expected to experience considerable blood loss may benefit from intentional or induced hypotensive anesthesia, using deep isoflurane, nitroprusside, nitroglycerin, labetalol, or ganglionic blockade techniques.[1]

ESTABLISHING A PATENT AIRWAY

For adult patients who are deemed unlikely to present the anesthetist with a difficult airway problem, a barbiturate or propofol induction after preoxygenation and succinylcholine relaxation is generally used for endotracheal intubation; however, occasionally unexpected difficulty is encountered and the anesthetist must be fully prepared both mentally and technically to properly gain control of the airway. Various sizes and types of face masks, laryngoscope blades, endotracheal tubes, oral and nasal airways, stylets, and a functioning suction are mandatory. If nasal intubation is planned, an acute-angle metal adapter should be inserted in the tube as a connector to anesthesia tubing to maintain a low profile on the forehead. Use of a nasal tube custom-trimmed to appropriate length and the acute angle connector helps prevent ischemia and necrosis of the tip of the nose. A nasal preformed (Rae) tube which is prebent as it exits the nose and crosses the forehead is also available.

Awake Oral Intubation

In patients who seem likely candidates for difficult intubation or for whom anesthesia prior to intubation may be dangerous, awake oral intubation is one alternative. After an intravenous infusion has been established, administration of light sedation with midazolam may be helpful to gain patient cooperation. Careful explanation of the necessity of the procedure and the steps involved greatly enhances its smoothness and markedly decreases the amount of midazolam that might otherwise be necessary.

The oral cavity and oral pharynx should be sprayed with 4 percent lidocaine. After several minutes a laryngoscope is partially inserted to retract the tongue. The posterior pharynx is sprayed repeatedly until the laryngoscope can be fully inserted without patient discomfort. A glossopharyngeal nerve block[2] at the posterior tonsillar pillar may be attempted bilaterally to inhibit gagging as an alternative or in addition to topical spray. Finally, the larynx and laryngopharynx are sprayed. While the patient is holding his or her breath after a full inspiration, 2 or 3 mL of 4 percent lidocaine is instilled via a 20-gauge needle through the cricothyroid membrane into the trachea. The violent coughing that results spreads the lidocaine and anesthetizes the trachea and larynx. After 2 minutes direct laryngoscopy is accomplished, and with the patient "panting like a dog" to help maintain an open glottis, the endotracheal tube is inserted and the cuff inflated. Induction of anesthesia may proceed as soon as the tube is checked for proper position and secured.

Awake Nasotracheal Intubation

Awake nasotracheal intubation can be used as an alternative to awake oral intubation.[3] It is usually better tolerated, particularly when accomplished blindly without the use of the laryngoscope. The same local anesthetic procedures used in the awake oral technique are used for the awake nasal intubation so that direct laryngoscopy can be accomplished if needed. Additionally, 4 percent cocaine or 0.5 percent phenylephrine followed by 4 percent lidocaine is sprayed into each nostril while the patient sniffs it in. The spray is more likely to spread throughout the entire surface of the nasal mucosa in this way than when applied with cotton-tipped applicators. Widespread vasoconstriction and subsequent shrinkage of nasal mucosal membranes decrease the incidence and severity of nasal hemorrhage and soft tissue trauma. A soft nasopharyngeal tube or nasal airway (trumpet) thickly coated with lidocaine ointment is gently inserted into the nostril that appears to be more patent or through which the patient feels he or she can best breathe. If there is no preference, the right side should be attempted first, as the smooth bevel on most tubes would then slide along the nasal septum and result in reduced frequency of turbinate or other nasal damage. If any resistance to the passage of this tube is encountered, the anesthetist should not hesitate to try the opposite side. The nasopharyngeal tube not only helps apply more topical anesthetic to the exact areas where the endotracheal tube will pass, but also provides insight into the patency of the passageway.

The maxillary division of the trigeminal nerve may also be blocked to provide profound anesthesia in the middle and posterior portions of the nasal passage. A 25-gauge, 1½-in. needle is inserted into the anterior palatine foramen and up the greater palatine canal, and 4 mL of 2 percent lidocaine is injected. The maxillary nerve block may also be attempted extraorally with the use of a 4-in. needle. It is inserted beneath the midpoint of the zygomatic arch and passes through skin, subcutaneous tissue, masseter and lateral pterygoid muscles, and finally through the pterygomaxillary fissure into the pterygomaxillary fossa. These procedures, also called a second-division nerve block, or V-2 block, are explained in detail in dental anesthesia sources.[4-6]

The nasoendotracheal tube is then lubricated and the tip is softened by the anesthetist's warm hand or by immersion in warm water for several minutes. Sterility during this process can easily be maintained if the tube is placed back in its sterile wrapper during warming.

After the nasopharyngeal tube is removed, the nasoendotracheal tube is inserted in the same manner and direction. The tube is twisted slightly so that the tip is directed toward the midline. With the patient's head elevated at the occiput into the sniffing position, the tube is slowly advanced while the anesthetist listens for breath sounds. The disappearance of breath sounds indicates that the tube has passed beyond the glottis and is in the esophagus, the vallecula, or the piriform recess. A bulge on either side of the neck produced by the tube may often be observed. The tube must be withdrawn at least 2 in. to clear the aryepiglottic fold; it is then slightly twisted toward the midline again and slowly advanced. If the tube is posterior to the glottis and advances into the esophagus, no bulge will appear. The head should be further extended so that the tip of the tube moves more anteriorly. Flexion of the head allows the tip to move posteriorly if it is projecting too far anteriorly. As the tube approximates the glottis, the breath sounds increase in volume and pitch and the tube is advanced into the trachea. If these techniques are not successful, direct laryngoscopy and manipulation of the tube with Magill forceps may be necessary.

Occasionally, the curve of the tube is such that the tip of the bevel may catch on the anterior commissure of the glottis. If excessive force is used to advance the tube, tracheal damage can result. By simply rotating the tube in a full circle while applying gentle forward pressure, the anesthetist can change the angulation of the tube and easily advance it unless tracheal stenosis or other pathology exists.

Nasal Intubation during General Anesthesia

Nasal intubation is necessary for many oral surgical procedures. The vast majority of these nasal intubations can be accomplished safely and comfortably after induction of general anesthesia.

Cocaine or phenylephrine nasal spray and a well-lubricated, presoftened endotracheal tube of proper diameter (7.0 mm in inner diameter and 27 cm in length for an average adult) are essential for an atraumatic procedure. The patient may be intubated under deep inhalation anesthesia with spontaneous respiration or may be induced with a barbiturate, relaxed with succinylcholine, and intubated

blindly or with direct laryngoscopy. The technique of blind intubation in the paralyzed patient uses observation or palpation of the tube in the neck instead of listening for breath sounds to guide the tube. In either case, if intubation is not accomplished within a reasonable amount of time, the tube may be partially withdrawn and positive-pressure ventilation accomplished by using it as a nasopharyngeal airway after the mouth and opposite nostril are closed. If ventilation is not satisfactory, the nasal tube should be removed and a full face mask applied for proper ventilation prior to a second nasal attempt.

Nasal intubation in the anesthetized, paralyzed patient using direct laryngoscopy involves a combination of twisting of the tube to orient it in the middle and flexion or extension of the head to move the tip in the proper anteroposterior position. Magill forceps may also be used to grasp the tube and place it into the glottis.

Nasal Intubation with the Fiberoptic Laryngoscope

The flexible fiberoptic laryngoscope is particularly useful in the patient who for one reason or another has not been able to be intubated by some other method.[6-8] Some anesthetists feel that it is the method of choice for awake nasal intubation. In addition to the advantage of directly viewing the patient's airway anatomy, the anesthetist can control the position of the tip of this device by rotating a knob for anteroposterior movement or by rotating the entire apparatus for side-to-side motion. Once the flexible tip is positioned in the trachea, the endotracheal tube is advanced over it in the same manner as a stylet is used in advancing an oral tube.

For successful use of the flexible fiberoptic laryngoscope, great attention to detail is very important. Inadequate vasoconstrictor use may result in subsequent nasal bleeding during fiberoptic intubation. The blood will cover or obscure the optical portion of the tip and interfere with the view. Premedication with drying agents such as atropine, antihistamines, and meperidine helps prevent accumulation of secretions on it. Antifogging solution may be applied to the tip to aid visualization. A soft nasal pharyngeal tube that has been cut lengthwise to facilitate rapid removal later may be inserted initially. The fiberoptic laryngoscope which has been preloaded with an appropriate-size endotracheal tube is then inserted into the nasal pharyngeal tube which acts as a guide toward the larynx. This also reduces trauma and bleeding of the nasal mucosa during repeated insertions of the scope. Once the scope is manipulated into the trachea and the carina is observed, the split nasal pharyngeal tube is quickly removed and the endotracheal tube is advanced into the nose, pharynx, and trachea over the fiberoptic scope.

Retrograde Intubation

When all other methods of intubation fail, the retrograde technique is usually successful. A convenient method is to introduce an epidural catheter through a needle placed through the cricothyroid membrane. The catheter is advanced through the larynx and into the mouth (or nasal passage). A suitable endotracheal tube is then passed over the catheter and into the trachea. The catheter is then removed from the neck and the tube advanced into proper position. Although the performance of retrograde intubation may produce complications, for example, tracheal damage, bleeding, infection, and false passage, it may be a safer alternative than elective or emergency tracheostomy.

Cricothyroidotomy

When endotracheal intubation cannot be accomplished and an acute respiratory emergency requires immediate ventilation, a cricothyroidotomy with insertion of a small endotracheal tube may be lifesaving. Advantages of the procedure include ease and rapidity and a lower complication rate than a "rapid" emergency tracheostomy. A horizontal incision through skin, subcutaneous tissue, fascia, cricothyroid ligament, and membrane is made with a scalpel, and a small (4.0- to 5.0-mm) endotracheal tube is inserted into the trachea. To check for proper placement, light compression of the chest produces airflow from the tube and positive-pressure ventilation can then be safely initiated.

An alternative procedure is to insert a 10-gauge catheter-over-needle through the cricothyroid membrane, remove the steel needle, and attach the connector from a No. 3 endotracheal tube to the hub. Although such an airway is of small diameter, the insufflation of 100 percent oxygen may sustain life for a few minutes until a more permanent airway can be established under more controlled conditions or until the anesthetized patient regains spontaneous ventilation and consciousness.

Tracheostomy

Tracheostomy may be performed as an emergency or elective procedure under local anesthesia or under general endotracheal anesthesia as an elective procedure. Conscious patients should be given oxygen and light sedation with verbal and tactile reassurance to decrease anxiety. For patients who are intubated, whether conscious or under general anesthesia, the anesthetist must usually back out the endotracheal tube to permit the surgeon to place the tracheostomy tube in the trachea. The endotracheal tube should not be entirely removed from the trachea until the surgeon and the anesthetist are satisfied that the patient is being properly ventilated via the new airway. If the surgeon is unable to properly insert the tracheostomy tube the anesthetist may need to advance the endotracheal tube past the surgical site to provide an adequate seal for ventilation. A postoperative chest film should be taken to rule out pneumomediastinum and pneumothorax.

INTRAOPERATIVE MAINTENANCE

When the anticipated duration of the surgery is at least 4 hours or when major blood loss is expected, additional preoperative preparation may include large-bore intravenous catheters, central venous pressure (CVP) measurement, intraarterial catheterization, urinary catheter, heating blanket, blood warmer units, and the use of humidified, heated, low-flow anesthetic gases. Head and neck cancer patients frequently have bronchitis and chronic obstructive pul-

monary disease. Preoperative and intraoperative blood gas analysis as well as hematocrit and electrolyte data may be extremely useful. The necessity of positive end-expiratory pressure (PEEP) valves placed on the expiratory limb of the anesthetic circuit should also be anticipated for such cases if the anesthetic machine does not already have PEEP capability. Extreme care must be used in installing PEEP valves as improper placement may lead to total blockage of ventilation. Bronchodilators such as terbutaline 0.25 mg subcutaneously, aminophylline intravenously, or albuterol by spray mist into the endotracheal tube may improve compliance.

Blood loss is often difficult to judge in head and neck surgery. Surgical assistants must keep careful records of the amounts of irrigation fluid used, and sponges may need to be weighed to more accurately evaluate blood loss. Large volumes of blood may also be "hidden" in the drapes and on the floor. Tachycardia, hypotension, and reduced central venous pressure and urine output signal the presence of hypovolemia, and corrective measures must be quickly instituted. Close cooperation with the hospital's blood bank is essential to ensure that an adequate supply of blood products is readily available.

SPECIAL CONSIDERATIONS FOR INDIVIDUAL OPERATIONS

The following sections discuss the types of surgical procedures performed by surgeons in the head and neck region and the special anesthetic considerations for each.

Parotidectomy with Facial Nerve Exploration and Reconstruction

The patient's head will be turned to the side, which may dislodge the endotracheal tube. Strong tape that will not stretch should be used to secure the position of the oral endotracheal tube. Additional adhesive such as tincture of benzoin applied to the skin helps the tape stick more firmly. Tubes that are positioned with sharp bends often collapse once they begin to warm and become soft. Sudden unexpected increases in airway resistance may not be caused by light anesthesia or bronchospasm but rather by a kinked tube. Coiled-wire or armored tubes are often used in such instances.

Skeletal muscle relaxation is usually not required and may inhibit the surgeon's ability to identify the facial nerve with an electric nerve stimulator. If neuromuscular relaxation is a necessary component of the anesthetic, a peripheral nerve blockade monitor must be used to ensure that the surgeon's nerve stimulator can function properly.

Nasal Surgery

Although many types of nasal surgery are performed with local anesthesia and sedation, general anesthesia with oral intubation is quite popular. Major blood loss may occur and is difficult to quantify in the conscious patient who may swallow a considerable amount. A cuffed endotracheal tube and a moistened gauze posterior pharyngeal pack are essential during general anesthesia to help prevent aspiration, postoperative nausea, and vomiting of blood swallowed intraoperatively during light anesthesia. Anterior and occasionally posterior nasal packs are placed to control hemorrhage. The position and number of posterior packs must be known as they may become dislodged during recovery and cause respiratory obstruction. Because epinephrine is frequently used by the surgeon, the anesthetist must plan the anesthetic technique to include agents compatible with the amount of epinephrine used. For plastic reconstructive nasal surgery the endotracheal tube should be secured in such a manner that excessive pull on tissues does not cause distortion of the face. An oral preformed (Rae) tube or an armored tube should exit the mouth in the midline over the lower central incisor teeth and be secured with a short piece of tape to the chin. For additional security, the anesthesia circuit tubes may be taped to the patient's chest.

After an adequate oxygenation period, extubation is usually performed after the patient can respond to verbal commands to ensure the return of protective reflexes. As application of the full face mask may cause distortion of the unstable nose, it should not be used unless absolutely necessary. It is the responsibility of both the surgeon and the anesthetist to be sure that the pharyngeal pack is removed and the pharynx suctioned prior to extubation. A large suture placed through the pharyngeal pack and extending out of the oral cavity may act as a visual reminder that the pack is still in place.

The patient who arrives in surgery from the emergency room with continual uncontrollable epistaxis presents several special problems. Ligation of the internal maxillary artery under general anesthesia is often required. The patient is usually uncomfortable, nauseated, extremely tired, agitated, tachycardic, hypovolemic, and anemic. Because much of the blood has been swallowed, the patient should be induced by rapid-sequence induction after rehydration via a large-bore intravenous infusion line. Alternatively, an awake oral intubation may be attempted, but the increased stress on this patient may increase the amount of hemorrhage. A large induction dose of anesthetic may produce severe hypotension if peripheral vascular resistance falls despite attempts at preinduction hydration.

Laryngoscopy and Bronchoscopy

The anesthetic considerations for laryngoscopy and bronchoscopy vary with the anticipated duration of the procedure, the type of equipment used by the surgeon, and the physical status of the patient. For procedures done only to take a quick look and lasting no more than 1 or 2 minutes, some anesthetists prefer a barbiturate induction and succinylcholine relaxation without insertion of an endotracheal tube or other means of ventilatory support. Hypoxia, hypercarbia, and arrhythmias may occur and have made this "apneic technique" somewhat archaic. The anesthetic is often a delicate balance between the surgeon's access requirements and proper ventilation. Laryngoscopy and bronchoscopy with ventilation are recommended.

Preoperative discussion with the surgeon and examination of x-rays may denote the size and location of the suspected pathology. Awake oral intubation by direct laryngoscopy may be necessary if the anesthetist suspects that the lesion might cause a soft tissue or ball-valve obstruction during relaxation and attempted positive-pressure ventilation by mask. A patient who exhibits stridor and dyspnea with exertion is expected to require a smaller endotracheal tube if it is to pass beside the area of the lesion. Stridor and dyspnea at rest combined with use of accessory muscles of respiration, sternal retraction, and flaring of the nares are best managed with a tracheostomy under local anesthesia without sedation, prior to other procedures.

Laryngoscopy and bronchoscopy are frequently performed under general anesthesia with a small (5- or 6-mm) endotracheal tube that can be manipulated by the surgeon for surgical access. If the cuff must be deflated during bronchoscopy, increasing gas flows will generally compensate for the leak. Ventilating laryngoscopes and bronchoscopes that connect to the anesthetic circuit are available and provide the patient with adequate gas exchange. High-frequency (jet) ventilation is discussed in Chapter 16.

Complications of laryngoscopy and bronchoscopy include trauma to teeth if a mouth guard is not used, tracheal tear, pneumothorax, laryngeal and epiglottal edema, thick copious secretions, hemorrhage, accidental extubation during removal of the endoscope, and laryngospasm. The well-oxygenated patient should be extubated when awake to ensure the return of protective reflexes and muscular tone. Provision should be made for immediate reintubation when necessary.

Postoperative stridor is not uncommon, particularly after a biopsy has been performed. The patient should be in a head-up position at approximately a 45-degree angle. Humidified oxygen should be delivered by face mask and the patient closely observed. Intravenous steroids and racemic epinephrine aerosol may be administered to decrease laryngeal edema. Thick copious secretions, bleeding, edema, and distorted anatomy may prevent reintubation if it is needed. Cricothyroidotomy or tracheostomy may be required.

Tonsillectomy and Adenoidectomy

Although adult patients are occasionally managed with local anesthesia and light sedation for tonsillectomy and adenoidectomy, such surgery is most often accomplished under endotracheal general anesthesia. Thiopental or propofol induction, oxygen, and nitrous oxide–narcotic–succinylcholine maintenance with an endotracheal tube are quite commonly used for adults. Oxygen–nitrous oxide–halothane inhalation induction followed by the insertion of an intravenous catheter for administration of succinylcholine, 1 to 2 mg/kg lidocaine, or both, with oral intubation is the most common anesthetic technique for children. Extremely large tonsils, particularly those that are abscessed, may produce upper airway obstruction on induction. Oral airways and endotracheal tubes must be inserted carefully as these enlarged tissues may be quite friable. Additionally, children between the ages of 5 and 12 are likely to have spontaneous shedding of deciduous teeth, which may be loosened and aspirated during laryngoscopy. As reflex bradycardia and preventricular contractions during light halothane anesthesia are quite common during tonsillectomy, the ECG should be monitored closely. Bradycardia may be treated by cessation of surgery and administration of atropine. Hyperventilation, deepening the plane of anesthesia, and possible intravenous lidocaine are recommended for the treatment of ventricular ectopy.

The anesthetist must recognize that the surgeon may move the endotracheal tube during his or her manipulations so that either endobronchial intubation or extubation can result.

Considerable bleeding may occur in a relatively short period, resulting in tachycardia and hypotension. Blood loss, particularly in small children, should be carefully measured throughout the procedure. In healthy children a pale skin color caused by peripheral vasoconstriction and tachycardia are early signs of hypovolemia; hypotension generally occurs later.

After surgery, the nose and throat should be carefully suctioned and the patient extubated when cough and swallowing reflexes return. Alternatively, in selected cases where bleeding is extremely well controlled, the patient may be extubated under deep halothane anesthesia. Children are placed in the lateral position with the head down to allow blood and other secretions to roll out the corner of the mouth.

Airway obstruction and continued bleeding are the two major problems of the recovery period. Airway obstruction generally responds to the usual methods of treatment, such as head positioning and humidified oxygen, and rarely requires the use of oral airways. Bleeding may be treated with a head-up position after the patient is awake. Calming the patient with reassuring words and a gentle touch may also be helpful.

The anesthetist may need to reanesthetize the patient so that the surgeon can obtain control of a severely bleeding operative site. The patient should be regarded as having a full stomach because of the excessive amount of blood swallowed after the initial surgery. After preoxygenation, a rapid-sequence induction of a relatively small dose of intravenous thiopental plus succinylcholine with cricoid pressure is recommended only after rehydration with crystalloid or blood. It is critical for the anesthetist to consider that a hypovolemic, vasoconstricted patient may experience severe hypotension during the induction, particularly if a "usual" dose of thiopental is administered. High-volume suction should be readily available to facilitate intubation. A large-bore gastric tube should be inserted to evacuate swallowed blood and then removed prior to extubation.

Thyroidectomy and Parathyroidectomy

Hyperthyroidism or Graves' disease frequently produces symptoms of tachycardia, arrhythmias, nervousness, weight loss, peripheral vasodilation, and heat intolerance. Surgery is usually considered after treatment with propylthiouracil and beta blockers or other antithyroid drugs that produce a drug-induced euthyroid state. Lack of control may predispose the patient to thyroid storm during the manipulation associated with thyroid surgery. The tachyarrhythmias may be treated with intravenous propranolol in increments of 0.5 mg. Postoperative stridor or obstruction after extubation may be caused by damage to one or both recurrent laryngeal nerves. Laryngoscopy should assist in differentiating the subsequent vocal cord paralysis from la-

ryngeal edema, tracheal compression by massive hematoma formation, or hypocalcemic tetany after inadvertent parathyroidectomy. Laryngeal edema may respond to vasoconstrictor (racemic epinephrine) nebulization, warmed moist oxygen mist, and steroids. A hematoma should be drained. Hypocalcemic tetany may be associated with hyperreflexia, muscle weakness, and low serum calcium levels. Slow and careful calcium replacement may be initiated by intravenous drip infusion until normal levels are reached. Reintubation in any of the aforementioned cases may be necessary.

Anesthesia considerations for parathyroid surgery differ from those for thyroid surgery only by the potential for high preoperative calcium levels, which may cause hypercontractibility of the heart and bradycardia. Proper medical management and recent laboratory analysis of serum calcium should be completed prior to parathyroid surgery.

Major Head and Neck Cancer Surgery

Extensive head and neck cancer surgery includes such procedures as supraglottic laryngectomy, total laryngectomy, pharyngectomy, radical neck dissection, mandibulectomy, maxillectomy with or without orbital exoneration, and tracheal resection.

Many of these patients have a history of alcohol or tobacco abuse, or both, and usually present with pulmonary and cardiovascular disease in addition to their cancer. Preoperative assessment may include pulmonary function tests, arterial blood gas analysis, chest radiographs, antibiotics for bronchitis, chest physiotherapy, and tomograms or magnetic resonance images of the tumor or lesion. Previous surgery such as a supraglottic laryngectomy, radiation therapy, or a large friable tumor may cause difficulty during intubation or airway obstruction.

Anesthetic techniques that allow spontaneous assisted ventilation with high concentrations of oxygen may be an advantage during laryngectomy when a sterile armored tube (coiled-wire tube) inserted into the transected trachea replaces the orotracheal tube. Controlled ventilation with or without PEEP may help prevent air embolism in more radical surgeries where large neck veins could be open. Sudden deterioration in vital signs accompanied by a millwheel murmur, pulmonary artery hypertension, and elevated central venous pressure are pathognomonic of an air embolism. The patient should be turned in a left lateral position with the head down after the wound is packed with moistened gauze. Hyperventilation with 100 percent oxygen and symptomatic treatment to improve vital signs should be initiated until air can be aspirated from the right atrium.

Major blood loss should be anticipated, particularly for the longer, more radical procedures. A Foley catheter is necessary for procedures lasting 4 or more hours, when large volumes of fluid replacement are anticipated, or to monitor kidney perfusion and urinary output especially in patients with severe cardiovascular or renal impairment.

Pressure or manipulation of the carotid sinus during neck dissections may cause significant bradycardia. Immediate cessation of surgical stimulation followed by infiltration of the adventitia at the bifurcation of the carotid artery with a local anesthetic is recommended. Intravenous atropine may also be helpful if the bradycardia is severe or accompanied by hypotension.

Ligation of the internal jugular vein frequently produces cyanosis and edema of the face until alternative venous drainage develops. Postoperatively, the patient should be placed in a head-up position; diuretics with fluid restrictions may also be necessary. Cerebral edema is a potential complication in severe cases, and careful evaluation of neurologic signs and frequent temperature measurements should be performed. A temperature rise about 12 hours after surgery may indicate cerebral edema and anoxia from compression.

Laser Excision and Vaporization

The laser (light amplification by stimulated emission) is frequently used in combination with suspension laryngoscopy for excision or vaporization of lesions in the pharynx, larynx, trachea, and bronchi. The surgeon's laryngoscope is suspended on a bracket or a Mayo stand which allows the surgeon to have both hands free to operate. The laser concentrates a high-energy monochromatic beam that is absorbed by tissue. The heat created may cause the desired, very controllable destruction of pathologic tissue while sparing adjacent healthy areas.

The laser most frequently used in the airway is the carbon dioxide laser. As its wavelength is in the infrared spectrum and thus invisible to the human eye, a helium–neon laser beam of very low energy that is visible is used with the carbon dioxide laser to enable the surgeon to precisely direct the beam to the lesion. The energy is highly absorbed by the water in the tissue and quickly boils, vaporizes, and eliminates the cells. Such surgery typically produces exceptional hemorrhage control postoperatively.

The argon laser emits energy in the visible part of the spectrum. It is poorly absorbed by water but highly absorbed by hemoglobin. Thus, with the argon laser, coagulation of blood vessels can occur without destruction of healthy tissue.

The safety of the patient and operating room personnel is of primary concern when lasers are used. All entrances to the operating room must warn of the use of the laser so that proper eye protection can be worn by all personnel entering the room. Because laser beams can reflect from metallic instruments, they may present a hazard to anyone near the patient. Damage to skin surfaces is unlikely, but corneas are very susceptible to carbon dioxide laser reflection. Goggles or glasses with side shields that absorb the beam are mandatory to prevent corneal injury. The anesthetized patient's eyes should also be lubricated, taped, and padded with moistened gauze pads. All other exposed areas of the patient's face should be covered with moistened towels to optimize protection.

The proper endotracheal tube must be chosen as the standard polyvinyl chloride tubes may be highly flammable, especially in an oxygen-enriched atmosphere, if inadvertent contact with the laser beam is made (Fig. 36–1). Because nitrous oxide can also support combustion, helium or nitrogen may be added to the anesthetic gas mixture to reduce the flammability somewhat. A flexible stainless-steel tube (Norton tube) is available, although the added rubber

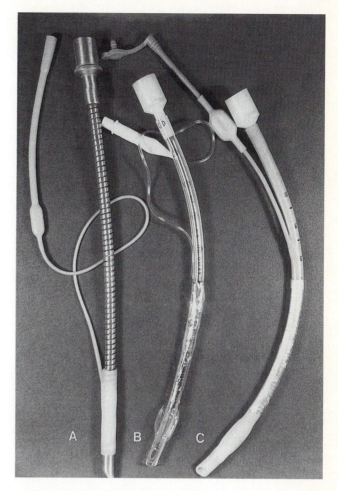

Figure 36–1. Three different types of tubes used for oropharyngeal laser surgery: **A.** Metal endotracheal tube with cuff. **B.** Red rubber endotracheal tube wrapped. **C.** Polyvinyl chloride endotracheal tube wrapped. All nonmetal tubes are wrapped with Radio Shack ¼-in. sensing foil.

cuff and pilot balloon are still fire hazards. The surgeon must pack off these areas with moist pledgets. A tube made of silicone and metallic particles offers some protection from fire because more energy is required for ignition; however, fire has been reported with this tube.[9] Alternatively, red rubber tubes may be wrapped with adhesive-backed aluminum tape (not Mylar or plastic-coated foil tape) to reflect laser beams (Fig. 36–2). Again, cuffs and pilot balloons must be protected, and cuffs may be filled with saline to help quench a fire if the cuff is accidentally ruptured. Jet ventilation without an endotracheal tube has been used but may introduce smoke and other debris into the lungs during laser surgery. It is imperative that all packs and pledgets be counted on insertion and removal to prevent aspiration at the end of the procedure.

Laser surgery for lesions in the trachea or bronchi may be accomplished with a small-diameter "protected" endotracheal tube in place and the surgeon's bronchoscope placed next to it. Ventilating bronchoscopes are available that have a proximal port for direct connection to the anesthetic circuit. This permits the patient to spontaneously

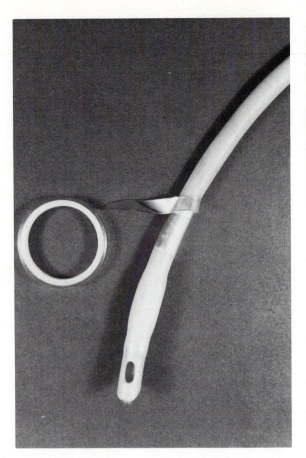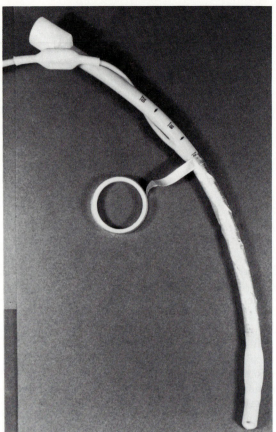

Figure 36–2. Method for wrapping a red rubber endotracheal tube with Radio Shack ¼-in. sensing foil.

breathe anesthetic gases while the surgeon operates; the paralyzed patient may be intermittently ventilated with positive-pressure from the anesthesia machine.

The anesthetist must not be lulled into a false sense of security with all these precautions. Should a fire occur, the lightly secured endotracheal tube must be immediately removed and any smoldering remains must be flooded with saline and removed. Bronchoscopy should be accomplished to see the extent of injury and to retrieve any remaining debris. The patient may need to be reintubated and ventilated depending on the damage. A tracheostomy may be necessary. Immediate consultation with a pulmonologist, particularly one with experience in treating burn victims, is essential.

Oral and Maxillofacial Trauma Surgery

Trauma to the face may produce fractures of the mandible, maxilla, zygoma, and associated structures. Additionally, skull fracture, intracranial hematoma, cervical spine injury, and laryngeal and tracheal damage may also be present. Preoperative assessment should include questioning about loss of consciousness; a neurologic examination; radiographs of the skull, cervical vertebrae, and chest; and identification of nasal secretions for possible cerebrospinal fluid leak.

The airway deserves careful examination. Upper airway obstruction may result from complete dislocation of the maxilla, blood, avulsed teeth, edema, and hematoma formation. Bilateral fracture of the necks of the mandibular condyles may allow the mandible and base of the tongue to drop posteriorly, causing airway obstruction. The tongue, mandible, maxilla, or all three, may need to be temporarily pulled forward until the airway can be stabilized. A towel clip placed through the body of the tongue may be a lifesaving method as it can be used to pull the tongue forward to treat airway obstruction in such cases. Unless contraindicated by severe nasal damage, a nasoendotracheal tube is preferred, as the application of arch bars and intermaxillary fixation with wires or elastic bands are commonly used to stabilize maxillary and mandibular fractures. Laryngeal and tracheal damage may be recognized by noting hoarseness, inspiratory stridor, inspiratory retraction, and submucosal emphysema or hematoma.

Patients who are likely to have swallowed large amounts of blood should be considered to have full stomachs and induced accordingly. A pharyngeal gauze pack should be placed following intubation to absorb blood and secretions and to keep the laryngeal pharynx clear of bone fragments, broken teeth, and other debris. Removal of the pack prior to intermaxillary fixation is mandatory. Failure to remove the pack and subsequent extubation of the patient whose jaws are wired together may be a fatal error.

Mandibular fractures are often accompanied by trismus, and pain is frequently the limiting factor in the patient's inability to open normally. If the inability to open is caused by a mechanical obstruction such as a depressed zygomatic fracture impinging on the coronoid process of the mandible or in the presence of a full stomach, an awake nasal intubation is necessary. Otherwise induction of general anesthesia and nasotracheal intubation may proceed as usual. Direct laryngoscopy is not contraindicated in most mandibular fractures and will not normally further damage the fracture site, although some additional bleeding may occur.

Maxillary fractures are classified as LeFort I, II, or III, depending on the extent of the injury.[10] A LeFort I fracture is a transverse fracture of the maxilla above the roots of the teeth. It produces a fracture segment that includes the alveolar process, portions of the maxillary sinus, the palate, and the lower portion of the pterygoid process of the sphenoid bone. It usually does not present the anesthetist with unusual problems. A LeFort II fracture involves the nasal bones, frontal process of the maxilla, lacrimal bones, inferior rim of the orbit, and the zygomaticomaxillary suture area. The lateral wall of the maxilla, the pterygoid plates, and the pterygomaxillary fossa are also included. A LeFort III fracture is synonymous with craniofacial dysjunction, which is the separation of the facial bones from their attachments to the cranium, including zygomaticofrontal, maxillofrontal, and nasofrontal sutures, orbital floors, ethmoid sinus, and sphenoid bones. Usually many other facial bones are also fractured. One side of the face may have one type of LeFort fracture and the other side may have another. A cerebrospinal fluid (CSF) leak may occur as a result of a dural tear in the cribriform area, and despite the administration of antibiotics to prevent meningitis and the surgical reduction of the fractures, some anesthetists prefer not to nasally intubate patients who have a CSF leak. A CSF leak, however, does not necessarily contraindicate a nasal intubation, particularly if early extubation is contemplated. LeFort II and III fractures may be associated with severe nasal damage, a contraindication to nasal intubation. If some doubt exists as to the extent of nasal damage, consultation with the surgeon and a very gentle attempt to pass a small, lubricated, soft nasopharyngeal tube may be helpful. The nasopharyngeal tube may be used to guide a small nasogastric tube or fiberoptic laryngoscope through it and into the oropharynx. The nasopharyngeal tube is removed over the nasogastric tube, which remains in the pharynx. The nasotracheal tube is then inserted through the nose using the nasogastric tube as a guide. Such a procedure may reduce the incidence of additional trauma and false passage. Obstruction to the passage of the nasopharyngeal tube or other evidence of severe nasal damage necessitates an oral intubation or tracheostomy. Occasionally oral intubation is chosen initially when patient cooperation is minimal. The nasal passages are then examined under general anesthesia and, if suitable, nasal intubation under direct vision is accomplished by removing the oral tube when the nasal tube is in close approximation to the glottis.

Nasal intubation should be through the naris on the side opposite a unilateral maxillary fracture, where packing of the maxillary sinus and support of the orbital floor with gauze is anticipated. For ease of removal, the end of the gauze is often placed through a surgically made nasoantral fistula in the anterior portion of the nasal floor on the side of the fracture.

Massive bleeding that is difficult to isolate and control may occur as a result of massive midface trauma or on attempts to reduce these maxillary fractures. One or more large-bore intravenous lines and pressure bags or 50-mL syringes to facilitate rapid volume replacement should be immediately available. Bags of packed red cells may be prewarmed in water prior to being hung to facilitate rapid infusion, even when an in-line blood warmer is being used. A large nasogastric tube (18 gauge), which is less likely to clot off with blood, should be inserted prior to intermaxillary fixation and its position checked by auscultation of air in the stomach. If the tube is placed after fixation of the jaws, it may curl in the pharynx and may even tie itself in a knot, preventing its removal through the nose.

Extubation of patients in intermaxillary fixation is most safely done when the patient is awake and is responsive to command. After a deep inspiration the tube is removed from the trachea. It may be used as a nasopharyngeal tube or may be entirely removed, with suction tubing applied directly to the connector to clear the pharynx and nasal passage of blood and secretions. It may become difficult or impossible to remove the endotracheal tube if a pin, wire, or Kirschner wire (which is drilled from a normal zygoma on one side through the nasal septum and through the fractured zygoma on the other side) pierces the tube and impales it.[11] Extubation may be delayed several days or longer for patients with severe midface (LeFort III) fractures. When prolonged intubation is anticipated, a low-pressure, high-volume cuffed endotracheal tube should be chosen preoperatively.

As mouth breathing is limited by the intermaxillary fixation and nasal breathing may be impaired by blood, edema, and the nasogastric tube, a soft nasopharyngeal tube may be helpful if increased respiratory effort is noted after extubation. This tube must be diligently cleaned every half-hour because clotted blood and mucus may plug the patient's only major source of air. Postoperative restlessness and agitation must initially be regarded as signs of airway obstruction and not pain or anxiety until proven otherwise. Only then should the judicious use of tranquilizers or narcotics be considered. The nasogastric tube should be left on continuous low-pressure suction and irrigated frequently until the return is clear, an indication that hemorrhage has ceased. The time for its removal is somewhat arbitrary, depending on the type and extent of surgery, the patient's ability to tolerate it, the presence of nausea, the patient's ability to swallow, and the surgeon's judgment.

Elective Oral and Maxillofacial Surgery

The spectrum of elective oral and maxillofacial surgery includes dentoalveolar, soft-tissue, temporomandibular joint, and orthognathic surgery and augmentation of bony ridges and clefts. Incision and drainage of an abscess may be considered elective or semielective. These procedures can be managed with the patient in a semireclined position with the head and upper body at a 30-degree angle and the legs elevated and flexed at the knees. This position is particularly advantageous for minor procedures such as tooth extraction in the conscious, sedated patient who receives local anesthesia or in the patient under general anesthesia where a nasal mask or nasopharyngeal tube and an oral gauze protective pack are used. When using the nasal mask the anesthetist positions the head in the sniffing position, extends the mandible with the fingers, and holds the mask in place with thumb traction on the inhalation tubes. The Bain circuit, which is designed for spontaneous unassisted ventilation with relatively high gas flows, is ideal for this procedure. A nasopharyngeal tube may be placed under the mask for additional airway support or may be connected directly to the anesthesia circuit with an acute-angle adapter. Proper positioning and support of the mandible by the anesthetist are necessary in either case.

Endotracheal intubation should be used in the following situations:

1. Ventilation is inadequate during nonintubated cases.
2. The surgical procedure is prolonged or complicated.
3. The surgeon requests greater access to the head area with the anesthetist positioned to the side.
4. The anesthetist or surgeon is inexperienced or uncomfortable without endotracheal control of the airway.

Nasotracheal intubation is most commonly used during major oral and maxillofacial surgery. Patients scheduled for temporomandibular joint surgery frequently have a mechanical limitation of jaw opening and may require awake nasal intubation. An anesthetic without skeletal muscle relaxant will permit the surgeon to electrically identify branches of the facial nerve during this extraoral procedure. Patients with a narrow palate frequently undergo rapid surgical expulsion or midpalatal split procedures. Such patients have narrow nasal passages, necessitating the use of small nasotracheal tubes or, less frequently, an oral intubation. The nasal intubation should first be attempted through the naris opposite the side of the nasal septum along which the surgeon plans to cut the palatal bone, so that burs or chisels are less likely to pierce the tube. Edentulous patients may sustain a fracture during forceful manipulation of the mandible, ventilation with a full-face mask, or intubation.

A LeFort I or II osteotomy for surgical repositioning of the maxilla may also expose the endotracheal tube to the hazard of inadvertent surgical puncture. Spontaneous assisted ventilation during this portion of the surgery is suggested should damage to the tube occur. If access to the damaged area exists, the tube can be taped or sutured. A long, large suture should be placed through the portion of the tube distal to the damage and extended through the nose onto the face. If the tube should break during extubation, the suture will permit retrieval of the distal portion. If absolutely necessary, the tube may be replaced after hemostasis is accomplished. After removal of the pharyngeal pack, a small nasogastric tube or epidural catheter is inserted into the trachea through the damaged tube, which is then removed over it, and another endotracheal tube is guided into position, usually with direct laryngoscopy.

As the maxilla is richly supplied with blood, the surgeon may wish to infiltrate the area with 1 : 100,000 or 1 : 200,000 epinephrine. The anesthetist may choose anesthetic agents compatible with epinephrine or consider deliberate hypotensive anesthesia techniques such as deep isoflurane, labetalol, nitroglycerin, or nitroprusside.[1,12–16] Major bleeding may occur acutely as a result of downfracture of the maxilla or chiseling of the pterygoid plates, possibly necessitating rapid replacement of volume through a large-bore intravenous line. A large nasogastric tube should be placed to help prevent nausea from blood swallowed during the recovery period. The patient should not be extubated until awake and responsive because intermaxillary fixation limits direct access to the airway. Some surgeons may use bone plates and screws for rigid fixation, which eliminates the need for intermaxillary fixation (wiring or banding the mandible to the maxilla).

A mandibular osteotomy may be a singular procedure or may be combined with maxillary surgery to treat either mandibular prognathia or retrognathia. Prognathic patients usually have a large tongue whereas retrognathic patients frequently have an anteriorly positioned larynx, which may make direct laryngoscopy and intubation difficult. If the patient is placed in intermaxillary fixation intraoperatively, he or she should be extubated when awake and responsive to commands; this anesthetic technique permits smooth awakening, helps prevent bucking, and attempts to open the mouth. Patients who are informed of what to expect in the immediate postoperative period will be better prepared to accept the tubes and fixation appliances on awakening. The anesthetist, recovery room nurses, and floor nursing personnel must be knowledgeable as to the number and location of wires used to fixate the mandible to the maxilla so that they may be cut, if necessary, for emergency access to the airway. Wire-cutting scissors should be taped to the head of the bed for immediate availability.

Incision and drainage of severe oral–facial infections are usually done under general anesthesia. Patients are normally febrile and severely dehydrated. Application of a tight-fitting full face mask prior to induction may cause excruciating pain. Trismus, large intraoral abscesses, and an elevated, swollen floor of the mouth may make ventilation or direct laryngoscopy impossible. Endotracheal tubes, oral airways, or the laryngoscope blade may cause massive intraoral drainage and aspiration of pus in the anesthetized patient. Consultation with the surgeon and examination of the patient for intraoral swelling make awake nasal intubation the safest alternative in such situations. Tracheostomy under local anesthesia may be necessary in life-threatening cases such as Ludwig's angina if a nasal tube cannot be passed successfully. In such cases when severe obstruction is evidenced by severe dyspnea, sternal retraction, inspiratory stridor, and inability to tolerate a supine position, even small amounts of sedatives or narcotics may markedly impair the patient's ventilatory capability and total obstruction may result.

SUMMARY

A complete preoperative evaluation of the patient's medical history, physical status, and extent of injury or disease, as well as an assessment of the controllability of the airway, is essential for the safe induction of anesthesia in head and neck surgeries of all types. Communication and close cooperation with the surgeon to establish a "game plan" are necessary. Diligent intraoperative monitoring of vital signs and functions and knowledge of the surgical procedures with their attendant complications make these cases quite challenging even for the most experienced anesthetist. Finally, postoperative management of the patient, with attention focused on the maintenance of a patent airway and adequate ventilation, may avert serious complications during this period when there is a natural tendency to relax "now that the serious part of the operation is over." Careful attention to detail and conservative, often time-consuming, anesthetic management increase the likelihood that both the anesthetist and the surgeon will reach their common goals.

REFERENCES

1. Anderson JA. Deliberate hypotensive anesthesia for orthognathic surgery: Controlled pharmacologic manipulation of cardiovascular physiology. *Int J Adult Orthod Orthognathic Surg.* 1986;1(2):133–159.
2. Barton S, Williams J. Glossopharyngeal nerve block. *Arch Otolaryngol.* 1971;93:186.
3. Kopman A, Wollman SB, Ross K, Surks SN. Awake endotracheal intubation. A review of 267 cases. *Anesth Analg.* 1975; 54:323–327.
4. Bennett RC. *Monheim's local anesthesia and pain control in dental practice.* 6th ed. St. Louis, MO: CV Mosby; 1978.
5. Baddour HM, Hubbard AM, Tilson HB. Maxillary nerve block used prior to awake nasal intubation. *Anesth Prog.* 1979;26: 43–45.
6. Triplett W, Ondrey J, McDonald JS. The use of the fiberoptic laryngoscope for nasotracheal intubation—A case report. *Anesth Prog.* 1979;26:49.
7. Raj PP, Forestner J, Watson T, et al. Technics for fiberoptic laryngoscopy in anesthesia. *Anesth Analg.* 1974;53:708–714.
8. Schwartz JD, Bauer RA, David NJ, Guralnick WC. Ludwig's angina: Use of fiberoptic laryngoscope to avoid tracheostomy. *J Oral Surg.* 1974;32:608–611.
9. Giffin B, Shapshay SM, Bellack GS, et al. Flammability of endotracheal tubes during Yd-YAG laser application in the airway. *Anesthesiology.* 1986;65:54.
10. LeForte R. (translated by Dr. P. Tessier). Experimental study of fractures of the upper jaw. *Plast Reconstr Surg.* 1963;30:6.
11. Lee C, Schwartz S, Mok MS. Difficult extubation due to transfixation of a nasotracheal tube by a Kirschner wire. *Anesthesiology.* 1977;46:427.
12. McNulty S, Sharifi-Azad S, Farole A. Induced hypotension with labetalol for orthognathic surgery. *J Oral Maxillofac Surg.* 1987;45:309–311.
13. Golia JK, Woo R, Farole A, Seltzer JL. Nitroglycerin-controlled circulation in orthognathic surgery. *J Oral Maxillofac Surg.* 1985;43:342–345.
14. Hegtvedt AK. Intraoperative and postoperative patient care (orthognathic surgery). *Oral and maxillofacial surgery clinics of North America.* 1990;2(4):857–868.
15. Davies RM, Scott JG. Anesthesia for major oral and maxillofacial surgery. *Br J Anaesth.* 1968;40:202.
16. Echenhoff JE. Deliberate hypotension. *Anesthesiology.* 1978;48:87.

Anesthesia for Plastic Surgery and the Thermally Injured Patient

Laura Wong

Advances in care of the burn patient have markedly decreased mortality in recent decades. In 1940, a total body surface area (TBSA) burn of 30 percent was associated with a mortality rate of 50 percent, and by 1980 an 80 percent TBSA burn was associated with a mortality rate of 50 percent.[1] This increase in survival has been attributable to improvements in antibiotic therapy, fluid resuscitation, nutritional support, and surgical treatment of the burn patient; however, 6000 persons continue to die yearly from burns.[2] Those patients of advanced age appear most susceptible to mortality from burns. Burn victims aged 60 to 74 have only a 53 percent survival rate after a 31 to 40 percent burn.[3] It has also been noted from morbidity and mortality statistics that inhalation injury is associated with a 61 percent mortality rate, a more reliable predictor of burn mortality than either percentage body burn or age.[4] Patients with major burns can sustain other traumatic injuries requiring surgical or medical intervention in addition to the multiple surgical operations often required for debridement and grafting. Planning anesthesia care for these patients requires substantial knowledge of emergency treatment including sophisticated airway management techniques, fluid resuscitation, modalities of treatment of pulmonary injury, and mechanics of dermal burn injury and awareness of the common complications associated with thermal injury.

ANESTHESIA FOR THE THERMALLY INJURED PATIENT

Inhalation Injury

The possibility of airway injury should be considered in all patients who present with an acute burn. Patients injured in an enclosed space are much more likely to have inhaled smoke and hot gases than those injured outdoors.[5] Oral and facial burns, singed nasal hairs, and soot in the nose or mouth are frequently associated with an upper airway burn.[6] Circumferential neck burns may produce airway compromise as a result of external compression of the airway by edematous tissues.[7] When any of these indicators are present, or when indications of airway obstruction, coughing, or respiratory distress such as mild hoarseness and wheezing are noted, the airway should be secured with an endotracheal tube before edema further compromises respiratory function. Delay can be fatal for the patient who develops severe edema of the face, neck, and airway making tracheotomy exceedingly difficult or impossible.

Patients who require intubation after a burn injury should be intubated with the largest possible endotracheal tube to facilitate bronchoscopy and long-term ventilatory support. An 8.0- or 8.5-cm endotracheal tube should be considered for most adult females and an 8.5- or 9-cm tube for most adult males. If possible, a nasotracheal intubation, with a tube usually 0.5 cm smaller than that chosen for the oral route, may be preferred because of its greater ease in anchoring and greater comfort for the patient. Nasotracheal intubation must be preceded by careful preparation of the nose to prevent excessive bleeding, as nasal mucosa is highly vascular and hemorrhage will complicate visualization during intubation. Cocaine liquid 2.5 percent via atomizer provides adequate vasoconstriction of the nasal mucosa. Neosynephrine has also been used successfully as a spray or topical application.

For the burn patient with signs of frank airway obstruction, intubation should not be delayed. An awake intubation is the technique of choice for intubation. Normal induction drugs such as sodium pentothol are usually avoided as the burn patient may be hypovolemic, and the depressant effects of this drug could cause cardiovascular impairment. In addition, should airway edema be present, no drug should be given that would further compromise airway patency in the spontaneously breathing patient until the airway is secured. It is also recommended that succinylcholine be avoided because of its propensity to result in dangerously high levels of extracellular potassium. All burn patients should be considered to have a full stomach; therefore, intubation is most safely done with a minimum of drugs or local anesthesia of the airway. In summary, intubation is most safely done without sedation or paralysis and without local anesthesia except of the nasal mucosa.

The definitive diagnosis of inhalation injury is made by bronchoscopy, which differentiates patients with upper airway edema from those with more distal pulmonary injuries. Xenon scanning can also be used to evaluate inhalation injury. Upper airway edema may resolve sufficiently within the first week of injury to permit extubation[8]; however, deep inhalation of smoke and hot gases produces injuries that may require prolonged ventilatory assistance.[9] In a recent series of 805 patients admitted to a regional burn unit, 14 percent were intubated. The median duration of intubation was 5 days; 40 percent of intubated patients (6 percent of all patients admitted) were given tracheostomies, which remained in place for a median of 28 days.[10]

Security of the airway via endotracheal tube is a crucial consideration for burn patients. The endotracheal tube should not be changed electively while significant edema of the face, neck, and upper airway persists. If a change is unavoidable, such as for failure of the endotracheal tube cuff, the change should be made using a fiberoptic bronchoscope to guide relocation of the glottic orifice, which may be completely obscured by edematous tissue. A variety of endotracheal tube sizes, as well as a tracheostomy set and an experienced surgeon, should be available should emergency tracheostomy be required. In the past, elective tracheostomy was associated with an increase in the incidence of pulmonary infection and the resulting mortality.[11] Studies have shown no difference in mortality between patients with an endotracheal tube and those with a tracheostomy.[10]

After edema subsides, an oral endotracheal tube may be electively exchanged for a nasotracheal tube in patients who require long-term ventilatory support and frequent pulmonary toilet. If required or requested by the surgeon or pulmonary consultant, the change to a nasotracheal tube should be done under controlled conditions by the anesthetist. This is often accomplished after induction of anesthesia for surgery. A tube of adequate internal diameter should be selected, usually 7.5 cm or larger for an adult. After induction of anesthesia, both nares should be prepared with a vasoconstrictive agent. A small nasal airway should be passed into the naris which provides easiest entry and successively larger nasal airways be passed to dilate the nare. Laryngoscopy should then be done to ensure good visualization of the glottis. With the patient paralyzed or breathing spontaneously, the nasotracheal tube is advanced to the posterior pharynx, which has been cleared of all secretions. The orotracheal tube is removed and the new tube is advanced into the trachea with Magill forceps under direct vision.

Various methods of anchoring endotracheal tubes in patients with facial burns have been described, including Velcro straps, umbilical tape, skin staples, and suture (Fig. 37–1).[12] A forehead splint which can stabilize both a nasotracheal tube and a nasogastric tube is recommended by Ward et al.[13] Whatever the method used, a piece of tape should be placed around the endotracheal tube to mark the depth of the tube at the nostril or teeth. Securing the endotracheal tube by piercing it with a safety pin and attaching ties to the pin is not recommended, as the pinholes can produce a significant loss of airway pressure or may damage the small tube to the cuff.

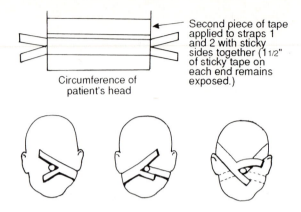

Figure 37–1. Anchoring method of the Shriners Burns Institute, Galveston, Texas. (*Reprinted, with permission, from Gordon.*[12])

Because of the recent trend toward early excision of the burn wound, many patients with recent inhalation injuries are undergoing surgery and anesthesia. Care of the patient with an inhalation injury is directed toward supportive interventions. The goal is to maintain adequate oxygenation via mechanical ventilation with positive-end-expiratory pressure (PEEP) until pulmonary damage has resolved. It is desirable to administer the lowest FIO_2 that maintains adequate oxygenation; however, high oxygen concentrations and levels of PEEP of 20 to 30 cm H_2O may be required to maintain acceptable blood oxygen content.

Bronchodilators may improve airflow in patients with inhalation injuries[14] and can be administered preoperatively or via the breathing circuit during anesthesia. Corticosteroids have not been found to be beneficial in the management of burn-associated airway edema and may increase susceptibility to infection, contributing to septic morbidity and mortality.[15] Humidification of ventilatory gases is recommended to prevent further drying of damaged airway tissues and to prevent evaporative heat loss. Damaged tracheobronchial mucosa may slough, producing airway obstruction requiring fiberoptic bronchoscopy and lavage for debridement.[16]

Inhalation of carbon monoxide produces further hypoxia in burn patients and is also an indicator of the severity of pulmonary injury.[17] The affinity of carbon monoxide for hemoglobin is 200 times that of oxygen. Breathing 0.1 percent carbon monoxide in room air rapidly produces a 50 percent carbon monoxide level, reducing blood oxygen-carrying capacity by 50 percent.[4] Carbon monoxide also shifts the oxyhemoglobin dissociation curve to the left, further limiting oxygen delivery to tissues. In burn patients, carboxyhemoglobin levels are often measured with other admission laboratory tests. A carboxyhemoglobin level greater than 10 percent is considered a significant elevation, although heavy cigarette smokers may have levels this high.[18] A carboxyhemoglobin level of 40 percent produces unconsciousness.[6] Carboxyhemoglobin levels fall rapidly in the period after injury if the patient is breathing supplemental oxygen. One hour of breathing 100 percent oxygen or 5 hours of breathing room air reduces carboxyhemoglobin levels by 50 percent.[16] If a patient brought to surgery immediately after multiple trauma may have inhaled smoke, it is important to remember that pulse oximeters will not differentiate carboxyhemoglobin from oxyhemoglobin.[19] Transcutaneous oxygen tension ($PtcO_2$) will be low in the presence of high levels of carboxyhemoglobin, reflecting reduced oxygen delivery to tissues; therefore, $PtcO_2$ may be a better continuous monitor of oxygenation for a patient with recent smoke inhalation than pulse oximetry.[18] Arterial PO_2 in the patient with smoke inhalation may be normal. Arterial blood gas analysis showing a measured oxyhemoglobin saturation much lower than expected relative to the measured PO_2 indicates a significant amount of carboxyhemoglobin.[20] Some laboratories calculate oxygen saturation from PO_2 rather than measure it directly, so that the only indicators of carbon monoxide poisoning on blood gas analysis are an acidemia and a base deficit, reflecting failure of oxygen delivery to tissues.[14] The treatment for carbon monoxide inhalation is ventilation with 100 percent oxygen.[6] Most patients with elevated carboxyhemoglobin levels also have elevated levels of cyanide, a combustion product of many materials; however, the half-life of cyanide in the blood is very short, about 1 hour.[17]

Fluid shifts and release of vasoactive substances from burned tissue may produce worsening of pulmonary function intraoperatively or in the immediate postoperative period. Therefore, the patient with unstable oxygenation requiring maximal or near-maximal ventilatory support should have anesthesia and surgery postponed until there is some improvement in pulmonary function.

Fluid Resuscitation of Patients with Burns

Damage to tissues by burning produces an increase in microvascular permeability, allowing movement of large amounts of electrolyte- and protein-containing body fluid into extravascular spaces, resulting in edema. This fluid movement may markedly deplete intravascular volume. Intravenous fluid resuscitation in the early postburn period replenishes intravascular volume, preventing tissue hypoperfusion and death from hypovolemic shock, which in past years was the primary cause of early mortality in patients with large burns.[21] An indwelling urinary catheter is indicated in patients with 20 to 30 percent or larger burns, to monitor volume status as reflected by urine output.

Isotonic, glucose-free crystalloid solutions are most commonly used for resuscitation and are satisfactory for maintenance of intravascular volume, but these solutions readily move out of the vascular space and increase burn edema.[22] Hypertonic saline solutions have been used successfully for resuscitation. Less volume is required than with isotonic solutions as reflected by urine output.[23] Edema of burned and unburned tissues may be reduced by resuscitation with hypertonic saline. Hypernatremia can occur and serum sodium levels should not be allowed to rise over 160 mEq/L.[21] Various colloid solutions have been used as a component of resuscitation with isotonic crystalloids.[24,25] Eight hours after burn injury, infused protein will remain in the intravascular space.[26] Restoration of intravascular protein content may help limit edema in unburned tissues and maintain a stable blood volume.[21]

The presence of an inhalation injury may increase fluid resuscitation requirements up to 50 percent.[27] Some authors

have suggested that commonly used fluid resuscitation formulas lead to excessive fluid administration, which can complicate inhalation injury, and recommend that fluids be given to achieve a urine output of 0.3 to 0.5 mL/kg/h.[7] Fluid requirements of burned children are not easily predicted; therefore, resuscitation of children should be titrated to urine output (1 mL/kg/h) rather than calculated by formula.[2] Two formulas for fluid resuscitation are described in Table 37–1.

Unless the burn patient has other life-threatening injuries requiring urgent surgical intervention, initial fluid resuscitation should be accomplished before induction of anesthesia. The burn patient who requires surgery too soon after injury to allow time for complete fluid resuscitation is likely to be significantly hypovolemic and reduction of vasomotor tone and cardiac output by anesthetic agents may result in profound hypotension. In this situation, rapid fluid administration should continue with induction using agents that support the sympathetic nervous system's responses to hypovolemia.

If the burn patient must undergo immediate surgery, it is useful to calculate estimated fluid requirements; however, surgery will likely increase the rate and volume of fluid required beyond initial estimates. As with other surgical patients, clinical indicators of volume status such as blood pressure, heart rate, and urine output guide fluid administration. Low urine output should be treated with rapid administration of warmed fluid while the patient is observed closely for signs of fluid overload. Diuretics are generally contraindicated for the burn patient.[28]

During fluid resuscitation of burns and prior to anesthesia, invasive monitoring of central venous pressures and potentially cardiac output is indicated if urine output does not improve with generous fluid administration. This is especially important if the patient develops signs of excessive preload or if the patient is elderly or has preexisting cardiovascular dysfunction. Progressive worsening of base deficits may indicate tissue anaerobic metabolism caused by hypoperfusion, from hypovolemia or other causes of low cardiac output. It should be noted that carbon monoxide poisoning also produces metabolic acidosis.[21] Inotropic medications may be required to optimize cardiac function and preserve renal and peripheral perfusion. In the measurement of central pressures, the goal should be a slightly low measured filling pressure combined with satisfactory tissue perfusion indicators such as measured cardiac output, urine output, or base deficit. Administration of fluids beyond that necessary for maintenance of adequate cardiac output increases edema.[22]

TABLE 37–1. FLUID RESUSCITATION OF BURNS

Formula	Solution	Time Postburn 0–8 h	8–24 h
Parkland	Lactated Ringer's	2[a]	2
Brooke	Crystalloid	0.75	0.75
	Colloid	0.25	0.25

[a] All values are expressed as mL/kg/% burn.

Fluid resuscitation after burn injury has not been found to increase lung water significantly in patients without pulmonary injury.[16,29] The risk of pulmonary edema related to fluid overload in the burn patient, with or without pulmonary bone injury, is overshadowed by the risk of hypovolemia and associated tissue hypoperfusion and acidemia. Should pulmonary edema and congestive heart failure present, they should be managed pharmacologically with inotropes and vasodilators and mechanically with positive-pressure ventilation and PEEP. Edema following resuscitation from burns is greatest 18 to 24 hours after injury.[21] Edema in unburned tissues is due to the hypoproteinemia produced by protein loss into the burn wound.[26]

Patients with inhalation injury may require approximately 2 mL/kg more isotonic crystalloid for resuscitation than patients with only cutaneous burns.[16] When the initial 24-hour period of resuscitation is complete, fluid maintenance requirements may be met with 5 percent dextrose in water, 2 mL/kg per %TBSA of burn, with supplemental potassium, 5 to 10 mEq/h. Albumin should be administered to maintain serum levels of 2.0 to 2.5 g/dL.[30]

Hypermetabolism and Sepsis

Burn injury produces a hypermetabolic and hyperdynamic state with large increases in oxygen consumption and cardiac output. Peripheral vascular resistance is low, and arterial pressure is typically normal.[31] This increase in metabolic rate is a characteristic of the burn wound and is not necessarily associated with burn wound sepsis.[32,33] Burn patients have alterations in intestinal permeability that may permit gut bacteria and endotoxins to enter circulation in the immediate postburn period.[34] This endotoxemia, originating in the intestine, has been postulated as the cause of the hypermetabolic state of the burn patient.[35]

Early enteral feedings help maintain the barrier function of the intestinal mucosa and may also attenuate the hypermetabolic response to burns.[36] Recognition of this protective effect has made enteral feeding by duodenal tube the standard method of providing nutritional support to burn patients. The calorie requirements of burn patients in recovery are extremely high and few are able to take in sufficient oral nourishment without supplementation via tube feeding. This high daily caloric intake and other alterations in the metabolism of the burn patient may produce insulin resistance and requirements for insulin supplementation.[37] When enteral and oral feedings are stopped in preparation for surgery, sufficient calories should be provided parenterally and the insulin dose adjusted to need. Preoperative and intraoperative serum glucose levels should be followed carefully, and postoperative enteral feeding resumed as early as possible.

Anesthesia using potent inhalation agents temporarily reduces cardiac output and oxygen consumption in burn patients; however, these will return to the hypermetabolic state after emergence.[31,38] Increased metabolic rates persist even when early excision and grafting of the burn wound are completed.[33,39] As such, the anesthetic care plan should incorporate oxygen concentrations sufficient to maintain adequate oxygen content and saturations.

Other Complications of Thermal Injury

Curling's ulcer, a stress-related gastric ulceration and hemorrhage, was a significant contributor to burn morbidity in the past[20]; however, administration of H$_2$-blocker drugs and antacids and enteral feeding have largely attenuated the incidence of this problem. The anesthetist must always institute appropriate prophylaxis for Curling's ulcer throughout the perioperative period.

Fluid resuscitation with hypotonic crystalloid solutions puts the burn patient at risk for dilutional hyponatremia, and the diuresis that accompanies resolution of edema may produce hypokalemia.[28] Burn patients often have reduced serum levels of total calcium, ionized calcium, and phosphorus and elevated magnesium levels.[40] Total serum hypocalcemia may be related to hypoalbuminemia.[41] Rapid administration of citrated blood products to burn patients has been shown to cause further reductions in ionized calcium levels which may produce hypotension.[42]

Acute cholecystitis,[43,44] pulmonary emboli,[45] rhabdomyolysis,[46] and the syndrome of inappropriate antidiuretic hormone secretion[47] are among the complications reported in burn patients. The understandable tendency to attribute all aspects of a burn patient's dysfunction to the burn wound can prevent correct identification of simultaneous injuries and disease processes, sometimes leading to death from untreated conditions.[48]

General Considerations for Debridement Procedures

Depending on the depth and extent of the burn sustained, debridement procedures can be carried out by the surgeon at the patient's bedside, in specialized treatment rooms with burned areas submerged in large water-filled tanks, or under general anesthesia in specially equipped operating rooms. The purposes of the debridement procedures are to cleanse the wound(s), remove nonviable tissue, and limit the extent of burn injury. Many of these procedures are scheduled within 24 to 48 hours of the acute injury or after initial stabilization of the patient. When general anesthesia is not required for debridement of minor burns, the surgeon or nurse usually administers narcotics or sedatives to patients prior to the procedure to minimize patient discomfort. For more extensive procedures, the administration of intramuscular ketamine may be required. A dose of 4 mg/kg provides about 20 minutes of analgesia, and the dose may be repeated as needed.[49] Ketamine dose requirements may increase over time,[50] as a result of tachyphylaxis.

Sequential tangential excision is well suited to areas of mixed burn depth in that viable dermis can be identified and salvaged during repeated minor debridements. Two to three weeks of weekly or biweekly debridements is usually required before grafting is done, if indicated.[51] Definitive treatment of the deep burn wound is surgical debridement and closure by autograft, homograft, or xenograft, as rapid wound closure improves patient survival.[52,53] Early tangential excision removes all devitalized tissue of deep burns within the first few days of injury, followed by immediate autografting. The procedure is done in the operating room usually under general anesthesia. Early tangential excision may be done for large areas and usually produces large blood losses. Topical thrombin, topical epinephrine, Gelfoam, and collagen pads may be used to limit blood loss.[51] Tourniquets should be used whenever possible.

Limitation of excision procedures to 2 hours, three times per week, is common in an attempt to control blood loss and other stresses associated with longer procedures of this type. A 2-hour procedure was found to permit excision and grafting of a 4.8 percent TBSA[54]; however, Foy et al did not find length of operation to be related to morbidity.[55] Included in this study were 77 procedures lasting an average of 4 hours with a mean excision of 14 percent TBSA, sometimes using two teams of surgeons. Primary excision to fascia involves less hemorrhage but results in a cosmetic defect because of the loss of all subcutaneous tissue.[56] Primary excision to fascia may be indicated in very deep or large burns.[51]

Preparation of the Burn Patient for Surgery

Because of the importance of enteral feeding to the integrity of the gut and prevention of sepsis in the burn patient, NPO (nothing by mouth) time should be kept to a minimum. Some burn centers stop tube feedings only 2 hours before surgery, then place the feeding tube to drainage to empty gastric contents to the extent possible.[54] Although this approach will likely be combined with a modified rapid-sequence induction with a nondepolarizing muscle relaxant and cricoid pressure to protect against aspiration of gastric contents, patients nevertheless remain at high risk for pulmonary aspiration.

Transport of the burn patient to the operating room is potentially hazardous and must be carefully planned. In cases where warranted, the persons transporting the patient should be licensed care providers skilled in airway management techniques and familiar with other unique needs of the burn patient. The patient should be transported with oxygen support systems sufficient to maintain oxygenation, especially if PEEP or continuous positive airway pressure has been used. Appropriate monitoring, especially pulse oximetry, should be continued during transport. Measures to prevent heat loss during transport should be considered, if necessary during protracted periods of transport. Premedication of the burn patient should provide control of the pain associated with moving the patient to the transport bed and onto the operating table. Narcotic analgesics and benzodiazepine anxiolytics are usually effective in doses similar to those being administered on the unit for pain control.[57] The patient's medication record should be reviewed to determine previously effective drug doses. If the patient arrives in the surgical area anxious or in pain, additional drugs should be given intravenously before anything else is done. Once in the operating room, consideration should be given to induction of anesthesia on the transport bed, before movement of the patient to the operating table.

Choice of Anesthetic Agents

Most common anesthetic induction and maintenance drugs in current use for the general surgical population are used in burn patients, subject to indications relative to coexisting medical problems. Etomidate,[58] however, has a relative contraindication for use in critically burned patients because of its property of adrenocortical suppression. As with other critically ill patients, titration of drug and careful monitoring are often as important for skillful anesthetic management as is drug selection.

Total intravenous anesthesia using propofol and alfentanil or fentanyl has been used in burn patients with satisfactory results. These drugs have the theoretical advantage of avoiding the potentially hepatotoxic effects of repeated exposures to halogenated inhalation agents.[59] If a nonnarcotic anesthetic technique is selected for the burn patient, sufficient narcotic should be given at the end of the procedure to provide analgesia when the patient awakens. A long-acting narcotic such as morphine, methadone, or hydromorphone is preferred.

In terms of inhalation agents, isoflurane remains the most popular, as it has less arrhythmogenic potential and fewer metabolites. Halothane is still used as an induction and maintenance agent, as its repetitive use in a large number of patients has not demonstrated an increased incidence of hepatitis.[60] Most practitioners, however, are prone to maintain low concentrations of the agent or switch to isoflurane for maintenance because of halothane's sensitization of the myocardium to catecholamines in the presence of epinephrine-soaked sponges used by the surgeon to control bleeding during debridement. High serum levels of epinephrine may be especially dangerous in patients with a history of hypertension, stroke, myocardial ischemia, or arrhythmias.[61] Adverse effects of epinephrine are usually transient; however, the sponges should be removed and the field irrigated if problems persist. Surgeons often substitute neosynephrine for epinephrine because of this problem.

Ketamine has been widely used for both induction and maintenance of anesthesia in burn cases. Because of its sympathomimetic effects, it may be preferable for use in patients who are at risk for hypotension secondary to the depressant effects of most induction and maintenance agents; however, even ketamine, when used for induction, can produce hypotension in some patients.[62] Emergence reactions after ketamine anesthesia can be reduced by administering moderate doses of benzodiazepine premedicants and by discussing with the patient the possibility of unusual dreams or mood alterations during the emergence period.[63] Induction doses of ketamine range from 1 to 1.5 mg/kg for 30 to 40 minutes of surgical anesthesia. Intramuscular ketamine can be given in the dose range 5 to 7 mg/kg, and maintenance by continuous infusion can be sustained up to 5 to 6 hours with a total dose of 1 to 1.5 g. Ketamine can be administered with oxygen, while the patient breathes spontaneously, as airway reflexes are usually intact in moderate doses. This drug can be supplemented successfully with narcotics or nitrous oxide. Premedication should include an antisialogogue, as salivation is often copious.

The effects of all neuromuscular blocking drugs are altered in the burn patient. Symptomatic, sometimes fatal hyperkalemia has been associated with the administration of succinylcholine, which causes the release of intracellular potassium from damaged cell membranes into extracellular circulation. This phenomenon has been reported in patients with small or large burns from 5 days to 3 months postburn.[64] Because it is not possible to predict with certainty the time of susceptibility to hyperkalemia, succinylcholine should not be given to patients with a significant acute burn. Likewise its use is contraindicated in infected burns or other acute trauma, especially that including suspected spinal cord involvement, a major breech of muscle mass, or infection.[65]

Nondepolarizing neuromuscular blocking drugs have a reduced potency in the burn patient. Resistance to neuromuscular block begins 6 to 7 days after burn injury and is more intense with larger burns, especially those greater than 20 percent TBSA.[66,67] This resistance is thought to be attributable to a proliferation in acetylcholine receptor density after burns. Atracurium 0.5 mg/kg produced a mean twitch depression of 66.1 percent in burn patients. In normal controls, this dose completely abolished the twitch response.[68]

When rapid-sequence induction is indicated, high doses (3 × ED95) of nondepolarizing neuromuscular blockers can be used to produce intubating conditions in less than 2 minutes.[69] The use of large doses of atracurium has the potential to produce hypotension related to histamine release; however, doses of atracurium that cause hypotension in nonburn surgical patients have not been found to alter blood pressure in burn patients.[70] Vecuronium has been studied in burned children and the effective doses are listed in Table 37–2.[71]

Regional anesthesia of all types can be used for procedures involving both donor and grafting sites. Regional anesthesia may be performed with or without general analgesia or anesthesia and has the advantage of providing postoperative analgesia.[72] Epidural and spinal anesthesia have the potential to produce hypotension in the immediate postburn period in patients who have not completed fluid resuscitation or have other causes of hypovolemia.[73]

Monitoring

The anesthetist must be resourceful in securing satisfactory intraoperative monitoring of the patient with a large burn. Surface electrodes may not function well over burned and edematous tissue and may need to be replaced with needle electrodes for electrocardiogram and twitch monitoring. An indwelling urinary catheter is essential for intraoperative monitoring of volume status as reflected by urine output.

TABLE 37–2. EFFECTIVE DOSES OF VECURONIUM IN PEDIATRIC PATIENTS WITH THERMAL INJURY

Percentage Burn	ED50 (µg/kg)	ED95 (µg/kg)
Controls	18	35
< 40% burn	34	68*
40–60% burn	55	111*
> 60% burn	65	129*

* P < 0.001 compared with controls.
Reprinted, with permission, from Mills and Martyn.[71]

Pulse oximetry is a satisfactory sole monitor of oxygenation during anesthesia in patients who have an unobstructed monitoring site and otherwise have no pulmonary dysfunction; however, constriction of extremities by burn eschar and edema or vasoconstriction resulting from hypothermia may limit the usefulness of the peripheral pulse oximeter as a monitor of total body oxygenation.[74] A warming pad wrapped around the extremity used for oximetry may improve the pulse signal.[75] Anesthesia equipment for the burn patient should include a full range of oximetry probes for ear, nasal bridge, and digits. Some disposable wraparound digit probes can be adapted for use on the ear.[76] The tongue has also been used as a site for pulse oximetry.[77] The pulse oximeter may also be helpful for evaluation of local tissue blood flow and need for escharotomy in potentially ischemic burned extremities.[78] In patients with pulmonary dysfunction, pulse oximetry provides important moment-to-moment information that can be used in conjunction with data obtained from arterial blood gas analysis.[79] Patients with known or suspected pulmonary burn injury or preexisting pulmonary disease should have intraoperative arterial blood gas monitoring as well as pulse oximetry.

Indirect measurement of blood pressure may be difficult in the burn patient. If blood pressure measurement via cuff methods is unsatisfactory, an arterial line should be placed before induction of anesthesia, but only after consideration that insertion of the line may provoke further problems with infection. Burn injury produces immune suppression and sepsis is a common cause of death in the burn patient.[80,81] The line should be placed using sterile technique and should not be placed through burned tissue, if other sites are available. As most excision and grafting procedures involve significant blood loss, at least one large-bore venous access site is always required.

Elderly patients and patients with cardiovascular problems may be managed most safely with a central venous pressure or pulmonary artery line, or both; however, when high levels of PEEP and high inspiratory pressures are required to maintain adequate oxygenation, elevated intrathoracic pressure may limit the usefulness of pulmonary artery occlusion pressure and central venous pressure as indicators of volume status. Martyn et al have advocated the use of a pulmonary artery catheter altered to permit thermodilution measurement of end-diastolic right ventricular volume and ejection fraction, which are unaffected by changes in intrathoracic pressure and ventricular compliance.[82,83] Disconnecting the patient from the ventilator to permit repeated measurements of vascular pressures is not recommended, as it may result in alveolar collapse and acute deterioration in oxygenation which may not be immediately reversible.

Surgical assistance may be needed to place peripheral and central lines in the burned patient; therefore, these lines should be identified to the surgeon before the start of operation. Each patient must be evaluated carefully to decide if invasive monitoring and lines for volume replacement should be placed before or after induction of anesthesia. The potential of the patient to become unstable during induction of anesthesia is the determining factor in the timing of line placement. Most patients without major cardiopulmonary dysfunction can have lines placed after induction and this may be preferable for patient comfort.

Intraoperative Replacement of Blood Components

Initial hematocrits are usually high in the burn patient, reflecting hemoconcentration caused by fluid shifts from the intravascular space. Red cell infusions are rarely if ever indicated in the immediate postburn period. In the first few days after the burn, loss of thermally injured red cells, blood loss during debridement, wound cleansing, dressing changes, and frequent blood sampling contribute to anemia in the burn patient. There is also evidence that the blood serum of burn patients contains a substance that inhibits erythropoiesis, limiting the capacity to replace lost red cell mass.[84] Although it is rarely possible to avoid transfusing the patient with a major burn, it is worth remembering that each additional unit of blood transfused represents an additional risk to the patient. Because blood loss can occur quickly, equipment for rapid replacement with large volumes of warmed crystalloid, colloid, and blood products must be set up prior to need. Two or more fluid warmers and pressure infusion devices should be ready. Availability of red cells and other blood components must be ascertained before the start of debridement.

In a study involving 20 patients with less than 40 percent burn undergoing a total of 36 operations, Burdge et al found that each procedure lasted an average of 2.25 hours, required 2 units of packed cells, and grafted 8 percent of TBSA.[3] In Cullen and colleagues' study of nine patients with an average burn of 46 percent TBSA, excision of a mean of 17 percent TBSA resulted in a loss of 64 percent of calculating blood volume.[85] In longer operations described by Foy et al, a mean of 14 percent TBSA was excised and grafted, requiring an average of 5 units of whole blood and 2.7 L of crystalloid.[56] In pediatric patients with greater than 30 percent burns, Desai at al reported that excision procedures between postburn days 2 and 16 involved an average blood loss of 0.75 mL/cm^2 (0.75 mL/cm^2 body surface area excised), but procedures done before day 2 or after day 16 produced blood loss of only 0.40 mL/cm^2.[57] The reduced blood loss during procedures in the early postburn period was probably due to the normal homeostatic mechanism of vasoconstriction present after acute burn injury.[57] Blood loss during surgery can be reduced by such measures as topical thrombin and epinephrine,[61] infusion of vasopressin,[86] and use of extremity tourniquets followed by compression dressings to extremity graft sites.[87]

In the first few days after burn injury, platelet, fibrinogen, and coagulation factors may be reduced.[88] In patients scheduled for tangential excision who were at least 7 days postburn, Cullen et al found significantly elevated preoperative levels of platelets, fibrinogen, and factor VIII. In this study, burn patients maintained normal platelet and fibrinogen levels even after intraoperative replacement of their entire red cell mass with transfused packed red cells. A control group of nonburn surgical patients had subnormal platelet and fibrinogen levels after about 75 percent red cell mass replacement.[85] Burn patients may be less likely than other surgical patients to require intraoperative administration of platelets and fresh-frozen plasma. The anesthetist should usually defer administering these blood components until indicated by objective measures, that is, platelet count, prothrombin time/partial thromboplastin time, fibrinogen levels, or excessive bleeding in the surgical field.[89]

Intraoperative Temperature Maintenance

Every possible means must be used to maintain normothermia of the burn patient, starting before the patient enters the operating room. Heat loss by evaporation from burned and debrided body surfaces can rapidly produce severe hypothermia in the burn patient. Warden et al found that 51 percent of patients undergoing debridement and grafting procedures lasting 120 minutes or longer had a postoperative temperature of less than 35C, although warming measures were taken.[90] The operating room should be warmed to 28 to 32C and an operating room table warming pad should be allowed to reach the preset temperature before patient transfer. Portable overhead heat lamps may be used to warm the patient prior to the start of surgery and should be constructed such that they can be used effectively during the procedure. Exposed body parts, not in the surgical field, should be wrapped to prevent heat loss. A clear plastic bag over the patient's skull is a useful insulator that does not interfere with observation of the patient's face. Passive heat and moisture exchangers combined with a low gas flow rate (3 L/min) have been shown to reduce the rate of heat loss in adult surgical patients.[91] Active warming and humidification of airway gases should be used for all burn patients, as this method can prevent hypothermia during anesthesia and surgery and may also be used to rewarm hypothermic patients.[92]

All fluids and blood components administered to burn patients intraoperatively should be warmed. Effective use of fluid warmers requires appreciation that warmed fluids will rapidly return to room temperature if there is a long section of tubing between the fluid warmer and the patient, especially if the flow rate is less than 30 mL/min.[93] Using high flow rates, employing a minimal length of tubing between the warmer and the patient, and wrapping the tubing between the warmer and the patient with cloth, plastic, or other insulating material improve the effectiveness of fluid warmers.[94]

Prevention of Positioning Injuries

Patients with burns of the face or severe facial edema should have frequent eye care with artificial tears or ointment and the eyes and ears should be inspected often for pressure points. The burned patient is positioned with extreme care to avoid loss of critical invasive lines and to prevent pressure on burned and recently grafted areas. At times, the distance between donor and graft sites requires considerable moving of the patient during the procedure. The usual precautions taken to prevent injury, including visual inspection, padding of potential pressure points, and palpation of pulses, must not be omitted when the patient is repositioned intraoperatively. If a positioning injury does occur, diagnosis may be difficult because of the many other causes of pain and dysfunction in the burn patient.[95]

Principles of Pain Management Outside the Operating Room

The anesthetist may serve as a member of the burn intensive care team to assist in the management of patients who are experiencing pain and agitation.[72] For instance, therapy for the agitated patient who struggles against the ventilator should first include adequate pain control. If administration of a sufficient quantity of analgesics does not improve patient compliance or result in clinical signs of pain relief, sedative-hypnotic drugs may be added. Midazolam by infusion may be used to facilitate mechanical ventilation without paralytic drugs.[96] Ketamine has also been used for sedation in the mechanically ventilated patient who may also benefit from the inotropic and bronchodilatory effects of this drug.[97] Etomidate should not be used as a sedative infusion because it produces adrenocortical suppression and has been reported to increase mortality among critically ill patients.[98] Sedative and analgesic drugs should be used cautiously in the hypovolemic immediate postburn period and at any time when vasodilation could produce cardiovascular instability.[73]

Adequate pain control and sedation usually facilitates an acceptable mechanical ventilatory pattern.[99] Use of paralytic drugs is required only in a small number of patients to reduce airway pressures and permit optimal oxygenation by mechanical ventilation. Paralytic drugs should be given in the minimum effective dosage and must never be administered without concomitant use of analgesics and sedatives,[73] as the unjudicious use of paralytics without benefit of amnestic agents has been reported in the literature.[100] The need for continued use of paralytic drugs should be reassessed every few hours.

The most significant impediment to effective pain control for the burn patient is the wide variation in degree of pain experienced and the individual variations in the response to analgesic drugs. Administration of safe and effective analgesic doses of narcotic requires time to make careful observations of the patient's condition and titrate the drug to effect. Drugs should be administered only after careful attention is given to the patient's state of hydration and proper central nervous system function so as not to precipitate hypotension or mask untoward signs of hypoxemia. Narcotics should never be withheld in the acute burn phase for fear of addiction.

Choiniere et al found that burn patients reported the pain of burn treatments such as dressing changes and wound cleansing to be more painful than the initial burn injury, even though they had received morphine prior to treatments.[101] Subjective pain scores, amount of analgesic medication received, and days postburn were all unrelated to requirements for pain relief. Patients with larger areas of first- and second-degree burns had more pain, an expected finding as third-degree or full-thickness burns destroy nerve endings and are classically described as painless. After the first week, however, severity of burn was not related to the amount of pain reported by the patients.

A number of methods of analgesic administration have been used in burn patients, including continuous infusion of narcotics.[72,102,103] Patient-controlled analgesia (PCA) using intravenous morphine has been reported.[104] In this study, as in studies of nurse-administered prn narcotics,[101] there was no relationship between burn size or body weight and narcotic requirements. In nonburn patients suffering postoperative pain, PCA produced high-quality pain control without the time lag and anxiety associated with waiting for a dose of analgesic to be administered and take effect.[105] The improved individualization of drug dosage that PCA permits is attractive for use in the burn patient. When intermittent analgesic dosing is used, contracting with patients to allow them more control over the timing and amount of analgesic administered may help ease patients' feelings of helplessness.[106] Pain and anxiety in burn patients may also be reduced by such nonpharmacologic interventions as hypnosis.[107] Narcotic analgesia may be supplemented with regional techniques in some patients. Continuous axillary block has been reported to provide satisfactory analgesia and motor block to facilitate success of hand grafting,[108] and epidural block may sometimes be useful for burn pain management.[72] Range-of-motion exercises help prevent contracture formation but can be limited by extreme pain produced in the burn wound. One center reported an increase in shoulder range of motion when exercises were done with the patient under anesthesia, just before operations for debridement and grafting.[109]

Anesthetic Conditions during Rehabilitation Phases

Safe airway management for the patient with limited neck or jaw mobility as a result of burn scar contracture requires careful preoperative assessment. Spraying the posterior pharynx and tongue with local anesthetic often permits brief direct laryngoscopy to be done at the time of the preanesthetic examination. If the glottis can be visualized, the patient can safely have a standard induction, provided the patient does not have tracheal stenosis. If the glottis is not seen during awake direct laryngoscopy, the airway should be approached conservatively and intubation accomplished awake with local anesthesia using a fiberoptic bronchoscope[110] or a lightwand.[111,112]

Attempts to place an endotracheal tube blindly in patients with burn scar contractures of the mouth and neck may produce bleeding in the airway with disastrous results. Blind attempts at awake nasotracheal intubation should be preceded by thorough application of topical vasoconstrictors and should be made with the utmost caution to avoid tissue injury.

An alternate safe approach to intubation of the patient with severe burn contractures of the neck and mouth requires preinduction release of the contractures in the operating room using local anesthesia.[113] Release of the contracting scar improves the chance of successful intubation but does not guarantee it; therefore, local anesthesia of the airway followed by awake laryngoscopy is still the recommended procedure after the scar has been incised.

The patient who has recovered from an airway injury may have tracheal stenosis as a result of scarring from the tracheal burn, from prolonged intubation, or from tracheostomy.[114,115] Stenoses are usually limited to the area just below the glottis but may occasionally involve the carina and mainstem bronchi.[116] Partial airway obstruction may develop early or late in the postburn period. Consequently, the patient should be questioned about any history or dyspnea on exertion or difficulty with respiratory secretions. Preoperative evaluation by tracheal radiograph, computed tomography scan, fiberoptic laryngoscopy, or inspiratory and expiratory flow–volume curves may be indicated.[117,118] If tracheal stenosis has not been ruled out, awake fiberoptic intubation is safest for these patients. Small endotracheal tubes should be available, as should equipment for emergency cricothyrotomy and tracheostomy.

Future advances in burn wound care will be made in the areas of improved resuscitation techniques, infection control, and early wound coverage. Measurement of serum levels of a lung hormone, immunoreactive calcitonin, may allow early screening for pulmonary burn injury without bronchoscopy.[119] Use of erythropoietin to increase red cell production may reduce the need for transfusion in burn patients, and cultured autologous epithelial tissue may be used to cover wounds in patients with extensive burns who have little available donor skin.[120,121] In addition, active participation in the care of burn patients by anesthesia providers will bring the newest pharmacologic and monitoring advances to enhance patient care and control pain.

ANESTHESIA FOR PLASTIC SURGERY

Preoperative Evaluation of the Patient

Operations to correct deformities or to improve physical appearance and function are undertaken in a variety of surgical settings. Today, most plastic surgery is done on an outpatient basis, whether in hospitals, surgery centers, or surgeon's offices. The plastic surgery patient receives the same preoperative evaluation as other types of surgical patients with similar risk factors. The patient may be interviewed initially by telephone or may visit a preoperative anesthesia clinic to be screened for any history of problems that would require further evaluation prior to surgery. Women of childbearing age should be informed about possible risks of anesthesia to the fetus and their acceptance of such risks should be documented on the patient record. The majority of plastic surgery patients can safely be anesthetized outside the hospital setting, but any potential for major perioperative problems must be carefully assessed. Nonhospital surgical facilities often limit themselves to American Society of Anesthesiologists (ASA) class 1 or 2 patients.[122,123]

Autologous Blood Banking

Some plastic procedures, particularly suction lipectomy and reduction mammoplasty, may involve substantial blood loss. Blood loss during suction lipectomy is estimated to be 20 percent of the tissue aspirated.[124] In patients undergoing reduction mammoplasty, the average blood loss is about 900 mL.[125,126] Moderate blood loss in this range is usually well tolerated and transfusion of donor blood is not indicated.[127] Losses of over 2000 mL have been suggested as a criterion for transfusion,[128] although this will be variable across patients. The risks of transfusion of donor blood are usually unacceptable for most elective plastic procedures

and can be reduced by the use of autologous blood. Autologous blood is not risk free, as there is always the slight possibility of contamination or of clerical error. Also, the cost of autologous donation is rarely justified for most plastic procedures by the small chance that a transfusion will be needed. Use of autologous blood may, however, permit two procedures, such as suction lipectomy and reduction mammoplasty, to be done on the same day, reducing the risk to the patient from a second anesthetic.[129]

Patients undergoing a procedure associated with significant blood loss should be informed of the possibility of mild symptoms of anemia postoperatively and the risks and benefits of autologous donation should be described. A simple, risk-free way to reduce symptomatic postoperative anemia in female premenopausal patients is to treat iron deficiency anemia preoperatively.[130] Similarly, any patient who makes an autologous donation should receive iron supplementation and preferably have enough time to return to a normal hematocrit after the donation.

The day before surgery the patient should be contacted for reinstruction about their NPO status and any medications to be taken on the morning of surgery. Oral diazepam is a popular premedication for outpatient plastic surgery.[122,131] The patient may be instructed to take the medications at home provided she or he will not be driving. It should never be assumed that the patient already knows what to do either before or after the operation. All instructions should be explicit, preferably in writing, and reinforced verbally at every opportunity.[124] Failure to do so exposes the patient to risk of injury and the anesthetist and surgeon to liability. On arrival at the surgical facility, the anesthetist should reconfirm the NPO status, conduct a complete head and neck exam for intubation problems, auscultate the chest, and assess vital signs.

Intravenous Sedation

Intravenous sedation for plastic surgery under local anesthesia is not a simple or casual undertaking for the anesthetist. Expert intravenous sedation should provide the patient with a safe, pain-free, anxiety-free surgical experience. From the surgeon's point of view, the ideal may be a motionless, silent patient who follows commands, maintains a clear airway, and has a rapid, trouble-free recovery. Meticulous attention to the patient's response to drugs is the only way to produce the conditions desired by both patient and surgeon.

Midazolam has largely replaced diazepam as a component of intravenous sedation, primarily because of midazolam's shorter half-life,[132] reduced incidence of pain and inflammation at the injection site,[133] and greater amnestic effects.[134] For intravenous sedation, the total dose given is about 0.1 mg/kg, titrated in small increments throughout the procedure.[132] Midazolam is often combined with ketamine to produce a brief period of profound analgesia while the operative area is injected with local anesthetic. Midazolam markedly reduces both the cardiovascular and the psychologic adverse responses to ketamine.[134] The initial doses used are 0.03 to 0.075 mg/kg for midazolam and 0.5 to 1.0 mg/kg for ketamine, followed by additional small doses as needed during the procedure.[122,134] Glycopyrrolate may be used to prevent the increase in salivation associated with ketamine.[135] Intravenous glycopyrrolate should be given 10 to 15 minutes before administration of ketamine to be effective.

Ketamine provides the advantage of producing less relaxation of upper airway structures than other agents at a comparable depth of anesthesia.[136] This property of ketamine allows the anesthetist to safely refrain from manipulating the head and neck to relieve airway obstruction while the surgeon is injecting local anesthetic into facial structures or operating on the face. In reports of large series of patients who received benzodiazepine premedication, a single dose of ketamine for analgesia during injection of local anesthetic was associated with a low or near-zero incidence of the unpleasant psychomimetic emergence reactions often attributed to ketamine anesthesia.[122,136–138] In diazepam-premedicated patients, Korttila et al found that ketamine 0.5 mg/kg produced no adverse effects; however, ketamine 1.5 and 3.0 mg/kg were associated with some postoperative anxiety and confusion.[139] Patients occasionally recall dreaming, sometimes colorfully, after receiving ketamine.[122,131,136,137] Patients should be informed preoperatively that they may remember dreams caused by this medication. Ketamine 0.5 mg/kg may also be preceded by small doses of methohexital to produce a brief period of sleep and profound analgesia. Methohexital attenuates dreaming produced by ketamine, and the ketamine increases upper airway tone and prevents airway obstruction caused by methohexital.

Administration of ketamine may be hazardous to some patients. Contraindications to ketamine are listed in Table 37–3. The cardiovascular stimulation caused by ketamine can be further augmented by absorption of epinephrine, and this combination has been associated with tachycardia, arrhythmia, and hypertension.[140] Glauber et al found the incidence of ventricular arrhythmias after IV ketamine and subcutaneous lidocaine with epinephrine to be 1.3 percent.[141] Hypertension resulting from intraoperative ketamine administration may increase bleeding, especially from mucosal surfaces, if epinephrine is not used to produce vasoconstriction. The bronchodilatory effects of ketamine make it a good choice for the patient with a history of bronchospastic disease.[63]

If it is desirable to avoid the use of ketamine, analgesia can be produced with narcotics. The disadvantages of narcotics include cardiovascular and respiratory depression and an increased incidence of nausea and vomiting.

TABLE 37–3. CONTRAINDICATIONS TO KETAMINE

Coronary artery disease
Congestive heart failure
Hypertension
Aneurysms
Cerebral vascular disease
Elevated intracranial pressure
Seizure disorder
Psychiatric disorder
Elevated intraocular pressure
Hyperthyroidism

Fentanyl has been combined with lorazepam[142] and with midazolam[131] to produce satisfactory sedation and analgesia for cosmetic procedures done with local anesthesia. The short-acting narcotic alfentanil may offer advantages over fentanyl in that a relatively large dose may be given for brief periods of strong stimulus, such as the initial injection of local, without producing excessive narcosis that lasts longer than the stimulus. Alfentanil 3 to 7 µg/kg given after a small dose of midazolam produces excellent analgesia for injection of local anesthesia for eye surgery, with the advantage that the patient remains responsive to command. Low-dose alfentanil (0.25 to 0.5 µg/kg/min) can be administered by infusion to produce a constant level of sedation and analgesia with a rapid recovery after the infusion is terminated. Like other narcotics, the effective dosage range of alfentanil is wide and dosage must be individualized. Alfentanil clearance is unrelated to body weight, choice of induction agent, duration of anesthesia, or use of inhalation agent.[143] In addition, there is large individual variation in alfentanil pharmacokinetics.[144]

A number of other drugs have been used for sedation of plastic surgery patients, including droperidol, various barbiturates, benzodiazepines, antihistamines, and phenothiazines.[145] A characteristic of many of these less frequently used agents is long duration of action, which may be an advantage only for lengthy procedures. Successful management of intravenous sedation requires precise drug selection and titration, with constant attention to the patient's responses. A precordial stethoscope is a very useful and sensitive monitor of the level of patient arousal because it allows the anesthetist to listen to rate and depth of respiration, detect swallowing, and note preliminary signs of airway obstruction.

Use of Epinephrine-Containing Solutions

A large amount of local anesthetic with epinephrine is often injected subcutaneously for plastic procedures. Transient tachycardia, sometimes with hypertension or arrhythmia, is often seen.[146] As an epinephrine-containing solution is injected subcutaneously, there is an initial brief period of systemic absorption, followed by local vasoconstriction which limits further absorption.[147] Attempts to treat tachycardia, hypertension, or arrhythmia caused by epinephrine absorption may result in the administration of a drug that takes effect after the epinephrine effect has ended, putting the patient at risk for iatrogenic hypotension or bradycardia. If the patient has risk factors such as dysrhythmia, coronary artery disease, or cerebral vascular disease that make epinephrine-induced tachycardia or hypertension hazardous, pretreatment with small amounts of an ultrashort-acting beta blockers may be considered, but the safest course is to avoid the use of epinephrine. Phenylephrine 1 : 50,000 has been recommended as a local vasoconstrictor for patients with contraindications to epinephrine. Onset of vasoconstriction is somewhat slower than for epinephrine, 15 to 20 minutes after injection.[148] Although tachycardia and arrhythmias are not produced by phenylephrine, it is a powerful vasoconstrictor that can produce a longer-lasting hypertensive response than epinephrine.[147]

Even with doses of local anesthetic in excess of recommended maximums, symptomatic local anesthetic toxicity is rare.[141] Gumucio et al studied patients under general anesthesia for augmentation mammoplasty who received an average of 8.5 mg/kg lidocaine with epinephrine. Serum lidocaine levels did not exceed 1 μg/mL.[149] Toxic effects were seen at 5 μg/mL or higher doses.[147,150] Although rare, toxicity resulting from absorption from subcutaneous sites may be prolonged compared with that associated with intravenous injection. A usual adult dose of local anesthetic may be toxic to a small child and maximal doses should be calculated for children to avoid overdosage.[151]

Regional Anesthesia

Intravenous regional anesthesia and brachial plexus blocks may be used for procedures on the hand and arm. Intravenous regional anesthesia has a very low complication rate and is a good choice for outpatients. Brachial plexus block has a higher incidence of complications but its use has been reported for outpatients in nonhospital settings without problems.[124] If the length of the procedure permits, choice of a short-acting local anesthetic for outpatients permits documentation of return of neuromuscular function before the patient goes home, without delaying discharge. This is desirable to prevent undetected residual deficits in the extremity.

Epidural anesthesia using a T-4 approach has been found satisfactory for outpatient submuscular breast augmentation.[152] The potential for dural puncture and the additional risks presented by a thoracic approach best limit this technique to the hospital setting and to those who have sufficient experience to minimize the likelihood of needle misplacement.

General Anesthesia

Although procedures on the trunk may be managed with or without an endotracheal tube, facial plastic procedures require intubation. Procedures in or around the oral cavity, maxillary and mandibular osteotomies, and some chin and neck procedures may require a nasotracheal tube.

Barbiturate induction followed by inhalation anesthesia allows for easy maintenance of spontaneous ventilation, an advantage in nonhospital settings where a mechanical ventilator may not be available. Methohexital is more rapidly metabolized and permits a more rapid recovery than thiopental.[153] Avoiding narcotics as a component of the anesthetic may reduce the incidence of postoperative nausea and vomiting. Because local anesthetics are often injected into the operative area, even when the patient is under general anesthesia, the patient may not need intraoperative narcotics to control pain in the immediate postoperative period.

Nonbarbiturate intravenous agents such as propofol and narcotics may be used for induction and maintenance of anesthesia with nitrous oxide or with low doses of potent inhalation agents. Administration of intravenous agents by infusion rather than intermittent bolus is recommended, because infusion reduces dose requirements and permits faster emergence and earlier readiness for discharge.[154,155] Emergence from propofol–nitrous oxide anesthesia is faster than pentothal–nitrous oxide or methohexital–nitrous oxide, although propofol produces more apnea and hypotension during induction.[156–158]

Fluid Administration

For procedures that involve substantial blood loss, such as reduction mammoplasty and suction lipectomy of large areas, it is advantageous to replace the patient's fluid deficit from fasting early in the operation. This reduces the likelihood of hypotension and tachycardia when rapid blood loss begins. Estimated blood losses should be replaced with crystalloid in the usual 3 : 1 ratio. Prior to suction lipectomy, it is important that the surgeon and anesthetist discuss preoperatively the amount of fat anticipated to be taken, so there is no disagreement about the acceptable blood loss. Some surgeons limit the amount of aspirated fat to 3000 mL during a single procedure. If the aspirated material is considered to be 20 percent blood, then the anticipated blood loss is 600 mL.[124]

Lengthy procedures under intravenous sedation call for more measured administration of fluids to prevent the patient from having a full bladder early in the operative course. A full bladder can cause the patient to be restless and uncomfortable and may even produce alterations in vital signs such as hypertension.[159] Attempts to overcome the powerful stimulus of a full bladder by administration of sedative and analgesic drugs may result in overdosage of the patient. Procedures such as rhytidectomy may involve steady but relatively slow bleeding over several hours. Therefore, it is reasonable to replace blood loss as it occurs. When long procedures are done in the office under general anesthesia, the patient may have a smoother emergence and be more comfortable in the immediate postoperative period if the bladder is emptied while the patient is still unconscious. A full bladder should always be part of the differential diagnosis of a restless, hypertensive patient who is heavily sedated or emerging from general anesthesia.

Occasionally an unexpected amount of bleeding occurs in areas injected with epinephrine-containing solutions. Epinephrine is readily degraded by air, light, and alkaline solutions.[147] For optimal vasoconstriction, it is recommended that epinephrine be added to local anesthetic solutions just prior to use.[159]

Equipment Requirements in the Office Setting

Standards for administration of anesthesia in a surgeon's private operating room are not different from standards in hospital operating rooms. Whenever gas mixtures are administered, an oxygen analyzer should be in service. ECG, blood pressure, breath sounds, and oxygen saturation should be monitored. End-tidal carbon dioxide analysis is desirable. Core temperature monitoring should be available. Unless only very brief procedures are to be done, the facility should stock equipment for catheterization of the bladder.

Plastic surgery of the head and neck under local anesthesia with intravenous sedation is unusual as it is often done without the provision of supplemental oxygen to the patient, permitting the surgeon full access to the area.

The sedated patient breathing room air is at greater risk of hypoxemia than the patient receiving supplemental oxygen and the pulse oximeter has added greatly to the safety of this type of anesthesia care. Transient hypoxemia is common during intravenous sedation of patients breathing room air. In studies by Singer and Thomas, 61 of 100 patients studied had saturations of less than 95 percent for 1 to 2 minutes, corrected by instructing the patient to breathe deeply. Sixteen had longer desaturations, usually corrected by chin lift, three required oral or nasal airways to maintain a saturation above 95 percent, and none were given supplemental oxygen.[160] The pulse oximeter allows detection of early desaturation, provides feedback on effectiveness of corrective measures, and prevents continued administration of sedation to a hypoxic patient who may exhibit restlessness as a symptom of poor oxygenation. Patients having cosmetic surgery of the head and neck under local anesthesia with intravenous sedation who are at risk for cerebral or myocardial ischemia should have supplemental oxygen, minimal sedation, or both to prevent hypoxemic episodes.

If general anesthesia is not planned, it is not necessary to have an anesthesia machine in the area where intravenous sedation will be administered. It is, however, necessary to have all equipment for resuscitation available, including airways, endotracheal intubation equipment, ventilating bag and masks, suction, defibrillator, and all drugs commonly used for advanced cardiac life support protocols. It is the anesthetist's responsibility to ensure readiness of this equipment as well as preparedness to solely undertake resuscitation of the patient outside the hospital setting.

Recovery from intravenous sedation or general anesthesia for cosmetic surgery may be conducted in the operating room itself or in a separate room equipped with similar monitors and emergency equipment in close proximity. Until the patient is free of serious risks related to the residual effects of the sedation or anesthesia, the anesthetist or a registered nurse should continually observe the patient. It is not within the standards of anesthetic care to conduct an anesthetic while observing another recovering patient, to conduct two simultaneous procedures requiring sedation or anesthesia, to require an operating room nurse to observe a recovering patient while also circulating or performing other duties, or to use nonnurse personnel to staff recovery areas. Until the patient is ready for discharge into the care of a responsible adult, the anesthetist is responsible for the safety of the patient.

Patients are ready for discharge when they can easily maintain an awake state, can ambulate with minimal assistance, and their vital signs are stable. If the patient is experiencing severe pain, small amounts of intravenous analgesics may be titrated until the pain is tolerable. Excessive pain medication is a hazard to the outpatient because it may prevent the patient from seeking assistance if a complication such as a hematoma develops. Mild oral analgesics are usually sufficient at home for most types of surgery.[124]

Amnesia produced by benzodiazepines and other drugs is desirable to prevent recall of unpleasant stimuli but may also prevent recall of postoperative instructions.[132,161] Postoperative instructions to outpatients should be given verbally and in writing to the person who will be caring for the patient in the 24-hour period following surgery. The anesthetist should contact the patient by telephone a few hours after discharge to check for the appearance of any late complications of anesthesia and to reinforce postoperative instructions.

For patients who need postoperative observation or assistance beyond that easily provided in the patient's home, there are several options. Some office surgical facilities have an area that can accommodate an overnight stay by a postoperative patient and a nurse.[162] Alternatively, the patient and nurse may lodge overnight in a nearby hotel. Some communities have specialized facilities that provide overnight nursing care to the plastic surgery patient at a cost below that of a night in the hospital.

Postoperative hospital admission may be warranted by the need to observe the surgical area closely in the immediate postoperative period, as for procedures involving grafts. Other indications for postoperative admission of the cosmetic surgery patient include a history of medical problems, such as poorly controlled diabetes mellitus or angina, or the occurrence of unexpected intraoperative or postoperative problems.

Intraoperative and Postoperative Complications

Venous air embolism resulting in cardiovascular collapse has been reported during elevation of a scalp flap in a child[163] and during mastectomy.[164] It is important to remain aware of the possibility of major intraoperative complications even among healthy patients undergoing "superficial" procedures. Phenol applied to the skin for chemical peeling is systemically absorbed and can produce cardiac arrhythmias.[165,166] Procedures involving osteotomies and wiring of the maxilla or mandible may damage the endotracheal tube intraoperatively.[167–169] The surgeon, while moving the patient's head, may inadvertently extubate the patient. The anesthetist must always be prepared to deal with emergent problems.

Patients undergoing reconstructive procedures of the head and neck with large pectoralis myocutaneous flaps have been found to have an increased incidence of postoperative pulmonary atelectasis, possibly related to chest constriction and pain in the area of the flap donor site.[170] Atelectasis may also complicate augmentation and reduction mammoplasty, mastopexy, and breast reconstruction.[124] Preoperative instruction in inspiratory exercises and adequate postoperative analgesia may help reduce this problem.

The most common postoperative problems of concern to the anesthetist are nausea and vomiting. Vomiting can increase edema and bleeding in operative areas, damaging the cosmetic result. A patient who is vomiting is not ready for discharge. Occasionally, intractable vomiting may require overnight admission to the hospital. An effective method to reduce nausea and vomiting in plastic surgery patients is to avoid using narcotics as a component of the sedation or anesthesia administered.[145] Emptying the stomach prior to emergence of patients from general anesthesia eliminates the emetic stimulus of gastric distension by air or nitrous oxide. Small doses of droperidol (0.625 mg) have a long lasting prophylactic antiemetic effect.[171] Metoclopramide is an effective antiemetic agent, but has a short duration of action. It should be given before emergence for best effect after a general anesthetic.[172]

If vomiting occurs, it may be treated with intravenous droperidol, metoclopramide, or one of the phenothiazine antiemetics. If the intravenous access has already been removed, an antiemetic suppository, prochlorperazine or trimethobenzamide, may be given. The anesthetist should be cautioned that dysphoria and extrapyramidal side effects may occur with antiemetic drugs. Diphenhydramine appears to be a useful treatment for these side effects.

REFERENCES

1. Alexander JW. Burn care: A specialty in evolution. 1985 Presidential Address, American Burn Association. *J Trauma.* 1986;26:1–6.

2. Herndon DN, Curreri PW, Abston S, Rutan TC, Barrow RE. Treatment of burns. *Curr Probl Surg.* 1987;24:341–397.

3. Burdge JJ, Katz B, Edwards R, Ruberg R. Surgical treatment of burns in elderly patients. *J Trauma.* 1988;28:214–217.

4. Herndon DN, Thompson PB, Traber DL. Pulmonary injury in burned patients. *Crit Care Clin.* 1985;1:79–96.

5. Vanacker B, Boeckx W, van Aken H, Gruwez JA. Current concepts of inhalation injury in burn victims. *Acta Anesthesiol Belg.* 1989;40:107–111.

6. Heimback DM, Waeckerle JF. Inhalation injuries. *Ann Emerg Med.* 1988;17:1316–1320.

7. Edlich RF, Nichter LS, Morgan RF, Persing JA, van Meter CH, Kenney JG. Burns of the head and neck. *Otolaryngol Clin North Am.* 1984;17:361–388.

8. Eliacher I, Moscona R, Joachims HZ, Hirshowitz B, Shilo R. The management of laryngotracheal stenosis in burned patients. *Plast Reconstr Surg.* 1981;68:11–17.

9. Deitch EA. Keys to early care of burn patients: Smoke inhalation injuries; metabolic and nutritional issues. *J Crit Illness.* 1990;5:1213–1222.

10. Clark WR, Bonaventura M, Myers W, Kellman R. Smoke inhalation and airway management at a regional burn unit: 1974 to 1983. II. Airway management. *J Burn Care Rehabil.* 1990;11:121–134.

11. Eckhauser FE, Billote J, Burke JF, Quinby WC. Tracheostomy complicating massive burn injury: A plea for conservatism. *Am J Surg.* 1974;127:418–423.

12. Gordon MD. Anchoring endotracheal tubes on patients with facial burns. *J Burn Care Rehabil.* 1987;8:233–237.

13. Ward CG, Gorham K, Hammond J, Varas R. Securing endotracheal tubes in patients with facial burns or trauma. *Am J Surg.* 1990;159:339–340.

14. Kinsella J. Smoke inhalation. *Burns.* 1988;14:269–279.

15. Levine BA, Petroff PA, Slade CL, Pruitt BA. Prospective trials of dexamethasone and aerosolized gentamicin in the treatment of inhalation injury in the burned patient. *J Trauma.* 1978;18:188–193.

16. Herndon DN, Barrow RE, Linares HA, et al. Inhalation injury in burned patients: Effects and treatment. *Burns.* 1988;14:349–356.

17. Clark CJ, Campbell D, Reid WH. Blood carboxyhemoglobin and cyanide levels in fire survivors. *Lancet.* 1981;1:1332–1335.

18. Barker SJ, Tremper KK. The effect of carbon monoxide inhalation on pulse oximetry and transcutaneous P_{O_2}. *Anesthesiology.* 1987;66:677–679.

19. Barker SJ, Tremper KK, Hufstedler S, Hyatt J, Zaccari J. The effects of carbon monoxide inhalation on noninvasive oxygen monitoring. *Anesth Analg.* 1986;65:S12. Abstract.

20. Vassallo SA, Martyn JAJ. Pathophysiology and anesthetic management of burn injury. *Semin Anesth.* 1989;8:275–284.

21. Demling RH. Fluid and electrolyte management. *Crit Care Clin.* 1985;1:27–45.

22. Monafo WW, Chuntrasakul C, Ayvazian VH. Hypertonic sodium solutions in the treatment of burn shock. *Am J Surg.* 1973;126:778–783.

23. Arturson G. Fluid therapy of thermal injury. *Acta Anaesthesiol Scand.* 1985;29:55–59.

24. Kramer GC, Perron PR, Lindsey DC, et al. Small-volume resuscitation with hypertonic saline dextran solution. *Surgery.* 1986;100:239–246.

25. Holcroft JW, Vassar MJ, Turner JE, Derlet RW, Kramer GC. 3% NaCl and 7.5% NaCl/dextran 70 in the resuscitation of severely injured patients. *Ann Surg.* 1988;206:279–288.

26. Demling RH, Kramer G, Harms B. Role of thermal injury-induced hypoproteinemia on fluid flux and protein permeability in burned and nonburned tissue. *Surgery.* 1984;95:136–143.

27. Navar PD, Saffle JR, Warden GD. Effect of inhalation injury on fluid resuscitation requirements after thermal injury. *Am J Surg.* 1985;150:716–720.

28. Hammond JS, Ward CG. Complications of the burn injury. *Crit Care Clin.* 1985;1:175–182.

29. Tranbaugh RF, Lewis FR, Christensen JM, Elings VB. Lung water changes after thermal injury: The effects of crystalloid resuscitation and sepsis. *Ann Surg.* 1980;192:479–490.

30. Deitch EA. Techniques for volume resuscitation in burn care: How to calculate the composition and volume of fluid needed. *J Crit Illness.* 1990;5:1225–1228.

31. Gregoretti S, Gelman S, Dimick A, Bradley EL. Hemodynamic changes and oxygen consumption in burned patients during enflurane or isoflurane anesthesia. *Anesth Analg.* 1989;69:431–436.

32. Aulick LH, Wroczyski FA, Coil JA, Mason AD. Metabolic and thermoregulatory responses to burn wound colonization. *J Trauma.* 1989;29:478–483.

33. Demling RH, Lalonde C. Effect of partial burn excision and closure on postburn oxygen consumption. *Surgery.* 1988;104:846–852.

34. Deitch EA. Intestinal permeability is increased in burn patients shortly after injury. *Surgery.* 1990;107:411–416.

35. Ziegler TR, Smith RJ, O'Dwyer ST, Demling RH, Wilmore DW. Increased intestinal permeability associated with infection in burn patients. *Arch Surg.* 1988;123:1313–1319.

36. Mochizuki H, Trocki O, Dominioni L, Brackett KA, Joffe SN, Aleander JW. Mechanism of prevention of postburn hypermetabolism and catabolism by early enteral feeding. *Ann Surg.* 1984;200:297–308.

37. Shangraw RE, Jahoor F, Miyoshi H, et al. Differentiation between septic and postburn insulin resistance. *Metabolism.* 1989;38:983–989.

38. Demling RH, Lalonde C. Oxygen consumption is increased in the post anesthesia period after burn excision. *J Burn Care Rehabil.* 1989;10:381–387.

39. Rutan TC, Herndon DN, Van Osten T, Abston S. Metabolic rate alterations in early excision and grafting versus conservative treatment. *J Trauma.* 1986;26:140–142.

40. Szyfelbein SK, Drop LJ, Martyn JAJ. Persistent ionized hypocalcemia in patients during resuscitation and recovery phases of body burns. *Crit Care Med.* 1981;7:454–458.

41. Vanholder R, Van den Bogaerde J, Vogelaers D, Colardyn F. Renal function in burns. *Acta Anaesthesiol Belg.* 1987;38:367–371.

42. Cote CJ, Drop LJ, Hoaglin DC, Daniels AL, Young ET. Ionized hypocalcemia after fresh frozen plasma administration to thermally injured children: Effects of infusion rate, duration, and treatment with calcium chloride. *Anesth Analg.* 1988;67:152–160.

43. Slater H, Goldfarb IW. Acute septic cholecystitis in patients with burn injuries. *J Burn Care Rehabil.* 1989;10:445–447.

44. Ross DC, Lee KC, Peters WU, Douglas LG. Acalculous chole-cystitis in association with major burns. *Burns.* 1987;13:488–491.

45. Purdue GF, Hunt JL. Pulmonary emboli in burned patients. *J Trauma.* 1988;28:218–220.

46. Pfeifer PM. Acute rhabdomyolysis following surgery for burns. *Anaesthesia.* 1986;41:614–619.

47. Potts FL, May RB. Early syndrome of inappropriate secretion of antidiuretic hormone in a child with burn injury. *Ann Emerg Med.* 1986;15:834–835.

48. Counce JS, Cone JB, McAlister L, Wallace B, Caldwell FT. Surgical complications of thermal injury. *Am J Surg.* 1988;156:556–557.

49. Demling RH, Ellerbe S, Jarrett F. Ketamine anesthesia for tangential excision of burn eschar: A burn unit procedure. *J Trauma.* 1978;18:269–270.

50. Khan MS, Bhatti AH. Ketamine tolerance. *Postgrad Med J.* 1988;64:833–834.

51. Achauer BM, Martinez SE. Burn wound pathophysiology and care. *Crit Care Clin.* 1985;1:47–58.

52. Scott-Conner CEH, Love R, Wheeler W. Does rapid wound closure improve survival in older patients with burns? *Am Surg.* 1990;56:57–60.

53. Tompkins RG, Burke JF, Schoenfeld DA, et al. Prompt eschar excision: A treatment system contributing to reduced burn mortality. A statistical evaluation of born care at the Massachusetts General Hospital (1974–1984). *Ann Surg.* 1986;204:272–281.

54. Lauwers LF. Anesthesia for burns. *Acta Anaesthesiol Belg.* 1987;38:363–366.

55. Foy HM, Pavlin E, Heimbach DM. Excision and grafting of large burns: Operation length not related to increased morbidity. *J Trauma.* 1986;26:51–53.

56. Lamb JD. Anaesthetic considerations for major thermal injury. *Can Anaesth Soc J.* 1985;32:84–92.

57. Desai MH, Herndon DN, Broemeling L, Barrow RE, Nichols RJ, Rutan RL. Early burn wound excision significantly reduces blood loss. *Ann Surg.* 1990;211:753–762.

58. Wagner RL, White PF. Etomidate inhibits adrenocortical function in surgical patients. *Anesthesiology.* 1984;61:647–651.

59. Reyneke CJ, James MFM, Johnson R. Alfentanil and propofol infusions for surgery in the burned patient. *Br J Anaesth.* 1989;63:418–422.

60. Martyn J. Clinical pharmacology and drug therapy in the burned patient. *Anesthesiology.* 1986;65:67–75.

61. Heimback DM. Early burn excision and grafting. *Surg Clin North Am.* 1987;67:93–107.

62. Stene JK, Grande CM. General anesthesia: Management considerations in the trauma patient. *Crit Care Clin.* 1990;6:73–84.

63. White PF, Way WL, Trevor AJ. Ketamine—Its pharmacology and therapeutic uses. *Anesthesiology.* 1982;56:119–132.

64. Gronert GA, Theye RA. Pathophysiology of hyperkalemia induced by succinylcholine. *Anesthesiology.* 1975;43:89–99.

65. Martyn J, Goldhill DR, Goudsouzian NG. Clinical pharmacology of muscle relaxants in patients with burns. *J Clin Pharmacol.* 1986;26:680–685.

66. Mills AK, Martyn JAJ. Evaluation of atracurium neuromuscular blockade in paediatric patients with burn injury. *Br J Anaesth.* 1988;60:450–455.

67. Dwersteg JF, Pavlin EG, Heimbach DM. Patients with burns resistant to atracurium. *Anesthesiology.* 1986;65:517–520.

68. Marathe PH, Dwersteg JF, Pavlin EG, Haschke RH, Heimbach DM, Slattery JT. Effect of thermal injury on the pharmacokinetics and pharmacodynamics of atracurium in humans. *Anesthesiology.* 1989;70:752–755.

69. Hagen J, Martyn J, Szyfelbein SK, Goudsouzian NG. Cardiovascular and neuromuscular responses to high-dose pancuronium-metocurine in pediatric burned and reconstructive patients. *Anesth Analg.* 1986;65:1340–1344.

70. Dwersteg JF, Pavlin EG, Haschke R, Heimbach DM, Macintyre PE. High dose atracurium does not produce hypotension in the burned patient. *Anesthesiology.* 1986;65:A293. Abstract.

71. Mills A, Martyn JAJ. Evaluation of vecuronium neuromuscular blockade in pediatric patients with thermal injury. *Anesth Analg.* 1987;66:S119. Abstract.

72. Wilson GR, Tomlinson P. Pain relief in burns—How we do it. *Burns.* 1988;14:331–332.

73. Mackersie RC, Karagianes TG. Pain management following trauma and burns. *Crit Care Clin.* 1990;6:433–449.

74. Giesecke AH, Grande CM, Whitten CW. Fluid therapy and the resuscitation of traumatic shock. *Crit Care Clin.* 1990;6:61–72.

75. Paulus DA, Monroe MC. Cool fingers and pulse oximetry. *Anesthesiology.* 1989;71:168–169.

76. Severinghaus JW, Naifeh KH. Accuracy of response of six pulse oximeters to profound hypoxia. *Anesthesiology.* 1987;67:551–558.

77. Hickerson W, Morrell M, Cicala RS. Glossal pulse oximetry. *Anesth Analg.* 1989;69:72–74.

78. Bardakjian VB, Kenney JG, Edgerton MT, Morgan FR. Pulse oximetry for vascular monitoring in burned upper extremities. *J Care Burn Rehabil.* 1988;9:63–65.

79. Barillo DJ, Mastropiere CJ, Cohen MB, Okunski W. How accurate is pulse oximetry in patients with burn injuries? *J Burn Care Rehabil.* 1990;11:162–166.

80. Ninnemann JL. Trauma, sepsis, and the immune response. *J Burn Care Rehabil.* 1987;8:462–468.

81. Deitch EA. The management of burns. *N Engl J Med.* 1990;323:1249–1253.

82. Martyn JAJ, Snider MT, Farago LF, Burke JF. Thermodilution right ventricular volume: A novel and better predictor of volume replacement in acute thermal injury. *J Trauma.* 1981;21:619–624.

83. Martyn JAJ, McKusick K, Strauss HW, Burke JF. Ventricular volume and ejection fraction in the diagnosis of the aetiology of low cardiac output in burned patients. *Anesthesia.* 1986;41:511–515.

84. Wallner S, Vautrin R, Katz J, Murphy J. The anemia of thermal injury: Partial characterization of an erythroid inhibitory substance. *J Trauma.* 1987;27:639–645.

85. Cullen JJ, Murray DJ, Kealey GP. Changes in coagulation factors in patients with burns during acute blood loss. *J Burn Care Rehabil.* 1989;10:517–522.

86. Achauer BM, Hernandez J, Parker A. Burn excision with intraoperative vasopressin. *J Burn Care Rehabil.* 1989;10:375–378.

87. Rosenberg JL, Zawacki BE. Reduction of blood loss using tourniquets and "compression" dressings in excising limb burns. *J Trauma.* 1986;26:47–50.

88. Simon TL, Curreri PW, Harker LA. Kinetic characterization of hemostasis in thermal injury. *J Lab Clin Med.* 1977;89:702–711.

89. Murray DJ, Olson J, Strauss R, Tinker JH. Coagulation changes during packed red cell replacement of major blood loss. *Anesthesiology.* 1988;69:839–845.

90. Warden GD, Saffle JR, Kravitz M. A two-stage technique for excision and grafting of burn wounds. *J Trauma.* 1982;22:98–103.

91. Haslam KR, Nielsen CH. Do passive heat and moisture exchangers keep the patient warm? *Anesthesiology.* 1986;64:379–381.

92. Stone DR, Downs JB, Paul WL, Perkins HM. Adult body temperature and heated humidification of anesthetic gases during general anesthesia. *Anesth Analg.* 1981;60:736–741.

93. Vaghadia H. Blood warming devices do not guarantee temperature homeostasis. *Anesthesiology.* 1986;65:237–238.

94. Russell WJ. A discussion of the problems of heat exchange blood warming devices. *Br J Anaesth.* 1969;41:345–351.

95. Hinton AE, King D. Anterior shoulder dislocation as a complication of surgery for burns. *Burns.* 1989;15:248–249.

96. Oldenhof H, de Jong M, Steenhoek A, Janknegt R. Clinical pharmacokinetics of midazolam in intensive care patients, a

wide interpatient variability? *Clin Pharmacol Ther.* 1988;43:263–269.

97. Park GR, Manara AR, Mendel L, Bateman PE. Ketamine infusion: Its use as a sedative, inotrope and bronchodilator in a critically ill patient. *Anaesthesia.* 1987;42:980–983.

98. Ledingham IM, Watt I. Influence of sedation on mortality in critically ill multiple trauma patients. *Lancet.* 1983;1:1270.

99. Miller Jones CMH. Paralysis or sedation for controlled ventilation? *Lancet.* 1980;1:312.

100. Parker MM, Schubert W, Shelhamer JH, Parrillo JE. Perceptions of a critically ill patient experiencing therapeutic paralysis in an ICU. *Crit Care Med.* 1984;12:69–71.

101. Choiniere M, Melzack R, Rondeau J, Girard N, Paquin M. The pain of burns: Characteristics and correlates. *J Trauma.* 1989;29:1531–1539.

102. Concilus R, Denson DD, Knarr D, Warden G, Raj PP. Continuous intravenous infusion of methadone for control of burn pain. *J Burn Care Rehabil.* 1989;10:406–409.

103. Denson DD, Concilus RR, Warden G, Raj PP. Pharmacokinetics of continuous intravenous infusion of methadone in the early post-burn period. *J Clin Pharmacol.* 1990;30:70–75.

104. Kinsella J, Glavin R, Reid WH. Patient-controlled analgesia for burn patients: A preliminary report. *Burns.* 1988;14:500–503.

105. White PF. Use of patient-controlled analgesia for management of acute pain. *JAMA.* 1988;259:243–247.

106. Simons RD, McFadd A, Frank HA, Green LC, Malin RM, Morris JL. Behavioral contracting in a burn care facility: A strategy for patient participation. *J Trauma.* 1978;18:257–260.

107. Van der Does AJW, van Dyck R, Spijker RE. Hypnosis and pain in patients with severe burns: A pilot study. *Burns.* 1988;14:399–404.

108. Randalls B. Continuous brachial plexus blockade: A technique that uses an axillary catheter to allow successful skin grafting. *Anaesthesia.* 1990;45:143–144.

109. Blassingame WM, Bennett GB, Helm PA, Purdue GF, Hunt JL. Range of motion of the shoulder performed while patient is anesthetized. *J Burn Care Rehabil.* 1989;10:539–542.

110. Larson SM, Parks DH. Managing the difficult airway in patients with burns of the head and neck. *J Burn Care Rehabil.* 1988;9:55–56.

111. Fox DJ, Castro T, Rastrelli AJ. Comparison of intubation techniques in the awake patient: The Flexi-lum™ surgical light (lightwand) versus blind nasal approach. *Anesthesiology.* 1987;66:69–71.

112. Stewart RD, Ellis DG. Lighted stylet and endotracheal intubation. I. *Anesthesiology.* 1987;66:851.

113. Tanzer RC. Burn contracture of the neck. *Plast Reconstr Surg.* 1964;33:207–212.

114. Calhoun KH, Deskin RW, McCracken MM, et al. Long-term airway sequelae in a pediatric burn population. *Laryngoscope.* 1988;98:721–725.

115. Flexon PB, Cheney ML, Montgomery WW, Turner PA. Management of patients with glottic and subglottic stenosis resulting from thermal burns. *Ann Otol Rhinol Laryngol.* 1989;98:27–30.

116. Timon CI, McShane D, McGovern E, Walsh M. Treatment of combined subglottic and critically low tracheal stenoses secondary to burn inhalation injury. *J Laryngol Otol.* 1989;103:1083–1086.

117. Bauer M, Balogh D, Hortnagl H, Kompatscher H. Clinical follow-up of burn patients after long-term mechanical ventilation. *Scand J Plast Reconstr Surg.* 1987;21:265–267.

118. Colice GL, Munster AM, Haponik EF. Tracheal stenosis complication cutaneous burns: An underestimated problem. *Am Rev Respir Dis.* 1986;134:1315–1318.

119. Skolnick A. Calcitonin assay may help identify burn patients at risk for respiratory distress. *JAMA.* 1990;264:565–566.

120. Teepe RGC, Kreis RW, Koebrugge EJ, et al. The use of cultured autologous epidermis in the treatment of extensive burn wounds. *J Trauma.* 1990;30:269–275.

121. Munster AM, Weiner SH, Spence RJ. Cultured epidermis for the coverage of massive burn wounds: A single center experience. *Ann Surg.* 1990;211:676–680.

122. Scarborough DA, Bisaccia E, Swensen RD. Anesthesia for outpatient dermatologic cosmetic surgery: Midazolam–low-dosage ketamine anesthesia. *J Dermatol Surg Oncol.* 1989;15:658–663.

123. Elliot DL, Tolle SW, Miller SH, et al. Medical considerations in ambulatory surgery. *Clin Plast Surg.* 1983;10:295–307.

124. Peacock EE. Major ambulatory surgery of the plastic surgical patient. *Surg Clin North Am.* 1987;67:865–879.

125. Mandel MA. Autotransfusion in elective plastic surgical operations. *Plast Reconstr Surg.* 1986;77:767–771.

126. Brown FE, Rawnsley HM, Lawe JE. The use of autologous blood in patients undergoing subcutaneous mastectomy or reduction mammoplasty. *Ann Plast Surg.* 1983;10:186–189.

127. Consensus Conference. Perioperative red cell blood cell transfusion. *JAMA.* 1988;260:2700–2703.

128. Kruskall MS. Autologous blood transfusions and plastic surgery: Comments concerning "other" "elective" procedures. *Plast Reconstr Surg.* 1990;86:163–165.

129. Uebel CO, Pohl P, Bahlis J. Autologous blood transfusion for combined plastic surgeries. *Aesthetic Plast Surg.* 1985;9:117–119.

130. Ploem JE, Bloem JAAM. Compensation for blood loss in plastic surgery with ferastral and autologous blood transfusions. *Scand J Haematol.* 1977;32(suppl):298–302.

131. Baker TJ, Gordon HL. Midazolam (Versed) in ambulatory surgery. *Plast Reconstr Surg.* 1988;82:244–246.

132. Reves JG, Fragen RJ, Vinik HR, Greenblatt DJ. Midazolam: Pharmacology and uses. *Anesthesiology.* 1985;62:310–324.

133. White PF, Vasconez LO, Mathes SA, Way WL, Wender LA. Comparison of midazolam and diazepam for sedation during plastic surgery. *Plast Reconstr Surg.* 1988;81:703–712.

134. Dion J, Power SJ, Grundy EM, et al. Sedation for local anaesthesia. Comparison of intravenous midazolam and diazepam. *Anaesthesia.* 1984;39:372–376.

135. White PF. Use of ketamine for sedation and analgesia during injection of local anesthetics. *Ann Plast Surg.* 1985;15:53–56.

136. Kryshtalskyj B, Direnfeld VN, Johnson TWG. Use of low dose ketamine hydrochloride in outpatient oral surgery. *Oral Surg Oral Med Oral Pathol.* 1990;69:413–419.

137. Cunningham BL, McKinney P. Patient acceptance of dissociative anesthetics. *Plast Reconstr Surg.* 1983;72:22–26.

138. Vinnik CA. An intravenous dissociation technique for outpatient plastic surgery: Tranquility in the office surgical facility. *Plast Reconstr Surg.* 1981;67:799–805.

139. Korttilla K, Levanen J. Untoward effects of ketamine combined with diazepam for supplementing conducting anaesthesia in young and middle-aged adults. *Acta Anaesthesiol Scand.* 1978;22:640–648.

140. Cabbage EB, Behbahani PM. Cardiovascular reactions associated with the use of ketamine and epinephrine in plastic surgery. *Ann Plast Surg.* 1985;15:50–52.

141. Glauber DT, Buffington CW, Hornbein TF, Hamacher EN. High dose lidocaine, ultradilute epinephrine and intravenous sedation for major plastic surgery. *Anesth Analg.* 1984;63:219. Abstract.

142. Colon GA, Gubert N. Lorazepam (Ativan) and fentanyl (Sublimaze) for outpatient office plastic surgical anesthesia. *Plast Reconstr Surg.* 1986;78:486–488.

143. Maitre PO, Vozeh S, Heykants J, Thomson DA, Stanski DR. The population pharmacokinetics of alfentanil: Quantitating the average dose–serum concentration relationship. *Anesthesiology.* 1986;65:A556. Abstract.

144. Burm AGL, Ausems ME, Stanski DR. Alfentanil pharmacokinetics during a variable-rate infusion in surgical patients. *Anesthesiology.* 1986;65:A557. Abstract.

145. Gordon HL. The selection of drugs in office surgery. *Clin Plast Surg.* 1983;10:277–284.

146. Dionne RA, Goldstein DS, Wirdzek PR. Effects of diazepam premedication and epinephrine-containing local anesthetic on cardiovascular and plasma catecholamine responses to oral surgery. *Anesth Analg.* 1984;63:640–646.

147. Gilman AG, Goodman LS, Gilman A, eds. *The pharmacological basis of therapeutics.* 6th ed. New York: Macmillan; 1980.

148. Graham WP. Anesthesia in cosmetic surgery. *Clin Plast Surg.* 1983;10:285–287.

149. Gumucio CA, Bennie JB, Fernando B, Young VL, Roa N, Kraemer BA. Plasma lidocaine levels during augmentation mammoplasty and suction-assisted lipectomy. *Plast Reconstr Surg.* 1989;84:624–627.

150. Alderman, EL, Kerber RE, Harrison DC. Evaluation of lidocaine resistance in man using intermittent large-dose infusion techniques. *Am J Cardiol.* 1974;34:342–349.

151. Alfano SN, Leicht MJ, Skiendzielewski JJ. Lidocaine toxicity following subcutaneous administration. *Ann Emerg Med.* 1984;13:465–467.

152. Nesmith RL, Herring SH, Marke MW, Speight KL, Efird RC, Rauck RL. Early experience with high thoracic epidural anesthesia in outpatient submuscular breast augmentation. *Ann Plast Surg.* 1990;24:299–303.

153. Hudson RJ, Stanski DR, Burch PG. Pharmacokinetics of methohexital and thiopental in surgical patients. *Anesthesiology.* 1983;59:215–219.

154. White PF. Use of continuous infusion vs. intermittent bolus administration of fentanyl or ketamine during outpatient anesthesia. *Anesthesiology.* 1983;59:294–300.

155. Cole AGH, Hinds CJ, Cole PV. Fentanyl by infusion—A method of total dose reduction. *Br J Anaesth.* 1980;52:229. Proceedings.

156. Henriksson BA, Carlsson P, Hallen B, Hagerdal M, Lundberg D, Ponten J. Propofol vs thiopentone as anaesthetic agents for short operative procedures. *Acta Anaesthiol Scand.* 1987;31:63–66.

157. O'Toole DP, Milligan KR, McCollum JSC, Dundee JW. A comparison of propofol and methohexitone as induction agents for day case isoflurane anaesthesia. *Anaesthesia.* 1987;42:373–376.

158. Mackenzie N, Grant IS. Comparison of the new emulsion formulation of propofol with methohexitone and thiopentone for induction of anaesthesia in day cases. *Br J Anaesth.* 1985;57:725–731.

159. Courtiss EH, Kanter MA. The prevention and management of medical problems during office surgery. *Plast Reconstr Surg.* 2990;85:127–136.

160. Singer R, Thomas PE. Pulse oximeter in the ambulatory anesthetic surgical facility. *Plast Reconstr Surg.* 1988;82:111–114.

161. Philip BK. Hazards of amnesia after midazolam in ambulatory surgical patients. *Anesth Analg.* 1987;66:97–98.

162. Elliott RA, Hoehn JG. The office surgery suite: The physical plant and equipment. *Clin Plast Surg.* 1983;10:225–246.

163. Roth AG, Dado DV. Venous air embolism during removal of tissue expander in a supine child. *Anesthesiology.* 1988;68:457–459.

164. Alexander JI, Lewis AAM. Air embolism during mastectomy. *Anaesthesia.* 1969;24:618–619.

165. Warner MA, Harper JV. Cardiac dysrhythmias associated with chemical peeling with phenol. *Anesthesiology.* 1985;62:366–367.

166. Truppman ES, Ellenby JD. Major electrocardiographic changes during chemical face peeling. *Plast Reconstr Surg.* 1979;63:44–48.

167. Fagraeus L, Angelillo JC, Dolan EA. A serious anesthetic hazard during orthognathic surgery. *Anesth Analg.* 1980;59:150–153.

168. Lee C, Schwartz S, Mok MS. Difficult extubation due to transfixation of a nasotracheal tube by a Kirschner wire. *Anesthesiology.* 1977;46:427.

169. Mosby EL, Messer EJ, Nealis MF, Golden DP. Intraoperative damage to nasotracheal tubes during maxillary surgery: Report of cases. *J Oral Maxillofac Surg.* 1978;36:963–964.

170. Seikaly H, Kuzon WM, Gullane PJ, Herman SJ. Pulmonary atelectasis after reconstruction with pectoralis major flaps. *Arch Otolaryngol Head Neck Surg.* 1990;116:575–577.

171. Korttila K, Kauste A, Auvinen J. Comparison of domperidone, droperidol, and metoclopramide in the prevention and treatment of nausea and vomiting after balanced general anesthesia. *Anesth Analg.* 1979;58:396–400.

172. Madej TH, Simpson KH. Comparison of the use of domperidone, droperidol and metoclopramide in the prevention of nausea and vomiting following gynaecological surgery in day cases. *Br J Anaesth.* 1986;58:879–883.

Anesthesia for Orthopedic Surgery

*Dana Lynn Grogan and
Thomas J. Grogan*

Orthopedic surgical procedures provide a wide variety of challenges for the anesthetist. Patient age varies from the infant to the centenarian, and the physiologic status may range from healthy to moribund. The dynamic nature of orthopedics demands that the anesthetist not only be adept in the basics of anesthesia but also keep abreast of innovative techniques in patient care. To facilitate reader comprehension, a glossary of orthopedic terms appears in the appendix at the end of this chapter.

PREOPERATIVE EVALUATION

Elective Surgery

The orthopedic patient requires careful preoperative evaluation to investigate past medical history and current physical status, especially as many are elderly.[1] As age advances, decreases in arterial oxygen tension, cardiac index, and gastrointestinal motility are common.[2,3] Confusion and disorientation, if present, influence the preoperative evaluation and may be either organic in nature or secondary to pain, hospitalization, or drug interactions. Old charts, when available, may be very informative. More detailed information on the geriatric patient can be found in Chapter 33.

Regardless of the patient's age, significant nonorthopedic disease processes may also be present.[4] The preoperative goal is to optimize the patient's status and anticipate the impact of the anesthetic and the operative procedure on the specific disease state.[5,6] In orthopedics, patients with osteoarthritis (OA), rheumatoid arthritis (RA), and ankylosing spondylitis deserve special attention.

Osteoarthritis. Osteoarthritis is a noninflammatory, degenerative disease of articular cartilage throughout the body.[7(p59)] Bony overgrowth of the joint surface also occurs.[8] The etiology is attributed to abnormal joint biomechanics secondary to a loss of water in the articular cartilage. Causative factors include aging, heredity, repetitive occupational stresses, trauma, and obesity.[7(p60),8] Patients often present with decreased joint motion and chronic pain, making intraoperative positioning potentially difficult. A systematic, careful assessment of temporomandibular joint function, neck extension, and airway anatomy is essential to identify patients at risk for difficult endotracheal intubation. Hoarseness and vocal weakness may indicate cricoarytenoid arthritis with associated glottic narrowing.[9,10]

Rheumatoid Arthritis. Rheumatoid arthritis is characterized by a chronic, immune-mediated synovitis of unknown origin.[11] As the disease advances, instability, deformity, and ultimately destruction of many joints occur. Involvement of the cervical spine, hips, shoulders, knees, elbows, ankles, wrists, and metacarpophalangeal joints is common.[12] Coronary insufficiency, cardiac dysrhythmias, conduction defects, valvular abnormalities, pericarditis, pleural effusions, pulmonary interstitial fibrosis, and anemia are also associated with rheumatoid arthritis and may be clinically significant.[8(pp172–174)]

Cervical ankylosis and instability, specifically atlantoaxial instability, may make endotracheal intubation difficult.[13–15] Atlantoaxial subluxation occurs when the alar ligaments at C-2 are invaded by rheumatoid pannus at the base of the odontoid process.[16,17] The odontoid is subsequently displaced, causing impingement on the cervical spine, medulla, or vertebral arteries.[18(p635)] Subjective symptoms include headache, neck pain, tingling, or numbness in the arms or legs with neck motion.[14] Acute subluxation can occur with flexion of the neck and may result in quadriparesis or sudden death. The goals of anesthetic management are to maintain cervical stability and to prevent neck flexion. Depending on the severity of cervical ankylosis and instability, anesthetic considerations should include awake fiberoptic endotracheal intubation with topical anesthesia, positioning of the patient while awake, or both. When appropriate, regional anesthesia with minimal sedation and neck stabilization may be an anesthetic alternative, as joints of the thoracic, lumbar, and sacral spine are rarely affected.[19]

Other technical concerns include flexion deformities of the wrist that make arterial line placement difficult and carpal tunnel syndrome, which precludes prolonged extension of the wrist.[20,21] Central venous access may be difficult because of cervical instability or fusion of the cervical spine.[22]

Ankylosing Spondylitis. Ankylosing spondylitis (Marie-Strumpell disease) is more common in men than women. Initially, it begins with ossification of ligaments at the site of bony attachment. The disease progresses to include the joint cartilage and disc space of the axial skeleton, resulting in bony ankylosis.[23,24] When this occurs awake fiberoptic intubation may be necessary. Arthritis and ankylosis may also be present in the costovertebral joints, shoulders, and hips.[23] As rigidity of the rib cage develops, lung function may be impaired. If there is diaphragmatic involvement, vital capacity will be reduced.[25] Aortic regurgitation and bundle branch block that require valve replacement or pacemaker insertion have also been reported in this patient population.[26] Sacroiliac and lumbar interspaces are usually fused, making lumbar epidural or spinal anesthesia difficult or impossible.[8(pp93-96)] As with rheumatoid arthritis, careful positioning while awake decreases the risk of spine fractures, joint dislocation or fractures, and problems associated with cervical instability.

Consideration must be given during preoperative evaluation for elective surgery to the medication regimen of each patient. In most instances, medications for control of cardiac, respiratory, or endocrine diseases should be continued up to the time of surgery. Patients with rheumatoid arthritis or other autoimmune diseases are frequently on steroid medications. To maintain adrenocortical stability augmentation with an exogenous steroid preparation is generally recommended.[27] Patients with osteoarthritis or rheumatoid arthritis may also be taking high-dose aspirin or nonsteroidal anti-inflammatory agents (NSAIAs) for symptomatic relief. These medications disrupt platelet aggregation which predisposes the patient to intraoperative bleeding.[28,29(pp245-246)] Preoperative assessment of the bleeding time will indicate the degree of platelet inhibition. To correct platelet inhibition and prolonged bleeding time, aspirin therapy should be discontinued 8 to 11 days prior to surgery[29(p242)]; however, the surgeon and the anesthetist must weigh the benefit of decreased blood loss against exacerbation of the patient's symptoms.

Emergency Surgery

Preoperative evaluation for the acutely traumatized patient requires the anesthetist to do a rapid overview of all injuries. Injuries may be singular or multiple, blunt or penetrating, hidden or easily visible. True orthopedic emergencies include traumatic posterior dislocation of the hip with disruption of blood supply, digital amputation for replantation, fractures with absent peripheral pulses, and compartment syndrome.[7(p496),8(p216),30,31] In multiple-trauma cases, the orthopedic injuries must be assessed in conjunction with systemic injuries. Initially, the anesthetist should conduct a complete assessment of the airway. Obstruction by dentures, teeth, laryngeal fracture, or an artificial airway is common. Evaluation of the mandible, maxilla, temporomandibular joint, and cervical spine for fractures is also cru-

cial. Identification of cervical fractures or dislocations helps the anesthetist to predict the success of orotracheal intubation, verify the need for fiberoptic intubation or tracheotomy, and prevent spinal cord damage. The cervical spine should be evaluated by lateral neck roentgenograms or through computerized axial tomography (CAT scanning) to ensure patency.[32]

Another critical area for the anesthetist to evaluate is potential blood loss. Bone is a very vascular tissue. Blood loss can be significant in open long bone fractures or if there is attendant vascular disruption. Bleeding may or may not result in hematoma formation and is often hidden from direct view. Table 38-1 lists various fractures and estimates of typical preoperative blood losses. Rapid access to the operating room for patients suffering from femoral, pelvic, and some open fractures can help reduce the amount of blood lost. Guidelines for assessment of blood loss include the stability of the blood pressure, tachycardia, peripheral color, capillary refill in the extremities, hemoglobin, hematocrit, and low central venous pressure if a central line has been placed. Correction of the volume deficit preoperatively with whole blood, packed red blood cells, fresh-frozen plasma, albumin, plasma expanders, or crystalloid is preferable.[33,34]

All trauma patients are considered to have a full stomach. Pain, stress, and narcotics are known to decrease gastric emptying time.[35] It is therefore important to determine not only what the patient last ate and drank but also the interval of time between oral intake and the onset of injury. Ileus also occurs. H_2 blockers that increase gastric pH such as ranitidine and cimetidine are appropriate if time allows.[36] Metoclopramide stimulates upper gastrointestinal motility and increases lower esophageal tone and may be beneficial.[37] It is contraindicated if there is the possibility of a bowel perforation or obstruction. Pediatric trauma victims may be uncooperative because of pain and fear, and all are considered to have full stomachs. For induction of general anesthesia, an awake intubation or rapid-sequence induction is the method of choice. A more detailed discussion of anesthesia for trauma surgery can be found in Chapter 42.

When life-threatening problems have stabilized, attention can then be turned toward the relief of severe pain. Intramuscular narcotics are not used in the emergency situation because of poor absorption in the hypotensive state

TABLE 38-1. ESTIMATES OF PREOPERATIVE BLOOD LOSS IN CLOSED FRACTURES IN THE ADULT[a]

Fracture Site	Blood Loss (mL)
Foot	< 250
Lower leg	500–1000
Femoral shaft	1000–2000
Intertrochanteric hip	800–1200
Intracapsular hip	50–100
Pelvis	2000–4000
Forearm	< 250
Humerus	< 500

[a] Estimates are based on 19 years of combined orthopedic and anesthetic experience.

and shunting of blood from the periphery to the central circulation. Intravenous opioids are most often used. Stabilization of fractures and immobilization help minimize pain and also decrease the incidence of a fat embolus.[38,39] A delay in taking the orthopedic trauma patient to the operating room is also associated with an increase in additional postoperative complications. Excessive tissue swelling makes closed reduction of a fracture more difficult and compartment syndrome more likely.[40] Recent evidence suggests that the risk of infection in severe open fractures increases as time passes from the onset of the injury.[41]

Pediatrics

Pediatric orthopedic patients place special demands on the anesthetist. The unique challenges of the pediatric patient include small airway diameter, cardiac output that is dependent on heart rate, high cardiac index, and the child's developmental level. In addition, the normal coping mechanisms and behaviors of a healthy child may be compromised in the face of acute injury, pain, or the unfamiliar hospital environment. More detailed discussions on the needs of the pediatric population can be found in Chapter 32.

Children who suffer from chronic illness such as cerebral palsy, polio sequelae, muscular dystrophy, and juvenile rheumatoid arthritis undergo repeated orthopedic procedures and may be emotionally distressed by another hospital visit. A calm approach to these patients may enable the anesthetist to develop some rapport and elicit cooperation from the child.[42]

Achondroplastic dwarfs exhibit abnormal growth patterns that may make mask fit difficult. Intubation, however, is usually accomplished without difficulty.[43] Atlantoaxial instability and foramen magnum stenosis may also be present, necessitating caution at intubation.[43–45] Kyphoscoliosis and a narrow epidural space make lumbar regional techniques technically difficult but not impossible.[46]

Children with cerebral palsy have static central motor deficits secondary to cerebral hypoxia or anoxia from a multitude of causes. Oftentimes, however, the etiology is unknown.[47] Mental retardation may or may not be present and many of these children often suffer from the residua of prematurity. Spasticity and muscle wasting frequently lead to contractures and joint deformities. Problems with positioning, hypothermia, delayed emergence, and poor gastroesophageal tone are a few common problems in this group.[18(p837)] Despite muscle wasting, succinylcholine administration has not been associated with potassium release in these patients.[48] A rapid-sequence induction technique is recommended for aspiration prophylaxis.

Children with Down syndrome (trisomy 21), in addition to systemic manifestations such as cardiac anomalies, may have atlantoaxial instability. If present, the child is at increased risk for spinal cord damage.[49] The anesthetic agents and techniques that are in routine use have all been successfully used in these children. When congenital cardiac lesions are present, however, the associated pathophysiology dictates the anesthetic agents.

Children with juvenile rheumatoid arthritis (JRA) often have ankylosis of the cervical spine and a hypoplastic mandible, making airway management difficult and routine intubation frequently impossible. Regional anesthesia may be difficult because of severe lumbar lordosis.[22,50] Central venous access may be difficult because of flexion of the neck and limited lateral neck movement.[22] These children also take aspirin, steroid preparations, and occasionally chemotherapeutic agents.

Mentally retarded children may or may not be cooperative. The choice of anesthetic technique must be individualized and flexible as children may be calm preoperatively yet uncontrollable when frightened or upset. No unusual sensitivity to drugs has been reported when retardation alone is present.[51]

Muscular dystrophy is a complex of diseases that results in painless degeneration and atrophy of skeletal muscles without denervation.[52,53] Cardiopulmonary involvement is common. Succinylcholine is contraindicated because of the exaggerated potassium release from skeletal muscle wasting.[54] Nondepolarizing muscle relaxants may exhibit prolonged effects. There is an increased incidence of malignant hyperthermia in this population and dantrolene should be available.[55,56]

Scoliosis, congenital or acquired, is characterized by lateral spinal curvature with vertebral rotation. Curvature greater than 40 degrees is most likely to be associated with moderate to severe cardiopulmonary derangements.[57–59] An increased incidence of malignant hyperthermia is also associated with scoliosis.[60] The details of management of malignant hyperthermia are discussed in Chapter 44 and scoliosis is discussed in depth at the end of this chapter.

SPECIAL CONSIDERATIONS FOR ORTHOPEDIC SURGERY

Pneumatic Tourniquet

The pneumatic tourniquet is an inflatable cuff in which the pressure is maintained by either compressed gas, a volatile refrigerant, or a dedicated pump. The primary advantage of the pneumatic tourniquet when applied to either upper or lower extremities is a bloodless operating field.[7(p112)] Disadvantages include a small but sudden increase in central blood volume on exsanguination of the limb and inflation of the pneumatic cuff. This is well tolerated in most patients but can be detrimental in patients with poor ventricular compliance.[61,62] The tourniquet also causes cellular acidosis that begins within 10 minutes of inflation. Hypoxia and acidosis subsequently cause the release of various intracellular contents including myoglobin, potassium, and thromboxane.[63–65] After 30 minutes of inflation, nerve conduction ceases from either nerve hypoxia or external pressure on the nerve itself from the tourniquet.[66,67] Tissue edema is common after 60 minutes of inflation time.[68]

Responsibilities for the pneumatic tourniquet rest with both the surgeon and the anesthetist. The anesthetist or the circulating nurse usually inflates and deflates the tourniquet at the surgeon's request; however, the anesthetist must monitor and record the time of inflation and pressure. The duration of safe inflation time is unknown.[69] Currently, the maximum recommended time is 90 minutes to 2 hours.[70,71] It is further recommended that the inflation time be decreased as the age of the patient increases. It is common practice to notify the surgeons at 60, 90, and 120 minutes of inflation time and every 10 minutes after.

The ideal inflation pressure is also unknown at this time. Current recommendations vary greatly. One source suggests 200 mm/Hg for the upper extremity and 250 mm/Hg for the lower extremity.[7(p112)] Another source recommends 100 mm/Hg greater than the systolic blood pressure for the thigh and 50 mm/Hg greater than the systolic blood pressure for the arm.[72] Another espouses two times the mean arterial pressure. Van Roekel et al[73] advocate using a formula relating limb circumference and systolic pressure.

Injuries from the pneumatic tourniquet are a function of both inflation pressure and duration.[69,74] Pressure appears to be more damaging than distal ischemia. Neuropraxia is most likely to occur if tourniquet time exceeds 2 hours.[75,76] Pneumatic tourniquets are generally contraindicated in patients with sickle cell disease, severe atherosclerotic heart disease, and severe peripheral vascular disease.

Vigilance by the anesthetist is warranted during deflation of the tourniquet. On deflation, there is reperfusion of the ischemic extremity and washout of the metabolic byproducts. Reactive hyperemia occurs in the extremity, leading to a loss of vascular volume from the central circulation. The subsequent drop in the blood pressure and the decrease in central pressures can cause mild to severe hypotension. This may progress to cardiac arrest if not treated with volume replacement or vasopressors.[64,77,78]

A unique effect of the pneumatic tourniquet is tourniquet pain, which occurs under regional and general anesthesia. Signs of tourniquet pain generally occur between 45 and 60 minutes after the onset of initial inflation.[79–81] Under regional anesthesia patients may complain of pain, and under general anesthesia the symptoms of hypertension and tachycardia can mimic signs of light anesthesia.[71] At this time there is no satisfactory explanation for the phenomenon of tourniquet pain. Current theories propose that it is due to cellular ischemia and the accumulation of cellular metabolites.[82] Pain fibers in the ischemic limb are stimulated and the pain is transmitted by either large myelinated fibers or small unmyelinated fibers to the central nervous system.[83–85] Treatment with narcotics or deepening of the anesthetic is not always successful and short-acting vasodilators may be needed.[71] The definitive treatment for tourniquet pain is deflation of the tourniquet; this should be done only at an appropriate time during the surgical procedure.

Orthopedic Fracture Table

Fracture tables used in the operating environment range from the simple to the complex. It is imperative that the operating team be familiar with the mechanics of each table preoperatively. Trendelenburg can be difficult to achieve with some tables and may make treatment of either aspiration or severe hypotension difficult.

The primary advantage of an orthopedic fracture table is the application of traction to the affected extremity to maintain reduction of the fracture. In addition, the table allows wider abduction of the legs to accommodate portable

x-ray machines and it facilitates application of plaster casts.[86(pp2–3)]

The primary disadvantage of the fracture table is a lack of padding. This may cause peripheral nerve injuries from pressure on bony prominences, especially in elderly, thin, or cachectic patients. Less common are peroneal paresthesias from the pressure exerted by the peroneal post.[86(pp10–11)] Because of the difficulty involved in positioning orthopedic patients on these tables, anesthesia is frequently induced in the bed and the patient is moved onto the fracture table once she or he is anesthetized and paralyzed and the airway is secure. This is less painful for the patient but there is increased risk for joint strains, dislocations, or fractures. It is the anesthetist's and surgical team's responsibility to move all patients carefully and prevent strain on the cervical spine and other joints. Also, the fracture table is not recommended if multiple teams are operating, if the patient is extremely unstable, or if cardiac arrest is imminent as access to the patient is restricted by the apparatus of most tables.

Infection Control

Infection that occurs after orthopedic surgery can have disastrous effects especially when prostheses have been inserted or if a deep bone infection occurs. The standard surgical wound infection rate is approximately 5 percent and, with special procedures, can be reduced to less than 1 percent.[87,88] Common sources of infection include the skin, the oropharynx, and airborne bacterial cross-contamination. Osteomyelitis occurs when the bone and marrow become infected. It can be acute or chronic. Eradication is expensive, time consuming, and can lead to loss of limb in some instances.[8(p116)] Efforts to decrease intraoperative and postoperative infections have included the use of perioperative antibiotics, laminar flow, personnel isolation suits, and ultraviolet light. These are not universally accepted precautions and use varies between institutions. It is recommended, however, that face masks be worn inside hoods to decrease bacterial contamination during prosthetic surgery.[89]

Laminar Airflow. Laminar airflow is used primarily to decrease the incidence of wound infections in total joint replacements. In a large study of greater than 8000 patients, laminar flow decreased the incidence of wound infection from 1.2 to 0.7 percent, and laminar flow plus antibiotics resulted in a decrease in infections from 0.7 to 0.3 percent.[90]

The main disadvantage of laminar airflow is the expense of installing the high-efficiency filters; therefore, the cost–benefit ratio to the hospital may be unacceptable.[91–94] Anesthetic concerns include noisy operating rooms and patient hypothermia from the constant flow of cold air across the field.

Personnel Isolation Suits. Self-contained personnel isolation suits similar to space suits are worn by the operating team to provide an infection-free environment for the patient.[87] They are not commonly used by the anesthesia personnel as the anesthetist is removed from close approximation to the operative area.

Ultraviolet Light Therapy. Continuous ultraviolet radiation of 25 µW cm^{-1} directed at the wound has been shown to reduce the infection rate.[95,96] During ultraviolet administration all personnel in the operating room and the patient require extensive protection with goggles, creams, and head gear to prevent skin and eye damage.

Positioning

A tremendous variety of positions are used during orthopedic procedures to facilitate exposure of joints and bones. The anesthetist is often challenged to find a balance between surgical exposure, cardiac and respiratory stability, and patient comfort and safety. In any position, improper positioning of the extremities may lead to stretch- or compression-induced neuropraxia. Tissue ischemia and necrosis can also occur from direct pressure on bony prominences.[97–99] These complications are exacerbated during hypotensive anesthesia or hypothermia. For these reasons, the anesthetist must take special care to ensure that adequate padding has been placed around all bony prominences and pressure points. A thorough discussion of patient positioning can be found in Chapter 13; however, a brief review of concerns specific to orthopedic patients is presented here.

Joint pain secondary to stretching of the joint is especially likely to occur in patients with osteoarthritis, rheumatoid arthritis, osteoporosis, or contractures. It is imperative that the anesthetist not move a joint beyond the patient's normal range of motion. Excessive neck flexion must be avoided in all patients as well. A team approach to positioning is essential to try and prevent injury.[100]

Venous obstruction in the arms can occur in the lateral position from axillary artery compression or mechanical devices to support the upper arm. Femoral vein obstruction can occur from the stabilizing post. Venous obstruction in any position may lead to compartment syndrome and necessitate further surgery. Arterial obstruction can also occur and, for this reason, it is imperative that the anesthetist check pulses in dependent extremities. Placement of the pulse oximeter on the dependent limb can provide continuous monitoring of arterial flow throughout the operation. An arterial line can also be used in this manner when the patient condition dictates use of this invasive monitor.

Air embolism is an infrequent but potentially devastating complication that can occur when the sitting position is used either for cervical spine surgery or, rarely, shoulder surgery. Transthoracic doppler, ETco$_2$, and a right atrial central venous line are beneficial in diagnosis and treatment.[101–103] Orthostatic hypotension is commonly seen in the sitting position and must be vigorously treated.

For surgery done in the prone position, the anesthetist must ensure adequate chest expansion for ventilation by the use of bolsters or one of a variety of frames such as the Wilson or Relton frame.[104,105] Proper prone positioning will not only allow the patient to be ventilated more easily but will also improve venous return, decrease epidural engorgement, and potentially decrease blood loss.[106,107] The arms must be folded at shoulder level or tucked at the sides, padded, and there should be no stretch on the brachial plexus. The anesthetist must check and periodically recheck for pulses in both arms, for pressure on the dependent eye and ear if the head is turned, and for orbital compression if the horseshoe headrest is used, and must ensure that all pressure points are padded.[97–99] Vigilance is of paramount importance.

INTRAOPERATIVE MANAGEMENT

Choice of Anesthetic Technique

The choice of anesthetic technique for an orthopedic case depends on various factors such as surgical site, intraoperative and postoperative patient needs, patient preference, patient's health status, anesthetist's skill, and surgeon's preference. Techniques range from simple to complex.

Repair of simple dislocations and fractures may require no anesthesia participation, especially if the surgeon is adept with local anesthetic injections.[108] This is frequently done in the office or emergency room.

Intravenous sedation and analgesia (monitored anesthesia care) is appropriate in certain procedures such as diagnostic arthroscopy, carpal tunnel, or trigger finger release. This technique requires a good working relationship between the surgeon and anesthetist and is most successful for short procedures, outpatient surgery, and patients with full stomachs as long as nitrous oxide is avoided and reflexes remain intact.

In many instances regional anesthesia may be the ideal choice for orthopedic procedures.[109] For surgery involving the upper extremities, intraoperative advantages include analgesia, muscle relaxation, immobility, abolition of sympathetic responses from the extremity, and minimal effects on the respiratory and circulatory systems.[109] Postoperative benefits include prolonged analgesia, immobility, and blockade of the sympathetic vasoconstrictor fibers, which is especially advantageous for digital replantation.[110,111] Depending on the surgical site, anesthesia can be achieved using various brachial plexus block techniques (interscalene or axillary), intravenous regional anesthesia (Bier block), or individual nerve blocks. Shoulder surgery can be done with an interscalene block and skin infiltration around the axilla if the incision extends that far.[112] Procedures on the elbow can be done with an axillary or interscalene block.[113] Intravenous regional technique is appropriate for procedures on the soft tissues of the hand, forearm, leg, or foot that last up to 90 minutes.[108] Longer procedures and those involving deep bone can be done with an axillary or interscalene block. Combined or individual blocks of the radial, ulnar, and median nerves can be performed by the anesthetist or surgeon depending on an individual's training.

Benefits of regional techniques on the lower extremities are similar to those on the upper limbs. Spinal anesthesia provides rapid onset, complete sensory and motor blockade, decrease in blood loss, postoperative analgesia, and normal respiratory function[114–117]; however urinary retention, spinal headache, hypotension, and prolonged sedation from intravenous adjuncts are potential drawbacks.[118] Epidural anesthesia has the advantages of no headache unless there is inadvertent dural puncture and slower onset of hypotension. Disadvantages of epidural anesthesia include a longer onset time for complete anesthesia; it often takes as long as 30 minutes to achieve ankle anesthesia.[119] Injection of local anesthetic with freshly added epinephrine at L5–S1 or L4–5 has been recommended by Galindo et al[119] to effect a complete blockade of nerve roots innervating the ankle. Spinal anesthesia and the less frequently used caudal anesthesia are options for patients with previous lumbar spine surgery. Individual nerve blocks are also viable choices. For example, ankle or midtarsal blocks can be used for surgery on the forefoot, and femoral and sciatic nerve blocks can be used for procedures on the thigh or leg.[120] The advantage of individual nerve blocks is the absence of hypotension, urinary retention, headache, nausea, and vomiting. These blocks may be ideal in the severely ill or unstable patient. The disadvantages are that these blocks are not universally taught and may be unreliable when attempted by the novice practitioner.

Regional anesthesia of any type is generally contraindicated when there is coagulopathy, infection at the placement site, multiple operative sites, or anatomic problems that prevent placement such as a herniated disc or when the patency of the airway is tenuous. In these situations, general anesthesia is recommended.

General anesthesia is indicated when the surgical procedure is not appropriate for regional or local techniques or when positioning a patient for a regional block is too painful. General anesthesia is also indicated whenever intubation is necessary. Intubation is preferable when the anesthetist is positioned at a distance from the head of the patient and regional anesthesia is not used. Situations that usually require intubation include the prone position; facial, neck, or shoulder surgery; procedures requiring muscle relaxation; extremely long surgeries; trauma; presence of a full stomach; vomiting or history of reflux; an unstable patient; or a tenuous airway.

Anesthesia can be induced either by mask inhalation or by intravenous injection depending on the needs of the patient. Awake fiberoptic, blind nasal, or oral intubation should be considered if the patient's airway is compromised by disease or trauma or if there is hemodynamic instability. Standard intravenous inductions for adults and mask inductions for children, however, can be used in the majority of cases. The choice of induction agents is dictated by the individual needs of the patient.

The maintenance phase of general anesthesia can be conducted with either nitrous oxide–narcotic or nitrous oxide–oxygen inhalation agents for stable patients. Inhalation agents provide a reduction in blood pressure that may decrease intraoperative bleeding. The advantage of a balanced technique is the provision of postoperative analgesia; however, it is important to keep in mind that nitrous oxide may not be tolerated in unstable patients and should not be used in patients with pneumothorax, bowel obstructions, or similar states with pathologic trapping of air. Muscle relaxants are occasionally required for fracture reductions and manipulations.

Prior to emergence, it is necessary to decide between extubation and the need for postoperative ventilation. A thorough evaluation of extubation criteria is imperative for all patients in whom airway patency is a major concern. This is especially applicable to patients with rheumatoid arthritis or ankylosing spondylitis, patients in halo traction,

patients with full stomachs, and trauma patients. It is also important for the patient to remain anesthetized until all casts are dry. Early emergence may result in distortion of the wet cast by patient movement, risking loss of fracture reduction, joint dislocation, or increased bleeding. After the patient has emerged and prior to transport to the postanesthesia recovery room, it is recommended that any operative extremities be elevated to retard swelling, decrease pain, and promote early healing. New intramuscular nonsteroidal anti-inflammatory medications such as ketolorac tromethamine (Toradol) may decrease postoperative swelling and provide initial pain relief when given 1 hour or more prior to emergence.[121]

Induced/Controlled Hypotension

In addition to other factors, blood loss is directly related to the level of the blood pressure. Hypotensive anesthesia may therefore be requested by the surgeons in an effort to decrease the intraoperative blood loss.[122] Hypotension should be induced only when the benefits outweigh the risks. The primary advantage of using a hypotensive anesthetic technique is a 30 to 50 percent reduction in intraoperative bleeding which subsequently decreases the need for transfusion.[123–125] Controlled hypotension has proven beneficial in both hip and scoliosis surgery.[124,126] It also should be considered in Jehovah's Witness patients who generally do not accept blood transfusions.[127] The limits of the reduction in blood pressure and the long-term efficacy have not been established.[128] Consequently this technique is contraindicated in unstable patients and in those with poor myocardial function, severe diabetes, or severe chronic obstructive pulmonary disease.

Hypotension has been induced and maintained by numerous techniques. In a comparative study by Rosberg et al,[122] inhalation agents and sodium nitroprusside in combination resulted in the greatest decrease in blood loss. Other practitioners have successfully used a variety of vasoactive agents such as nitroprusside, esmolol, propranolol, labetalol, trimethaphan, captopril, and nitroglycerin.[126,129,130] Insertion of an arterial line is usually considered mandatory in these cases for moment-to-moment blood pressure observation. Finally, inhalation agents can be used as either a primary or an adjunctive hypotensive agent to decrease blood loss. They have a slower onset and recovery than most intravenous and vasoactive agents. Another alternative is regional anesthesia since the pharmacologic sympathectomy results in pooling of blood, thereby decreasing blood loss by 30 to 50 percent.[124,125]

Transfusion Therapy

Bone is quite vascular and, overall, receives a significant proportion of the cardiac output. All bony procedures conducted without a tourniquet are associated with chronic oozing. Major orthopedic procedures may elicit blood losses that approach the patient's total blood volume.[131] Hidden bleeding is always a possibility, especially when pooling occurs in deep spaces. Severed arteries or veins can create precipitous bleeding and it is important to remember that, in spinal surgery, the aorta, vena cava, and iliac arteries lie adjacent to the anterior aspect of the intravertebral disc.[132] In addition, patients often have postoperative drains and continue to ooze for the first 24 to 48 hours. Table 38–2 describes typical ranges for blood loss in various surgical procedures.

The use of autologous or designated donor blood for transfusions has risen in popularity because of increased public awareness of the dangers of hepatitis and acquired immunodeficiency syndrome from transfusions of anonymous donor blood.[133,134] Also, patients who are on nonsteroidal anti-inflammatory medications or aspirin have a greater tendency to bleed. The objectives during the operative procedure are to maintain an adequate level of hemoglobin that provides for optimum oxygen content and transport and a normal circulating volume for tissue perfusion.

Hemodilution has also been advocated as a strategy to reduce transfusions. In this technique, blood is drawn from the patient just prior to the operative procedure and replaced with crystalloid fluid. The blood is then retransfused after the surgical blood loss is finished.[135,136] Others have advocated the use of the cell saver. The presence of bone chips, debris, and fat from the bone marrow has limited widespread use of this technique in general orthopedics. Scoliosis surgeons, however, have reported successful use of this therapeutic modality.[137]

Evaporative losses need to be replaced in orthopedic patients as incisions are usually moderate in size and exposed surfaces are vascular. Third-space fluid losses are usually small compared with those of abdominal surgery, except in the thoracic approach to a laminectomy.

X-ray Therapy

Orthopedic procedures result in frequent exposure to radiation from the use of C-arm fluoroscopy or flat-plate x-rays. Current recommendations are for personnel in the room to use the standard lead shield precautions for the body and thyroid and lead glasses for eye protection.[138,139] In addition, many institutions advocate the use of radiation badges to quantitate total radiation exposure over time. The anesthetist should also shield the patient from unnecessary exposure to radiation whenever possible.

Monitoring

In conjunction with the standard monitoring employed for any anesthetic, arterial cannulation should be considered in

TABLE 38–2. ESTIMATES OF BLOOD LOSS IN SPECIFIC SURGERIES[a]

Surgical Procedure	Blood Loss (mL)
Hip pinning	200–500
Scoliosis/spinal surgery	500–3000
Total hip replacement	800–2500
Revision total hip replacement	1500–7000
Total knee replacement (± tourniquet)	100–1000
En bloc resection	1000–5000

[a] Estimates are based on 19 years of combined orthopedic and anesthetic experience.

long, complex operations. Examples include patients who will be exposed to large fluid shifts, massive blood loss, or induced hypotension or patients whose individual health history dictates the use of cannulation, as in patients with severe hypertension or chronic obstructive pulmonary disease. When the procedure is done in the lateral position, the dependent arm should be used for pulse oximetry and arterial cannulation to evaluate the adequacy of circulation to that limb.

A central venous pressure line or pulmonary artery catheter is indicated for patients undergoing procedures with large volume shifts who have poor ventricular function. The absolute value of numbers obtained from the pulmonary artery catheter and central venous pressure line is questionable in the lateral position; however, following trends can be quite beneficial.

The current recommendation in prosthetic surgery is that a urinary catheter should not be placed.[140] There is an increased risk of gram-negative infection with these catheters and infection in the joint prosthesis can be devastating.

SPECIAL PROCEDURES IN ORTHOPEDICS

Amputations

Amputation of part or all of an extremity can be done for congenital anomalies, tumors, or osteomyelitis. Most often, however, the procedure is done because of insufficient blood supply as a result of peripheral vascular disease, diabetes, or trauma. The choice of anesthesia for these procedures is frequently dictated by the physical status of the patient. In the patient with severe systemic disease, lower extremity amputations occasionally can be done under local anesthesia but are usually done under spinal anesthesia. This technique has demonstrable advantages within the first 24 hours.[141] The surgeon may or may not use the tourniquet during these cases. If the tourniquet is not used, it enables the surgeon to identify viable tissue more easily and avoid damage to sclerotic vessels.

Arthroscopy

In the last 10 years arthroscopy has become one of the most prevalent and profitable orthopedic procedures. Initially this procedure was developed for examination of the knee joint, and now has been expanded to include ankles, shoulders, elbows, wrists, and temporomandibular joints. Arthroscopies can be done under local, regional, or general anesthetic techniques.[142-144] The choice of anesthesia depends on the operative site, the patient's physical status, and the preferences of the surgeon, the patient, and the anesthetist. A diagnostic arthroscopy can be of brief duration. More advanced procedures such as anterior cruciate ligament reconstruction can be done partially through the arthroscope and are often quite lengthy.

Bone Grafting

Bone grafting is done in conjunction with other procedures such as spinal fusions, leg lengthening, joint reconstructions, repair of fractures, and tumor resections. The bone graft acts either as a source of bone inductive material or as a mechanical support.[7(p77)] Bone grafts are usually harvested from the iliac crest. These procedures are bloody, and patients can lose up to one unit of blood intraoperatively.[145] Postoperatively the bone harvest site is usually a persistent source of pain for the patient, necessitating adequate pain management.

Closed Reduction of Fractures/Dislocations

Closed reductions of fractures or dislocations are also short procedures that require intense analgesia and occasionally require skeletal muscle relaxation. Regional techniques, heavy sedation with midazolam, and general anesthesia via mask or endotracheal tube have all been used. Patients scheduled for these procedures may arrive in the operating suite in a sedated state from medications given in the emergency room during initial attempts to reduce the fracture or dislocation.

Examination under Anesthesia

Examinations under anesthesia can range from evaluation of joint range of motion to joint manipulation in which the surgeon attempts to break up adhesions. Examinations under anesthesia tend to be very short, lasting from 5 to 20 minutes. Unless there is a history of reflux or a full stomach, these patients can usually be anesthetized using a face mask. The intraoperative course is generally uneventful. If adhesions have been broken during joint manipulation, the pain is usually intense in the immediate recovery period.

Fractures of the Hip

One of the most common operations done in orthopedics is repair of a hip fracture. These patients are often elderly; half of all hip fractures are in persons 80 years of age or older.[7(p75)] In one study of over 200 patients, 91 percent had significant nonorthopedic findings that required treatment or correction prior to surgery.[4] Careful preoperative evaluation with attention to the details identified previously in this chapter is therefore important.[6]

Repair of a hip fracture can be on an urgent or semi-urgent basis. Orthopedic data have shown a fourfold increase in morbidity and mortality for patients whose operative repair is delayed longer than 24 hours, compared with patients who receive earlier fixation.[146] Patients with intracapsular fractures of the hip have an increased incidence of avascular necrosis if repair is delayed. This tendency toward necrosis of the head of the femur is due to swelling and bleeding into the enclosed space.[8(p198)] Intertrochanteric fractures are associated with greater blood loss and the patients are at increased risk for hypovolemic shock as time passes.[8(p198)] Complicating factors that should be corrected preoperatively include dehydration, anemia, shock, heart failure, and pneumonia. Dehydration from bedrest, bleeding, and NPO status can result in a 500- to 1000-mL deficit, and anemia from the bleeding can result in decreased oxygen-carrying capacity. The hematocrit may appear to be within normal limits if the patient is dehydrated.

Pneumonia is a major cause of morbidity and mortality after a hip fracture.[8(p198)] The respiratory insult may not improve until the fracture is stabilized, the pain is decreased, and the patient becomes ambulatory. Consequently, early mobilization is attempted whenever possible. In addition, pain from the fracture itself can inhibit coughing and deep breathing which increases atelectasis and exacerbates the compromise of the respiratory system. Preoperatively, it is important to achieve maximum ventilatory function with intermittent positive-pressure breathing treatments, hand-held nebulizer treatments, or deep breathing exercises.

The ideal anesthetic for repair of a fractured hip has been, and still is, controversial.[6,147] Regional techniques have been advocated by many.[114,116,148] When a spinal anesthetic is chosen, the patient should be gently positioned with the fractured extremity down for a hyperbaric spinal or with the fractured extremity up if a hypobaric solution is used. The choice of local anesthetic depends on the anticipated length of the procedure. It is important to remember that positioning can be painful for the patient. The pain can be minimized with the judicious use of narcotics while traction is maintained on the fractured extremity.[149] The logistical problems associated with regional anesthesia in hip fractures dictate that this technique be used by experienced practitioners. Continuous spinal technique has also been advocated to provide extended anesthesia for longer cases as well as for postoperative pain management.[114,150] Femoral nerve blocks are an alternative anesthetic choice. They provide less hemodynamic disruption than a spinal or epidural sympathetic blockade while maintaining adequate analgesia.[151]

General anesthesia is a viable alternative for patients with hip fractures. Overhead traction is often used to maintain alignment of the fracture and should not be removed prior to induction. The induction is usually carried out with the patient in the hospital bed. The patient is then transferred and positioned on the operating room table. The logistical difficulties of moving and positioning an awake patient who is in pain on the operating table are therefore avoided. Gastric emptying time is delayed in these patients from the combination of trauma, pain, and age. Therefore, the risk of aspiration on induction is increased. The choice of induction agents and the type of general anesthetic must be individualized and based on the patient's physical status, medication regimen, and health history. If the patient is extremely unstable, light sedation can be used for positioning. Induction is then delayed to minimize the anesthetic exposure; however, this can be done only when the patient is supine on a regular operating room table, as positioning an awake patient on most fracture tables is uncomfortable and unwieldy. For elderly patients, the anesthetist can usually decrease the dosages of narcotics, inhalation agents, and muscle relaxants during the maintenance phase of the anesthetic.

Hypotension from hypovolemia is a frequent complication associated with hip fractures. Hypovolemia may be caused by blood loss from the fracture itself, dehydration, orthostatic changes during positioning, or excess anesthesia. To aid hemodynamic stability, it is advisable to judiciously preload the patient with fluids prior to anesthetizing and positioning. Vascular emboli from venous stasis and a poorly defined hypercoagulopathy may also occur. Prophylaxis usually consists of low-dose heparin, antiembolism stockings, or both. Emboli that travel to the pulmonary system are the most common cause of death pre-, intra-, and postoperatively in patients with hip fractures.[152]

Pelvic Fractures

The majority of pelvic fractures do not need operative fixation for stabilization. An acetabular fracture is a less common pelvic fracture that always requires operative fixation. These cases are usually bloody and muscle relaxation is necessary to dislocate the hip and expose the socket.[153,154]

Replantation of Digits/Limbs

Surgery to reimplant traumatically severed digits or limbs provides several challenges for the anesthetist. These procedures are done with microsurgical anastomoses and require fine attention to detail on the part of the surgeon; the procedure is also quite lengthy.[110,111] A combined regional and general approach has been advocated that is advantageous in several areas. The general anesthetic provides patient comfort for the long duration of the surgery, and the sympathectomy from the regional blockade improves blood flow to the digit or limb that is being reanastomosed. Hypothermia should be avoided whenever possible because of the undesirable effects of vasoconstriction and shivering during the emergence and postanesthetic phases of the patient's recovery.

Shoulder Operations

Shoulder operations are done for shoulder instability, recurrent dislocations, torn rotator cuff, joint manipulation, or shoulder replacement. The anesthetic technique of choice is usually general anesthesia because of the proximity of the patient's head to the operative site. Regional anesthesia with an interscalene block supplemented by a supraclavicular block or a paravertebral block can provide adequate anesthesia but patient hearing is acute and sedation is often warranted.[155]

Spinal Column Surgery

Indications for surgery on the spinal column include laminectomy, spinal fusion, tumor excision, and scoliosis correction. Prior to surgery it is important for the anesthetist to review the etiology of the case. This information and that found in the preoperative workup assist in planning a safe anesthetic. Regional or general anesthesia can be used alone or in combination for spinal surgery.[156–158] Under general anesthesia, the surgeon may occasionally opt to test nerve function directly. In these situations, muscle relaxation should be minimized or avoided. Communication with the surgical team preoperatively will clarify whether or not this technique will be used.

Occasionally a laminectomy is done under local anesthesia, but the majority of cases are done under general anesthesia. A laminectomy is usually done to remove a herniated disc or decompress the lamina. Laminectomies can be done on the lumbar spine, thoracic spine, or cervical spine. The patient is usually in the prone position, although for thoracic and cervical laminectomies, the patient may be supine or lateral when the surgeon uses an anterior approach.[159,160] Major concerns for laminectomy include blood loss and positioning. Patients undergoing a cervical laminectomy need careful airway attention and monitoring. An awake blind nasal or an awake fiberoptic intubation is the preferred technique for patients who are in a halo jacket, have limited range of neck or jaw motion, or have an unstable neck.[161]

Spinal fusion is usually done to stabilize the vertebral column. The lamina are often fused with a bone graft harvested from the iliac crest. Positioning and blood loss are major concerns during these procedures.

Documentation of the preoperative neurologic status is important in patients with spinal cord tumors. Neurologists frequently consult on these patients and the anesthetist should be familiar with the neurologic exam. If neurology is not involved, it is imperative that the anesthetist conduct and document a detailed preoperative assessment of neurologic deficits to provide a baseline for postoperative comparison.

Patients with scoliosis come to the operating room for either anterior or posterior spinal fusion, with or without instrumentation. The scoliotic curve can range from mild to severe. The operative goal is to prevent progression of the curvature, maintain posture, and arrest any decline in pulmonary and cardiac status.[162] Scoliosis can be congenital, acquired, or secondary to neuromuscular disorders such as muscular dystrophy and polio.

In addition to the usual considerations, it is important to carefully assess the pulmonary status of scoliotic patients preoperatively. As the compressed hemithorax approaches residual volume these patients develop the pattern typically seen in pulmonary restrictive disease. The mechanical defect results in increased pulmonary vascular resistance, decreased compliance, restricted rib expansion, decreased vital capacity, and decreased total lung capacity. In addition, there is increased ventilation–perfusion mismatch, increased physiologic shunting, increased dead space, decreased arterial oxygen tension, and increased arterial carbon dioxide tension.[57] If the spinal curve is greater than 90 degrees, it can be expected that the forced expiratory volume at 1 second (FEV_1) will be less than 25 percent of predicted.[58] Whenever the respiratory symptoms or the curvature is significant, pulmonary function testing and arterial blood gases should be done.

The spinal curvature may limit range of motion of the neck and make intubation difficult. It is important that this be assessed prior to induction. Intubation options include awake oral intubation with local anesthesia, awake blind nasal intubation, and awake fiberoptic intubation especially if the spine is severely compromised or unstable.[162]

Cardiac problems in this patient population are usually secondary to progression of the scoliotic curve. Right ventricular hypertrophy and cor pulmonale commonly occur. This patient population also has an increased incidence of malignant hyperthermia and a family history of previous anesthetics should be obtained.[60] Blood loss is moderate to large in these cases and blood should be available.

Frequently, the patients have autologous or designated donor units.[137]

Paresthesias and paralysis are always possible complications from manipulation of the spinal cord as the surgeon tries to straighten the spine. Two methods are commonly used to assess function of the cord. One is the intraoperative wakeup; the other is the use of somatosensory evoked potentials.[163,164] As the spine is distracted, anterior spinal artery flow may be compromised, leading to ischemia and motor weakness in the lower extremity. This may or may not be detected by evaluation of somatosensory evoked potentials; therefore, some surgeons still use the intraoperative wakeup procedure.[165]

An intraoperative wakeup requires the anesthetist to awaken the patient while intubated, with the incision open, and request him or her to move the feet. The anesthetic most commonly used is a short-acting narcotic infusion with nitrous oxide and a muscle relaxant.[166] It is important to avoid rapid reversal of the narcotic and muscle relaxant which could cause sudden alertness and dangerous movement. The muscle relaxant is allowed to ebb to two twitches on the train-of-four, the narcotic infusion is decreased, and the nitrous oxide is discontinued. Within 3 to 5 minutes, most patients respond to verbal commands and move their feet. Once movement is detected, anesthesia can be reintroduced. Other institutions have successfully used potent inhalation anesthetics for the intraoperative wakeup test. Neuromuscular blockade is again allowed to ebb to two twitches, the inhalation agent is decreased, and a small amount of narcotic is given to blunt laryngeal reflexes. With this technique, it can take up to 15 minutes for the patient to become alert enough to move the feet. With either technique, the incidence of recall is minimal. An intraoperative wakeup test is not foolproof, however, and false-negative results have been reported.[167]

Somatosensory evoked potentials (SSEPs) are used to assess the neural outflow from the posterior spinal cord on a continuous basis. Changes in the latency and amplitude of the evoked potentials alert surgeons to spinal cord dysfunction.[168] Evoked potentials are affected by temperature, blood pressure, acidosis, and inhalational anesthetics. The goal for the anesthetist is to keep all factors stable and minimize changes; any variation in the SSEPs is then attributed to the surgical procedure. Inhalation agents decrease the amplitude of the SSEPs and are generally avoided. Muscle relaxants have no direct effect on SSEPs. Nitrous oxide–narcotic with muscle relaxation is the anesthetic of choice for spinal surgery with SSEPs.[164] Whether intraoperative wakeup or SSEPs are used, rapid emergence at the end of the case is desirable to assess possible cord deficits.

Spinal surgery is associated with continuous blood loss from bony surface oozing, necessitating close attention to the patient's volume status. Severed arteries or veins can result in sudden, rapid blood loss. A patient undergoing scoliosis repair is also at risk for increased bleeding because of the proximity of the aorta, vena cava, and iliac arteries to the intervertebral disc space.[132] To decrease the blood loss, deliberate hypotension may be requested by the surgeons.[126,129,169,170] In addition, surgeons also frequently use local anesthetics with epinephrine to help control the blood loss. The anesthetist should calculate the maximum doses of epinephrine and local anesthetics. The surgeon should be informed of these limits, especially when inhalation agents are used.

Patients having anterior spinal fusions will have an open chest, and the lung will need to be compressed to aid in surgical exposure. Ventilation and perfusion abnormalities both intra- and postoperatively can be expected. Ventilatory support in the immediate postoperative period is often necessary as transient deterioration in lung function is not uncommon.[57] It is important that the anesthetist follow arterial blood gases and pulse oximetry closely. Patients with anterior fusions will also have chest tubes postoperatively.

Total Joint Replacements

Hips. Total hip replacements are done for a variety of reasons including osteoarthritis, rheumatoid arthritis, ankylosing spondylitis, congenital anomalies, failed repair of fractures, hip dysplasias, failed total hip replacements, and neoplasms. A significant subset of these patients are elderly and arthritic. A thorough preoperative evaluation is essential. These patients often have a limited ability to exercise because of pain or joint dysfunction, making assessment of cardiovascular and respiratory reserves difficult. Primary hip replacements differ from revision hip replacements. Revision total hip replacements are associated with increased blood loss and patients have an increased need for transfusions.[171]

Patients for total hip replacements can benefit from adequate premedication. Narcotics are appropriate if the airway is not compromised and the hemodynamic profile is stable. A light dose of a benzodiazepine is an alternative for patients with moderate to severe systemic disease; no narcotic should be administered if there are any doubts.

Regional anesthesia, general anesthesia, and a combined technique have all been successfully used for hip replacements. Regardless of the technique chosen, consideration of a fluid challenge prior to induction and positioning is warranted. The fluid helps maintain hemodynamic stability, especially if the patient is dehydrated. Cautious fluid loading is recommended in the elderly patient. Under general anesthesia, intubation is usually mandatory because of lateral positioning after induction. Occasionally, muscle relaxation is necessary to enable the surgeon to dislocate the hip intraoperatively. For all techniques, it is recommended that the blood pressure and electrocardiogram be monitored closely and all fluids be warmed.

The prostheses used in total hip replacements fall into two categories, cemented and porous ingrowth implants. The porous ingrowth prosthesis is the newest of the implants and was initially considered superior as cement was not needed. The porous ingrowth implants have a titanium mesh or beads that allow bone to grow into the implant itself. Consequently, revisions of ingrowth implants can be very bloody. Cemented implants, which had fallen into disfavor in the recent past, are regaining popularity as a result of improved techniques.[172] The cement used is polymethylmethacrylate, an acrylic compound. It is a space-filling mortar used to transmit compressive loads between the bone and prosthesis.[173] The surgeon may ask for deliberate hypotension to decrease bleeding and facilitate a dry interface between bone and cement.[122,124–125,130] This helps make a dry seal and prevents loosening of the prosthesis and subsequent pain.

Polymethylmethacrylate is associated with several serious complications. Hypotension is the most common and occurs in some, but not all, patients.[174,175] There is variability in the onset, duration, and degree of hypotension.[176] The onset can be as soon as 30 to 60 seconds after insertion of the cement or can be delayed for up to 10 minutes. The duration is approximately 5 minutes. The exact cause of the hypotension is not known. One theory attributes the hypotension to a monomer in the cement that is a myocardial depressant or a vasodilator.[176–178] It has also been postulated that the hypotension is due to fat and bone marrow emboli that are released into the circulation as the cement is forced down the femoral canal.[179–181] A third theory identifies thermal necrosis as the culprit. The hot cement heats marrow and red blood cells which triggers the release of thrombotic and vasoactive substances.[182] The hypotension is most severe after the femoral component is cemented as compared with cementing of the acetabular component. Ultimately, if not treated, the hypotension may lead to cardiovascular collapse.[177,179,180,183] Whenever possible, anesthesia should be lightened and the patient should be given fluids by bolus. In addition, careful monitoring of the blood pressure should be initiated prior to insertion of the cement.

Respiratory compromise may also occur during cemented polymethylmethacrylate replacements; the etiology is unclear. The partial pressure of arterial oxygen decreases after insertion of the cement into the femoral shaft. This decreased arterial oxygen content may last up to 5 days.[115,176] Clinically, an increase in pulmonary vascular resistance, an increase in airway resistance, as well as fat, blood, and bone marrow emboli, have been documented. Emboli from the fat and bone marrow can lead to hypoxemia and an increased incidence of pulmonary edema, as well as deterioration of the ventilation–perfusion ratio.[115,176,183–186] Some practitioners advocate discontinuing any nitrous oxide 1 to 3 minutes prior to insertion of the cement and then leaving it off until the cement has set for 5 minutes. This maximizes oxygen content and transport prior to any hypoxia or hypotension.

Hemorrhage is an ever-present potential problem especially during total hip replacements. It is most likely to occur during reaming of the femoral canal.[187] As blood loss in these cases may be sudden and considerable, it is recommended that the volume status be kept within 10 percent of the normal blood volume at all times. In general, porous ingrowth replacement surgery tends to elicit more bleeding while the polymethylmethacrylate in a cemented hip prosthesis helps stop the bleeding.

Knee. Prosthetic knee replacements are indicated for the relief of pain, most commonly related to osteoarthritis or rheumatoid arthritis. In addition, these patients are often obese and it is believed that the extra weight exacerbates cartilage damage and increases pain.[7(p586)] The prosthesis can be either cemented or porous ingrowth. Regional anesthesia is ideal for this group of patients; however, general anesthesia is also used frequently. A tourniquet is usually used intraoperatively to decrease blood loss and pro-

vide a dry operating field. Postoperatively, drains can put out as much as 500 to 1000 mL during the first 24 hours, which may necessitate transfusion therapy. These patients are usually placed in either passive motion devices or long leg casts. The trend toward early movement of the knee results in increased postoperative pain, leading to difficult pain management in some cases.[188]

Other Joints. Shoulder replacements are being done with increasing frequency. The prosthesis is cemented and currently showing good results. Elbow joint replacements are not often done at this time as the prosthesis has not been perfected. Prosthetic ankle replacements, also known as tibial–talus joints, are done infrequently as fusions work equally as well and the patient avoids an implanted foreign body. Finger joint replacements, specifically for the interphalangeal joint or metacarpophalangeal joint, have been done for years with very good results. These are also known as Swanson arthroplasties. These cases are ideal for regional anesthesia but may be done under general as well. Of all the joint replacements, knees, hips, and fingers are the most commonly done.

Tumor Resection

Surgical repair is indicated for tumors in which the defect in the bone is greater than 2.5 cm or when greater than 50 percent of the cortical strength of a long bone is destroyed.[189(p47)] Metastatic cancers are the number one reason for tumor resection by the orthopedist; renal cell cancer produces the bloodiest tumor. The most common type of primary tumor for resection is a myeloma followed by osteogenic sarcoma.[189(p41)] Treatment usually consists of curettage or resection with subsequent fixation by a plate, intramedullary rodding, cementing of the defect in the long part of the bone, or en bloc resection.[189(pp115–141)] With metastatic disease, surgical treatment is advocated for fracture prophylaxis or for symptomatic pain control.

Allografts, either living or cadaveric, are older techniques that provide stabilization to the tumorless bone after resection.[190,191] Vascularized fibular grafts or autografts were widely used in the past but their popularity in current clinical practice is waning.[192,193] A more aggressive approach to bony tumors that enables limb salvage is the en bloc resection with custom prosthesis.[194] These are usually done in major medical centers and occasionally in community hospitals. En bloc resections are associated with large blood losses.[7(p129)] The patient may require as many as 6 to 10 units of blood. These resections are frequently quite long, requiring aggressive warming measures and a urinary drainage catheter for fluid management. Regional narcotics are useful for postoperative pain relief because of the extensive operative area.

The anesthetist should be aware of any prior radiation and chemotherapeutic regimens that the patient has received. Various chemotherapeutic agents have direct interactions with anesthetic medications. Examples include cardiomyopathy from adriamycin exposure and susceptibility to oxygen toxicity after bleomycin administration. Prior radiation therapy is associated with an increased incidence of bleeding during surgical excision of the affected area.

POSTOPERATIVE CONSIDERATIONS

Fat Embolism

Fat embolism is a common complication after bone trauma, especially when the long bones are affected.[195] Fat emboli can occur anytime between the first hour of surgery and 96 hours postoperatively. Symptoms include dyspnea, tachycardia, restlessness, and hypoxia. Less obvious symptoms include mild fever, petechiae, bilateral patchy infiltrates on chest x-rays, shunting patterns on arterial blood gases, and low saturations on the pulse oximeter.[196,197] If the patient has a known fat embolus preoperatively, it is recommended that elective surgery be postponed 5 days. Treatment for fat emboli is generally supportive. Intubation with positive end-expiratory pressure is used only when absolutely necessary. Other treatment regimens for fat emboli that have been tried include steroids, heparin, dextran, and intravenous alcohol.[197,198] Currently oxygen therapy, appropriate fluid management, and prevention of hypoxemia constitute the most widely accepted approach.[195,199]

Deep-Vein Thrombosis

Deep-vein thrombosis (DVT) is a postoperative complication that can occur after any orthopedic procedure. Fatal pulmonary embolism from deep-vein thrombosis is a major cause of death in total joint replacement surgery with rates as high as 3.5 percent.[200] After total hip or total knee arthroplasty, up to 70 percent of the patients may develop DVT and rates in excess of 75 percent have been reported after fractures of the femoral head.[201] It is believed that the initial thrombus forms intraoperatively as a result of venous stasis and, in conjunction with changes in the coagulation system, thrombus development occurs.[202] Regional anesthetic techniques that enhance lower extremity blood flow have been advocated in an effort to avoid DVT[203,204]; however, studies such as that by Modig et al[205] have reported rates of DVT as high as 50 percent under epidural anesthesia. The reported incidence of DVT under regional anesthesia is quite variable, leading some to propose a multifactorial pathway. Other contributory factors that are postulated include decreased cardiac output, controlled hypotension, excessive blood loss, and hypothermia. Prophylaxis against DVT can be achieved by administration of anticoagulants preoperatively, perioperatively, or both. Antiembolism stockings are another widely used form of DVT prophylaxis and are pneumatic or elastic in nature.

Pain Control

Postoperative pain management for orthopedics has benefited greatly from the recent advances in this field. New techniques include patient-controlled analgesia, continuous intravenous narcotic infusions, epidural infusions of narcotics and local anesthetics, and transcutaneous electric nerve stimulation (TENS).[206–209] The judicious use of an appropriate pain management modality allows for early ambulation and the prevention of postoperative muscle atrophy or pulmonary compromise from immobility.[147] Epidural anesthesia in the immediate postoperative period appears to provide the most complete resolution of pain.[210]

Medications used for epidural administration include morphine, fentanyl, sufentanil, local anesthetics, and combinations of a local anesthetic and a narcotic. It is important to remember that delayed-onset respiratory depression can occur with epidural narcotics. Caution must be used in patients with rheumatoid arthritis, ankylosing spondylitis, and halo traction and in anyone with a compromised airway. Epidural pain management is appropriate in the immediate postoperative period only, as ambulation is not advisable with this technique because of possible motor weakness. In our institution, it is common to maintain epidural narcotics for the first 24 hours and then change over to patient-controlled analgesia to facilitate early ambulation. A more thorough discussion of pain management techniques can be found in Chapter 48.

REFERENCES

1. Banks HH. Symposium on care of the critically ill orthopedic patient. *Orthop Clin North Am.* 1978;9:3.
2. Jeffers FC. The science of gerontology. In: Jeffers FC, ed. *Proceedings of seminars.* Durham, NC: Duke University Press; 1959–1961:123.
3. Ellison N, Mull TD. Unique anesthetic problems in the elderly patient coming to surgery for fracture of the hip. *Orthop Clin North Am.* 1974;5:493.
4. Haljamae H, Stefansson T, Wichkstrom I. Preanesthetic evaluation of the female geriatric patient with hip fracture. *Acta Anaesth Scand.* 1982;26:393.
5. Allen HL, Metcalf DW. Fractured hip: A study of anesthesia in the aged. *Anesth Analg.* 1965;44:408.
6. Davie IT, MacRae WR, Malcolm-Smith NA. Anesthesia for the fractured hip: A survey of 200 cases. *Anesth Analg.* 1970;49:165.
7. Poss R, ed. *Orthopaedic knowledge update 3.* Park Ridge, IL: American Academy of Orthopaedic Surgeons; 1990.
8. Mercier LR, Pettid FJ. *Practical orthopedics.* Chicago: Year Book Medical; 1980:168.
9. Marbach JJ, Spiera H. Rheumatoid spondylitis and systemic lupus erythematosus with temporomandibular joint changes. *NY State Med.* 1969;69:2908.
10. Phelps JA. Laryngeal obstruction due to cricoarytenoid arthritis. *Anesthesiology.* 1966;27:518.
11. McCarthy DJ. Pathology of rheumatoid arthritis and allied disorders. In: McCarthy DJ, ed. *Arthritis and allied conditions.* 11th ed. Philadelphia: Lea & Febiger; 1989:647.
12. Canale ST. Miscellaneous affections of bones and joints. In: Edmonson AS, Crenshaw AH, eds. *Campbell's operative orthopaedics.* 6th ed. Saint Louis, MO: CV Mosby; 1980:1169–1181.
13. Santavirta S, Slatis P, Kankaanpaa J, et al. Treatment of the cervical spine in rheumatoid arthritis. *J Bone Joint Surg.* 1988; 70A:658.
14. Ranawat CS, O'Leary PK, Pellicci PM, et al. Cervical spine fusion in rheumatoid arthritis. *J Bone Joint Surg.* 1979;61A:1003.
15. Breeveld FC, Algra PR, Veilvoye JC, Cats A. Magnetic resonance imaging in the evaluation of patients with rheumatoid arthritis and subluxations of the cervical spine. *Arthritis Rheum.* 1987;30:624.
16. Rana NA, Hancock DO, Taylor AR, Hill AGS. Atlantoaxial subluxation in rheumatoid arthritis. *J Bone Joint Surg.* 1973;55B:458.
17. Rana NA, Hancock DO, Taylor AR, Hill AGS. Upward translocation of the dens in rheumatoid arthritis. *J Bone Joint Surg.* 1973;55B:471.
18. Stoelting RK, Dierdorf SF, McCammon RL, eds. *Anesthesia and co-existing disease.* 2nd ed. New York: Churchill Livingstone; 1988.

19. Stevens JM, Kendall BE, Crockard HA. The spinal cord in rheumatoid arthritis with clinical myelopathy: A computed myelographic study. *J Neurol Neurosurg Psychiatry.* 1986;49:140.

20. Chamberlain MA, Corbett M. Carpal tunnel syndrome in early rheumatoid arthritis. *Ann Rheum Dis.* 1970;29:149.

21. Chamberlain MA, Corbett M. Rheumatoid neuropathy. Clinical and electrophysiological features. *Ann Rheum Dis.* 1970; 29:609.

22. McCarthy DJ. Juvenile rheumatoid arthritis. In: McCarthy DJ, ed. *Arthritis and allied conditions.* 11th ed. Philadelphia: Lea & Febiger; 1989:913.

23. McCarthy DJ. Ankylosing spondylitis. In: McCarthy DJ, ed. *Arthritis and allied conditions.* 11th ed. Philadelphia: Lea & Febiger; 1989:934.

24. Munson ES, Cullen SC. Endotracheal intubation in a patient with ankylosing spondylitis of the cervical spine. *Anesthesiology.* 1965;26:365.

25. Feltelius N, Hendenstrom H, Hillerdall G, Hallgreen R. Pulmonary involvement in ankylosing spondylitis. *Ann Rheum Dis.* 1986;45:736.

26. Bukley BH, Roberts WC. Ankylosing spondylitis and aortic regurgitation. Description of the characteristic cardiovascular lesion from study of eight necropsy patients. *Circulation.* 1973;48:1014.

27. Symreng T, Karlberg BE, Kagedal B, Schildt B. Physiological cortisol substitution of long-term steroid treated patients undergoing major surgery. *Br J Anaesth.* 1981;53:949–953.

28. Smith JB, Willis AL. Aspirin selectively inhibits prostaglandin production in human platelets. *Nature.* 1971;231:235–237.

29. Stoelting RK. *Pharmacology and physiology in anesthetic practice.* Philadelphia: JB Lippincott; 1987.

30. Pietrafesa CA, Hoffman JR. Traumatic dislocation of the hip. *JAMA.* 1983;249:3342.

31. Milford L. The hand. In: Edmonson AS, Crenshaw AH, eds. *Campbell's operative orthopaedics.* 6th ed. Saint Louis, MO: CV Mosby; 1980:268.

32. Harris JH Jr, Edeiken-Monroe B, Kopaniky DR. A practical classification of acute cervical spine injuries. *Orthop Clin North Am.* 1986;17:15–30.

33. Shires GT. Management of hypovolemic shock. *Bull NY Acad Sci.* 1979;55:139.

34. Gallagher TH, Banner MJ, Barnes PA. Large volume crystalloid resuscitation does not increase extravascular lung water. *Anesth Analg.* 1985;64:323.

35. Nimmo WS. Effects of anaesthesia on gastric motility and emptying. *Br J Anaesth.* 1984;56:29.

36. Francis RN, Kwik RSH. Oral ranitidine for prophylaxis against Mendelson's syndrome. *Anesth Analg.* 1982;61:130–132.

37. Murphy DF, Nally B, Gardiner J, et al. Effect of metoclopramide on gastric emptying before elective and emergency cesarean section. *Br J Anaesth.* 1984;56:1113.

38. Bone LB, Johnson KD, Weigelt J, et al. Early versus delayed stabilization of femoral fractures: A prospective randomized study. *J Bone Joint Surg.* 1989;71A:336–340.

39. Johnson KE, Cadambi A, Seibert GB. Incidence of adult respiratory distress syndrome in patients with multiple musculoskeletal injuries: Effect of early operative stabilization of fractures. *J Trauma.* 1985;24:375–384.

40. Bone L, Bucholz R. The management of fractures in the patient with multiple trauma. *J Bone Joint Surg.* 1986;68A:945–949.

41. Godina M. Early microsurgical reconstruction of complex trauma of the extremities. *Plast Reconstr Surg.* 1986;78:285–292.

42. Stehling L. Anesthesia for children requiring orthopaedic surgery. *Anesthesiol Rev.* 1978;5:19.

43. Mayhew JF, Katz J, Miner M, et al. Anaesthesia for the achondroplastic dwarf. *Can Anaesth Soc J.* 1986;33:216–221.

44. Kalla GN, Fening E, Obiaya MD. Anaesthetic management of achondroplasia. *Br J Anaesth.* 1986;58:117–119.

45. Reid CS, Pyeritz RE, Kopits SE, et al. Cervicomedullary compression in young patients with achondroplasia: Value of comprehensive neurologic and respiratory evaluation. *J Pediatr.* 1987;110:522–530.

46. Cohen SE. Anesthesia for cesarean section in achondroplastic dwarfs. *Anesthesiology.* 1980;52:264–266.

47. Nelson KB, Ellenberg JH. Antecedents of cerebral palsy. *N Engl J Med.* 1986;315:81–86.

48. Dierdorf SF, McNiece WL, Rao CC, et al. Effect of succinylcholine on plasma potassium in children with cerebral palsy. *Anesthesiology.* 1985;62:88–90.

49. Williams JP, Somerville GM, Miner ME, Reilly D. Atlanto-axial subluxation and trisomy-21: Another perioperative complication. *Anesthesiology.* 1987;67:253–254.

50. Hensinger RN, DeVito PD, Ragsdale CG. Changes in the cervical spine in juvenile rheumatoid arthritis. *J Bone Joint Surg.* 1986;68A:189–198.

51. Stiles CM. Anesthesia for the mentally retarded. *Orthop Clin North Am.* 1981;12:45.

52. Smith PEM, Calverley PMA, Edwards RHT, et al. Practical problems in the respiratory care of patients with muscular dystrophy. *N Engl J Med.* 1987;316:1197–1204.

53. Smith CL, Bush GH. Anaesthesia and progressive muscular dystrophy. *Br J Anaesth.* 1985;57:112–118.

54. Seay AR, Ziter FA, Thompson JA. Cardiac arrest during induction of anesthesia in Duchenne's muscular dystrophy. *J Pediatr.* 1978;93:88–90.

55. Rosenberg H, Heiman-Patterson T. Duchenne's muscular dystrophy and malignant hyperthermia: Another warning. *Anesthesiology.* 1983;59:362.

56. Brownell AKW, Paasuke RT, Elash A, et al. Malignant hyperthermia in Duchenne's muscular dystrophy. *Anesthesiology.* 1983;58:180–182.

57. Levin DB. Pulmonary function in scoliosis. *Orthop Clin North Am.* 1979;10:761.

58. Weinstein SL. Idiopathic scoliosis: Natural history. *Spine.* 1986;11:780–783.

59. McCollough NC III. Non-operative treatment of idiopathic scoliosis using surface electrical stimulation. *Spine.* 1986;11: 802–804.

60. Kafer ER. Respiratory and cardiovascular function in scoliosis and the principles of anesthetic management. *Anesthesiology.* 1980;52:339–351.

61. Valli H, Rosenberg PH. Effects of three anaesthesia methods on hemodynamic responses connected with the use of thigh tourniquet in orthopaedic patients. *Acta Anaesthiol Scand.* 1985;29:142.

62. Bradford EMW. Haemodynamic changes associated with the application of lower limb tourniquets. *Anesthesiology.* 1969; 24:190.

63. Ikemoto Y, Kobayashi H, Usui M, Ishii S. Changes in serum myoglobin levels caused by tourniquet ischemia under normothermic and hypothermic conditions. *Clin Orthop.* 1988; 234:296.

64. Lynn AM, Fisher T, Brandford HG, Pendergrass TW. Systemic responses to tourniquet release in children. *Anesth Analg.* 1986;65:865.

65. Lelcuk S, Alexander F, Valeri CR, et al. Thromboxane A_2 moderates permeability after limb ischemia. *Ann Surg.* 1985;202:642.

66. Benzon HT, Toleikis JR, Meagher LL, et al. Changes in venous blood lactate, venous blood gases, and somatosensory evoked potentials after tourniquet application. *Anesthesiology.* 1988; 69:677.

67. Dery R, Pelletier J, Jacques A, et al. Metabolic changes induced in the limb during tourniquet ischaemia. *Can Anaesth Soc J.* 1967;12:366.

68. Wilgis EFS. Observations of the effects of tourniquet ischemia. *J Bone Joint Surg.* 1971;53A:1343.

69. Klenerman L. Tourniquet time—How long? *Hand*. 1980;12:231.

70. Heppenstall RB, Scott R, Sapega A, et al. Comparative study of the tolerance of skeletal muscle to ischemia. *J Bone Joint Surg*. 1986;68A:820.

71. Kaufman RD, Walts LF. Tourniquet induced hypertension. *Br J Anaesth*. 1982;54:333.

72. Kallos T, Smith TC. Anesthesia and orthopedic surgery. In: Barash PG, Cullen BF, Stoelting RK, eds. *Clinical anesthesia*. Philadelphia: JB Lippincott; 1989:1168.

73. Van Roekel HE, Thruston AJ. Tourniquet pressure: The effect of limb circumference and systolic pressure. *J Hand Surg*. 1985; 10B:142–144.

74. Hurst LN, Weinglein O, Brown WF, et al. The pneumatic tourniquet: A biomedical and electrophysiologic study. *Plast Reconstr Surg*. 1981;67:648.

75. Miller SH, Price G, Buch D, et al. Effects of tourniquet ischemia and postischemic edema on muscle metabolism. *J Hand Surg*. 1979;4:547.

76. Patterson S, Klenerman L. The effect of pneumatic tourniquets on ultrastructure of skeletal muscle. *J Bone Joint Surg*. 1979; 61B:178–183.

77. Klenerman L, Biswas M, Hulands GH, et al. Systemic and local effects of the application of the tourniquet. *J Bone Joint Surg*. 1980;62A:385.

78. Kahn RL, Marino VG, Urquhart B, Sharrock NE. Hemodynamic changes associated with tourniquet use under epidural anesthesia for total knee arthroplasty. *Anesthesiology*. 1989; 71A:77.

79. Bridenbaugh PO, Hagenouw RRPM, Gielen MJM, Edstrom HH. Addition of glucose to bupivacaine in spinal anesthesia increases incidence of tourniquet pain. *Anesth Analg*. 1986; 65:1181.

80. Valli H, Rosenberg PH, Kytta J, Numinen M. Arterial hypertension associated with the use of a tourniquet with either general or regional anesthesia. *Acta Anaesthesiol Scand*. 1987;31:279.

81. Rocco A, Concepcion MA, Desai S, et al. The effect of general and regional anesthesia on tourniquet induced blood pressure elevation. *Region Anaesth*. 1987;12:174.

82. Sapega AA, Heppenstall RB, Chance B, et al. Optimizing tourniquet application and release times in extremity surgery. *J Bone Joint Surg*. 1985;67A:303.

83. Egbert LD, Deas TC. Cause of pain from a pneumatic tourniquet during spinal anesthesia. *Anesthesiology*. 1962;23:287.

84. Egbert LD. Tourniquet pain. *Anesthesiology*. 1964;25:247.

85. DeJong RH. Tourniquet pain during spinal anesthesia. *Anesthesiology*. 1962;23:881.

86. Edmonson AS. Surgical techniques. In: Edmonson AS, Crenshaw AH, eds. *Campbell's operative orthopaedics*. 6th ed. Saint Louis, MO: CV Mosby; 1980.

87. Grogan TJ, Dorey F, Rollins J, et al. Deep knee sepsis following total knee arthroplasty: Ten-year experience at the University of California at Los Angeles Medical Center. *J Bone Joint Surg*. 1986;68A:226–234.

88. Cruse RJ, Ford R. A five-year prospective study of 23,649 surgical wounds. *Arch Surg*. 1973;107:206.

89. Ha'eri GB, Wiley AM. The efficacy of standard surgical face masks: An investigation using "tracer particles." *Clin Orthop*. 1980;148:160.

90. Lidwill OM, Lowbury EJ, Whyte W, Blowers R, Stanley SJ, Lowe D. Effect of ultra clean air in operating rooms on deep sepsis in the joint after total hip or knee replacement: A randomized study. *Br Med J*. 1982;285:10–14.

91. Allander C, Abel E. Investigation of a new ventilating system for clean rooms. *Med Res Engl*. 1968;7:28.

92. Charnley J, Eftekhar N. A sterile-air operating theatre enclosure. *Br J Surg*. 1964;51:195.

93. Ha'eri GB, Wiley AM. Total hip replacement in a laminar flow environment, with special reference to deep infections. *Clin Orthop*. 1980;148:163.

94. Haslam KR. Laminar air-flow air conditioning in the operating room: A review. *Anesth Analg*. 1974;53:194.

95. Hart D. Bacterial ultraviolet radiation in the operating room. Twenty-nine-year studies for control of infections. *JAMA*. 1960;172:1019.

96. Howard JM, Barker WF, Culbertson MR, et al. Postoperative wound infections: The influence of ultraviolet radiation on the operating room and various other factors. *Ann Surg*. 1964; 160S:1.

97. Epps CH Jr. *Complications in orthopedic surgery*. Philadelphia: JB Lippincott; 1986:59.

98. Anderson JM, Keen RI, Neave R. *Positioning the surgical patient*. London: Butterworth; 1988.

99. Leffert RD. *Brachial plexus injuries*. New York: Churchill Livingstone; 1985.

100. Martin JT. Complications associated with patient positioning. *Anesth Analg*. 1988;67(suppl 4S):106.

101. Brechner VL, Bethune RWM. Recent advances in monitoring pulmonary air embolism. *Anesth Analg*. 1971;50:255.

102. Michenfelder JD. Central venous catheters in the management of air embolism: Whether as well as where. *Anesthesiology*. 1981;55:339.

103. Michenfelder JD, Miller RH, Gronert GA. Evaluation of an ultrasonic device (Doppler) for the diagnosis of venous air embolism. *Anesthesiology*. 1972;36:164.

104. Relton JES, Hall JE. An operation frame for spinal fusion: A new apparatus designed to reduce hemorrhage during operation. *J Bone Joint Surg*. 1957;49:327.

105. Smith RH. One solution to the problem of the prone position for surgical procedures. *Anesth Analg*. 1974;53:221.

106. Fielding JW, Rothman RH, eds. Symposium on the lumbar spine II. *Orthop Clin North Am*. 1977;8:3.

107. Smith RH, Gramling ZW, Volpitto PP. Problems related to the prone position for surgical operations. *Anesthesiology*. 1961; 22:189.

108. Harkess JW. Principles of fractures and dislocations: In: Rockwood CA Jr, Green DP, eds. *Fractures*. Philadelphia: JB Lippincott; 1975:78.

109. McKenzie PH, Loach AB. Local anesthesia for orthopaedic surgery. *Br J Anaesth*. 1986;58:779–789.

110. Bird TM, Strunin L. Anaesthetic considerations for microsurgical repair of limbs. *Can Anaesth Soc J*. 1984;31:51.

111. MacDonald DJF. Anaesthesia for microvascular procedures. *Br J Anaesth*. 1985;57:904.

112. Conn RA, Cofield RH, Byer DE, Lindstromberg JW. Interscalene block anesthesia for shoulder surgery. *Clin Orthop*. 1987;216:94.

113. Sanborn KV, Sharrock NE. Axillary brachial plexus block provides reliable anesthesia for elbow surgery. *Anesthesiology*. 1989;71:S727.

114. Kallow T, Smith TC. Continuous spinal anesthesia with hypobaric tetracaine for hip surgery in lateral decubitus. *Anesth Analg*. 1972;51:766.

115. Mebius C, Hedestierna G. Airway closure and gas distribution during hip arthroplasty. *Acta Anaesth Scand*. 1982;26:72.

116. Davis FM, Laurenson VG. Spinal anaesthesia or general anaesthesia for emergency hip surgery in elderly patients. *Anaesth Intensive Care*. 1981;9:352.

117. Scott DB, Schweitzer S, Thron J. Epidural block in postoperative pain relief. *Region Anesth*. 1982;7:135.

118. Katz J, Aidinis SJ. Complications of spinal and epidural anesthesia. *J Bone Joint Surg*. 1980;62:1219.

119. Galindo A, Hernandez J, Benavides O, et al. Quality of spinal extradural anesthesia: The influence of spinal nerve root diameter. *Br J Anaesth*. 1975;47:41.

120. Riou B, Barriot P, Viars P. Femoral nerve block in fractured shaft of femur. *Anesthesiology*. 1988;69:A375.

121. Brown CR, Wild VM, Bynum L. Comparison of intravenous ketolorac tromethamine and morphine sulfate in postoperative pain relief. *Clin Pharmacol Ther*. 1988;43:142.

122. Rosberg B, Fredin H, Gustafson C. Anesthetic techniques and surgical blood loss in total hip arthroplasty. *Acta Anaesth Scand*. 1982;26:189.

123. Lambert DH, Deane RS, Mazuzan JE. Anesthesia and the control of blood loss in patients with spinal cord injury. *Anesth Analg*. 1982;61:344.

124. Thompson GE, Miller RD, Stephens WC, Murray WR. Hypotensive anesthesia for total hip arthroplasty. *Anesthesiology*. 1978;48:91.

125. Vazeery AK, Lunde O. Controlled hypotension in hip surgery. *Acta Orthop Scand*. 1979;50:433.

126. McNeil TW, DeWald RL, Kuo KN, et al. Controlled hypertensive anesthesia in scoliosis surgery. *J Bone Joint Surg*. 1974; 56A:1167.

127. Nelson CL, Bowen WS. Total hip arthroplasty in Jehovah's Witnesses without blood transfusions. *J Bone Joint Surg*. 1986;68A:350.

128. Donald JR. Induced hypotension and blood loss during surgery. *J R Soc Med*. 1982;75:149.

129. Knight PR, Lane GA, Nichols MG, et al. Hormonal and hemodynamic changes induced by pentolinium and propranolol during surgical correction of scoliosis. *Anesthesiology*. 1980; 53:127.

130. Bernard JM, Pinaud M, Carteau S, et al. Hypotensive actions of diltiazem and nitroprusside compared during fentanyl anesthesia for total hip arthroplasty. *Can Anaesth Soc J*. 1986;33:308.

131. Gardner RC. Blood loss in orthopedic operations: Comparative studies in 19 major orthopedic procedures utilizing radioisotope labeling and an automatic blood volume computer. *Surgery*. 1970;68:489.

132. Vanden Brink KD, Edmonson AS. The spine. In: Edmonson AS, Crenshaw AH, eds. *Campbell's operative orthopaedics*. 6th ed. Saint Louis, MO: CV Mosby; 1980:2112.

133. AAOS Task Force on AIDS and Orthopaedic Surgery. *Recommendations for the prevention of human immunodeficiency virus (HIV) transmission in the practice of orthopaedic surgery*. Park Ridge, IL: American Academy of Orthopaedic Surgeons; 1989.

134. Kruskall MS, Umlas J. Acquired immunodeficiency syndrome and directed blood donations: A dilemma for American medicine. *Arch Surg*. 1988;123:23–25.

135. Rakower SR, Worth MH, Lackner H. Massive intraoperative autotransfusion of blood. *Surg Gynecol Obstet*. 1973;137:633.

136. Messmer K, Sunder-Plassman L, Jesch F, et al. Oxygen supply to the tissues during normovolemic hemodilution. *Res Exp Med*. 1973;159:152.

137. Bailey TE, Mahoney OM. The use of autologous blood in patients undergoing surgery for spinal deformity. *J Bone Joint Surg*. 1987;69A:329.

138. Cullings HM, Hendee WR. Radiation risks in the orthopaedic operating room. *Contemp Orthop*. 1984;8:48.

139. Miller ME, Davis ML, MacClean CR, et al. Radiation exposure and associated risks to operating room personnel during use of fluoroscopic guidance for selected orthopaedic procedures. *J Bone Joint Surg*. 1983;65:1.

140. Jinnah RH, Amstutz HC, Tooke SM, et al. The UCLA Charnley experience: A long-term follow-up study using survival analysis. *Clin Orthop*. 1986;211:164–172.

141. Mann RAM, Bisset WLK. Anaesthesia for lower limb amputation. *Anaesthesia*. 1983;38:1185.

142. Eriksson E, Haggmark T, Saartok T, et al. Knee arthroscopy with local anesthesia in ambulatory patients. *Orthopaedics*. 1986;9:186.

143. Patel NJ, Flashburg MH, Paskin S, et al. A regional anesthetic technique compared to general anesthesia for outpatient knee arthroscopy. *Anesth Analg*. 1986;65:185.

144. Besser MI, Stahl S. Arthroscopic surgery performed under local anesthesia as an outpatient procedure. *Arch Orthop Trauma Surg*. 1986;105:296–297.

145. Edmonson AS. Surgical techniques. In: Edmonson AS, Crenshaw AH, eds. *Campbell's operative orthopaedics*. 6th ed. Saint Louis, MO: CV Mosby; 1980:24.

146. Sisk DT. Fractures. In: Edmonson AS, Crenshaw AH, eds. *Campbell's operative orthopaedics*. 6th ed. Saint Louis, MO: CV Mosby; 1980:616.

147. Davis FM, Woolner DF, Frampton C, et al. Prospective, multicenter trial of mortality following general or spinal anaesthesia for hip fracture surgery in the elderly. *Br J Anaesth*. 1987;59:1080.

148. Nightingale PH, Marstrand T. Subarachnoid anaesthesia with bupivacaine for orthopaedic procedures in the elderly. *Br J Anaesth*. 1981;53:369.

149. Birks RIS, Edbrooke DL, Mundy JVB. Etomidate as a sedative agent in patients undergoing hip surgery under epidural anaesthesia. *Anaesthesia*. 1983;38:295.

150. Underwood RJ. Experiences with continuous spinal anesthesia in physical status group IV patients. *Anesth Analg*. 1969;47:18.

151. Howard CB, Mackie IG, Fairclough J, et al. Femoral neck surgery using a local anesthesia technique. *Anaesthesia*. 1983;38:993.

152. Groucke CR. Mortality following surgery for fracture of the neck of the femur. *Anaesthesia*. 1985;40:578.

153. Matta J, Merritt P. Displaced acetabular fractures. *Clin Orthop*. 1988;230:83–97.

154. Mayo KA. Fractures of the acetabulum. *Orthop Clin North Am*. 1987;18:43–57.

155. Peterson DO. Shoulder block anesthesia for shoulder reconstruction surgery. *Anesth Analg*. 1985;64:373.

156. Willis DG. Anaesthetic management of posterior lumbar osteotomy. *Can Anaesth Soc J*. 1985;32:248.

157. Rosenberg MK, Berner G. Spinal anesthesia in lumbar disc surgery: Review of 200 cases, with a case history. *Anesth Analg*. 1965;44:419.

158. Matheson D. Epidural anesthesia for lumbar laminectomy and spinal fusion. *Can Anaesth Soc J*. 1960;7:149.

159. Pearce DJ. The role of posture in laminectomy. *Proc R Soc Med*. 1957;50:109.

160. Taylor AR, Gleadhill CA, Bilsland WL, et al. Posture and anaesthesia for spinal operations with special reference to intervertebral disc surgery. *Br J Anaesth*. 1956;18:213.

161. Ovassapian A, Land P, Schafer MF, et al. Anesthetic management for surgical correction of severe flexion deformity of the cervical spine. *Anesthesiology*. 1983;58:370.

162. Harrington PR. Treatment of scoliosis. *J Bone Joint Surg*. 1962;44A:591.

163. Waldman J, Kaufer H, Hensinger RN, et al. Wake-up technique to avoid neurologic sequelae during Harrington Rod procedure: A case report. *Anesth Analg*. 1977;56:733.

164. Grundy BL, Nash CL, Brown RH. Deliberate hypotension for spinal fusion: Prospective random study with evoked potential monitoring. *Can Anaesth Soc J*. 1982;29:452.

165. Brown RH, Nash CL Jr. Current status of spinal cord monitoring. *Spine*. 1979;4:466.

166. Pathak KS, Brown RH, Nash CL Jr, et al. Continuous opioid infusion for scoliosis fusion surgery. *Anesth Analg*. 1983;62:841.

167. Diaz JH, Lockhart CM. Postoperative quadriplegia after spinal fusion for scoliosis with intraoperative awakening. *Anesth Analg*. 1987;66:1039.

168. Wilber RG, Thompson GH, Shaffer JW, et al. Postoperative neurologic deficits in segmental spinal instrumentation: A

study using spinal cord monitoring. *J Bone Joint Surg.* 1984;66A:1178.

169. Mandel RJ, Brown MD, McCollough NC III, et al. Hypotensive anesthesia and autotransfusion in spinal surgery. *Clin Orthop.* 1981;55:277.

170. Marshall WK, Bedford RF, Arnold WP, et al. Effects of propranolol on the cardiovascular and renin–angiotensin systems during hypotension produced by sodium nitroprusside in humans. *Anesthesiology.* 1981;55:277.

171. Sharrock NE, Mieo R, Go G. The value of autologous blood donation and hypotensive anesthesia in reducing homologous blood requirements for total hip replacement. *Anesth Analg.* 1989;68:S257.

172. Poss R, Brick GW, Wright J, et al. The effects of modern cementing techniques in the longevity of total hip arthroplasty. *Orthop Clin North Am.* 1988;19:591.

173. Combs SP, Greenwald AS. The effects of barium sulfate on the polymerization temperature and sheer strength of surgical simplex P. *Clin Orthop.* 1979;145:287.

174. Gooding JM, Smith RA, Weng JT. Is methylmethacrylate safer than previously thought? *Anesth Analg.* 1980;59:542.

175. Modig J, Busch C, Olerud S, et al. Arterial hypotension and hypoxemia during total hip replacement: The importance of thromboplastic procedures, fat embolism and acrylic monomers. *Acta Anaesth Scand.* 1975;19:28.

176. Ellis RH, Mulvein J. The cardiovascular effects of methylmethacrylate. *J Bone Joint Surg.* 1974;56:59.

177. Johansen I, Benumof JL. Methylmethacrylate: A myocardial depressant and peripheral dilator. *Anesthesiology.* 1979;51:S77.

178. Peebles DJ, Ellis RH, Stide SDK, et al. Cardiovascular effects of methylmethacrylate cement. *Br Med J.* 1972;1:349.

179. Duncan JAT. Intra-operative collapse or death related to the use of acrylic cement in hip surgery. *Anaesthesia.* 1989;44:149.

180. Anderson KH. Air aspirated from the venous system during total hip replacement. *Anaesthesia.* 1983;38:1175.

181. Weissman BN, Sosman JL, Braunstein EM, et al. Intravenous methylmethacrylate after total hip replacement. *J Bone Joint Surg.* 1984;66A:44.

182. Bengtson A, Larsson M, Gammer W, et al. Anaphylatoxin release in association with methylmethacrylate fixation of hip prostheses. *J Bone Joint Surg.* 1987;69A:46.

183. Herndon JH, Bechtol CO, Crickenberger DP. Fat embolism during total hip replacement. *J Bone Joint Surg.* 1974;56A:1350.

184. Orsini EL, Byrick RJ, Muller JBM, et al. Cardiopulmonary function and pulmonary microemboli during arthroplasty using cemented and non-cemented components. *J Bone Joint Surg.* 1987;69A:822.

185. Byrick RJ, Kay JC, Mullen JB. Capnography is not as sensitive as pulmonary artery pressure monitoring in detecting marrow microembolism. *Anesth Analg.* 1989;68:94.

186. Sevitt S. Fat embolism in patients with fractured hips. *Br Med J.* 1972;2:257.

187. Byrick RJ, Forbes D, Wardell JP. A monitored cardiovascular collapse during cemented arthroplasty. *Anesthesiology.* 1986;65:213.

188. Morrey BF, Adams RA, Ilstrup DM, et al. Complications and mortality associated with bilateral or unilateral total knee arthroplasty. *J Bone Joint Surg.* 1987;69A:484–488.

189. Asher MA, ed. *Orthopaedic knowledge update I.* Park Ridge, IL: American Academy of Orthopaedic Surgeons; 1984.

190. Mankin HJ, Gebhardt MC, Tomford WW. The use of frozen cadaveric allografts in the management of patients with bone tumors of the extremities. *Orthop Clin North Am.* 1987;18:275.

191. Springfield D. Massive autogenous bone grafts. *Orthop Clin North Am.* 1987;18:249.

192. Sowa DT, Weiland AJ. Clinical applications of vascularized bone autografts. *Orthop Clin North Am.* 1987;18:257.

193. Mankin HJ, Doppelt S, Tomford W. Clinical experience with allograft implantation: The first ten years. *Clin Orthop.* 1983;174:69.

194. Sim FH, Beauchamp CP, Chao EY. Reconstruction of musculoskeletal defects about the knee for tumor. *Clin Orthop.* 1987;221:188–201.

195. Gossling HR, Pellegrini VD. Fat embolism syndrome: A review of the pathophysiology and physiological basis of treatment. *Clin Orthop.* 1982;165:68.

196. Peltier LF. The diagnosis and treatment of fat embolism. *J Trauma.* 1971;11:661.

197. Wilson FR, McCarthy B, LeBlanc LP, et al. Respiratory and coagulation changes after uncomplicated fractures. *Arch Surg.* 1973;106:395.

198. Gossling JR, Ellison SE, Degraff AC. Fat embolism: The role of respiratory failure and its treatment. *J Bone Joint Surg.* 1974;56A:1327.

199. Dyson A, Henderson AM, Chamley D, Campbell ID. An assessment of postoperative oxygen therapy in patients with fractured neck of femur. *Anesth Intensive Care.* 1988;16:405.

200. Coventry MB, Nolan DR, Bechenbaugh RD. "Delayed" prophylactic anticoagulation: A study of results and complications in 2,012 total hip arthroplasties. *J Bone Joint Surg.* 1973;55A:1487.

201. Salzman EW, Hirsch J. Prevention of venous thromboembolism. In: Coleman RW, Hirsch J, Marder V, Salzman EW, eds. *Hemostasis and thrombosis.* Philadelphia: JB Lippincott; 1987:1252.

202. Hirsch J, Salzman EW. Pathogenesis of venous thromboembolism. In: Coleman RW, Hirsch J, Marder V, Salzman EW, eds. *Hemostasis and thrombosis.* Philadelphia: JB Lippincott; 1987:1199.

203. Davis FM, Laurenson VG, Gillespie WJ, et al. Leg blood flow during total hip replacement under spinal or general anesthesia. *Anesth Intensive Care.* 1989;17:136.

204. Thornburn J, Louden FR, Vallance R. Spinal and general anesthesia in total hip replacement: Frequency of deep vein thrombosis. *Br J Anaesth.* 1980;52:1117.

205. Modig J, Borg T, Karlstrom G, et al. Thromboembolism after total hip replacement: Role of epidural and general anesthesia. *Anesth Analg.* 1983;62:174.

206. Owen H, Mather LE, Rowley K. The development and clinical use of patient-controlled analgesia. *Anaesth Intensive Care.* 1988;16:437.

207. Allen PD, Walman T, Concepcion M, et al. Epidural morphine provides postoperative pain relief in peripheral vascular and orthopedic surgical patients: A dose–response study. *Anesth Analg.* 1986;65:165.

208. Kalso E. Effects of intrathecal morphine, injected with bupivacaine, on pain after orthopedic surgery. *Br J Anaesth.* 1985;55:415.

209. Arvidsson I, Eriksson E. Postoperative TENS pain relief after knee surgery: Objective evaluation. *Orthopedics.* 1986;9:1346.

210. Raj PP, Knarr DC, Vigdorth E, et al. Comparison of continual epidural infusion of a local anesthetic and administration of systemic narcotics in the management of pain after total knee arthroplasty. *Anesth Analg.* 1987;66:401.

APPENDIX: GLOSSARY OF ORTHOPEDIC TERMS AND ABBREVIATIONS

Ankylosis: Bony or fibrous bridging on two bones across a joint; results in fusion.

Atlantoaxial: C1–2 articulation.

Arthroplasty: Joint reconstruction or replacement.

Dislocation: Complete misalignment of the continuity of a joint.

Distraction: To separate and straighten, as in the spine.

En bloc resection: Large segmental resection of bone and soft tissue.

Fx: Fracture.

Kyphosis: Curvature of the spine in the anteroposterior plane; posterior curve is convex; a hunched state.

Lordosis: Curvature of the spine in the anteroposterior plane; anterior curve is convex; bending backward.

Neuropraxia: Transient disruption of nerve function as a result of stretching or compression.

ORIF: Open reduction and internal fixation.

Pannus: Chronic or acute lymphocytic inflammation of the lining of the joint, caused by a rheumatoid process.

Reduction: Open or closed resolution of a fracture or dislocation.

Scoliosis: Curvature of the spine in the sagittal plane.

Spondylitis: Inflammation of the spine.

Spondylolisthesis: Slippage of one vertebra on an adjacent vertebral body.

Subluxation: Partial or incomplete misalignment of a joint.

Synovitis: Inflammation of the lining of the joint.

THR: Total hip replacement.

TKR: Total knee replacement.

Anesthesia for Neurosurgery

Barbara Shwiry

New diagnostic and monitoring techniques have improved patient outcome when surgical intervention is indicated in patients with neurologic disease. Computerized tomography and magnetic resonance imaging provide rapid initial identification of pharmacologically or surgically treatable lesions such as tumors, abscesses, hematomas, and edema without significant hazard to the patient because of delayed diagnosis, mechanical complications, or expansion of residual ventricular air from pneumoencephalography. Electrophysiologic monitoring of the brain via electroencephalogram (EEG) and multimodality evoked potentials readily detects abnormal neuronal function in the presence of brain ischemia. In selected cases, intracranial pressure (ICP) monitoring has also proved to be an essential guide to initiation and efficacy of therapy as well as a prognostic indicator of outcome, especially after head trauma.

Expanded care of comatose patients and the introduction of barbiturates for control of intracranial hypertension and brain protection from ischemic injury have necessitated unique life support measures in the neurologic intensive care unit. This specialized care is initiated before surgery and continued into the postoperative period, as ICP, cerebral blood flow, and the formation of edema are affected by alteration of arterial blood pressure, central venous pressure, inspiratory airway pressure, arterial oxygen pressure (Pa_{O_2}), carbon dioxide tension (Pa_{CO_2}), and hydrogen ion concentration (pH). Close attention to cardiopulmonary dynamics in patients with poor intracranial compliance will improve survival significantly. Consideration of the effect of cardiopulmonary parameters and pharmacokinetics on intracranial dynamics in conjunction with new diagnostic and monitoring techniques, has contributed greatly to improved management and outcome of the neurosurgical patient.

CEREBRAL PHYSIOLOGY

Global cerebral blood flow (CBF) through the brain is 44 to 50 mL/100 g per minute in adult humans. This approximates 750 mL/min or 15 percent of cardiac output. Cerebral blood flow is sensitive to chemical, myogenic, and neurogenic factors and is closely related to the cerebral metabolic requirement for oxygen (CMR_{O_2}) and other critical substrates. Although global CBF is relatively stable, alterations in regional CBF (rCBF) occur frequently and rapidly, varying from 20 to 80 mL/100 g per minute. At regional levels, variations in metabolic activity produce an increased oxygen demand that is met by an increased oxygen supply to that specific area. As the number of brain cells involved in such shifts in rCBF is small, compared with total brain mass, global CBF does not change; however, CMR_{O_2}-related changes in rCBF are vital to neuronal function, and regional ischemia can quickly cause marked neurologic deficits. The regulation of rCBF is thought to be mediated by local changes in pH, increased extracellular concentrations of H^+ and K^+, and decreased extracellular Ca^{2+}. In situations where cortical activity is depressed, such as in barbiturate anesthesia or hypothermia, rCBF remains under metabolic influence; that is, the reduction in CBF parallels the reduction in CRM_{O_2}. In situations such as brain injury or during use of inhalational anesthetics, there may be an uncoupling of the CMR_{O_2}/CBF relationship and a relative hyperemia is observed.

Myogenic regulation of CBF, commonly referred to as autoregulation, is a control process whereby CBF is maintained relatively constant over a wide range of arterial pressures, provided changes in systemic arterial pressure (SAP) are not precipitous. Autoregulation is thought to be a stretch receptor response of arteriolar smooth muscle which, on distension of the vessel because of increased SAP, induces cerebral arteriolar constriction in a negative feedback loop. This produces a subsequent decrease in flow to the capillaries. Decreased SAP reduces cerebral arteriolar muscle tone, causing capillaries to dilate to augment flow. Impairment of autoregulation may result from hypoxia, ischemia, acidosis, volatile anesthetics, and trauma. Impaired autoregulation can cause cerebral vasomotor paralysis which results in arteriolar dilation and renders the capillary bed vulnerable to hypertensive insult or ischemia.

Cerebral perfusion pressure (CPP) is an estimate of the pressure gradient between the internal carotid artery and the subarachnoid veins, that is, the pressure gradient across the entire brain. Cerebral perfusion pressure is equal to the difference between the mean arterial pressure (MAP) and the ICP (CPP = MAP – ICP). In functioning autoregulation, CPP ranges from 85 to 95 mm Hg and may be narrowed by either a fall in MAP or an increase in ICP. Cerebral perfusion pressure is maintained by autoregulation when MAP ranges between 50 and 150 mm Hg in normotensive patients. Below this level, CBF is directly related to the mean arterial pressure and progressive cerebral ischemia may ensue. Above the limit of autoregulation or when MAP exceeds 150 mm Hg, high blood flow at this pressure overwhelms the arteriolar constrictor response, injuring endothelial cells of the capillary bed (the blood–brain barrier) and impairs their normal semipermeability. The resultant increase in transudation of fluid and protein across damaged capillaries and into the cerebral extracellular spaces produces edema.

With chronic arterial hypertension of more than 2 to 3 months' duration, the autoregulatory curve is displaced to the right. Cerebral vessels adapt to higher pressure levels and upper and lower limits of autoregulation are increased. In awake patients with hypertension (MAP between 125 and 180 mm Hg), the lower limit of autoregulation ranges from 90 to 125 mm Hg. In these patients, clinical signs of cerebral ischemia may occur with a MAP range of 35 to 80 mm Hg.

Changes in Pa_{CO_2} can significantly affect CBF. As the blood–brain barrier is permeable to CO_2 and essentially impermeable to bicarbonate, the P_{CO_2} of cerebrospinal fluid (CSF) is largely determined by Pa_{CO_2} and bicarbonate concentrations are controlled by cerebral metabolic processes. Bicarbonate and P_{CO_2} become the primary determinants of environmental pH, to which cerebral arterial smooth muscle is extremely responsive. Variations in Pa_{CO_2} from 20 to 80 mm Hg produce direct changes in CBF of about 2 percent for every 1 mm Hg change in Pa_{CO_2}. Hypercapnia causes periarteriolar acidosis and marked cerebral vasodilation, thereby increasing cerebral blood volume (CBV) and CBF. Hypocapnia-induced periarteriolar alkalosis causes constriction of cerebral vessels, thus decreasing CBF and CBV. Consequently, in patients with intracranial hypertension, hyperventilation becomes a useful therapeutic maneuver to decrease cerebral blood flow. Marked hypoxia ($Pa_{O_2} < 50$ mm Hg) causes progressive lactic acidosis of brain tissue which has a potent dilatory effect on arterioles. Marked hypoxia significantly increases CBF and is capable of overriding hypocarbia.

Neurogenic control of cerebral vessels through autonomic innervation plays a relatively minor role in determining arteriolar tonus. Sympathetic innervation to the larger cerebral arteries and arterioles is derived from the superior cervical ganglion. Parasympathetic innervation is from the greater petrosal branch of the facial nerve. Maximum autonomic stimulation alters CBF by 5 to 10 percent. The major contribution of neurogenic influences on CBF is seen during

hemorrhagic or hypovolemic hypotension which is often accompanied by a marked adrenergic vasoconstrictor response. In the brain, this sympathetic vasoconstriction is superimposed on myogenic vasoconstriction, tending to produce maximum vasoconstriction at a higher MAP. In these circumstances, autoregulation fails at a higher threshold, as in chronic hypertension. Controlled hypotension does not appear to induce the sympathetic vasoconstrictor response seen with hemorrhagic shock and is better tolerated than hemorrhagic shock as less cerebral lactic acidosis occurs.

High flow in excess of metabolic need, referred to as luxury perfusion, results from vasomotor paralysis of vessels in tissue surrounding ischemic, infarcted, or other areas surrounding tumor. The low pH, resulting from accumulation of lactic acid and acid metabolites, is the primary factor responsible for the loss of normal vascular responsiveness. Should hypercapnia cause dilation of surrounding responsive arterioles, blood is directed away from the zone of vasomotor paralysis to normal areas because the affected arterioles cannot dilate further. This is known as the *steal phenomenon*. Conversely, hypocarbic vasoconstriction of normal vessels can direct more blood to the bed of paralyzed, maximally dilated vessels, which do not constrict in response to hypocarbia. This is known as the *Robin Hood effect* or *inverse steal phenomenon*.

In summary, physiologic control of CBF is a multifactorial system in which the cerebral arterioles respond with varying intensity to a variety of stimuli including (1) the acid–base or chemical determinants of arteriolar tonus, which operate primarily through the effect of Pa_{CO_2} on the pH of interstitial fluid as well as those effects from lactic acidosis (acidosis, whether secondary to hypercarbia or ischemia, has a potent dilatory effect on arterioles); (2) autoregulation, a property inherent in arteriolar smooth muscle, which causes constriction in response to stretch forces; (3) cerebral metabolic rate, which determines arteriolar tonus by an undefined mechanism; (4) and neurologic control

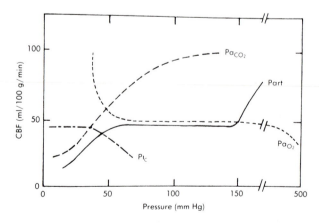

Figure 39–1. Variation of cerebral blood flow (CBF) with changes in systemic arterial pressure Pa_{CO_2}, Pa_{O_2}, and intracranial pressure (P_{IC}). "Part" represents limits of autoregulation. (*Reprinted, with permission, from Shapiro HM. Intercranial hypertension: Therapeutic and anesthetic considerations. Anesthesiology. 1975;43:445.*)

through autonomic innervation of the cerebral vessels, which plays a relatively minor role in determining arteriolar tonus. Each determinant of CBF has a characteristic response curve (Fig. 39–1).

INTRACRANIAL PRESSURE

Intracranial contents including the brain, intra- and extracellular water, CSF, blood, and meninges, generate an ICP of 8 to 12 mm Hg. As the skull is relatively rigid, a change in volume of one of these intracranial constituents must be accompanied by a reciprocal change in one of the other constituents, if increased ICP is to be avoided. If these reciprocal changes do not occur, the craniospinal compartment is said to be noncompliant or "tight." Normal intracranial compliance permits limited expansion of intracranial volume without increasing ICP. Patients with low compliance poorly tolerate increases in intracranial volume (Fig. 39–2).

Initially, spatial compensation is accomplished by shift of CSF into the distensible subarachnoid space, increased absorption of CSF across the arachnoid villi, and translocation of intracranial blood volume systemically, as a result of pressure exerted on thin-walled cerebral veins. As much as 1 mL of CSF per minute can be expressed from the cranial space in the presence of increased intracranial pressure. If rapid spatial compensation were not possible, rapid expansion of even small masses would be incompatible with life. When the ability of CSF to act as the ICP buffer has been exhausted and further spatial compensation cannot be achieved by further reductions in intracranial blood volume, displacement of brain structures through midline shifts and herniation, collapse of CSF cisterns, and compression of the arachnoid villi occur (Fig. 39–3). The management of intracranial hypertension is aimed at reducing intracranial volume, improving cerebral perfusion, and

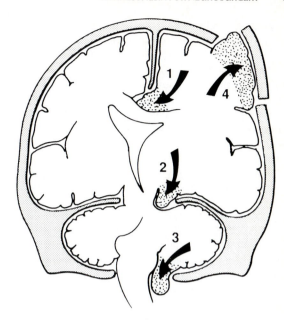

Figure 39–3. Areas of potential brain herniation: (**1**) cingulate, (**2**) temporal (uncal), (**3**) cerebellar, (**4**) transclival (postoperative or traumatic). Intracranial component (intracranial pressure) normally comprises the meninges, brain tissue, intra- and extracellular water, blood, and cerebrospinal fluid. Intracranial masses (tumor, hematoma, or abscess) and edema expand these components and increase intracranial pressure. (*Reprinted, with permission, from Fishman RA. Brain edema.* N Engl J Med. *1975;293:706–711.*)

ensuring optimal metabolic function. Therapy may include the use of osmotic and loop diuretics, corticosteroids, hyperventilation, systemic barbiturates, sedatives, muscle relaxants, hypothermia, CSF diversion, and surgical decompression to alleviate increased ICP.

METHODS OF INTRACRANIAL PRESSURE REDUCTION

Although a common method of rapidly reducing ICP involves manipulation of respiratory parameters as previously discussed, other pharmacologic and surgical interventions may be undertaken in certain situations to affect these decreases.

Diuretics

Osmotherapy is a mainstay of treatment for increased ICP in the presence of brain edema. Reductions in ICP of greater than 10 percent can be obtained by osmotherapy. After osmotic intervention, ICP returns to the pretreatment level within 45 minutes to 11 hours; however, rebound of ICP to levels higher than the pretreatment level can occur with all osmotic drugs. Several mechanisms may be responsible for this rebound phenomenon. Diffusion of the osmotic agent into brain interstitial space and CSF causes the interstitial osmolarity to be higher than the plasma level, as the osmotic agent is excreted renally. Disruption of the blood–brain barrier after trauma also permits rapid diffusion of the osmotic agent into the interstitial space. Brain

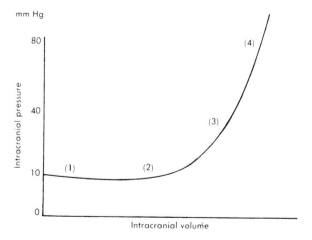

Figure 39–2. Interrelation of intracranial volume and intracranial pressure (ICP) within the closed cranium. As volume expands progressively, compliance is reduced so that each increment in volume (points 1, 2, and 3) causes a more marked rise in ICP. When ICP is already elevated (point 3), even a small increase in intracranial volume may cause ICP values to surge tremendously (point 4). (*Adapted, with permission, from Shapiro HM. Intercranial hypertension: Therapeutic and anesthetic considerations.* Anesthesiology. *1975;43:445.*)

cells generate their own osmotic molecules as well, and these in part balance the osmotic gradient favoring cellular dehydration. The identity of these molecules is not clear, but some appear to be amino acids, which constitute up to 50 percent of the intracellular solute 7 days after the induction of experimental hypernatremic hyperosmolarity. The significance of these idiogenic osmoles in blunting acute osmotherapeutic maneuvers is probably not great, but they do appear to reduce the effectiveness of chronic or long-term administration of hyperosmolar drugs.

Mannitol, a naturally occurring polyhydric alcohol, is the most widely used osmotic diuretic. With a molecular weight (MW) of 182.17, it is neither metabolized nor reabsorbed by the renal tubules. The usual intravenous dose of mannitol is 0.25 to 1.5 g/kg administered as an infusion over 15 to 30 minutes. Onset of action is within 20 minutes, maximal effect is reached within 1 to 2 hours, and duration of action is 6 hours. Needlelike crystals of the drug may precipitate with cool storage and must be dissolved by heating before use.

Rapid administration of mannitol rapidly expands circulatory volume and may precipitate left ventricular failure, especially in patients with preexisting cardiovascular disease. This acute volume expansion, coupled with hypertonic cerebral vasodilation and increased CBF, will increase ICP. Therefore, osmotic diuretics should be administered slowly to patients with increased ICP. Increased CBF may be beneficial to those patients with ischemic cerebrovascular disease; however, osmotherapy is relatively contraindicated in patients with cerebrovascular lesions such as aneurysms and arteriovenous malformation. It must be used with caution in elderly patients in whom sudden shrinkage of brain mass can rupture bridging veins and cause subsequent intracranial hemorrhage. If intracranial bleeding is suspected, shrinkage of brain tissue, which may have been acting as a tamponade, may cause expansion of the hematoma. Repeated or long-term administration of mannitol may induce electrolyte imbalance, especially hyponatremia and hypokalemia, in addition to renal dysfunction in doses beyond therapeutic levels. Mannitol can increase ICP and cerebral edema in the presence of a disrupted blood–brain barrier, because it can diffuse into brain tissue and reverse the osmotic gradient.

Several techniques have been suggested to reduce the undesirable effects of mannitol osmotherapy. A lower dose range of 0.25 to 0.5 g/kg appears to reduce the risk of acute expansion of intravascular volume and interstitial hyperosmolarity while producing reductions in ICP equal to those attained with larger doses, although the effect is shorter in duration. The administration of furosemide 1 mg/kg before or concomitant with mannitol may reduce the incidence and severity of ICP rebound. Rebound elevations of ICP may also be minimized by restricting fluid replacement to one-half to two-thirds the volume of urine produced by the osmotic diuresis.

Urea is a smaller molecule that diffuses through tissues more rapidly and has a short duration of action and a purportedly greater rebound effect. Glycerol may have advantages over mannitol or urea as 80 percent is metabolized by the liver, thereby reducing the potential for rebound. Glycerol should be infused initially at 5 mg/kg per minute for 30 minutes and then at 3 mg/kg per minute for the next 90 minutes. Experiments with rat brain suggest that glycerol may exacerbate ischemic cerebral edema.

The loop diuretics, such as furosemide (Lasix) and ethacrynic acid (Edecrin), have been used to control brain edema associated with tumor and head injury. Furosemide has recently been used for reduction of ICP in patients with aneurysmal subarachnoid hemorrhage. The diuretic effect of furosemide is due to inhibition of sodium absorption in the proximal and distal tubules and in the loop of Henle. Furosemide effects a reduction in ICP by systemic diuresis, relaxation of capacitance vessels, and inhibition of astroglial chloride and water transport, and reduces CSF production through carbonic anhydrase inhibition. Furosemide reduces ICP without significant osmolar or electrolyte change and can be given as a primary (1 mg/kg) or adjuvant (0.15 to 0.30 mg/kg) diuretic. Furosemide given prior to mannitol may attenuate the increase in ICP seen with mannitol. Furosemide may be considered as a substitute for mannitol in neurosurgery in those patients presenting with increased ICP, an altered blood–brain barrier, or increased pulmonary water content, as well as for those patients who have preexisting cardiac and electrolyte abnormalities.

Diuretic therapy should be monitored by serum and urine osmolarity and electrolytes, especially during chronic administration. Ideally, ICP should be measured to ascertain the effectiveness of treatment and adjust the dose and frequency of diuretic administration.

Steroids

In 1961, Galilich and colleagues introduced the use of steroids for reduction of edema associated with brain tumors. The effect of steroids is presumably due to their ability to stabilize membranes, inhibit lysosomal enzyme release, and scavenge free radicals. The effectiveness of steroids, particularly dexamethasone and methylprednisolone, in decreasing the vasogenic edema associated with brain tumor abscess is undisputed. With increase of intracranial compliance, the level of consciousness frequently improves and neurologic deficits resolve before ICP is reduced. Operative and postoperative cerebral edema is also reduced by steroids.

Steroids appear to be less effective in treating cytotoxic edema associated with ischemia, hyposmolarity, asphyxia, and hypoxia. The results of steroid therapy for experimental and clinical ischemic cerebral edema are inconclusive. Membrane stabilization may not, however, be crucial to the effect of steroids in reducing cerebral edema, because accumulation of water in ischemic cerebral edema peaks before significant alteration in the permeability of the blood–brain barrier occurs. Clinical use of steroids for control of ischemic cerebral edema has met with varied success.

The role of steroids in the treatment of head-injured patients remains controversial. Although steroids in low doses (10 mg IV initially, followed by 4 mg every 6 hours) have been ineffective, studies indicate that therapy with steroids in high doses (0.5 to 15 mg/kg) may improve the quality of life as well as prolong survival after craniocerebral trauma; however, patients with severe structural derangement die early despite treatment with steroids. Attempts to determine the efficacy of steroids in reducing edema after head injury may be complicated by the fact that the initial brain swelling following trauma is due to vascular engorgement from an increase in CBF rather than to formation of edema. The increase in ICP as a result of this augmentation of CBV may actually serve to counteract edema formation. Computerized tomography scans of head-injured patients substantiate an initial absence of edema, the increased density suggesting blood rather than water. This may explain the lack of early response to steroid therapy in patients with head trauma; however, resolution of subsequently formed edema is enhanced by a reduction in ICP, which facilitates bulk flow of edema fluid from the interstitium to the ventricles.

Cerebrospinal Fluid Diversion

When intracranial CSF pathways are obstructed, shunts are inserted to reduce ICP by providing a low-resistance pathway for CSF. Ventriculoperitoneal shunts are most commonly used and ventriculoatrial shunts are avoided because of the risk of introducing an infection to the heart. A direct ventricular tap or spinal subarachnoid catheter may be placed intraoperatively to relieve brain tension prior to dural opening and to increase operative space.

Surgical Decompression

Internal and external surgical decompression may be done for uncontrollable brain swelling, especially in patients with severe craniocerebral trauma. Internal decompression in-

volves removal of intracranial tissue. This decreases ICP, and reduces midline shift, brain herniation, and brainstem displacement. External decompression involves removal of part of the skull, usually for evacuation of epidural or subdural hematomas. External decompression can actually increase brain tissue distortion and neurologic deterioration. Decompressive surgery is generally considered a last resort for persistent intractable cerebral edema.

ANESTHETIC PHARMACOLOGY

The objective in anesthetizing patients for neurosurgical procedures is to sustain neurologic function at a level equal to or greater than that present preoperatively. Of utmost importance is the maintenance of CPP in the presence of potentially deranged autoregulation, impaired response to changes in Pa_{CO_2}, abnormal rCBF, and decreased intracranial compliance. Selection of anesthetic techniques is governed by the effects of anesthetic drugs on CBF, CBV, cerebral compliance, ICP, and CMR_{O_2} (Table 39–1).

Inhalation Agents

The inhalation anesthetics halothane, enflurane, and isoflurane all decrease cerebral vascular resistance, causing vascular dilation and dose-dependent impairment of autoregulation. These agents also promote increases in CBF, CBV, and ICP. CMR_{O_2} appears to be decreased. Halothane at 0.5 minimum alveolar concentration (MAC) causes minimal disturbance to cerebral dynamics; however, at 1.6 MAC,

TABLE 39–1. EFFECTS OF ANESTHETIC AGENTS ON INTRACRANIAL DYNAMICS

Agent	Cerebral Blood Flow	CMR_{O_2}[a]	Intracranial Pressure	Cerebral Perfusion Pressure
Halothane	↑↑	↓	↑	↓
Enflurane	↑	↓	↑	↓
Isoflurane	↑	↓	↑	↓
Nitrous oxide	↑	↑↓	↑	↓
Nitrous oxide with thiopental for narcotics	↓	↓	↓	↑
Ketamine	↑↑↑	↑	↑↑↑	↓
Morphine with hypocarbia	↓	↓	↓	↑
Meperidine with hypocarbia	↓	↓	↓	↑
Fentanyl	↓	↓	↓	↑
Droperidol	↓	↓	↓	sl ↓[b]
Innovar	↓	↓	↓	↑
Diazepam	↓	↓	↓	↑
Thiopental	↓↓	↓↓	↓↓	↑
Midazolam	↓	↓	↓	↑
Etomidate	↓	↓	↓	sl
Lidocaine	↓	↓	↓	↑
Succinylcholine	Z	Z	? ↑	Z
d-Tubocurarine	↑	NC	↑	
Pancuronium	NC	NC	NC	NC
Vecuronium (Norcuron)	Z	Z	NC	NC
Atracurium	?	Z	NC	NC

[a] CMR_{O_2}, cerebral metabolic requirement for oxygen.
[b] sl, slightly; NC, no change; Z, effects of agents on these parameters have not been established.

CBF triples. Enflurane and isoflurane at 1.6 MAC double CBF. The resultant rise in ICP as a result of an impairment of autoregulation during an anesthetic-induced reduction in MAP can severely compromise CPP and cause focal or generalized ischemia or even brain herniation. As CO_2 responsiveness is retained with all three inhalation anesthetics, the elevation in ICP that occurs with these agents may be attenuated by prior hyperventilation and barbiturates; however, there are reports of an increase in ICP despite institution of these therapies. This increase may arise from the impairment of vascular CO_2 responsiveness that accompanies extensive intracranial disease. The intracranial volume increases with halothane were primarily from increases in cerebral blood flow, and those with enflurane, from CSF. When isoflurane, fentanyl, or thiopental was used, the CSF pressure-lowering effect of hypocarbia was sustained.

Additionally, halothane has been found to alter brain water and electrolyte distribution as well as permeability of the blood–brain barrier, thus contributing to the formation of cerebral edema. Enflurane has been associated with convulsant activity noted on EEG, especially during deep anesthesia and in the presence of hypocarbia. If an inhalational anesthetic is to be used, low-dose isoflurane combined with hypocarbia may be the most advantageous choice. In a study involving normotensive, normocarbic subjects, CBF did not increase using isoflurane up to 1 MAC. At 1.1 MAC, CBF did increase, and at 1.5 to 2.0 MAC, frank alterations in autoregulation occurred (Fig. 39–4). Gordon et al demonstrated that as long as hyperventilation is used and MAP is not greatly depressed (thereby maintaining CPP), isoflurane in concentrations of up to 1 percent is a suitable adjunct to a balanced narcotic technique. Comparative animal studies demonstrate that increases in ICP and edema were greatest with the inhalation anesthetics and least with barbiturate and neuroleptic anesthetics. Furthermore, an acute rise in blood pressure has been

shown to cause more damage to the blood–brain barrier in animals anesthetized with inhalation agents than in those given thiopental.

Nitrous oxide (N_2O), when used with oxygen only, will increase CBV and ICP by cerebral dilation. The cerebral vasoconstrictive effects of hyperventilation, barbiturates, and narcotics counteract the dilatory effect of N_2O when used concomitantly. Hartung and Cottrell compared the effective cerebral protective effect of barbiturates with and without simultaneous N_2O administration in hypoxic and anoxic mice. Their findings indicated that N_2O offsets thiopental's protective effect on the brain during hypoxia and significantly diminishes that effect during anoxic periods.

Induction Agents

Barbiturates are potent cerebral vasoconstrictors and as such increase cerebrovascular resistance (CVR) while reducing $CMRO_2$, CBF, CBV, and ICP. The reduction in $CMRO_2$ parallels the reduction in CBF. Because of these effects, thiopental is a drug of choice for patients with poor cerebral compliance. In addition, barbiturates may improve operative results after temporary periods of focal ischemia, such as before clip ligation of an aneurysm. Etomidate decreases CBF, $CMRO_2$, and ICP. CO_2 reactivity is maintained. The minimal cardiovascular effects of this agent result in an unchanged or mildly increased CPP. Major objections to the use of this agent are the reportedly high incidence of nonpurposeful movements and thrombophlebitis. Ketamine is not recommended for neurosurgical patients. Ketamine causes profound cerebral vasodilation and greatly increases central nervous system (CNS) activity (see Table 39–1 for effects of anesthetic agents on intracranial dynamics). Recent studies of the effects of propofol on intracranial dynamics are yet unclear. Ravussin and colleagues found that although CSF pressure and MAP were decreased, CPP was maintained at doses of 1.5 mg/kg with fentanyl in moderate doses. Herregods et al found significant decreases in ICP and CPP when 2 mg/kg propofol were used.

Muscle Relaxants

Pancuronium bromide 0.06 to 0.1 mg/kg has been the muscle relaxant of choice for intubation and maintenance of neurosurgical patients as it has no significant effect on ICP. The mild tachycardia seen with pancuronium usually has no deleterious effect on systemic or intracranial pressures. Pancuronium 0.15 to 0.20 mg/kg may be used for patients requiring rapid-sequence induction, as onset approaches that of succinylcholine when large doses are used. Tubocurarine, because of its histamine-releasing property, causes transient decreases in MAP and CPP and increases in CBF, CBV, and ICP. Atracurium is not recommended for use in neurosurgical patients because of its potential for releasing histamine. Vecuronium appears to be a safe alternative to pancuronium. Vecuronium has a shorter onset and duration of action than pancuronium, and maintains hemodynamic and intracranial stability. Doses of 0.07 to 0.10 mg/kg provide complete muscle relaxation. Vecuronium may also be used for intubation or in patients requiring rapid-sequence induction. A small subparalyzing primary dose of 0.01 mg/kg 4 minutes prior to the intubating dose

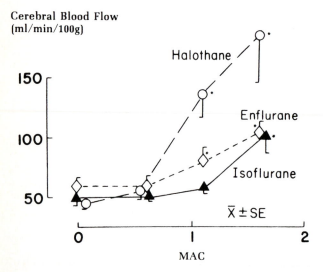

Cerebral Blood Flow
(ml/min/100g)

Figure 39–4. Measurement of cerebral blood flow in volunteers receiving minimum alveolar concentrations (MAC) for halothane, enflurane, and isoflurane. $Paco_2$ and mean arterial pressure were kept at normal levels. (*Reprinted, with permission, from Eger EL II. Isoflurane: A compendium and reference, 1981. Madison, WI: Anaquest, BOC; 1981.*)

of 0.07 to 0.15 mg/kg will allow safe intubation within 90 seconds. Succinylcholine has been noted to increase ICP regardless of whether or not the patient fasciculates (Fig. 39–5). The increased ICP is attributed to sympathetic stimulation and increased serum norepinephrine. Succinylcholine is contraindicated in paretic or paralyzed patients who have denervated muscle or are chronically immobilized because of the potential for cardiac arrest from hyperkalemia.

Narcotics

Morphine, meperidine, and fentanyl maintain CO_2 responsiveness and autoregulation. Formation of edema in response to injury is also reduced. The mild cardiovascular changes associated with narcotics are due primarily to bradycardia and venous dilation which produce a mild decrease in MAP. Morphine and meperidine cause dose-dependent, parallel decreases in CVF and $CMRo_2$. As ICP decreases more than MAP, CPP is increased. Fentanyl decreases CBF with less of a decrease in $CMRo_2$.

In high doses, seizure activity and an increased $CMRo_2$ have been demonstrated with fentanyl and sufentanil in animal models. Sufentanil, as with other narcotics, can precipitate decreases in both CBF and $CMRo_2$ of over 50 percent. A clinical comparison of alfentanil, fentanyl, and sufentanil showed no major differences across variables including brain condition at dural opening, duration of intubation at completion of the procedure, or level of consciousness postoperatively. It was noted that the alfentanil group did require ephedrine more frequently before intubation.

Sedatives and Anesthesia Adjuncts

Because of its alpha-adrenergic blocking effect, droperidol may decrease MAP and increase CPP with little effect on CBF and $CMRo_2$. Reactivity to CO_2 is maintained with droperidol. The effects on autoregulation have not been determined. The combination of droperidol and fentanyl (Innovar) has not been associated with significant change in CBF or $CMRo_2$ in human subjects. Diazepam and lorazepam reduce CBF and $CMRo_2$ with little or no effect on

the cardiovascular system. Droperidol, diazepam, and lorazepam might best be used in small doses as CNS depression persists many hours and may mask signs of intracranial events.

Midazolam maleate, a water-soluble benzodiazepine, has been shown to maintain better hemodynamic stability than thiopental when administered to patients with intracranial mass lesions. In these patients, MAP was better maintained and CPP did not decrease when compared with similar patients anesthetized with thiopental.

Fluid Management

Patients undergoing elective neurosurgical procedures who show no evidence of increased ICP will generally have a normal intravascular volume. Many patients, however, present with depleted intravascular volume as a result of aggressive diuretic therapy, restriction of intravenous fluids, and abnormalities of antidiuretic hormone release. Poor oral intake may be the result of deliberate restriction, decreasing level of consciousness, or nausea and vomiting from increased ICP. In the otherwise healthy accident victim hypovolemia may be masked by a compensating vascular system and by arterial hypertension, which often occurs with intracranial damage. Traumatic head injury is often associated with peripheral injury. In these cases, blood losses of 500 to 1500 mL may be sequestered, for example, in the retroperitoneum or tissue surrounding fracture sites of long bones. Blood loss from open wounds often tends to be underestimated and as such, an adequate circulating blood volume is necessary to prevent severe hypotension at induction. Measurement of CVP or pulmonary capillary wedge pressure (PCWP) may provide a useful guide for fluid therapy. Over hydration must be avoided as it can rapidly lead to cerebral edema because the blood–brain barrier is disrupted by trauma and surgery.

Unless there are signs or symptoms of hypovolemia, it is not necessary to replace overnight losses. Maintenance fluids consist of Ringer's lactate and other balanced salt solutions given at a rate of 1.0 to 1.5 mL/kg per hour. Volume replacement is usually accomplished with Ringer's lactate

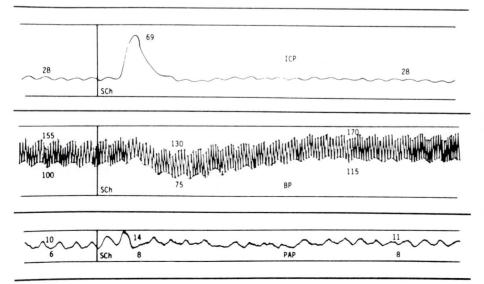

Figure 39–5. Tracing of intracranial pressure (ICP), blood pressure (BP), and pulmonary arterial pressure (PAP) for approximately 100 seconds. The vertical line indicates the injection of succinylcholine (Sch) 1.5 mg/kg (from cat 10, initial ICP increased). (*Reprinted, with permission, from Cottrell JE, Hartung J, Givvin JP, et al. Intracranial and hemodynamic changes after succinylcholine administration in cats. Anesth Analg. 1983;62:1006–1009.*)

or blood. Whenever possible blood loss should be replaced with blood. Rapid volume expansion with isotonic salt solution should be avoided as this can elevate ICP. Large volumes of dextrose solutions should also be avoided because the available free water of the solution plus the water from oxidation of glucose add to the potential for cerebral edema. Although hypertonic dextrose solutions initially decrease ICP, there will be a rebound increase in ICP from glucose metabolism. In addition, there is evidence that cerebral ischemia may be worsened by higher-than-normal serum glucose levels. The use of albumin is controversial. A disrupted blood–brain barrier is highly permeable to most fluids including albumin. Experimentally, when the plasma concentration of albumin falls, the albumin in brain tissue remains elevated. This creates an osmotic gradient favoring cerebral edema. Other fluids are more easily mobilized from the interstitial space than is albumin.

Inadequate fluid volume is indicated by tachycardia, hypotension, sensitivity to vasodilators or inhalational anesthetics, and an inspiratory–expiratory variation in blood pressure when peak expiratory pressure exceeds 20 mm Hg. If the patient is undergoing surgery for cerebral aneurysm, careful attention to fluid administration is required. Aneurysm rupture can occur as a result of overhydration and resultant hypertension. In this case, deliberate hypotension is often required immediately prior to clip ligation of the aneurysm. A decreased circulating volume may make the patient response to vasodilators unpredictable. After ligation of the aneurysm, most neurosurgeons feel that volume replacement and mildly increased blood pressure (about 10 percent above normal) will reduce the risk of vasospasm. A CVP of 12 mm Hg or a PCWP of 18 mm Hg is considered optimal. Arterial blood gases, hematocrit, and serum potassium, chloride, sodium, and glucose should be frequently assessed perioperatively to further assess the effects of fluid administration.

ANESTHETIC MANAGEMENT AND TECHNIQUE

Preoperative Evaluation

The preoperative anesthetic visit includes evaluation of the patient's general medical condition and state of intracranial tension. Assessment should be made of any peripheral sequelae associated with the intracranial lesion, and in the case of traumatic head injury, careful examination for multiple injuries, especially those of the chest and abdomen, should be made. Those patients exhibiting altered states of consciousness should be assessed for aspiration pneumonitis, making chest x-ray and arterial blood gases valuable assessment tools. Assessment of intravascular volume and electrolyte balance is essential, especially in those patients treated with diuretics. Patients with lesions of the pituitary should be evaluated for endocrine abnormalities. All neurologic deficits should be noted on the patient's chart preoperatively.

The extent of intracranial tension determines the use of premedicants. In all cases, those drugs that cause respiratory depression, hypotension, nausea, vomiting, or significant alteration in consciousness should be avoided. These include narcotics, butyrophenones, and, in the case of cere-

bral aneurysms, atropine because of the increased heart rate and MAP. Glycopyrrolate may be used to protect against excessive secretions and vagal reflexes. Hydroxyzine or diazepam may be used to sedate awake, anxious patients. Hydroxyzine has antiemetic and sedative affects with little effect on ICP. Diazepam has amnesiac, antiseizure activity and decreases CBF with minimal effect on the cardiorespiratory system. Lethargic, obtunded patients should not usually receive premedication.

Monitoring in Intracranial Procedures

Physiologic monitoring during neurosurgical procedures affords opportunity for prompt identification of potential complications such as increased ICP, extensive blood loss, venous air embolism, cardiac arrhythmias, fluctuations in blood pressure, pulmonary abnormalities, and fluid balance. All patients should receive basic monitoring equipment outlined in the American Association of Nurse Anesthetists' *Monitoring Standards.* In addition, other monitors should be used depending on the position of the patient, his or her medical history, and the type and extent of the surgery planned.

Monitoring of intraarterial blood pressure should be instituted prior to induction whenever possible and maintained through the postanesthetic period. Arteries suitable for short-term cannulation are the radial, brachial, axillary, and dorsalis pedis. Before an arterial catheter is placed, collateral circulation should be ascertained by palpation or doppler. Prior to cannulation of the radial artery and in cooperative patients, patency of the palmar arch may be determined by a modified Allens test. The arterial transducer should be zeroed at the highest point of the skull to accurately assess CPP. Intraarterial pressure is a valuable monitor to assess CPP, especially in the presence of wide fluctuations in blood pressure attendant to some procedures or for assessment of venous air embolism. The ECG should be monitored continuously as it has been found to be a reliable indicator of brainstem compression. Posterior fossa dissection and venous air embolism frequently produce bradycardia and arrhythmias. Myocardial ischemia, if present, will be demonstrated in the precordial leads.

Maintenance of appropriate anesthetic depth and adequate muscle relaxation is necessary to prevent straining and coughing, especially while the dura is open. A peripheral nerve stimulator helps to assess the extent of muscle paralysis and guides supplemental dosing of muscle relaxant to prevent movement during microdissection of vital structures. Measurement of urinary output provides an indication of intravascular volume. Knowledge of the exact urinary output is important after administration of osmotic and loop diuretics and in patients with diabetes insipidus or abnormalities of antidiuretic hormone secretion. Decreased urinary output during induced hypotension may indicate decreased renal perfusion and the need to increase blood pressure. Body temperature is best measured by an esophageal or nasopharyngeal thermistor as core temperatures are usually more accurate, especially during hypothermia. Body temperature can be raised intraoperatively by warmed blankets, increased ambient temperature, warmed intravenous solutions, and decreased flow of anesthetic gas.

Chlorpromazine is an effective antipyretic and will prevent shivering by hypothalamic suppression.

A primary determinant in the selection of monitoring equipment relates to their uses for detection of venous air embolism (VAE). This is a complication most often encountered when the patient is in the sitting position but may also occur with the patient in the lateral, supine, or prone positions. The precordial doppler is still the most relied on device for detection of venous air emboli. The doppler is placed over the right atrium, from the fourth to the sixth intercostal space, to the right of the sternum. Correct positioning of the doppler in relation to the tip of the central venous catheter is ascertained by injecting a 10-mL bolus of crystalloid solution through the catheter. The resultant turbulence and micro-air bubbles generate sounds similar to those of air in the right heart. The doppler may not be as effective in patients who have distortion in intrathoracic structure, as with scoliosis or following pneumonectomy. A transesophageal doppler, yet reserved primarily to the research laboratory, may attenuate problems of precordial doppler positioning. Transesophageal echocardiography can detect air bubbles, provide a visualization of air in the right and left sides of the heart, and detect paradoxical air emboli.

As reliance on a single method of monitoring for VAE is inadvisable, other measures have been employed including the esophageal stethoscope, pulse oximetry, mass spectrometry, end-tidal CO_2, right-sided heart catheterization, and pulmonary artery catheterization. The least effective appears to be the esophageal stethoscope. The $ETCO_2$ analyzer and mass spectrometer is a noninvasive method that demonstrates a precipitous drop on VAE. Although its sensitivity to these events is secondary to the doppler, $ETCO_2$ changes should occur prior to the onset of major vascular effects. Because of potential delays in mass spectrometry readings because of rotational site sampling, a separate monitor should be used unless sampling delays are less than 1 minute. Likewise, when more than six sites are used, a separate oxygen analyzer should be used.

A right heart catheter may be helpful to confirm placement of a doppler and for providing a method of extracting air from the right heart, if properly placed and confirmed by x-ray or by P-wave on ECG. This is accomplished by connecting the saline-filled catheter to the V lead of the ECG by means of a metal stopcock, converting the catheter into an ECG lead. Characteristic ECG changes are observed as the catheter is advanced into the right atrium. A biphasic P-wave indicates that the catheter tip is in proper position. Caution must be exercised that faulty equipment is not connected to the patient, as the catheter can now act as an electroconductor directly into the heart. The optimal position of the catheter tip is at the junction of the superior vena cava and the right atrium.

The right-sided heart catheter is usually introduced via the basilic, subclavian, internal, or external jugular vein. A multiorificed catheter may allow for maximal air aspiration, eliminating the possibility of suction adhesion to the chamber wall, and not compromising catheter efficiency from clot formation. Balloon-tipped, flow-directed thermodilution catheters for measuring pulmonary artery pressure (PAP) and PCWP are helpful for detecting air emboli, reliably measuring intravascular volume, and monitoring pa-

tients with severe myocardial dysfunction. An acute increase in PAP suggests air embolus. With resolution of the embolus by extraction or absorption, PAP values should return to normal affording some diagnostic evidence of clearance.

Noninvasive electrophysiologic monitoring of the central nervous system is accomplished with the intraoperative use of the electroencephalogram (EEG) and with evoked potentials. The EEG is useful for detection of compromised cerebral perfusion or oxygenation and drug effects during anesthesia. Evoked potentials (EPs) can be used to monitor a sensory pathway at risk during neurosurgical manipulation. Application of a stimulus to a peripheral nerve elicits voltage changes in the EEG. If the stimulus applied to one part of the nervous system elicits a recordable response in another part of the nervous system then it can be assumed that the pathway between stimulus and response is functioning properly.

The most frequently used EPs are somatosensory EPs (SSEPs) which are monitored during procedures on the spine, spinal cord, or vasculature. Brainstem auditory evoked responses (i.e., potentials) are used to monitor function of the auditory pathway between the eighth cranial nerve and the brainstem. Surgical retraction and manipulation of structures in the posterior fossa can impede impulse transmission along this pathway. Visual evoked responses (VEPs) are monitored in the operating room using flash stimulation through opaque goggles over closed eyes. Monitoring of VEP is useful for surgery on the anterior vasculature, sphenoid wing, optic chiasm, pituitary, and occipital poles. Functional areas of the brain can be localized using sensory evoked potentials recorded from the surface of the brain or from deeper within the tissue with probes. Cortical evoked potentials are sensitive to global insults such as hypoxia or anesthetic overdose.

Intracranial pressure is monitored by inserting a subdural screw, an epidural fiberoptic transducer or cup catheter, or an intraventricular catheter (Fig. 39–6). The greatest risk for this procedure is an increase in the incidence of infection when the dura is punctured. Other hazards of ICP monitoring include nerve tissue damage and hematoma formation. This is often seen with the use of intraventricular catheters in patients in whom brain tissue distortion alters position of vital structures and ventricles; however, an intraventricular catheter has the advantage of permitting CSF drainage thus directly decreasing ICP. With all forms of monitors, distorted ICP readings occur if brain herniates against the monitor.

Normal ICP is a pulsatile pressure that varies with cardiac impulse and respiration. Normal ICP is 10 mm Hg. It is considered slightly increased at 11 to 20 mm Hg, moderately increased at greater than 21 to 40 mm Hg, and severely increased at 40 mm Hg. At pressures greater than 40 mm Hg, compromise of cerebral perfusion may occur. Intracranial pressure can be normal in the presence of an intracranial mass; however, compliance can be significantly decreased. Compliance can be evaluated by injecting 1 mL of saline through the intraventricular catheter, the subdural screw, or the epidural transducer and noting the resultant rise in ICP (see Fig. 39–2). If an increase greater than 2 mm Hg occurs, compliance is impaired and care must be taken to avoid fur-

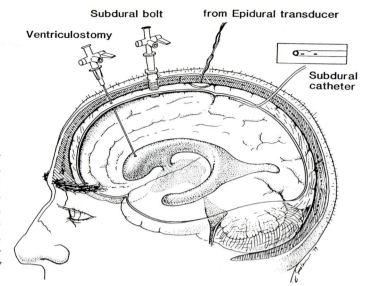

Figure 39–6. Commonly employed sites and techniques for monitoring intracranial pressure. For the epidural technique, an epidural transducer is inserted into the epidural space. Pressure is monitored subdurally using either a subdural bolt or subdural catheter. Ventriculostomy permits monitoring of intraventricular pressure and allows aspiration of cerebrospinal fluid. (*Reprinted, with permission, from Shapiro, HM. Neurosurgical anesthesia and intracranial hypertension. In: Miller RD, ed: Anesthesia, 3rd ed. New York, Churchill Livingstone, 1991:1749.*)

ther increases in intracranial content. Treatment is indicated when ICP reaches 20 mm Hg. Severe elevation of ICP to 40 to 50 mm Hg for more than 4 to 8 minutes is associated with significantly increased morbidity and mortality.

In studies of neurosurgical patients with a wide variety of intracranial pathology (excluding craniocerebral trauma), three distinct, spontaneous pressure wave fluctuations were noted: A-waves, which are high-amplitude plateau waves; B-waves, which are small-amplitude nonplateau, 1-minute waves; and C-waves, which are small-amplitude, 6-minute waves. B- and C-waves were of limited clinical usefulness. B-waves were associated with Cheyne–Stokes respirations but did not appear to be a prodromal sign. C-waves were associated with blood pressure waves. Both B- and C-waves were associated with natural and pathologic depressions in level of consciousness. A-waves (plateau waves) were clini-

cally significant, varying in amplitude and duration. Plateau waves occurred with elevations of ICP greater than 20 mm Hg and were frequently associated with overt symptoms of increased ICP (Fig. 39–7).

Positioning

The sitting position affords excellent surgical access and reduces bleeding and intracranial pressure by gravitational drainage of blood and CSF from the cranium. The disadvantages of the sitting position include an increased incidence of venous air embolism, hypotension as a result of peripheral pooling of blood, impaired venous return, and decreased cardiac output, especially in elderly, debilitated, or dehydrated patients. Cerebral ischemia may go undetected, as blood pressure at the level of the brain is 2 mm Hg less

Figure 39–7. Recordings showing that plateau waves (A-waves) are associated with a simultaneous increase in regional cerebral blood volume (rCBV). The increase in rCBV is thought to be the etiology of the plateau wave. VFP, ventricular fluid pressure. (*Reprinted, with permission, from Risberg J, Lundberg N, Ingrav DM. J Neurosurg. 1969; 31:303.*)

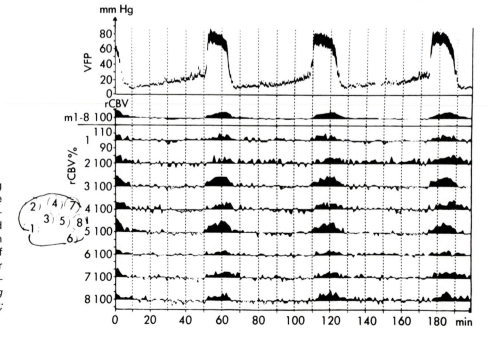

for every inch the head is elevated above the heart. The transducer is therefore placed at the level of the head. For patients in poor physical condition, the lateral decubitus or prone position is appropriate.

In the correct sitting position, the back forms a 60-degree angle with the horizontal, the hips are flexed, and the knees are elevated to heart level to facilitate venous return. Postural hypotension accompanying position change is minimized by ensuring an adequate circulating blood volume, by wrapping the legs with ace bandages, and by moving the patient to the sitting position gradually, while blood pressure and heart rate are continuously monitored. The patient's head is supported in a three-point pin head holder. To avoid pressure necrosis of the skin, increase in ICP, and ischemic damage to the cervical spinal cord, flexion of the neck must leave at least 2 cm between the mandible and sternum at the peak of inspiration. A soft bite block is recommended instead of an oropharyngeal airway to avoid obstruction of venous and lymphatic drainage by compression of oral soft tissue.

The lateral decubitus position offers wide exposure of the lateral posterior fossa structures and the temporal region. To prevent jugular compression, increased venous bleeding, and elevated ICP, excessive lateral flexion of the head on the dependent shoulder is avoided. Pillows or blankets cushion the arms and legs, and the feet rest on foam pads. Inserting a towel roll under the dependent axilla protects the brachial plexus from compression injury. In addition, the adequacy of circulation is tested by transducing or palpating the radial pulse in the downside arm. The prone position provides access to midline and lateral structures. Venous air embolism is less likely in this position. To ensure adequate gas exchange and decrease vena caval compression, ventilation is controlled and bolsters are placed under the patient on each side from shoulder to thigh.

Airway Management

Maintaining a patent airway is critical for the neurosurgical patient as obstruction will increase intrathoracic pressure and exacerbate intracranial hypertension. In the presence of obstruction, accumulation of CO_2 dilates cerebral vessels and increases CBF and CBV. Obstruction may worsen the patient's oxygenation if preexisting medical conditions exist that have already compromised ventilation. Both improved oxygenation and adequate ventilation are achieved by proper airway control.

The decision to intubate a comatose patient depends on the depth of coma. When there is airway obstruction, loss of reflexes, or inability to clear secretions, the patient should be intubated to ensure oxygenation and prevent aspiration. If the patient exhibits purposeful movement in response to a painful stimulus, the protective reflexes are probably intact. Rather than immediate intubation, close observation may be indicated; however, one must remain aware that the patient's neurologic status is dynamic and may deteriorate precipitously.

There are potential difficulties related to airway management and intubation of patients with suspected or known cervical spinal fractures, cervical spine fixation, head and neck trauma, or impaired mandibular motion. The ne-

cessity of avoiding flexion and extension of the neck may make airway maintenance impossible after an anesthetic-induced loss of muscle tone and airway reflexes. For this reason, intubation is most often accomplished with the patient awake or mildly sedated. Awake tracheal intubation may be facilitated by local anesthetic blockade of the upper airway via topical application to the nose and mouth, to the trachea via cricothyroid puncture, and to the larynx via bilateral superior laryngeal nerve block. An absolute contraindication to this technique would be a full stomach because of the risk of aspiration through the anesthetized larynx. In addition, infection or tumor in the area of the block would be a contraindication to its use. This technique can be used in patients already intubated who require ventilatory support, attenuating discomfort of the tube. Lidocaine 1 mg/kg administered intravenously may be substituted for the transtracheal method. Patients who cough and strain on the endotracheal tube despite local anesthesia require sedation to prevent elevation of ICP and deficits in rCBF. In ventilated patients, muscle relaxation may be required, as poor synchronization with the ventilator and inadequate muscle relaxation may also raise ICP. The practitioner should also consider that in cases of head trauma, nasal intubations should be avoided so as not to exacerbate potential CSF leaks.

Damage to the respiratory center or to the ninth, tenth, and twelfth cranial nerves from trauma or during posterior fossa exploration may cause central impairment of respiration. The possibility of operative trauma requires cautious assessment of airway and swallowing after extubation and during the first feeding. Complete inability to cough or swallow effectively may necessitate tracheostomy, but patients eventually compensate for unilateral paralysis of the vagus nerve. Dissection or hemorrhage in the area of the posterior fossa can directly compress the inspiratory center. Perifocal edema associated with tumor, trauma, or surgery may increase ICP, causing brainstem compression. Compression impairs pharyngeal reflexes and may lead to airway obstruction. Such occurrences may be preceded by a period of ataxic respiration, especially after an interval of wakefulness and adequate spontaneous ventilation. Prompt reintubation and mechanical hyperventilation are indicated, especially as hyperventilation can reduce brain volume and control edema formation. Computerized axial tomography or magnetic resonance imaging will identify surgically removable hematomas.

Whenever any respiratory treatment modality is instituted, possible effects on CBF, CPP, and ICP must be taken into consideration. Suctioning during tracheal toilet will significantly increase ICP by producing an arousal response or, in the apneic patient, by causing accumulation of CO_2. The arousal response can be mitigated by prior sedation with intravenous lidocaine followed by instillation of lidocaine in the tube. Moving the head to the left or right can increase ICP by altering cerebral venous outflow. It is advisable to avoid rotation of the head during tracheal suctioning and transport. Elevation of the head to 30 degrees above the horizontal helps to control ICP as this facilitates cerebral venous drainage. The 30-degree head-up position is helpful in counteracting the elevation of ICP produced by positive end-expiratory pressure (PEEP). Repeated lowering of the head of the bed for tracheal suctioning or measurement of CVP or PCWP must be minimized.

Mechanical positive-pressure ventilation significantly affects CBF, CPP, and ICP. Controlled mechanical ventilation (CMV) eliminates the negative intrathoracic pressure of normal inspiration, thus decreasing venous return. If this reduction in preload is superimposed on preexisting hypovolemia, arterial hypotension may quickly follow institution of CMV and significantly affect CBF, especially in the presence of increased ICP. In addition, the intrathoracic positive pressure generated during the inspiratory phase of CMV is transmitted to the great veins and contributes to increasing ICP by increasing CVP. Maintenance of normovolemia and the 30-degree head-up position improve central venous outflow and is therefore indicated during CMV. The use of PEEP for treatment of refractory hypoxemia with increased intrapulmonary shunt and decreased functional residual capacity produces similar cardiovascular changes that may elevate ICP. Positive end-expiratory pressure should be instituted at low pressures and decreased gradually as oxygenation improves, as sudden reductions increase cardiac output, causing an increase in CBF and ICP.

Intermittent mandatory ventilation (IMV) is a useful technique for supplying supplemental ventilation to the spontaneously breathing patient who requires assistance to maintain an acceptable Pa_{CO_2}. This mode reduces the risk of hypotension or decreased cardiac output in the presence of increased ICP. Modern ventilators have internal IMV circuits with mandatory breath cycles timed so that breaths occur at the beginning of the spontaneous inspirations. This is referred to as synchronized IMV (SIMV). If spontaneous ventilation is borderline, IMV will decrease the work of breathing, thus providing a useful alternative to the combination of CMV plus sedation in the patient who tolerates the ventilator poorly.

Controlled, or therapeutic, hyperventilation is a major nonoperative technique for decreasing ICP. Reduction of Pa_{CO_2} to 25 to 30 mm Hg constricts cerebral vessels and decreases CBF, CBV, and ICP, with minimal risk of cerebral ischemia. Cerebral blood flow and CSF pH normalize after a few days of hypocarbia, and may have a diminished effect during prolonged use. Although the duration of ICP reduction may be limited, hyperventilation is a rapid and effective method of decreasing ICP. A Pa_{CO_2} below 20 mm Hg may be associated with ischemia as a result of extreme cerebral vasoconstriction. The ideal level of hypocarbia is difficult to define as variations in CBF are not usually monitored; however, if the patient hyperventilates spontaneously, ventilator assistance should be adjusted to maintain the spontaneously achieved level of hypocarbia.

Induction of Anesthesia

Implementing the principles of neurophysiology and considering the effects of anesthetic agents on intracranial dynamics, the anesthetist should carefully devise an anesthetic plan for each patient. Again, noninvasive monitoring should be applied prior to induction of all patients regardless of pathology. These include blood pressure cuff, modified V_5 ECG, PCS, PNS, pulse oximetry, ET_{CO_2} or mass spectrometry. Ideally, invasive monitors such as an arterial line, CVP line, Swan-Ganz catheter, EEG, and EP monitor should also be placed prior to induction. In the overly anxious patient, however, it may be wiser to wait until the patient has been sedated or anesthetized.

Induction of anesthesia should proceed smoothly and carefully, while attempting to avoid large variations in MAP. The patient should be preoxygenated with 100 percent oxygen via face mask. Sedation with small amounts of benzodiazepines and, in selected cases, a butyrophenone or incremental narcotics are titrated according to the patient's vital signs and estimation of clinical effect. Induction can proceed with combinations of intravenous and inhalation agents that are sufficient to anesthetize and intubate the patient, yet avoid excessive catecholamine release or clinical effects that may increase ICP. Although succinylcholine for intubation is not contraindicated, vecuronium or pavulon is a safe alternative. Systemic and intracranial hypertension during laryngoscopy and intubation is prevented by additional thiopental, narcotic, or intravenous lidocaine 1 minute prior to laryngoscopy, especially if a protracted induction time has been used to facilitate uptake of inhalation agent. Lidocaine spray may also be applied topically to the larynx and trachea. An armored endotracheal tube (anode tube) may be used if positioning requires extreme rotation or flexion of the head. Care must be taken to secure all endotracheal tube connections as the patient's airway may be out of view and repositioning of the head during surgery can cause disconnection or accidental extubation.

Anesthesia is maintained with continuous administration of oxygen and nitrous oxide and intermittent doses or continuous pump infusion of narcotic, muscle relaxant, and barbiturate. As intubation, application of the head pins, drilling through bone, and insertion of the Gigli saw guide are highly stimulating, intravenous lidocaine may be used to prevent an increase in ICP from noxious stimuli without altering cardiovascular parameters. Low concentrations of isoflurane or drugs affecting the autonomic nervous system may be used as necessary to control blood pressure. After adequate depth of anesthesia is established, ventilation is adjusted to keep the arterial Pa_{CO_2} between 25 and 30 mm Hg. Although the rate, rhythm, and depth of spontaneous respiration have been used to assess brainstem integrity intraoperatively, blood pressure and cardiac rate and rhythm are sufficiently sensitive as their control centers are sufficiently close to respiratory areas to indicate compromise of respiratory centers during controlled ventilation.

Smooth emergence from anesthesia requires that the patient neither cough nor strain on the endotracheal tube, as systemic pressure and ICP will rise and compromise hemostasis. Muscle relaxation should be reversed with anticholinesterase and anticholinergic drugs. Stable, responsive patients with adequate spontaneous respiration are extubated in the operating room. Narcotic reversal should be avoided if increased MAP is undesirable. Patients to be ventilated postoperatively because of trauma, cerebral edema, or poor preoperative status may remain asleep and paralyzed.

Portable ECG and blood pressure monitoring equipment may accompany the patient from the operating suite to the recovery room, where monitoring is continued. With the exception of cerebral vascular surgery, hypocarbia is maintained during the immediate postoperative period. Laboratory tests, including determinations of arterial blood gases, complete blood count, glucose, serum electrolytes, and osmolality, urine specific gravity, chest roentgenogram, and an ECG, are performed in the recovery room as soon as the patient's vital signs have stabilized. Unless otherwise contraindicated, the patient is maintained in a semi-Fowler's position.

MANAGEMENT OF SPECIFIC NEUROLOGIC PROCEDURES

Trauma

In the United States, more than 600,000 people annually sustain epidural or subdural hematomas or cerebral lacerations. Deaths from vehicular accidents involving head injuries number 33,000 annually. As 50 percent of deaths from head injury occur within the first 2 hours, optimal management requires effective emergency treatment at the site of the accident and rapid transport to care facilities. The initial management of acutely injured patients is aimed at rapid reduction of intracranial volume to decrease ICP, improve cerebral perfusion, and balance metabolic supply and demand. Aggressive management with hyperventilation, dehydrating agents, and sedatives has been effective in reversing impending brain herniation. Steroids, muscle relaxants, and, in certain cases, barbiturates can significantly improve the prognosis of patients with head injury. Temperature control is essential in all patients with head injury. Hyperthermia may result from blood in the subarachnoid space, especially in the area of the posterior fossa. Hypothermia may also be problematic in the trauma patient, especially in those who have been unattended at the accident site and for those whom the practitioner suspects alcohol intoxication.

Frequently, trauma patients spontaneously hyperventilate and may be hypertensive. Hyperventilation is centrally induced by the acidic cerebral metabolites that accumulate in the area of injury. Cerebral vascular reactivity to P_{CO_2} may be impaired in areas of injury; however, reactivity should remain in the surrounding tissue. Hyperventilation stimulates restoration of normal cerebral pH, thereby limiting development of secondary injury caused by acidosis and hypoxia, and aiding in the preservation of viable brain tissue. Hyperventilation may also be a useful maneuver prior to the therapeutic effect of corticosteroids. Systemic hypertension accompanying acute head injury is a compensatory mechanism to maintain CPP. Attempts to decrease MAP should not be instituted until medical or surgical measures to decrease ICP and improve compliance have been instituted. Often, MAP decreases spontaneously as compliance improves. If MAP remains elevated despite reduction in ICP and improvement in compliance, antihypertensive agents should be considered.

Patients with depressed skull fractures and acute epidural, subdural, and intercerebral hematomas frequently require craniotomy. Chronic subdural hematomas are often evacuated through burr holes. Occasionally, cerebral contusion may require removal of contused brain tissue and subtemporal decompression. The majority of patients who undergo surgical procedures are unconscious preoperatively and usually remain so postoperatively. Treatment involves a coordinated approach to respiratory care, maintenance of hemodynamic stability, fluid and electrolyte balance, as well as specific measures to control CBF and ICP.

Removal of an acute subdural hematoma is frequently followed by significant postoperative elevations in ICP. ICP monitoring and other treatment modalities to reduce ICP should be continued during the recovery period. Studies on patient mortality from severe head injury report a reduction in deaths from 70 to 30 percent in adults and to as low as 7 percent in children when timely alleviation of elevated ICP is achieved. Traumatically injured patients should always be evaluated for concomitant head injury. Conversely, patients with obvious head injury should also be evaluated for other injuries, especially those of the spinal column, chest, and abdomen.

Carotid Endarterectomy

Carotid endarterectomy for stenosis or ulcerated plaques of the internal carotid artery may be performed under regional or general anesthesia. Regional anesthesia affords the advantage of an awake patient, facilitating intraoperative monitoring of the neurologic state. Changes in mental status and the occurrence of aphasia, paresis, or loss of consciousness can be observed immediately. General anesthesia affords superior physiologic control, especially for maintenance of acceptable arterial blood gases, and limits the patient's discomfort, anxiety, and problems with aspiration. Many of these patients have attendant coronary artery disease where anxiety and increases in rate–pressure product may increase the likelihood of developing myocardial ischemia or infarction intraoperatively.

Anesthetic agents and techniques that maintain blood pressure and CPP should be selected. It is most desirable to decrease CMR_{O_2} while maintaining CBF, without hypotension and myocardial ischemia. Induction and intubation should be slow and smooth, devoid of hypertension or tachycardia. Inhalation agents, which decrease CMR_{O_2} and increase CBF, may be preferable to neuroleptanesthesia, which generally produces parallel reductions in CMR_{O_2} and CBF. Blood pressure should be kept at or 10 percent above normal levels and normocarbia maintained. Intraoperative bradycardia and hypotension may result from surgical manipulation at the carotid bifurcation. This response can be treated with intravenous atropine or by local infiltration with 1 percent Xylocaine. Emergence should be smooth and prompt to allow assessment of neurologic studies. Special monitoring should include an electrophysiologic measure of brain function, such as EEG. Stump pressure and jugular bulb oxygen tension do not correlate well with the development of postoperative neurologic deficits.

Direct blood pressure monitoring should be continued during transport to the recovery room. Hyper- or hypotensive episodes occur in 40 percent of patients in the immediate postoperative period. Hypotension may result from temporary impairment of carotid sinus baroreceptor reflexes. As these patients are unable to raise their pressure, any decrease must be treated promptly to prevent ischemic insult to the brain. Therapy includes placing the patient in the supine or Trendelenburg position and administering crystalloid or colloid solution if the CVP is low or vasopressors if the response to volume loading is inadequate. Hypertension in the 24 hours following surgery may reflect a transient increase in sympathetic tone, as occurs after posterior fossa procedures. Loss of cerebral autoregulation, cerebral edema, and stroke may ensue. If blood pressure is elevated above the preoperative level, a variety of adrenergic blockers may be used for control. Marked blood pressure elevations greater than 25 percent above preoperative levels are best managed by intravenous infusion of short-acting vasodilators such as sodium nitroprusside, nitroglycerin, or trimethaphan.

Carotid body function may be affected after bilateral carotid endarterectomy, with the loss of normal cardiorespiratory responses to hypoxia, including an increase in pulse, blood pressure, and ventilation. These patients may experience severe hypoxia without ventilatory or circulatory response. When conditions known to provoke hypoxemia emerge, the potential loss of carotid body function can be averted by means of adequate supplemental oxygen, blood gas monitoring, and close observation. An uncommon but potentially catastrophic cause of acute respiratory distress after carotid endarterectomy is tracheal compression by cervical hematoma, which requires immediate evacuation. Other causes of acute respiratory distress after carotid endarterectomy are tension pneumothorax and vocal cord paralysis.

Intraoperative or postoperative acute myocardial infarction is reported to be the second most frequent cause of morbidity and death after carotid endarterectomy. Mortality rates ranging from 9.6 to 16 percent have been reported for patients with a history of heart disease who undergo this procedure. Preexisting cardiovascular disease appears to be the major predisposing factor. For such patients, intraoperative administration of vasopressors during clamping of the carotid artery increases the incidence of acute myocardial infarction. The use of intracarotid shunts, rather than induced hypertension, has been recommended when carotid clamping is not tolerated. Appropriate therapy such as nitroglycerin should be instituted if ischemia occurs.

Cerebral Revascularization

Blood flow to ischemic areas of the brain in patients with cerebrovascular insufficiency secondary to occlusion distal to the cervical portion of the internal carotid artery is restored by creation of microvascular extracranial-to-intracranial (EC–IC) anastomoses. The anastomosis is achieved between the anterior circulation of the superficial temporal artery (STA) and the middle cerebral artery (MCA). Connections are also created posteriorly between the occipital artery and the posterior inferior cerebellar artery. Continuing refinements in microsurgical techniques and the use of the operative microscope have enhanced the success of these procedures. Long-term patency rates greater than 90 percent have been reported with an operative mortality of 1.7 percent. Although patients with a local reduction in CBF benefit most from EC–IC bypass, it is not clear whether the increase in CBF after EC–IC bypass will prevent infarction in the acutely ischemic cortex. Opinion suggests that cerebral revascularization may be of benefit to patients with small infarctions rather than large ones.

Patients selected for EC–IC bypass are typically male and in their sixth decade. They frequently have a number of risk factors for stroke and heart disease, including a history of transient ischemic attacks or partial stroke, hypotension, smoking, previous vascular surgery, and associated pulmonary or renal disease. Monitoring during anastomosis is the same as for other craniotomies. Blood pressure is maintained at mildly elevated levels to ensure cerebral perfusion and prevent thrombosis. As the procedure is superficial and performed through a small craniotomy, reduction of brain volume with hyperventilation or osmotic diuretics is not indicated. Ventilation is adjusted to keep the Pa_{CO_2} between 35 and 40 mm Hg. Minimal movement of the brain during respiratory excursion is achieved by the use of low tidal volumes and increased rate.

Cerebral Vascular Disease

Anesthetic techniques are selected that maintain CPP, limit cerebral oxygen requirements, sustain systemic arterial pressure, and render the patient awake and responsive at the conclusion of the operation to permit immediate assessment of neurologic status. The CMR_{O_2} is reduced by either barbiturates or inhaled agents. As barbiturates constrict cerebral arteries, low-dose inhalation agents may be advantageous by providing a measure of vasodilation. Combinations of thiopental and narcotic with low concentrations of halothane, enflurane, or isoflurane are appropriate. The prime concern in postoperative care after EC–IC bypass is augmentation of blood flow through the new anastomosis by maintaining blood pressure in the high normal range and expanding intravascular volume by administration of colloid or low-molecular-weight dextran at 50 to 100 mL/h. Neurologic assessment should be performed frequently.

Cerebral Aneurysm. Cerebral aneurysms are abnormal, localized dilations of the arteries within the skull. They are classified as congenital (berry), mycotic, traumatic, dissecting, neoplastic, and arteriosclerotic. Rupture of an intracranial aneurysm is one of the leading causes of subarachnoid hemorrhage (SAH). Signs and symptoms of intracranial aneurysms are usually those of SAH or of an intracranial mass. The presence of blood after SAH impairs consciousness and produces signs of meningeal irritation such as headache, meningismus, and photophobia. Patients present with convulsions, nausea, vomiting, dizziness, paresthesia or paralysis, alterations in consciousness, or neurogenic pulmonary edema. Signs such as cranial nerve paresis and impairment of brainstem function may result from direct pressure of the aneurysm on adjacent neural structures. Neurologic dysfunction may also occur as a result of an elevation of ICP caused by disruption of the brain parenchyma by an associated hematoma, by cerebral vasospasm or infarction, or by the mass effect of the aneurysm itself. Diagnosis of a cerebral aneurysm is based on clinical history, general physical and neurologic examinations, examination of CSF obtained via lumbar puncture, computerized axial tomography scanning, and complete angiographic studies. The most important guide to diagnosis and recovery is the clinical condition of the patient at the time therapy is initiated (Table 39–2).

The natural history of the untreated intracranial aneurysm is such that mortality during the first week after initial SAH is 27 percent, and during the first month, 49 percent. Ninety percent of patients who die within 72 hours of SAH have an associated intracerebral, intracerebellar, or subdural hematoma. Rebleeding occurs within 1 month of the first SAH in 23 percent of cases. There is a 40 percent mortality rate during the first year after the rupture of a single aneurysm. Mortality from the second SAH approaches 78 percent. The risk of rebleeding is greatest during the first 24 hours after SAH.

Preoperative management of patients after SAH is directed toward minimizing complications, preventing rebleeding, and facilitating recovery from the initial insult. The patient is monitored closely in a tranquil environment including complete bed rest, sedation, analgesia, administration of corticosteroids to reduce cerebral edema, maintenance of normal fluid and electrolyte balance, as well as attention to respiratory function. Blood pressure is maintained in the patient's high normal range to minimize ischemia from vasospasm. ε-Aminocaproic acid (Amicar) has been used to prevent recurrent SAH from ruptured cerebral aneurysms, although its efficacy is still in question. The timing of surgery is an important factor in determining prognosis, but the optimal interval has not yet been established. Classically, surgery is delayed 1 to 3 weeks after a bleed so that the patient can recover from the acute effects of SAH which include disrupted autoregulation and edema; however, risk of rebleed and significant ischemia from vasospasm is high. Most damage from rebleeding occurs 1 to 2 weeks after SAH. Treatment of vasospasm includes enhancing circulatory volume and moderate hypertension. In the patient with an unclipped aneurysm, this treatment can significantly increase the risk of rebleed. The highest incidence of vasospasm occurs within 5 to 9 days of SAH.

Surgery is usually scheduled after vasospasm on pre-operative angiogram has subsided and no infarction with mass effect is seen on computerized axial tomography scan. Vasospasm can produce profoundly severe ischemia and possible infarct. Mass effect on computerized axial tomography scan would illustrate less than optimal surgical conditions, as the brain would be edematous and vital structures distorted and shifted. Unless the situation is life threatening, the presence of vasospasm and its mass effect require postponement of surgery. Some institutions do not perform preoperative angiography because they believe the degree of spasm does not correlate well with the clinical picture. Instead, they take the patient to the operating room and induce hypotension with the patient awake. If a neurologic deficit such as aphasia or hemiparesis develops, the MAP is increased to normal levels, resolution of the deficit demonstrated, and surgery postponed for several days. If no deficit develops, the pressure is allowed to return to normal values, the patient is induced, and surgery ensues.

Many surgeons do not operate on stuporous patients who have hemiparesis, decerebrate rigidity, or vegetative disturbances, unless they have a life-threatening intracerebral hematoma. The mortality rate for operations that remove such hematomas is high and the prognosis poor. Although many patients with intracranial hematomas can be stabilized so that their surgery for clot evacuation and aneurysm clip ligation can be performed electively, the decision to perform evacuation of a hematoma is based on the rapidity of neurologic deterioration, the location and size of the hematoma, anatomic characteristics of the aneurysm, and the patient's age and clinical grade. Important considerations for these patients are maintenance of blood pressure and intravascular volume and improvement of intracranial compliance. As aneurysms are space-occupying lesions, their effect on intracranial compliance must also be recognized.

Surgical treatment of aneurysms has been refined considerably by the development of microsurgical instrumentation and techniques permitting small exposure and precise dissection. Minimized retraction and consequent trauma to the brain also prevent premature rupture. Clipping the neck of the aneurysm is the treatment of choice in the majority of cases. Large aneurysms and those with anatomic features that preclude safe clip ligation may be reinforced with muslin. This causes intense scarring, which in time strengthens the wall of the aneurysm. "Giant" aneurysms are treated by induction of a thrombus by direct or stereotactic insertion of a fine wire through the aneurysm wall to reduce the risk of recurrent hemorrhage or pressure-induced deficit. The only definitive therapy, however, is clip ligation. The same precautions necessary to prevent aneurysmal rupture during induction of anesthesia are indicated during emergence from anesthesia after the aneurysm has been clipped.

Anesthetic Considerations for Aneurysm Repair. Preoperative evaluation is the same for these patients as for any other neurosurgical patient. Careful assessment of the extravascular volume is essential because of the precarious relationship of vasospasm to large variations in systemic blood pressure. Antihypertensive agents or vasopressors

TABLE 39–2. THE HUNT CLASSIFICATION[a]

Grade 0	Unruptured
Grade 1	Asymptomatic or minimal headache, slight nuchal rigidity
Grade 1A	Stable, residual neurologic deficit, past the period of further cerebral reaction
Grade 2	Moderate to severe headache, nuchal rigidity, no deficit except palsy of cranial nerve III
Grade 3	Drowsiness, confusion, mild focal deficit
Grade 4	Stupor, hemiparesis
Grade 5	Deep coma, decerebrate rigidity, moribund

[a] Prognosis after subarachnoid hemorrhage is closely related to the patient's initial condition. The Hunt Classification is one of the systems that is used to grade patients on admission and that allows for comparison among various studies.

should be continued until the time of surgery. Direct arterial monitoring is essential; a pulmonary artery line may be valuable for monitoring myocardial function and vascular dynamics. If the patient is to be in a sitting position, a precordial doppler, central venous line, and $ETCO_2$ analyzer (in the absence of pulmonary artery catheter) are essential. Selection of anesthetic agents is governed by patient status, with consideration given to avoiding extreme changes in blood pressure and providing improvement in cerebral oxygenation and protection in the event of focal ischemia.

Osmotic dehydrating agents may be avoided during aneurysm surgery or used in smaller doses in conjunction with spinal drainage. Spinal drainage of CSF may be used to produce a slack, easily retractable brain and thus improve operating conditions. Spinal drainage is accomplished with indwelling subarachnoid catheters or malleable needles inserted through the lumbar interspace at L3–4 or L4–5. Two catheters are usually placed in case one occludes. Care must be taken to avoid excessive loss of CSF on lumbar puncture, as the sudden decrease in pressure can cause hemorrhage or herniation. The catheter may be attached to a transducer and a calibrated drip chamber receptacle and closed with a clamp. Drainage is not begun until the dura is opened to prevent the development of pressure gradients across the brain. Cerebrospinal flow should be passively drained, approximately 5 mL/min. As much as 150 mL may be withdrawn, as required for adequate surgical exposure. Drainage is stopped when dural closure begins and the catheters are removed at the end of surgery. During anesthetic maintenance, arterial blood gases are monitored frequently to maintain $PaCO_2$ at preoperative levels. If hypocarbia is necessary to allow dissection, normocarbia is restored before controlled hypotension is induced. The combined effects of vasoconstriction and hypotension can cause severe ischemia and infarct.

Fluids such as lactated Ringer's are given to replace urine loss and maintain hourly requirements. Packed cells or whole blood is given to replace blood loss. An additional one or two units of blood may be given to augment intravascular volume and counteract potential vasospasm after ligation of the aneurysm. MAP is maintained in a high normal range. Controlled hypotension is frequently used to decrease blood loss and operative time and to facilitate dissection and clipping of the aneurysm. Normotensive patients can usually tolerate a reduction in MAP to 50 mm Hg at normocarbia. Chronically hypertensive patients have higher limits of autoregulation and do not tolerate as low a reduction as normotensive patients. A 30 percent reduction in MAP is usually tolerated. ECG and urine output should be carefully monitored for signs of ischemia or decreased renal blood flow. Controlled hypotension can be achieved with sodium nitroprusside, nitroglycerin, or trimethaphan in the manner previously described.

Cerebral Vasospasm. Vasospasm is the clinical syndrome of neurologic deterioration that follows rupture or attempted surgical treatment of narrowing cerebral vessels. This arterial narrowing results in impaired cerebral perfusion and secondary infarction of the brain. Rarely detected until 2 to 3 days after SAH, vasospasm may be severe for 2 to 4 weeks. Surgery is frequently postponed until there is

clinical and angiographic evidence that the spasm has resolved. Vasospasm also occurs postoperatively, with onset in a matter of hours or several days. The incidence of radiographically identified vasospasm has been correlated with the location of the aneurysm, number and severity of hemorrhages, catecholamine levels in the blood, and intraoperative employment of hypothermia.

Delayed or recurrent spasm which develops 3 to 7 days after hemorrhage is usually responsible for any ischemic damage to the brain. This recurrent spasm is more intense than that occurring immediately after surgery, involves vessels distal to the site of rupture, and may last days or weeks. Direct trauma to vessels or mechanical distortion or displacement produces localized, short-term spasms. Extravasated blood may produce severe vasospasm from the products of hemoglobin breakdown. Platelet concentrations of serotonin are also capable of producing vascular muscle contraction in vitro. Other circulating prostaglandins have been implicated as an etiologic source.

Therapeutic efforts directed toward alleviating spasm have met with limited success (Table 39–3). Physiologic measures include elevation of blood pressure and expansion of intravascular volume. This approach is based on demonstration of a passive increase in rCBF after hypertension in the ischemic hemispheres of animals with vasospasm. Because of the risk of rebleeding, both hypertension and hypervolemia are used cautiously in the period preceding surgical correction by clip ligation; however, patients with aneurysms frequently receive intraoperative transfusion, despite unremarkable blood loss, to augment intravascular volume and prevent vasospasm.

Most of the drugs known to dilate cerebral vessels produce significant systemic hypotension before cerebrovascular relaxation occurs. As a direct smooth muscle relaxant, sodium nitroprusside has been used in combination with dopamine to achieve relief of spasm without causing sys-

---

TABLE 39–3. VASOSPASM TREATMENT MODALITIES

Augmentation of blood pressure and intravascular volume

Vasodilation and blood pressure support
  Sodium nitroprusside
  Dopamine

Topical alpha antagonism
  Phentolamine
  Phenoxybenzamine

Beta agonism and antiarrhythmics
  Isoproterenol
  Lidocaine

Phosphodiesterase inhibition
  Aminophylline
  Theophylline

Serotonin and catecholamine reduction
  Reserpine
  Kanamycin

Calcium entry blocking drugs
  Nimodipine[a]

[a] Of the various pharmacologic methods used to treat vasospasm, nimodipine is the most recent addition. It is considered to be cerebral selective in its effects.

temic hypotension. The alpha-adrenergic antagonists phentolamine and phenoxybenzamine reduce or abolish spasm only when applied topically. Isoproterenol produces vasodilation through stimulation of adenylate cyclase, which activates phosphorylase by means of cyclic adenosine monophosphate (cAMP), resulting in increased calcium permeability and relaxation. Isoproterenol, in combination with lidocaine to counteract ventricular irritability, has produced encouraging results.

Arteriovenous Malformation. In patients with arteriovenous malformation, there may be, in addition to the mass effect from the lesion itself and associated hematomas, a steal phenomenon in which blood is shunted away from healthy brain to the arteriovenous malformation, resulting in neurologic deficit. To avoid exacerbating this problem, maintenance of blood pressure during anesthesia is critical. The size of the arteriovenous malformation and the flow through its feeding arteries may be decreased by selective preoperative embolization with particulate matter or rapidly polymerizing glue. During this procedure, patients are sedated yet awake to permit frequent neurologic evaluation. Although surgical resection is facilitated and blood loss reduced by neuroradiologic vascular occlusion, intracranial hemorrhage and stroke are potential complications.

NEURODIAGNOSTIC TECHNIQUES

Neurodiagnostic techniques include magnetic resonance imaging, positron emission tomography, computerized axial tomography, cerebral angiography, pneumoencephalography, ventriculogram, and myelogram. These are frequently performed without anesthesia; however, there are certain situations when anesthesia standby or general anesthesia may be required. Testing in pediatric, elderly, debilitated, uncooperative, and decompensating or severely injured patients may best be done under conscious sedation or general anesthesia. The principles of neuroanesthesia should be maintained throughout all procedures. Careful, continuous observation of vital signs and respiration is mandatory, especially when conscious sedation is used. Technical difficulties may also arise from inadequate diagnostic facilities that should properly accommodate anesthesia equipment, but often do not. Anesthesia and monitoring systems often must be transported to the diagnostic area. In addition, suites are often dark, which impairs assessment of the patient's skin color and respiration and makes it difficult to read the dials and numeric displays on equipment. Airflow turnover may be inadequate, thereby increasing the levels of gases in the environment. Proper maintenance and function of the diagnostic equipment require that the suite be maintained at 60F to 65F. Control of body temperature, especially in babies, small children, and the elderly, is an important consideration.

Radiopaque iodine-containing contrast media may be injected into arteries, veins, or CSF spaces. Careful observation during injection of these dyes is necessary as they can cause allergic reactions ranging from mild skin rashes to anaphylactic shock. Seizures and cardiovascular reactions may also occur. A burning sensation and flushing during injection constitute a fairly common reaction during angiography. If the patient has a history of allergy to iodine, steroids should be given several hours before the study and diphenhydramine hydrochloride (Benadryl) immediately before the contrast dye is given.

Gas Studies. Pneumoencephalogram and ventriculogram, rarely used today, involve the incremental removal of up to 70 mL of CSF and replacement of that volume with air, oxygen, or nitrous oxide injected into the spinal subarachnoid space or directly into the ventricles. The patient is securely positioned in a special chair which allows a variety of positions and complete somersaulting to aid passage of the gas through the ventricles and subarachnoid space. Usually, mild sedation and local anesthesia are sufficient for gas encephalogram. When general anesthesia is required, care must be taken to support the patient's head. An anode tube may be useful to prevent kinking with position changes. If nitrous oxide is used as the contrast agent, then it may be incorporated into the anesthetic technique. If air or oxygen is used, nitrous oxide is not recommended as it will rapidly equilibrate into the gas-filled ventricle or subarachnoid space and add unmeasurably to the intracranial volume. Air embolus is a distinct possibility especially if the patient has a patent ventricloatrial CSF shunt. Nitrous oxide is reabsorbed from the ventricles and the subarachnoid space in about 1 hour. Air takes approximately 1 week for complete reabsorption. For this reason, general anesthesia planned within 1 week of gas studies should avoid nitrous oxide unless complete reabsorption of the nitrous oxide is confirmed by skull roentgenogram. Poststudy headache and nausea and vomiting are usually due to air remaining in the ventricles. Appropriate analgesics and antiemetics can provide comfort to the patient until the air is completely reabsorbed. Occasionally, the nausea and vomiting are due to postural hypotension and may be relieved by maintenance of a normal MAP and Trendelenburg position.

Myelogram. Myelograms are usually performed under local anesthesia, possibly with mild sedation. If general anesthesia is necessary, consideration must be given to the fact that lumbar and cervical myelograms are usually done in prone position. Cervical myelograms may involve hyperextension and flexion of the neck. Complications of myelogram are due to the use of contrast medium and may include local infection at the site of needle puncture, bacterial or aseptic meningitis, venous extravasation of contrast medium, headache, adhesive arachnoiditis, and allergic reaction. Pantopaque is an oil-base contrast medium, and as such it is nonabsorbable and must be removed after the study.

Metrizamide (Amipaque) is a water-soluble, iodinated contrast material whose benefits include decreased incidence of headache, nausea, vomiting, hypotension, arachnoiditis, and seizures. Amipaque does not need to be withdrawn after the study because it is quickly diluted by the CSF and absorbed into the bloodstream. For this very reason, studies must be completed in a much shorter period. A major drawback of metrizamide is that it cannot be used in patients receiving medications that lower the seizure threshold. These drugs include phenothiazines, monoamine oxidase inhibitors, antihistamines, tricyclic antidepressants, central nervous system stimulants, and psychoactive drugs encompassing analeptics, major tranquilizers, and antipsychotic drugs. The synergistic action between metrizamide and any of these drugs can precipitate epileptic seizures. These medications should be discontinued 24 hours prior to the study. Clearly, as antihistamines cannot be used, metrizamide must be avoided in patients with a history of allergy to iodinated compounds.

Computerized Axial Tomographic Scanning

Computerized axial tomography (CT) scanning is a noninvasive technique that gives an anatomic depiction of a transverse section of the head. The scanning device rotates around the patient's head in a 180-degree arc. The anatomic images are depicted on a cathode-ray screen and can be processed as a hard-copy x-ray film. Abnormalities can be identified by differences in density or by displacement of normal structures. Contrast medium may be used for greater differentiation. Radiation exposure to the patient in the area being scanned is approximately equal to that received with conventional skull x-ray per half-hour scan. Skin dose to the anesthetist is many times less than that. Anesthesia or intravenous sedation may be required when patient movement threatens to invalidate the scan.

Magnetic Resonance Imaging

Magnetic resonance imaging (MRI) is a painless, noninvasive technique that uses magnetic fields and radio frequency pulses for the production of its images. Magnetic resonance imaging is superior to CT scan in differentiating between white and gray matter; displaying images in sagittal, coronal, or axial planes with equal ease; reflecting the chemical environment as well as the elemental structure of tissue; and visualizing the posterior fossa. Indications for anesthetic intervention during MRI are similar to those for CT scan. MRI poses one unique problem for anesthetic equipment. Any equipment affected by a magnetic field would be affected by the MRI unit. All anesthetic equipment within 20 ft of the unit must be nonmagnetic. Some machines are now using aluminum replacement parts for the magnetic steel to avoid this problem.

In positron emission tomography radiation emitted as a consequence of radioactive decay is used to reconstruct an image or to produce spatially identified digital data. This device is used primarily for in vivo study of cerebral metabolic activity and drug interactions. Unless anesthetic agents are the materials under study, no anesthetic intervention should be required.

Therapeutic Neuroradiology

Embolization techniques performed in the radiology suite treat a variety of intra- and extracranial vascular and brain tissue pathologies. For carotid–cavernous sinus fistula, aneurysm, intra- or extracranial fistula, angioplasty, and intracranial thrombolysis, these treatments may be curative. For tumor, arteriovenous malformation, and test occlusion of the carotid, the treatment decreases flow to the lesion thus facilitating other interventions or decreases operative time, risk, and morbidity, or both. Most patients require only monitored anesthesia care with minimal intravenous sedation, providing comfort while still rendering them arousable and appropriately responsive. Patients who are at the extremes of age are restless or uncooperative, or present with spinal arteriovenous malformation may require general anesthesia, the latter of which can be exquisitely painful. Neuroanesthetic management principles should be considered in relationship to concomitant systemic problems. For example, children presenting with arteriovenous fistula, intracranial arteriovenous malformation, or vein of Galen fistula may be in congestive heart failure and pulmonary edema induced by the high-flow circuit. Another example demonstrates that neurofibromatosis has been found in association with extracranial arteriovenous fistula.

Anesthetic monitoring beyond the basics is dictated by the patient's physical status. EEG and, often, CBF are monitored during these procedures. The anesthetist must be in constant communication with personnel administering radioactive intravenous xenon which is used to measure CBF. The elimination of xenon is solely through ventilation, most of which occurs on the first pass. The patient respires through a tight-fitting scavenger mask which takes the waste through a charcoal filter into a lead-lined container. The amount of radiation received by the patient per CBF measurement is less than one-quarter that received during conventional chest x-ray. The level of radiation in the environment is less than that and is carefully monitored. Lead shields are used to protect personnel.

The patient's preoperative regimen may include steroids, Ca^{2+} channel blockers, and Nitropaste. Steroids are used to decrease the inflammatory effect of the embolic material and to reduce swelling of tumors. Perioperative supplementation will be required. Nimodipine is a Ca^{2+} channel blocker that preferentially dilates cerebral vessels, increasing flow around the lesion. The systemic vasodilation, decreasing SVR, and myocardial depressant effects of Nimodipine may be potentiated by anesthetic agents. Nimodipine or Nitropaste may be used to prevent vasospasm. This spasm is not the typical clinical vasospasm seen after vessel rupture. Spasm occurs in the smaller vessels and can prevent the catheter from being placed.

A path to the lesion is established using a coaxial catheter, usually through the femoral artery. Because of the large dead space in these catheters, there is significant risk of forming emboli; therefore, the patient and the flush are both heparinized. The anesthetist must be prepared to reverse the heparin in the event of vessel rupture. Nonionic contrast medium is used for vascular visualization. Although there is less risk of allergic reaction, there is a risk of kidney damage in long procedures. This contrast medium is excreted by the kidneys. It is also an osmotic diuretic. Urinary output should be monitored and a Foley catheter should be considered for longer procedures.

Sodium amytal is often used for test occlusion of arteriovenous malformation. The radiologist injects this medication through the microcatheter so that it is deposited directly into the vessel serving the lesion. Sodium amytal produces a temporary, discrete depression in neuronal activity, thereby helping to determine if normal territory will be affected by permanent occlusion of the lesion. Small coils, silk threads, balloons, particles of various synthetic compounds, and liquid polymerizing agents are some of the materials used for embolization. Any of these materials can migrate from the cerebral circulation to systemic circulation and, eventually, to the lungs. At the very least, the Sao_2 will decrease. At worst, pulmonary infarction will occur. Coughing is a telltale sign that material has migrated to the lungs. If baseline pulmonary reserve is decreased, then even small amounts of migrating material can be significant.

When tumors are embolized, the ensuing ischemia can cause the tumor to swell, producing a potentially dangerous increase in ICP. Ischemia in adjacent tissue can occur if more is blocked than was anticipated. When a high-flow shunt is embolized, normal perfusion pressure breakthrough can occur in which CBF and CBV are increased across the brain. The vessel adjacent to the shunt, which is already maximally vasodilated and cannot autoregulate, can rupture. The radiologist can monitor vessel pressures through the catheter and be warned of impending danger. In the event of a hyperemic crisis, the patient may exhibit symptoms of increased ICP. Inadvertent embolization of venous outflow requires rapid blood pressure control to prevent rupture of the aneurysm or arteriovenous malformation. In many cases, induced hypotension may be instituted prophylactically rather than therapeutically.

INTRAOPERATIVE PROBLEMS

Hypertension

Hypertension can occur with light anesthesia or with surgical manipulation and retraction of the brainstem and cranial nerves. Beta blockade with propranolol may be used to treat hypertension with tachycardia that is not associated with surgical manipulation and that does not respond to deepening anesthesia. Other neurosurgical procedures associated with cardiac arrhythmias include orbital decompression, carotid ligation, sudden intracranial decompression, and manipulation of the vagus and trigeminal nerves. The perturbations caused by surgical manipulation usually resolve with cessation of stimulation and deepened anesthesia. If persistent stimulation of the brainstem or cranial nerves is necessary because of the location of the lesion and deepened anesthesia does not ameliorate the response to stimulation, the surgeons can apply local anesthetic directly to the area. Small amounts of intravenous atropine may be used to block persistent vagal stimulation.

Venous Air Embolism

Venous air embolism can occur whenever a gradient of 5 cm or more exists between the wound and the right side of the heart. Although the incidence of air embolism is 25 to 35 percent among patients operated in the sitting position, air has also entered during operations in the lateral, supine, and prone positions. Air is entrained most often during the early part of the operation when the bone flap is elevated and the dura opened, less frequently during conclusion of the operation, and least frequently during the surgery. The head pin site may also be a source of entrained air. This may be prevented by wrapping the pins and covering the site with Vaseline gauze after insertion of the pins.

Pathophysiologic effects of entrained air include hypotension, arrhythmias, hypercarbia, hypoxia secondary to reflex bronchoconstriction and pulmonary edema, and asystole. These sequelae follow accumulation of more than 50 mL of air because of obstruction of right ventricular and pulmonary arterial outflow, which increases pulmonary artery and wedge pressure and $Paco_2$ and decreases cardiac output, Pao_2, and end-tidal CO_2. Paradoxical air emboli may occur in which air passes directly through the pulmonary circulation or through right-to-left intracardiac shunts to reach the coronary and cerebral circulation. Death in these instances results from air occlusion of coronary arteries and ventricular fibrillation.

Early diagnosis of air embolism is essential to successful treatment. The mass spectrometer and Doppler ultrasonic unit are the most sensitive methods for detection of air embolism. Air is "heard" because the air–blood interface is a much better acoustical reflector than blood alone, producing a noise of characteristic frequency. In addition to monitoring $ETco_2$, a measurement of ETn_2 indicates air entrained from surgical sites or intravenous access. Sources of Fin_2 are due to mechanical failure such as leaks in ventilators, connecting tubing, partial endotracheal tube disconnections, and mask fit. Table 39–4 summarizes the cardiopulmonary changes associated with air emboli.

As soon as a change in Doppler signal or monitored parameters occurs, nitrous oxide is turned off and ventilation continued with 100 percent oxygen to avoid increasing the size of embolic bubbles. The anesthetist aspirates the right atrial catheter while the surgeon occludes possible sites of air entry by irrigating the wound with saline and waxing the bone edges. It has been found that the proximal and distal lumens on the Swan-Ganz catheter are usually too narrow to adequately aspirate air. If a pulmonary artery catheter is used, a separate, large-bore right atrial catheter should also be placed to allow optimal aspiration. The anesthetist performs a Valsalva maneuver and adds PEEP to demonstrate bleeding points and reduce negative pressure in the venous sinuses. Pulmonary artery or $ETco_2$ measurements aid in calculating the amount of air and the duration of its presence in the pulmonary vasculature. No change in

AIR EMBOLI

Parameter	Change
PAP[a]	Increases
PCWP	Increases
CVP	Increases
Cardiac output	Decreases
ECG	Arrhythmias
MAP[b]	Decreases
$Paco_2$	Increases
Pao_2[b]	Decreases
ETn_2	Measurable
Doppler sounds	Turbulent
Cyanosis[b]	Present
Neck vein congestion[b]	May occur

[a] PAP increases in proportion to the volume of air embolized and corresponds to the change in $ETco_2$.
[b] These relatively late-occurring changes precede cardiovascular collapse.

PAP or ETco$_2$ with reintroduction of nitrous oxide indicates resolution of the air and safe continuation of surgery. Massive air embolism or inability to arrest air entry necessitates placement of the wound at or below heart level and termination of the operation.

Postoperative Complications

Neurosurgical patients are frequently hypertensive in the recovery room, particularly after neurovascular and posterior fossa procedures. Although this usually resolves within 12 hours of surgery, the danger of hematoma formation or hemorrhagic infarction requires that hypertension be treated immediately. When analgesics in small doses are not effective, sodium nitroprusside (SNP), nitroglycerin (NTG), trimethaphan, labetolol, apresoline, or propranolol is indicated for rapid control. SNP, NTG, and trimethaphan are included in the discussion on deliberate hypotension. Elevation of temperature in the immediate postoperative period is usually due to blood irritation of the meninges.

DELIBERATE HYPOTHERMIA

Reduction of core temperature is the most common situation requiring hypothermic techniques in anesthesia. Hyperthermia increases CBF and CMRo$_2$ by 7 percent per degree elevation over 37C. These effects can obviously be deleterious in the neurology patient. Indications for induced hypothermia, specific to neurosurgery, include operations on cerebral vessels which may result in prolonged cerebral ischemia, for instance, during clipping of aneurysms. During hypothermia, cerebral metabolism is reduced 7 percent for each degree decrease below 37C. CBF and ICP are also reduced. Slowing of cerebral edema formation, decreased inflammatory reaction to injury, and decreased CSF secretion may also occur. Among the complications of induced hypothermia are cardiac arrhythmias and shivering during cooling and rewarming which increases CMRo$_2$ by 50 to 200 percent. Decreased cardiac output, increased blood viscosity, and immobilization may also predispose the patient to venous thrombosis and subsequent embolism. If continued through the postoperative period, temperature suppression, especially with steroid therapy, will mask signs of infection. Cooling may be induced primarily with chilled intravenous fluids and exposure of the patient to ambient room temperatures. Caution must be given to careful monitoring during intentional hypothermia and cooling procedures should be stopped when the patient reaches 34C, as temperature will continue to drift down another several degrees before stabilization or rewarming is instituted.

DELIBERATE HYPOTENSION AND ANTIHYPERTENSIVE THERAPY

During neurosurgical procedures, blood pressure is reduced to treat hypertension and to facilitate clipping of aneurysms and resection of arteriovenous malformation and vascular tumors such as meningiomas and hemangioendotheliomas. In addition, pharmacologically decreasing MAP reduces blood loss and, by affording better surgical conditions, decreases operative time. Adjuvant techniques to complement the primary action of the hypotensive drug and to aid in achieving precise blood pressure control include alterations of position or airway pressure or addition of other vasoactive drugs.

Ideally, induction of hypotension should decrease CPP without significantly reducing CBF. This is accomplished by maintaining a normal circulating blood volume and cardiac output as cerebral vascular resistance falls. Increased intrapulmonary shunting accompanies the use of vasodilators. To avoid ischemia, it is critical to ensure adequate Pao$_2$ during a reduction in CPP. Hypocarbia to 30 mm Hg when MAP is less than 50 mm Hg in normotensive patients may produce ischemia. It is best to maintain a Paco$_2$ of 35 to 40 mm Hg when inducing hypotension. In most patients, MAP may be safely reduced to 50 mm Hg without causing ischemic depletion of brain energy substances or accumulation of acid metabolites. Higher pressure levels are required in patients with chronic arterial hypertension and during altered autoregulation in brain regions compressed by masses. In chronic arterial hypertension, the lower limits of autoregulation are shifted to the right, which means that a higher MAP is necessary to prevent ischemia. Unless EEG and CBF are monitored it is difficult to determine the level to which MAP may be safely reduced. MAP is usually not decreased more than 30 percent from baseline.

In addition to disturbances of the blood–brain barrier and autoregulation, patients in the acute phase of subarachnoid hemorrhage may also present with a range of cardiac problems, decreased blood volume, or both. Recent myocardial infarction (within 6 months) is an absolute contraindication to induced hypotension. A history of cardiac, pulmonary, renal, or hepatic disease is a relative contraindication. At the very least, continuous intraarterial MAP monitoring and frequent analysis of Pao$_2$, Pvo$_2$, and Paco$_2$ or ETco$_2$ are necessary whenever MAP is manipulated.

Sodium Nitroprusside

Sodium nitroprusside is currently the most widely used hypotensive drug because it is easy to control and has a short duration of action. Despite the reduction in blood pressure, caused by decreased afterload, CBF continues to be adequate as cerebral vascular resistance is reduced and cardiac output remains near normal. This arteriolar dilation increases CBV and ICP, especially in patients who have impaired intracranial compliance. For this reason, SNP is not administered until the dura is opened or until compliance has improved. Sodium nitroprusside should be dissolved in 5 percent dextrose and water; however, in solution SNP is photosensitive and should be protected from light by wrapping the solution container and tubing in aluminum foil. Once in solution, SNP is stable for no more than 4 hours. Infusion is begun at 0.2 to 1.0 µg/kg per minute and titrated to 10 µg/kg per minute to maintain the desired MAP. It is easiest and most accurate to use a volumetric pump to administer SNP. Onset is within 30 seconds and duration is 2 to 4 minutes. Sodium nitroprusside should be used with caution in patients with hepatic or renal insufficiency as the hepatic enzyme rhodanese mediates conversion of cyanide to thiocyanate which is excreted by the kidneys. The adverse effects associated with SNP administration include increased ICP, rebound hypertension, cyanide and thiocyanate toxicity, hypothyroidism, and blood coagulation abnormalities.

Rebound hypertension occurs after abrupt discontinuance of SNP. It is especially dangerous in patients with neurovascular disorders as the upper limits of autoregulation may be exceeded and formation of cerebral edema enhanced. Rebound hypertension results from increased plasma renin activity, possibly because of renal artery dilation or renal ischemia. Renin has a plasma half-life of 30 minutes; SNP has a biologic half-life of 2 minutes. Discontinuation of SNP over 30 to 60 minutes or administration of propranolol, 20 mg orally preoperatively or small amounts intravenously intraoperatively, may be effective in preventing rebound hypertension because it decreases renin release.

The major disadvantage of SNP is the toxicity caused by its metabolic decomposition to cyanide (Fig. 39–8). Cyanide reacts in mitochondria to form a cyanide–cytochrome oxidase complex that inhibits cellular respiration and produces cellular hypoxia. Signs of toxicity include tachyphylaxis, tachycardia, metabolic acidosis, and cardiovascular collapse. The total amount of SNP administered should not exceed 0.7 µg/kg over 2 to 3 hours as the blood cyanide level correlates directly with the total dose. Administration of intravenous hydroxocobalamin together with SNP will decrease the blood cyanide concentration. Thiosulfate also decreases blood cyanide by increasing urinary excretion of thiocyanate. If the patient develops acidosis or tachyphylaxis, SNP should be discontinued and another hypotensive drug substituted. Thiocyanate also inhibits uptake and binding of iodine by the thyroid; thus hypothyroidism can be induced. Blood coagulopathies may occur after SNP-induced platelet disintegration and inhibition of platelet aggregation.

Nitroglycerin

Nitroglycerin acts primarily by relaxing capacitance vessels, decreasing preload, which in return decreases venous return, stroke volume, and MAP. As NTG reduces MAP by acting on the peripheral circulation, there is no direct effect on the normal heart. Nitroglycerin has a short duration of action, is easy to control, and does not cause tachyphylaxis, production of toxic metabolites, or rebound hypertension; however, ICP increases as blood accumulates and pools in the cranium faster than it can exit through the rigid venous channels. As with SNP, NTG should not be administered to patients with intracranial hypertension until the dura is opened or intracranial compliance has improved. Nitroglycerin may fail to induce adequate hypotension in younger patients, especially those under balanced narcotic anesthesia, necessitating the use of alternate drugs. Parenteral nitroglycerin (Tridil) is absorbed by polyvinyl chloride solution bags and intravenous administration sets. The amount of drug absorbed and, therefore, the amount actually administered to the patient cannot be calculated. Tridil should be diluted in *glass* containers of D_5W or 0.9 percent sodium chloride and administered through the nonabsorbing tubing supplied with Tridil. When diluted in glass containers the solution is stable for up to 48 hours at room temperature and 7 days under refrigeration. Nitroglycerin is not light sensitive.

Administration should be made with a volumetric pump. Infusion should start with 1 to 2 µg/kg per minute and titrated for desired MAP levels. Nitroglycerin has a biologic half-life of 1 to 4 minutes. Adverse reactions including severe tachycardia or paradoxical bradycardia are rare. Toxic effects have not been described. Nitroglycerin should be used with caution in patients with hepatic or renal disease, as the drug is metabolized by the liver and excreted by the kidneys.

Trimethaphan

Trimethaphan (Arfonad) induces hypotension by occupying sympathetic and parasympathetic ganglionic receptor sites and stabilizing the postsynaptic membrane against acetylcholine. Depression of parasympathetic activity causes tachycardia, mydriases, cycloplegia, decreased gas-

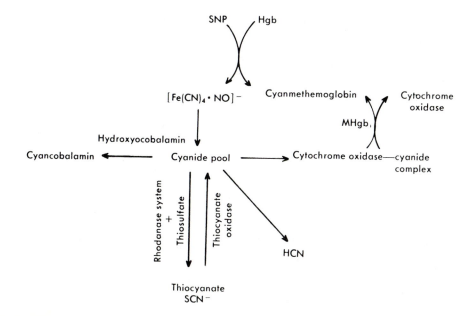

Figure 39–8. Biotransformation of sodium nitroprusside (SNP). Hgb, hemoglobin; MHgb, methemoglobin; SCN, thiocyanate; HCN, hydrogen cyanide. (*Reprinted, with permission, from Cottrell JE, Van Aken H, Gupta B, Turndorf H. Induced hypertension. In: Cottrell JE, Turndorf H, eds: Anesthesia and neurosurgery.* 2nd ed. St. Louis, MO: CV Mosby; 1986:421.)

trointestinal tone and motility, and urinary retention. In addition to ganglionic blockade, Arfonad decreases MAP by histamine release and direct vasodilation. Because it is rapidly inactivated by plasma cholinesterase and excreted by the kidneys, trimethaphan has a short duration of action. It is easy to control and does not increase ICP because autoregulation remains intact as MAP decreases. Arfonad should probably be used to treat intraoperative hypertension that occurs before the dura is opened, and should be avoided when hypotension to MAP of 50 mm Hg is required. At an MAP of 50 mm Hg, the drug has direct cerebral toxic effects. Signs of this include burst suppression; slowing, high-voltage waves on EEG; and elevation of brain lactate levels. Tachyphylaxis, histamine-induced bronchospasm, and myoneural blockade have been associated with the use of Arfonad. At high doses or after prolonged use (several hours) cycloplegia, fixed dilated pupils, can occur and may interfere with postoperative neurologic assessment. Arfonad can be diluted in D_5W and, at room temperature, is stable in solution for 24 hours. It is not light sensitive. Infusion through a volumetric pump should be started at 30 to 50 µg/kg per minute and titrated to the desired MAP (Table 39–5).

Hydralazine Hydrochloride (Apresoline)

Hydralazine hydrochloride (Apresoline) is a direct-acting, predominant arteriolar vasodilator. Diastolic pressure is usually decreased more than systolic. Heart rate, stroke volume, and cardiac output are increased. Tachycardia following hydralazine is often significant. Unless the drop in MAP is severe, CBF is increased. Hydralazine is best used in neurosurgical patients after intracranial compliance has improved. Parenteral hydralazine may be given without dilution. Onset of action is within 10 to 20 minutes. Although 20 to 40 mg is the recommended dose, our experience has been such that much smaller doses are usually adequate. Control of hypertension can be accomplished with 5 mg intra-

venously every 20 minutes until effect; this may be followed by 10–20 mg intramuscularly.

Volatile Anesthetics

Administered in high concentrations, the volatile anesthetics produce hypotension by causing myocardial depression and direct vasodilation. As these agents also decrease CVR and raise CBF, ICP is increased, cerebral perfusion reduced, and the likelihood of edema formation enhanced. Therefore, the volatile anesthetics should be avoided for induction of hypotension during neurosurgical procedures.

CONSIDERATIONS IN PEDIATRIC NEUROANESTHESIA

With few exceptions, the principles of neuroanesthetic management for adult patients apply to the pediatric population. These differences are related to the anatomic, physiologic, and pharmacokinetic characteristics common to premature babies, neonates, infants, and children. Premature babies are generally classified as those born less than 37 weeks after conception. Low-birth-weight babies are those who weigh less than 2500 g at birth. Any alterations in response typical of the full-term, normal-birth-weight baby will be increasingly obvious with greater deficits in age and weight.

Cerebral vasculature and the central nervous system are very immature in premature babies. Intracranial hemorrhage, both subependymal and intraventricular, occurs in 40 to 50 percent of sick premature infants. There is an increased incidence of intracranial hemorrhage with stress from traumatic delivery and hypoxia. Aggressive correction of metabolic acidosis with sodium bicarbonate may cause hyperosmolarity and may lead to intracranial hemorrhage. For this reason, bicarbonate administration should be accomplished slowly and cautiously, perhaps in less than the calculated dosage. These children are also subject to seizure and apneic spells.

TABLE 39–5. DELIBERATE HYPOTENSION: ADMINISTRATION AND HEMODYNAMIC AND TOXIC EFFECTS OF THE MOST COMMONLY USED AGENTS

Drug	Dosage	Onset/Duration	CO[a]	PCWP	SVR	CVR	CBF	ICP	CPP	Toxic Effects
Trimethaphan	2–4 mg/min; titrate to desired MAP	1–2 min/4–8 min	↓[b]	↓	↓	0	0	0	0	Direct cerebral toxicity (MAP < 50 mm Hg)
Nitroprusside[c]	0.2–1.0 µg/kg per min; titrate to 10 µg/kg per min; max 0.7 µg/kg over 3–4 h	30 s/2–4 min	0	↓	↓	↓	↑	↑	↓	Cyanide toxicity rebound hypertension, ↓ Pao_2
Nitroglycerin[c]	2.4–5.0 µg/kg per min; titrate to desired MAP	1–2 min/10 min	0	↓	↓	↓	↑	↑	↓	↓ Po_2

[a] CO, cardiac output; PCWP, pulmonary capillary wedge pressure; SVR, systemic vascular resistance; CVR, cerebral vascular resistance; CBF, cerebral blood flow; ICP, intracranial pressure; CPP, cerebral perfusion pressure; MAP, mean arterial pressure.
[b] ↑, increase; ↓, decrease; 0, no change.
[c] Should not be used until the dura is open or measures have been taken to improve intracranial compliance.

Autoregulation is often absent in the premature infant but present in the neonate. The blood–brain barrier, if present, is immature. Cerebral vessels are not well developed. Vascular tone, CVR, and $Paco_2$ responsiveness are decreased. Considering the lower MAP, CPP is also much lower in proportion to the age and weight of the child. $CMRo_2$ is 5 to 6 mL/100 g per minute, gradually increasing to adult levels. In general, physiologic functions reach adult levels by 1 year of age. Intracranial hypertension is usually not a problem in neonates and infants, owing to the open sutures and fontanels. The exception would be those infants born with craniosynostosis and severe hydrocephalus. The posterior and coronal fontanels close by 3 months of age, and the anterior fontanel by 18 months. The sagittal, coronal, and lambdoidal sutures usually close by 1 year.

Hydrocephalus

Hydrocephalus refers to a group of conditions characterized by enlarged ventricles usually secondary to blockage of normal CSF circulation or failure of normal CSF reabsorption. ICP is normal or elevated depending on the pathology involved. Hydrocephalus is categorized as communicating or noncommunicating. In the former, obstruction is distal to the fourth ventricle outlets, at the arachnoid villi, or within the arachnoid surface over the brain. Communicating hydrocephalus may be caused by adhesion, obstruction of basilar or surface subarachnoid spaces from hemorrhage, infection meningitis, development failure of arachnoid villi, or overproduction of CSF from choroid plexus papilloma. Noncommunicating hydrocephalus is an intraventricular obstruction, usually where the pathways are narrow. Noncommunicating hydrocephalus may be caused by aqueductal maldevelopment or stenosis between the third and fourth ventricles, atresia, mass lesion obstruction, hemorrhage, infection, arachnoiditis, or Dandy–Walker syndrome. Management involves removal of the cause, although this is not always possible. CSF shunting, ventriculoatrial, or, more commonly and with less hazard, ventriculoperitoneal shunt is the mainstay of therapy. General anesthesia is usually required for insertion of these shunts.

Other Congenital Defects

Various birth defects involving the central nervous system may bring the neonate to the operating room within the first hours or days of life. Systemic complications are often associated with the neurologic defect. Cerebrovascular defects such as vein of Galen aneurysms may present with congestive heart failure, high-output failure, and cranial bruits. Spina bifida is a developmental defect of the vertebrae in which the canal fails to close normally. The defect may be limited to bony malformation (spina bifida occulta) or may include herniation of the meninges (meningocele) and nerve roots and spinal cord (myelomeningocele). Neurologic and systemic symptoms are associated with the spinal cord level involved. Meningitis is always a threat with meningocele and myelomeningocele. These same defects may occur over the cranium. Cranium bifidum is a defect of fusion of the cranial bone. Meningocele and encephalocele, which is a protrusion of meninges and brain tissue, may accompany cranium bifidum. Meningocele, myelomeningocele, and encephalocele usually require excision of the sac and its contents, with dural closure very early in life. If large amounts of nervous tissue are present in the sac, normal developmental prognosis is usually poor. Hydrocephalus commonly occurs with many of these conditions or follows surgical closure of the sac. Tumors tend to occur more frequently in older children and have a tendency to present in the posterior fossa.

Craniosynostosis. Craniosynostosis involves premature closure of the sutures with malformation of the skull and may produce secondary effects on the brain and eyes. This defect may be present at birth or may not be evident until the child is a few months old. Correction of craniosynostosis is usually performed during the first few months of life. If there are no other central nervous system defects, outcome is usually good, with no retardation or neurologic deficit. On occasion, correction of craniosynostosis is purely for cosmetic reasons. A major anesthetic concern during correction of this defect is the large blood loss that occurs because of the removal of a large amount of cranial bone. Blood loss is carefully measured and replaced as lost, from the beginning of the case.

Arnold–Chiari Malformation. Arnold–Chiari malformation is a congenital defect involving projection of the medulla and cerebellum through the foramen magnum and into the cervical spinal canal. It is thought to develop during fetal life, with fixation of the lower spinal cord or nerve roots exerting a downward pull on the upper cervical cord and brainstem. It may be associated with spina bifida, hydrocephalus, and other defects of bone, meninges, and nervous tissue. Treatment during infancy, childhood, or early adulthood involves decompression of the posterior fossa and, on occasion, correction of hydrocephalus. In older children and adults, pheochromocytoma occasionally coincides with Arnold–Chiari malformation and must be ruled out before surgery is scheduled.

Platybasia. Platybasia is a deformity of the occipital bone and upper cervical spine. Compression of the medulla and obstruction of the subarachnoid space and hydrocephalus occur. Treatment involves decompression of the foramen magnum, freeing of adhesions, and possible amputation of cerebellar tonsils.

Anesthetic Considerations

Anesthetic management is based on the child's age, weight, clinical status, and surgical lesion. All indications for drug selection and monitoring for adults apply to children as well. Perhaps the most difficult and controversial aspect of anesthesia involves the technique of induction. Although an inhalational induction may appear outwardly smooth, the effects of inhalation agents on ICP can be just as detrimental in children as they are in adults. In a well-sedated child, it may be possible to start an intravenous route without problem and proceed with a balanced narcotic anesthetic. Rectal thiopental or intranasal midazolam may offer a safe alternative to preoperative sedation in the child in whom intracranial compliance may be compromised. Thiopental 25 to 30 mg/kg, either solution or suppository, may be given rectally in the operating suite to sedate the child; then an intravenous line may be started. Preoperative colon evacuation may minimize the problem of unpredictable absorption of the drug. Midazolam 0.5 to 0.7 mg/kg may be given intranasally or orally. Pancuronium bromide should be used with caution in the sick premature child. The combination of increased heart rate and increased MAP from light anesthesia may stress the delicate intracranial vessels and cause hemorrhage. Vecuronium may be a safer alternative for muscle relaxation. Temperature control is particularly important in neonates and infants. Hypothalamic temperature regulation does not mature until about 6 months of age.

CONCLUSION

Perioperative anesthetic management significantly affects the prognosis of the patient undergoing a neurosurgical procedure. Recent advances in neuroanesthesia have contributed significantly to the greater safety and success of neurosurgical procedures. Improved understanding of the intracranial effects of pharmacologic and mechanical interventions during anesthesia and intensive care have diminished secondary traumatic and operative injury by providing means for enhancement of cerebral perfusion and reduction of cerebral edema. Increasingly sophisticated technological developments in the practice of neurosurgery have been fostered by parallel progress in the technology of monitoring, neuroradiology, and the surgical microscope. It is these technical and conceptual refinements that have enabled neurosurgeons and neuroanesthetists to undertake more intricate operations and achieve decreased mortality and improved outcomes.

The author thanks Dr. Gary Duckweiler, Assistant Professor, Endovascular Therapy/Neuroradiology, UCLA School of Medicine; Dr. Scott Foster, Associate Professor of Clinical Anesthesiology, UCLA School of Medicine; Dr. Eduardo Rubenstein, Professor of Anesthesiology, UCLA School of Medicine; and Ellen Jackson, SUNY Downstate Medical Center, for their very generous gifts of time and knowledge.

BIBLIOGRAPHY

Physiology and Pharmacology

Adams RW, Gronert GA, et al. Halothane, hypocapnia, and cerebrospinal fluid pressure in neurosurgery. *Anesthesiology.* 1972;37:510–517.

Alexander SC, Lassen NA. Cerebral circulatory response to acute brain disease. Implications from anesthetic practice. *Anesthesiology.* 1970;32:60.

Artru AA. Effects of anesthetics. II. Reduction of cerebrospinal fluid pressure by hypocapnia: Changes in cerebral blood volume, cerebrospinal fluid volume and brain tissue water and electrolytes. *J Cerebral Blood Flow Metab.* 1988;8(5):750–756.

Basta SA, Savarese JJ. Comparative histamine-releasing properties of vecuronium, atracurium, tubocurarine, and metocurine. Clinical experience with Norcuron. *Excerpta Med Curr Clin Pract Ser.* 1983;11:183–184.

Bedfore RF, Pesing JA, et al. Lidocaine or thiopental for rapid control of intracranial hypertension. *Anesth Analg.* 1980;59:435–437.

Brown EM, Krishnaprasas D, Smiler BG. Pancuronium for rapid induction technique for tracheal intubation. *Can Anaesth Soc J.* 1979;26:489.

Cottrell JE, Casthely P, Brodie JD, et al. Prevention of nitroprusside-induced cyanide toxicity with hydroxocobalamin. *N Engl J Med.* 1978;298:809–811.

Cottrell JE, Giffin JP, Hartung J, et al. Intracranial pressure during nifedipine-induced hypotension in cats. *Anesth Analg.* 1983; 62:245.

Cottrell JE, Giffin JP, Lim K, Milhorat T, Stein S, Shwiry B. Intracranial pressure, mean arterial pressure, and heart rate following midazolam or thiopental in humans with intracranial masses. In: *ABA abstracts, 1982 annual meeting.*

Cottrell JE, Hartung J, Givvin JP, et al. Intracranial and hemodynamic changes after succinylcholine administration in cats. *Anesth Analg.* 1983;62:1006–1009.

Cottrell JE, Patel K, et al. Nitroprusside tachyphylaxis without acidosis. *Anesthesiology.* 1978;49:141–142.

Cottrell JE, Robustelli A, et al. Furosemide- and mannitol-induced changes in intracranial pressure and serum osmolality and electrolytes. *Anesthesiology.* 1977;47:28–30.

Cottrell JE, Turndorf H. Intravenous nitroglycerin. *Am Heart J.* 1978;96:550–553.

Donegan M, Bedfore FR, Dacey R. IV lidocaine for prevention of intracranial hypertension. *Anesthesiology.* 1979;51:S201.

Fitch W, Barker J, et al. The influence of neuroleptanalgesic drugs on cerebrospinal fluid pressure. *Br J Anaesth.* 1969;41:800–806.

Fitch W, McDowall DG. Effect of halothane on intracranial pressure gradients in the presence of space-occupying lesions. *Br J Anaesth.* 1971;43:904–911.

Forster A, Van Horn K, et al. Influence of anesthetic agents on blood–brain barrier function during acute hypertension. *Acta Neurol Scand [Suppl].* 1977;64:60–63.

From RP, Warner DS, Todd MM, Sokoll MD. Anesthesia for craniotomy: A double-blind comparison of alfentanil, fentanyl and sufentanil. *Anesthesiology.* 1990;73:896–904.

Gagnon RL, Marsh ML, et al. Intracranial hypertension caused by nitroglycerin. *Anesthesiology.* 1979;51:86.

Giffin JP, Hartung J, et al. Effect of vecuronium on intracranial pressure, mean arterial pressure, and heart rate in cats. *Br J Anaesth.* 1986;58:441–443.

Gordon E, et al. The effects of isoflurane on cerebrospinal fluid pressure in patients undergoing neurosurgery. *Acta Anesth Scand.* 1988;32:108–112.

Harp JR, Wollman H. Cerebral metabolic effects of hyperventilation and deliberate hypotension. *Br J Anaesth.* 1973;45:256.

Hartung J, Cottrell JE. Nitrous oxide reduced thiopental-induced prolongation of survival in hypoxic and anoxic mice. *Anesth Analg.* 1987;66:47–52.

Henriksen HT, Horgensen PB. The effect of nitrous oxide on intracranial pressure in patients with intracranial disorders. *Br J Anaesth.* 1973;45:486.

Herregods L, Verbeke J, Rolly G, Colardyn F. Effect of propofol in elevated ICP. Pulmonary results. *Anesthesia.* 1988;43(suppl):107–109.

Hochwald G. Cerebrospinal fluid mechanisms. In: Cottrell JE, Turndorf H, eds. *Anesthesia and neurosurgery.* St. Louis, MO: CV Mosby; 1980:37–53.

Javid M, Gilboe D, Cesario T. The rebound phenomenon and hypertonic solutions. *J Neurosurg.* 1964;21:1059–1066.

Kelly PJ, Gorten RJ, et al. Cerebral perfusion, vascular spasm, and outcome in patients with ruptured intracranial aneurysms. *J Neurosurg.* 1977;47:44–49.

Lall NG, Jain AP. Circulatory and respiratory disturbances during posterior fossa surgery. *Br J Anaesth.* 1969;41:447–449.

Lassen NA. Cerebral blood flow and oxygen consumption in man. *Physiol Rev.* 1959;39:183–235.

Lewelt W, Moszynski K, Kozniewska H. Effects of depolarizing, nondepolarizing muscle relaxants and intubation on the ventricular field pressure. In: Beks JW, Bosch DA, Brock M, eds. *Intracranial pressure.* New York: Springer-Verlag; 1976:215–218.

Lundburg N, et al. Non-operative management of intracranial hypertension. In: Kerayenbuhl H, ed. *Advances and technical standard in neurosurgery.* New York: Springer-Verlag; 1974;1:1–59.

MacCarthy E, Bloomfield SS. Labetalol: A review of its pharmacology, pharmacokinetics, clinical uses and adverse effects. *Pharmacotherapy.* 1983;3:193–219.

Marsh ML, Dunlap BJ, et al. Succinylcholine—Intracranial pressure effects in neurosurgical patients. *Anesth Analg.* 1980;59:550–551. Abstract.

McDowal DG. The effects of clinical concentrations of halothane on the blood flow and oxygen uptake of the cerebral cortex. *Br J Anaesth.* 1967;39:186–196.

McKay RD, Sundt TM, Michenfelder JD, et al. Internal carotid artery stump pressure and cerebral blood flow during carotid endarterectomy: Modifications by halothane, enflurane, and Innovar. *Anesthesiology.* 1976;45:390–399.

McQueen JD, Jeanes LD. Dehydration and rehydration of the brain with hypertonic urea and mannitol. *J Neurosurg.* 1964;21:118–128.

Michenfelder JD, Theye RA. Effects of fentanyl, droperidol, and Innovar on canine cerebral metabolism and blood flow. *Br J Anaesth.* 1971;43:630–636.

Miller RD, Tausk HC. Prolonged anesthesia associated with hypotension induced by trimethaphan (Arfonad). *Anesthesiol Rev.* 1974;1:36–37.

Misfeldt BB, Jorgensen PB, Rishos M. The effect of nitrous oxide and halothane upon the intracranial pressure in hypocapnic patients with intracranial disorders. *Br J Anaesth.* 1974;46:853–858.

Munson ES, Merrick HC. Effects of nitrous oxide on venous air embolism. *Anesthesiology.* 1966;27:783–787.

Murphy FL Jr, Kennell EM, et al. The effects of enflurane, isoflurane, and halothane on cerebral blood flow and metabolism in man. In: *Abstracts of scientific papers, annual meeting of American Society of Anesthesiologists.* 1974:61–62.

Newman B, Gelb AW, Lam AM. The effect of isoflurane-induced hypotension on cerebral blood flow and cerebral metabolic rate of oxygen in humans. *Anesthesiology.* 1986;64(3):307–310.

Pierce EC Jr, Lambertsen CJ, Deutsch S, et al. Cerebral circulation and metabolism during thiopental anesthesia and hyperventilation in man. *J Clin Invest.* 1962;41:1664–1671.

Ravussin P, Gunard JP, Ralley F, et al. Effect of propofol on cerebrospinal fluid pressure and cerebral perfusion pressure in patients undergoing craniotomy. *Anesthesia.* 1988;43(suppl):37–41.

Rottenberg DA, Posner JB. Intracranial pressure control. In: Cottrell JE, Turndorf H, eds. *Anesthesia and neurosurgery.* St. Louis, MO: CV Mosby; 1980:89–113.

Schettini A, Furniss WM. Brain wave and electrolyte distribution during the inhalation of halothane. *Br J Anaesth.* 1979;51:1117.

Shapiro HM, Wyte SR, Harris AB. Ketamine anesthesia in patients with intracranial pathology. *Br J Anaesth.* 1972;44:1200.

Shapiro HM, Wyte SR, et al. Acute intraoperative intracranial hypertension in neurosurgical patients: Mechanical and pharmacologic factors. *Anesthesiology.* 1972;37:399–405.

Shapiro HM, Yoachim J, Marshall LF. Nitrous oxide challenge for detection of residual intravascular pulmonary gas following venous air embolism. *Anesth Analg.* 1982;61:304.

Siesjo BK, Norberg K, et al. Hypoxia and cerebral metabolism. In: Gordon E, ed. *A basis and practice of neuroanesthesia: Monographs in anesthesiology.* New York: Elsevier; 1975;2:47–83.

Smith AL, Marque JJ. Anesthetics and cerebral edema. *Anesthesiology.* 1970;45:64–72.

Steffey EP, Gauger GE, Eger EI II. Cardiovascular effects of venous air embolism during air and oxygen-breathing. *Anesth Analg.* 1974;53:599–604.

Stoyka WW, Schutz H. The cerebral response to sodium nitroprusside and trimethaphan controlled hypotension. *Can Anaesth Soc J.* 1975;22:275–283.

Strandgaard S, Oleson J, Skinhoh E, et al. Autoregulation of brain circulation in severe arterial hypertension. *Br Med J.* 1973;1:507–510.

Vandesteen A, Tremport V, Engleman E, et al. Effect of propofol on CBF and metabolism in man. *Anesthesia.* 1988;43(suppl):42–43.

Weir DL, Goodchild CS, Graham DJ. Propofol: Effects on indices of cerebral ischemia. *J Neurosurg Anesth.* 1989;1(3):284–290.

Therapeutic and Diagnostic Neuroradiology

Duckweiler G. Detailed personal communication on therapeutic neuroradiology. Los Angeles: Endovascular Therapy/Neuroradiology, UCLA School of Medicine; January/February 1991.

Saidman LJ, Eger EL II. Change in cerebrospinal fluid pressure during pneumoencephalography under nitrous oxide anesthesia. *Anesthesiology.* 1965;26:67–71.

Anethestic Techniques

Albin MS, Babinski M, et al. Anesthetic management of posterior fossa surgery in the sitting position. *Acta Anaesthesiol Scand.* 1976;20:117–128.

Dahlgren BE, Gordon E, Steiner L. Evaluation of controlled hypotension during surgery for intracranial arterial aneurysms. In: *Progress in anesthesiology.* New York: Excerpta Medica; 1970:1232.

Fitch W. Anaesthesia for carotid artery surgery. *Br J Anaesth.* 1976;48:791–796.

Fitch W, McDowal DG. Hazards of anesthesia in patients with intracranial space-occupying lesions. *Int Anesthesiol Clin.* 1969;7:639–662.

Lassen NA, Tweed WA. A basis and practice of neuroanesthesia. In: Gordon E, ed. *Monographs in anesthesiology.* New York: Elsevier; 1975;2:113–133.

McDowell DG. The influence of anesthetic drugs and techniques on intracranial pressure. In: Gordon E, ed. *A basic practice of neuroanesthesia.* New York: Excerpta Medica; 1975;2:135–170.

Rich NW, Hobson RW. Carotid endarterectomy under regional anaesthesia. *Am Surg.* 1975;41:253–259.

Samuels SL. Anesthesia for supratentorial tumor. In: Cottrell JE, Turndorf H, eds. *Anesthesia and neurosurgery.* St. Louis, MO: CV Mosby; 1980:150–167.

Shapiro HM. Intracranial hypertension: Therapeutic and anesthetic considerations. *Anesthesiology.* 1975;43:445–471.

Shwiry B, Josephs S, Sullivan CA, Gotta AW. A method of intubation for cervical spine injured patients. *AANA J.* 1983;51:403–405.

Monitoring and Equipment

Albin MS. Resuscitation of the spinal cord. *Crit Care Med.* 1978;6:170.

Bunegin L, Albin MS, et al. Positioning the right atrial catheter: A model for reappraisal. *Anesthesiology.* 1981;55:343–348.

Cottrell JE, Van Aken H, Gupta B, Turndorf H. Induced hypotension. In: Cottrell JE, Turndorf H, eds. *Anesthesia and neurosurgery.* 2nd ed. St. Louis, MO: CV Mosby; 1986:421.

Furuya H, Suzuki T, et al. Detection of air embolism by transesophageal echocardiography. *Anesthesiology.* 1983;58:124.

Grundy BL. Electrophysiologic monitoring: Electroencephalography and evoked potentials. In: Newfield P, Cottrell JE, eds. *Handbook of neuroanesthesia: Clinical and physiologic essentials.* Boston: Little, Brown; 1983:28–59.

Jones TH, Chiappa KH, et al. EEG monitoring for induced hypotension for surgery of intracranial aneurysms. *Stroke.* 1979;10:292.

Lundberg N. Monitoring of the intracranial pressure. In: Critchley M, O'Leary JL, Jeannett B, eds. *Scientific foundations of neurology.* Philadelphia: FA Davis; 1972:356–371.

Maroon JC, Goodman JM, et al. Detection of minute venous air emboli with ultrasound. *Surg Gynecol Obstet.* 1964;127:1236–1238.

Marshall WK, Bedford RF. Use of a pulmonary artery catheter for detection and treatment of venous air embolism. *Anesthesiology.* 1980;52:131.

Munson ES, Paul WL, et al. Early detection of venous air embolism using a Swan-Ganz catheter. *Anesthesiology.* 1975;42:223–226.

Neigh JL, Garman JK, Harp JR. The electroencephalographic pattern during anesthesia with ethrane: Effects of depth of anesthesia, Pa_{CO_2}, and nitrous oxide. *Anesthesiology.* 1971;35:482–487.

Rae EC. Anesthesia machine for use during magnetic resonance imaging. *Anesthesiology.* 1990;73:1054–1055.

Anesthesia for Thoracic Surgery

Cathy Mastropietro

The anesthetic management of the patient undergoing thoracic surgery can be very complex. Often, isolation of one lung is required which presents particular challenges to the anesthetist in maintaining adequate ventilation and perfusion. Pulmonary anatomy, physiology, and pathophysiology are discussed in relation to preoperative evaluation and intraoperative management. Anesthetic techniques for a number of thoracic surgical procedures with particular emphasis on one lung anesthesia are presented in this chapter.

PULMONARY CIRCULATION AND PHYSIOLOGY

Pulmonary Circulation

The pulmonary circulation is unique in that it has a double arterial supply from the pulmonary arteries and the bronchial arteries. The circulation begins at the right and left pulmonary arteries, which transfer mixed venous blood from the right side of the heart to the pulmonary capillaries for gas exchange. The arteries, veins, and bronchi initially run close together. Toward the periphery of the lung, the veins move away to pass between the lobules, whereas the arteries and bronchi travel down the centers of the lobules to the terminal bronchioles.[1] At this point they branch into capillaries that form a dense network in the walls of the alveoli (Fig. 40–1). The capillaries are just wide enough to accommodate a red blood cell and form a continuous sheet of blood in the alveolar wall.[1]

The pulmonary artery receives the entire output of the right side of the heart; however, the resistance in this system is low. Each red cell spends approximately 1 second in the capillary network crossing two to three alveoli. The anatomy for gas exchange is so efficient that this short second allows for complete equilibrium between oxygen and carbon dioxide, between alveolar gas and capillary blood.[1] In addition to the circulation provided by the pulmonary arteries, the bronchial arteries carry arterial blood from the conducting airways to the terminal bronchioles. The right

lung has one bronchial artery, whereas the left usually has two.

The oxygenated blood is carried from the pulmonary capillary bed by small pulmonary veins, which emerge as four large veins to drain into the left atrium. The azygos and hemiazygos veins may absorb some of the venous drainage from the bronchi. The flow through the bronchial circulation is a small fraction of that which flows through the pulmonary circulation, and the lung can function fairly well without it, as is seen with lung transplantation.[2]

Pulmonary Physiology

Pressures in the pulmonary circulation are very low. The mean pressure in the main pulmonary artery is only about 15 mm Hg; the systolic and diastolic pressures are about 25 and 8 mm Hg, respectively, implying a pulsatile flow.[1] The systemic pressures, on the other hand, are much higher (mean aortic pressure 100 mm Hg) to direct the flow of blood to various organs. The pulmonary circuit is not concerned with the distribution of blood from one area to another and requires pressures sufficient only to provide adequate gas exchange. In other words, even though the lung accepts the entire cardiac output, the work of the right side of the heart is minimized because the only blood that it directs is that supplying the lung itself.

Unique to the pulmonary circulation is the fact that the capillaries are surrounded by gas and easily collapse or expand, depending on the pressures in and around them. The pressures within the capillaries are very close to alveolar pressures but can succumb to rises in alveolar pressures and collapse.[3] The pressure difference between the inside and outside of the vessels is called the transmural pressure.[1]

The pressure around the pulmonary arteries and veins is less than alveolar pressure; therefore, the pulmonary arteries are capable of increasing their diameter as the lung expands. The capillaries and blood vessels (alveolar and extraalveolar) differ markedly in terms of their ability to change caliber. Alveolar vessels include capillaries, arterioles, and venules; their calibers depend on the alveolar pressure and the pressures within them. Extraalveolar ves-

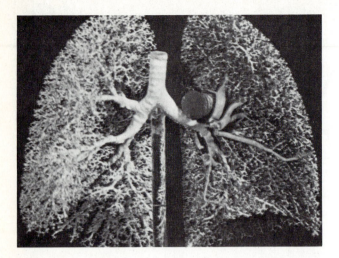

Figure 40–1. The pulmonary circulation. (*Reprinted, with permission, from Shields TW.* General thoracic surgery. *Philadelphia: Lea & Febiger; 1972.*)

sels, arteries and veins, run through the lung parenchyma; their caliber is dependent on lung volumes.[1]

The amount of vascular resistance that occurs in the pulmonary circulation is one-tenth that of the systemic system and measures 1.7 mm Hg/L per minute or approximately 100 dyn. Vascular resistance is defined as (input pressure – output) divided by pressure blood flow. The pulmonary vascular resistance is low, once again, because of the small area to which blood is distributed compared with the systemic circulation. Even though this resistance is small, it has the capability of becoming smaller as the pressure within the pulmonary circulation rises. According to

West,[1] this fall in pulmonary resistance is produced by two mechanisms: (1) recruitment and (2) distension.

Increasing pressure within the pulmonary vessels begins the flow of blood through capillaries that are closed or have no blood flow. With increased blood flow, the overall resistance is decreased; this is known as recruitment. Distension occurs when pressure rises, the caliber of the vessels increases, and resistance is lowered.[1] Large lung volumes lower vascular resistance, whereas low lung volumes reduce caliber and increase vascular resistance. Distensibility is influenced strongly by the presence of smooth muscle in the vascular walls and anything that influences contraction of smooth muscle increases pulmonary resistance. Drugs such as serotonin, histamine, and norepinephrine vasoconstrict the vascular walls when lung volumes are low. Relaxation of bronchial smooth muscle is seen with acetylcholine and isoproterenol.[3,4]

Distribution of Blood and Ventilation

The distribution of blood flow in the lung is unequal. This distribution varies with position and is highly influenced by gravity.[5] West divides perfusion to the lungs into three zones (Fig. 40–2).[5] Zone 1 encompasses the apex of the lung where no flow exists; zone 2 is the middle portion of lung with increased flow; and zone 3 is the base of the lung, which has maximum flow. Distribution of ventilation is also dependent on gravity. Blood flow per unit volume decreases rapidly up the lung, but the change in ventilation is not nearly so marked.[5] Change of posture from the erect to the supine position abolishes this uneven distribution.

The areas of the lung being ventilated need not necessarily be perfused and vice versa. This inequality of ventilation to perfusion can be expressed as the $\dot{V}/\dot{Q}$ the ventilation–perfusion ratio. The normal value is 0.85 derived from 5 L/min total ventilation and 6 L/min total blood flow. This

Figure 40–2. Model explaining the uneven distribution of blood flow in the lung based on the pressures affecting the capillaries. (*Reprinted, with permission, from West JB, Dollery CT, et al.* J Appl Physiol. *1964;19:713.*)

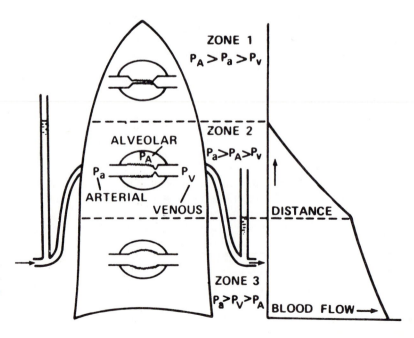

ratio describes the degree of overperfusion or underventilation and determines the gas exchange in any lung unit.[5]

Hypoxic Pulmonary Vasoconstriction

Hypoxic pulmonary vasoconstriction (HPV) is a local compensatory mechanism peculiar to the lungs whereby contraction of the smooth muscle of the arterioles occurs in the presence of a decline in Po_2. HPV is due either to a direct action of alveolar hypoxia on the pulmonary vasculature or to an alveolar hypoxia-induced release of vasoactive substance.[6] This diversion of blood flow enhances gas exchange by bypassing unoxygenated regions and adjusting regional ventilation–perfusion ratios. Hypoxic ventilation or atelectasis of one lung or one lobe generally causes a 30 to 40 percent or 50 to 60 percent diversion of blood from the hypoxic to the nonhypoxic lung.[7] This is vital in minimizing the transpulmonary shunt during disease of one lung, one-lung anesthesia, or inadvertent intubation of a mainstem bronchus.[3,8] HPV is inhibited by several factors. Certain inhalation agents, such as nitrous oxide, halothane, methoxyflurane, enflurane, and isoflurane, inhibit HPV.[9] All systemic vasodilatory drugs probably inhibit HPV.[10] Large hypoxic compartments[11] and decreases in Pco_2 below 30 mm Hg[12] inhibit HPV. Infections, hypothermia, and clinical conditions that increase pulmonary vascular pressure such as mitral stenosis, volume overload, vasopressors, and ligation of pulmonary vessels all inhibit HPV.[7,11,13]

PREOPERATIVE EVALUATION

The primary purpose of the preoperative evaluation and preparation of the patient is to avoid or at least lessen the incidence of postoperative complications. There is a strong correlation between preoperative respiratory dysfunction and postoperative complications.

Of all thoracotomies performed, 40 to 60 percent are associated with respiratory complications and overall mortality can be as high as 15 percent.[3] The risk factors associated with thoracic surgery are age, obesity, and underlying heart and lung disease. The severity of lung disease must be determined to provide some clues as to the likelihood of development of complications. The assessment of respiratory function should begin with a thorough medical history and physical examination. A tobacco history is one of the most important predictors of postoperative pulmonary difficulty.[13] This can be determined by calculating the number of pack-years. A pack-year is determined by multiplying the number of packs smoked per day by the number of years smoked.[14] Any increase in pack-years will obviously increase the risk for chronic lung disease as well as malignancy. Smoking should be stopped as early as possible before surgery to reduce small-airway abnormalities. A significantly noticeable improvement in small-airway function, sputum production, and mucociliary transport is usually evident after 6 to 14 weeks of smoking cessation.[15] Cessation for 48 hours has been shown to decrease carboxyhemoglobin levels.[16]

The electrocardiogram (ECG) not only detects rhythm disturbances but also can show chronic obstructive pulmonary disease by demonstrating clockwise rotation, right-

axis deviation, or right ventricular hypertrophy. The anteroposterior diameter of the chest is usually increased on roentgenogram and fibrotic changes or increased vascular markings are common. Tracheal deviation or obstruction, detected by chest radiograph, provides information about potential difficulty with intubation. Potential ventilatory problems can exist with pleural effusions, pulmonary edema, or lung consolidation. Spread of infection must be a concern in the presence of an abscess or infected bullous cyst. The chest radiograph may not be diagnostic as it can be normal even in the severely obstructed patient. As many as 10 percent of patients with chronic diffuse infiltrative lung disease may have normal chest roentgenograms.[17] The cardiac status of the patient must also be evaluated. Chronic medications should be reviewed and either continued or withheld depending on the stability of the disease process. Patients with preexisting infections should be treated with antibiotic or antimicrobial therapy. Elective surgery should be delayed until the infection is adequately treated. Overt respiratory failure associated with body water imbalance should be corrected by the use of diuretic therapy. Conversely, dehydration, which results in interstitial or intracellular water loss, needs to be corrected by enteral or parenteral fluid therapy because dehydration may compromise the efficiency of the mucociliary host defense system.

Patients with esophageal obstructive tumors may demonstrate abnormalities in serum potassium, calcium, or chloride values as a result of excessive vomiting. Elective surgical procedures should be postponed until these values are corrected to normal limits, which may take approximately 12 to 48 hours after treatment.

Obesity, especially morbid obesity, is a problem that cannot be corrected easily or rapidly. Rapid sudden weight loss may compromise respiratory function by reducing vital capacity. Normally, the obese patient suffers from chronic hypoxemia resulting from a lowered functional residual capacity (FRC).[18] Anesthesia further compounds hypoxemia by decreasing FRC by as much as 10 to 25 percent.[19]

The degree of pulmonary disease can be ascertained by the use of pulmonary function studies. Routine spirometry, particularly forced expiratory volume in 1 second (FEV_1) and lung volumes with residual volume/total lung capacity (RV/TLC), is a sensitive indicator of the likelihood of perioperative difficulty. Patients with an FEV_1 below 2 L or a RV/TLC greater than 40 percent should stop smoking, receive bronchodilator therapy for at least 48 to 72 hours, and then be retested.[3]

Chronic Lung Disease

Chronic lung disease can be determined by the presence of chronic productive cough, dyspnea, wheezing, or asthmalike attacks. Chronic respiratory insufficiency results in an inability to maintain adequate Pao_2 and $Paco_2$ at normal activity and may be either nonrespiratory or respiratory in origin. Nonrespiratory causes include (1) central nervous system disorders caused by drugs, infection, and trauma; (2) peripheral nervous system diseases such as polio or Guillain–Barré syndrome; (3) myopathies, which include myasthenia gravis and multiple sclerosis; or (4) chest wall abnormalities from obesity, surgery, or scoliosis.[2] Respiratory causes include (1) upper airway obstruction, (2) chronic bronchitis, (3) parenchymal diseases such as emphysema, (4) vascular problems such as congestive heart failure and pulmonary embolism, and (5) chronic pleural inflammation.[2] Of these, emphysema and chronic bronchitis are the most common causes of chronic respiratory insufficiency.

Emphysema. Emphysema is an irreversible condition characterized by abnormal enlargement of air spaces distal to the terminal bronchioles; it is also associated with destructive changes of the interalveolar septal walls. Destruction of the connective tissue responsible for much of the elastic recoil of the lung results in large alveolar sacs with little elastic recoil.[20] A resultant increase in residual volume with small-airway changes leads to increased airway resistance.[20] Many types of emphysema are classified according to the area of the acinus involved. Centrilobular emphysema involves the respiratory bronchioles in the proximal portions of the acinus and is usually found only in smokers. Other classifications include paraseptal, panlobular, and irregular emphysema.

Asthma. Asthma is usually a reversible respiratory condition characterized by an acute episodic respiration from bronchial smooth muscle constriction, mucosal edema, and accumulation of bronchial secretions.[2] The pathophysiology is a result of a lack of adenylcyclase from the cell membrane, leading to a reduction in the formation of 3′,5′-cyclic adenosine monophosphate from adenosine triphosphate. A beta blockade occurs, with resultant hyperirritability of the bronchial tree.[2]

Chronic Bronchitis. Chronic bronchitis is characterized by a chronic increase in mucous secretions of the tracheobronchial tree. Edema and ciliary dysfunction also occur. The underlying pathology is associated with smoke and air pollution, infection, and allergies.

The physiologic effects of chronic obstructive pulmonary disease (COPD) are many. They include metabolic alkalosis, pulmonary hypertension, polycythemia, and hepatic congestion. Chest roentgenogram reveals fiberoptic changes, increased anteroposterior diameter, and increased vascular markings. ECG may show right-axis deviation and right ventricular hypertrophy. The effects on ventilation are due to a gaseous alveolar distension and are as follows: increased FRC, decreased expiratory reserve volume (ERV), decreased inspiratory reserve volume (IRV), and decreased vital capacity (VC). Alveolar dead space is increased, resulting in an increased carbon dioxide retention and a decreased PaO_2.[2,20] Carbon dioxide levels above 70 mm Hg inactivate the respiratory center's response to $PaCO_2$, and respiration becomes hypoxic drive dependent.

The metabolic effects associated with COPD are the result of hypercarbia and hypoxia. Compensatory metabolic alkalosis is most frequently seen. The increased carbon dioxide retention increases chloride excretion and bicarbonate reabsorption by the kidneys. The circulatory changes include pulmonary hypertension and right-sided heart failure or cor pulmonale. Pulmonary hypertension develops because of an increasing constriction of the pulmonary arterioles and a reduction in pulmonary capillary bed size.[2,7] The

physical signs of right ventricular failure and pulmonary hypertension include right ventricular heave, palpable pulmonary artery pulsation, accentuated pulmonary component of the second heart sound, peripheral edema, hepatomegaly, jugular vein distension, and hepatojugular reflex.[21] Wide fluctuations in stroke volume and blood pressure may occur during the respiratory cycle as a result of forced expirations.[2]

Polycythemia develops from chronic hypoxia. If the hematocrit reaches above 55 percent, the tendency to develop thrombosis within the pulmonary arterial tree increases. Leukocytosis may indicate active infection. Congestive heart failure may cause elevations of blood urea nitrogen and serum creatinine and accompanying hepatic congestion may cause abnormal liver function tests.[21]

Bronchodilator Therapy

The tracheobronchial tree is supplied by both sympathetic and parasympathetic nerves. If the sympathetic nerves are stimulated, bronchial relaxation occurs, whereas the opposite effect, bronchoconstriction, is evidenced with parasympathetic stimulation. The sympathetic nervous system is believed to accomplish bronchodilation by releasing epinephrine at the receptor site, stimulating beta-2 receptors and causing relaxation of bronchial muscle (Fig. 40–3). On the other hand, alpha receptors mediate vasoconstriction and may be involved in bronchoconstriction (Fig. 40–4). Pharmacologic manipulation of bronchial smooth muscle

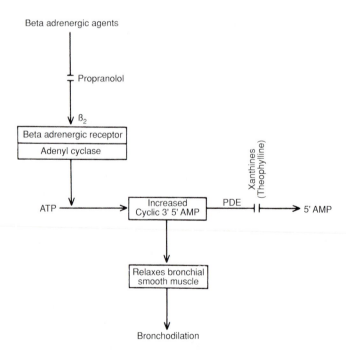

Figure 40–3. Beta-adrenergic pathways through which cyclic AMP is increased in the bronchial smooth muscle cell, leading to bronchodilation. AMP, adenosine monophosphate; ATP, adenosine 5′-triphosphate; PDE, phosphodiesterase. (*Reprinted, with permission, from Webb-Johnson DC, Andrews JL Jr. Drug therapy: Bronchodilator therapy. N Engl J Med. 1977; 297(9):476–482.*)

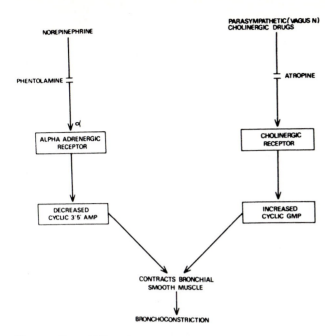

Figure 40–4. Alpha-adrenergic and cholinergic pathways through which cyclic AMP is decreased, or cyclic GMP is increased, in bronchial smooth muscle cell, thus causing bronchoconstriction. AMP, adenosine monophosphate; GMP, ganosine monophosphate. (*Reprinted, with permission, from Webb-Johnson DC, et al.* N Engl J Med. *1977;297:476–482.*)

TABLE 40–1. CLASSIFICATION OF BRONCHODILATORS

I. Bronchoactive autonomic drugs
  A. Sympathomimetics
    1. Catecholamines
      a. Epinephrine
      b. Isoproterenol
      c. Isoetharine
      d. Ephedrine (indirect acting)
    2. Resorcinols (not metabolized by catechol-O-methyl transferase [COMT]; beta-2 specificity)
      a. Terbutaline
      b. Metaproterenol
    3. Saligenin
      a. Salbutamol (beta-2 specificity)
    4. Others
      a. Protokylol Ventaire
      b. Ethyl norepinephrine (Bronkephine)
      c. Methoxyphenamine (Orthoxine)
  B. Parasympatholytic
    1. Anticholinergic
      a. Atropine
      b. Ipratroprium (SCH-1000)
II. Methylxanthines
  A. Phosphodiesterase inhibitors
    1. Theophylline ethylenediamine (aminophylline)
III. Antimediator drugs
  A. Glucocorticoids
    1. Hydrocortisone
    2. Methylprednisolone
    3. Declomethasone
    4. Triamcinolone
    5. Betamethasone
  B. Antihistamines
  C. Bischromes
    1. Cromolyn
IV. Prostaglandins

Reprinted, with permission, from Kaplan JA. Thoracic anesthesia. *New York: Churchill Livingstone; 1983.*

tone involves specific intervention at various points of the complex neurohumoral mechanism controlling muscle tone.[22]

The smooth muscle cells of the tracheobronchial tree contain an intracellular messenger nucleotide called 3′,5′-cyclic adenosine monophosphate (cAMP). Increased levels of this nucleotide catalyze a series of chemical events that result in relaxation of muscle fibers. Bronchodilating drugs cause an increase in cAMP levels, either by increased production or decreased breakdown.[22] In general, catecholamines increase the production of cAMP and other bronchodilators decrease the breakdown of cAMP.[21] Table 40–1 identifies bronchodilating agents by classification.

It is essential that appropriate bronchodilator therapy be instituted several days preoperatively to maximize pulmonary function, by promoting mobilization of secretions and a more effective cough.

Premedication

The preoperative use of anticholinergics remains controversial for management of patients with difficult airway or COPD. Some studies reveal complications such as laryngospasm and coughing associated with excessive secretions. Conversely, other investigators feel that the drying effects of anticholinergics increase complications by decreasing the transportability of bronchial mucus because of increased viscosity.[3] Generally speaking, the amount of secretion is thought to be increased in those who are obese and those who smoke.

Atropine dilates air passages, the larger ones more than the smaller, and reduces airway resistance. Atropine also improves airway conductance in COPD and in allergic states because there is intrinsic bronchoconstriction in these situations that is mediated by the parasympathetic nervous system.[23] Glycopyrrolate produces the same drying effects with less incidence of cardiac dysrhythmia, is twice as potent as atropine, and causes little central nervous system stimulation. Opiates in large doses can increase the incidence of postoperative respiratory depression and, therefore, are eliminated from the protocol for thoracic surgery. Benzodiazepines are useful premedicants. They produce mild depression of the respiratory system while providing relief of anxiety. Cardiovascular effects are minimal, and the amnesic effect is certainly advantageous.

ANESTHESIA TECHNIQUES

Airway Access

When there is a need to anesthetize a patient for a diagnostic thoracic procedure the anesthetist must determine whether or not the vocal cords can be visualized. This can be decided by using the standard techniques of airway evaluation such as Mallampati's classification, determination of mandibular depth and whether or not the normal physiologic airway (sniffing position) can be assumed.

If there is concern as to the degree of visualization of the vocal cords, fiberoptic bronchoscopy and intubation can be performed. To adequately perform the procedure the patient's airway must be adequately anesthetized with a topical spray (0.5 percent tetracaine with 1 : 200,000 epinephrine) through an atomizer.[24] In addition, bilateral superior laryngeal nerve blocks can be performed. An airway intubator is inserted. The bronchoscope is inserted into an endotracheal tube, then through the airway intubator, vocal cords, and into the trachea. Once the bronchoscope is in the trachea, the endotracheal tube is advanced and inserted in place. The intubator is removed, the tube secured, and general anesthesia administered. Oxygen should be insufflated through the suction port of the bronchoscope throughout the procedure.[24]

If a nasal fiberoptic intubation is performed the nose must be adequately anesthetized topically. A well-lubricated nasal endotracheal tube is advanced into the pharynx. The bronchoscope is advanced, and then the endotracheal tube is advanced to its proper position and general anesthesia is instituted.

A retrograde intubation technique can also be performed.[24] The airway is anesthetized as previously discussed. The technique involves puncturing the cricothyroid membrane with a needle. A long flexible wire is passed through the needle into the pharynx and out through the mouth. If visualization is impaired by blood or secretions, a central venous pressure or epidural catheter can be used. Air is injected to identify the tip of the catheter. The endotracheal tube is then passed over the guidewire into the trachea. The tube may need to be rotated 90 degrees to guide the tube to the trachea.

Tracheal jet ventilation is a method used to ventilate the patient who cannot be ventilated by mask or tube. A large intravenous catheter is inserted through the cricoid membrane. After the catheter enters the trachea, it is pointed cephalad at a 30-degree angle. As it is advanced the stylet is removed. No matter what jet system is attached to the hub of the catheter, it is important to remember that the oxygen source must be near 50 psi to be of benefit when using the catheter.[24] The only method by which jet-inspired air can be exhaled is via the natural airway and thus this airway must be maintained.[24]

Anesthetic Agents

Each of the inhalation anesthetics exerts its own specific effects on the respiratory system, and this raises concern for the patient undergoing thoracic surgery. The major parameters of an agent's influence on the respiratory centers are tidal volume (V_T), respiratory rate, minute volume, and effective alveolar ventilation.[25]

Nitrous Oxide.   Nitrous oxide (N_2O) in analgesic doses exerts little effect on the respiratory center. The tidal volume, respiratory rate, and minute volume are unaffected. Effective alveolar ventilation is decreased.

Because of its weak anesthetic properties, nitrous oxide must be supplemented with opiates and other anesthetic

agents so that perioperative awareness is avoided. Nitrous oxide is rapidly taken up by the alveoli. Oxygen administered with it will be concentrated (concentration effect) as the nitrous oxide enters the blood, leaving relatively more oxygen in the alveoli and raising the PaO_2, thereby improving oxygenation.[26]

On emergence from anesthesia the reverse is true. Nitrous oxide will rapidly dilute the oxygen left in the alveoli and, if patients are not properly oxygenated, diffusion hypoxia may be produced.[27] Nitrous oxide depresses the respiratory response to hypoxia and can aggravate the diffusion hypoxia syndrome.[3,28]

Nitrous oxide appears to produce little or no effect on bronchial musculature but does depress mucociliary flow in the trachea, which may increase airway resistance because of the accumulation of secretions.[3]

The untoward effect of nitrous oxide that causes the most concern is its ability to trap in gas-enclosed spaces. Nitrous oxide is thus contraindicated in procedures in which it can potentiate an increased volume such as pulmonary blebs, cysts, pneumothorax, and even hemothorax. Mediastinal shift results if the volume expansion is significant. After a pneumonectomy, the hemithorax contains free air. The possibility of mediastinal shift exists if a chest tube is not used or is dysfunctional.

Halothane.   Halothane rapidly obtunds laryngeal and pharyngeal reflexes. Secretory activity of the glands lining the respiratory tract is depressed, as is ciliary activity. Bronchial relaxation occurs, resulting in a reduction in airflow resistance and an increase in conductance, which is an advantage in those patients with increased bronchial tone such as asthmatics. Halothane decreases tidal volume in a dose-related fashion. Minute volume and effective alveolar ventilation are also decreased. Respiratory rate is increased, possibly because of sensitization of the stretch receptors in the lungs.[25]

A depression of the ventilatory response to hypoxemia occurs at concentrations as low as 0.1 minimum alveolar concentration (MAC) and, when it occurs in those patients who are hypoxic drive dependent, is a cause for concern postoperatively.[29] At concentrations of 1.0 to 1.5 percent, the apneic threshold rises and, as anesthetic depth increases, the $PaCO_2$ rises causing a release of catecholamines.[3,30]

It is believed that halothane depresses HPV resulting in a venous admixture.[31] This may be of clinical significance during one-lung anesthesia, because if HPV is depressed in the nondependent lung, increased shunting of blood is probable.[3] The degree of shunting can be significant. Even though this HPV does occur, Kaplan suggests that the use of halothane is acceptable in one-lung anesthesia provided inspired oxygen (FiO_2) of 1.0 is used.[3]

Enflurane.   Enflurane is a profound respiratory depressant that may produce respiratory acidosis with increasing doses. There is a reduction in tidal volume and alveolar ventilation in the absence of assisted or controlled ventilation. Respiratory rate increases and mucociliary flow is depressed. Enflurane is thought to relax constricted airways and therefore conductance, but cases of bronchospasm have been reported. The ventilatory response to hypoxia is also greatly depressed by enflurane, more so than with halothane.[32] The effects on HPV are similar to those of halothane; it inhibits HPV in anesthetic ranges.

Isoflurane. Isoflurane is also a profound respiratory depressant. It reduces tidal volume, minute volume, alveolar ventilation, and respiratory rate. Mucociliary activity is also depressed. Depression of the ventilatory response to Pa_{CO_2} increases or Pa_{O_2} decreases is apparent with isoflurane, as with other inhalation agents. Depression is evident at 0.1 MAC. Lung compliance and FRC are thought to decrease slightly and pulmonary resistance increases. HPV is significantly decreased by isoflurane in animal studies.[3] Addition of nitrous oxide to isoflurane decreases the degree of respiratory depression, secondary to a dilutional effect.

Intravenous Anesthetics. Fentanyl and related compounds produce potent respiratory depressant effects. Both tidal volume and respiratory rate are decreased. This decline in respiratory rate is opposite the effect observed with inhalation agents where a compensatory increase in rate occurs. There is no apparent effect on HPV. In addition to the depressant effects produced by narcotics, lung compliance is decreased and truncal rigidity may occur. The occurrence and degree of truncal rigidity are accentuated by the rapidity of injection.

Ketamine produces minimal respiratory effects. It has bronchodilating properties, which are thought to be caused by beta-adrenergic stimulation secondary to increased catecholamine levels. Ketamine is thought to increase both pulmonary artery pressure and pulmonary vascular resistance and may be contraindicated in pulmonary hypertension.[3,33]

ONE-LUNG ANESTHESIA

Indications

The absolute indications for one-lung-ventilation anesthesia are prevention of cross-contamination by infected material or blood between lungs, as with lung cysts, or bronchopleural fistula, for one-sided bronchopulmonary lavage and for differential bronchospirometry.

The relative indications for the use of one-lung anesthesia are facilitation of surgical exposure in repair of thoracic aneurysm, pneumonectomy, and upper lobectomy (the most difficult lobe to remove); however, this technique is advantageous in procedures such as segmental resections, removal of other lobes, or esophageal surgery.[3]

Physiology

In one-lung ventilation, the nondependent lung (up lung) is nonventilated. Blood flow to this lung becomes shunt flow, in addition to whatever shunt flow might exist in the dependent lung (down lung).[3] The term *shunt* refers to blood that goes to the arterial system without going through ventilated areas of lung.[1] One-lung ventilation creates an obligatory right-to-left transpulmonary shunt through the nondependent lung, and this is not present during two-lung ventilation.[3]

Pa_{O_2} measurements in one-lung ventilation are lower than measurements during two-lung ventilation, but carbon dioxide levels do not appear to be affected. A single over-ventilated lung can eliminate enough carbon dioxide but cannot take up enough oxygen to compensate for the nonventilated lung. In addition, there is a great disparity between venous-to-arterial oxygen and carbon dioxide tension differences and a shunt will cause a larger change in Pa_{O_2} than in Pa_{CO_2}.

Although the benefits of one-lung anesthesia in terms of isolation of a diseased lung or optimization of surgical exposure are obvious and often mandatory, a large alveolar-to-arterial oxygen pressure difference (PA_{O_2}–Pa_{O_2}) is a consequence of this intervention.[34] The greatest reason for this difference is that the transpulmonary shunt continues because there is perfusion to nonventilated lungs. The venous blood of the nonventilated lung mixes with oxygen from the ventilated lung, lowering the arterial oxygen tension. This degree of hypoxemia varies with the amount of perfusion to the nonventilated lung.[34,35]

Several factors influence the degree of perfusion to the deflated lung. These include the condition of the dependent lung; the degree of HPV; the degree of a manual insult, such as compression or retraction of the atelectatic lung; and the method used to ventilate the dependent lung. If the dependent lung has pathology, such as COPD, alterations in both ventilation and perfusion may occur depending on the degree of surgical trauma. Perfusion to the deflated lung is also influenced by the degree of HPV. HPV minimizes the amount of transpulmonary shunting by diverting blood flow. The dependent lung may become diseased intraoperatively from long periods in the lateral decubitus position, leading to fluid accumulation or atelectasis secondary to extended periods of low FRC and low tidal volume and to hydrostatic effects.

The method by which the dependent lung is ventilated influences the degree of perfusion of the deflated lung. The influence of positive end-expiratory pressure (PEEP) and Fi_{O_2} affects HPV and the degree of atelectasis. If a positive pressure is maintained during expiration, the FRC will increase. This effect is desired to prevent atelectasis but may not be welcome when its effects on blood flow are considered. If FRC is low and then increases to a normal value, pulmonary vascular resistance decreases with a resultant increase in blood flow. But if a normal FRC increases, pulmonary vascular resistance increases and a considerable amount of blood is shunted through the ventilated lung. Other factors such as diminished cardiac output and an inadequately functioning endotracheal tube can also lead to hypoxemia.

The minute volume plays a major role in controlling the carbon dioxide value during one-lung anesthesia, whereas several factors control oxygenation. These include the efficiency of the ventilated lung, the amount of residual gas in the nonventilated lung, the cardiac output, and the inspired oxygen tension.

The degree of efficiency of the ventilated lung is vital to maintenance of adequate oxygenation. A large tidal volume (10 mL/kg) with 100 percent oxygen during anesthesia usually improves ventilation. In some instances, however, oxygenation with 100 percent oxygen does not provide adequate oxygenation because of the cumulative effects of shunting in the ventilated lung and increase in blood flow through the nonventilated lung. The amount of residual gas left in the unventilated lung is usually absorbed within several minutes, provided blood flow is present. Thus, there is little effect on the shunt fraction after the first 10 minutes. Low cardiac output and low FiO$_2$ will, for obvious reasons, influence the degree of oxygenation.

The patient undergoing a thoracic procedure may suffer some consequences from the nature of the surgery itself. Among these are the insult from a general anesthetic, which is complicated by a lateral decubitus position, an open pleural space, and one-lung ventilation. Collapse of the operated lung provides easier exposure to intrathoracic structures, limiting the damage to lung tissue from excessive traction.[36] Atelectasis in one lung is usually tolerated well in the majority of patients because of pulmonary vascular adaptation, but the risk of hypoxia is always present.

Positioning

The major alterations in ventilation and perfusion that cause arterial oxygen desaturation and increased intrapulmonary shunting during one-lung ventilation are largely influenced by position and position changes.[36]

Awake Supine Closed Chest. When the awake patient assumes the supine position, the FRC decreases as a result of the pressure of the abdominal contents against the diaphragm. When this position is changed to the lateral decubitus position, the FRC decreases more in the lower lung than in the upper lung. This occurs because the dome of the lower diaphragm is pushed higher into the chest than the upper diaphragm which is more sharply curved. As a result, the lower diaphragm is able to contract more efficiently during spontaneous respiration and thus the lower lung is always better ventilated than the upper lung (Fig. 40–5). Gravitational pull provides better perfusion to the lower lung. The preferential ventilation to the upper lung then is matched by its increased perfusion so that ventilation–perfusion ratios of the two lungs are not greatly altered when the awake patient assumes the lateral decubitus position.[37]

When the patient is turned from supine to lateral, the cardiac output may drop because of a diminished venous return secondary to pooling in the dependent lung.

Anesthetized Closed Chest. When the anesthetized patient is positioned in the lateral decubitus position, the dependent lung receives more perfusion than the nondependent lung because of gravitational influences. Significant changes in ventilation also occur. In this position, the upper lung in the spontaneously ventilated anesthetized patient receives most of the tidal volume. This major change is due to (1) a decrease in FRC bilaterally and loss of lung volume, (2) interference with the contracting diaphragm by muscle relaxants, (3) impeding of lower lung expansion by the mediastinum, (4) the weight of the abdominal contents pushing against the diaphragm, and (5) methods to improve operative access such as supporting rolls that may jeopardize lower lung expansion.[3] The nondependent lung is well ventilated and poorly perfused, and the dependent lung is well perfused but poorly ventilated, indicating ventilation–perfusion mismatch. Ventilation to the dependent lung can

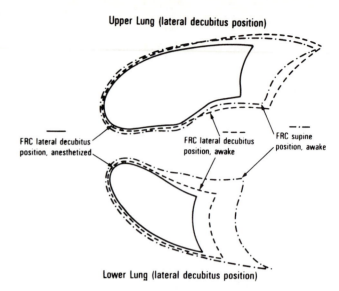

Figure 40–5. Schematic of the lungs at functional residual capacity (FRC) during supine position, awake; lateral decubitus position, awake; and lateral decubitus position, anesthetized. Note the greater loss in FRC in the lower lung in the lateral decubitus position when awake and anesthetized. (*Reprinted, with permission, from Miller.*[21])

be improved by adding PEEP to both lungs.[38] Consideration should be given to the fact that PEEP can also increase the shunt fraction.

Anesthetized Open Chest. Opening of the pleural cavity causes the lung to collapse and the mediastinum to shift toward the dependent lung, decreasing ventilation.[39] This can be prevented by intermittent positive-pressure ventilation, which maintains airway and alveolar pressure above atmospheric.[36] When the chest is open, pulmonary blood flow remains the same as in the closed chest position; however, ventilation can no longer be spontaneous and must be accomplished by positive-pressure ventilation. Opening of the chest wall and pleural space affects the distribution of the positive-pressure ventilation and perfusion.[3] If the upper lung is no longer restricted by the chest wall, it will easily be overventilated. Conversely, the dependent lung continues to be poorly ventilated and overperfused.

It must be emphasized that spontaneous breathing during open chest surgery can cause a mediastinal shift. With the chest open, atmospheric pressure in the chest cavity on the nondependent lung exceeds the negative pressure in the dependent hemithorax, causing an imbalance of the pressure in the mediastinum.[3] This condition is augmented with inspiration and reversed with expiration (Fig. 40–6). The tidal volume in the dependent lung is decreased by an amount equal to the inspiratory displacement caused by mediastinal movement.[3]

Technique

The most common way to administer one-lung anesthesia is by way of the double-lumen endotracheal tube. The advantage of this method is that it is possible to ventilate either one or both lungs independently. One lumen reaches

EXPIRATION

Pneumothorax

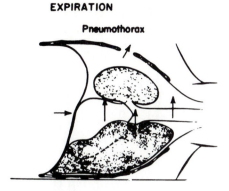

INSPIRATION

Pneumothorax

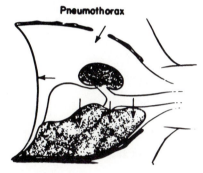

Figure 40–6. Schematic representation of mediastinal shift in the spontaneously breathing open-chest patient in the lateral decubitus position. During inspiration, negative pressure in the intact hemithorax causes the mediastinum to move downward. During expiration, relative positive pressure in the intact hemithorax causes the mediastinum to move upward. (*Reprinted, with permission, from Tarhan and Muffit.*[39])

into one of the main bronchi; the other descends only as far as the trachea. Leakage of gas during positive-pressure ventilation is prevented by a cuff placed above the shorter lumen. Separation of gas flow and infected material can be accomplished by use of a cuff placed above the longer lumen.

Endobronchial Tubes. The tubes most commonly used today are the Carlens, White, Bryce–Smith, and Robertshaw. The Carlens tube, the first double-lumen tube to be used, is designed for a left-sided intubation and a right thoracotomy, and it has a carinal hook for ensuring proper placement. It ranges in size from 35 to 37 French for females or young adults to 39 and 41 French for males (Fig. 40–7).

The White tube is a modification of the Carlens and is used for right main bronchus intubation (left thoracotomy). The bronchial cuff is slotted to provide ventilation to the right upper lobe. It is available in 37, 39, and 41 French.

The Bryce–Smith also is a modification of the Carlens tube and can be used for intubation of the right or left main bronchus. It does not have a carinal hook (Fig. 40–8).

The Robertshaw tube is the most commonly used double-lumen endotracheal tube.[40] Because it has large lumens, airway resistance is minimized and suctioning is facilitated. It is available in both right- and left-sided tubes and has no carinal hook (Fig. 40–9).

Placement. When isolation of the left lung is required, either a left- or right-sided tube may be used. If a right-sided tube is used for left lung isolation, the right upper lobe may be inadequately ventilated if there is no opening in the endobronchial cuff to permit right upper lobe ventilation. Consequently, some practitioners prefer to use only left-sided tubes for left lung isolation. Generally speaking, it is advisable to intubate the bronchus of the dependent nonoperative lung.[3]

Prior to insertion of a double-lumen tube, the cuffs and connections must be checked for proper performance. The tube and stylet must be adequately lubricated. If the Carlens or White tube is used, the carinal hooks should be down when inserted through the cords. Once through the cords, the hook should be rotated to pass through the glottis, then rotated 90 degrees to enter the appropriate bronchus. It is then advanced slowly until the hook engages the carina. Because carinal hooks can cause laryngeal trauma, these tubes must be inserted carefully.

The Robertshaw tube is passed with the distal curvature concaved anteriorly, then rotated 90 degrees so that the proximal curve is concave anteriorly to allow for endobronchial intubation.[37] Once resistance is met, passage of the tube should be stopped. Once the tube is inserted, both lungs should ventilate with inflation of either cuff. Slow inflation of the endobronchial cuff with the tracheal limb clamped confirms position in the appropriate bronchus.

With the tracheal cuff inflated, both lungs should ventilate. Next, one connecting tube should be clamped and the

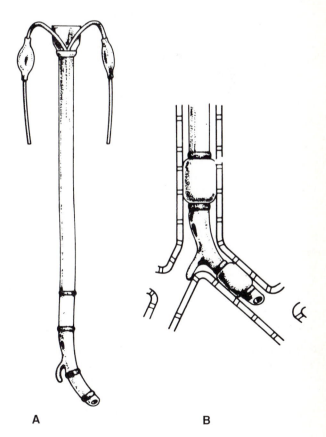

A   **B**

Figure 40–7. A. Carlens double-lumen endotracheal tube. **B.** Placement at the carina. (*Reprinted, with permission, from Miller.*[21])

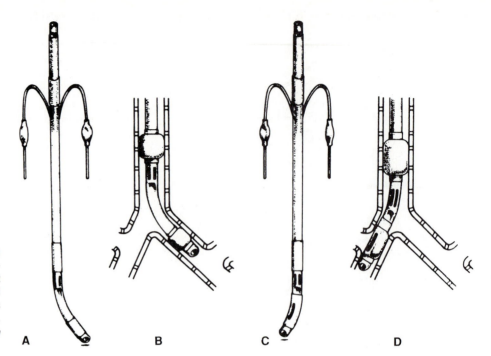

Figure 40–8. Left (**A**) and right (**C**) Bryce–Smith double-lumen endotracheal tubes. **B, D.** Placement at the carina. In (**C**), note the slotted endobronchial cuff, which inflates primarily on the medial side. (*Reprinted, with permission, from Miller.*[21])

disappearance of breath sounds on that side noted. Breath sounds should be audible on the unclamped side. This procedure is then repeated on the opposite side. Proper placement of the endobronchial tube should be ensured by use of a flexible fiberoptic bronchoscope. Malposition is the most common cause of inadequate gas exchange.

Once placement has been evaluated, the tube must be secured to avoid dislodgement during positioning of the patient. When the lateral decubitus position is assumed, the head must be kept in a neutral or slightly flexed position because head extension causes movement of the tube cepha-

lad.[41] The positioning of the tube should be verified once again by bronchoscopy.

Management of One-Lung Ventilation

Even though atelectasis of one lung is tolerated well in most instances, hypoxemia still occurs in some subjects. Several steps can reduce the incidence or degree of hypoxemia during one-lung anesthesia. First, two-lung ventilation should be maintained as long as possible. Once one-lung ventilation begins, a tidal volume of 8 to 10 mL/kg should be used

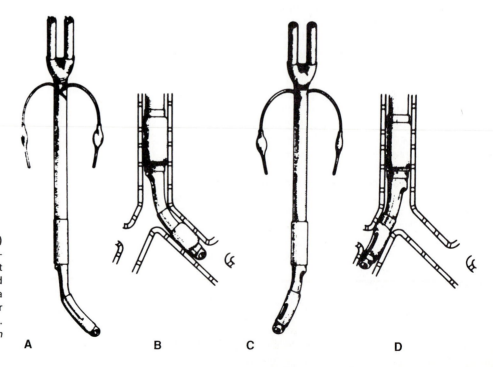

Figure 40–9. Left (**A**) and right (**C**) Robertshaw double-lumen endotracheal tubes. **B, D.** Placement at the carina. In (**C**), note the slotted endobronchial cuff, which has a relatively large proximal area for inflation to provide a better seal. (*Reprinted, with permission, from Miller.*[21])

and the rate adjusted to maintain a $Paco_2$ of 40 mm Hg. High Fio_2 with frequent blood gas sampling is recommended.

If severe hypoxemia develops, down-lung PEEP can be used. Caution must be taken because even though PEEP can improve ventilation–perfusion ratios in the down lung, it may also increase down-lung pulmonary vascular resistance and shunt blood flow up the nonventilated nondependent lung, resulting in no change or even a decrease in Pao_2.[42]

Complications to the Use of Double-Lumen Tubes

In addition to hypoxemia, other complications can occur with the use of double-lumen tubes. These include laryngitis, soft tissue injury, suturing of the tube to a pulmonary vessel, tracheobronchial laceration or rupture, inability to deflate the nondependent lung, and improper positioning or misplacement.[3] Such complications may develop because of inadequate tube size, requiring overinflation of the bronchial cuff; malposition of the tip of the tube; or too rapid inflation of the distal cuff.[3]

MANAGEMENT OF THORACIC PROCEDURES

Mediastinoscopy

Mediastinoscopy is a frequently performed diagnostic procedure used to determine the presence of mediastinal lung tumors. During this procedure, a small incision is made above the suprasternal notch and the mediastinoscope is inserted into the mediastinal cavity. This can cause serious problems if the patient is breathing spontaneously. Because of development of a negative intrathoracic pressure during inspiration, venous air embolism may occur. Controlled positive-pressure ventilation is indicated to minimize the risk of air embolism. Coughing should be controlled by muscle relaxants to avoid venous engorgement or trauma to surrounding structures by the mediastinoscope.

Another serious complication of this procedure is massive blood loss from accidental trauma to a major vessel from the biopsy instrument. Blood loss can be rapid and often is not controllable by direct pressure on the bleeding site necessitating a thoracotomy. Should hemorrhage originate from a superior vena caval tear, intravascular volume replacement and drug therapy may be lost in the surgical field unless these drugs are administered via a peripheral intravenous line placed in the lower extremity.[43] During biopsy, the mediastinoscope can exert pressure on the innominate artery, causing diminished flow to the right carotid and right subclavian arteries. A transient cerebral ischemia and hemiparesis may occur. To prevent occlusion of the innominate artery blood pressure should be measured in the left arm and the right radial artery pulse should be monitored closely during this procedure by constant palpation. Some clinicians encourage the placement of a blood pressure cuff on both arms to rapidly assess compression of the innominate artery. The size of the mediastinal tumor must be evaluated preoperatively and a decision made as to whether the supine position and general anesthesia will cause major problems with ventilation and circulation.

Pneumothorax is also a potential problem that can occur postoperatively. It usually does not require a chest tube, provided respiratory compromise is not evident or is less than 5 to 10 percent.

Bronchoscopy

Bronchoscopy, either rigid or flexible, is a valuable diagnostic tool and, in most instances, can be performed under local anesthesia. The most common complications are bronchospasm, pneumothorax, and hemorrhage. If the hemorrhage is severe, the patient should be placed in the lateral decubitus position with the bleeding side down to avoid spillage into the opposite lung. A double-lumen tube may be necessary to occlude the bleeding bronchus and resection should be instituted if bleeding is not controlled by tamponade.

Tracheostomy

Indications for tracheostomy include (1) upper airway obstruction, (2) access for tracheal toilet, (3) administration of positive-pressure ventilation, and (4) airway protection from aspiration of gastric contents.[3] Tracheostomy is usually performed under local anesthesia with some sedation. These patients are usually intubated and it is the responsibility of the anesthesia provider to slowly withdraw the endotracheal tube so that the tracheostomy tube can be inserted. The most common complications include hemorrhage and failure to cannulate the trachea. A tracheostomy is usually performed between the second and third tracheal rings. Pulsation of a tracheostomy tube indicates pressure on the innominate artery; erosion can occur if the tube is not positioned properly.

Lobectomy

The anesthetic considerations for a lobectomy are related to principles of the insertion of a double-lumen tube and to assumption of the lateral decubitus position. The right upper lobe is the most frequently resected lobe, followed by the left upper lobe.[3]

Provided that the patient is in good general health, this procedure is usually well tolerated. Intraoperative arrhythmias in the form of supraventricular rhythms such as atrial fibrillation and flutter are frequent during major pulmonary resections (5 to 15 percent).[3,44,45]

When a lobe of a lung is resected, a portion of the total alveolar, bronchial, and vascular mass is removed and an overinflation of the contralateral as well as the remaining ipsilateral lung occurs. There is increased perfusion to the remaining lung tissue. Although there is an increase in the ratio of dead space to total lung volume, the decrease in dead space occurs with respect to tidal volume. There can be loss of membrane diffusion capacity and overventilation and underperfusion of remaining lung tissue.[45]

Pneumonectomy

Patients undergoing pneumonectomy experience a high degree of surgical stress. This procedure should be performed only in patients with sufficient cardiopulmonary reserve.[3] Total removal of the lung is indicated for bronchial carcinoma, multiple lung abscesses, or extensive bronchiectasis. Three positions on the operating table may be employed to facilitate this procedure: lateral, posterior, and anterior. The lateral position, using a posterolateral incision in which the fifth rib is resected, provides the best access to the hilum of the lung.[46]

Problems in the intraoperative period center on operative exposure, methods of controlling bronchial closure, and hemostasis. Proper closure of the bronchial stump is extremely important to avoid bronchopleural fistula and infection. The incidence of dysrhythmias is higher than with lobectomies (25 to 40 percent).[3]

After pneumonectomy, the pulmonary artery and right ventricular pressures rise temporarily and a transient change in cardiac output occurs. In addition, the depth and rate of breathing increase. An increase in the ratio of tidal volume to FRC leads to an improved mixing of inspired gases, and compliance is reduced. Once the remaining lung adjusts to the new volume, it hyperinflates, resulting in a 10 to 30 percent increase in vital and total capacities.[45] The pulmonary artery pressure may be normal at rest or during mild exercise because a normal lung can adjust by doubling its blood flow. But with moderate or strenuous exercise, the pulmonary artery pressure increases.

If the remaining lung is diseased, the FRC and tidal volume are decreased. This capacity is determined by the expansibility of the remaining vascular bed, and when the limit of the bed is reached or exceeded, persistent pulmonary hypertension occurs with the development of cor pulmonale.[45]

Esophageal Surgery

Patients with esophageal tumors or strictures are usually debilitated because of dysphagia and inability to take both solids and liquids. In addition, they are prone to regurgitation and aspiration during the induction of anesthesia. Poor nutritional status produces metabolic changes that can be challenging to the anesthetist. These include dehydration and hypovolemia, which lead to hypotension; hypoalbuminemia resulting from decreased protein intake, which will affect the degree of drug binding; and decreased hemoglobin and electrolytes, resulting in shifts in the oxyhemoglobin curve and cardiac dysrhythmias, respectively.[3] These abnormal values should be corrected preoperatively. Hypovolemia and dehydration can cause perioperative hypotension; decreased protein intake can cause hypoalbuminemia, affecting drug binding, immune mechanisms, and wound healing; reduction in hemoglobin and shifts in oxygen dissociation can lead to desaturation and hypoxemia; and fluid shifts and electrolyte abnormalities can lead to cardiac dysrhythmias, congestive heart failure, and pulmonary edema.

During the induction of anesthesia, there must be emphasis on the high probability of a full stomach and possibility of gastric juice aspiration. Preoperatively patients with large hiatal hernias or esophageal tumors should receive clear antacids, H_2 antagonists, metoclopramide, and

the choice of either an awake intubation or a rapid-sequence induction–intubation procedure.

The location of the tumor determines the type of incision and the type of endotracheal tube. Tumors of the upper or lower third of the esophagus can be reached without thoracotomy incisions and can be managed with a standard endotracheal tube. Interthoracic esophageal tumors must be approached by thoracotomy, and use of a double-lumen tube provides optimal exposure for the surgeon.

Intraoperative complications include hypotension from blood loss or from inferior vena caval obstruction during the dissection of the lower end of the esophagus. The carotid sinus reflex can be stimulated, causing bradycardia and hypotension, and the trachea may be ruptured during midesophageal resection.[3] If tracheal rupture occurs, endobronchial intubation is necessary to provide ease of access to the trachea for repair. This can be accomplished by advancing the endotracheal tube into the trachea. It is advisable not to shorten the length of an endotracheal tube prior to induction in the event an endobronchial intubation should be necessary.

Bronchopleural Fistula

A bronchopleural fistula may arise as a result of a ruptured lung abscess or bulla, a carcinomatous erosion, suture line separation after pulmonary resection, or trauma. The most common occurrence is after pulmonary resection for carcinoma.[3]

A bronchopleural fistula interrupts airflow in the lung by providing an alternate pathway in which air bypasses the lungs. A gas escape across the bronchopleural fistula develops. This abnormal external communication may result in contamination of the lung, loss of air, or development of a tension pneumothorax during positive-pressure ventilation.[3]

Treatment is aimed at reducing the flow of gas over the fistula, thereby promoting healing. If the lung is intact on the affected side, an effort is made to expand the lung fully and eliminate the gas in the pleural space. This is first attempted by a chest tube with negative pressure. Once the chest tube is inserted, hypoventilation usually occurs because of loss of tidal volume through the fistula.[3] An increase in negative pressure or the application of positive pressure serves only to worsen the condition by increasing flow across the fistula, and a reduction in rate and tidal volume is recommended.[3] If the ventilatory status does not improve, selective endobronchial intubation and differential treatment of the lungs may permit diminution or cessation of flow across the bronchopleural fistula on the affected side while promoting adequate support of ventilation on the unaffected side.[3,37] Insertion of this long-term endobronchial tube is usually performed under local anesthesia if the physical status of the patient is poor or if tolerated, under general anesthesia spontaneous breathing, with the head-up position.[37]

High-frequency positive-pressure ventilation (driving pressure 35 psi, rate 115 breaths per minute, inspiratory : expiratory ratio 1 : 2, gas flow 15 L/min) has been successfully used to provide adequate oxygenation and carbon dioxide removal in a patient with a large bronchopleural fistula.[46]

Aspiration presents a major risk to these patients. Sudden drainage of pus, with contamination of the healthy lung, can cause severe ventilatory problems or even death. The patient should be transported in the sitting position, lying toward the affected side, to avoid spillage into the contralateral lung. Bronchoscopy before intubation is recommended to determine the degree of impairment or to delineate problems with intubation. Surgery is performed with the patient in the lateral position with the contaminated lung dependent. The pleural space should be aspirated as completely as possible.

Bronchopulmonary Lavage

The technique of bronchopulmonary lavage is used to remove the lipoproteinaceous material from the alveoli of patients with pulmonary alveolar proteinosis.[47]

Lung lavage is performed under general anesthesia with the use of a double-lumen tube. Mild sedation can be used as a premedicant followed by oxygen by mask to avoid hypoxemia. Volatile inhalation anesthetic agents that do not induce bronchoconstriction are recommended. Muscle relaxation should be maintained to prevent coughing during the procedure. The left lung Robertshaw double-lumen tube, a clear plastic, high-volume, low-pressure tube, should be used.[3] This left lung double-lumen tube is desirable because the cuff inflates asymmetrically, providing a secure seal, whereas the right lung cuff inflates asymmetrically to avoid obstruction of the right upper lobe.[3] Appropriate placement is absolutely essential to ensure separation of the lungs. The cuff must be inflated to a pressure high enough to withstand the peak airway inspiratory pressure and lavage pressures (the left endobronchial lumen should just begin to invaginate).[3,37] Fiberoptic bronchoscopy and chest radiograph should be performed to confirm placement.

Once the endobronchial tube is inserted, a spirometer can be placed in the expiratory limb to measure tidal volume. A volume ventilator should be used to deliver high inflation pressure to noncompliant lungs (10 to 15 mL/kg). Prelavage compliance of both lungs and then each lung separately should be recorded.[3]

Bilateral lung involvement is common, and lavage should be performed on the most severely affected lung first so that gas exchange can be provided from the less affected lung. The procedure takes several hours, and it is recommended that these patients be placed on a warming blanket to prevent hypothermia from lavage fluid temperature.

Baseline arterial gases and frequent intraoperative values should be assessed to monitor oxygenation. The lung to be treated should not be ventilated for several minutes before lavage to allow complete oxygen extraction and to augment the effectiveness of lavage.[21]

Warm saline, 500 to 1000 mL, is used as the lavage fluid and is instilled by gravity from 30 cm above the midaxillary line.[3] After the lavage fluid ceases to flow, it is drained by a line to a collection bottle 20 cm below the midaxillary line.[3] A total of 10 to 20 L of lavage fluid is generally used.

During lavage, the fluid infusion pressure exceeds pulmonary pressure, causing nonventilated lavaged lung blood flow to be diverted to the ventilated lung.[48,49]

As the lung drains, the pulmonary artery pressure exceeds the lavaged lung alveolar pressure, and lavaged lung blood flow, which is transpulmonary shunt flow, is reestablished.[48,49] Thus, the degree of hypoxemia is greatest during lung drainage and gases should be monitored carefully during this time.[47–49] The nonaffected lung should be auscultated frequently to ensure that the lungs are still ventilated separately. The presence of air bubbles in the drainage fluid may represent a leak. The volume of fluid introduced into the lung should equal that of the drainage. If not, the presence of a leak should be suspected.

Insertion of a pulmonary artery catheter is strongly recommended. If the tip of the catheter is located in the pulmonary artery of the lung being lavaged, inflation of the balloon during lung drainage diverts blood flow away from the nonventilated lung and improves oxygenation.[50]

Once lavage is completed, the lung should be suctioned, positive pressure (15 to 20 mL/kg) applied to reexpand alveoli (15 to 20 mL/kg), and chest wall percussion initiated to improve lung compliance. This procedure is repeated until the compliance returns to the prelavage value. Muscle relaxation should be maintained until this process is completed. The patient is extubated if blood gases are normal and peak inspiratory force is greater than – 20 cm H_2O. If not, an endotracheal tube should replace the endobronchial tube and the patient should be placed on PEEP or continuous positive airway pressure (CPAP) with intermittent mandatory ventilation (IMV).[3]

Tracheal Resection

Lesions of the trachea may be congenital, neoplastic, or traumatic. Traumatic injuries may be the result of direct injury or may be caused by endotracheal or tracheostomy tubes. Lesions may also result from infections.

The clinical symptoms generally consist of dyspnea, especially with effort; wheezing, which may present as frank stridor; difficulty in clearing secretions; and eventually, airway obstruction from inability to clear mucus or from tumor enlargement.[3,51]

A careful history is important to the diagnosis of these lesions because they often go undetected until the severe stages of respiratory obstruction. Symptoms are frequently inappropriately considered as an advancement of a preexisting cardiopulmonary problem or frequently this process is misdiagnosed as asthma and not properly assessed until the routine corrective measures for asthma fail.

The existence of a tracheal lesion is detected by pulmonary function tests and radiologic study. Bronchoscopy should be deferred until the time of surgery to avoid precipitation of airway obstruction secondary to edema or hemorrhage.[3] The anatomic structure of the upper airway should be analyzed carefully, with attention to jaw motion or problems associated with the fit of the mask to prevent unnecessary episodes of hypoxia. Baseline blood gases can be drawn, although they are seldom abnormal in the presence of pure airway stenosis.[3]

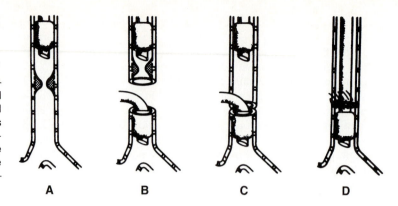

Figure 40–10. Airway management and surgical procedure for resection of a high tracheal lesion. **A.** Initial intubation above the lesion. **B.** Second endotracheal intubation distal to the lesion after the trachea has been opened. **C.** Placement of sutures for the posterior anastomosis. **D.** The second endotracheal tube has been removed and the original endotracheal tube advanced distal to the anterior anastomosis. (*Reprinted, with permission, from Geffin et al.[52]*)

A   B   C   D

The use of premedicants is controversial. There are some concerns that sedative and drying agents may augment respiratory difficulty. These patients may be treated with steroids to reduce edema, and administration should be continued intraoperatively.

Four approaches have been used to provide adequate ventilation during tracheal resection: standard orotracheal intubation, insertion of a tube into the opened trachea distal to the area of resection, jet ventilation through the stenotic area, and cardiopulmonary bypass.[20]

Routine monitoring modalities measures should be employed. Arterial catheters should be placed in the left radial artery because the right artery pulse is often lost by compression of the innominate artery which crosses the trachea.[3] Routine induction techniques can be employed in those patients with minimal airway obstruction. If the obstruction is severe, however, a slow inhalation induction should be used. Muscle relaxants should be avoided because a successful intubation may not be readily accomplished. Inhalation should proceed until it is determined that laryngoscopy can be performed without undue stress on the patient. The larynx should be anesthetized with a topical spray and bronchoscopy then performed. Careful analysis of the lesion must be made at this time. Its exact location and size should be determined. Lesions involving the upper third of the trachea, especially those in the subglottic area, pose special problems with placement because of cuff position. A lesion that is located high in the airway, where the tube cannot be passed through the lesion because of a limited opening, will not allow the cuff to pass below the cords and results in inability to attain a complete seal of the airway.

Lesions in the mid and lower thirds of the trachea are less problematic with respect to position but must be considered in view of the need to pass the tube through the lesion itself to maintain adequate ventilation until the trachea is resected or dilated.[3] The bronchoscopy and intubation must be as gentle as possible to prevent serious bleeding or dislodging of the tumor, resulting in further obstruction. The inhalation agent of choice and oxygen are used as maintenance agents. Muscle relaxants should be avoided. Nitrous oxide may be used if arterial gases are within normal limits.

The location of the lesion will necessitate special anesthetic interventions during surgical reconstruction. For lesions of the upper half of the trachea, ventilation can be managed by one of two means. A standard endotracheal tube can be inserted above the lesion and then advanced through the stenosis during resection. Second, intubation can be performed proximal to the lesion and then the surgeon can insert an additional endotracheal tube into the open trachea distal to the site of the lesion, requiring an additional anesthesia machine (Fig. 40–10).[52,53] Anesthetic considerations for upper airway lesions should include the following: (1) In those patients who are not intubated through the lesion, release of the supporting structure of the trachea may result in complete airway obstruction. (2) If nitrous oxide is being used, it should be discontinued at the time of the resection. (3) When anastomosis of the trachea begins, the endotracheal tube cuff should be deflated so that it is not damaged by the surgical needle. (4) Flexion of the head is required for tracheal approximation, and care must be taken so as not to advance the endotracheal tube into the

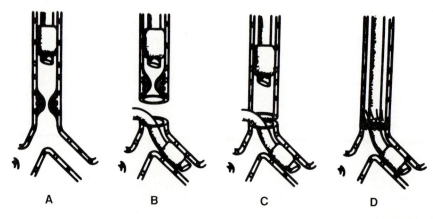

Figure 40–11. Airway management and surgical procedure for resection of a low tracheal lesion. **A.** Initial intubation above the lesion. **B.** Endobronchial intubation distal to the lesion after the trachea has been opened. **C.** Placement of sutures for the posterior anastomosis. **D.** The endobronchial tube has been removed and the original endotracheal tube advanced distal to the anterior anastomosis into an endobronchial position. (*Reprinted, with permission, from Geffin et al.[52]*)

A   B   C   D

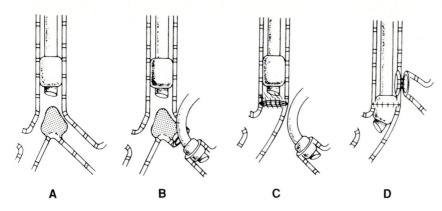

A   **B**   **C**   **D**

Figure 40–12. Airway management and surgical procedure for resection of a carinal lesion. **A.** Initial intubation above the lesion. **B.** Left endobronchial intubation distal to the lesion after the left mainstem bronchus has been severed. **C.** The trachea is anastomosed to the right of the mainstem bronchus. **D.** The left endobronchial tube has been removed to allow anastomosis between the trachea and the left mainstem bronchus. Ventilation during (**D**) is accomplished via the original endotracheal tube. (*Reprinted, with permission, from Geffin et al.*[52])

right mainstem bronchus. (5) With the patient spontaneously breathing, extubation should proceed in the surgical suite so that reintubation, if necessary, takes place in a controlled environment.[3,50,54]

Reconstruction of the lower trachea or carina is facilitated by right thoracotomy incision and may require an endobronchial intubation if there is not enough distance between the tracheal lesion and the carina (Fig. 40–11).[20,53] Figure 40–12 demonstrates the surgical approach and airway management for carinal lesions. Anesthetic considerations for reconstruction of the lower trachea include the following: (1) The endotracheal tube must be long enough to enter the mainstem bronchus. (2) Positive-pressure ventilation or high inspired oxygen concentrations are required to provide additional oxygen to compensate for periods of obstruction or tube displacement. (3) Left mainstem intubation is necessary to provide adequate oxygenation once the trachea is divided, because the tracheal stump is short and cannot hold the endotracheal tube cuff, making it extremely difficult to ventilate both lungs. (4) Additional right mainstem intubation may be necessary if adequate ventilation cannot be maintained with one-lung ventilation; this requires a second gas machine and sterile tubing to provide positive pressure to the independent lung. (5) Once the repair has been established, an endotracheal tube can be passed through the anastomotic site and endobronchial tubes removed. (6) Extubation is dependent on whether or not preexisting lung disease is present. (7) Frequent blood gas analysis is mandatory.[3,51,53,54]

In addition to the aforementioned techniques, jet (high-flow) ventilation through small-bore endotracheal catheters has been used.[55] This technique appears to ventilate adequately, while providing little interference from the surgical standpoint because of the small tube size. Carinal resections have also been managed by means of cardiopulmonary bypass, but the risk of intrapulmonary hemorrhage from heparinization limits its use.[52]

Postoperative Pain Control

The recommended technique to control postoperative pain after thoracic surgery is the administration of epidural narcotics. Profound analgesia can be produced without sympathetic block or motor loss. The catheter is inserted during the preinduction period and then dosed during surgical wound closure. The patients can be extubated on comple-

tion of the procedure. Significant increases in postoperative ventilatory parameters secondary to the analgesia effects have been obtained using this technique.

REFERENCES

1. West JB. *Respiratory physiology.* Baltimore: Williams & Wilkins; 1974.
2. Wilson R. *Principles and techniques of critical care.* Kalamazoo, MI: Upjohn Co.; 1976.
3. Kaplan J. *Thoracic surgery.* 2nd ed. New York: Churchill Livingstone; 1991.
4. Miller RD, ed. *Anesthesia.* 3rd ed. New York: Churchill Livingstone; 1990.
5. West JB. *Ventilation/blood flow and gas exchange.* 3rd ed. Oxford: Blackwell; 1977.
6. Bohr D. The pulmonary hypoxic response. *Chest.* 1977; 71:244–246.
7. Zarslow MA, Benumoff JL, Trousdale FR. Hypoxic pulmonary vasoconstriction and the size of the hypoxic compartment. *Anesthesiology.* 1981;35(1):379.
8. Grant JL, Naylor RW, Crandall WB. Bronchial adenoma resection with relief of hypoxic pulmonary vasoconstriction. *Chest.* 1980;77:446–449.
9. Benumoff JL, Wahrenbock EA. Local effects of anesthetics on regional hypoxic pulmonary vasoconstriction. *Anesthesiology.* 1975;43:525–532.
10. Benumoff JL. Hypoxic pulmonary vasoconstriction and sodium nitroprusside infusion. *Anesthesiology.* 1979;50:481–483.
11. Benumoff JL, Mathers JM. Inhibition of hypoxic pulmonary vasoconstriction by decreased Pv_{O_2}: A new indirect mechanism. *J Appl Physiol.* 1981;51:871–874.
12. Benumoff J, Pirlo A. Cyclic hypoxic pulmonary vasoconstriction induced by concomitant carbon dioxide changes. *J Appl Physiol.* 1976;41:446–469.
13. Finlayson D. *Pharmacology for the anesthesiologist.* 16th annual postgraduate course, Atlanta, GA; 1980.
14. Ayres SM. Cigarette smoking and lung diseases: An update. *Basics Respir Dis.* 1975;3(5):1–6.
15. Buist AS, Sexton GV, Nagy JM, Ross BB. The effect of smoking cessation and modification on lung function. *Am Rev Respir Dis.* 1976;114(1):115–122.
16. Davies JM, Lotto IP, Jones JG, Veale A, Wardrop CA. Effects of stopping smoking for 48 hours on oxygen availability from the blood: A study of pregnant women. *Br Med J.* 1979; 2(6186):355–356.
17. Epler GR, McLoud TC, Gaensler EA, Mikus JP, Carrington CB. Normal chest roentgenograms in chronic diffuse infiltrative lung disease. *N Engl J Med.* 1978;298(17):934–939.
18. Stalnecker MC, Suratt PM, Chander JG. Changes in respiratory

function following small bypass for obesity. *Surgery.* 1980;87: 645–651.

19. Marshall BE, Wyche MQ Jr. Hypoxemia during and after anesthesia. *Anesthesiology.* 1974;37:178–209.

20. Shapiro BA, Harrison RA, Trout CA. *Clinical application of respiratory care.* Chicago: Yearbook Medical; 1975.

21. Miller RD, ed. *Anesthesia.* 2nd ed. New York: Churchill Livingstone; 1986.

22. Nadel JA. Autonomic control of airway smooth muscle and airway secretions. *Am Rev Respir Dis.* 1977;115:117–126.

23. Butler J, Caro CG, Alcala R, DuBois AB. Physiologic factors affecting airway resistance in normal subjects and in patients with COPD. *J Clin Invest.* 1960;39:584–591.

24. Benumoff JL. *Management of the difficult/impossible airway, Parts I and II.* San Antonio, TX: 37th Annual Dannemiller Memorial Education Foundation; 1990.

25. Stoelting RK, Eger E. Additional explanation for the second gas effect: A concentrating effect. *Anesthesiology.* 1969;30:273–277.

26. Sheffer L, Stefferson JG, Birch AA. Nitrous oxide induces diffusion hypoxia in patients breathing spontaneously. *Anesthesiology.* 1972;37:436–439.

27. Yacoub O, Doell D, Kryger MH, Anthonisen NR. Depression of hypoxic ventilatory response by nitrous oxide. *Anesthesiology.* 1976;45(4):385–389.

28. Eckenoff JE, Helrich M. The effect of narcotics, thiopental and nitrous oxide upon respiration and respiratory response to hypercarbia. *Anesthesiology.* 1985;19:240–253.

29. Gelb AW, Knell RL. Subanesthetic halothane: Its effects on regulation of ventilation and relevance to recovery room. *Can Anaesth Soc J.* 1977;25:813–816.

30. Hickey RF, Fourcade E, Eger EI II, Larson CP Jr, Bahlman SH. The effects of ether, halothane and forane on apneic thresholds in man. *Anesthesiology.* 1971;35(1):32–37.

31. Weinreich AI, Silvay G, Lumb PD. Continuous ketamine infusion for one-lung anesthesia. *Can Anaesth Soc J.* 1980;27:485–490.

32. Knell RL, Manninen PH, Clement J. Ventilation and chemoreflexes during enflurane sedation and anesthesia in man. *Can Anaesth Soc J.* 1979;26:353–360.

33. Gooding JM, Dimick AR, Tavakoli M, Corssen G. A physiologic analysis of cardiopulmonary response to ketamine anesthesia in noncardiac patients. *Anesth Analg.* 1977;56(6):813–816.

34. Torda TA, McCullock CH, O'Brien HD, Wright JS, Horton DA. Pulmonary venous admixture during one-lung anesthesia. The effect of inhaled oxygen tension and respiration rate. *Anesthesia.* 1974;29(3):272–279.

35. Kerr JH, Smith AC, Prys-Roberts C, Meloche R, et al. Observations during endobronchial anesthesia. Vol. II, Oxygenation. *Br J Anaesth.* 1974;46(2):84–92.

36. Peltola K. Central hemodynamics and oxygenation during thoracic anesthesia. *Acta Anesthesiol Scand.* 1983;77:1–51.

37. Miller RD, ed. *Anesthesia.* New York: Churchill Livingstone; 1981.

38. Rheder K, Weathe FM, Sessler AD. Function of each lung during mechanical ventilation with ZEEP and with PEEP in man anesthetized with thiopental–meperidine. *Anesthesiology.* 1973;39:597–606.

39. Tarhan S, Moffit EA. Principles of thoracic anesthesia. Symposium on surgery of the chest. *Surg Clin North Am.* 1973;53(4):813–826.

40. Pappin JC. The current practice of endobronchial intubation. *Acta Anesthesiol Scand.* 1983;77:1–51.

41. Conrady PA, Goodman RA, Lainge F, Singer MM. Alteration of endotracheal tube position: Flexion and extension of the neck. *Crit Care Med.* 1976;4(1):7–12.

42. Tarhan S, Lundborg RO. Effects of increased expiratory pressure on blood gas tensions and pulmonary shunting during thoracotomy with use of the Carlens catheter. *Can Anaesth Soc J.* 1970;17(1):4–11.

43. Roberts JT, Gesson AJ. Management of complications encountered during anesthesia for mediastinoscopy. *Anesthesiol Rev.* 1979;6:31.

44. Mowry F, Reynold E. Cardiac rhythm disturbances complicating resectional surgery of the lung. *Ann Intern Med.* 1974;61:688.

45. Shields TW, Ujiki GT. Digitalization for prevention of arrhythmias following pulmonary surgery. *Surg Gynecol Obstet.* 1968;126:743.

46. Carlon GC, Ray C Jr, Klain M, McCormack PM. High-frequency positive-pressure ventilation in management of a patient with bronchopleural fistula. *Anesthesiology.* 1980;52(2):160–162.

47. Busque L. Pulmonary lavage in the treatment of alveolar proteinosis. *Can Anaesth Soc J.* 1977;24:380.

48. Rogers RM, Tantam KR. Bronchopulmonary lavage. A new approach to old problems. *Med Clin North Am.* 1970;54:755.

49. Rogers RM, Szidan JP, Shelburne J, Neigh JL, Shuman JF. Hemodynamic response of the circulation to bronchopulmonary lavage in man. *N Engl J Med.* 1972;286(23):1230–1233.

50. Alfrey DD, Zamost BG, Benumoff JL. Unilateral lung lavage: Manipulation of pulmonary blood flow. *Anesthesiology.* 1980;53:53–81.

51. Grillo HC. Resection of the trachea. Experience in 100 consecutive cases. *Thorax.* 1973;28:667–679.

52. Geffin B, Bland J, Grillo C. Anesthetic management of tracheal resection and reconstruction. *Anesth Analg.* 1969;48:884.

53. Bayan PC, Privitera PA. Resection of stenotic trachea: A case presentation. *Anesth Analg.* 1976;55:191.

54. Ellis RH, Hinds CJ, Gadd LT. Management of anesthesia during tracheal resection. *Anesthesia.* 1976;31:1076–1080.

55. Lee P, English ICW. Management of anesthesia during tracheal resection. *Anesthesia.* 1974;29:305.

Anesthesia for Cardiac and Peripheral Vascular Surgery

Cathy Mastropietro

The surgical intervention and anesthetic principles of management for cardiovascular and peripheral vascular surgery are the focus of this chapter. Pertinent anatomy, physiology, and pathophysiology are discussed and related to the preoperative assessment of the patient. Anesthesia for cardiac surgery for coronary artery disease and valvular disease as well as numerous peripheral vascular procedures including aortic surgery is considered. Some congenital anomalies are presented, but the emphasis of this chapter is adult patient management. The principles underlying the anesthetic management of patients with cardiac disease are the same for cardiac and noncardiac surgery. This factor is especially important because of the prevalence of heart and vascular disease in the general population.

CORONARY ARTERY DISEASE

Etiology

When symptoms occur from inadequate oxygen delivery to the myocardium, the result is said to be ischemic coronary heart disease. In a vast majority of patients, the cause is an atherosclerotic narrowing of the coronary arteries, and in the remainder the cause is embolism, inflammatory changes, or vasospasm.

The incidence of coronary artery disease (CAD) is vastly increasing. It has been estimated that 600,000 individuals develop CAD annually. It has been the major cause of deaths between the ages of 45 and 54 and the most common cause of death in males between the ages of 35 and 44. The increase in incidence, sudden onset of symptoms, and tragic nature of the disease has warranted concern by both the medical profession and the public.

Several risk factors are associated with the development of coronary artherosclerosis. These include (1) genetic susceptibility, (2) obesity and carbohydrate tolerance, (3) hemodynamic and local arterial factors, and (4) stress (Table 41–1).

Extensive coronary artery narrowing can exist without symptoms. Asymptomatic individuals are classified as the coronary atherosclerotic, whereas those who present with symptoms are classified as the coronary artery diseased.[1]

Atherosclerosis refers to a thickening and hardening of medium- or large-sized arteries. The disease process rarely involves small arteries and should not be confused with the term *arteriosclerosis,* which seldom has notable clinical effects. The feature that sets atherosclerosis apart from other forms of arteriosclerosis is the lipid component, which in the advanced plaque is often represented by a central necrotic core that is rich in cholesterol esters and is often accompanied by visible cholesterol crystals.[2] This part of the lesion, which on gross examination is usually soft and grumous, is responsible for the name of the disease process, derived from the Greek stem *athera,* meaning "gruel" or "porridge."[2]

Atherosclerotic plaques more frequently involve the abdominal aorta, especially around the ostia of its major branches. Renal arteries are usually spared from plaque except at their ostia; coronary arteries show the most intense involvement within the first 6 cm.

Plaques are composed of plaque cells, arterial smooth muscle cells, and lipid. Several theories have been proposed to explain the pathogenesis of plaques. The most accepted one is the insudation theory which suggests that there is increased passage and accumulation of plasma constituents from the arterial lumen into the intima promoting a type of low-grade inflammatory edema. Elevated serum lipoproteins assist in carrying cholesterol, in the form of low-density lipoprotein, into the arterial system; chronically elevated levels are always associated with progressive atherosclerosis. Endothelial injury often plays a major part in accelerating atherosclerosis because it results in encrustation of platelets and monocytes, which in turn exposes the intimal and medial arterial smooth muscle cell to the peptides that stimulate cell proliferation.[2]

Clinically, the formation of plaque produces symptoms resulting from stenosis caused by its space-occupying tendencies or because of its embolic properties. Ulceration in the area of the plaque leads to thrombus formation; its oc-

TABLE 41–1. RISK FACTORS ASSOCIATED WITH THE DEVELOPMENT OF CORONARY ATHEROSCLEROSIS

Genetic susceptibility: inherited traits

Obesity, carbohydrate tolerance: hypercholesterolemia, hypertriglyceridemia, diabetes mellitus

Hemodynamic and local arterial factors: hypertension, cigarette smoking

Stress: psychologic and personality factors (type ''A'' personality)

currence in the coronary system results in occlusion or infarction. In larger vessels, such as the aorta, occlusion is not the problem. Weakening of the aortic wall occurs, resulting in aneurysm formation and embolization to distal arteries.

Educating the public on how to reduce risk factors has resulted in some decline in statistics; however, the incidence and mortality rates remain high. Prevention, early detection, and medical or surgical intervention are essential to longevity.

Pathophysiology

When atherosclerosis becomes symptomatic, the disease is usually extensive, because a 75 percent stenosis is required before flow is decreased. Lesions may be found in one or several vessels. Generally, the left anterior descending (LAD) and circumflex arteries are affected in their proximal areas, whereas the right coronary artery (RCA) lesion can be proximal or distal. Whether a lesion is proximal or distal in the LAD artery is important because of its anatomic structures. The LAD artery gives rise to its major branches as it descends. Conversely, the main right coronary artery branches are in its periphery and proximal or distal lesions are less compromising. (Fig. 41–1 illustrates a coronary arteriogram with triple-vessel disease.)

The LAD artery is most commonly affected, followed by the right, the left circumflex, and the left main coronary arteries.[1] The subendocardial region of the left ventricle is more prone to ischemic damage because of ventricular contraction and compression of subendocardial vessels. The coronary vessels are initially epicardial, perforate the myocardium,

and then become subendocardial arterioles. Perfusion to subendocardial areas depends on diastolic time. If left ventricular end-diastolic pressure (LVEDP) is greatly increased or diastolic pressure decreased, the gradient declines and subendocardial ischemia occurs. Tachyarrhythmias shorten diastolic time and decrease subendocardial perfusion. Figure 41–2 illustrates zones of predilection of atherosclerotic lesions.

History of Coronary Artery Bypass

The impact of coronary artery bypass surgery on the survival of patients with CAD has been a subject of debate since its inception. The first coronary bypass procedure was performed in the late 1960s. Now, approximately 300,000 revascularization procedures are performed annually. The setting in which bypass grafting is performed certainly influences the statistical analysis of this debate. Successful intraoperative management reflected by low rates of mortality, perioperative infarction, and other postoperative complications and short hospital convalescence depends not only on surgical skill and judgment, but also on the availability of competent anesthesia personnel, efficient extracorporeal support, the best possible myocardial preservation techniques, and a minimal period of myocardial ischemia consistent with optimal revascularization.[3]

The consensus is that in those patients with angina pectoris and a 50 percent narrowing of the left main coronary artery, bypass surgery results in better survival than medical treatment. In patients with chronic angina pectoris who undergo bypass surgery, 60 to 70 percent obtain complete anginal relief and 80 to 90 percent note symptomatic improvement in the early postoperative period.[4]

Larrieu published statistics on the current status of coronary bypass surgery.[5] His results show that patients with left main coronary artery stenosis who had surgical intervention had survival rates of 86 to 88 percent at 3 years postoperatively, those with triple-vessel disease had quite similar statistics, and those with double-vessel disease ranged from 69 to 96 percent. No supportive data exist reflecting increased survival rates in patients surgically treated for single-vessel disease, unless severe left main lesions are present. Medical treatment for single-vessel disease allowed for a 90 percent survival rate.

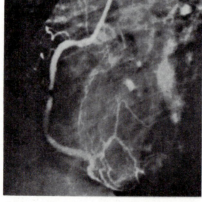

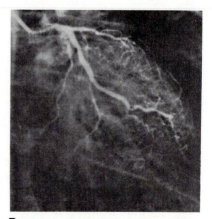

Figure 41–1. A. Right coronary arteriogram. There is significant stenosis of the midportion of the right coronary artery. **B.** Left coronary arteriogram. There is profound disease of the anterior descending coronary artery followed by a stenosis; the circumflex origin is also stenosed.

A   B

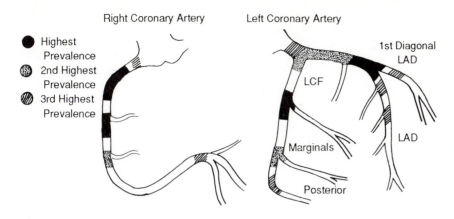

Figure 41–2. Zones of predilection of the atherosclerotic lesion in the left and right coronary arteries. LAD, left anterior descending artery; LCF, left circumflex artery. (*Reprinted, with permission, from Vanden Belt et al.*[1])

PREOPERATIVE INTERVIEW

The preoperative interview, imperative for all surgical procedures, has a tremendous impact on the cardiac patient. Persistent preoperative anxiety can be detrimental to these patients, and as mentioned previously catecholamine release with a concomitant hypertension and tachycardia increases myocardial oxygen demand. A detailed, unhurried explanation of the preoperative, intraoperative, and postoperative events is of paramount importance because the fear of anesthesia is just as great as the fear of the actual surgery. It is not uncommon for anginal attacks, with increased blood pressure and heart rate, to occur immediately during the preinduction period. The incidence of such attacks can be reduced by informing the patient and family of upcoming events.

The preoperative evaluation begins by taking a thorough history, because it is imperative to determine the pathologic condition of cardiac and other organ systems. The specific inquiries and laboratory examinations should be designed to determine the kind of functional impairment that the patient suffers with regard to the heart and peripheral vascular system, oxygen-carrying capacity, pulmonary exchange, renal and hepatic function, and body compartment volumes. (Table 41–2 lists the minimum preoperative studies required to evaluate the cardiac patient.)

Angina

There are various forms of angina pectoris. Classic angina is described as either stable or unstable. Angina pectoris is regarded as stable when it has not changed in frequency, duration, or time of appearance of precipitating factors during the preceding 60 days. Stable angina may be (1) mild (of brief duration, not markedly interfering with the patient's life-style) or (2) disabling (occurring at less than the usual daily activity level but not at rest).[6]

Unstable angina (preinfarction angina) describes a whole group of syndromes varying from the above definition.[6] These patients experience chest pain; however, serum enzyme evidence is lacking. With acute coronary insufficiency anginal pain has a duration of 20 minutes or longer without relief from vasodilators. Variant angina (Prinzmetal's) is the term used to describe pain that occurs at rest with a concomitant elevation in the ST segment.

TABLE 41–2. MINIMAL PREOPERATIVE STUDIES USED IN EVALUATING THE CARDIAC PATIENT

Function	Factors to Consider
Angina	Type
	Severity
	Medication
	Dosage
Electrocardiogram	Presence of arrythmias
	Myocardial ischemia
	Cardiac catheterization report
Left ventricular	Ejection fraction
	Left ventricular end-diastolic pressure
	Cardiac output
	Cardiac index
Peripheral vascular	Carotid stenosis
	Aortic disease
	Renal vascular disease
Respiratory	Pulmonary function studies
	Arterial blood gas analysis
	Chest x-ray
Renal/hepatic	Blood urea nitrogen
	Serum creatinine
	Prothrombin time
	Partial thromboplastin time
	Platelet and bleeding times
Fluid compartment volume	State of hydration
	Electrolyte values
	Pulmonary artery pressure
	Pulmonary wedge pressure
	Pulmonary mean pressure
Chronic medications	Type
	Dosage
	Side effects
General appearance	Dyspnea
	Exercise tolerance
	Retinopathy
	Xanthoma

The interviewer must determine the type of angina that presents, if it is relieved by medication, and the dosage needed for relief. Shortness of breath, exercise limitations, arrhythmias, and signs of pulmonary hypertension should be looked for. Xantheloma or retinopathy are common. An S_4 gallop is often present in angina patients. The patient with valvular heart disease should be evaluated carefully for the degree of cardiac impairment. Symptoms such as chest pain, arrhythmias, and syncope indicate difficulties with oxygen balance; dyspnea, edema, and orthopnea point to a failing myocardium.

Electrocardiogram

The electrocardiogram (ECG) should be evaluated for rate and rhythm disturbances, axis, conduction disease, chamber enlargement, and electrolyte or drug effect. ST depression greater than 2 mm is often indicative of CAD. Electrocardiogram findings may not be conclusive. Nonspecific R-ST segment or T-wave abnormalities are common. Typically, during myocardial ischemia, a horizontal or downsloping depression of the R-ST segment is present that is worse prognostically than upsloping segments.

Left Ventricle Function

The degree of left ventricular function must be determined. Previous myocardial infarction or evidence of congestive heart failure should cause the clinician to question the degree of ventricular function. The ejection fraction ([end-diastolic volume minus end-systolic volume] divided by end-diastolic volume) is a useful measure of ventricular function and is currently the most reliable. A normally contracting ventricle will eject 67 percent of end-diastolic volume with each beat. Ejection fractions of 0.40 to 0.55 are common in patients with previous infarction who are asymptomatic. When the values range between 0.25 and 0.40, symptoms occur with exercise, and when less than 0.25, symptoms occur at rest.[6]

Another useful method of assessing ventricular function is evaluating wall motion, which is determined by echocardiography or cardiac catheterization. Ventricular wall abnormality is classified as either hypokinetic (decreased motion), akinetic (absent motion), or dyskinetic (paradoxical motion). Resting LVEDP is also an indicator of ventricular function. The normal value is 12 mm Hg, and levels above 18 usually indicate poor ventricular function.

Cardiac output and index provide some knowledge of ventricular function. Indexes less than 2 L min/m$_2$ indicate impaired function. Cardiac output is the best indicator of overall cardiac performance. Abnormally low values indicate cardiac decompensation.

Patients scheduled for revascularization procedures can be divided into two groups: (1) those with good left ventricular function (hyperdynamic ventricles) evidenced by normal cardiac output, LVEDP less than 12 mm Hg, and ejection fraction greater than 0.55; and (2) those with poor ventricular function (hypodynamic ventricles) evidenced by decreased cardiac output, LVEDP greater than 19 mm Hg, ejection fraction less than 0.40, and symptoms of congestive heart failure. These patients have had previously detected infarctions.

Peripheral Vascular Disease

One should automatically assume that peripheral vascular disease accompanies coronary atherosclerosis. Carotid stenosis is common and higher-than-usual systemic pressures may be desirable in patients with carotid artery disease. The management of combined carotid stenosis and coronary bypass remains controversial; however, the neurologic status of these patients must be evaluated and managed accordingly.

The presence of aortoiliac disease should be determined before bypass in the event that use of the intraaortic balloon becomes necessary.

Respiratory Status

The most common respiratory insult is chronic obstructive lung disease, and symptoms are surgically compounded by large doses of crystalloid therapy and hemodilution, hypothermia, and cardiopulmonary bypass itself. Pulmonary function studies and arterial blood gas analysis should be performed preoperatively to provide a baseline for reference. It is an advantage to have baseline pulmonary artery pressures to evaluate the origin of abnormal values during the preoperative period. The oxygen content of arterial blood is dependent on the amount of hemoglobin, the amount of 2,3-diphosphoglycerate, and a normal acid–base status. Any abnormalities in these areas should be corrected before elective surgery begins.

Renal and Hepatic Function

Renal vascular disease causes ischemic kidneys and presents problems with urinary output. Also, vast fluctuations in blood pressure can be expected with renal artery lesions. Renal function can be determined by blood urea nitrogen and serum creatinine levels. Abnormally high levels may indicate renal impairment and should be further evaluated.

Coagulation Function

Coagulation studies are mandatory preoperative assessment screening studies. The prothrombin (PT), partial thromboplastin time (PTT), platelet count, and bleeding time should be evaluated.

Fluid Compartment Volume

Special attention should be paid to the patient's hydration. Patients in congestive heart failure have peripheral pooling of water and pulmonary congestion. They are usually taking diuretics, which may induce electrolyte imbalance. In addition, diuretics reduce plasma volume which has been altered by hypertension and volume expansion may be necessary prior to induction.

Infection

Provided the patient's condition can tolerate surgical delays, any preexisting infection should be treated. The reticuloendothelial system functions poorly in post-cardiopulmonary bypass patients, and they are predisposed to infections. Preoperative prophylactic use of antibiotics is essential.

Chronic Medications

The cardiac patient is usually taking several medications to provide stability and comfort. These may include beta blockers to reduce myocardial contractility, heart rate, and systemic hypertension; nitroglycerin for angina relief; calcium channel blockers for arrhythmias; diuretics; vasodilators; cardiac glycosides; angiotensin converting enzyme (ACE) inhibitors; and sedatives. The general rule of thumb is to maintain blood levels of these medications preoperatively, so as not to interfere with the supply : demand ratio.

ANESTHETIC MANAGEMENT

Preoperative Phase

Preoperative Medication. The goal of preoperative medication in patients with CAD is to provide enough sedation to obtund heightened anxiety levels for the patient arriving in the operating room suite. The anxiety experienced by these patients is often unexpressed and frequently denied, accentuating angina or the possibility of myocardial infarction. The heightened sympathetic response associated with stress must be obliterated. The ultimate goal is to prevent intraoperative infarction.

Silent ischemia can account for a significant percentage of ischemic episodes. The incidence rises significantly in patients who have heart rates greater than 110 beats per minute. Hypertensive or hypotensive episodes do not appear to increase the incidence. The occurrence of silent ischemia is greatest from the preinduction phase until the onset of cardiopulmonary bypass (CPB) and has been fingered as a significant cause of perioperative myocardial infarction and unfavorable outcome.[7]

Obviously, rapid heart rates increase myocardial oxygen requirements, coronary flow, and oxygen delivery. Elevated systolic pressures, on the other hand, increase myocardial oxygen requirements, but this is compensated for by improved perfusion through sclerotic coronary arteries which have become pressure dependent.

Unlike the heavy sedation that is required for the patient with CAD, light premedication is preferred in patients with valvular disease. Because of the limited cardiac reserve, these patients are very susceptible to cardiac and respiratory depressant drugs.

Premedication should be avoided on the hypodynamic patient. Belladonna administration must be minimal, so that the cardioaccelerator effect of these drugs is avoided.

Preinduction. The ideal anesthetic induction provides comfort to the patient, stability of circulatory dynamics, and absence of excitement. Regardless of the technique selected, it is imperative that these patients be in surgical planes of anesthesia prior to stimulation to prevent tachyarrhythmias and hypertension. The anesthetist must remember that patients with low cardiac outputs will have a decreased circulation time and thus a delayed onset of action of intravenous agents. On the other hand, in the presence of low cardiac output, inhalation agents will rapidly come into equilibrium with alveolar gas and onset of anesthesia will be more rapid.

Monitoring

Changes in oxygen supply–demand balance caused by alterations in circulatory dynamics can be determined by using the appropriate monitoring devices. Effective monitoring alerts the anesthetist when something goes awry, provides some clue to the reason, and may help determine the appropriate treatment.

Minimal monitoring for the patient undergoing coronary revascularization should include electrocardiogram, esophageal temperature, direct arterial pressure, central venous pressure, serum electrolytes and pH, and urinary output. In addition, cardiac output, pulmonary artery pressure, wedge pressures, and venous oxygen saturation have become accepted monitoring parameters for cardiac surgery to determine hemodynamic alterations (Table 41–3).

Electrocardiogram. The ECG readily alerts the anesthetist to changes in rate, rhythm, or segment. It can also provide some information about myocardial ischemia. A five-lead system reflects leads I, II, III, aVR, aVF, aVL, and V_2. Table 41–4 lists the areas of myocardial ischemia as reflected by the ECG.[8] Arrhythmias are best determined in lead II, whereas ischemia is more readily detected in V_5. Lead II parallels the P-wave vector, thus differentiating ventricular from supraventricular arrhythmias. The presence or absence of the P-wave is especially important in the assessment of the hemodynamic effect of the atrial kick.[9]

Lead V_5 monitors the myocardium in areas most susceptible to ischemic change. Typically, the ECG change noted in ischemia is a downsloping depression of the R-ST

TABLE 41–3. NORMAL VALUES FOR MEASURED AND CALCULATED HEMODYNAMIC PARAMETERS

Parameter	Value
Central venous pressure	10–15 mm Hg
SVO_2	75%
Cardiac output	4–8 L min
Systemic vascular resistance	800–1600 units (dyn)
Pulmonary vascular resistance	75–200 units (dyn)
Rate–pressure product	12,000
Triple index	150,000
Stroke volume	60–100 mL/beat
Cardiac index	2.5–4.0 L min m^2
Left ventricular stroke work index	45–75 g/m^2 per beat
Right atrial pressure	0–7 mm Hg
Right ventricular pressure	Systolic: 15–25 mm Hg Diastolic: 0–8 mm Hg
Pulmonary artery pressure	Systolic: 15–25 mm Hg Diastolic: 8–15 mm Hg Mean: 10–20 mm Hg
Pulmonary capillary wedge pressure	6–12 mm Hg
Left ventricular end-diastolic pressure	8–12 mm Hg
Left atrial pressure	5–10 mm Hg

TABLE 41–4. AREA OF MYOCARDIAL ISCHEMIA AS REFLECTED BY THE ELECTROCARDIOGRAM

Electrocardiogram Lead	Coronary Artery Responsible for Myocardial Ischemia	Area of Myocardium That May Be Involved
II, III, aVF	Right coronary artery	Right atrium Sinus node Atrioventricular node Right ventricle
V_3-V_5	Left anterior descending coronary artery	Anterolateral aspects of the left ventricle
I, aVL	Circumflex coronary artery	Lateral aspects of the left ventricle

Reprinted, with permission, from Stoelting RK, Miller RD. Basics of anesthesia. 2nd ed. New York: Churchill Livingstone; 1989:263.

segment of 1 mm and 0.08-second duration. The electrophysiology of the ST segment changes in myocardial ischemia has not been completely clarified, but an altered ion transport across the myocardial cell membrane apparently is the underlying cause of the change in current responsible for the ST segment shift induced by ischemia.[2] The use of transesophageal echocardiography (TEE) is also available for continuous cardiac monitoring. This device allows for viewing of the chambers, the ascending and descending aorta, as well as the pericardium, and readily provides information about filling valvular function, contractility, shunting, aortic dissection, and air emboli.

Central Venous Pressure. Central venous pressure values represent right-sided heart filling pressure. Radiographic examination should be used to assess proper placement. A sudden increase in venous pressure may indicate obstruction of cannula drainage and requires immediate correction. The central venous pressure does not directly indicate left-sided heart filling pressure, and it may not be reliable in patients with left ventricular dysfunction, but can be used as a rough estimate of this measure.

Pulmonary Artery (Swan-Ganz) or Oximetric Catheter. Primary indications for use of oximetric or Swan-Ganz catheters are ventricular dysfunction, recent myocardial infarction, altered chamber pressures, and whenever there is an anticipated alteration in preload or afterload.[9] In patients with CAD, two distinct situations exist in which LVEDP (pulmonary capillary wedge pressure [PCWP]) can be evaluated: (1) myocardial ischemia causing left ventricular dysfunction, resulting in elevated LVEDP; (2) elevated LVEDP causing increased myocardial oxygen consumption.

Measurements of SVO_2 are valuable in early detection of hemodynamic disturbances and prediction of the adequacy of the body's cardiac output in meeting oxygen demands, thus avoiding irreversible stages of metabolic acidosis. It should be remembered that patients with abnormal cardiac anatomy such as those with ventricular or septal defects should not have pulmonary artery lines inserted. Complications can occur after the use of pulmonary

arterial catheters. These include balloon rupture, endocarditis, pulmonary artery perforation, thrombosis, and intracardiac knotting. Complications can be minimized by a sound background knowledge and skill in the use of these catheters.

The myocardial oxygen demand should also be monitored closely. Since Rohde demonstrated, in 1912, that MVO_2 varies directly with the heart rate times peak developed pressure, extensive investigation into the relative effects of pressure, stroke volume, and heart rate on oxygen consumption has been carried out.[6] Rohde theorized that the rate–pressure product (systolic blood pressure times heart rate) correlates with MVO_2. A value greater than 12,000 increases oxygen demand, and even though it is a crude estimate it offers a quick reference to MVO_2.[6]

Triple index (systolic pressure times heart rate times PCWP) and the tension time index (heart rate times area under the systolic portion of the aortic pressure curve) have also been used to determine oxygen demand, but the rate–pressure product (RPP) seems to be more reliable.

Perioperative Phase: Induction of Anesthesia

Choice of anesthesia for coronary revascularization should be made on the basis of the patient's left ventricular function, that is, good versus poor cardiac performance. If normal ventricular function is present with CAD, the incidence of reflex response to stimulation, that is, hypertension or tachycardia, is increased. Controlled myocardial depression is necessary to prevent sympathetic nervous system activity and subsequent increases in myocardial oxygen requirements. If left ventricular function is depressed, the induction technique must prevent a further depression in hemodynamic status. Patients with left coronary disease are especially vulnerable during induction. When selecting anesthesia for the patient with valvular disease, the anesthetist should be concerned with control of heart rate, regulation of intravascular volume, and regulation of stress imposed on the circulatory system.

Cardiac output is determined by two factors, heart rate and stroke volume, and control of output is essential. Because heart rate is one of the major determinants of MVO_2, maintenance of a normal heart rate is important because there is a decrease in myocardial oxygen delivery. Tachycardia will decrease the total time for diastole, thus decreasing the time for ventricular filling. A reduction in cardiac output follows. Selection of an anesthetic technique that does not interfere with heart rate is imperative. This is of particular concern when a muscle relaxant is being selected. Propranolol or digitalis may be necessary for optimal control of heart rate.

Selection of the induction agent varies according to vital sign lability and user preference. Commonly used nonnarcotic drugs are thiopental, etomidate, diazepam, lorazepam, midazolam, and propofol. Thiopental sodium possesses myocardial depressant properties and vasodilating effects. Therefore, hypotension may ensue, and doses large enough to prevent contact stimulation may not be achievable. For this reason, thiopental is frequently used in conjunction with sedatives or narcotics.

Etomidate is a unique nonbarbiturate hypnotic agent

that provides excellent cardiorespiratory stability. It produces little cardiovascular depression and the effect of MVO_2 is minimal. Another advantage to its use is that there is no histamine release.

Diazepam possesses transient cardiovascular depressor effects and no peripheral autonomic blocking action, thus providing somnolence with minimal hemodynamic changes. Diazepam also produces antegrade amnesic effects by affecting the storage period of memory—the stage during which information is encoded and entered into memory.

Lorazepam also has antianxiety and sedative effects. Doses of 2 to 4 mg intravenously provide somnolence, relief of preoperative anxiety, and lack of recall of events related to the day of surgery.

Midazolam shares the same pharmacologic properties as the other benzodiazepines. Dosage is 1 to 5 mg intravenously. Duration of action is shorter than with lorazepam. All of the benzodiazepines are used in conjunction with other induction agents.

Should the patient be unable to tolerate any degree of myocardial depression, a narcotic can be used. Fentanyl in doses of 50 to 100 μg/kg is commonly used. The advantage to this dose range is that there are minimal effects on myocardial performance. The pharmacokinetics of fentanyl is discussed later.

As mentioned previously, the goal of induction is to provide the patient some degree of relaxation, progressing to a surgical plane of anesthesia that will, on noxious stimulation, propagate minimal hemodynamic change.

Muscle relaxation must be adequate before endoscopy. Because of the length of cardiac surgery, long- or intermediate-acting muscle relaxants are the drugs of choice. This is not to say that a short-acting relaxant, such as succinylcholine, cannot be used for induction particularly if a difficult intubation is suspected; however, if used, the dosage should be large enough to prevent the need for additional drug, because the risk of arrhythmias is increased with consecutive doses.

Pancuronium bromide is very popular as a muscle relaxant for these procedures. The degree of muscle relaxation is profound and effects are of long duration. Pancuronium-induced tachycardia and hypertension must be avoided. The cardiovascular effects of pancuronium are thought to result from inhibition of vagal tone and a direct or indirect beta-adrenergic effect. This does not seem to be as problematic with narcotic inductions as with other techniques, with the exception of sufentanil, which does not appear to protect the heart against adverse tachyarrhythmias. The narcotic-induced bradycardia appears to override the tachyarrhythmic effects of pancuronium. If pancuronium is used to provide skeletal muscle relaxation for intubation, doses of 0.06 to 0.1 mg/kg are recommended. The onset and duration of action are dose dependent.

Doxacurium chloride and pipecuronium bromide are long-acting muscle relaxants similar to pancuronium. Doxacurium appears to be two to three times as potent as pancuronium; however, this drug lacks aberrant cardiovascular effects. One disadvantage of this drug may be its slow onset of action. Pipecuronium bromide appears to be equipotent to pancuronium but is devoid of tachycardia or hypotensive-like effects.[10]

Metocurine is an intermediate-acting muscle relaxant that structurally resembles d-tubocurarine. Its effects are at the myoneural junction, but it does not produce autonomic ganglionic blockade as does d-tubocurarine. Histamine release occurs less frequently. Intubation doses appear adequate at 0.2 to 0.4 mg/kg, followed by 0.5 to 1 mg for maintenance. The main excretory pathway for metubine is via the kidneys; thus caution must be exercised with those patients who have coexisting renal disease.

Atracurium besylate is an intermediate-acting, nondepolarizing skeletal muscle relaxant. The duration of blockade is approximately one-third to one-half that of pancuronium, metubine, or tubocurarine in equipotent doses. An intubation dose of 0.4 to 0.5 mg/kg produces relaxation of 35 to 45 minutes' duration. There are no adverse clinical effects on the heart; however, some histamine may be released with larger doses, so caution should be used in patients in whom an exaggerated response may be anticipated. Neuromuscular blockade is enhanced with the use of inhalation anesthetic agents as with other nondepolarizing relaxants. It should be remembered that because the rate of degradation of atracurium is dependent on temperature (Hoffman elimination) and pH, significant reductions in body temperature will affect the half-life. Flynn and Hughes found that a reduction in temperature from 37C to 23C increased the half-life at least twofold.[11]

The depth of anesthesia and degree of muscle relaxation can be assessed during urinary catheter insertion. If no change in hemodynamics occurs with insertion, the patient is ready for intubation. The patient is preoxygenated during the entire preparatory period. A bolus of lidocaine 1 to 1.5 mg/kg is injected prior to endoscopy. The use of laryngeal tracheal anesthesia spray is optional.

The competent anesthetist will have adjunctive drugs on hand such as nitroglycerin, nitroprusside, or propranolol to counteract any hypertension or tachycardia associated with endotracheal intubation.

MAINTENANCE OF ANESTHESIA

When significant myocardial depression is a desired response, as in the case of patients who have normal ventricular function, the inhalation anesthetics are the drugs of choice. All inhalation anesthetics in significant concentrations depress myocardial function. Potent inhalation anesthetics suppress reflex response to noxious stimulation, provide muscle relaxation, and allow for early extubation.

Inhalation Agents

Eger suggests that enflurane and halothane produce a dose-related depression of contractility, whereas isoflurane and nitrous oxide do not. When selecting an inhalation agent, or any agent for that matter, the reader should remember that the young surgical patient usually responds to stress by increasing heart rate, whereas the elderly one usually responds by elevating arterial pressure.[12]

Halothane. Halothane is a haloethane that produces significant myocardial depression. In a study performed by Hilfiker et al,[13] halothane–nitrous oxide anesthesia was associated with significant decline in oxygen consumption of the left ventricle, together with a corresponding decrease in coronary blood flow, both of which decreased the hemodynamic load on the myocardium and decreased contractility. Even though coronary perfusion was decreased, myocardial lactate (index of myocardial ischemia) was not measurable.

Halothane seems to prevent disturbances in myocardial oxygen balance mainly by attenuating or preventing tachycardia, hypertension, and sympathetic hyperactivity caused by noxious stimuli during anesthesia and surgery.[13] It has been suggested that data concerning the effects of halothane on the ischemic myocardium are inconsistent, and controversy exists as to whether anesthesia with myocardial depressants is beneficial for the ischemic heart.[14]

Enflurane. Enflurane is a halogenated ether that dilates both resistance vessels and coronary vessels and in this sense is more potent than halothane. Enflurane decreases mean arterial pressure and reflexly increases heart rate to maintain cardiac output. Left ventricular filling pressure decreases because of a reduction in afterload. Enflurane also reduces coronary perfusion pressure. There is a critically low perfusion pressure at which coronary autoregulation is lost. In patients with normal coronary arteries, this occurs at a mean aortic pressure of approximately 60 mm Hg. In patients with coronary atherosclerosis, autoregulation may be lost at a higher perfusion pressure because of the pressure fall over a stenosis.[15] Delaney et al[16] compared the myocardial function of halothane and enflurane and concluded that both agents decrease arterial pressure, but by different mechanisms. Halothane decreases cardiac output and systemic vascular resistance (SVR), whereas enflurane decreases only SVR. Halothane increases both PCWP and central venous pressure (CVP), but enflurane does not, suggesting greater myocardial depression with halothane. Halothane decreases the contractile state, heart rate, and afterload and so presumably decreases MVO_2, while slightly increasing preload; on the other hand, enflurane reduces afterload only.[16]

Isoflurane. Isoflurane also is a halogenated ether. Ethers generally increase stability of cardiac rhythm. It has been reported that cardiac output is sustained with isoflurane by an increase in heart rate, which compensates for a reduction in stroke volume. This increase in heart rate is probably due to beta-adrenergic stimulation. Cardiac responses that occur with isoflurane represent an imbalance between autonomic sympathetic and parasympathetic influences on the heart.[17] Isoflurane causes depression of both preganglionic sympathetic and vagal nerve activity, with a greater effect on the vagus.[17] There is a marked decrease in pulmonary vascular resistance (PVR), with only a slight decline in mean arterial pressure. The sympathoadrenal responses associated with isoflurane are elevated plasma epinephrine levels in conjunction with increased heart rate and decreased plasma norepinephrine levels, with decreased SRV. The efficiency of the heart (the ratio of MVO_2 to external work) appears to be greater with enflurane and halothane than with isoflurane.[12] Because halothane decreases arterial pressure by reducing cardiac output without a decrease in PCWP, and isoflurane reduces arterial pressure by decreasing SVR, some authors feel that isoflurane is superior to halothane in controlling intraoperative hypertension.

Nitrous Oxide. Nitrous oxide can be used as a supplement to both inhalant and narcotic anesthetics. Generally, the depressant effects of nitrous oxide are mild; however, in the patient with poor cardiac performance, the degree of myocardial depression and hypotension can be severe. The use of nitrous oxide also carries the risk of expanding air spaces. If cardiac chambers or saphenous grafts are not devoid of air, these spaces can expand with the use of nitrous oxide. Nitrous oxide potentiates truncal rigidity induced by narcotic analgesics and limits the inspired oxygen concentration to the extent of its own concentration in the inspired gas mixture.[18]

Inhalation anesthetics do have disadvantages, the most severe of which is postoperative shivering, with a concurrent increase in oxygen demand, caused by heat loss from vasodilation. In addition, they provide very little analgesia in the postanesthesia period. A summary of the hemodynamic effects of inhalation agents is given in Table 41–5.

Intravenous Agents

The patient with poor ventricular function is unable to tolerate minimal myocardial depression. Anesthetic techniques based on the opiates as primary agents produce min-

TABLE 41–5. HEMODYNAMIC EFFECTS OF INHALATION AGENTS[a]

	Preload	Afterload	Contractility	CO	O₂ Consumption	MAP	HR	SVR	PCWP	CVP
Halothane (1.25 MAC)	↓	↓	↓	↓	↓	↓	↓	↓	↓	↑
Enflurane (1 MAC)	—	↓	↓	+↓	↓	↓	↑—	↓	—	↑
Isoflurane (2 MAC)	—	↓	↓	↓	↓	↓	↑	↓	—	—
Nitrous oxide (50%)	↑ —	↑	↓	↓	↓	—	—↓	↑	↑	—↑

[a] Note MAC differences.

CO, Cardiac output; CVP, central venous pressure; HR, heart rate; MAC, minimal alveolar concentration; MAP, mean arterial pressure; PCWP, pulmonary capillary wedge pressure; SVR, systemic vascular resistance.

imal cardiac depression and this remains popular for those patients with reduced myocardial function. The first narcotic to be used for these procedures was morphine sulfate. One major disadvantage to its use is histamine release, which produces some change in hemodynamic status. Morphine, although still in use, has given way in popularity to fentanyl, which is ten times more potent and produces less histamine release.

Fentanyl. Fentanyl was introduced in 1968 as the first synthetic morphinomimetic. At equianalgesic doses, side effects are minimal because fewer fentanyl molecules are available to reach sites other than intended opiate receptors. Protection against stress, more rapid recovery, and a shorter duration of respiratory depression are the major advantages of fentanyl. Fentanyl is highly lipophilic, rapidly penetrating cell membranes. Peak brain levels occur in minutes. With intravenous administration, the initial concentration of fentanyl in plasma is directly proportional to dose. The highest concentration is produced immediately but declines rapidly because of tissue uptake and biotransformation. Even though the plasma concentrations fall rapidly after a single injection, tissue concentration remains high. Because the tissues already contain some fentanyl, they take up a smaller proportion of subsequent doses during the distribution phase. Hence, plasma levels decline less during the distribution phase, and they remain above the threshold concentration for progressively longer times after each dose because of their slow decline during the elimination phase. Therefore, repeated intravenous bolus doses of the same size should produce progressively more intense and prolonged effects.[19]

When attenuation of the response to surgical stress is desired, doses of 50 to 100 µg/kg (0.05 to 0.1 mg/kg or 1 to 2 mL/kg) in an intravenous drip are administered with oxygen and a muscle relaxant until surgical planes are reached. The primary advantage of this technique is protection of the myocardium from excess oxygen demand. Some authors do report an increase in arterial pressure and SVR during stimulation, thus increasing the potential of myocardial ischemia. In doses of such magnitude, truncal rigidity can occur, and it is best to anticipate this side effect. There have been several reports documenting such large doses. It may be necessary to supplement with nitrous oxide or an inhalant at this time, not only to decrease the stress response but also to obliterate intraoperative awareness. Fentanyl decreases cardiac output and mean arterial pressure. There is no change in SVR. Fentanyl does not control hormonal releases while on pump. Elevated cortisol, antidiuretic hormone, and catecholamine levels have been reported.

Sufentanil. Sufentanil citrate, a synthetic opioid analgesic, is five to ten times as potent as fentanyl but has the same duration of action and a much greater margin of safety. Sufentanil has an immediate onset of action, with limited accumulation. There is rapid elimination from tissue storage, which allows for a more rapid recovery compared with fentanyl. Sufentanil decreases cortisol and antidiuretic hormone levels but produces the same effect on catecholamine as fentanyl. Dosage for coronary artery bypass procedures is 20 to 25 µg/kg. Recovery ranges from 3 to 6 hours.

De Lange et al[20] compared the effects of fentanyl with those of sufentanil for coronary artery surgery. Their study concluded that sufentanil had properties similar to those of fentanyl but, in addition, appeared more effective in preventing intraoperative hypertension and tachycardia, reducing MVO_2, and producing less postoperative depression, indicating that sufentanil provides greater protection against the stress response. Sufentanil increases the incidence of chest rigidity and this effect is proportional to the speed of administration. The recurrence of narcotics in the circulation during the recovery period has been reported. Causes of recurrence include elevated central nervous system activity and elevated plasma concentrations from intestinal reabsorption or shift from muscle to circulation.

Alfentanil. Alfentanil is a short-acting narcotic that is structurally related to fentanyl but with only one-third its potency and duration. The use of alfentanil during coronary artery surgery has been studied. Episodes of intraoperative hypertension, primarily during sternotomy or sternal spread, were common, probably because of the extremely short duration of action of alfentanil, suggesting that a continuous drip, supplementation with other agents, or both may be necessary to eliminate this hazard. Lofentanil is also an analgesic analog of fentanyl. It is 50 times more potent and has a long duration of action. It possesses strong respiratory depressant properties and for this reason is desirable when prolonged respiratory support is indicated. The desirability of its use in coronary artery surgery has not been confirmed.

The role of chronic propranolol therapy on cardiovascular dynamics and narcotic requirements has been studied. The findings suggest that patients on preoperative beta-blocking agents require less narcotic and supplements than those who are not. Also, these patients appeared to exhibit a lower incidence of hypertension and tachycardia than those not receiving beta-blocking drugs.[21]

EXTRACORPOREAL CIRCULATION AND CARDIOPULMONARY BYPASS

The ultimate objective of extracorporeal circulation in open heart surgery is to provide essentially normal organ perfusion while the surgeon has optimal conditions for cardiac procedures of indefinite duration.[22] The concept of extracorporeal circulation is more than 150 years old, but it was not until 1951 that it was used with open heart surgery.

Extracorporeal circulation involves the diversion of venous blood through an external device that returns the blood to the arterial side of the circulation. In its most advanced form, the device consists of a pump to provide the motive force, an oxygenator to add oxygen and remove carbon dioxide, a heat exchanger to promote hypothermia or normothermia, filters to trap bubbles and debris, and pressure transducers to monitor its function.[3] Basically, extracorporeal bypass reroutes all the blood returning to the right atrium away from the heart and lungs.

For total cardiopulmonary bypass, that is, when the lungs are completely bypassed, the entire systemic venous return to the heart must be collected and delivered to an oxygenator via gravity drainage. After heparinization, a 32-

and 36-French cannula or two 51-French single cannulas, depending on surgeon preference, are used to cannulate both the superior and inferior vena cava. Cannulation of the superior vena cava is performed using the right atrial appendage as access. The apex of the appendage is excised and the cannula introduced into the right atrium and directed into the superior vena cava approximately 2 to 3 cm. A similar procedure is used for the inferior vena cava. Once both cannulas are secured, they are connected to a ½-in. Y connector and then to a ½-in. venous tubing leading to the oxygenator. These cannulas are clamped during insertion of the aortic cannula.

Cannulation of the ascending aorta (antegrade flow) is the most common technique for patients undergoing total cardiopulmonary bypass; however, if previous surgery was performed, or if there are anatomic problems with the aorta, the femoral artery can then be cannulated (retrograde flow). If this method is used, perfusion to that extremity is minimal and complications secondary to decreased perfusion and retrograde flow can occur. The most common problem with femoral artery cannulation is dissection of the artery. When cannulating the ascending aorta for cardiopulmonary bypass, a vascular clamp first is applied longitudinally to the ascending aorta and an aortotomy is performed; the cannula is then inserted and secured. Air is evacuated from the cannula and from the arterial line leading to the pump. The clamps on the venous lines are released and blood flows by gravity to the oxygenator, which is a minimum of 30 cm below the level of the heart. After equilibrium between drainage and inflow is achieved, snares are applied to occlude blood flow to the lungs, and total bypass begins. The use of a sump suction to further empty the heart is optional. The time bypass began, mean pressure, CVP, temperature, arterial and venous gases, and activated clotting times should be recorded.

Principles of Cardiopulmonary Bypass

Equipment. The pump component of the extracorporeal circuit should provide the equivalent of a basal cardiac output. Early on, these were designed to provide a pulsatile flow imitating physiologic flow through the circulatory system; however, the size of the cannulas and connectors altered this flow, and as a result, the pulsing was ineffective. Consequently, pulsatile flow, although considered essential for long-term isolated organ perfusion, has not been thought to be essential for routine cardiopulmonary bypass.[23] To date, the use of a continuous-flow nonpulsatile pump is common. The roller head pumps are driven in a circular motion, milking the blood-filled pump tubing. This tubing is securely attached so that there is no net movement of the tubing. It is this compression of the tubing that drives the blood forward. These rollers may also be used to aspirate blood from the surgical field. Three to four pumps are necessary: one for arterial inflow, one to vent or empty the heart, and one to two to maintain a dry surgical field. Venous blood is drained by gravity. Figure 41–3 illustrates the pump roller head system and the entire cardiopulmonary bypass circuit.

The integrity of the red cell is usually well maintained with the roller pump because of the low-pressure nonturbulent flow. Red cell damage can be attributed to the negative pressure provided by the pump suction. Thus, the amount of hemolysis depends on the amount and duration of suction used. Tissue lysosomes and blood left in the pericardial cavity for prolonged periods also contribute to cell damage.[6]

The oxygenator not only supplies oxygen, as the name implies, but also eliminates carbon dioxide. Two main types of oxygenators are in existence today. The first is the bubble oxygenator, which provides a gas interface; the other is the membrane oxygenator, which lacks a gas interface. It should be mentioned that the membrane oxygenator is

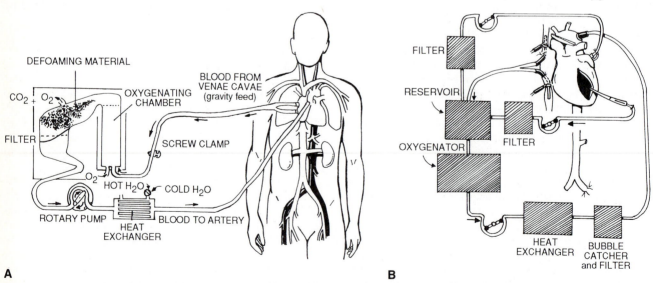

A **B**

Figure 41–3. A. Blood is drained from the vena cava by gravity. As it enters the oxygenator, a mixture of carbon dioxide and oxygen is implemented. The process of deforming, debubbling, heating, or cooling then occurs. Propulsion is obtained by a rotary pump, and the blood is returned antegrade via the aorta. **B.** Blood loss is kept to a minimum by returning all blood to a filtered cardiotomy reservoir via a pericardial suction vent to assist in further drainage of the heart.

somewhat more sophisticated and more physiologic because it causes less damage to red blood cells. Its main disadvantage is that it is not economical.

In the bubble oxygenator, ventilating gases, oxygen and carbon dioxide, are passed through multiple perforations in a diffusing plate, giving rise to bubbles that exit into the venous blood at the bottom of what is usually a columnar reservoir.[24] This produces turbulence, which drives the blood into a "debubbling section." The perforations in the diffusing plate and the bubble size are controlled so that bubbles are just the right size for appropriate gas transfer.

Oxygenation in the bubbler is not membrane limited as in the normal lung or membrane oxygenator but depends on the gas–blood surface contact area, the thickness of the film, the mean red cell transit time, and the partial pressure of oxygen used.[25] The gas–blood interface surface contact area is usually in the range of 15 m^2.[26] Large bubbles are used to provide a more efficient, thicker film. The red cells' mean transit time is usually 1 to 2 seconds (normally 0.1 to 0.75 second). Thus, the flow of gas should equal the flow of blood to allow for carbon dioxide elimination and oxygen uptake.

The bubble oxygenator, by means of gravity, conducts venous blood to the bottom of the reservoir where a stream of bubbles passes over it. The bubbles produce turbulence and froth, which increases the gas–bubble contact, leading to increased gas exchange. An exhalation port at the debubbling site allows for exhaust gases to escape, especially inhalation anesthetics. When gas exchange is complete, the blood descends into the heat exchanger and finally into the arterial system.

Oxygenators are ventilated with 100 percent oxygen, but controversy exists over the detrimental effects of such high oxygen tensions, suggesting that physiologic oxygen tensions are less traumatic with regard to enzyme systems and the degree of hemolysis.

In the membrane oxygenators, instead of the blood–gas interface, blood passes between layers of membrane with the gas phase on the other side. The membrane oxygenator is lobular because of its increased efficiency. There are two types, hollow fiber and microporous (thin Teflon or polypropylene sheets). Gas exchange through a membrane device is limited by the characteristics of the membrane and the degree of mixing of blood on either side.[26] Silicone membranes have carbon dioxide : oxygen transfer capacities of 5:1 to 6:1 rather than lower ratios and thus more closely resemble the lung.[6] There is less risk of disruption of red blood cell integrity; however, once again this is influenced by the rigorous nature of the sump suction and by pericardial suctioning.

Volatile anesthetic agents can be added to the oxygenators by incorporating a flow- and temperature-compensated vaporizer into the gas line. It should be kept in mind that hemodilution, hyperthermia, and low flows all alter the expected response, and concentrations must be adjusted accordingly.

The tubing used in the circuit should have the following characteristics. It should be clear, chemically inert, and pliable and should accommodate small priming volumes. In addition, it should be thrombus resistant. In essence, the tubes must withstand prolonged assault by the roller pump and also provide optimal physiologic conditions, such as minimal overhydration from priming solutions and safety from thrombi formation.

The filter, placed on the arterial side, is designed to trap the smallest of particles. This may include red blood cells, platelets, and leukocytes, fat, silicone, air, and any other debris. The introduction of filters has contributed significantly to the reduction of organ dysfunction.

The heat exchanger is a system in which blood and water (housed in a stainless-steel or aluminum container) flow in opposite directions. The cooling and warming are provided by a hot and cold water system that changes the temperature of the blood as it passes over it. The pump flow rates vary somewhat from team to team, with an average rate of about 2400 mL/m^2 per minute. This is roughly 50 to 70 mL/kg per minute. Although the tissue oxygen need may be considered the most basic requirement, it is calculated in terms of blood flow. Basal cardiac output is approximately 3000 mL/m^2 of body surface per minute. This provides for a full oxygen uptake at an average arteriovenous oxygen difference of about 4.4 volume percent.[22] If blood flow is low, blood flow redistribution with resultant ischemia to some organs may occur. Therefore, the adequacy of extracorporeal flow should be determined by monitoring blood gases and acid–base balance.

Priming. Solutions used to prime the heart–lung machine vary with the institution. Some use a dextrose and water solution; others use a balanced electrolyte solution with a plasma expander, such as dextran or hetastarch, and an osmotic diuretic like mannitol. Hetastarch is an artificial colloid derived from amylopectin with colloidal properties similar to those of albumin. An all-blood priming solution may still be used in a few institutions. The total amount of solution ranges between 1500 and 2400 mL and should be as close to extracellular fluid composition as possible so as not to increase the patient's metabolic requirement. It is believed that the priming solutions that provide hemodilution are most physiologic.

The trend is to add blood only if the patient is severely anemic, having the circuit maintain only a 30 to 40 percent blood volume of the patient. The hematocrit levels should not be below 20 to 25 percent because lower values result in severe hypotension caused by changes in blood viscosity. A reduction in oxygen-carrying capacity accompanies hematocrit reduction; however, this is compensated for by the use of hypothermia during bypass.

Hemodilution does not proceed without some ill effects. Oncotic pressure changes, caused by alterations in serum protein, can expand the extracellular fluid compartment. This is in accordance with Starling's hypothesis that fluid balance (absence of flow in either direction) is achieved when osmotic and hydrostatic forces at the compartment membrane are equal. If these are not equal, fluid moves in the direction of the superior force.

Changes in electrolyte values can occur. Low serum potassium levels are a common occurrence, partly because of hyperventilation. Serum potassium levels should be monitored frequently during cardiopulmonary bypass. Reductions in calcium, magnesium, phosphate, and zinc can accompany hemodilution. Changes in calcium levels may be significant in altering mean arterial pressure, and calcium administration may be necessary to overcome hypotension, particularly at the outset of perfusion.

Anticoagulation. Heparin should always be administered through a well-functioning central line. Heparin works by producing a thrombin–antithrombin complex, which in the presence of the cofactor deactivates thrombin. Heparin is protein bound and thus is readily distributed in the plasma volume. The effects of heparin vary from individual to individual both in onset and in half-life. Factors that affect the pharmacologic action of heparin are age, body temperature, and lean body mass.

The method of calculation of heparin dosage is still a matter of controversy. Some institutions use a fixed-dose technique, that is, 3 to 4 mg/kg or 90 mg/m^2; others use a dose–response method based on the activated clotting time (ACT). Calculation by the dose–response method appears to be more accurate and is used by the majority of institutions today. This method allows for individualized heparin and protamine dosage calculations. A baseline ACT is drawn prior to heparin administration and immediately after administration and every 15 to 30 minutes thereafter.

The procedure for constructing and using the dose–response curve is illustrated in Figure 41–4. As depicted, the heparin dose in mg/kg is on the vertical axis and the ACT in seconds is on the horizontal axis. Three graphs are plotted: (1) the preheparin ACT, (2) the ACT immediately postheparin, and (3) the ACT prior to protamine administration. By plotting the curves, dosages can be determined, eliminating excessive anticoagulation or heparin reversal.[27] The ACT, drawn every 15 to 30 minutes, should have a value above 480. If not, additional heparin should be given. It should be remembered that the ACT is temperature and heparin dependent, so during the hypothermic period and with hemodilution, the ACT may increase unreliably; however, if the bypass procedure does not exceed 2 or 3 hours, additional heparin should not be necessary. The rapid infusion of crystalloid with resultant hemodilution can significantly lengthen ACT. The effect is usually transient, lasting only the first 30 minutes of bypass.[27]

The dosage for heparin reversal with protamine sulfate is also determined by the ACT. Because of its hypotensive tendency, protamine should be given slowly, over a 30-minute period, and not before stability of vital signs is ensured. The current practice of protamine administration is to administer smaller doses over a longer period. It is suggested that this dose should be less than the first heparin dose. Successive doses may be administered if necessary. Protamine injection should be slow to avoid a hypotensive episode. This decline in arterial pressure may be associated with the release of vasoactive drugs such as histamine and serotonin. Severe anaphylactic reactions have been documented with protamine administration.

On Bypass. Once the circuit has been primed, the patient appropriately heparinized, and surgical access attained, bypass commences. The anesthetist immediately notes and records ACT levels, mean arterial pressure, heart rate, uri-

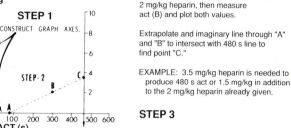

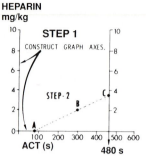

STEP 2

Determine initial act (A) and administer 2 mg/kg heparin, then measure act (B) and plot both values.

Extrapolate and imaginary line through "A" and "B" to intersect with 480 s line to find point "C."

EXAMPLE: 3.5 mg/kg heparin is needed to produce 480 s act or 1.5 mg/kg in addition to the 2 mg/kg heparin already given.

STEP 3

After required heparin has been given, measure act. Plot point "D."
If point "D" does not superimpose on point "C," then a dose response curve is drawn from "A" to a point midway between "C" and "D."

STEP 4

After 60 min, measure the act. Determine amount of heparin in patient's circulation from the dose response curve.

EXAMPLE: Assume an act of 350 s: The heparin level would be 2.8 mg/kg. To return to 480 s, 1.2 mg/kg of heparin is needed.

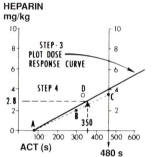

STEP 5

To reverse anticoagulation circulating heparin level is determined as in STEP 4. The neutralizing dose of protamine is heparin level mg/kg x 1.3.

EXAMPLE: Act of 325 s is measured. Heparin level 2.6 mg/kg, and 3.4 mg/kg protamine is required.

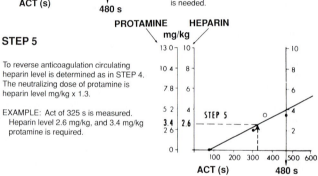

Figure 41–4. Dose–response curve for heparin and protamine dosage calculations. ACT, activated clotting time. (*Reprinted, with permission, from Bull et al.*[27(p686)])

nary output, and CVP. Depth of anesthesia, degree of muscle relaxation, and pupil size should also be evaluated.

The perfusionist and anesthetist must work very closely to maintain desired hemodynamics. If drug administration is necessary, it is done via the pump. Drugs needed would most likely be additional heparin, anesthetic, vasopressor, and a vasodilator. Mean atrial pressure is usually maintained between 60 and 80 torr. Increases or decreases can be altered by changes in flow or alterations in total peripheral resistance, as mean pressure equals cardiac output times total peripheral resistance.

Pump flow is maintained at 2 to 2.5 L/min per square meter of body surface area (BSA) but can be varied according to blood gases or temperature. The CVP should be very low or at zero when on bypass. The CVP catheter should be placed in the superior vena cava above the venous return line so that obstructed venous return from the head can be determined,[22] because persistent elevated venous pressure can lead to cerebral edema. PCWP, pulmonary artery pressure, and left atrial pressure also should be at zero. Elevations suggest left ventricle distension. If the pulmonary artery pressure rises above 15 mm Hg while on bypass, there is cause for concern. Appropriate measures must be taken to decompress distended ventricles.

The patient's urinary output during bypass should be maintained above 1 mL/kg per hour. Careful observation should be made for hemolysis of red blood cells. If this is noted, the urinary output should be maintained at a higher level with diuretics or by alkalinization with tromethamine or bicarbonate; however, with the hybrid oxygenators in use today, hemolysis is seldom seen.

Several blood studies are performed routinely during cardiopulmonary bypass, usually at 15-minute intervals. These include arterial blood gases, hematocrit, venous oxygen, electrolytes, blood sugar in diabetics, and ACT. The hematocrit is maintained between 20 and 30 percent. Arterial gases should be at normal range while on bypass. Venous P_{O_2}, obtained from the oxygenator, ranges from 40 to 45 torr. Causes of abnormal values were discussed above. Electrolyte values can change abruptly because of hemodilution and the use of cardioplegic solutions that are hyperkalemic. Any alterations in electrolytes should be remedied.

Revascularization of coronary arteries requires a quiet, dry operative field. Many methods can be used to stop heart motion. A normal contracting myocardium can be slowed or fibrillated by core and topical cooling. If spontaneous fibrillation does not occur, this can be achieved by electric current, but is best avoided because of increased oxygen consumption and possible muscle destruction.

The most commonly used method of obtaining circulatory arrest of the heart is aortic cross-clamping. This procedure produces a static heart with no flow through its arteries. The disadvantage of aortic cross-clamping is anoxia to the myocardium. The time frame for anoxia can be reduced under the hypothermic conditions produced by core and surface cooling. Oschner and Mills state 7 minutes of core cooling, achieved by progressively lowering the perfusate temperature in increments of 1, 2, and 3 minutes, and concomitant surface cooling with a cold isotonic solution at 7C probably allows more than 40 minutes of myocardial protection.[28]

Hypothermia. Adequate myocardial preservation remains the key determinant of successful cardiac procedures. Although myocardial ischemia can occur at any time intraoperatively, the most common cause is inadequate preservation during cardiopulmonary bypass. One of the key elements in maintaining myocardial protection is maintaining myocardial temperature below 15C during ischemic arrest. This is accomplished by systemic hypothermia plus the direct application of cold cardioplegia.

The heart is relatively more active metabolically at any given temperature level than other major organs, including the brain. The working myocardial cell maintains a high coupling between energy production and energy utilization; thus adenosine triphosphate (ATP) is produced relative to need, whereas oxygen and substrate are consumed in the precise amounts needed to resynthesize ATP. In the normal myocardial cell, the three main reactions using ATP are (1) myosin ATPase involvement in the development of wall tension, (2) calcium and magnesium ATPase involvement in the sequestration of calcium that is liberated from the sar-

coplasmic reticulum in the activation of contractile protein, and (3) sodium plus potassium ATPase involvement in sodium efflux.[29]

Approximately 50 to 60 mol of ATP is produced per minute per gram of heart during these three reactions; the value increases tenfold during moderate cardiac effort.[29] A reduced flux of adenosine diphosphate (ADP) in the mitochondria is associated with reduced flux of citric acid cycle intermediates, high citrate levels (which inhibit glycolysis), high levels of nicotinamide adenine dinucleotide (NADH) (as electron transport is slowed), and elevated acetyl-CoA levels, resulting in a limiting effect on fatty acid beta oxidation. During cardioplegia, glucose utilization and pyruvate dehydrogenase activity are decreased, so metabolite formation is inhibited.

The production of systemic hypothermia decreases oxygen consumption and metabolic requirements. It has been estimated that oxygen consumption is decreased by 50 percent at 30C and 85 percent at 20C. Profound hypothermia is provided by perfusing cold blood, followed by the infusion of a cold cardioplegic solution and then topical cooling. Perfusion cooling is performed rapidly, dropping the temperature to 22C or 25C. Once the heart fibrillates, the aorta is cross-clamped and cardioplegic infusion into the aortic root is begun at 4C and a volume of 10 mL/kg. In addition, the heart is bathed in a cold solution at 4C.

Although these methods are very successful in reducing myocardial consumption, they are not without side effects. Hypothermia causes several physiologic manifestations. There is a reduction of 6.7 percent in cerebral blood flow for each degree of temperature decrease.[3] Nerve impulse conduction and neuromuscular transmission are reduced, thus affecting the dosages of muscle relaxant. (Nondepolarizing drug dosage should be decreased.) The oxyhemoglobin curve shifts to the left; thus the partial pressure of oxygen in tissues must fall before hemoglobin gives up oxygen. Systemic blood pressure decreases. Renal blood flow is decreased, with a concomitant decrease in urinary output. Splanchnic flow is impaired, resulting in decreased drug metabolism. Clotting factors are impaired, and hypothermia increases blood viscosity.

Chemical cardioplegia protects the myocardium against inadequate cooling. The cardioplegic solution must be at 2C to 4C to be effective. The composition of chemical cardioplegic solutions varies somewhat, but most often the agent responsible for cardioplegia is potassium chloride in concentrations of 12 to 30 mEq/L. Table 41–6 lists various solutions in use.

The use of cardioplegic solutions is based on the following principles:

- Rapid asystole to prevent breakdown of high-energy phosphate groups
- Hypothermia to lower energy demands without inducing cold injury
- Membrane stabilization to prevent breakdown of sodium–potassium and calcium membrane pumps
- Hyperosmolarity to prevent intracellular edema
- Acid buffering to counteract intracellular acidosis from anaerobic metabolism[29]

TABLE 41–6. VARIOUS CARDIOPLEGIC SOLUTIONS IN USE

Solutions		Components		Quantities	
Sodium	120.0 mEq	Lactated Ringer's	1000 mL	Lactated Ringer's	1000 mL
Potassium chloride	16.0 mEq	Potassium chloride	20 mEq	Potassium chloride	25.0 mEq
Magnesium	32.0 mEq	Procainamide	1 g	Sodium chloride	152.0 mEq
Calcium	2.4 mEq	Dextrose 50%	30 mL	Magnesium sulfate	20.0 mEq
Chloride	160.0 mEq	Regular insulin	20 U	Calcium chloride	4.5 mEq
Sodium bicarbonate	10.0 mEq			Dextrose	2.0 g
				Sodium bicarbonate	25.0 mEq

Rapid asystole is produced by potassium chloride. Potassium causes asystole during diastole by depolarizing the cell membrane. The amount of potassium required to produce asystole appears to be directly proportional to the myocardial temperature.[29] Hyperosmolarity (provided by glucose or mannitol) in the range 350 to 400 mOsm appears to combat myocardial swelling associated with the sodium ion shifts secondary to ischemia during aortic cross-clamping.[29] Buffers such as tromethamine, bicarbonate, and histidine are necessary to overcome the effects of inhibited glycolysis, thus allowing some ATP formation, and to prevent decreased enzymatic activity caused by variant pH ranges.

Once myocardial temperature reaches 10C to 12C, asystole occurs within seconds. Myocardial temperature and ECG activity must be monitored so as to recognize increases in metabolic demands caused by an upward shift in temperature. These values are checked every 15 to 20 minutes and reinfusion of cardioplegic solution is begun if necessary, usually at the completion of each distal anastomosis. Clinical studies indicate that despite the infusion of large volumes of hyperkalemic cardioplegic solution, serum potassium levels rarely exceed 5.5 mEq/L because increased urinary excretion of potassium rapidly compensates for the exogenous administration.[29]

Some problems that may occur during chemical cardioplegia administration include a solution that is not cold enough, insufficient delivery to the myocardium because of valvular disease or coronary artery stenosis, and heat gain from environmental influences. Some studies have also demonstrated nonhomogenous cooling, incomplete protection, and delayed reperfusion when significant coronary stenosis is present. It is wise to use a myocardial temperature probe to monitor temperature to be certain that the solution is achieving proper cooling.

There are some proponents of cold-blood cardioplegia who urge that this technique provides oxygenation and substrate delivery during aortic cross-clamping. Blood cardioplegia should be administered at 20C; otherwise, red cell sludging and possible activation of cold agglutinins can occur. (Patients should have a cold agglutinin test preoperatively if blood cardioplegia is used.) Studies have determined that the myocardial preservation is equivalent to that provided by crystalloid solutions; however, patients with abnormal left ventricular function (ejection fraction below 40 percent) or prolonged aortic cross-clamp seem to have more favorable results with cold blood than crystalloid. It must be emphasized that the temperature must be 20C because lower temperatures interfere with oxygen delivery.[30]

Revascularization. The approach to revascularization depends on coronary artery distribution, that is, whether or not there is left dominance, right dominance, or a balanced system. With right coronary dominance, circulation is provided to both right and left ventricles posteriorly and to the interventricular septum via a descending artery. With left dominance, the posterior left ventricle and interventricular septum are supplied by the circumflex. With a balanced system, one descending branch from each coronary provides the circulation. There is no limit to the number of bypass grafts that can be performed, but the most frequent is the triple bypass, that is, to the right coronary artery, to the LAD artery, and to the obtuse marginal branch of the circumflex artery. This should supply enough blood flow to the left ventricle and interventricular septum.

The greater saphenous vein is preferred for supplying graft material and is prepared as the sternum is being opened. Once the site of anastomosis is determined and the graft cut to size, the distal end is sewn, followed then by the proximal end of each graft. Air should be evacuated from the grafts as the clamp on the aorta is released.

Once revascularization has been completed, the patient is rewarmed. Approximately 5 minutes before aortic clamp removal, the perfusion temperature is raised to 30C. After the clamp is removed, the temperature is raised to 38C and the room is warmed. Bypass continues until the esophageal temperature is 37C.

Removal of the aortic clamp allows oxygen, blood, and substrate to fill the myocardium. During aortocoronary bypass, myocardial ATP levels may be very high, but once the heart starts its own beat, the ATP levels fall rapidly, probably because of energy requirements for contraction.

There has been some evidence that mitochondrial distortion may occur after reperfusion to ischemic hearts. Possible causes of this injury include loss of magnesium and increase in mitochondrial calcium uptake, decrease in ATP levels critical to enzymatic performance, accumulation of long-chain fatty acid acetyl-CoA esters, and loss of critical enzymes from the postischemic cell.[29]

Usually, once the patient's temperature reaches 37C, the heart will resume its normal beat. If not, the patient is defibrillated. Pump flow is gradually reduced, and arterial pressure, ECG, and heart size are carefully watched. The adequacy of volume replacement is usually determined by each of these parameters, plus left atrial pressure, central venous blood gases, acid–base status, and serum potassium levels. Because of the large volumes of cardioplegic solution, it may be necessary to give sodium bicarbonate or calcium chloride through the pump to resume myocardial function.

Withdrawal from cardiopulmonary bypass should be slow (approximately 15 to 20 minutes) and stability of vital signs sustained before cannulas are removed. Reinstitution of anesthetic agents and muscle relaxants may be necessary at this time. Depressant agents should be avoided as should nitrous oxide because of air embolism potentials.

As cardiovascular dynamics are restored, reversal of anticoagulation is instituted. The protamine dosage is calculated according to the dose–response curve described earlier. At this time, the sump tubing should be removed so as not to suction protamine into the remaining pump volume.

Postvascularization. Low output states may be present after revascularization procedures. Symptoms include low arterial pressure and cardiac output. Initial treatment should be a fluid challenge to determine if hypovolemia is the underlying cause. If cardiac output does not increase with adequate preload, left ventricular failure must be assumed, provided normal pH, Pa_{CO_2}, and cardiac rhythm exist.

The pharmacologic treatment of ventricular failure is twofold: (1) reduce the workload of the heart and (2) increase myocardial contractility.[9]

There are relatively standard regimens of drug administration for the patient who does not wean from bypass easily. As previously noted, there are four major determinants of myocardial performance: preload, afterload, heart rate, and contractility or the inotropic state. Preload and inotropic properties determine myocardial contractile performance, whereas afterload and heart rate are mechanical factors that affect myocardial performance.[31]

Circulatory supportive measures should be directed at alterations in ventricular preload, ventricular afterload, or ventricular contractility. In discussion of preload, several terms can be used interchangeably. *Preload* refers to the venous side of the circulatory system. It is synonymous with left ventricular volume. Other terms that correlate with preload are left ventricular end-diastolic pressure (LVEDP) and diastolic filling pressure. When calculating preload, one is essentially measuring left atrial pressure or capillary wedge pressure. The normal value is 14 to 16 mm Hg. Preload is, therefore, determined by Swan–Ganz catheter or left atrial pressure.

Afterload, on the other hand, reflects the arterial side of the circulatory system and is synonymous with resistance, that is, how much effort the ventricle must work against to obtain a functional cardiac output. Afterload, or systemic vascular resistance (SVR), is also calculated by means of a Swan-Ganz catheter. In determining SVR, it must be remembered that the CVP is measured in centimeters of water and must be changed to millimeters of mercury. (To convert cm H_2O to mm Hg, multiply the CVP by 10 and then divide by 13.)

Referring to Starling's law, a maximally dilated ventricle will eject the entire volume that it holds, so whether the volume be 10 mL or 200 mL, it will be totally ejected, provided the heart can do so. The cardiac output, or left ventricular ejection volume, is altered by (1) a failing ventricle that lacks enough force to pump, (2) aortic resistance that the ventricle must overcome (SVR), or (3) volume depletion.

It is essential to know the underlying pathophysiology

behind the decreased cardiac output before treatment is instituted so as not to complicate the problem. A failing left ventricle, that is, one with poor contractile properties, is best treated with an inotropic agent such as epinephrine, dobutamine, or isoproterenol. The inotrope should be selected on the basis of its pulmonary effects. Norepinephrine dramatically increases pulmonary artery pressure and pulmonary vascular resistance, whereas isoproterenol or dobutamine reduces pulmonary artery pressure and pulmonary vascular resistance.

Aortic resistance, or afterload, is best decreased by the use of a vasodilator such as nitroglycerin that decreases SVR and concomitantly increases stroke volume. Alterations of aortic pressure affect cardiac function because of the resistance it places on the left ventricle during emptying. These aortic pressure changes result in changes in strength and duration of the left ventricular ejection and stroke volume.

If the cardiac output is low because of volume depletion (decreased preload), then volume expanders are used judiciously. If preload is increased, treatment with a vasodilator, a diuretic, or both is also recommended.

Post Bypass

The incidence of abnormality in heart rate and rhythm is common at the end of cardiopulmonary bypass. Table 41–7 lists the therapeutic interventions for various arrhythmias.[30] Low output states may be present after cardiac procedures. Symptoms include low arterial pressure and low cardiac output. Initial treatment should be a fluid challenge to determine if hypovolemia is the underlying cause. If cardiac output does not increase with adequate preload provided normal pH, Pa_{CO_2} and cardiac rhythm exist, left ventricular failure must be assumed.[32] Table 41–8 lists the pathologic effects on cardiac dynamics.

Vasodilating Drugs. Vasodilators are able to improve cardiac performance because of their ability to dilate peripheral arteries and veins. Five factors that determine the hemodynamic and clinical responses to vasodilator drugs have been identified: (1) the direct vascular effects of the drug; (2) the activation of endogenous neurohumoral mechanisms by peripheral vasodilation; (3) the response of the left ventricle to a decrease in venous return and peripheral resistance; (4) the regional distribution of the improved peripheral blood flow; and (5) the physiologic response during exercise. It is obvious that vasodilator therapy is successful only after careful scrutiny of the patient's pathophysiologic condition. Treatment must be individualized to each patient's specific cardiac performance.

Perioperative hypertension is a common phenomenon that is associated with coronary artery bypass as well as other types of vascular operations, particularly carotid endarterectomies and aortic aneurysm resections. Hypertension is usually defined as blood pressure that exceeds 20 percent of the patient's normal range during hospitalization.

As previously discussed, control of intraoperative hypertension must be a major concern in patients who have myocardial dysfunction. Kaplan and Jones[33] have found this is best accomplished with nitroglycerin. Their studies conclude that the use of nitroglycerin has several advantages

TABLE 41-7. THERAPY OF ABNORMAL HEART RATE AND RHYTHM AT END OF CARDIOPULMONARY BYPASS

Diagnosis	Therapeutic Steps
Asystole or heart block resulting from potassium cardioplegia, surgery (trauma to nodal and conducting tissue or preoperative pathophysiology)	Calcium chloride 1–2 g Sodium bicarbonate 50 mEq Insulin 10 units regular ± glucose 25 g Pacemaker: atrial, ventricular, atrioventricular sequential Temporary epicardial pacing wires for postoperative use Isoproterenol 1–10 µg/min Atropine, incremental doses up to total of 2–2.5 mg/70 kg over 5–10 minutes
Supraventricular tachyarrhythmia	Increase core temperature to 37C Correct arterial pH, Pco_2, and hematocrit Correct electrolyte abnormalities (K^+, Mg^{2+}) Cardioversion (internal paddles, 5–10 watt-seconds) Overdrive atrial pacing Ouabain 0.1–0.2 mg or digoxin 0.25–1.0 mg Propranolol 0.5–3 mg, esmolol 25–75 mg bolus, 5–200 µg/kg per minute infusion Check position of central venous pressure or other monitoring catheters
Recurrent ventricular tachycardia or fibrillation	Increase core temperature to 37C Correct arterial pH, Pco_2, Po_2, and hematocrit Correct electrolyte abnormalities (K^+, Mg^{2+}) Defibrillation (internal paddles, 10–60 watt-seconds) Lidocaine 1–2 mg/kg bolus, 3–4 mg/min infusion Maintain satisfactory blood pressure, pulmonary artery pressure, and cardiac output Check position of pulmonary artery catheter

Reprinted, with permission, from Ream.[49]

over the use of nitroprusside, and is the drug of choice in 90 percent of their bypass procedures. Kaplan also suggests that use of nitroglycerin during cardiopulmonary bypass is less effective in reducing blood pressure in hypertensive patients than in normotensive patients and that additional doses may be required to lower mean pressure.[8] Nitroglycerin is especially useful in patients with increased PCWP and hypotension; however, if the nitroglycerin brings about an excessive decline in systemic pressure, then simultaneous supplemental doses of phenylephrine can be used.[34]

The use of intravenous nitroglycerin is advantageous to the anesthetist because of ease of titration and ability to control hemodynamic parameters. The most frequent use is for acute hypertension. During valvular surgery, nitroglycerin is useful in the treatment of pulmonary hypertension or to reduce systemic afterload.[8]

TABLE 41-8. PATHOPHYSIOLOGIC EFFECTS ON CARDIAC INDEX, RIGHT ATRIAL PRESSURE, AND PULMONARY CAPILLARY WEDGE PRESSURE

	Cardiac Index	Right Atrial Pressure	Pulmonary Capillary Wedge Pressure
Normal	2.3–3.5	1–5 mm Hg	6–12 mm Hg
Hypovolemia	↓	↓	↓
Pump or heart failure	↓	↑	↑
Tamponade	↓	↑	↑

Failure to Terminate Cardiopulmonary Bypass

Intraaortic Balloon Pump. If termination of cardiopulmonary bypass remains impossible after the administration of various drug combinations, insertion of an intraaortic balloon pump (IABP) may be necessary to provide circulatory support with minimal increase in afterload.

The use of the IABP had its inception in 1969 to treat patients with left ventricular failure. Technical advances and catheter simplification have expanded its use to patients suffering from myocardial ischemia. The two primary effects of IABP therapy are increased coronary perfusion and decreased afterload. Reduction of afterload is achieved during counterpulsation by deflating the IABP prior to ventricular ejection.

The IABP is used frequently after open heart surgery to enhance ventricular function, after acute myocardial infarction, and in cardiogenic shock secondary to myocardial infarction.

The intraaortic balloon is usually inserted via the femoral artery and positioned with the tip of the balloon just below the subclavian artery and its base just above the renal arteries. The balloon, once properly positioned, is then connected to a gas-driven pump, which inflates and deflates the balloon at different phases of systole and diastole (Fig. 41–5).

When appropriately set, that is, when the timing of inflation and deflation is correct, the balloon serves to augment myocardial oxygenation and reduce cardiac workload. Therefore, coronary perfusion is increased and afterload decreased. To understand the theory behind the use of intraaortic balloon therapy, the cardiac cycle must be understood. Figure 41–6 demonstrates the normal cardiac cycle. The most common method of activating the pump is

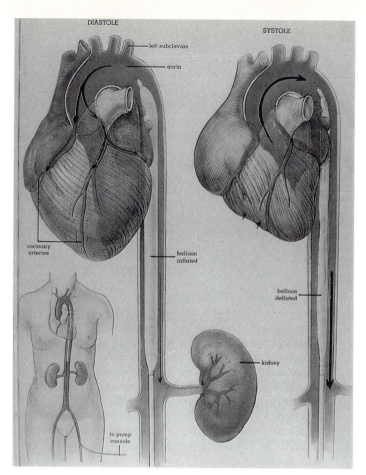

Figure 41–5. The balloon should inflate at the beginning of diastole–aortic valve closure. The balloon should deflate just prior to systole to allow the left ventricle to eject blood without interference. (*Reprinted, with permission, from Purcell J, Pippin L, et al. IAPB therapy. Am J Nurs.* 1983; 83(5):788.)

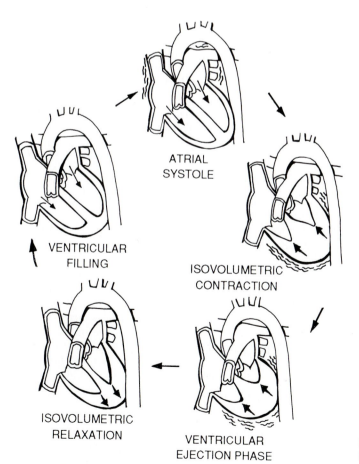

Figure 41–6. The cardiac cycle. (Courtesy of the Datascope Corporation.)

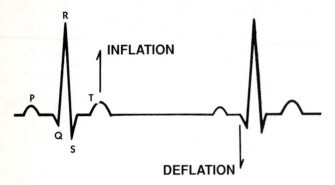

Figure 41–7. Electrocardiogram (ECG) demonstrating optimal inflation and deflation timing. The ECG lead should be one that maximizes R-waves and minimizes other wave forms. (*Reprinted, with permission, from Purcell J, Pippin L, et al. IAPB therapy. Am J Nurs. 1983;83(5):778.*)

to trigger the machine according to the R-wave on an ECG. The pump inflates the balloon in the middle of the T-wave or diastole, and deflates just prior to the QRS complex, or systole. Figure 41–7 shows an ECG with inflation and deflation patterns. Because systole and diastole cannot be observed from an ECG, an arterial waveform must be used. Balloon inflation (diastolic augmentation) should occur at the beginning of diastole, which occurs on the dicrotic notch when arterial pressure is being measured at the aortic root. Diastolic augmentation should exceed or at least equal the patient's systolic pressure.

Deflation should occur during the time of isovolumetric contraction, that is, the beginning of systole, prior to opening of the aortic valve. During isovolumetric contraction, the left ventricle must overcome aortic root end-diastolic pressure before it can eject its volume. Because deflation occurs just prior to systole, blood fills the area vacated by the deflated balloon, decreasing aortic root end-diastolic pressure. The ventricle does not need to work as hard to empty, and peak ventricular systolic pressure is reduced (Figs. 41–8 and 41–9).

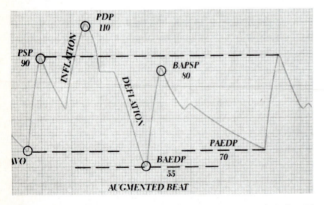

Figure 41–8. Changes in arterial pressure associated with properly timed balloon inflation and deflation. AVO, aortic valve opening; BAPSP, balloon-assisted peak systolic pressure; BAEP, balloon-assisted end-diastolic pressure; PAEDP, patient's aortic end-diastolic pressure; PDP, peak diastolic pressure; PSP, peak systolic pressure. (*Reprinted, with permission, from Purcell J, Pippin L, Mitchell M. IAPB therapy. Am J Nurs. 1983;83(5):778.*)

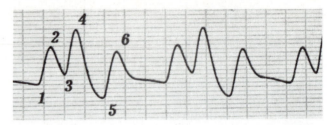

Figure 41–9. **1.** Aortic valve opening (unassisted end-diastolic pressure). **2.** Peak systolic pressure (unassisted). **3.** Dicrotic notch (balloon inflation). **4.** Maximum pressure generated by balloon. **5.** End-diastolic pressure associated with balloon deflation (assisted end-diastolic pressure). **6.** Peak systolic pressure assisted by balloon (assisted systolic pressure). (*Reprinted, with permission, from Purcell J, Pippin L, Mitchell M. IAPB therapy. Am J Nurs. 1983;83(5):779.*)

The use of IABP therapy is not without complications. Limb ischemia occurs in 4 to 8 percent of the patients. Excessive bleeding may occur at the insertion site. Thrombocytopenia with a rapid decrease in platelets is also seen. Catheter migration is common.

Ventricular Assist Device. Occasionally the heart does not function optimally with drugs and IABP. Devices that pump blood and bypass either ventricle are necessary. The impairment of cardiac function is usually temporary and is the myocardial response to the surgical insult. Ventricular support allows the heart time to revive. Very often, mechanical support for one ventricle unmasks unrecognized failure in the other, necessitating additional intervention.[35]

SURGICAL REPAIR OF VALVULAR HEART DISEASE

Valvular heart disease in its earliest stages is identified by a murmur. Most murmurs are caused by obstruction or regurgitation in a cardiac valve. Obstruction, as evidenced in aortic stenosis, produces a pressure overload, whereas mitral or aortic regurgitation produces a volume overload.

Indications for Valve Replacement

The proper selection of patients about to undergo valvular surgery must be made with the patient's history in mind. Clearly, those patients who have aortic stenosis and suddenly develop symptoms should be operated on immediately to avoid rapid deterioration and high mortality. Braunwald[2] suggests that a drop in the mortality rate of patients with aortic stenosis from 50 to 5 percent or less has been achieved with timely aortic valve replacement. Patients with aortic regurgitation may have severe left ventricular dysfunction and yet be devoid of symptoms, so it is imperative that these patients be evaluated frequently to determine the best time for replacement. Generally speaking, cardiac catheterization is indicated in patients with LVEDP exceeding 5 mm Hg or more on two successive echocardiograms and replacement is recommended at this time because the majority of patients usually develop symptoms in 2 to 3 years.[36]

In patients with mitral regurgitation, the presence of symptoms is a strong indication that replacement may be necessary. The degree of ventricular dysfunction may be misleading in these patients. If the ejection fractions are evaluated, a moderate reduction may indicate significant dysfunction. The full extent of the dysfunction may be apparent only postoperatively when the afterload imposed on the left ventricle increases as mitral competence is restored. Mortality rates higher than average should be expected for patients with advanced left ventricular dysfunction, as well as for those undergoing mitral valve replacement on emergency basis, such as patients with ruptured chordae tendinae caused by bacterial endocarditis, mitral valve prolapse, trauma, postinfarction rupture of a papillary muscle, or intractable infective endocarditis.[37]

Mitral stenosis, on the other hand, is not as rapidly progressive as regurgitation and can be treated medically for long periods. If possible, commissurotomy should take preference to replacement if surgery is required. Replacement is required if the valvular opening is significantly reduced.

Aortic Regurgitation

Approximately three fourths of all patients with pure aortic regurgitation are males. The disease is caused primarily by rheumatic fever, which causes shortened valve cusps resulting in improper closure during diastole. It is also a result of endocarditis or ascending aortic aneurysms.

Pathophysiology. In contrast to mitral regurgitation, in which a fraction of the left ventricular stroke volume is delivered into the low-pressure left atrium, in aortic regurgitation the entire left ventricular stroke volume must be ejected into a high-pressure zone, the aorta.[38] Although the low aortic diastolic pressure facilitates ventricular emptying during early systole, an increase in the left ventricular end-diastolic volume constitutes the major hemodynamic compensation of aortic regurgitation, and the total stroke volume is augmented primarily through the operation of the Frank Starling mechanism.[38]

Aortic insufficiency results in ventricular hypertrophy and dilation (Fig. 41–10). As left ventricular function diminishes, the ejection fraction and stroke volume decrease. There is a decreased aortic diastolic pressure and shortened isovolumetric contraction. Cardiac output is reduced slightly and pulmonary wedge, arterial, and left atrial pressures are elevated. Coronary perfusion is decreased and myocardial ischemia ensues.

Symptoms. The interval between the first episode of acute rheumatic fever and the development of hemodynamically significant aortic regurgitation averages approximately 7 years, and this period is followed by an asymptomatic interval of approximately 10 to 20 years, during which the severity of the regurgitation usually increases.[38] Symptoms include palpitations, sinus tachycardia, and premature ventricular beats. Dyspnea, orthopnea, and diaphoresis are common, along with symptoms of left ventricular failure (Table 41–9). Angina, unaffected by nitroglycerin, is common to advanced stages as is systemic fluid retention.

Surgical intervention must be instituted at the appropri-

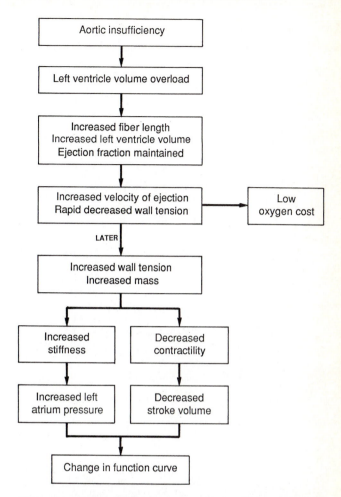

Figure 41–10. Pathophysiology of aortic insufficiency. LA, left atrium; LV, left ventricle. (*Reprinted, with permission, from Thomas SJ, Lowenstein E. Anesthetic management of the patient with valvular heart disease,* Int Anesthesiol Clin. *1979;17:67.*)

ate time. It should be considered in patients with symptom-free aortic regurgitation who do not respond to medical treatment.

Management. Patients with mild-to-moderate aortic insufficiency should have a slightly elevated heart rate to reduce ventricular distension by decreasing LVEDP and to reduce oxygen consumption.[17] Bradycardia should be avoided because it predisposes to ventricular distension and subsequent pulmonary congestion.[17] Blood pressures are very labile and unresponsive to vasoactive agents. Vasodilator therapy can be used if it is done judiciously and, in fact, is desirable to decrease ventricular afterload, increasing forward cardiac output and decreasing regurgitant volume (Table 41–10). Caution should be exercised to avoid vasoconstriction and increased SVR, which will reduce effective cardiac output.

Aortic Stenosis

Aortic stenosis occurs in about one fourth of all patients with chronic valvular heart disease. It is most frequently found in adult males. The normal aortic valve has three

TABLE 41–9. DIFFERENCES BETWEEN ACUTE AND CHRONIC AORTIC REGURGITATION

	Clinical Features	
	Acute	*Chronic*
Congestive heart failure	Early and sudden	Late and insidious
Arterial pulse		
Rate per minute	Increased	Normal
Rate of rise	Normal	Increased
Systolic pressure	Normal to decreased	Increased
Diastolic pressure	Normal to decreased	Decreased
Pulse pressure	Near normal	Increased
Contour of peak	Single	Bisferiens
Pulsus alternans	Common	Uncommon
LV impulse	Near normal to moderately displaced, not hyperdynamic	Displaced hyperdynamic
Auscultation		
S_1	Soft to absent	Normal
Aortic component of S_2	Soft	Normal or decreased
Pulmonic component of S_2	Normal or increased	Normal
S_2	Common	Uncommon
S_4	Consistently absent	Usually absent
Aortic systolic murmur	Grade 3 or less	Grade 3 or more
Aortic regurgitant murmur	Short, medium-pitched	Long, high-pitched
Austin Flint	Middiastolic	Presystolic, mid-diastolic, or both
Peripheral arterial auscultatory signs	Absent	Present
Electrocardiogram	Normal LV voltage with minor repolarization abnormalities	Increased LV voltage with major repolarization abnormalities
Chest roentgenogram		
Left ventricle	Normal to moderately increased	Markedly increased
Aortic root and arch	Usually normal	Prominent
Pulmonary venous vascularity	Increased	Normal

	Hemodynamic Features	
	Acute	*Chronic (Without Left Ventricular Failure)*
LV compliance	Normal	Normal or increased
Regurgitant volume	Increased	Increased
LV end-diastolic pressure	Markedly increased	Normal or increased
LV ejection velocity (*dP/dt*)	Not significantly increased	Markedly increased
Aortic systolic pressure	Not increased	Increased
Aortic diastolic pressure	Normal to decreased	Markedly decreased
Systemic arterial pulse pressure	Slightly to moderately increased	Markedly increased
Ejection fraction	Normal or decreased	Normal
Effective stroke volume	Decreased	Normal
Effective cardiac output	Decreased	Usually normal
Heart rate	Increased	Normal
Peripheral vascular resistance	Usually increased	Normal

	Echocardiographic Features	
	Acute	*Chronic*
Mitral valve		
Closure point	Premature	Normal
Opening point	Delayed	Normal
E-F slope	Decreased	Normal
Fluttering	Usually present	Usually present
Left ventricle		
Internal dimension (end diastole)	Normal	Increased
Septal and free wall thickness	Normal	Normal
Septal and free wall motion	Normal	Increased
Left ventricular mass	Normal	Increased

LV, left ventricular.

Morganroth J, Perloff JK, Zeldis SM, Dunkman WB. Acute severe aortic regurgitation. Pathophysiology, clinical representation, and management. Ann Intern Med. *1977; 87(3):223–232.*

TABLE 41–10. AORTIC INSUFFICIENCY: IMPORTANT CONSIDERATIONS

Pathophysiology
  Left ventricular volume overload
  Left ventricular hypertrophy and dilation
  Low aortic diastolic pressure (with coronary flow)
  Increased left ventricular output and work
Management
  Hypertension increases regurgitation; avoid hypertension
  Decreased peripheral resistance decreases regurgitation
    (beneficial)
  Avoid bradycardia
    Lower diastolic pressure during regurgitation
    Increased intraventricular volume and pressures
    Decreased coronary flow
  Keep "full"!

cusps that are thin and movable. Disease processes affect the valve structure by causing a thickened or calcified area, which causes commissural fusion.

Pathophysiology. The primary insult with aortic stenosis lies in obstruction to the left ventricular outflow, resulting in a pressure gradient between the left ventricle and aorta during systolic ejection, which produces pressure overload on the left ventricle. The causes may be congenital, rheumatic fever that affects the aortic valve, or calcification of the aortic cusps. Besides aortic valvular stenosis, three other lesions may be responsible for obstruction to left ventricular outflow: (1) idiopathic hypertrophic subaortic stenosis, characterized by marked left ventricular enlargement; (2) discreet congenital subvalvular stenosis, caused by a fibrous ridge below the aortic valve; (3) supravalvular aortic stenosis, which is a congenital anomaly produced by narrowing of the ascending aorta.[3] Aortic stenosis overloads the left ventricle but does not cause dilation, that is, if there is low ventricular compliance.[3] There are two major consequences of decreased ventricular compliance: (1) higher filling pressures are needed for optimal cardiac performance, leading to pulmonary congestion if too high, and (2) normal sinus rhythm helps maintain adequate ventricular filling because the atrial kick may account for up to 40 percent of ventricular filling.[3]

Hemodynamic values such as cardiac output and stroke volume are normal in severe stenosis at rest. As the disease progresses, cardiac output and stroke volume decrease and elevations of the mean left atrial, pulmonary wedge, and pulmonary artery pressures are seen.

Symptoms. Murmurs usually precede onset of symptoms by several years. Aortic stenosis is rarely of hemodynamic or clinical importance until the orifice has narrowed to one third of normal.[33] In contrast to mitral stenosis, severe aortic stenosis may be present for years before clinical symptoms appear. When symptoms do occur, they include dyspnea, syncope, and angina. Dyspnea occurs from elevation of LVEDP, syncope from hypotension secondary to vasodilation from fixed cardiac output, and angina from myocardial oxygen supply–demand imbalance. Terminal symptoms include orthopnea, pulmonary edema, right ventricular fail-

ure, systemic venous hypertension, hepatomegaly, atrial fibrillation, and tricuspid regurgitation.[33]

Aortic stenosis and mitral stenosis can exist simultaneously. If so, the symptoms of mitral stenosis prevail. Surgical intervention should be undertaken prior to the development of left ventricular failure, but not before the patient is symptomatic.

Management. Patients who exhibit symptoms of aortic stenosis are usually considered high risks. Normal heart rate helps maintain ventricular filling and normal cardiac output. Adequate ventricular filling becomes increasingly dependent on sufficient intravascular volume and maintenance of normal sinus rhythm.

These patients may be on diuretic therapy and thus suffer from reduced intravascular volume. Adequate hydration is essential to avoid hypotensive episodes. Also, they are especially at risk from peripheral vasodilation, which can produce sudden and profound hypotension, thus impairing both cerebral and coronary perfusion.[6,17]

Any hemodynamic change that causes myocardial ischemia, such as tachyarrhythmias and hypotension, must be avoided. Bradycardia must also be avoided, once again, because it limits stroke volume (Table 41–11). Table 41–12 identifies the steps of the surgical procedure for aortic valve replacement.

Mitral Regurgitation

The mitral valve has several anatomic structures that are responsible for closure of the valve during ventricular systole. These include the anterior and posterior mitral leaflets, the chordae tendinae, the papillary muscles, the left ventricular myocardium, and the mitral annulus. Mitral regurgitation may result from a defect in any one of these; specific disease states tend to center on certain components. Mitral regurgitation is caused by chronic ischemic heart disease, endocarditis, and mitral valve prolapse.

Mitral regurgitation caused by involvement of the valve leaflets occurs most commonly in rheumatic heart dis-

TABLE 41–11. AORTIC STENOSIS: IMPORTANT CONSIDERATIONS

Pathophysiology
  Outflow obstruction with left ventricular pressure overload;
    essentially fixed cardiac output
  Left ventricular hypertrophy, not dilation
  Decreased left ventricular compliance
  Thickened ventricular wall with relative subendocardial
    ischemia (even with normal coronary arteries)
  High myocardial oxygen demand
Management
  Keep mean systemic pressure at or above awake baseline;
    use vasopressors if necessary
  Ensure that patient is full but not overfull
  Avoid inotropic stimulation unless below inotropic baseline
  Avoid tachycardia; faster ejection increases oxygen demand and increases gradient
  Deterioration can occur with loss of atrial kick; be prepared to cardiovert if loss of sinus rhythm

TABLE 41–12. SURGICAL PROCEDURE FOR CORRECTION OF AORTIC VALVE PATHOLOGY

Median sternotomy

Transverse aortotomy incision above right coronary artery

Traction sutures placed at the three commissural points

Interrupted sutures are placed, marking three groups of sutures for each cusp

Valve holder removed after valve is seated

Sutures tied

Aortotomy repair

Reprinted, with permission, from Cooley and Norman.[43]

ease and is seen more frequently in males than females.[2] It is a consequence of shortening, rigidity, deformity, and retraction of one or both cusps of the mitral valve as well as shortening and fusion rupture of the chordae tendinae.[2] If the leaflets are strictured by excessive tissue, the valves will prolapse into the left atrium.

Papillary muscle fibrosis, if present, will cause inadequate shortening of the papillary muscle during systole, with prolapse of the leaflets into the atrium, and regurgitation ensues. The papillary muscles receive their blood supply from the coronary vessels, so any insult to coronary perfusion can cause ischemia to the papillary muscles, with concurrent dysfunction. If severe enough, papillary muscle necrosis can occur and result in mitral regurgitation. Papillary muscle ischemia can also be caused by anemia, shock, coronary arteritis, or left ventricular aneurysm.

The chordae tendineae may be abnormal at birth or may rupture because of rheumatic fever, trauma, endocarditis, or left ventricular regurgitation. If this abnormality exists, acute regurgitation ensues. Emergency surgery may be required for those patients who suffer from ruptured papillary muscle or chordae tendinae secondary to myocardial infarction or those reasons previously cited.

Calcification of the mitral annulus results in dilation of this opening and severe dilation of the left ventricle. Normally during systole, the annulus constricts and plays a very important role in valve closure. When it is calcified, mitral regurgitation occurs. This condition presents with severe myocardial dysfunction, and these patients may not improve after valve replacement because of the increase in left ventricular afterload, which occurs with dilation of the regurgitation leak.[2]

Left ventricular function can be determined by evaluating the end-systolic volume. Braunwald et al found that patients with normal end-systolic volume retained normal ventricular function postoperatively, whereas marked enlargement of the end-systolic volume usually correlated well with postoperative mortality.[2]

The combined left atrial and pulmonary venous bed compliance is an important determinant of the hemodynamic and clinical picture in mitral regurgitation.[2] Three major subgroups have been identified: (1) normal or reduced compliance, in which there is little enlargement of the left atrium but marked elevation of the mean left atrial pressure, with prominent systems of pulmonary congestion; (2) moderately increased compliance, which is the most common and consists of patients with variable atrial enlargement and

significant elevation of left atrial pressure; and (3) markedly increased compliance, which within the adult population frequently is secondary to high ventricular pressure.

Pathophysiology. In patients with mitral regurgitation, the resistance to left ventricular emptying is reduced. As a result, the left ventricle decompresses itself rapidly into the left atrium early during ejection, and with a marked reduction in left ventricular size there is a rapid decline in left ventricular tension.[33] Therefore, a greater proportion of the contractile activity of the left ventricle is expanded in shortening, and the cardiac output may be maintained for long periods.

The initial compensation to mitral regurgitation consists of more complete systolic emptying of the left ventricle; however, a progressive increase in left ventricular end-diastolic volume occurs as the severity of the regurgitation increases and the left ventricular function declines.[33] Significant mitral regurgitation is progressive, because enlargement of the left atrium places tension on the posterior mitral leaflet, pulling it away from the mitral opening. Dilation of the left ventricle increases the regurgitation, which further enlarges the left atrium and ventricle, resulting in a vicious cycle.[33]

Mitral regurgitation produces volume overload of the left ventricle. The volume of mitral regurgitance flow depends on the size of the regurgitant orifice as well as the pressure gradient between the left ventricle and the left atrium. Left ventricular systolic pressure and thus left ventricular–left atrial gradient are dependent on SVR and forward stroke volume. Thus, increases in both preload and afterload and depression of contractility increase left ventricular size and enlarge the regurgitant orifice. If regurgitation is caused by something other than a diseased valve, the volume of flow is affected by left ventricular dimensions, which in turn affect orifice size.[2]

Ejection fractions must be closely examined in these patients. Values may be at normal levels and yet myocardial function may be impaired. If ejection fractions are reduced, severe myocardial dysfunction may be present. An ejection fraction under 40 percent in patients with mitral regurgitation represents massive enlargement of the left atrium.[2]

Symptoms. The symptoms that present depend on the pressure in the left atrium and the cardiac output. The left atrial pressure determines the pulmonary venous pressure and the severity of dyspnea.[1] Symptoms include fatigue, dyspnea, orthopnea and nocturnal dyspnea, weight loss, exhaustion, and cachexia. Right-sided failure and associated symptoms can be seen with patients who have pulmonary vascular disease and regurgitation. Figure 41–11 summarizes the hemodynamic and physiologic changes that occur with mitral regurgitation.

Management. The patient who develops acute mitral regurgitation is at considerable risk from sudden, significant changes in hemodynamic status. Of prime importance is the degree of pulmonary involvement that may occur secondary to increased left atrial pressure. If these changes do exist, the same principles of pulmonary protection apply as do for mitral stenosis.

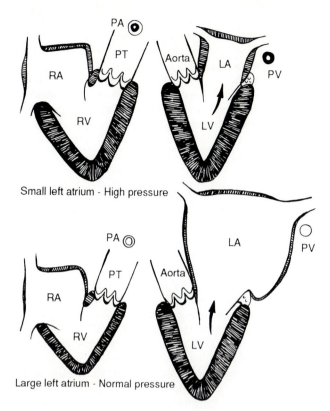

Small left atrium - High pressure

Large left atrium - Normal pressure

Figure 41–11. The extremes of the syndrome of mitral regurgitation. **Top:** Mitral regurgitation into small, hypertrophied left atrium results in pulmonary vascular changes and right ventricle hypertrophy. **Bottom:** Mitral regurgitation into large, thin-walled left atrium results in little or no changes in pulmonary vessels or right ventricle. LA, left atrium; LV, left ventricle; PA, pulmonary artery; PT, pulmonary trunk; PV, pulmonary vein; RA, right atrium; RV, right ventricle. (*Reprinted, with permission, from Roberts WC, Perloff JK. Mitral valvular disease. Ann Intern Med. 1972;77:939.*)

Compensatory increases in sympathetic nervous system activity exist with right-sided heart failure. Tachycardia and increased SVR increase the regurgitant flow.[8] Chronic mitral regurgitation has little effect on the pulmonary vasculature, and heart failure develops only late in the disease process.

The anesthetist should strive for (1) maintenance of normal heart rate, (2) afterload reduction with vasodilators to increase cardiac output and reduce SVR (3) reduction of heart size with inotropic agents if necessary, and (4) avoidance of cardiac depressant drugs (Table 41–13).

Mitral Stenosis

The incidence of mitral stenosis after rheumatic fever is high; it is estimated that roughly 40 percent of all patients with a past history will develop mitral stenosis. Mitral stenosis is more prevalent in women.

Pathophysiology. Valve leaflets become thickened and fibrous or impeded by calcified deposits, the chordae tendi-

nae shorten, the cusps become rigid, and the apex of the valve narrows. Rheumatic fever results in four types of fusion of the apparatus, leading to stenosis: (1) commissural, occurring in 30 percent; (2) cuspal, occurring in 15 percent; (3) chordal, occurring in 10 percent; and (4) combined, occurring in 45 percent.[6] The stenotic mitral valve is usually funnel-shaped, and the orifice is frequently shaped like a fish mouth or buttonhole, with calcium deposits in the valve leaflets. The deposits sometime extend to involve the valve ring, which may become quite thick.

The basic problem in tight mitral stenosis is getting blood out of the blocked left atrium and into the left ventricle during diastole. The price of moving blood rapidly is inevitably an increase in left atrial pressure, which must be shared by the left pulmonary venous reservoir. Two events contribute to the left atrial pressure and hence to the important task of squeezing blood through the stenotic valve into the left ventricle: (1) atrial systole is an active effort but is quite brief. It does not greatly shrink the atrium. Its major role may be during exercise and tachycardia. (2) More important is the leftover force of right ventricular contraction, dampened more or less by transmission through the pulmonary vascular bed.[39] For this to be of any benefit in stenosis, the pressure in the pulmonary bed must be very high, limiting left atrial pressure and consequently blood flow.

Normally, the orifice of the mitral valve is 4 to 6 cm^2. With mild stenosis, this is reduced to 2 cm^2. In these circumstances, blood flows from the left atrium to the left ventricle only by abnormally high pressure gradients. In patients with severe stenosis (opening reduced to 1 cm^2) an even higher gradient is required to maintain a normal cardiac output. Pulmonary capillary and venous pressures are elevated and dyspnea results. Any episodes of tachycardia will augment the pressure gradient and result in an increased left atrial pressure. Thus, it is obvious that tachyarrhythmias must be avoided in these patients.

The severity of mitral obstruction influences the elevation of left atrial pressure, which, in turn, determines the extent of the pulmonary congestive symptoms of dyspnea and orthopnea. The following hemodynamic changes are associated with mitral stenosis: Left ventricular diastolic pressure is normal with pure stenosis and elevated if regurgitation is present; ejection fraction is usually normal or somewhat re-

TABLE 41–13. MITRAL INSUFFICIENCY: IMPORTANT CONSIDERATIONS

Pathophysiology
  Left ventricular volume overload
  Left atrial enlargement
  Backward transmission of high pressures
  Right-sided heart failure and pulmonary edema
  Atrial fibrillation
  Left ventricle used to lower afterload
Management
  Hypertension increases regurgitation; decreased peripheral resistance decreases regurgitation (use nitroprusside)
  Keep full
  Bradycardia increases regurgitation; avoid
  Left ventricle may need inotropic support

duced in moderate stenosis and subnormal even at rest in the severely stenosed patient.

The clinical and hemodynamic pictures of mitral stenosis are dictated largely by the level of the pulmonary artery pressure. Pulmonary hypertension results from (1) the passive backward transmission of the elevated left atrial pressure; (2) arteriolar destruction, which is presumably triggered by left atrial and pulmonary venous hypertension; and (3) organic obliterative changes in the pulmonary vascular bed.[38]

Symptoms. The most common symptoms associated with mitral stenosis are dyspnea and episodes of pulmonary edema caused by chronic pulmonary congestion. Orthopnea and paroxysmal nocturnal dyspnea also occur, especially in the recumbent position, as a result of rapid redistribution of blood from the periphery to the lungs. Pulmonary edema develops if there is a sudden increase in flow through the mitral orifice. Arrythmias in the form of atrial abnormalities are common when moderate stenosis is present. These include premature atrial beats, flutter, fibrillation, and paroxysmal atrial tachycardia. Hemoptysis occurs in those patients with increased left atrial pressures.

Symptoms of a more serious nature include (1) thrombi, particularly as a result of atrial fibrillation, with emboli to brain, kidneys, and spleen; (2) pulmonary emboli, particularly in those patients with increased pulmonary vascular resistance; (3) bacterial endocarditis; and (4) pulmonary infections.

Unless there is a specific contraindication, operative treatment is indicated in the symptomatic patient with pure mitral stenosis whose effective orifice is less than 1.5 cm². Mitral commissurotomy has been an excellent operation in patients without significant mitral regurgitation and without severe valvular calcification. Before commissurotomy is begun, the atrial cavity should be examined closely for thrombi. It is common practice to tie off the atrial appendage from the left atrium to avoid embolization from chronic atrial fibrillation. Emboli frequently occur when there are sudden changes from atrial fibrillation to sinus rhythm and the atria begin to contract. Valvular replacement with a prosthetic valve may be done in those cases in which commissurotomy may not be helpful, particularly in those patients with coexisting mitral regurgitation or heavy valvular regurgitation.[40]

Management. The following are anesthetic considerations: (1) Control of heart rate is of paramount importance and drug therapy may be necessary to keep the rate within normal limits. (2) Ventricular filling pressures must be maintained; however, it must be remembered that both PCWP and left atrial pressure are greater than LVEDP in the presence of mitral stenosis because of the pressure gradient across the mitral valve.[6] (3) If pulmonary hypertension exists, the deleterious effects of anesthetics on the pulmonary circulation must be considered. Pulmonary vasoconstriction induced by anesthetic agents causes right ventricular strain or failure and must be avoided. The use of nitrous oxide should be avoided in patients where there is suspected or determined pulmonary hypertension because of the tendency of nitrous oxide to increase pulmonary artery pres-

sure. The use of vasodilators may be considered. (4) Changes in position, especially to the Trendelenburg, are poorly tolerated because of increased blood flow to the lungs, which can result in impaired oxygenation or pulmonary edema. (5) Ventricular contractility is usually not of clinical significance.[8] Table 41–14 lists important considerations in the management of mitral stenosis. The procedure for mitral valve replacement is described in Table 41–15.

Mitral Valve Prolapse

Mitral valve prolapse has become one of the most common valvular abnormalities, affecting roughly 6 to 17 percent of the population, with the highest incidence in females. This increase in occurrence is probably due more to advanced diagnostic technique than to an actual increase in prevalence. Several names have been given to this syndrome: midsystolic click-murmur syndrome, Barlow's syndrome, floppy valve syndrome, and redundant cusp syndrome. A number of diseases can predispose the patient to mitral valve prolapse including rheumatic endocarditis, congestive cardiomyopathy, myocarditis trauma, lupus erythematosus, Wolfe–Parkinson–White syndrome, and coronary artery disease; however, this list is not all inclusive.

General symptoms include systolic clicks and a late systolic murmur. Clinically, these patients are asymptomatic; however, if the prolapse is severe enough, palpitations, chest discomfort, or any symptoms indicative of mitral regurgitation may present. Palpitations are often caused by arrhythmias, which may be secondary to autonomic dysfunction. The arrhythmias may be atrial or ventricular in nature; they may be premature beats, ventricular tachyarrhythmias, or bradyarrhythmias. The exact cause of the

---

TABLE 41–14. MITRAL STENOSIS: IMPORTANT CONSIDERATIONS

Pathophysiology
    Obstruction to left ventricular filling; essentially fixed cardiac output
    Left atrial pressure and volume overload
    Backward transmission of increased pressures
    Pulmonary hypertension
    Right ventricular failure (pressure overload)
    Atrial fibrillation

Management
    Tachycardia to be avoided; decreased left ventricular filling
    Bradycardia may be dangerous, lower cardiac output
    A narrow range of acceptable right-sided pressures and fixed low cardiac output require slow changes, even in correct direction (as rate of induction, rate of fluid infusion)
    Inotropic stimulation rarely helpful unless contractility is below awake baseline and may be harmful
    Rarely, vasopressors may be necessary to ensure adequate aortic root diastolic pressure for coronary perfusion
    Control fast atrial fibrillation with digoxin
    Keep full but not to point of pulmonary edema
    May require prolonged ventilatory assistance
    May be very sensitive to postural changes (Trendelenberg, turning on side)

TABLE 41–15. SURGICAL PROCEDURE FOR CORRECTION OF MITRAL VALVE PATHOLOGY

Median sternotomy

Left atriotomy performed

Valve excised with chordae tendinae and apices of papillary muscle

Prosthesis is sutured for tying into atriotomy

Valve lowered into annulus

Valve holder removed, sutures tied

Cannulas removed and pericardium closed

Reprinted, with permission, from Cooley and Norman.[43]

arrhythmias is not definite, but some theorize that they may be caused by stretch of the leaflets. By far the most common arrhythmia is paroxysmal supraventricular tachycardia. This is probably related to the existence of atrioventricular bypass tracts.

The pathophysiology of mitral valve prolapse is similar to that of mitral regurgitation; thus, similar hemodynamic changes are seen. The mitral valve leaflets are myxomatous, weakening the valves' ventricular surface and thus allowing the valve to protrude toward the atrium. In most cases there is no apparent cause and consequently the prolapse is idiopathic.[1] If progressive mitral regurgitation occurs and becomes severe enough, valve replacement is necessary. Surgical correction of mitral valve prolapse without mitral regurgitation, but with cardiac arrhythmias, has also been reported to be of benefit.[2]

Ventricular Septal Defect

Ventricular septal defect (VSD) occurs in the adult as a complication to myocardial infarction. The incidence is 1 to 2 percent.[41] VSD is a communication that allows blood to be shunted from the left to the right ventricle. Its size determines the physiologic alterations that occur. Ventricular septal defects are categorized as either restricted or nonrestricted. A restricted VSD is one in which the amount of blood that is shunted is regulated by the size of the defect; in the nonrestricted VSD it is not.[41] The direction and degree of the shunt across a VSD depend on the size of the defect and the pressure gradient that occurs during the various phases of the cardiac cycle.[41] When the defect is small, it offers considerable resistance to flow, and slight variations in the size of the defect are accompanied by large variations in the rate of flow (or shunting).[2] If the defect is large, it offers little resistance to flow, and small pressure differences between left and right ventricle result in shunting.[2]

When left-to-right shunting exists, pulmonary blood flow is increased above normal. Both left and right ventricles are overworked, resulting in hypertrophy. As a result of elevated left atrial pressures and pulmonary venous pressures, pulmonary resistance increases and pulmonary hypertension results. The severity of increased resistance can be defined by the level of the pulmonary vascular resistance ([mean pulmonary arterial pressure minus left atrial pressure] divided by cardiac index) or by the level of total pulmonary resistance (mean pulmonary arterial pressure divided by cardiac index). If the pulmonary resistance is severely elevated, the flow across the septal defect is usually bidirectional and of about equal magnitude in both directions.[2]

Because the occurrence of VSD in the adult is rapid, it is usually seen in conjunction with cardiogenic shock. It is best to manage these patients medically until the hemodynamic parameters are stable and then to proceed with surgical intervention. The surgical procedure is described in Table 41–16. The anesthetic management consists of maintenance of these normal hemodynamic parameters with anesthetic agents and techniques that do not decrease ventricular function or increase the workload of the myocardium.

Multivalvular Disease

Multivalvular disease is common, particularly in patients with rheumatic heart disease, and a variety of clinical and hemodynamic syndromes can be produced by different combinations of valvular abnormalities.[2]

Mitral Stenosis and Aortic Regurgitation. If mitral stenosis and aortic regurgitation coexist, the mitral stenosis and its sequelae usually mask the presence of aortic stenosis. It is important to recognize the presence of hemodynamically significant aortic valvular disease preoperatively in patients about to undergo surgical correction of mitral stenosis, because isolated mitral commissurotomy may be hazardous in such patients; this operation can impose a sudden hemodynamic load on the left ventricle that may lead to acute pulmonary edema.[2]

Aortic Stenosis and Mitral Regurgitation. The presence of aortic stenosis and mitral regurgitation produces complications that are life-threatening. Obstruction to left ventricular outflow, on the one hand, augments the volume of mitral regurgitant flow, and the presence of mitral regurgitation, on the other, diminishes the ventricular preload necessary for maintenance of left ventricular stroke volume in aortic stenosis.[2] Significant reductions in cardiac output and symptoms of venous hypertension ensue.

Aortic Regurgitation and Mitral Regurgitation. The combination of aortic regurgitation and mitral regurgitation is frequent, and the symptoms of aortic regurgitation usually manifest. When both leaks are severe, blood may reflux from the aorta all the way through both chambers of the left heart into the pulmonary veins.[2]

TABLE 41–16. SURGICAL PROCEDURE FOR CORRECTION OF VENTRICULAR SEPTAL DEFECT

Median sternotomy

Area of infarction excised along with necrotic septal tissue creating interventricular communication

Dacron patch is used to repair the septum and is placed on the left ventricular side of the septum

Felt pledgets are sutured to margins of the ventricular incisions

Ventriculorrhaphy closed

Reprinted, with permission, from Cooley and Norman.[43]

Idiopathic Hypertrophic Subaortic Stenosis. Idiopathic hypertrophic subaortic stenosis (IHSS) is an obstruction to left ventricular outflow that results in asymmetric hypertrophy of the interventricular septum. During systole, the hypertrophied outflow tract muscle often narrows sufficiently to obstruct left ventricular ejection.[42] The etiology behind IHSS has not been fully determined. The incidence is higher in men than women. There is no ventricular filling, and wall stiffness and MVo_2 increase. The obstruction usually becomes severe enough to cause left ventricular failure. Symptoms include dyspnea, angina, fatigue, and syncope.

Approximately two thirds of patients respond to propranolol therapy and require no surgical intervention. Propranolol reduces oxygen consumption and prevents the increase in outflow obstruction that occurs with physical activity. If beta blockade is not successful in relieving symptoms, surgical intervention is necessary. The goal is to relieve obstruction, and this may be accomplished by reducing the hypertrophied myocardium or by replacing the mitral valve.

With left septectomy, care must be taken not to damage the anterior leaflet of the mitral valve and to avoid injury to major conduction bundles in the ventricular system.[43] Left bundle branch block is a common complication to this procedure.

The procedure for mitral valve replacement in IHSS is the same as that required for other pathologic conditions.

Tricuspid Regurgitation. Tricuspid regurgitation is commonly associated with rheumatic heart disease; therefore it may accompany other valvular diseases. The venous pressure is frequently elevated. Atrial fibrillation is present because of mitral stenosis. These patients have murmur over the lower left sternal border. Because of cardiac cirrhosis, splenomegaly, jaundice, and pain in the right upper quadrant may develop. The most common problem is right ventricular failure and pulmonary hypertension.

Replacement of severely leaking tricuspid valves is determined by the patient's hemodynamic status. Once the left-sided lesion is repaired, symptoms may be alleviated, but this may not be determined until the time of surgery.

When it is impossible for a postoperative patient to get along without the pump oxygenator the cause may be secondary to an acute increase in tricuspid regurgitation. There is difference of opinion about how often the minimally diseased but severely leaking tricuspid valve needs to be replaced, but there is no doubt that such replacements may sometimes be lifesaving.[39]

Pericarditis. Pericarditis is an inflammation of the visceral or parietal pericardium or both. Some of the causes of pericarditis include acute rheumatic fever, infection, acute myocardial infarction, trauma, metastatic tumor, uremia, and tuberculosis.

When the pericardium is subject to infection or trauma an inflammatory response occurs with exudate formation and effusion. If the involvement is extensive, enough fluid may accumulate in the pericardial space to restrict ventricular filling. Slow fluid accumulation usually does not present a problem because the pericardium is able to accommodate to the stretch. Rapid fluid accumulation, on the other hand, can produce tamponade, which will restrict blood flow to the ventricle and cause a decrease in cardiac output. Other symptoms may include elevated venous pressure and decreased arterial pressure.

As the pericardium heals, it becomes thickened and scarred, resulting in a decrease in ventricular filling. Pericardial friction rub, venous distension, peripheral edema, and hepatomegaly ensue with this "constrictive" pericarditis.

Electrocardiographic changes include ST segment elevation similar to that associated with myocardial infarction. Atrial arrhythmias, such as premature atrial contraction or atrial fibrillation, are common, especially with acute pericarditis. Pericardial effusion is noted on chest radiograph.

Constrictive pericarditis is best treated surgically. If the ventricular involvement is minimal, a pericardectomy can be performed. The operative procedure can usually be performed satisfactorily without the use of cardiopulmonary bypass; however, pump standby is recommended.

COMPLICATIONS OF VALVE REPLACEMENT

The complications of valve replacement are generally the same regardless of the type of valve used.

Thromboembolism

The threat of thromboembolus formation with mechanical valves is ever present; however, the incidence is rare with the tissue valve. Long-term anticoagulation therapy is required for all patients with mechanical valves, whether aortic or mitral, and should not be interrupted for elective surgical procedures of any nature. Tissue valves are generally nonthrombogenic and usually do not require anticoagulation therapy. If, however, the patient has an increased susceptibility to thromboembolism, such as atrial fibrillation, large left atrium, clots detected intraoperatively, or low cardiac output states, anticoagulation therapy should be instituted, especially if mitral valve replacement is being considered.[37]

Endocarditis

The average incidence of prosthetic valve endocarditis is 1 to 4 percent and is not significantly different in mechanical or tissue valves.[37] Between 36 and 53 percent of these cases are documented within 2 months of surgical implantation and are described as early prosthetic valve endocarditis.[44] The organisms most commonly involved are *Staphylococcus aureus* and *S. epidermidis. Streptococcus* and gram-negative organisms are less commonly noted. The infection usually involves the suture line and is highly virulent, with reported mortality rates as high as 87 percent, regardless of the mode of therapy employed.[45] Those patients who develop late endocarditis, especially with a streptococcal infection, fare better, with mortality significantly decreased.

Tissue valve endocarditis has a higher success rate for treatment, which is believed to result from the location of the infection. Mechanical valve endocarditis usually involves the subvalvular cardiac tissue, whereas tissue valve infection is frequently limited to the cusps of the prosthesis.[45]

Hemolysis

Formed blood element destruction is a complication of all mechanical cardiac valves and occasionally leads to the development of anemia. The incidence is related to turbulence of blood flow across the prosthesis. Laboratory evidence of hemolysis is noted more frequently in patients with aortic stenosis than with mitral stenosis, especially if a paravalvular leak is present.[45]

Flow Obstruction

The incidence of flow obstruction is greatest in the caged disk valve design and least with the tissue valve. Roberts has demonstrated significant intimal proliferation in the aortic root of patients with the caged disk design and fibrous tissue deposition in the coronary ostia.[44]

Regurgitation

The volume of backflow varies with the particular valve design. Backflow associated with prosthetic heart valves falls into two categories: (1) closure backflow, which is required to close the valve; and (2) leakage backflow, which occurs after the valve is closed.[46] Regurgitation is dependent on heart rate and cardiac output. During tachycardia, closure backflow dominates, whereas during bradycardia, leakage backflow dominates. Regurgitation varies inversely with cardiac output.[46] Tachycardia and decreased cardiac output increase the energy expended tremendously, and a valve designed to reduce energy requirements by low-closure backflow is desirable. The bradycardic patient requires a valve with little or no leakage backflow because the total backflow may be as high as 75 percent with leakage.

Prosthetic Cardiac Valves

The first insertion of a valve in the mitral position was performed by Albert Starr in 1960.[37] Since that time, several valves have been designed to improve hemodynamics. Currently there are four functional categories of prosthetic heart valves: (1) caged ball, (2) caged disk, (3) tilting disk, and (4) tissue valves (Fig. 41–12). Selection of the type of valve is influenced by several factors. These include age, sex, heart size, hemodynamics, and contraindications to anticoagulation therapy. Several broad guidelines are suggested for valve selection.[47]

Tissue valves are suitable for (1) patients with absolute contraindications to anticoagulation therapy, such as those with bleeding tendencies, athletes, patients who will not reliably take anticoagulants, and women of childbearing age; and (2) patients with short life expectancies. Mechanical valves are suitable for (1) patients with a long life expectancy, (2) patients with no contraindications to coagulation therapy, (3) patients with small left ventricles or aortic root, (4) children, and (5) patients with chronic renal disease or altered calcium metabolism.

ANESTHESIA FOR CONDUCTION ABNORMALITIES

Etiology of Conduction Abnormalities

Abnormalities of electrical conduction can occur for many reasons. The conduction can be affected either directly or indirectly by disease processes, drug effect, or electrolyte imbalance or as a complication of open heart surgery.

The sinoatrial node is perfused by the right coronary artery in 60 percent of the population and by the left circumflex artery in 40 percent, so any disturbance in perfusion in these areas compromises blood flow to the sinoatrial node causing atrial dysrhythmias.

Because of its location, the sinoatrial node is vulnerable to the inflammatory process that is associated with pericarditis. Lupus may cause inflammatory changes that affect the sinoatrial node.

Pharmacologically induced vagal stimulation can be responsible for bradyarrhythmias. The sinoatrial node can be responsible for bradyarrhythmias. The sinoatrial node can also be damaged during cannulation procedures for aortocoronary bypass.

If the right coronary artery is occluded, disturbances will be seen in the atrioventricular node, bundle of His, and bundle branches. The right coronary artery supplies the atrioventricular node in 90 percent of hearts, whereas the remaining 10 percent is supplied by the left circumflex artery.

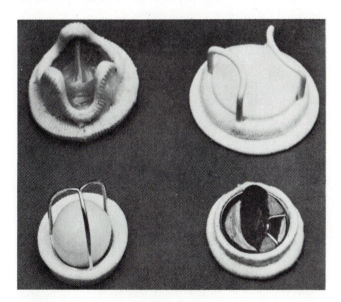

Figure 41–12. Four prosthetic heart valves. From upper left clockwise: **1.** Porcine xenograft (pig aortic valve fixed in glutaraldehyde attached to sewing ring) used for aortic, mitral, or tricuspid valve replacement. **2.** Caged disk (Beall) valve used for mitral valve replacement. The lower cloth ring is designed for suturing in the atrioventricular annulus. **3.** Tilting disk semicentral flow valve (Bjork-Shiley) used for mitral or aortic valve replacement. The disk is shown in the full open position. Sutures are placed in the lower cloth ring. **4.** Caged ball valve with Silastic poppet (Starr–Edwards Model 1260) used for aortic valve replacement. With some modification, this valve is used in the mitral position as well. The porcine, Beall, and Starr–Edwards valves are shown in the closed position. (*Reprinted, with permission, from Vanden Belt et al.*[1])

The sequence of events (sinus bradycardia, nausea and vomiting, and atrioventricular block) frequently seen with inferior myocardial infarction can be linked to ischemia or edema of the atrioventricular node when the right coronary artery is occluded.[48] The block is usually transient and may be treated pharmacologically, but if residual block occurs, artificial pacing may be necessary.

Valvular disease, primarily in the form of calcification, may intrude on normal conduction tissue and cause dysrhythmias. The location of the atrioventricular node and the distal conduction system relative to the tricuspid valve, aortic valve, and mitral annulus make it vulnerable to disease processes in these structures.[48] Tumors, sarcoidosis, myocarditis, and syphilis have all been known to affect normal conductivity.

Primary heart block is a degenerative disease process that is fibrotic or sclerotic in nature and is usually seen in patients over 60 years of age.[48] Heart block is frequently induced after open heart surgery, especially after ventricular septal defect repair or aortic and tricuspid replacement because of edema or damage to the atrioventricular node. Pacing may be required to alleviate symptoms.

Conduction defects caused by drug toxicity or electrolyte imbalance can usually be treated by withdrawing the drug or correcting the imbalance.

Cardiac Mapping

Cardiac mapping procedures are performed to correct electrophysiologic disorders. The procedure is performed on patients with preexcitation syndromes such as Wolfe–Parkinson–White (WPW) syndrome or on those with intractable ventricular tachyarrhythmias.

Preexcitation of ventricular muscle occurs when other than normal critical pathways are used, producing early ventricular depolarization. These pathways have various anatomic configurations and names (Fig. 41–13): Kent bundle, fiber of Brechennacher, Mahaim fiber, and Lown–Ganong–Levine pathway.[49] The most common example of preexcitation via an abnormal pathway is seen in WPW syn-

drome[48] (Fig. 41–14). Surgical correction of WPW syndrome involves interruption of the abnormal pathway by epicardial mapping techniques (Fig. 41–15).

Anesthetic and surgical considerations include minimization of electrical interference from monitoring or cautery, maintenance of normothermia, hemodynamic support, maintenance of MAP at 70 to 90 torr, avoidance of tachyarrhythmias, and avoidance of catecholamine release.[49]

When mapping is performed for intractable ventricular arrhythmias the considerations are somewhat different. The etiology in these patients is usually secondary to anatomic and physiologic abnormalities that include ischemic heart disease, ventricular aneurysm, cardiomyopathy, or previous ventriculotomy.[49] The earliest electrical focus is identified and the area is resected along with any aneurysm.[48]

Ventricular tachycardia is induced during mapping and lidocaine may interfere with the ventricle's response. A minimum amount of lidocaine should be used for local infiltration and intravenous and intratracheal lidocaine should be avoided.[49] The lidocaine level that can impair electrophysiologic studies is in the range 1 to 1.2 μg base/mL.[50] This range is easily exceeded with laryngotracheal lidocaine. Bypass is performed at normothermic levels. Adequate coronary blood flow must be maintained (MAP 70 to 90 torr) as the heart remains perfused during mapping. Table 41–17 lists postmapping considerations. Arrhythmias are common after mapping. Table 41–18 lists rhythm conditions and suggestions for treatment.

Treatment of Conduction Abnormalities

Conduction disorders that cannot be controlled by medication may need pacemaker generation for relief of symptoms as pacemakers provide the rhythm that the heart is incapable of producing. Pacing systems may be either temporary or permanent.

The use of cardiac pacemakers has increased significantly and certainly has improved the quality of life for patients with conduction disturbances. A wide variety of pac-

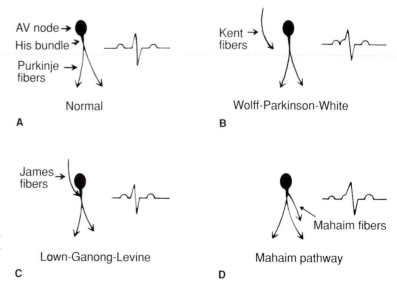

Figure 41–13. Preexcitation syndromes—types of accessory pathways. Conduction in the (**A**) normal, (**B**) Wolfe–Parkinson–White, (**C**) Lown–Ganong–Levine, and (**D**) Mahaim pathways. (*Reprinted, with permission, from Sadowski AR, Moyers JR. Anesthetic management of the Wolfe–Parkinson–White syndrome. Anesthesiology. 1979;51:553–556.*)

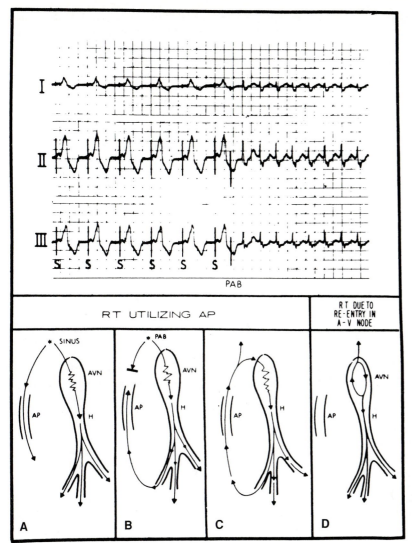

Figure 41–14. Reentry and reciprocating tachycardia (RT). Mechanisms of tachycardia in Wolfe–Parkinson–White syndrome. **A.** Normal sinus rhythm (NSR) fusion. **B.** Premature beat dissociates normal and accessory pathways. **C.** Reentry established antegrade conduction over atrioventricular node (AVN). **D.** Reentry confined to atrioventricular junction wth reciprocation. (*Reprinted, with permission, from Gallagher JJ, Pritchett ELC, Sealy WC, et al. The preexcitation syndromes.* Prog Cardiovasc Dis. *1978;20:285–327.*)

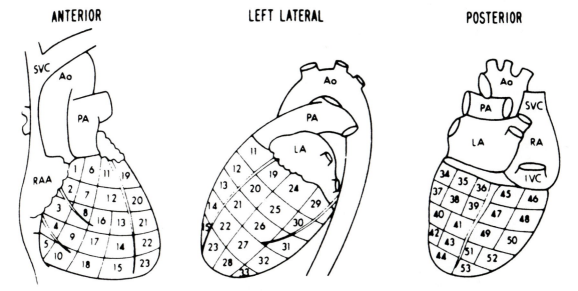

Figure 41–15. Epicardial mapping grid. There are 53 areas from which activation data are recorded. Surface landmarks serve as references. (*Reprinted, with permission, from Gallagher JJ, Kase J, Sealy WC, et al. Epicardial mapping in the Wolfe–Parkinson–White syndrome.* Circulation. *1978;57:854–866.*)

TABLE 41–17. GUIDING PRINCIPLES AND GOALS FOR POSTMAPPING MANAGEMENT

Maintain thorough effective monitoring, all variables, to where benefit exceeds risk.

Maintain myocardial oxygen supply–demand.

Maintain cardiac output sufficient for total body needs.

Maintain heart rate at 90–130 beats per minute: sinus rhythm.

Optimize preload for best cardiovascular function.

Maintain cardiac output by adjusting vascular volume, vascular resistance, and then contractility.

Maintain renal function by adequate cardiac output and volume status; diuretics only as a secondary concern.

Maintain coagulation status within normal limits: protamine, platelets, fresh-frozen plasma, factor IX concentrate.

Plan to have packed cell volume in early postop period above 30 percent.

Return rectal temperature, if possible, to normal, at ≥ 35C.

Maintain serum potassium at 5.0–5.5 mEq/L.

Maintain serum ionized calcium in normal range.

Anticipate the inconceivable, and plan!

Transport with electrocardiogram monitoring, defibrillation equipment, and cardiopulmonary resuscitation drugs.

Reprinted, with permission, from Ream.[49]

ing generators are available, but they all function on the same basic principle. The two most important components are the pulse generator and the pacing electrode. The generator senses electrical activity and will send impulses via the electrode to the myocardium if necessary. The electrode serves to carry stimuli to the heart and to transmit an electrogram retrograde to pacemaker amplifier circuits.[49]

Mechanics of Pacing

The artificial pacing system stimulates cardiac contraction by passing current between electrodes that have been positioned in the myocardium. The system is designed to produce electrophysiologic changes similar to the normal heart. The electrical field created between the two electrodes causes hyperpolarization of the membrane nearest the anodal electrode and reduction of the membrane potential in that portion nearest the cathode.[49]

A pacing threshold (that energy at which depolarization is initiated) is determined. There are three basic determinants of threshold: (1) the intrinsic excitability of the myocardium, (2) current density at the electrode–myocardial cell surface, and (3) pulse duration.[48] The threshold usually remains stable provided the electrode is well placed. Pathologic states that may alter the level of threshold are acidosis, hypoxia, electrolyte imbalance, antiarrhythmic agents, exercise, and position changes.

Pacemakers are either temporary or permanent and are usually inserted transvenously. Epicardial pacers are frequently used in open heart surgery. Transthoracic pacers are also being used. These require the use of skin electrodes which are designed to be either unipolar or bipolar. A unipolar design means that the anode is not in contact with the myocardium, but is within the generator or attached to

the skin. Bipolar refers to that design in which both the anode and cathode are in touch with heart muscle. The precise criteria for the use of temporary or permanent cardiac pacemakers vary slightly from institution to institution and from physician to physician.

TABLE 41–18. ARRHYTHMIA MANAGEMENT POSTMAPPING

Rhythm Condition	Treatment
Sinus rhythm	0
Nodal rhythm	0
Sinus bradycardia	Atropine
	Isoproterenol or dopamine
	Atrial pacemaker
Sinus tachycardia	Chronotropic drugs
	Vascular volume
	Evaluate anesthetic status
	Switch to dobutamine
	Consider cardiac glycosides/propranolol
	Arterial pacemaker overdrive
Premature atrial contractions	0
Premature nodal contractions	0
Premature ventricular contractions	Check ventilation (and arterial blood gases)
	Give KCl 1–2 mEq/min
	Magnesium sulfate 1–2 g (8–16 mEq)
	Lidocaine 1 mg/kg IV; infusion 2 mg/min, if needed
	Bretylium
	Procainamide
	Quindine
Atrioventricular dissociation	Isoproterenol
Second-degree atrioventricular block	Atrioventricular sequential pacemaker
Third-degree atrioventricular block	Ventricular pacemaker
SVT	Cardioversion
Atrial fibrillation	Digitalis glycosides
Atrial flutter	Verapamil
	Atrial pacemaker overdrive?
	Atrioventricular sequential pacemaker
Recurrent ventricular fibrillation	? Ischemia
Ventricular fibrillation	Lidocaine 2 mg/kg; IV infusion 3–4 mg/kg
Ventricular tachycardia	KCl 2 mEq/min until K⁺ ≥ 6.0 mEq/L
	Intraaortic balloon pump
	Magnesium sulfate 1–2 g IV (8–16 mEq)
	Bretylium 8–10 mg/kg IV
	Procainamide
	Quinidine
	Propranolol?
	Experimental antiarrhythmic agents?
	Defibrillation

a Treat only if hemodynamically significant, or if runs of premature ventricular contractions.
Reprinted, with permission, from Ream.[49]

Types of Pacemaker Generators

Asynchronous. The asynchronous pacemaker generator is responsible only for the formation of electrical impulses and is used safely in patients who have no intrinsic ventricular activity. If used in those patients with ventricular activity, it may compete with the patient's own conduction system. If such competition occurs during the supranormal period of repolarization, ventricular tachycardia can result.

Synchronous. The synchronous pacemaker generator contains two circuits: one forms impulses, and the other acts as a sensor. When activated by an R-wave, the sensing circuit either triggers or inhibits the pacing circuit. These are classified as triggered or inhibited pacemakers. The inhibited is the most frequently used pacemaker because it eliminates competition and is energy sparing.

Sequential. Sequential pacing facilitates a normal sequence between atrial and ventricular contraction, promoting the normal atrial kick.

Programmable. The programmable pacemaker generator is the newest type of pacemaker and, as the name implies, it is programmable as well as operable on a fixed-function basis. Rate, output, and R-wave sensitivity are the most common programmed areas. An advantage to the use of this type of generator is that it can overcome the interference caused by the electrocautery machine.

Three- and five-letter code systems have been devised to simplify the naming of pacemaker generators. The letters used in these codes are listed in Tables 41–19 and 41–20.

1. AOO and VOO are asynchronous generators that pace the atrium and ventricle, respectively.
2. VVI is a synchronous generator that paces and senses in the ventricle. As implied, this generator is inhibited if a sinus or escape beat occurs.
3. DVI is used for atrioventricular sequential pacing in which both atria and ventricles are paced.

Ventricular Pacing

Temporary Ventricular Pacing. Temporary ventricular pacing is indicated in short-term conduction defects until

TABLE 41–19. THREE-LETTER PACEMAKER CODE

Letter 1	Chamber paced
A	Atrium
V	Ventricle
D	Dual (both A and V)
Letter 2	Chamber sensed
A	Atrium
V	Ventricle
D	Dual (both A and V)
O	Asynchronous, or does not apply
Letter 3	Response to sensed signal
I	Inhibition
T	Triggering
O	Asynchronous, or does not apply

Reprinted, with permission, from Zaidan JR. Pacemakers. Anesthesiology. 1984;60(4):321.

TABLE 41–20. FIVE-LETTER PACEMAKER CODE

Letter 1	See Table 41–22
Letter 2	See Table 41–22
Letter 3	Responses to sensed signal
T	Triggered
I	Inhibited
O	Asynchronous
D	Dual (triggering and inhibition)
R	Reverse functions (activation of the generator by rapid heart rates rather than slow heart rates
Letter 4	Programming
O	No programming
P	Programming only for output and/or rate
M	Multiple programmable
Letter 5	Tachyarrhythmia functions

Reprinted, with permission, from Zaidan JR. Pacemakers. Anesthesiology. 1984;60(4):321–323.

symptoms are abolished. It may be used in acute myocardial infarction when the patient exhibits conduction absences or conduction delays, to suppress tachyarrhythmias, and after open heart surgery.

Transvenous pacing electrodes can be inserted into the subclavian, jugular, and basilic veins through the superior vena cava into the right atrium, and through the tricuspid valve into the right ventricle. Once proper positioning has been verified, the electrode is connected to its power source and pulses are generated.

Once the electrode is in place, a stimulation threshold must be determined. Threshold is defined as the minimum amount of electrical current necessary to produce a consistent cardiac depolarization when the inherent heart rate falls below a predetermined rate.[48] If a ventricular response to stimulation is not observed on the ECG, then the current is of too low a magnitude.

Rate is predetermined according to the patient's need. If the rate falls below this predetermined figure, the demand mode will kick in and begin to pace. Figure 41–16 demonstrates unipolar and bipolar ventricular pacing patterns.

Permanent Ventricular Pacing. Permanent ventricular pacing is indicated for patients who suffer from congestive heart failure with associated dysrhythmias, postmyocardial infarction whereby the conduction system is permanently damaged, sinus arrest or sinus bradycardia with symptoms, Stokes–Adams syndrome, and fascicular block.

Atrial Pacing

Atrial pacing is designed for those patients with pure atrial arrhythmias or with ventricular tachyarrhythmias (Fig. 41–17). It is also of benefit to those patients with heart disease in that it provides the atrial kick, thus increasing cardiac output. The atrial kick is lost with ventricular pacing because the atrial and ventricular contractions may not be sequential.

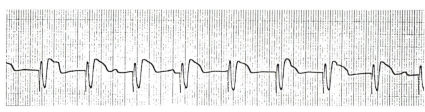

A

Figure 41–16. Ventricular pacing (**A**) with a unipolar catheter and 100 percent capture and (**B**) with a bipolar electrode. Note that pacer artifact in the bipolar tracing (indicated by arrows) is much more difficult to see than obtained with a unipolar electrode. (*Reprinted, with permission, from Jones.*[48])

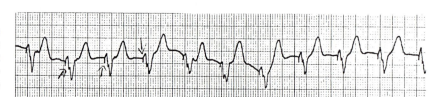

B

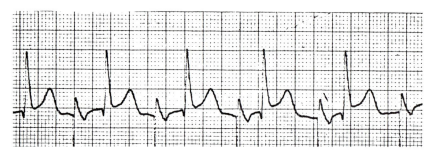

Figure 41–17. Atrial pacer firing 100 percent with 100 percent capture. (*Reprinted, with permission, from Jones.*[48])

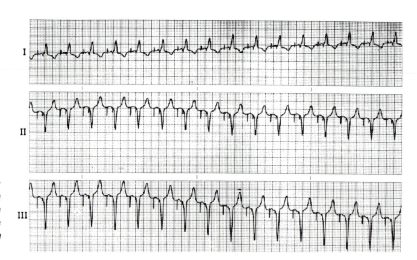

I

II

III

Figure 41–18. Bifocal demand pacemaker (sequential atrioventricular) rhythm. Note that there are two sets of artificial pacemaker spikes: one precedes the P-waves, and the other precedes the QRS complex. (*Reprinted, with permission, from Chung.*[51])

A major problem associated with atrial pacing is electrode instability. Because of the anatomic structure of the atrium (lack of trabeculae) the electrode cannot be secured and has a tendency to float, causing inconsistent pacing. This plus inability to achieve a consistent atrial "demand" function and the unpredictable appearance of atrioventricular conduction defects have limited the use of pure atrial pacing.[51] Consequently, an atrioventricular sequential pacemaker was developed.

Atrioventricular Sequential Pacemaking

The atrioventricular sequential pacemaker can be used on both a temporary basis and a permanent basis. The sequential pacemaker consists of two stimulators, which are recycled by the sensing of the ventricular R-wave but fire at a preset escape interval.[51] The ventricular bipolar electrode subserves the dual function of sensing and stimulating, whereas the atrial bipolar electrode subserves stimulation only.

By separately programming the two stimulators, the pacemaker is made to remain dormant while the electric R-R interval is shorter than the two escape intervals; it functions as an atrial pacer when the R-R interval is greater than the atrial escape interval, as an atrioventricular sequential pacer when a block renders the atrioventricular conduction period longer than the pacemaker's sequential interval, or as a ventricular pacer when the atrial electrode is not functioning, avoiding the danger of asystole from loss of control of the atrial electrode (Fig. 41–18).[51]

Permanent pacemakers may be inserted either transvenously or transthoracically. The most serious complication of pacemaker insertion or implantation is ventricular fibrillation, especially in the asynchronous type of generator, because of the R-on-T phenomenon.

The pacer may malfunction as a result of broken or displaced electrodes or loss of generator power. Malfunctioning pacers may cause acceleration of pacing, deceleration of pacing, irregular pacing, or failure to sense and pace.

TABLE 41–21. INDICATIONS FOR TEMPORARY PACING

1. Symptomatic second-degree, high-degree, and complete atrioventricular block
2. Symptomatic bradyarrhythmias caused by any mechanism as a result of acute myocardial infarction
3. Acute bifascicular or trifascicular block as a result of acute myocardial infarction
4. Sick sinus syndrome and brady/tachyarrhythmia syndrome
5. Symptomatic digitalis-induced bradyarrhythmias
6. Drug-resistant tachyarrhythmias
7. Carotid sinus syncope
8. Ventricular standstill
9. Before or during implantation of a permanent pacemaker
10. Therapeutic trial for intractable congestive heart failure, cardiogenic shock, and cerebral or renal insufficiency
11. Prophylactic pacing during and immediately after major cardiac surgery

Reprinted, with permission, from Chung.[51]

TABLE 41–22. INDICATIONS FOR PERMANENT PACING

Sick sinus syndrome and brady/tachyarrhythmia syndrome

Mobitz type II atrioventricular block

Complete or advanced atrioventricular block
  As a result of trifascicular block
  Congenital in origin
  Surgically induced (irreversible)
  Lasting more than 2–3 weeks in acute myocardial infarction

All other chronic and symptomatic atrioventricular blocks

Symptomatic bilateral bundle branch blocks

Bifascicular block or incomplete trifascicular block with intermittent complete atrioventricular block as a result of acute myocardial infarction

Carotid sinus syncope

Recurrent ventricular standstill

Recurrent drug-resistant tachyarrhythmias benefited by temporary pacing

Intractable congestive heart failure and cerebral or renal insufficiency benefited by temporary pacing

Reprinted, with permission, from Chung.[51]

The newer pacemaker generators are lithium-powered and should survive for 5 years.

Anesthetic Considerations

Both transvenous and transthoracic pacemakers can be inserted under local anesthesia with monitored anesthesia care. Several factors modify pacer function: (1) Sympathomimetic amines may increase myocardial irritability. (2) Quinidine or procainamide toxicity may cause failure of cardiac capture. (3) Hyperkalemia, advancement of heart disease, or fibrosis around the electrode may cause failure of cardiac capture.

The primary considerations for the anesthetist are patient comfort and control of dysrhythmia during insertion. Mild sedation with an intravenous dose of a benzodiazepine is helpful in reducing anxiety. A lidocaine bolus and an isoproterenol infusion should be available to treat arrhythmias. Patients with incomplete heart block can be placed in complete block during the pacer insertion. Atropine may be used for blocks that occur at the atrioventricular node. With transvenous pacing hemorrhage, cardiac perforation pneumothorax, and severe cardiac arrhythmias may occur.

Patients who present with pacemakers intact require special attention. The ECG should be observed for pacemaker malfunction. If temporary pacers are in place the generator should be protected to prevent microshock. This can be accomplished with the use of a rubber sheet or glove.

Permanent pacemakers can have electromagnetic interference from cautery, causing demand pacemakers to be in fixed mode. A magnet placed over the generator can convert this. Cautery pads should be placed as distant as possible from the generator. The indications for temporary and permanent pacing are listed in Tables 41–21 and 41–22.

PERIPHERAL VASCULAR OCCLUSIVE DISEASE

Diseases of Abdominal Aorta

Abdominal Aortic Aneurysm. True aneurysms or athero-sclerotic occlusive disease can occur along the aorta or in any of its branches. A true aneurysm is one whose walls, although dilated and deformed, contain elements of the original vessel wall. The process usually affects middle-aged or elderly people and is thought to be the result of congenital defects, degenerative changes, dissection aortitis, or trauma.[34]

Aneurysms confined to the infrarenal abdominal aorta are the most common aortic aneurysm and true aneurysms of this area result almost entirely from atherosclerosis.[52] The natural course of this disease has been well established as one that progresses to rupture and death in about half of the patients within a year of diagnosis and in 91 percent at unpredictable times within 5 years.[52] Surgical intervention, when electively performed, provides for mortality ranges of 3 to 5 percent[53] secondary to myocardial infarction and renal or cardiac failure.

Early detection and surgical interventions are the keys to successful treatment. These patients generally present with abdominal or back pain and a pulsating abdominal mass. Diagnosis is confirmed by aortogram (Fig. 41–19). Once diagnosis has been established, replacement graft should be considered. Generally speaking, replacement is indicated when the aneurysm is twice the size of the distal or proximal uninvolved aorta.[53] Aneurysms that are 5 cm in diameter or larger are at risk of rupture. Abdominal

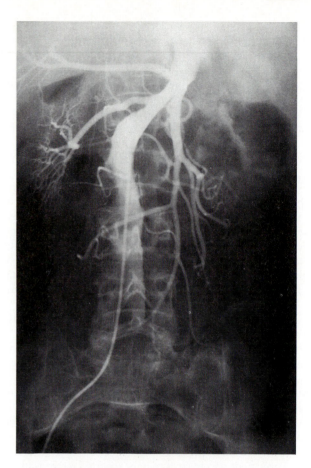

Figure 41–20. Ruptured abdominal aortic aneurysm.

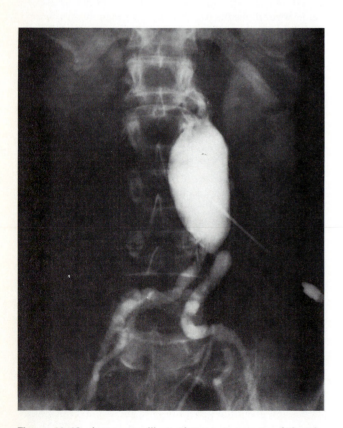

Figure 41–19. Aortogram illustrating an aneurysm of the abdominal aorta.

aneurysms frequently rupture and are a source of emboli, leading to lower extremity ischemia (Fig. 41–20). In 60 percent of cases, the aneurysms are located 2 to 5 cm below the origin of the renal arteries and extend down to, but do not include, the aortic bifurcation.[34] In 40 percent of patients, the common iliac arteries are involved either by aneurysmal disease or by associated atherosclerotic occlusive disease.[34] Approximately 15 percent of patients undergoing aneurysm resection have associated narrowing of iliac vessels.

Aortoiliac Occlusive Disease. Atherosclerotic occlusive disease is a common cause of ischemic symptoms in the lower extremities. Initially, symptoms include intermittent claudication of muscles of the thigh, hips, buttocks, and calf and progress to impotence and diminished pulses. The risk factors for these patients are the same as for other atherosclerotic processes, that is, smoking, diabetes, hypertension, and elevated serum cholesterol levels.

The initial lesions of aortoiliac occlusive disease appear to begin at the terminal aorta and the proximal portion of the common iliac arteries or at the bifurcation of the common iliacs and progress slowly. The ultimate anatomic result of progressive aortoiliac atherosclerosis is occlusion of the distal abdominal aorta, with progression of a thrombus up to the level of the renal arteries (Fig. 41–21).[34]

The indications for surgery are disabling claudication and ischemia at rest, manifested by rest pain in the foot, ischemic ulceration, or pregangrenous skin changes.[34]

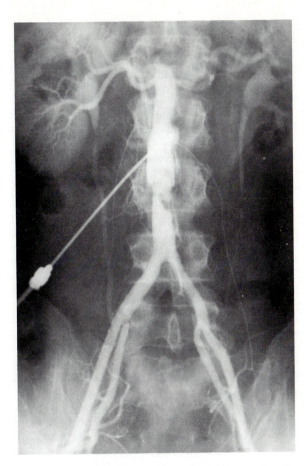

Figure 41–21. Abdominal aorta with severe atherosclerotic occlusive disease.

Preoperative Assessment. The anesthetic evaluation includes adequate assessment of other systems. Generally speaking, these patients should be managed as though occlusive disease exists in all arterial systems. Because these patients are older, impairment of renal, cardiac, and respiratory systems is common and the possibility of complication is high. Some institutions routinely perform a cardiac catheterization preoperatively. An effective noninvasive method of determining the degree of coronary artery disease is dipyridamole thallium imaging. It assesses both hypoperfused areas and infarcted areas of the myocardium.

Most of these patients present with extremely labile blood pressures preoperatively, demonstrating the need for adequate antihypertensive regimens. Chronic hypertension presents several problems to the anesthetist in major procedures such as this. Patients with uncontrolled hypertension, when anesthetized, suffer a greater reduction in systemic vascular resistance and a marked fall in mean arterial blood pressure and are subject to a higher incidence of arrhythmias and ischemia.[32]

Patients with diastolic hypertension usually have a reduced plasma volume, leading to lability of blood pressure under anesthesia. In addition to antihypertensive agents, diuretics are common for the patient with elevated arterial pressure. Electrolyte imbalance may accompany their use. Except in the case of an emergency procedure, electrolyte imbalances, intravascular volume depletion, and hypertension should be corrected preoperatively.

The most common cause of death after elective vascular surgery of the aorta or its major branches is myocardial infarction,[32] and 33 to 49 percent of the deaths are secondary to an infarction that occurs perioperatively.[54] Careful preoperative assessment of myocardial status is indicated.

Renal status is another area of importance in the preoperative evaluation. Careful analysis of renal laboratory studies should be made to determine if a prerenal condition exists. Several causal factors are associated with postoperative renal failure in these patients: (1) arterial dye studies, (2) mechanical occlusion of renal vessels during surgery, (3) renal trauma, and (4) dehydration. If laboratory values are borderline, special precautions to protect the kidneys should be taken, such as adequate hydration and diuresis. Dialysis may be necessary in the renally impaired patient.

Anesthetic Technique. Standard monitoring techniques for these procedures include a precordial V_5 lead, arterial line, esophageal stethoscope, pulse oximeter, capnograph, urimeter, and Swan-Ganz catheter. The pulmonary artery catheter is used to optimize intravenous fluid administration and detect hemodynamic changes during cross-clamping. The presence of an abnormal V-wave in the PCWP trace may indicate ischemia.

The use of a combined general/epidural anesthetic appears to have risen in popularity as the choice of management for patients undergoing peripheral vascular surgery. This combined technique has several advantages: there is a reduction in inhalation and narcotic anesthesia requirements, there is a reduction in SVR with cross-clamping, the stress response is altered by blocking different impulses from reaching the central nervous system and efferent reflex response to pain, there is a lower incidence of hypertension, and airway reflexes are preserved. In addition the incidence of postoperative thromboembolism, confusion, and ventilator dependence is reduced. These advantages are secondary to the physiologic effects of the regional anesthetic. These include decreased afterload, increased peripheral sympathetic blockade, muscle relaxation, and prolonged postoperative analgesia.[55] The most commonly used are lidocaine, chloroprocaine, and bupivacaine. The catheter is left in place and postoperative analgesia is provided with epidural morphine or fentanyl.

There are at least three indications for administration of large volumes of intravenous fluid in vascular surgery: (1) elimination of discrepancies between the volumes of circulating blood and blood in the vascular bed caused by large blood loss or release of an occluding clamp, (2) dilution of radiopaque dyes, and (3) prevention of postoperative oliguria.

Some advocate the use of crystalloid solutions whereas others advocate the use of hypertonic sodium solutions. Proponents of hypertonic sodium solutions feel that sodium, being largely confined to the extracellular compartment, in hypertonic solution will expand the extracellular fluid space by extracting water from cells.[56] Several authors have postulated that, in addition to its role in the restoration of the functional extracellular fluid space, sodium itself has a beneficial effect on oxidative phosphorylation in the shock state.

The pulmonary artery catheter has been a major breakthrough for monitoring under anesthesia. Besides providing pulmonary artery and right arterial pressures, this instrument has made possible monitoring of left ventricular filling pressure (via pulmonary artery wedge pressure) and, thus, left ventricular function as well as cardiac output determinations on a moment-to-moment basis.[32] Furthermore, measurements of pulmonary or mixed venous oxygen tension are an extremely sensitive index of the adequacy of cardiac output for total body metabolic needs.[57] The pulmonary artery catheter also provides a central venous line for administration of vasoactive drugs, heparin, and electrolytes.

The primary concern of the anesthetist throughout the surgical procedure should be adequate hydration. As mentioned previously, such factors as chronic hypertension, arteriography, age, and poor nutrition predispose these patients to inadequate intravascular volumes.

The pulmonary artery catheter provides information about the hydration of the patient. The need for volume replacement can be assessed before surgical insult. It is essential to maintain "patient normal" volume replacement or slightly above because of the hemodynamic changes associated with aortic occlusion and release. Furthermore, blood loss during these operations can be significant and poorly tolerated by the patient with marginal myocardial function. The most critical part of the surgical procedure is the time during aortic occlusion and release. Aortic occlusion produces a variety of changes in the cardiovascular status of the patient. The degree of change is dependent on several variables. These include intravascular volume status, myocardial function, degree of collateral circulation around the occlusion, the anesthetic agent, and metabolic status of the patient. Infrarenal occlusion above and below an abdominal aneurysm generally produces a change in arterial pressure because the vascular bed proximal to the occlusion still constitutes 70 percent of the total circulatory bed, including circulation to all major organs.[58] Backflow of blood from the severed distal aortic segment usually appears, indicating the presence of collateral circulation. Ischemia of the lower extremities can therefore be expected only with prolonged occlusion and with lumbar artery involvement.[58] On occlusion of the aorta, a transient rise in arterial blood pressure (10 to 20 percent) and pulse rate, reduction in stroke volume and cardiac index and a sharp rise in SVR, decreased venous return, and elevated LVEDP can be expected.

Systemic and pulmonary pressures usually return to normal after 10 to 20 minutes of cross-clamp time. It should be noted that fewer hemodynamic changes occur when cross-clamp is performed with aortoocclusive disease than on patients with abdominal aortic aneurysm. The increased hemodynamic stability is thought to result from the development of good collateral circulation with occlusive disease.

In an effort to reduce myocardial afterload during clamping, to permit fluid volume loading of the patient, and to avoid declamping hypotension, the use of nitroglycerin or nitroprusside is advocated before and during aortic cross-clamping. Vasodilation with nitroprusside can reverse hypertensive episodes and decreases in cardiac output. Recent studies propose that nitroglycerin in doses ranging from 0.25 to 1.0 μg/kg per minute may improve subendo-

cardial blood flow and prevent ischemia. Vasodilators should be discontinued before unclamping. Because aortic cross-clamping can produce hemodynamic changes consistent with ischemia, the V_5 lead should be used, it being the most sensitive to ischemic changes. Aortic occlusion results in absence of circulation to the lower extremities and distal organs, producing metabolic acidosis that becomes evident when the clamps are removed. Lactic acid and end products of metabolism accumulate in the lower extremities. Analysis should be performed at regular intervals to evaluate the metabolic state of the patient. Metabolic acidosis is due to accumulation of nonvolatile acids.

If left untreated, several processes can evolve: the myocardium becomes depressed, reducing cardiac output; peripheral vasoconstriction may occur; the oxyhemoglobin curve is shifted to the right; the respiratory center is stimulated; hyperkalemia occurs; and response to sympathetic stimulation, whether direct or indirect, decreases. Acidosis also interferes with normal enzymatic activity and can produce changes at the cellular levels.

Severe acidosis should be corrected to provide normal hemodynamic and cellular function. Corrective treatment should be aggressive and immediate using sodium bicarbonate. The dosage of bicarbonate can be calculated as follows: dose (mEq) = base excess × body weight in kilograms divided by 3. One-half of the calculated dose should be given slowly and samples drawn to determine correction. The administration of bicarbonate to correct a metabolic acidosis presents a carbon dioxide load for the lungs to excrete, and efficient buffering of a metabolic acidosis depends on adequate pulmonary ventilation. The use of bicarbonate to correct acidosis has become a controversial issue because it is postulated that it increases the intracellular concentrations of carbon dioxide.

Aortic occlusion is associated with a reduction in renal blood flow. The exact mechanism by which renal cortical blood flow is reduced has not been well defined. Several theories exist regarding its etiology. Flow may be impaired by arterial pressure changes, direct trauma, or embolization of plaque or because of a renin–angiotensin response.

Even with judicious care, transient oliguria or renal failure may occur and can be a major cause of death after successful surgery.[58] Oliguria may be the result of preoperative dehydration, effects of anesthetics and related pharmacopeia, and hypovolemia, all of which play a role in increasing secretion of antidiuretic hormone.

The kidney may be protected by administration of large volumes of balanced salt solution just before clamping and by administration of a diuretic such as mannitol 0.5 to 1 g/kg or furosemide 10 to 20 mg prior to clamping. Renal doses of dopamine are also recommended during aortic cross-clamp. The urinary output should be maintained at 1 to 2 mL/kg per hour.

Mannitol is completely excreted by the kidney, together with a volume of obligatory water of about 5 mL/g mannitol.[59] Because it requires water for excretion, mannitol should not produce diuresis in dehydrated patients, nor should it dehydrate patients in whom sufficient volumes of obligatory water are available or supplied by infusion.[60] The erythrocyte is most sensitive to changes in osmotic pressure, and it is suggested that one-half of obligatory water comes from this source.[61] The fall in hematocrit, without change in hemoglobin or red blood cell count, leads to a reduction in viscosity, a decrease in renal vascular resistance, and an increase in renal blood flow.[58]

Excessive blood loss can create serious problems for the anesthetist, particularly when rapid transfusion is necessary. The risk of throwing these elderly patients into frank congestive failure is ever present. Generally speaking, blood should be replaced volume for volume. The cell saver devices currently available allow for intraoperative autotransfusion during sudden excessive blood loss. Intraoperative autotransfusion has obvious advantages: immediate availability, normothermia, and none of the hazards inherent to use of homologous bank blood.[62] Autotransfused blood contains only washed, packed red cells suspended in saline solutions and is essentially devoid of other blood components. Coagulation factors must be replenished and heparin-neutralized when large volumes of salvaged red blood cells are transfused. Autotransfusion is not without complication. Air embolism and hemolysis with associated renal dysfunction and microembolism have been reported.[62]

Excessive administration of stored whole blood always risks reaction and decreased coagulation function. After administration of four to five units of whole blood, fresh-frozen plasma should be considered to enhance coagulation function. The administration of calcium with massive transfusion remains a controversial issue. It may be necessary to infuse a vasodilatory agent to improve the efficiency of volume replacement. Elevated SVR may prevent adequate hydration, and if tolerated, dilation should be concomitant with replacements.

Once reconstruction of the aorta has been performed, circulation to the lower extremities can be reestablished. When the aortic occlusion clamp is released, vasoactive metabolites are liberated and a hypotension phenomenon may occur. "Declamping shock" has been attributed to many factors including the duration of occlusion, the amount of acid metabolites generated during occlusion, abruptness of declamping, sympathetic tone of the venous system, lack of sufficient collateral blood flow during cross-clamp, anesthetic agents and depth of anesthesia, presence of associated cardiorespiratory problems, actual blood loss before and during cross-clamp, and inadequacy of left ventricular filling pressure before cross-clamp.[63]

The most common cause of hypotension after release of the clamp appears to be an inadequate circulating volume. This can be avoided by increasing left ventricular filling pressure. One approach is to infuse lactated Ringer's solution in a volume significant enough to increase PCWP 3 to 4 mm Hg above preanesthetic values during cross-clamping.[63]

Aortic Dissection. Aortic dissection refers to aneurysmal dilation of the false lumen of the aorta and may result in compression of the true lumen of the aorta or rupture and death. Mortality rates are in the range 75 to 90 percent. Aortic dissections can be classified as types A and B. Type A dissection involves the ascending aorta and type B dissection begins distal to the left subclavian artery. Approximately 57 percent begin in the proximal aorta, 28 percent begin distal to the left subclavian, and 10 percent begin proximal to the innominate artery. Type A dissections usu-

ally require surgery unless neurologic symptoms are worsening. Symptoms associated with dissections include back and shoulder pain, substernal ecchymosis, heart block, dyspnea, neck vein distension, hematuria, Horner's syndrome, hoarseness, and a pulsating neck mass. Aortic regurgitation is present in 50 percent of type A dissections.[64]

As previously mentioned, the majority of the total blood volume is proximal to the occlusion, and excessive blood loss can occur without being reflected by hemodynamic changes. Hypovolemia is also due to evisceration of bowel necessary for aortic exposure; the small bowel dilates and significant fluid loss occurs.[58] Thus, when aortic occlusion is discontinued, a smaller blood volume is available to fill the vascular bed.

Overhydration will contract the vascular bed, eliminating decreases in cardiac output and venous return. Even after satisfactory replacement of the vascular volume as determined by pulmonary artery pressure, hypotensive episodes frequently occur in the postoperative period because of third-space shift. It may take several hours for stabilization of fluid compartments. Hypothermia is also a common problem with aortic surgery. Every effort should be made to keep the patient normothermic. The effects of hypothermia can be severe: increased myocardial contractility, raised oxygen consumption, coagulopathy, and fibrillation can occur. All fluids should be warmed, inspired gases humidified, and room temperature raised in an effort to conserve heat. Warm saline irrigation may also be of benefit.

In addition to the complications mentioned throughout this discussion spinal cord injury may occur from aortograms or surgical intervention. The incidence of spinal cord damage/paralysis is highest with thoracic aneurysm repair because of position of the clamp.

Ruptured Abdominal Aneurysm. The mortality rate for a ruptured or leaking aneurysm is approximately 50 percent. Because of the highly lethal nature of a ruptured aneurysm, the key to resuscitation is speed. These patients present with frank circulatory collapse and rapid cessation of blood loss is imperative. This is accomplished only by aortic clamping and it is not until clamping occurs that beneficial results from resuscitative measures can be seen.

Induction of anesthesia is on an emergency basis, with care taken to avoid cough, strain, or fasciculation and aspiration. Once muscle relaxation has been established additional bleeding may occur from removal of the tamponade caused by a rigid abdominal wall.

Rapid replacement of fluids and blood to expand the vascular bed is essential to prevent death in these patients. Although hypotension or circulatory collapse exists, contraction of the vascular bed with vasoconstrictors should be avoided in an effort to provide for maximum volume replacement.

Blood loss usually proceeds at a rate faster than availability or replacement can occur. Volume expanders and crystalloid solutions are recommended until adequate blood replacement can occur. Rapid massive blood administration is not without consequence and all principles governing massive transfusion should be followed.

Even though all resuscitative measures may be taken, the rate of mortality is high for this group of surgical pa-

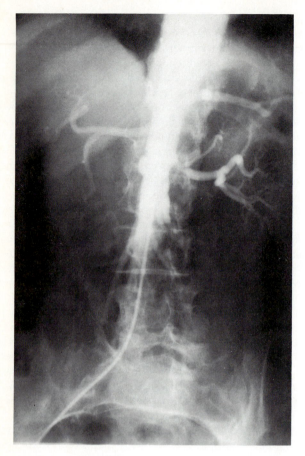

Figure 41–22. Renal artery stenosis.

tients. These patients succumb to massive blood loss, myocardial failure or infarction, irreversible hypotension, renal failure, and hypothermia.

Renal Artery Revascularization. Occlusion or stenosis of the renal arteries results in hypertension and renal failure (Fig. 41–22). Renovascular hypertension is thought to account for 5 to 10 percent of the hypertensive population. The presence of renovascular hypertension should be sus-

pected when severe hypertension that is uncontrolled by drug therapy exists. This form of hypertension usually affects the young adult and usually there is no familiar history of hypertension.

The most common cause of renal vascular hypertension is atherosclerotic narrowing of the renal artery. Reduced pulse pressure distal to a stenotic lesion in the main or segmental artery activates the renin–angiotensin system, resulting in increased renin production by the ischemic kidney.[61] The macula densa and juxtaglomerular apparatus are the two intrarenal sites that exert control on blood pressure. The macula densa is the intrarenal sensor of sodium concentration and thereby exerts a control in renin production in the juxtaglomerular apparatus.[61] The juxtaglomerular cells are sensors of intraarteriolar perfusion pressure. Reduced perfusion pressure causes an increased release of renin by these cells[34] and the renin–angiotensin system is activated (Fig. 41–23).

Theory suggests that there are three mechanisms whereby renin release is regulated: (1) According to the intrarenal arteriolar baroreceptor mechanism, renin secretion increases when the intraarteriolar pressure at the juxtaglomerular cell decreases. (2) The macula densa theory postulates that renin secretion is inversely proportional to the rate of sodium transport across this area of distal tubule. (3) The sympathetic nervous system increases renin secretion by increasing circulatory catecholamines and by stimulating renal sympathetic nerves. Diagnosis is made not only by a demonstrable lesion but also by selective renal vein renin production. A renal vein : renin ratio of 1:1.5 is considered positive.[61] Surgical correction of these lesions provides good results in correction of hypertension. Preferred methods of surgical revascularization include aortorenal bypass, splenorenal bypass, hepatorenal bypass, and renal endarterectomy.

Anesthetic considerations for these procedures are the same as for any major abdominal vascular surgery, with special attention to preservation of renal tissue.

Antihypertensive therapy must be continued to the time of surgery. α-Methyldopa appears to be the drug of choice, producing little effect on hemodynamics when combined with anesthesia. It reduces both central and peripheral norepinephrine levels and is known to interact with

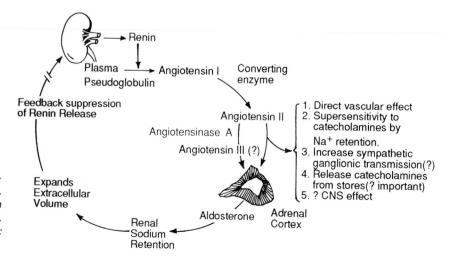

Figure 41–23. Summary of renin–angiotensin aldosterone pharmacology. CNS, central nervous system. (*Reprinted, with permission, from Brenner BM, Rector FC. The kidney. Philadelphia: WB Saunders; 1976;2.*)

anesthetic agents by lowering the minimal alveolar concentrations (MACs) of anesthetics required for analgesia.[61]

Because the aortic occlusion clamp is placed above the renal arteries, special precautions need to be taken for kidney preservation. Local hypothermia may be applied. Mannitol or furosemide is given to promote diuresis and to overcome the renin–angiotensin response. In addition, some centers use a renal perfusion fluid consisting of chilled Ringer's lactate, mannitol, heparin, and methylprednisolone.[61]

Manipulation of the stenosed artery may cause a renin–angiotensin response, and drugs should be available to overcome this reaction. Although most inhalation agents are to some extent biotransformed and the products of metabolism often eliminated by the kidney, these drugs do not rely on renal excretion for reversal of their therapeutic effects; thus all inhalants, with the exception of methoxyflurane and enflurane, can be used in mild or moderate renal failure.[30]

The action of narcotics is intensified with renal disease. The only drugs absolutely contraindicated for muscle relaxation are gallamine and decamethonium, which are excreted almost entirely by the kidney.

Patients suffering from renal disease and those on antihypertensive therapy are generally hypovolemic and caution must be taken not to cause a reduction in arterial pressure. The best therapy for hypotensive episodes is volume expansion, because all vasopressors result in some degree of renal compromise.

Ultrashort-acting barbiturates produce few side effects in the patient with renal compromise. Belladonna alkaloids such as atropine and hyoscyamine are excreted unchanged by the kidneys and should be avoided or the dosage modified. Hyoscine is almost entirely metabolized and is the drug of choice if a belladonna is indicated.

Aortoduodenal Fistula. Aortoduodenal fistula is characterized by gastrointestinal bleeding, which can be exsanguinating. Rupture usually occurs on the left side into the retroperitoneal space, but it can occur on the right into the retroperitoneal space, duodenum, vena cava, or iliac vein.[34] Treatment consists of control of bleeding by graft replacement and repair of the duodenum.

These patients are septic, with all of the sequelae that accompany this shocklike state. Blood loss is usually excessive and requires massive transfusions. Swan-Ganz catheters are beneficial in determining hemodynamic status.

Hepatodecompression. Portal hypertension is the result of obstruction to splanchnic blood flow. Diagnosis is usually made on the basis of a past history of cirrhosis accompanied by esophageal varicocele bleeding. About 30 percent of patients with varices will bleed. Approximately 70 percent who have bled from varices die within 1 year and 60 percent rebleed massively in 1 year.[30] The pathogenesis of esophageal varices relates to the development of collateral vessels between the high-pressure splanchnic circulation and the low-pressure systemic circulation.[34] A number of collateral pathways develop in an attempt to decompress the portal system, but regardless of their number and size, they are rarely able to bring about complete portal decompression.[34]

Ascites is very common in portal hypertension and is due to redistribution of fluid between plasma and extracellular fluid and also to excessive renal reabsorption of salt and water.[34] Abnormal laboratory findings include elevated lactic dehydrogenase, serum glutamic–oxaloacetic transaminase, serum glutamic–pyruvic transaminase, globulin, bilirubin, and prothrombin time. Hypoalbuminuria exists. Hypersplenism, if present, is accompanied by decreases in white cell count and platelets. Anemia is also common.

To date, surgical intervention is not the treatment of choice in the management of these patients, but if selected, the following procedures may be used: (1) Portal caval shunt (anastomosis of portal vein to inferior vena cava) to shunt blood away from the portal system is indicated only when esophageal hemorrhage is present. (2) Mesocaval shunt (anastomosis of the superior mesenteric vein to the inferior vena cava) is indicated in emergency management of varicocele bleeding. (3) Distal splenorenal shunt, or the Warren shunt (anastomosis of splenic vein to the left renal vein), was developed in an effort to avoid total diversion of portal blood flow.

Although ideally bleeding is controlled before surgery, emergency surgery to control bleeding may be necessary. Tamponade with an inflatable tube is usually necessary and remains in place until after induction. Even with the tube inserted, these patients must be treated as a full stomach patient. Awake intubation is strongly encouraged.

Blood loss is extreme and, if possible, only fresh blood should be given to provide the clotting factors needed. Hypertonic salt solutions should be avoided because these patients conserve sodium. Large volumes of crystalloid and plasma expanders should be on hand. Generally, because of poor nutritional habits, these patients are anemic, which predisposes them to thrombocytopenia or granulocytopenia. Vitamin K, potassium, glucose, and protein usually need to be replenished.

Anesthetic agents that will not further compromise the liver should be employed, limiting choices to nonmetabolized inhalation agents or to intravenous agents. Muscle relaxants that are not metabolized via the liver should be used.

Because these patients are prone to bleeding, induction should be as atraumatic as possible to avoid oral and pharyngeal bleeding. Bony prominences should be padded to prevent ecchymosis from pressure areas.

Thoracoabdominal Aortic Aneurysm. Aneurysms of this type are becoming more prevalent; it has become apparent that many patients with aneurysms of the thorax have abdominal extension of the disease or have separate lesions located in the abdomen (Fig. 41–24).[65]

Aneurysms that involve segments of both the descending thoracic and abdominal aorta in continuity, that is, true thoracoabdominal aortic aneurysms, are considered with abdominal aortic aneurysms that involve the upper segment from which visceral vessels arise, because they pose similar problems in treatment.[34] Visceral artery reconstruction may be necessary because over 20 percent of patients have occlusive disease in these arteries.

The causes of aneurysms of this nature are chronic dissection, arteriosclerosis, and medial degenerative disease,

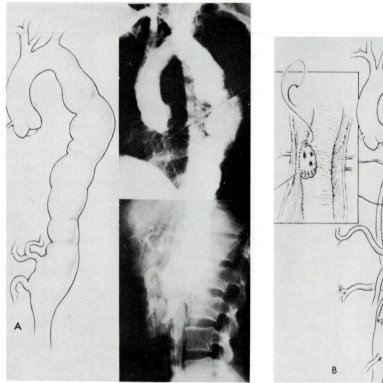 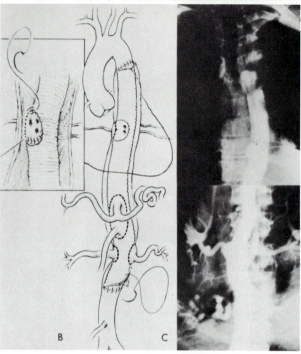

Figure 41–24. Treatment of fusiform degenerative thoracoabdominal aortic aneurysm by graft. **A.** Aortogram made before operation showing nature and extent of aneurysm. **B.** Technique of graft replacement. **C.** Aortogram made after operation showing graft in place. (*Reprinted, with permission, from Crawford and Saleh.*[66])

with the latter two being the most common.[34] They occur more commonly in the middle-aged and elderly, with high incidence of associated coronary artery, pulmonary, and renal disease. The treatment is graft replacement.

The preoperative and anesthetic regimen described is that used by the Baylor College of Medicine. Hydration is very important in these patients, and in an effort to minimize renal dysfunction, 5 percent dextrose with Ringer's lactate solution with 25 g mannitol/1000 mL is given at 150 mL per hour for 12 hours before and after aortography.[34] Blood urea nitrogen and creatinine levels should be within normal limits. All patients are placed on digitalis. Electrolytes, serum blood gases, and arterial pressures should be within normal limits.

Routine monitoring plus a Swan-Ganz catheter, right atrial catheter, and two radial artery lines to evaluate cardiac hemodynamics, blood gases, electrolytes, acid–base balance, and plasma colloidal osmotic pressure are indicated.[66] Four peripheral lines are used. A double-lumen tube is used to aid in operative exposure and to avoid pulmonary or cardiac injury.

The patient is placed on the right side at a 60- to 80-degree angle. The abdominal component of the thoracoabdominal incision is midline and is curved across the costal arch into intercostal space, appropriately located according to the extent of the descending thoracic aorta involvement.[34]

CVP, PCWP, and cardiac output are kept within normal limits. Mannitol 25 g is given postinduction. Blood re-

placement is by component technique, using packed red cells, fresh-frozen plasma platelets, and albumin. A unit of albumin and two units of fresh-frozen plasma are given at the onset of surgery. A unit of fresh-frozen plasma is given after the third transfusion and then alternated with two units of red cells. Fresh platelets 10 to 16 units are given rapidly when flow is restored through the graft.[66] Sodium nitroprusside is used to maintain normal cardiac hemodynamics during aortic clamping.

After visceral vessel anastomosis, the head of the operating room table is lowered, the graft is filled with blood to expel air, and the aorta is reclamped.[65] Restoration of circulation is slow, and once achieved, the table is elevated to its original position.

Extraanatomic Arterial Reconstruction. Although conventional aortic reconstruction for occlusive disease is in most instances performed with low mortality, extraanatomic vascular reconstruction may be necessary for life or limb salvage when conventional approaches cannot be used.

These procedures are considered for the severely debilitated, the septic, or the patient with an infected vascular prosthesis. Patients with occlusions of the distal aorta or proximal iliac arteries may then be treated with femoral-to-femoral, axillofemoral, or iliofemoral reconstruction. With proper patient and donor vessel selection, operative mortality rates are low; nevertheless patency rates decline after a 5-year period.

The protocol for anesthetic management of these patients depends on the physiologic status of the patient and his or her general overall presentation. The surgical procedure itself is less taxing because the aorta is not occluded.

Blood loss may be significant, particularly if there is anatomic difficulty in exposure. The general condition of these patients may necessitate the need for Swan-Ganz monitoring, which allows for ease of administration of large volumes of fluid or blood without fear of subjecting the patient to congestive heart failure.

Lower Extremity Procedures: Femoral–Popliteal–Tibial Occlusive Disease

Arteriosclerosis may involve the common femoral artery and its branches, the above-the-knee or below-the-knee popliteal artery, any of the infrapopliteal arteries including their terminal branches, or any combination of these arteries[34] (Fig. 41–25).

Primary considerations for the anesthetist focus on the selection of an anesthetic agent. Surgical procedures of this nature become longer in duration the further distal the reconstruction becomes. The goal of the anesthetist is to provide optimal anesthesia with the lowest concentrations possible. Fluid replacement should be carefully monitored, taking into account the insensible loss during such long

cases. Blood loss usually is not excessive, unless unforeseen developments occur.

Endovascular Surgery

Recent advances in the treatment of peripheral arterial occlusive disease include a number of specialty procedures categorized as endovascular surgery. These include balloon angioplasty, laser angioplasty, and mechanical atherectomy. These procedures provide for alternatives and replacement of conventional vascular procedures. The indications for peripheral vascular angioplasty include (1) intermittent claudication; (2) pain at rest; (3) ischemic tissue changes (ulceration, gangrene); (4) impaired distal wound healing; (5) simplification of surgical revascularization; and (6) limb salvage.[67] The advantages include less surgical trauma, reduced anesthesia time, regional versus general anesthesia, reduced hospital stay, and lowered morbidity and mortality rates.

Percutaneous Transluminal Angioplasty. With percutaneous transluminal angioplasty, a flexible guidewire is percutaneously introduced into an artery proximal to the area of occlusion. Under fluoroscopy or intraoperative arteriography a Teflon balloon-tipped catheter or balloon-tipped wire is passed to the area of occlusion. Once the occluded area is transversed the balloon is intermittently inflated,

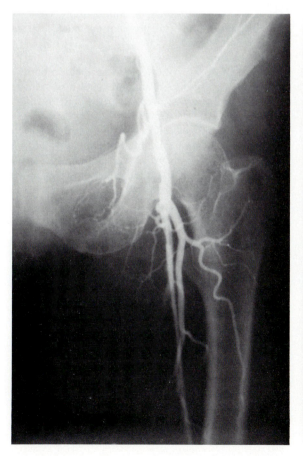
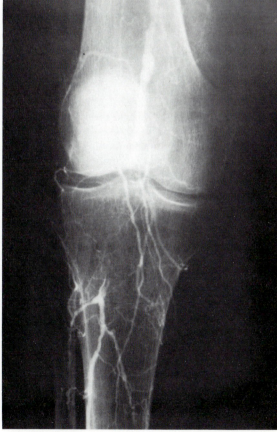

Figure 41–25. Femoral–popliteal occlusive disease.

TABLE 41–23. COMPLICATIONS OF PERCUTANEOUS TRANSLUMINAL ANGIOPLASTY

Arterial dissection

Arterial perforation

Hematoma

Embolization

Hypotension

Contrast reactions

Contrast renal failure

Pseudoaneurysm

Infection

with predetermined pressures and time limits, until the desired degree of dilation occurs. A variety of catheter sizes are available for various-size arteries. The complications of angioplasty are listed in Table 41–23.

Laser-Assisted Balloon Angioplasty. The word *laser* is an acronym derived from "light amplification by the simulated emission of radiation." The amplification of the simulated emission of radiation is the actual physical process that goes on within the laser device.[68] Different kinds of lasers are identified by the type of material inside the device. There are four categories of lasering materials: solid, gas, liquid, and semiconductor. Solid lasers include the ruby and Nd:YAG (neodynium:yttrium–aluminum–garnet). Gas lasers include helium–neon, argon, and carbon dioxide lasers. Liquid lasers use dyes, and the semiconductors use two layers of a semiconductive material such as gallium.

Laser light is a form of energy that is characterized in terms of power, is measured in watts, and is subject to a number of physical laws beyond the scope of this discussion. Basically, the laser light is absorbed by the tissue producing a local thermal event, which vaporizes plaque. The goal of laser angioplasty is to accomplish atheroma ablation without damaging surrounding normal artery wall or without causing perforation especially in a totally occluded vessel. This is best accomplished by the hot-tip laser and hybrid spectraprobe which creates a smooth wall without excessive arterial wall heating.[69] This in combination with

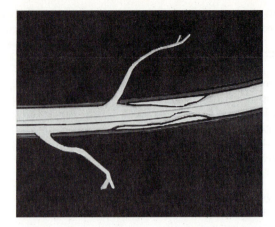

Figure 41–27. Placement of wire through lasered channel.

the balloon provides a greater increase in arterial lumen size (Figs. 41–26, 41–27, and 41–28).

Mechanical Atherectomy. In mechanical atherectomy, a special catheter with a rotary tip is slowly advanced in the artery, pulverizing plaque.

Anesthetic Technique. Local anesthetics are less than ideal for these procedures because the amount of narcotic and sedative needed results in a state of uncontrolled general anesthesia. In addition, vasospasm in the unanesthetized patient precludes adequate fluoroscopic visualization and technique. This problem is obviated by the use of epidural anesthesia.

Measures to prevent renal failure from contrast medium must be instituted. These include both pre- and perioperative hydration and prevention of administration of excessive contrast medium in the renal-insufficient patient.

All patients should be treated with preoperative and postoperative antiplatelet medication. Therapeutic anticoagulation has not been proven to be beneficial in these patients. These procedures should be performed in an operating room setting so that complications such as dissection,

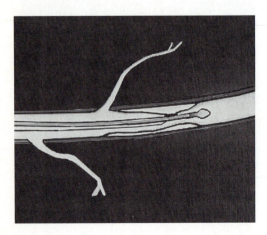

Figure 41–26. Laser probe traversing occlusion.

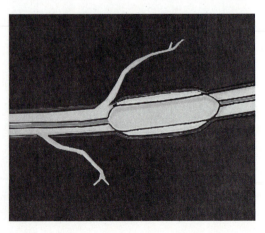

Figure 41–28. Balloon angioplasty procedure.

perforation, hemorrhage, and thrombosis can be swiftly managed.

Future Technologies. Endovascular surgery, the ability to "fix" arteries from the inside, was given its impetus by the advent of laser angioplasty. Recognizing first-generation technology, future technologies will enhance this technique with its lessened morbidity and mortality. These future technologies include lasers of different wavelength (holmium) to obviate the problem of thermal injury, guidance systems including intraarterial ultrasonography, the use of intraarterial stents, angioscopy, and thrombolysis.[67]

REFERENCES

1. Vanden Belt RJ, Ronan JA, Bedynek JL. *Cardiology: A clinical approach.* Chicago: Yearbook Medical; 1979.
2. Braunwald E. *A textbook of cardiovascular medicine.* 3rd ed. Philadelphia: WB Saunders; 1988.
3. Orkin FK, Cooperman LH. *Complications in anesthesiology.* Philadelphia: JB Lippincott; 1983.
4. Smith HC, Frye RL, Piehler JM. Does coronary bypass surgery have a favorable influence on the quality of life? *Cardiovasc Clin.* 1983;13(1):253–264.
5. Larrieu HJ. Current status of coronary bypass. *Bol Assoc Med Pr.* 1981;10:473–478.
6. Kaplan JA. *Cardiac anesthesia.* 2nd ed. New York: Grune & Stratton; 1987.
7. Slogoff S. Perioperative ischemia. *Semin Anesth.* 1990;9(1):1–7.
8. Kaplan JA. *Cardiac anesthesia: Cardiovascular pharmacology.* New York: Grune & Stratton; 1983;2.
9. Naples J. *Management of ventricular dysfunction.* Presented at Baylor College of Medicine Anesthesia and Surgery for Ischemic Heart Disease, Houston, TX; 1981.
10. Waugaman WR, Foster SD. New advances in anesthesia. *Nurs Clin North Am.* 1991;26:451–461.
11. Flynn PJ, Hughes R, Walton B. Use of atracurium in cardiac surgery involving cardiopulmonary bypass with induced hypothermia. *Br J Anaesth.* 1984;56(9):967–972.
12. Eger EI. Cardiovascular effects of inhalation anesthesia. *ASA Refresher Course Lectures.* 1983.
13. Hilfiker O, Larsen R, Sonntag H. Myocardial blood flow and oxygen consumption during halothane–nitrous oxide anesthesia for coronary revascularization. *Br J Anaesth.* 1983;55(10):927–932.
14. Merin RG. Effects of anesthetics and anesthetic adjuvants on the heart. *Contemp Anesth Pract.* 1980;2:1–18.
15. Reiz S. Effects of enflurane–nitrous oxide anesthesia and surgical stimulation on regional coronary hemodynamics in a patient with LAD bypass. *Acta Anaesthesiol Scand.* 1983;27(5):417–420.
16. Delaney TJ, Kistner JR, Lake CL, Miller ED Jr. Myocardial function during halothane and enflurane anesthesia in patients with coronary artery disease. *Anesth Analg.* 1980;59(4):240–244.
17. Balasoraswathi K, Glisson SN, El-Etr AA, Mummaneni N. Haemodynamic and catecholamine response to isoflurane anaesthesia in patients undergoing coronary artery surgery. *Can Anaesth Soc J.* 1982; 29(6):533–538.
18. Miller RD, ed. *Anesthesia.* New York: Churchill Livingstone; 1981.
19. Hug CC Jr. *The pharmacokinetics of fentanyl.* Janssen Pharmaceutical Product Information; 1981.
20. de Lange S, Stanley TH, Boscoe MJ. Alfentanil–oxygen anesthesia for coronary artery surgery. *Br J Anaesth.* 1981;53(12):1291–1296.
21. Stanley TH, de Lange S. Propranolol therapy for heart disease. *Can Anaesth Soc J.* 1982;29(4):319–324.
22. Pierce EC. *Extracorporeal circulation for open heart surgery.* Springfield, IL: Charles C Thomas; 1969.
23. Dunn J, Kirsch MN, Harness J, et al. Hemodynamic, metabolic, and hematologic effects of pulsatile cardiopulmonary bypass. *J Thorac Cardiovasc Surg.* 1974;68(1):138–147.
24. Hammond GL, Barley WW. Bubble mechanics in oxygen transfer. *J Thorac Cardiovasc Surg.* 1974;68:138.
25. Dorsen WJ Jr, Larsen KG, Elgas RI, Voohees ME. Oxygen transfer of blood: Data and theory. *Trans Am Soc Artif Intern Organs.* 1971;17:309–316.
26. Barlett RH, Galletti PM, Drinker PA, et al. *Mechanical devices for cardiopulmonary assistance.* Basel: S. Karger; 1971.
27. Bull BS, Hyse WM, Brauer FS, Korpman RA. Heparin therapy during extracorporeal circulation. *J Thorac Cardiovasc Surg.* 1975;69(5):685–689.
28. Oschner JL, Mills NH. *Coronary artery surgery.* Philadelphia: Lea & Febiger; 1978.
29. Engeilman RM, Levitsky S. *Textbook of clinical cardiology.* New York: Futura; 1981.
30. Benumoff Kadis LB, Katz J. *Anesthesia and uncommon diseases.* 2nd ed. Philadelphia: WB Saunders; 1981.
31. Smith JJ, Kampine JP. *Circulatory physiology.* Baltimore: Williams & Wilkins; 1980.
32. Miller RD. *Anesthesia.* New York: Churchill Livingstone; 1990.
33. Kaplan JA, Jones EL. Vasodilator therapy during coronary artery surgery: Comparison of nitroglycerin and nitroprusside. *J Thorac Cardiovasc Surg.* 1979;77:301–309.
34. Moore WS, ed. *Vascular surgery: A comprehensive review.* Orlando, FL: Grune & Stratton; 1983.
35. Barash PG. *Clinical anesthesia.* Philadelphia: JB Lippincott; 1989.
36. Henry WL, Bonon RO, et al. Observation on the optimum time for operative intervention for aortic regurgitation. I. Evaluation of the results of aortic valve replacement in asymptomatic patients. *Circulation.* 1980;61:471–483.
37. Arfan A. Prosthetic cardiac valves—1983. *Conn Med.* 1983; 47(10):619–625.
38. Isselbacher KJ, Adams RD, Braunwald E, Petersdorf RG, et al (eds.). *Harrison's principles of internal medicine.* 9th ed. New York: McGraw-Hill; 1980.
39. Hurst JW, Logue RB. *The heart.* 2nd ed. New York: McGraw-Hill; 1970.
40. Goodman LS, Gilman A. *The pharmacological basis of therapeutics.* 8th ed. New York: Macmillan; 1990.
41. Gilboney GS. Ventricular septal defect. *Heart Lung.* 1983;12:3.
42. Paulson DB. Cerebral apoplexy (stroke): Pathogenesis, pathophysiology, and therapy as illustrated by regional blood flow measurement in the brain. *Stroke.* 1971;2:327.
43. Cooley DA, Norman JC. *Techniques in cardiac surgery.* Houston, TX: Medical Press; 1975.
44. McClung JA, Stein JH, Ambrose JA, Herman MV, Reed GE. Prosthetic heart valves: A review. *Prog Cardiovasc Dis.* 1983;26(3):237–270.
45. Ferrans VJ, Boyce SW, Billingham ME, Spray TL, Roberts WC. Infection of glutaraldehyde-preserved porcine valve heterografts. *Am J Cardiol.* 1979;43(6):1123–1136.
46. Dellsperger KC, Wieting DW, Baehr DA, et al. Regurgitation of prosthetic heart valves. Dependence on heart rate and cardiac output. *Am J Cardiol.* 1983;51(2):321–328.
47. Guyton A. *Human physiology and mechanics of disease.* 5th ed. Philadelphia: WB Saunders; 1992.
48. Jones P. *Cardiac pacing: Continuing education in cardiovascular nursing.* East Norwalk, CT: Appleton-Century-Crofts; 1980.
49. Ream AK. *Acute cardiovascular management. Anesthesia and intensive care.* Philadelphia: JB Lippincott; 1982.
50. Nattel S, Rinkenberger RL, Lehrman LL, Zipes DP. Therapeutic blood lidocaine concentration after local anesthesia for

cardiac electrophysiologic studies. *N Engl J Med.* 1979;301(8): 418–420.

51. Chung EK. *Artificial cardiac pacing: A practical approach.* Baltimore: Williams & Wilkins; 1978.

52. Szelagyi DE, Elliot JP, Smith RF. Clinical fate of the patient with asymptomatic abdominal aortic aneurysm and unfit for surgical treatment. *Arch Surg.* 1972;104(4):600–606.

53. Crawford ES, Saleh SA, Babb JW 3d, et al. Infrarenal abdominal aortic aneurysm: Factors influencing survival after operation performed over a 25-year period. *Ann Surg.* 1981;193(6):699–709.

54. Morris GC Jr, DeBakey ME. *Renal arterial hypertension.* In: Brest AN, Moyer JH (eds). *Cardiovascular disorders.* Philadelphia: Davis; 1968:989–1000.

55. Rosner H. Optimal anesthesia for vascular surgery. Regional anesthesia is the answer. *Anesthesiol Rep.* 1989;1(3):356–363.

56. Earley LE, Bartoli E, et al. *Sodium metabolism.* In: Maxwell MH, Kleeman CR (eds). *Clinical disorders of fluid and electrolyte metabolism.* 2nd ed. New York: McGraw-Hill; 1972.

57. Stanley TH, Isern AJ. Periodic mixed venous oxygen tension analysis as a measure of the adequacy of perfusion during and after cardiopulmonary bypass. *Can Anaesth Soc J.* 1979;21:454.

58. Sabawala P, Strong MJ, Keats AS. Surgery of the aorta and its branches. *Anesthesiology.* 1970;33(2):229–259.

59. Wylie WD, Churchill-Davidson HC. *A practice of anesthesia.* 5th ed. Chicago: Yearbook Medical; 1984.

60. Barry KG, Berman AR. The acute effect of intravenous infusion of mannitol on blood and plasma volume. *N Engl J Med.* 1961;264:1085.

61. Brewster D. *Surgical management of renovascular disease.* Harvard Postgraduate Course in Vascular Surgery; 1984.

62. Duncan SE, Edwards WH, Dale WA. Caution regarding autotransfusion. *Surgery.* 1974;76(6):1024–1030.

63. Lunn JK, Dannemiller FJ, Stanley TH. Cardiovascular responses to clamping of the aorta during epidural and general anesthesia. *Anesth Analg.* 1979;58:372–376.

64. Phillips RE. *Cardiovascular therapy: A systemic approach to circulation.* Philadelphia: WB Saunders; 1979.

65. Crawford ES, Cohen ED. Acute aneurysm: A multifocal disease. *Arch Surg.* 1982;117:1393.

66. Crawford ES, Saleh SA. *Operative techniques in vascular surgery.* Orlando, FL: Grune & Stratton; 1980.

67. Pesa F. *An analysis of 500 cases of laser angioplasty.* Presented at DeBakey Society Meeting, Japan, 1990.

68. Yang Y, Hashizume M, Arbutina D. Argon laser angioplasty with a laser probe. *J Vasc Surg.* 1987;6(1):60–65.

69. White R. *Laser angioplasty.* Philadelphia: JB Lippincott; 1989.

Anesthesia for the Trauma Patient

Karen L. Zaglaniczny

The impact of trauma on health care has increased significantly in recent years. Statistics indicate that trauma is the fourth leading cause of death in the United States, surpassed only by heart disease, cancer, and stroke.[1] Trauma is the leading cause of death in the first three decades of life.

Recent advances in emergency medical care have greatly improved survival rates. Rapid evaluation and aggressive resuscitation measures by a competent trauma care team can be initiated on the patient's arrival to the emergency room. Survival depends on age, prior health status, extent of injury, and the rapidity with which adequate therapy is instituted.

Traumatic injuries can result from motor vehicle accidents, knives, guns, hatchets, and other objects. The insult may result in single- or multiple-organ damage. The type and severity of injury determine guidelines for initial and subsequent management. Priorities of trauma management include securing a patent airway and support of the circulation.

This chapter focuses on the general guidelines for optimal management of a trauma patient. Effective interaction with trauma team members is essential to facilitate the anesthetic process.

PHYSIOLOGIC RESPONSE TO TRAUMA

The physiologic responses that occur after a traumatic insult are adaptive mechanisms of the neuroendocrine and cardiovascular systems. The neuroendocrine responses are (1) activation of the autonomic nervous system with release of endogenous catecholamines, (2) renin–angiotensin–aldosterone secretion, (3) vasopressin secretion, and (4) stimulation of adrenocorticotropic hormone (ACTH) activity.[2]

The cardiovascular system responds by attempting to maintain adequate perfusion to the vital organs. The degree of response is proportional to the amount of hemorrhage and area of injury, and if inadequately treated, cardiovascu-

lar collapse occurs. A 10 to 15 percent loss of circulating blood volume can be tolerated by most patients. The blood pressure is normal with slight elevation of the heart rate. Intravascular volume can be restored with fluid therapy.

A 20 to 25 percent loss of circulating blood volume results in a decrease in cardiac output, hypotension, and tachycardia. Peripheral vascular resistance increases in an attempt to restore an effective circulating volume. Fluid and blood therapy is required to regain hemodynamic stability.

Loss of greater than 30 percent of vascular volume produces an acute insult to major organ systems. Myocardial, cerebral, and renal function are endangered by the presence of persistent hypotension and shock states.[3] Aggressive resuscitation with fluid and blood therapy, correction of acid–base and electrolyte abnormalities, and control of hemorrhage are goals of treatment. The pathophysiologic events of hemorrhagic shock are described in Figure 42–1.

Initial stabilization of the patient occurs in the emergency room. If life-threatening hemorrhage is imminent, the severely injured patient may be quickly transported to the operating room for immediate surgical intervention and resuscitation.

PREOPERATIVE ASSESSMENT

Preoperative evaluation of the trauma patient may be limited by the urgency of the impending surgery and the condition of the patient. The anesthetist should perform a rapid comprehensive assessment and examination of the patient. Further information can be obtained from the patient's chart, family, and surgeon.

The history and physical examination should include the following information:

1. Preexisting diseases
2. Current medications
3. Allergies
4. Previous anesthetic experience
5. Recent fluid and food intake
6. Alcohol and drug ingestion
7. Extent of traumatic injury

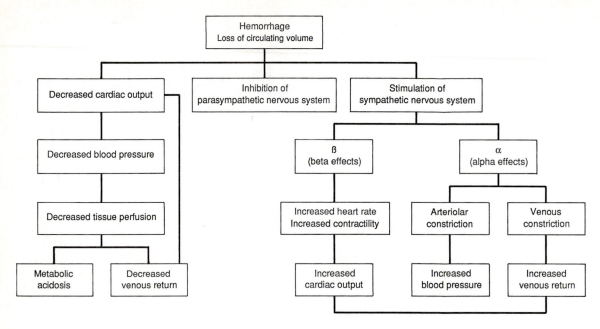

Figure 42-1. Pathophysiologic events of hemorrhagic shock.

Preexisting Disease

Trauma patients with major systemic preexisting diseases have a 5 to 10 percent increase in morbidity and mortality rates. It is essential to determine the existence and severity of any major disease process.[4] A systems approach facilitates the rapid evaluation of the patient (Table 42-1).

It is important to ascertain whether the trauma patient is taking any medications that might influence the course of

the anesthetic. The time and dosage of most recent intake should be identified. The potential for drug interactions and exaggerated responses to pharmacologic agents used during the anesthetic management is present.

Allergies

The patient is questioned for known allergies pertinent to the administration of anesthesia. These can include drugs

TABLE 42-1. SYSTEMS REVIEW

System	Major Disease	Assessment/History
Respiratory	Chronic obstructive pulmonary disease Asthma Bronchitis	Respiratory rate and rhythm Chest expansion Patency of airway Smoking Chest x-ray Arterial blood gases
Cardiovascular	Coronary artery disease Myocardial infarction Hypertension Congestive heart failure Peripheral vascular disease	Range of blood pressure Episodes of hypotension Pulse rate Jugular vein distension Electrocardiogram Cardiac reserve Incidence of angina
Neurologic	Stroke Transient ischemic attack Seizures Head injury Skull fracture	Level of consciousness Pupil size and reaction Movement of extremities
Metabolic	Diabetes Hepatitis Pancreatitis	Jaundice Hypoglycemia–hyperglycemia Lab values—enzymes, blood sugar
Renal	Acute renal disease Chronic renal disease Glomerulonephritis	Urine output Blood urea nitrogen, creatinine, electrolytes Urinalysis

and other substances such as iodine or intravenous x-ray dyes.

Previous Anesthetic Experiences

The date, type, and course of past anesthetic experiences are recorded. A familial history of previous anesthesia administration is also noted.

Recent Food and Fluid Intake

All trauma patients are assumed to have a full stomach. Gastric emptying ceases or is greatly diminished at the time of injury. The type and amount of recent food intake as well as the presence of nausea or vomiting should be determined. A nasogastric tube may be in place to remove secretions but it will not remove large particles of food. The hazards associated with regurgitation and aspiration of gastric contents are always present in the trauma patient. Aspiration pneumonitis can occur with as little as 0.4 mL/kg gastric fluid with a pH of less than 2.5. Although some practitioners recommend the administration of agents (ranitidine, metoclopramide, antacids) to reduce the acidity and volume of gastric contents, this practice is not universally accepted.[5] All appropriate measures must be used to reduce the risk of aspiration during the induction of anesthesia. These include an awake intubation or rapid-sequence induction with cricoesophageal pressure.

Alcohol and Drug Ingestion

Alcohol and illicit drug use have been documented to be significant factors in accidental and violent crime-related injuries.[6,7] The intoxicated patient may be belligerent, uncooperative, and combative. The drug abuse patient will exhibit symptoms of excitability or depression depending on the type of drug ingested. Knowledge of the possible physiologic alterations and drug interactions associated with substance abuse is fundamental to the appropriate anesthetic management.

Extent of Injury

The severity of the injury should be determined and evaluated. Episodes and duration of hypotension and estimation of initial blood loss should be noted. The amount of blood and fluid therapy used for initial emergency room resuscitation provides a guide for further replacement.

The chart can provide valuable information if the patient is unable to respond to questions. When available, laboratory data may include hemoglobin, hematocrit, electrolytes, blood urea nitrogen, creatinine, glucose, blood alcohol level, and urinalysis. Radiographic studies and an electrocardiogram may be helpful. All major trauma patients should be typed and cross-matched and there should be sufficient blood available for transfusion prior to the start of the surgical procedure, if time permits.

The information obtained from the preoperative evaluation should be integrated with the patient status and discussed with the surgeon to formulate the optimal anesthetic plan. If the patient has sustained a life-threatening injury, little time will be available for chart review and patient assessment. For these patients, the anesthetist can consult with the surgeon and other health care team members to organize the priorities for management.

PREMEDICATION

Pharmacologic agents employed for routine premedication can exhibit profound cardiovascular and respiratory depressant effects in the trauma patient. The narcotics, barbiturates, and other hypnosedatives should be used judiciously or not at all to avoid undesirable effects. Anticholinergic agents such as atropine and glycopyrrolate may be administered to reduce secretions and suppress vagal reflexes. As stated previously, agents may be used to raise gastric pH or reduce gastric volume; however, the efficacy of this treatment varies in the trauma patient.

Intramuscular injection of any preoperative medication is avoided to prevent possible delayed interactions with the anesthetics. All agents should be administered intravenously with cognizant monitoring of the patient.

PREPARATION OF ESSENTIAL EQUIPMENT

The operating room must be equipped with the necessary drugs and supplies prior to the patient's arrival. Valuable time can be saved if equipment and supplies are readily available and functioning. Frequently, trauma centers designate one or more operative suites that are always prepared for emergency patients. Adherence to departmental infection control policies including the implementation of universal precautions is vital when providing anesthesia care.[8]

All routine equipment must be functional, including the gas machine, electrocardiac monitor, ventilator, oxygen analyzer, pulse oximeter, end-tidal carbon dioxide monitor, blood pressure cuff, temperature monitor, and suction apparatus. Drugs to be administered during anesthesia must be prepared and labeled. Other essential supplies such as airway equipment, precordial and esophageal stethoscopes, blood warmers, micropore filters, blood infusion pumps, and intravenous fluids must be available. A hypothermia/hyperthermia blanket is placed on the operating room table. An arterial line and pressure transducer can be prepared and calibrated. An emergency cart with resuscitative drugs and defibrillator must be available.

MONITORING

Monitoring of the trauma patient requires continuous clinical assessment and accurate interpretation of data obtained from available monitoring devices. Use of routine and specialized monitoring equipment complements the senses of the anesthetist to provide information concerning the patient.

Routine monitoring devices—a blood pressure cuff, electrocardiograph, precordial stethoscope, pulse oximeter, end-tidal carbon dioxide, and peripheral nerve stimulator—are immediately applied on patient arrival to the operating room. Further information related to the major organ systems can be obtained from additional monitoring devices.

Continuous arterial pressure readings are obtained

through the use of an intraarterial catheter and pressure monitoring apparatus. A 20- or 22-gauge nontapered, Teflon catheter can be inserted into one of the peripheral arteries. The radial artery is usually selected because of its ease of cannulation and accessibility. The arterial line also provides an available route to obtain blood samples for arterial gases and other laboratory determinations.

The central venous pressure (CVP) measurement is a reflection of the blood volume, venous tone, and right ventricular pressures. In trauma patients receiving large volume replacements, the CVP can be a valuable guide. Serial measurements are obtained and interpreted to determine the adequacy of volume replacement. The external jugular or internal jugular veins can be cannulated for CVP monitoring.

Pulmonary artery pressure monitoring can provide information about left-sided heart function. The pulmonary artery pressure (PAP), pulmonary capillary wedge pressure (PCWP), and cardiac output are measured via a pulmonary artery (Swan-Ganz) catheter. It is not a routine procedure to insert pulmonary artery catheters in trauma patients because of the time and specialized equipment required. The pulmonary artery catheter can be inserted postoperatively in critically injured patients for serial hemodynamic measurements.

The temperature is continuously monitored through an esophageal stethoscope or other available route. Trauma patients can be rapidly cooled through large incisions, cold operating rooms, the effect of anesthetic agents, and the administration of cold blood. During the first hour of anesthesia, the temperature can decrease 1C to 3C.[9] Table 42–2 lists the available methods that can be implemented to maintain or increase body temperature.

Urine output measurements from a Foley catheter are a guide for adequacy of (1) renal perfusion, (2) volume replacement, and (3) transfusion reactions. The urine output should be maintained at a minimum of 1 to 2 mL/kg per hour.

Respiratory status is monitored for adequacy of ventilation, oxygenation, and respiratory dysfunction. A precordial or esophageal stethoscope allows continuous assessment of the breath sounds. The pulse oximeter provides continuous evaluation of oxygen saturation. Monitoring end-tidal carbon dioxide allows visual analysis of ventilation and other factors that can affect the respiratory system. Observation of the inspiratory pressure reflects changes in lung compliance. Arterial blood gas determinations provide information about acid–base status, arterial oxygenation, and adequacy of ventilation.

Serial determinations of laboratory values provide useful data related to blood replacement, electrolytes, and acid–base status. Arterial blood gases, hemoglobin, hematocrit, and electrolytes should be measured and correlated to the clinical status. Coagulation studies are measured in patients receiving ten or more units of blood.

All of the information obtained must be integrated with the clinical assessment of the patient. One must not depend on the monitoring apparatus alone but incorporate the anesthetist's own assessment skills to recognize and correct problems. Prompt interventions must be initiated to prevent a deterioration of the patient's condition.

INDUCTION

Choice of induction technique depends on the hemodynamic status and area of traumatic injury. Anesthetic guidelines for specific areas of injury are discussed later in this chapter. The most important initial consideration is airway management. The risks of regurgitation and aspiration in the trauma patient dictate the use of an awake intubation or rapid-sequence induction. The technique that is safest for the patient and most familiar to the anesthetist should be chosen.

Awake intubation is considered the best approach in the cooperative patient and those patients with severe maxillofacial or neck trauma. This technique should not be used in patients who have neurologic or penetrating eye injuries. Guidelines for the awake intubation technique are listed in Table 42–3.

A rapid-sequence induction is employed in the intoxicated, confused, restless, or uncooperative trauma patient. Guidelines for this technique are listed in Table 42–4.

If the initial attempt at intubation is unsuccessful, the anesthetist should gently ventilate with the mask while maintaining cricoesophageal pressure and proceed with laryngoscopy. In the event of failed intubation, alternative airway management techniques are quickly instituted. These include allowing the patient to regain conscious, fiberoptic laryngoscopy, retrograde intubation, cricothyrotomy, and tracheostomy. Oxygenation and ventilation of the patient must be ensured throughout the process of establishing a patent airway.

The choice of induction agent depends on the hemodynamic status of the patient. In some trauma patients the blood pressure may be falsely elevated as a result of restlessness, pain, or anxiety and a large dose of an induction agent may induce a precipitous fall in blood pressure. Of

---

TABLE 42–2. INTRAOPERATIVE WARMING METHODS

Plastic/thermal wrap to head

In-circuit humidifier (Conchatherm)

Blood/fluid warmers (Level-One, Hamilton)

Warming blanket (Bair Hugger)

Operating room temperature of 22C

Infusion of heated intravenous solutions

TABLE 42–3. GUIDELINES FOR AWAKE INTUBATION

1. Administer a topical vasoconstrictor nasally for a nasal intubation.
2. Administer local anesthetic topically into oral cavity.
3. Supplement low doses of intravenous agents if patient is hemodynamically stable.
4. Proceed with technique of nasal or oral intubation.
5. Inflate endotracheal tube cuff.
6. Auscultate breath sounds and assess end-tidal carbon dioxide measurement.
7. Administer induction agent.

TABLE 42–4. GUIDELINES FOR RAPID-SEQUENCE INDUCTION

1. Preoxygenate for 3 to 5 minutes with mask.
2. Connect nasogastric tube to suction (if in place).
3. Administer a small dose of nondepolarizing muscle relaxant intravenously 3 minutes prior to succinylcholine to minimize fasciculations.
4. Intravenously administer the induction agent: ketamine 0.25 to 0.75 mg/kg, thiopental 2 to 3 mg/kg, etomidate 0.2 mg/kg, or midazolam 0.05 mg/kg.
5. Immediately follow with succinylcholine 1–2 mg/kg intravenously.
6. Apply cricoesophageal pressure immediately after loss of consciousness and continue until the cuff is inflated.
7. Do not ventilate.
8. Intubate the trachea.
9. Inflate the cuff.
10. Ventilate.
11. Assess breath sounds and evidence of end-tidal carbon dioxide measurement.

the available intravenous induction agents, thiopental 2 to 3 mg/kg and ketamine 0.25 to 0.75 mg/kg are most frequently selected for major trauma. Etomidate 0.2 to 0.3 mg/kg is an alternative induction agent for patients with hemodynamic instability. The inhibition of adrenal steroidogenesis that has been shown with single bolus injections of etomidate has influenced its acceptance for use in trauma patients. Midazolam 0.05 mg/kg intravenously can be considered for induction, although the onset of action may not be as rapid as with the other agents.

ANESTHETIC MANAGEMENT

Immediately after the induction, hemodynamic stability is assessed prior to the introduction of additional anesthetic agents. Two general principles are considered for optimal management. First, the patient is resuscitated with fluid and blood therapy, and then anesthesia is carefully titrated according to need. Second, minimal amounts of anesthetic agents are administered until the severity of the injury is determined and cardiovascular stability is present.

The severely injured patient will require the administration of oxygen, blood, fluids, and a nondepolarizing muscle relaxant, such as vecuronium or pipecuronium. As soon as cardiovascular stability is restored other general anesthetic agents can be administered.

The inhalational agent isoflurane has several advantages in the trauma patient. Low concentrations (0.25 to 0.5 percent) can be slowly introduced, permitting careful observation of the hemodynamic effect. If the blood pressure falls, the agent can be easily eliminated. A high inspired oxygen concentration can be delivered with this agent.

Nitrous oxide (N_2O) has depressant effects in the hypotensive or hypovolemic patient. Low concentrations can be titrated and the hemodynamic effect observed. Adequate oxygenation must be ensured prior to the introduction of this agent.

Narcotics, tranquilizers, and ketamine can be administered in small incremental intravenous dosages. The nondepolarizing muscle relaxants (vecuronium, atracurium, pan-

curonium, pipecuronium) are usually used as adjunct agents to provide optimal relaxation. Vecuronium and pipecuronium are most commonly selected for trauma because of their minimal cardiovascular depressant effects.

A concern in trauma anesthesia is patient recall. This concept is usually attenuated when dealing with the injured patient who has experienced shock. Incremental intravenous dosages of the benzodiazepines (midazolam, lorazepam) can be titrated to provide amnesia. The priorities of anesthesia management are to ensure adequate oxygenation and restore hemodynamic stability before the administration of anesthetic agents.

MAJOR PROBLEMS

Major problems that may be encountered during the anesthetic management of the trauma patient include persistent hypotension, cardiovascular collapse, pulmonary edema, and hypothermia. If the patient cannot be adequately resuscitated with blood and fluid therapy adjunct cardiovascular drugs are carefully administered. Vasopressors can increase the blood pressure transiently but can also increase the severity of tissue acidosis. These drugs should be used to treat hypotension after appropriate volume replacement. Inotropic agents (dopamine, dobutamine, calcium chloride) can be used to restore perfusion and improve myocardial contractility.

Pulmonary edema can result from massive infusion of fluids and blood. Prompt recognition and aggressive treatment are imperative to maintain adequate oxygenation and effective ventilation. Symptoms during anesthesia include rales, increased airway pressure, and large amounts of secretions. Treatment includes frequent suctioning, restriction of fluids, and possible low dosages of diuretics and cardiac glycosides.

Hypothermia (temperature less than 33C) can cause severe impairment of the physiologic functions of the major organ systems.[10] Myocardial depression, inadequate tissue perfusion, and coagulation abnormalities complicate resuscitation efforts. Several outcome studies have revealed that hypothermia is related to the mortality rates in severely injured patients.[11,12] Therefore, efforts to maintain normothermia need to be initiated as soon as the patient arrives in the operating room to reduce the severity and consequences of hypothermia.

FLUID AND BLOOD THERAPY

Guidelines for fluid and blood replacement therapy are correlated to the severity of the injury and the amount of blood loss. The goals of volume therapy are to restore circulating blood volume, maintain adequate oxygen delivery to all tissues, and ensure hemodynamic stability.

The physiologic responses to acute blood loss include alterations in cell membrane stability and transcapillary fluid shifts. Body fluids from the interstitial space replace those lost from the plasma space.[13] Therefore, expansion of both the plasma and interstitial fluid space is required. Initial resuscitation begins with the infusion of balanced electrolyte solutions (BESs) until blood components are available. It is essential to secure at least two large-bore (14-

or 16-gauge) intravenous lines for rapid fluid administration. Advantages of BESs include physiologic components, availability, ease of administration, cost effectiveness, and long shelf-life. BESs with dextrose are not advocated as they may cause hyperglycemia and an osmotic diuresis. The plasma glucose level in trauma patients is elevated as a result of the injury and catecholamine release.

Monitoring of blood pressure, pulse pressure, heart rate, central venous pressure, pulmonary capillary wedge pressure, and urine output guides volume replacement. BESs are administered until hemodynamic stability is attained or until blood is available. During the initial resuscitation period, BESs are infused at a 3:1 ratio, that is, 3 mL of fluid for every 1 mL of blood loss.[14] Clinical judgment individualizes volume therapy for the different types of trauma.

Blood therapy is initiated when the hematocrit is less than 30 percent or in the presence of obvious large losses of blood. Replacement should be with blood products that have been typed and cross-matched if possible. Cases of extreme emergency may warrant the infusion of type-specific or low-titer O-negative non-cross-matched blood.

Recent trends in blood banking now advocate component therapy rather than whole blood administration. Whole blood, when available, is indicated for transfusion in massive trauma. Component therapy with packed red blood cells and fresh-frozen plasma may be administered to maintain a hemoglobin level of 8 to 10 mg/100 mL or a hematocrit of 28 to 30 percent.

One unit of packed red blood cells has an oxygen-carrying capacity similar to that of 1 unit of whole blood. The hematocrit of each unit is 60 to 70 percent. Each unit may be diluted with 100 to 200 mL of intravenous solution to facilitate rapid transfusion. One unit of fresh-frozen plasma can be administered for every 4 to 6 units of packed cells during massive transfusion. Fresh-frozen plasma contains many of the clotting factors except platelets. Platelets can be transfused if the platelet count falls below 65,000/mm^3.

Several storage and delivery problems can arise during blood administration. Changes in stored blood are listed in Table 42–5. The longer the blood is stored, the greater the accumulation of cellular debris, which may cause microemboli to be deposited in the respiratory system, leading to respiratory dysfunction. All blood must be warmed prior to administration to minimize hypothermia and arrhythmias. Micropore filters remove aggregates in stored blood.

Electrolyte, acid–base, and coagulation disorders are

TABLE 42–5. CHANGES IN STORED BLOOD

	Normal Blood	Bank Blood
pH	7.40	6.7
Hematocrit (%)	45	41
K$^+$ (mEq/L)	4.5	7–30
Ca^{2+} (mg/100 mL)	5	0.5
Pco$_2$ (mm Hg)	40	130
Platelets (mm^3)	230,000	0
Factors V and VII (%)	100	20–50
2,3-Diphosphoglycerate (μmol/mL)	13	< 1

TABLE 42–6. TRANSFUSION REACTIONS

Hemolytic reactions
  Clinical symptoms
    Hypotension
    Tachycardia
    Hemoglobinuria
    Ooozing at operative site
    Increase in temperature
  Treatment
    Stop transfusion
    Administer fluids
    Administer diuretics
    Administer bicarbonate
    Administer steroids
    Support hemodynamic status
Allergic reactions
  Clinical symptoms
    Laryngeal edema
    Bronchospasm
    Urticaria
    Hives
  Treatment
    Stop transfusion
    Administer an antihistamine
    Administer bronchodilator
    Administer steroids

associated with the rapid transfusion of blood that is 1.5 times the patient's estimated blood volume.[15] The changes in serum potassium levels are related to the rate and volume of blood administration. Hypokalemia and hyperkalemia have been reported in trauma patients.[16,17] The treatment of hyperkalemia includes slowing the rate of blood infusion and administering calcium, insulin, bicarbonate, and glucose intravenously.

Controversy about the administration of sodium bicarbonate and calcium chloride exists. These drugs should not be administered routinely. Frequent arterial blood gas determinations can guide sodium bicarbonate replacement to correct metabolic acidosis. A guideline for calculation of bicarbonate replacement is patient weight in kilograms times the base deficit times 0.3. One half to two thirds of the calculated dose is given intravenously and the arterial blood gases are repeated.

The ionized calcium levels may be dramatically lowered during transfusion. Calcium chloride 1 g can be slowly administered intravenously to the severely injured patient for its inotropic effect.

Transfusion reactions can occur in any patient receiving blood. Prompt recognition and treatment is important. The clinical symptoms and treatment of allergic and hemolytic transfusions are listed in Table 42–6.

Volume therapy requires close monitoring of the patient's blood pressure, pulse, urine output, central venous pressure, pulmonary capillary wedge pressure, and serial laboratory data. Blood components and BESs must be readily available and administered in proper amounts to avoid pathologic alterations in organ function. Effective communication with the surgeon and other health care team members facilitates prompt volume restoration and hemodynamic stability.

SPECIFIC AREAS OF INJURY

The major areas of injury are discussed, with focus on the anesthetic guidelines for each type of patient. All patients require the same priorities of management—airway and cardiovascular stabilization—regardless of the type of injury.

Thoracic Trauma

Statistics indicate that 25 to 30 percent of all injuries involve the thorax. Injuries can include damage to the heart, lung, diaphragm, and great vessels. Major problems that can result from thoracic injuries are pneumothorax, hemothorax, flail chest, and cardiac tamponade.[18]

Pneumothorax is the accumulation of air within the pleural cavity. Intrapleural pressure is increased, resulting in collapse of lung tissue on the affected side and decreased effective ventilation. Venous return is diminished by a mediastinal shift and the effects of positive pressure. The most common clinical signs include respiratory distress and the absence of breath sounds on the affected side. Subcutaneous emphysema and a deviated trachea may also be present. Treatment includes insertion of a chest tube. Under anesthesia a pneumothorax can be detected by an increased airway pressure, low compliance, absence of breath sounds, hypotension, low arterial oxygen saturation, and low arterial blood oxygen content. If a tension pneumothorax is present, a chest tube or large-bore needle should be immediately inserted into the second or third intercostal space in the midclavicular line. Adequate reexpansion of the lung and ventilation are observed. A chest x-ray is performed postoperatively.

Hemothorax is the accumulation of blood in the pleural cavity as a result of injury to the great vessels or thoracic organs. The clinical signs are similar to those of pneumothorax, although if blood loss is significant, rapid deterioration of vital signs may occur. Treatment includes insertion of a chest tube, close monitoring of chest tube drainage, and institution of resuscitation measures. Assessment of the amount of blood loss in the chest drainage tube and hemodynamic stability is important prior to the selection of anesthesia techniques.

Flail chest results from two segmental fractures in each of three adjacent ribs. The injured segment causes paradoxical movement of the chest wall, leading to ventilation–perfusion abnormalities. Treatment includes maintenance of effective ventilation, stabilization of the flail segment, and administration of pain medication.

Cardiac tamponade is the rapid accumulation of blood in the pericardial sac. The rate and amount of blood accumulation determine the pathophysiologic response. The increase in intrapericardial pressure causes impairment of diastolic ventricular filling and reduces cardiac output. The heart rate and peripheral vascular resistance increases as compensatory mechanisms; however, as the intrapericardial pressure continues to increase, cardiovascular collapse ensues. Clinical symptoms include increased central venous pressure, jugular vein distension, pulsus paradoxus, muffled heart sounds, tachycardia, and hypotension. Treatment involves cardiovascular support, pericardiocentesis, and,

possibly, thoracotomy. Anesthetic management of the patient consists of careful titration of anesthetic induction agents. Ketamine (0.25 to 0.75 mg/kg) is usually the agent of choice for a rapid-sequence induction. The surgeon must be ready to perform a thoracotomy immediately if cardiac arrest occurs during the induction. Once the tamponade is released, and cardiovascular stability returns, additional anesthetic agents may be administered.

Cardiac contusions should be suspected in the patient with blunt chest injuries. The most common presenting symptom is arrhythmias. The electrocardiogram may not initially reflect evidence of myocardial damage. Anesthetic consideration for these patients includes prevention of myocardial depression and close monitoring of heart rate and rhythm.

Thoracic aortic injuries are associated with significant mortality rates. The primary goal of anesthetic management is to maintain cardiovascular stability until the surgeon can repair the injured area. Large amounts of blood and fluid should be administered to maintain an effective vascular volume and perfusion pressure.

One-lung anesthesia may be required to aid in control of bleeding and surgical exploration of the thoracic injury. Endobronchial intubation with a Carlens or Robertshaw tube can be performed using a rapid-sequence induction technique. Close monitoring of the adequacy of ventilation and oxygenation is imperative, as is maintenance of hemodynamic stability. Knowledge of the physiologic alterations induced by one-lung anesthesia is mandatory. Any patient with significant lung injury should be mechanically ventilated postoperatively until adequate respiratory function is restored.

Abdominal Trauma

Blunt or penetrating abdominal injuries can cause single- or multiple-organ damage. Most injuries involve the liver, spleen, and small intestine.[19] In severe injuries, bleeding into the abdominal cavity occurs, causing a tense, distended abdomen and creating a tamponade. Symptoms of hemorrhagic shock can be present, requiring aggressive resuscitation with blood and fluid therapy and immediate surgical intervention.

A rapid-sequence induction is followed by the administration of minimal depressant agents until the extent of injury is determined and the bleeding is controlled. When the abdomen is opened, a precipitous drop in blood pressure can occur from the release of the tamponade. The anesthetist must be prepared to immediately infuse large volumes of fluid and blood to maintain an adequate perfusion pressure. Further management guidelines include accurate assessment of blood loss, correction of acid–base abnormalities, and careful titration of anesthetic agents.

Maxillofacial Injuries

Over 72 percent of persons involved in motor vehicle accidents sustain injury to the head and neck area. Other sources of injury are gunshot and stab wounds.[20] The most important priority for successful management is establishment of a patent airway. Depending on the severity and nature of the injury, endotracheal intubation or cricothyrotomy is performed. Endotracheal intubation may be accomplished in several ways: awake oral or nasal, asleep oral or nasal, or by the use of a fiberoptic bronchoscope. The choice of technique depends on the area and severity of injury. Direct visualization of oropharyngeal structures may be necessary in the presence of large amounts of bleeding or complex facial fractures. Nasal intubation is avoided in any patient with suspected communicating facial and neurologic injury. Consideration of cervical spine injury warrants neck stabilization and immobilization during intubation. Control of bleeding, cardiovascular support, and elevation of injuries are other goals of initial management.

The patient transported to the operating room for surgical exploration must be carefully assessed to determine the extent of airway difficulty caused by the injury. Prior planning of airway management prevents catastrophic situations such as inability to ventilate or intubate, leading to episodes of hypoxia. If a question arises as to whether successful asleep intubation can be accomplished, an awake intubation or tracheostomy is performed. After surgical explorations of the injury, the patient is closely observed and carefully assessed prior to extubation.

Management of the trauma patient who has sustained an ocular injury poses several conflicting problems. Prevention of increase in intraocular pressure and guarding against aspiration are the goals of management. A rapid-sequence intravenous induction with vecuronium 0.07 to 0.10 kg or atracurium 0.4 to 0.5 mg, thiopental 3 to 5 mg/kg, and lidocaine 1 to 1.5 mg/kg is advocated by many practitioners. Other authorities recommend the following technique: pretreatment with a nondepolarizing muscle relaxant, thiopental 3 to 5 mg/kg and succinylcholine 1 to 2 mg/kg intravenously. Conflicting reports exist as to whether succinylcholine does increase intraocular pressure during induction.[21] Ketamine should be avoided in these patients. Awareness of the factors that may raise intraocular pressure is essential. These factors include light planes of anesthesia, hypertension, and coughing. Emergence and extubation are potentially difficult because of the conflicting desire to have the patient fully awake to guard against aspiration and yet in a plane of anesthesia deep enough to prevent coughing on the endotracheal tube. Establishment of priorities guides individual judgment.

Head Trauma

Successful anesthetic management of the patient with acute head injuries incorporates the basic principles of neuroanesthesia and trauma. Priorities include airway patency, cardiovascular support, and measures to decrease intracranial pressure.[22] Endotracheal intubation and hyperventilation are usually initiated in the emergency room. Once the patient is transported to the operating room, essential monitoring is applied, and controlled hyperventilation is continued.

If the patient is not intubated prior to surgery, a rapid-sequence intravenous induction with thiopental 3 to 5 mg/kg, vecuronium 0.07 to 0.10 mg/kg, or succinylcholine 1 to 2 mg/kg and lidocaine 1 to 2 mg/kg is advocated. Controversy exists regarding the use of succinylcholine in head trauma, but the prior administration of a low-dose,

nondepolarizing muscle relaxant and high dose of thiopental aids in preventing any increase in intracranial pressure. Ketamine is avoided. Further anesthetic agents and fluid and blood replacement are titrated depending on hemodynamic stability. Controlled ventilation is used to maintain a Pa_{CO_2} of 28 to 30 torr. Postoperatively, management depends on the severity of intracranial injury and the overall status of the patient.

Multiple Injuries

The trauma patient who has sustained multiple-organ injuries presents an anesthetic challenge. Multiple injuries most frequently include head trauma, with major abdominal or thoracic organ involvement. Initial management focuses on prompt recognition and accurate diagnosis of all injuries. Adequate oxygenation and stabilization of the blood pressure are of the utmost importance. Priorities are then established to maintain adequate support of the major organ systems.

Anesthetic guidelines follow those already mentioned in the previous discussion.

POSTOPERATIVE CONSIDERATIONS

Close observation of major system function continues in the postoperative period. Mechanical ventilation is indicated for any patient who has sustained life-threatening injuries. Assessment of the patient's respiratory function is essential prior to extubation. Hemodynamic stability is monitored, with proper fluid, blood, and drug therapy instituted as needed. Serial laboratory determinations are evaluated. Effective communication with the surgical staff and recovery room personnel is essential to promote optimal postoperative care of the trauma patient.

CARDIOPULMONARY RESUSCITATION

Cardiopulmonary resuscitation (CPR) in the operating room setting involves the principles of advanced cardiac life support (ACLS). Anesthesia providers must be knowledgeable and able to quickly implement the current standards of resuscitation. ACLS includes six components:

1. Basic life support
2. Use of adjunctive equipment and special techniques for establishing and maintaining effective ventilation and circulation
3. Electrocardiographic monitoring and arrhythmia recognition
4. Establishment and maintenance of intravenous access
5. Employment of therapies (including drug and electrical therapies) for emergency treatment of patients with cardiac and respiratory arrests and for stabilization in the postarrest phase
6. Treatment of patients with suspected or overt acute myocardial infarction[23]

The initial approach to patients in cardiopulmonary arrest is to establish a patent airway, ventilate (10 to 12 per

TABLE 42–7. DRUG THERAPY FOR RESUSCITATION

Drug	Dose
Atropine	0.5–1 mg IV
Bretylium	Initial dose: 5 mg/kg Maximum dose: 30 mg/kg
Calcium chloride	2–4 mg/kg
Dopamine	Initial dose: 2–5 µg/kg/min Maximum dose: 20 µg/kg/min
Dobutamine	2.5–20 µg/kg/min
Epinephrine	0.5–1.0 mg IV Infusion: 1–4 µg/min
Lidocaine	Initial dose: 0.5–1.5 mg/kg Infusion: 2–4 mg/min
Sodium bicarbonate	1 mEq/kg; check arterial blood gases
Verapamil	0.075–0.15 mg/kg Maximum dose: 10 mg

minute), and restore perfusion to the vital organs through cardiac compressions (80 to 100 per minute). Prompt recognition and treatment of rhythm disturbances observed on the electrocardiogram monitor is based on an understanding of cardiac electrophysiology and pharmacology. The most frequently used agents for resuscitation are listed in Table 42–7.[24]

Electrical therapy may be necessary to treat ventricular fibrillation, ventricular tachycardia, and asystole. Initial defibrillation of 200 joules is recommended for asystole with subsequent shocks delivered between 200 and 300 joules. Treatment of ventricular and supraventricular tachycardia with cardioversion requires 25 to 100 joules. During open chest resuscitation, defibrillation with 5 joules is used initially up to a maximum of 100 joules.[23] Combined pharmacologic and electrical therapies may be required to restore cardiac rhythm.

Resuscitative measures are implemented after careful assessment and accurate interpretation of the patient's findings. The outcomes of cardiopulmonary resuscitation are determined by the prompt restoration of oxygenation and circulation.

REFERENCES

1. Trunkey DD. Trauma: A public health problem. In: Moore EE, ed. *Early care of the injured patient.* Philadelphia: BC Decker; 1990:3.
2. Lilly PM, Gann DS. The neuroendocrine response to injury. In: *Blunt multiple trauma: Comprehensive pathophysiology and care.* New York: Dekker; 1990:165–190.
3. Berne RM, Levy MN. Interplay of central and peripheral factors in the control of the circulation. In: *Physiology.* St. Louis, MO: CV Mosby; 1988:566–571.
4. Taylor RW, Dellinger RP. Preexisting medical problems in the trauma patient: Do they matter? In: Kirby RR, Brown DL, eds. *Anesthesia for trauma. International anesthesiology clinics.* Boston: Little, Brown; 1987;25:143–161.
5. Branch RA, Wood M. Histamine and histamine H₁ and H₂ receptor antagonists; 5-hydroxytryptamine, kinins, and the carcinoid syndrome; angiotensin and the renin–angiotensin system. In: Wood M, Wood A, eds. *Drugs and anesthesia, pharmacology for anesthesiologists.* Baltimore: Williams & Wilkins; 1990:614–623.
6. Lindenbaum GA, Carroll SF, Daskal I, Kapusnick R. Patterns of alcohol and drug abuse in an urban trauma center: The increasing role of cocaine abuse. *J Trauma.* 1989;29:1654–1658.
7. Soderstrom CA. Alcohol and trauma: Perspectives and clinical issues. In: Maull KI, ed. *Advances in trauma.* Chicago: Yearbook Medical; 1989:211–239.
8. Fay MF. Anesthesia: Employee health and safety. In: *Reviving asepsis: Criteria for the 90's anesthesia today.* Philadelphia: Comed Communications; 1991;2:1–5.
9. Morris RH. Operating room temperature and the anesthetized, paralyzed patient. *Arch Surg.* 1971;102:95–97.
10. Kalish MA. Hypothermia and hyperthermia in trauma patients. In: Stene JK, Grande CM, eds. *Trauma anesthesia.* Baltimore: Williams & Wilkins; 1991:340–351.
11. Jurkovich GJ, Greiser WB, Luterman A, Currieri PW. Hypothermia in trauma victims, an ominous predictor of survival. *J Trauma.* 1987;27:1019–1024.
12. Luna GK, Maier RV, Pavlin EG, Anardi D, Copass MK, Oreskovich MR. Incidence and effect of hypothermia in seriously injured patients. *J Trauma.* 1987;27:1014–1018.
13. Lucas CE. Hemorrhagic shock, crystalloids, colloids and the interstitial space matrix. *Panam. J Trauma.* 1989;1:48–55.
14. Gieseke AH, Grande CM, Whitten CW. Fluid therapy and the resuscitation of traumatic shock. In: Grande CM, Stene JK, eds. *Critical care clinics: Overview of trauma anesthesia and critical care.* Philadelphia: WB Saunders; 1990;6:61–72.
15. Miller RD. Complications of massive blood transfusion. *Anesthesiology.* 1973;39:82–93.
16. Linko K, Tigerstedt I. Hyperpotassemia during massive transfusions. *Acta Anaesth Scand.* 1984;28:220–221.
17. Wilson RF, Mammen E, Walt AJ. Eight years of experience with massive blood transfusion. *J Trauma.* 1971;11:275–285.
18. Hood MR. Early definitive diagnosis and management. In: Hood MR, Boyd AD, Culliford AD, eds. *Thoracic trauma.* Philadelphia: WB Saunders; 1987:35–66.
19. Anderson CB, Ballinger WF. Abdominal injuries in the management of trauma. In: Luidema GD, Rutherford RB, Ballinger WF, eds. *The management of trauma.* Philadelphia: WB Saunders; 1987:449–504.
20. Kline SN. Maxillofacial trauma. In: Kreis DJ, Gomex GA, eds. *Trauma management.* Boston: Little, Brown; 1989:131–145.
21. Cunningham AJ, Barry P. Intraocular pressure—physiology and implications for anesthetic management. *Can Anaesth Soc J.* 1986;33:195–207.
22. Head trauma. In: *Advanced trauma life support program.* Chicago: American College of Surgeons; 1989:131–155.
23. Adult advanced cardiac life support. In: Standard and guidelines for cardiopulmonary resuscitation and emergency cardiac care. *JAMA.* 1986;255:2933, 2942–2943.
24. Cardiovascular pharmacology I and II. In: *Textbook of advanced cardiac life support.* 2nd ed. Dallas: American Heart Association; 1990:97–127.

Anesthesia for Organ Transplantation

Carol Boetger Mann

This chapter covers the anesthetic management of the organ donor, kidney transplant procedures, and non-transplant surgery for patients who have previously received organ transplants. Multiorgan donor management is addressed initially and encompasses general considerations for all donors. Donation of some organs requires alterations in the multiorgan guidelines and these considerations are addressed in the appropriate section. Pancreatic transplants are not commonly performed, nor do they enjoy a high graft survival rate compared with the success of other organ transplants. Heart, heart–lung, and liver transplant procedures are highly specialized fields in anesthesia that the nurse anesthetist does not usually encounter unless this area of specialization is specifically pursued. Suggested readings are cited in the text for liver, heart, and heart–lung procedures.

Modern methods of organ preservation and the sophisticated transportation network for donated organs make any medical facility with surgical capabilities a potential site for an organ harvest. This fact places responsibility on every anesthetist to be well informed regarding the proper anesthetic management of the donation procedure for one or more organs. Appropriate and competent anesthetic management of organ donors and recipients is a key link in the chain of events that culminates in successful transplantation.

ORGAN DONATION

There is a great need for donated kidneys and other organs in the United States, not only for the eventual convenience of the recipient but also to reduce soaring medical costs associated with hemodialysis, chronic illness, and prolonged hospital care. Cost analysis by the Health Care Financing Administration (HCFA) has shown that between $30,000 and $66,000 would be saved over a 5-year period for each suitable hemodialysis patient who receives an organ transplantation. More than 6000 kidneys were transplanted in 1984; however,

with improved immunosuppressive regimens, it is estimated that as many as 18,000 individuals per year could benefit from kidney transplantation.[1] The Centers for Disease Control (CDC) concluded that between 12,000 and 27,000 patients die each year who otherwise would have benefited from transplantation of viable organs.[2]

Wasted potential organ donations are attributable to various factors including reluctance to approach the family regarding donation during a period of intense grief, fear of legal ramifications, lack of awareness of existing organ shortages, lack of enthusiasm for organ donation, and lack of information regarding donor criteria and procedures for retrieval on the part of medical personnel. These and other factors consume 80 percent of the potential organ donations, causing viable, scarce, and lifesaving organs to be buried rather than transplanted into needy recipients.[1]

Several laws have been passed both to educate the public and the medical community about the need for organ donors and to facilitate harvest in a timely manner. The organ donor card is a legal document allowing removal of organs, without the consent of the family, under the provisions of the Uniform Anatomical Gift Act. The major benefit of the donor card has been to educate the public regarding organ donation; however, it does not significantly increase organ acquisitions. Frequently the cards are not available at the time of death, and family consent is often sought despite the presence of a signed card. Canada's experience is that 49 percent of donor card information is unusable and in some U.S. states, less than 2 percent of the residents have signed their cards.[1,3] Many U.S. states have enacted "required request" legislation, which requires an organ donation request, once brain-death criteria have been met, before the patient can be declared legally dead; however, preliminary results of this legislation seem to be rather disappointing. Many countries (the United States not included) have enacted a "presumed consent" law which assumes consent to donate organs unless the person has specifically stated preferences to the contrary. In June of 1986, Belgium enacted a law based on "presumed consent" and realized a subsequent increase of 140 percent in the number of kidneys, hearts, and livers that were transplanted within 5 years.[4]

The Uniform Determination of Death Act, recommended in 1981 by the President's Commission for the Study of Bioethics in Medicine, has been passed by several state legislatures. This facilitates the diagnosis of brain death for physicians and provides more liberal criteria for the determination of brain death than the Harvard group recommended more than 20 years ago.[5] The President's Commission reduced the observation time to 6 hours in some cases, as cardiac death usually occurs within 48 to 72 hours of brain death,[6] making a delay in diagnosis potentially disastrous for the viability of harvested organs. Noninvasive bedside tests are being developed that are easily performed and interpreted by an intensivist. These tests are inexpensive, sensitive, and adequately represent physiologic death.[1,7]

The National Transplant Act of 1984 has prohibited the buying and selling of human organs, eliminating a potential controversy associated with the lack of supply of donated organs.[1] The United Network for Organ Sharing (UNOS) was set up in 1978 to coordinate organ donors and recipients in the United States. The emergence of the donor coordinator, interfacing with families, physicians, nurses, operating rooms, and anesthesia providers, has greatly facilitated successful acquisition and timely transplant of donated organs. Nevertheless, it has been reported that up to 20 percent of kidneys that are harvested for transplant have been discarded for a variety of reasons despite this level of coordination.[8] S. L. Youngner writes that we cannot legislate society's ambivalence regarding organ transplantation. By asking for organ donations, medical science has challenged deeply held emotional ties and religious beliefs. Giving life from someone who is losing it to someone who will die without the gift makes the goals of organ procurement worthy and just; however, Youngner advises the medical community to be patient with society as it contemplates these issues and develops norms for dealing with new ethical challenges.[9]

ANESTHETIC MANAGEMENT OF THE ORGAN DONOR

The Multiorgan Donor

Donor organs from one successful harvest will determine the quality of life for as many as seven critically ill recipients. The community donor pool consists of any appropriate patient in any medical facility, with surgical capabilities, that is accessible to the recipient institution within the period of time the organ can be preserved. Therefore, virtually any anesthesia provider should be prepared to administer optimum donor support during an organ harvest. Common medical problems presented to the anesthetist by the donor include diabetes insipidus, neurogenic or cardiogenic pulmonary edema, hypotension, arrhythmias, hypovolemia, hypothermia, hypoglycemia, and electrolyte disorders. These problems exist in addition to the vigilance required to avoid bacterial transfer and subsequent infection in the immunosuppressed recipient. Consequently, strict guidelines of sterile technique should always be followed. For information beyond the scope of this chapter, an excellent review of the perioperative management of the multiorgan donor by Robertson and Cook[10] should be read.

Multiple surgical transplant teams, each from their respective facility and each focusing on the needs of their own target organ, are frequently present in the operating room simultaneously to accomplish a multiorgan harvest. Conflicts regarding donor management may arise because of differing institutional practices as well as the predicament that optimal management of one organ may directly contradict optimal management of another organ when both are designated for retrieval. For example, lung surgeons want the donor to be kept relatively dry and renal transplant surgeons prefer ample hydration. Liver transplant teams prefer desmopressin (DDAVP) over vasopressin, which is acceptable to the heart team; however, renal transplant surgeons prefer not to use either agent, in most cases. Multiple-organ management becomes a dilemma for the anesthetist attempting to optimize the conditions for all organs to be harvested. When conflicts in management are encountered, discussion between the surgical teams and with the transplant coordinator should delineate priorities for optimal protection of the organs to be procured.

In some institutions, it may be appropriate for anesthesia personnel to assist with transport of the donor to the operating room, because of the inherent instability of the brain-dead patient and the potential compromises in ventilation, blood pressure, and temperature that may take place during transport. Preoperatively, the anesthetist must ensure that appropriate determination of brain death, certification of death, and consent for the organ donation have been documented in the chart. Cadaveric donors are usually young, previously healthy patients who have sustained irreversible catastrophic neurologic damage. Table 43–1[10] identifies the expected sequelae of brain death and suggested management in the intensive care unit (ICU). This support should extend into the intraoperative phase with an emphasis on optimum target organ perfusion and oxygenation. Recent arterial blood gases, complete blood count with differential, electrolytes, glucose, blood urea nitrogen (BUN), creatinine, serum glutamic–oxaloacetic transaminase (SGOT), serum glutamic–pyruvic transaminase (SGPT), lactate dehydrogenase (LDH), creatine kinase, total and direct bilirubin, chest x-ray, and electrocardiogram should be on the chart preoperatively.[11]

Intraoperative monitors for the cadaveric donor should include electrocardiogram, central venous pressure (CVP), urine output, temperature, esophageal stethoscope, oxygen saturation, end-tidal carbon dioxide, and an arterial catheter to monitor blood pressure during sequential organ removal. The arterial catheter should be placed in an upper extremity and greatly assists in the maintenance of a systolic blood pressure greater than 100 mm Hg (mean arterial pressure greater than 70 mm Hg) as well as the hourly monitoring of arterial blood gases, hematocrit, electrolytes, and glucose.

Although analgesics and anesthetics are not necessary when operating on a brain-dead patient, the anesthetist should be prepared for some physiologic response by the patient to stimulation. Spinal reflexes remain intact and may cause complex movements of the limbs and trunk. Pancuronium should be administered in a high dose (0.15 mg/kg) to avoid these unpredictable movements.[12,13] Incision may elicit tachycardia or increased blood pressure, presumably from the remaining brainstem or spinal re-

TABLE 43–1. NORMAL SEQUELAE OF BRAIN DEATH

Sequela	Cause	Management
Hypotension	Neurogenic shock; hypovolemia	Maintain intravascular volume; provide inotropic support, in order of preference: dopamine ≤ 10 µg/kg per minute; dobutamine ≤ 15 µg/kg per minute; epinephrine ≤ 0.1 µg/kg per minute; norepinephrine and dopamine 2–4 µg/kg per minute
Arrhythmia–bradycardia	Central nervous system injury; hypothermia; abnormal electrolytes or blood gases; myocardial ischemia	Atropine resistant; use chronotropic drugs or temporary venous pacing
Hypoxemia	Central or pulmonary	Pa_{O_2} = 100–150 mm Hg; Pa_{CO_2} = 35–45 mm Hg; pH = 7.35–7.45; PEEP ≤ 7.5 cm H_2O^a; F_{IO_2} ≤ 0.40 (heart–lungs)
Diabetes insipidus	Pituitary or hypothalamic dysfunction	Volume replacement; vasopressin (0.1 U/min infusion) or DDAVP (0.3 µg/kg IV) to maintain a urine output of 1.5–3 mL/kg per hour; correct electrolyte disorders; provide inotropic support
Hypothermia	Loss of hypothalamic temperature regulation	Early aggressive warming to maintain the temperature above 34C
Anemia	Hemorrhage; hemodilution	Transfuse to keep hematocrit > 30%

^{a} PEEP, positive end-expiratory pressure; DDAVP, desmopressin acetate.
Reprinted, with permission, from Robertson and Cook.[10]

flexes, or catecholamine release from the adrenal gland mediated by spinal reflexes.[14–17] Wetzel et al have documented a reflex pressor response to nociceptive stimuli in brain-dead patients.[14] To avoid damage to the renal grafts or excessive operative blood loss secondary to hypertension, venodilation, or a reduction in afterload and is suggested using nitroglycerin or nitroprusside as the preferable agents; however, isoflurane is probably the most convenient agent to effect these changes.[10]

Arterial blood gases should be kept within normal limits as indicated in Table 43–1 and arterial saturation should be greater than 95 percent. The effects of trauma and prolonged ventilatory support may decrease pulmonary compliance and impede alveolar gas exchange. A normal tidal volume (10 to 12 mL/kg) should be combined with a ventilatory rate that maintains Pa_{CO_2} between 35 and 45 mm Hg. Some degree of respiratory acidosis (Pa_{CO_2} ≥ 45 mm Hg) may optimize organ perfusion by employing the direct vasodilatory effects of hypercapnia and avoiding arterial vasospasm. Mild hypercapnia may also increase cardiac output as a result of direct stimulation of the sympathetic nervous system.[10] Oxygen consumption and carbon dioxide production will be reduced as compared to normal patient levels. This requires a decrease in the expected minute volume to avoid respiratory alkalosis. Positive end-expiratory pressure (PEEP) should be limited to ≤ 7.5 cm H_2O to avoid barotrauma and decreased cardiac output. The F_{IO_2} should be increased to 1.0 prior to transport to the operating room and during surgery.

Endocrine disorders become apparent in brain death. The two most important regarding transplant success include diabetes insipidus (DI) and hypothyroidism. Donor management in the ICU frequently includes triiodothyronine (T_3) replacement. Although somewhat controversial,[18,19] it is felt that T_3 supplementation may offset the natural course of deterioration of the brain-dead patient, allowing more time for organ retrieval, as well as improving cardiac and renal functional stability in the recipient.[20] Monitoring electrolytes and glucose at least every hour is essential especially if DI has been diagnosed in the donor. As many as 87 percent of organ donors will be diagnosed with DI[21] due to lack of secretion of antidiuretic hormone, which results in production of up to 1000 mL of urine per hour. Antidiuretic hormone works specifically by increasing sodium and water reabsorption from the distal tubule of the nephron. This massive urine output leads to serum hyperosmolarity, hypernatremia, hypermagnesemia, hypokalemia, hypophosphatemia, hypocalcemia, and hypovolemia if not treated properly.[22] If DI is not promptly arrested, this decreased intravascular volume and electrolyte imbalance lead to hemodynamic instability and cardiac dysrhythmias. Titrating the urine output and free water clearance against the serum electrolytes and glucose requires careful fluid and electrolyte replacement with the goal of maintaining the serum sodium below 155 mEq/L, serum potassium above 3.5 mEq/L, and hematocrit above 30 percent. Other electrolytes and intravascular volume should be kept as close to normal as possible. Vasopressin or desmopressin acetate may be used as suggested in Table 43–1. Inotropic support may also be necessary in severe cases.

Vasopressin (antidiuretic hormone) causes generalized systemic vasoconstriction and increased smooth muscle activity which can decrease the eventual viability of the organ graft. Desmopressin (DDAVP) is a synthetic analog of vasopressin and exhibits enhanced antidiuretic potency, diminished pressor activity, and prolonged duration of action as compared with the natural hormone. Debelak et al found no difference in the rates of posttransplant acute tubular necrosis (ATN) when either of the two drugs was used and suggested that DDAVP may have some advantages over vasopressin.[21] DDAVP can be given either intravenously or subcutaneously. The subcutaneous dose is 2 μg.[23] Subcutaneous administration produces an onset of action within 30 to 40 minutes and a duration of 12 hours.[24] The benefits of treating polyuria to avoid the sequelae outweigh the potential for ischemic end-organ injury secondary to drug administration.[10] Urine output should be controlled to 100 mL/h.

Hypotension and hemodynamic instability secondary to lack of central sympathetic outflow, neurogenic shock, and hypovolemia should be anticipated in all donors.[10,25] This problem extends into the intraoperative period and, if uncontrolled, can be quite deleterious to organ grafts. Major causes of preoperative hypovolemia include therapeutic dehydration, hemorrhage, DI, inadequate fluid replacement, and osmotic diuresis as a result of hyperglycemia, mannitol, and radiocontrast dye.[10] Major intraoperative causes of hypotension are due to surgical manipulation during sternotomy; manipulation of the heart, lungs, and liver; and intraperitoneal dissection of the inferior vena cava. Hypotension can also be the result of increased intracranial pressure with cerebellar herniation leading to acute spinal cord shock. Rapid infusion of iced preservation solution into the portal system causes precipitous hypothermia and cardiovascular instability as well[10]; however, infusion of iced preservation solution, which is accomplished for all target organs simultaneously, coincides with clamping of the aorta and anesthesia supportive measures become no longer necessary.

Hypotension is best corrected with warmed fluids, either crystalloid, colloid, or albumin according to the preferences of the anesthesia provider and the organs to be harvested. Very large volumes of fluid administration can be anticipated, therefore a large intravenous line is necessary and warming of the fluid is imperative. Brain-dead donors are poikilothermic and a core temperature of less than 32C can result in dysrhythmias, cardiovascular instability, decreased renal function, and a left shift in the oxyhemoglobin dissociation curve.[10] A warming blanket and heated humidifed inspiratory gases are also indicated. Anemia may be profound, due to traumatic injuries, hemodilution, and prolonged dissection procedures incurring large surgical losses. Packed red blood cells should be used to maintain a hematocrit greater than 30 percent to facilitate oxygen transport to the target organs. Although controversial, administration of blood to the donor may improve organ graft survival in nonrelated donors.[26] Disseminated intravascular coagulation (DIC) and primary fibrinolysis may persist despite appropriate measures due to factors released by necrotic brain tissue.[27,28] In this case, early organ harvest is accomplished.

If pressors are necessary, preferable agents are listed on Table 43–1; the use of pure alpha-agonist vasopressor agents is discouraged. Dopamine at doses below 10 μg/kg per minute is usually the preferred pressor. All pressor agents should ideally be discontinued prior to the organ procurement procedure, but not at the cost of cardiovascular collapse immediately prior to organ retrieval. Administration of dopamine to infants may require doses significantly higher than those necessary to maintain adequate perfusion pressures in adults.[29] A dose of 15 μg/kg per minute does not seem to harm kidney function in pediatric donors.[30] Isoproterenol may be especially useful in pediatric donors because the increase in heart rate may improve their rate-dependent cardiac output. In addition, the anesthesia provider may be requested to administer steroids, diuretics, antibiotics, prostaglandins, alpha antagonists, and calcium channel blockers[31,32] by either the surgeon or the transplant coordinator with the intent of maximizing the chances of graft survival.

A central venous pressure of 8 to 12 cm H_2O, systolic arterial pressure above 100 mm Hg, and a heart rate less than 100 beats per minute are desirable. Hypervolemia may predispose to donor organ edema; however, augmentation of the cardiac output, by increasing the circulating fluid volume, has been shown to be more important for oxygen transport than the blood viscosity or the hemoglobin concentration.[33] Although pulmonary artery catheters have been reported to cause right-sided endocardial lesions,[34] they remain valuable for monitoring pulmonary capillary wedge pressure (10 ± 3 mm Hg), mean pulmonary arterial pressure (15 ± 4 mm Hg), cardiac output (4 to 8 L/min), and mixed venous saturation (> 75 percent).

Electrocardiographic abnormalities that can be anticipated in the organ donor are many and varied. Electrocardiographic changes such as ST-T segment and enzyme changes, indicating myocardial damage, may be seen with traumatic head injury and bleeding. These are usually not significant unless the donor has a pretraumatic history of myocardial ischemia.[10,35,36] Conduction blocks and atrial or ventricular arrhythmias occur with varying frequency.[37] Bradycardia is not considered a problem unless it is contributing to hypotension. Bradycardia is atropine resistant because of the loss of the vagal motor nucleus. While the arrhythmia is managed, the case should be determined and eliminated by monitoring electrolytes and arterial blood gases (see Table 43–1). Bradycardia can be treated with dopamine, dobutamine, isoproterenol, or temporary cardiac pacing. Ventricular fibrillation is usually the terminal arrhythmia in adult brain-dead donors, whereas bradycardia and asystole are more common in pediatric donors.[38] In the event of cardiac arrest or inadequate cardiac activity, resuscitation measures should be initiated to maintain adequate circulation to the target organs. Preservation and procurement of the liver and kidneys should proceed rapidly after cardiac arrest has occurred.

Multiple organ harvest is a sterile surgical procedure lasting approximately 3 to 4 hours depending on the number of organs to be retrieved. After usual surgical positioning and preparation, a midline incision from the suprasternal notch to the pubis and a sternal split are accomplished. Each team of surgeons examines and isolates their target organ. Immediately prior to aortic occlusion, the anesthetist may be requested to administer several agents to preserve the organs such as prostaglandins or free oxygen radical scavengers, like mannitol and allopurinol.[39] When all the organs to be harvested are isolated, the surgical occlusion of the proximal aorta is accomplished and the in situ flushing of organs with cold preservation solution is begun. Rapid cooling is facilitated by slush over the entire field. At this point, anesthetic support is no longer necessary. The time of proximal aortic cross-clamp and infusion of cardioplegia solution should be recorded to document the beginning of cold ischemia time for the transplantable organs. Monitoring and other supportive measures should be discontinued at this point to minimize emotional distress for operating room personnel.[10]

The Living Kidney Donor

Thirty percent of transplanted kidneys in the United States are obtained from living donors who are related to the recipient. Living related donor kidneys improve the chances of immediate transplanted organ function to 95 percent because of well-matched tissue and a short ischemic time. Major complications for the donor occur in less than 5 percent of cases and include primarily deep vein thrombosis and pulmonary embolus.[1] One case of fatal halothane-induced hepatitis has been reported[40]; however, the overall morbidity and mortality are extremely low. It is of utmost importance that all potential risks be eliminated from the healthy live related donor volunteer undergoing unilateral nephrectomy.

The preoperative visit usually reveals a generally healthy individual especially with respect to good kidney function bilaterally. Laboratory tests appropriate for the patient's age and history should be accomplished. Premedication can be administered in the usual manner to manage the patient's anxiety level. An intravenous infusion of balanced salt solution should be initiated the night before surgery and administered at the appropriate rate to maintain optimal hydration. Routine monitors are used in accordance with the current nationally accepted standards. The method of induction and maintenance of general anesthesia with endotracheal intubation does not appear to be critical.[41] Halothane might be avoided to decrease unnecessary risk to the donor[40] and drugs that are eliminated solely by the kidney should be avoided as the donor is losing 50 percent of his or her renal tissue. Although one kidney is sufficient for normal excretory function, renal homeostasis may be temporarily disrupted by spasm of renal vessels caused by vascular manipulation or by sudden hemorrhage.[42] Intravascular volume should be well maintained and the use of vasoactive agents should be limited to dopamine and avoided if possible because of effects on renal blood flow, especially in doses greater than 10 µg/kg per minute. Pneumothorax on the side of the nephrectomy is a concern that may limit the use of nitrous oxide. Maintenance of arterial carbon dioxide at near-normal levels will further ensure adequate renal blood flow in that either hypocapnia or hypercapnia may have a deleterious effect.[43] The anesthetist should be prepared for transfusion, if necessary, with adequate intravenous access and blood available. The administration of mannitol and furosemide is accomplished prior to cutting the ureter and heparin may be given prior to clamping the renal artery.[44] The procedure may be accomplished in either the supine or lateral position.

The Brain-Dead Kidney Donor

The Multiorgan Donor section of this chapter delineates general anesthetic management for all brain-dead donors. Specific considerations for cadaveric kidney donation are similar to those previously mentioned for the live kidney donor. Hypotension is best supported by increasing the intravascular volume with warmed balanced salt solutions and colloid, if necessary. The use of vasopressors should be avoided to ensure adequate renal blood flow. Dopamine is the pressor of choice to maintain a systolic blood pressure greater than 100 mm Hg (see Table 43–1). Pienaar et al[45] report that dopamine, used to support blood pressure, should be administered concurrently with T_3 to further ensure post-transplant renal function. Schneider et al[46] reported that kidneys obtained from donors supported with dopamine and pitressin demonstrated a higher incidence of acute tubular necrosis (ATN) after transplant and a lower rate of graft survival. The use of a central venous pressure (CVP) line and arterial pressure line is advised to monitor arterial blood pressure and intravascular volume, maintaining the CVP between 8 and 12 cm H_2O.[42] In the absence of DI, management of the kidney to be harvested should be directed toward optimizing filling pressures (CVP) and maintaining an adequate urine output between 100 and 200 mL/h. The use of dopamine 2 to 5 µg/kg per minute, mannitol, and furosemide may enhance glomerular filtration rate, increase renal blood flow, and increase urine output as well as increase protection from injury due to preservation procedures. Mannitol is thought to inhibit oxygen free radicals which serves to decrease hypoxic injury to the organ. Pharmacologic intervention initiated just prior to aortic cross-clamping includes agents such as dopamine, mannitol, furosemide, thorazine, heparin, and lidocaine[47] with the objective of extending organ viability.[10]

The Heart and Heart–Lung Donor

Care of the donor for heart or heart–lung organ retrieval should include all of the previously discussed concerns for multiorgan harvest with a few additional management priorities incorporated. Only 10 to 15 percent of referred heart donors meet the criteria for heart–lung transplantation. Heart–lung transplant recipients have a 25 percent mortality rate attributed directly to organ failure. With these odds against successful grafts, the responsibility lies with the anesthetist to identify and prevent those factors under anesthesia's control that may lead to deterioration of organ function before removal from the donor.[24]

After transport of the donor to the operating room, the lung harvest team accomplishes a bronchoscopy to establish the predicted viability of the lung. Less than one in ten potential lung donors have suitable organs for transplant.[48] During dissection, the pericardium and pleura are frequently left intact until the abdominal organs for retrieval have been dissected, although this sequence can vary between transplant surgical teams. The heart and lungs are harvested first because of the shortest acceptable cold ischemia time before transplant.

As with all organ donors, hypotension and fluid resuscitation are primary concerns, although lung donors should be fluid restricted as much as possible due to the possibility of pulmonary edema, either neurogenic, cardiogenic, or as a result of fluid overload. Crystalloid has a propensity to diffuse out of the vascular compartment and accumulate in the lungs; therefore, colloid is recommended for fluid resuscitation during lung harvest.[49] Twenty percent human albumin solution is preferable for heart–lung donors.[24] A large-bore intravenous line should be placed in an upper extremity, as the inferior vena cava (IVC) is clamped during this procedure. For lung harvest, the radial artery catheter should be placed on the left side and the CVP catheter on the right side.[11] This placement is necessary because the right subclavian artery and the brachiocephalic vein are divided early in the donor operation, with subsequent loss of monitoring and access from the right-sided arterial and left-sided venous cannulas.[24] If the heart is the only organ to be retrieved, which is unusual, the best choice of an inotrope would be an alpha-adrenergic agent such as metaraminol, phenylephrine, or norepinephrine. These agents maintain coronary perfusion pressure while limiting increases in myocardial oxygen consumption, and decreasing changes in coronary artery flow induced by increased heart rates.[10] Some institutions involved in heart transplantation feel that dopamine should be avoided for donor management based on two theoretical concerns: an iatrogenic catecholamine-induced donor cardiomyopathy,[50] and catecholamine depletion of the myocardium through endogenous release of norepinephrine[51]; however, if other organs are also targeted, dopamine is once again the agent of choice, as alpha-adrenergic vasopressors cause severe peripheral vasoconstriction.[52] Division of the mediastinal pleura and dissection of the trachea from the aorta and esophagus with manipulation of each lung separately out of the mediastinum may require an increase in the dose of dopamine to maintain a mean arterial pressure of 60 mm Hg[10] (see Table 43–1). This mechanical manipulation may also result in difficulties with ventilation and oxygenation. Large-volume losses should be anticipated and as much as 8 L of replacement fluid may be required in the form of colloid or blood.[24]

Sterility of the airway must be maintained with proper endotracheal suctioning techniques and the use of sterile breathing circuits and sterile PEEP valves even during transfer to the operating room. Endotracheal tube position should be confirmed with the heart–lung transplant surgeons to minimize mucosal injury to the harvested portion of the trachea.[10] Oxygen toxicity and barotrauma become issues when accomplishing heart–lung or lung retrieval. The lungs are ventilated with an FIO_2 of less than 0.40 and a normal tidal volume with peak inspiratory pressures below 30 cm H_2O. Low levels of PEEP (≤ 7.5 cm H_2O) may be employed to maintain a PaO_2 greater than 100.[53] The anesthetist should closely observe the lungs for areas of atelectasis and collapsed segments (collapsed and/or cyanotic) and attempt to reinflate these areas periodically by manual ventilation, in coordination with the surgeon's activities.[24]

Subsequent to the infusion of cold potassium cardioplegia into the heart, the lungs are flushed as well. During this infusion, the lungs should be manually ventilated at 4 breaths per minute to ensure distribution throughout both lungs. Prostaglandin E_1 (PGE_1) may be injected into the pulmonary artery by the surgeons just prior to cooling which

may cause significant hypotension, although it is known as a selective pulmonary vasodilator.[54] PGE_1 may also be contained in the preservation solution.[10,11] When ventilatory support is discontinued, the mouth and airway are suctioned and the endotracheal tube is removed to facilitate division of the trachea and removal of the heart and lungs from the chest cavity.[10]

The Liver Donor

Incorporating the general considerations identified under The MultiOrgan Donor, liver retrieval presents very few additional considerations for the anesthetist. Although most hepatic procurements have occurred in heart-beating, brain-dead donors, it is possible to harvest a viable graft from a non-heart-beating donor. Effective and viable procurement can be compatible with 15 to 30 minutes of cardiac arrest, which requires rapid efforts by the operating room and anesthesia personnel. Prior to the acceptance of the brain death laws in the United States in 1968 almost all livers where harvested in this manner, but improved methods of rapid cooling and organ preservation have increased the overall viability of the graft.[55]

Approximately 20 percent of liver transplant recipients are in the intensive care unit immediately prior to transplantation and are gravely ill. When the liver is grafted, no backup support such as hemodialysis is available to the recipient. The liver graft must function properly and immediately for a successful transplantation. Preoperatively, the donor liver is evaluated by the surgical team for the presence of infectious agents and function, that is, a total bilirubin of 2.0 mg/dL and an SGOT and SGPT below 400 U/L. Intraoperatively, the PO_2 should be kept above 70 mm Hg and the CVP should be maintained at a value less than 15 cm H_2O and preferably less than 10 cm H_2O to avoid edema in the liver.[56] When the donor has DI, liver transplant surgeons prefer the use of DDAVP over vasopressin. Hypotension may occur during liver dissection as a result of compression of the inferior vena cava[24]; however, as dopamine interferes with portal vein flow, a serious effort should be made to discontinue dopamine, or at least reduce the dose.[56]

Liver transplant surgery is lifesaving and many recipients are able to return to normal life-styles. Scantlebury et al[57] described 17 post-liver-transplant women who have successfully delivered 20 babies. There was an increased incidence of prematurity and cesarean birth over the normal population. One mother died 4 years after transplantation and 2.5 years after delivery; however, 16 of the 17 mothers are alive from 2 to 18 years after transplantation and all children are normal and healthy.

THE IMMUNE SYSTEM AND IMMUNOSUPPRESSIVE DRUGS

Pharmacologic control of the immune system is another key link in organ graft survival. The history of such agents is extremely short in that azathioprine (Imuran), a primary agent, has only been in clinical use since 1962.[58] Being somewhat unsatisfactory when used as the sole agent, corticosteroids were added in 1963 which caused an additive and synergistic effect.[59] The first major clinical experience with cyclosporine (Cyclosporin A) was reported in 1979 as a sole agent for immunosuppression.[60] Many centers are currently using a combination of cyclosporin A, corticosteroids, and azathioprine for their immunosuppressant regimens. The monoclonal antibody Orthoclone OKT3 was introduced in 1983 and approved by the Food and Drug Administration (FDA) in 1987 and is used during acute rejection of the transplanted organ.[61,62] Before discussing these drugs, a summary of the components of the immune system responsible for rejection of transplanted tissue is given.

Immune System Review

Unless the transplanted organ is from an identical twin, proteins on the cell surface identify the organ as foreign tissue and cause toxic reactions resulting in transplant rejection. Recipients must be chronically maintained on antirejection medication after transplantation, balancing the need to prevent immune system responses from injuring the transplanted organ with the need to protect against bacterial infection and the proliferation of malignant cells. Drugs such as OKT-3 are reserved for short-term therapy to reverse the processes of acute rejection. The following terms will assist in understanding the immune system.

Antigen. Molecular structure unfamiliar to the host's immune system, usually on a bacterial cell surface, and perceived as foreign by the host's immune system.

B lymphocytes. White blood cells producing antibodies.

Antibody. Protein produced by B lymphocytes that binds to a specific antigen. Also known as immunoglobulin (Ig) of various types (e.g., IgA). After binding to an antigen, antibodies activate the complement system and promote ingestion of bound material by macrophages.

Complement system. A series of enzymes activated by the antigen–antibody interaction that cause lysis of cells containing antigen.

Macrophages. Cells that attack substances (bacteria or tissue) that have been coated with antibody. Macrophages activate lymphocytes by (1) concentrating antigen on their surface, allowing lymphocytes to interact with antigen, and (2) releasing **interleukin-1,** which activates helper T cells.

T lymphocytes. Thymus-dependent white blood cells consisting of helper T, cytotoxic T, and suppressor T cells.

Helper T cells. Assists B lymphocytes in producing antibody and releases **lymphokines** (protein mediators) from sensitized lymphocytes which include the following:

- **Blastogenic factor** causes lymphocytes not sensitized to antigen to replicate, thereby increasing their population at the site of the antigen reaction.
- **Transfer factor** converts lymphocytes not sensitized to antigen to lymphocytes sensitized to a specific antigen at the site of the antigen reaction.
- Factor (no name) attracts phagocytic cells to site of reaction.
- Factor (no name) activates phagocytic cells.
- **Leukocyte migration inhibition factor** and **macrophage migration inhibition factor** keep cells at the site of reaction.
- **Skin reactive factor** releases histamine from mast cells to increase vascular permeability and allow immune system cells to enter tissue.

Cytotoxic T cell. Directly binds to antigens; releases **lymphotoxin,** which causes lysis of cells bound to the cytotoxic T cells.

Suppressor T cell. Suppresses responses of B and T lymphocytes.

OKT and **Leu.** Surface markers on helper T cells that are identical among individuals. Each designates a series of antibodies produced in mice that specifically react to surface markers (antigens) of specific (human) immune system cells. For example, OKT3 reacts with all T lymphocytes, OKT4 reacts with helper T cells, and Leu2 reacts with cytotoxic and suppressor T cells.

K cell. Attaches to antibody (IgG) that has interacted with antigen and releases a lymphotoxin. This is antibody-dependent cellular cytotoxicity.

Natural killer (NK) cell. Attacks malignant host cells by an unknown mechanism.

ABO and **HLA.** Cell surface proteins that are present on all tissue cells, but differ between individuals; may become antigens after transplantation. Close matching of ABO and HLA types will decrease the incidence and severity of immune system responses against the transplanted organ.

Immunosuppressants

Drugs used for immunosuppressive management of posttransplant patients have a variety of side effects that must be considered when these agents or an anesthetic is administered to such patients. The four main agents in current use are described. When dealing with an immunosuppressed patient, strict aseptic technique must be observed as infection is a major cause of mortality.

Corticosteroids. Corticosteroids are administered for their anti-inflammatory effects resulting from stabilization of the lysosomal membranes. The concentration of peripheral blood leukocytes (lymphocytes, monocytes, and basophils) decreases within 4 to 6 hours of the dose. Corticosteroids inhibit T-lymphocyte growth factor, causing T lymphocytes to lose their ability to proliferate. Antibody production is suppressed with high doses over a long period.[63] Chronic steroid therapy causes adrenal suppression which requires perioperative stress doses of corticosteroid. A variety of regimens are used.[11] Other side effects include the following: electrolyte and metabolic changes, osteoporosis, peptic ulcer disease, skeletal muscle myopathy, central nervous system dysfunction, peripheral blood changes, inhibition of normal growth, and increased susceptibility to infection.[64]

Azathioprine (Imuran). Purine analogs act by multiple mechanisms, including effects on purine nucleotide synthesis and metabolism as well as alterations in the synthesis and function of RNA and DNA, leading to decreased immune cell proliferation.[64] The exact mechanism of action of azathioprine is not fully understood.[63] Azathioprine may cause some resistance to muscle relaxants[65] and can also cause leukopenia and suppress antibody formation.

Cyclosporin A (Cyclosporine). In contrast to azathioprine, cyclosporine causes suppression of T-cell-mediated cellular immunity without causing major effects on the antibacterial defenses of the body.[66] Early heart transplant graft arteriosclerosis can be attributed to cyclosporine.[67–70] High doses can also be associated with hepatotoxicity and renal failure, even in the post renal transplant patient.

Muromonab CD-3 (Orthoclone OKT3). Muromonab CD-3 is a monoclonal antibody that has been shown to be effective during allograft rejection. OKT3 binds to all mature T lymphocytes and blocks function of the cell.[63] The acute administration of the drug may cause hemodynamic instability, fever, diarrhea, encephalitis, and possibly pulmonary edema. Ongoing treatment with OKT3 should not affect anesthetic management,[11] keeping in mind that the grafted organ may not be functioning normally because of acute rejection.

ANESTHETIC MANAGEMENT OF THE RENAL TRANSPLANT RECIPIENT

General Principles

The preoperative assessment of the renal transplant recipient should be appropriate for the patient's age and history, keeping in mind that chronic uremia may cause a variety of cardiovascular complications including hypertension, accelerated atherosclerosis, cardiomegaly, pericarditis, and impaired left ventricular function resulting in congestive heart failure.[43] Additionally, examination of the most recent dialysis record should indicate that dialysis was accomplished within 24 hours of surgery to ensure a safer surgical course by correcting abnormalities in fluid or electrolyte balance. The dialysis record should be examined to note changes in vital signs and body weight before and after dialysis and to determine if blood was administered. An increase in the hematocrit that is disproportionate to the amount of blood administered along with loss of 1 kg or more of body weight should alert the anesthetist that the patient may have a decreased intravascular volume predisposing to potential hypotension, especially during induction.[41]

Postdialysis electrolytes, complete blood count (CBC), calcium, phosphorus, magnesium, platelet count, prothrombin time, partial thromboplastin time, room air arterial blood gases, chest X-ray, and electrocardiogram are recommended[43] to guide the anesthetist's anesthetic plan as well as ensure that there is no need for further dialysis prior to elective surgery. Anemia and bleeding abnormalities from abnormal platelet aggregation are common in these patients. The issue of preoperative blood transfusion has yet to be fully resolved, the concern being that transfusions may lead to either increased or decreased incidence of graft rejection.[71,72] Hemoglobin levels are rarely greater than 9 to 10 g/100 mL; therefore, the necessity for preoperative transfusion should be determined on the basis of the patient's preoperative hematocrit, other significant history, and institutional policy. Coagulation studies should be normal and serum potassium should be in the range 4.0 to 5.5 mEq/L. Acid–base balance should be normal and serum calcium is usually low, 7 to 8 mg/10 mL. Hypertension should be improved over predialysis values and serum creatinine and BUN concentrations should be below 10 and 60 mg/100 mL, respectively.[41] The preservation time for cadaver kidneys has been extended to 36 to 48 hours which allows ample time to optimize a patient preoperatively.[72]

If renal failure patients require emergency surgery without preoperative dialysis, a full set of electrolytes should be obtained. Hyperkalemia greater than 5.5 to 6.0 mEq/L can be managed with a solution of 5 percent dextrose in water with 2 units of regular insulin added for every 5 g of dextrose. A glass bottle may be preferable to prevent absorption of the insulin into the walls of a plastic intravenous bag. Flushing of the intravenous tubing with 60 mL of solution will serve to saturate insulin-binding sites of the tubing,[73] although it has been shown that the small amount of insulin that binds to the tubing and container walls may be clinically insignificant.[74] Infusing this solution at a rate of 3 to 5 mL/min facilitates transfer of serum potassium into the intracellular compartment. Calcium gluconate 2 g/100 mL can be added to this solution to antagonize the cardiac effects of hyperkalemia. If moderate to severe acidosis is present, bicarbonate rather than lactate should be used as the latter may be poorly metabolized. Administered blood should be deionized to reduce its potassium content.[41]

Premedication

Common premedications can be used in ordinary doses for patients not severely debilitated or physiologically compromised. Benzodiazepines and narcotics may have exaggerated effects in renal failure patients; however, these recipients have frequently had multiple surgical procedures which may significantly increase their anxiety and preexisting hypertension. Ranitidine and metoclopramide should be administered if the patient has the potential for regurgitation even though metoclopramide has antidopamine activity and may necessitate the use of dopamine intraoperatively to encourage graft function.

Anesthetic Management

General anesthesia is usually employed to accomplish renal transplantation although regional anesthesia may be considered if contraindications to general anesthesia exist. As the procedure is entirely extraperitoneal and in the lower abdomen, a regional block maintained at a low thoracic dermatome level will provide adequate anesthesia. Regional anesthesia also avoids intubation, iatrogenic respiratory infection, the use of muscle relaxants, and the depressant effects of general anesthetics; however, the procedure requires at least 4 hours which necessitates either a high single administration block or the use of a continuous regional anesthetic technique with supplemental intravenous sedation. Many of these patients have a preoperative history of abnormal platelet aggregation[43] and the common use of intraoperative heparinization may contraindicate the use of a continuous regional technique.[75] In addition, the depressant effects of 4 hours of intravenous sedation cannot be disregarded.

Advisable monitors during renal transplantation include accepted protocols. The anesthetist should avoid using the extremity containing the arteriovenous shunt for blood pressure cuffs, monitoring devices, or intravenous lines. Additional monitors include a central venous pressure (CVP) line to monitor fluid balance in a potentially hypovolemic or hypervolemic patient. Carlier et al[76] suggested the routine use of a pulmonary artery catheter to maintain a pulmonary artery diastolic pressure above 15 mm Hg, with intent to avoid acute tubular necrosis. Gallo et al[43] stated that hydration status can be adequately monitored in the absence of left ventricular failure by following the CVP. An arterial catheter is not routinely recommended; however, if one is placed, the extremity containing the arteriovenous shunt should not be used.

Induction of general anesthesia may be accomplished with sodium thiopental and a supplemental opioid analgesic in appropriate doses to blunt the response of instrumenting the airway and endotracheal intubation. Succinylcholine remains widely used for the characteristic rapid onset of action; however, the use of succinylcholine may increase the serum potassium level in a patient who may already be hyperkalemic and the subsequent generation of dysrhythmias is extremely common.[43] The use of either atracurium or vecuronium (short-acting nondepolarizing muscle relaxants) for intubation is a preferable technique.[77–79] Muscle relaxants can be continued throughout the procedure with the same nondepolarizing agent and should be antagonized at the end of the case. An oral, as opposed to nasal, intubation is performed because epistaxis from nasal intubation may be difficult to control in the renal failure patient due to abnormal platelet aggregation.

Isoflurane appears to be the agent of choice for maintenance in addition to supplemental doses of opioid analgesics. Cyclosporine, a widely used immunosuppressant known to reduce kidney function, may compromise renal function and reduce the ability of the kidney to excrete fluoride ions produced via the biotransformation of enflurane to inorganic fluoride.[80,81] Halothane was reported to possibly modulate reperfusion injury at a cellular level and, therefore, inhibit the recovery of a cold ischemic kidney.[82] The clearance of alfentanil (Alfenta) is unchanged by renal failure,[83] although the imposition of diabetes on renal failure significantly increases the clearance time.[84]

Fluid management during the case is pivotal to the success of the graft. Suspected hypovolemia is confirmed by a greater than expected acute fall in arterial and central venous pressures after induction. If hypotension does occur, centrally acting pressors are recommended, such as dopamine (which has been shown to increase renal blood flow),[85] although isoproterenol may also be beneficial. Vasoconstricting agents such as phenylephrine should be avoided because of the decrease in renal blood flow. Hypervolemia is diagnosed by a rise in central venous pressure and signs of pulmonary congestion. Central venous pressure, heart rate, arterial pressure, and auscultation of the chest should all be used to guide fluid management. Adequate hydration should ensure a rapid diuresis after the graft is unclamped if the ischemic time has been less than 30 minutes.

Immunosuppressive therapy is begun at the time of the procedure requiring the anesthetist to administer large doses of drugs such as antibiotics, steroids, azathioprine, cyclosporine, and OKT3. Antibiotics are administered simultaneously as immunosuppressive therapy causes the patient to be more susceptible to infection. Naloxone has been reported to cause improved organ survival and kidney function after severe ischemic injury in a preliminary animal model.[86] Calcium channel blockers have been shown to protect against ischemic injury of the graft when administered to the donor and recipient.[31,32] Low-dose dopamine, 2 to 5 µg/kg per minute, furosemide, and mannitol may also be necessary if the ischemia time has been longer than 30 minutes and there is no immediate brisk diuresis from the graft of up to 1 L/h.[41] The potential for toxic drug interactions is readily apparent with the simultaneous administration of multiple agents.

A high incidence of peripheral vascular disease and left ventricular dysfunction requires the anesthetist to anticipate episodes of either hypotension or hypertension. Glucose and electrolytes should be followed closely. If the donor kidney was perfused with Collin's solution, there may be an acute hyperkalemia when the kidney is unclamped in addition to a sudden transient episode of hypertension secondary to the release of renin by the ischemic kidney.

Renal function after transplantation can take one of three courses. An excellent result is immediate brisk diuresis including adequate excretion of waste products. The major postoperative problems in these patients are hypovolemia and electrolyte imbalance. The second course is a pattern similar to acute tubular necrosis (ATN) exhibited by diuresis without excretion of metabolic products. A recovery phase follows rapidly enough to avoid hemodialysis. Third, a pattern of oliguria and anuria followed by a diuretic phase and then subsequent recovery of kidney function may be seen. Postoperative care includes usual intensive care criteria with special attention to fluid and electrolyte balance. Avoiding fluid and electrolyte imbalance is imperative. Hemodialysis may be required initially to support the graft in eliminating the toxic waste products of metabolism.

ANESTHETIC MANAGEMENT OF THE HEART AND HEART–LUNG RECIPIENT FOR NONTRANSPLANT SURGERY

Anesthetic management of the heart and heart–lung transplant is undertaken by specialized cardiac anesthesia teams, discussion of which is beyond the scope of this text; however, these patients present problems similar to those faced when anesthetizing any patient, adult or pediatric, with severe cardiomyopathies or ischemic heart disease. Effectively dealing with these clinical situations should be familiar and comfortable to any cardiac anesthesia provider. An excellent chapter covering the anesthetic management of these patients has been written by Baum[11] and is suggested as further reading for management of heart and heart–lung transplantation procedures.

Heart transplantation has been shown to effectively restore patients to a level of general health that is comparable to the general population,[87] making the postheart or postheart–lung transplant patient a likely candidate for nontransplant surgery. The management of these patients presents unique clinical problems as the denervated heart and lungs and the side effects of immunosuppressive therapy present physiologic responses that are not normally expected. Both regional and general anesthesia have been used extensively.[88–93] As long as the physiology is appreciated, many different agents and techniques can be employed.

The transplanted human heart has a higher resting heart rate (90 to 120 beats per minute), reflecting lack of vagal innervation. The maintenance of arterial blood pressure is preload dependent. Intrinsic responses to an increase in preload cause increases in stroke volume when the denervated heart responds to stress from either exercise or surgical stimuli. Increases in contractility and heart rate occur within 5 to 6 minutes as a result of increased circulating catecholamines,[94–97] since cardiac adrenergic receptors are intact and respond normally.[98] Therefore, an increase in heart rate is a poor guide to estimate depth of anesthesia or fluid status. Vasodilation caused by regional anesthesia, histamine-releasing drugs, and vasodilating agents may cause a precipitous fall in cardiac output as a result of inadequate preload. Myocardial depressants, such as inhalation agents, may cause a greater decrease in blood pressure than normally expected as cardiac output is affected by increases in stroke volume rather than heart rate. The human heart remains denervated[99–101] and requires direct-acting agents such as isoproterenol and phenylephrine to correct bradycardia and hypotension. Dysrhythmias, both atrial and ventricular, are more common during the first 6 months after transplantation and during episodes of rejection.[90,101,102] These dysrhythmias, except bradycardia, are treated in the same manner as for nontransplanted patients, keeping in mind that the negative inotropic effects of antiarrhythmic agents are enhanced in the transplanted heart.[92] Painless ischemia, diagnosed by ECG, is a concern in heart transplant patients as immunosuppressive therapy with cyclosporine is associated with early graft atherosclerosis.[67–70]

Lung transplantation results in loss of innervation, bronchial artery blood flow, and lymphatic drainage. The clinical implications of these losses are not yet completely clear; however, within 4 months of transplant, blood gases are normal, rate and rhythm of breathing are normal, appropriate increases in ventilation occur in response to exercise, and collateral circulation restores bronchial blood flow.[103] Loss of lymphatic drainage raises the possibility that there is greater susceptibility to fluid overload; therefore, the CVP is kept as low as possible. Oxygen toxicity also remains an issue so it is recommended that inspired oxygen concentrations be adjusted to minimum levels, maintaining an arterial P_{O_2} between 80 and 100 mm Hg. Damage to the recurrent laryngeal nerve is possible during the transplantation procedure, causing the patient to be at greater risk of aspiration.[43]

Monitors for nontransplant procedures for these patients consist of appropriate monitors employed for any patient undergoing a similar surgical procedure. As transplanted heart function is usually good, unless acute rejection is present, invasive cardiac monitoring is dictated by the planned operative procedure. As always, strict aseptic technique must be maintained for all immunosuppressed patients as infection is a major cause of mortality, accounting for at least 32 percent of deaths in a recent report.[104] Invasive monitoring and all forms of instrumentation, including intubation, should be kept to a minimum. If the anesthetic plan requires endotracheal intubation, use of a sterile intubation tray[43] and sterile gloves is recommended. Exposing the patient to a minimum of attendants also re-

duces the risk of infection.[105] The patient should be extubated as early as possible, preferably in the operating room.[11]

Heart–lung transplant patients require additional observation because of late posttransplant pulmonary dysfunction. One year after transplantation, oxygenation is usually normal and the alveolar–arterial oxygen gradient is only slightly increased.[106] Nearly 50 percent of transplanted patients develop late pulmonary complications after a year of good function. These complications include recurrent pulmonary infections and bronchiolitis obliterans. The ratio of forced expiratory volume at 1 second to forced vital capacity (FEV_1/FVC) decreases from 92 to 55 percent and the $FEV_{25–75}$ decreases from 70 to 9 percent of predicted values.[107,108] The denervation of the pulmonary stretch receptors, which are felt to be responsible for the sensation of dyspnea, may alter signs of respiratory distress.[11] If the patient has progressed to pulmonary dysfunction, regional anesthesia should be considered if appropriate for the planned surgical procedure.

For preoperative anesthetic planning to be comprehensive, it is important to know which organs have been transplanted into the patient and, in some cases, what approach was used. Single-lung transplantation patients do not seem to be as susceptible to pulmonary deterioration from bronchiolitis obliterans.[93] Triantafillou et al[109] reported that a bilateral lung transplant with bronchial attachments may be an improvement over the single tracheal attachment for long-term durability. Bilateral or single-lung transplant preserves innervation of the heart which simplifies intraoperative cardiac management.[109]

ANESTHETIC MANAGEMENT FOR SURGERY AFTER RENAL TRANSPLANT

The 1-year survival rate of renal transplant patients is between 80 and 90 percent. The 3-year survival rate is about 70 percent, and the 6-year survival rate decreases to 51 percent. This early, initial success is attributed to the introduction of cyclosporine, yet some believe the decline in survival rates is ultimately due not only to late rejection, but also to cyclosporine.[110] Immunosuppression pharmacology is relatively new and various regimens and combinations are being implemented in different centers; however, the nephrotoxicity of cyclosporine remains a concern. Renal transplantation in children less than 4 years old as well as in patients greater than 60 has become much more common. The major causes of death in renal transplant patients include myocardial infarction, infection, and neoplasias.[111] These major causes of mortality, the excellent survival rate, the wide age range of patients, and the complications of immunosuppression greatly increase the potential for encountering the post-renal-transplant patient for other types of surgical procedures. The commonsense approach for these procedures includes strict maintenance of sterile technique to avoid infection in the immunosuppressed patient. Typically, a renal consult is obtained regarding steroid preparation, maintenance of immunosuppression perioperatively, and evaluation of current renal function. Presenting conditions that were present prior to the transplant frequently remain, including diabetes and hypertension. Posttransplant renal function is not uniformly good because of repeated episodes of rejection, continued presence of preexisting disease, and immunosuppressive therapy (Raybould D. Personal communication). Serum creatinine has been shown to underestimate renal impairment.[112]

The anesthetic technique should focus on maintenance of existing renal function as well as the management of other complicating preexisting conditions. Maintenance of adequate renal perfusion is essential, balancing fluid load and blood pressure and avoiding the use of agents that compromise renal blood flow. Renal artery stenosis may be present as a side effect of immunosuppressant therapy, but there is no evidence that transplanted kidneys have an increased susceptibility to hypotensive acute tubular necrosis over native kidneys. Maintenance of adequate hydration to protect kidney graft function is dependent on renal function. Monitoring urine output is accomplished when appropriate, but the risks of infection should be weighed against the value of this information. Kidneys function better with high normal central venous pressures. Diuretics, to improve urine output, should be used after adequate fluid status is established. When the patient is being positioned, the presence of arteriovenous shunts should be considered, as should avoidance of the shunt-containing extremity for other lines and monitors. The presence of probable cardiovascular disease brings attention to myocardial oxygen supply and demand during the perioperative period. Anesthetic drugs and techniques commensurate with the presenting conditions and level of renal function should be used, probably avoiding enflurane (Raybould D. Personal communication).

ANESTHETIC MANAGEMENT OF SURGERY AFTER LIVER TRANSPLANT

Anesthesia for orthotopic liver transplantation challenges the anesthesia provider's skills and knowledge of physiology to the fullest during a very dynamic and lengthy case. It is a complex situation requiring management of massive blood loss and major pathologic changes secondary to profound liver failure. Three operative phases of the transplant begin with the initial dissection which involves rapidly changing fluid and electrolyte balance and a partially functioning liver. The anhepatic phase excludes the presence of liver function combined with tremendous venous congestion in the inferior vena cava and portal system, even if venovenous bypass is used. Reperfusion of the grafted liver, when the new liver is beginning to establish function, presents further challenges. Kang et al provides an excellent chapter to which the reader is referred for further information.[113]

As liver transplant recipients enjoy a 5-year survival rate of 65 percent, they may very well present for nontransplant surgery. Essentially, all organ systems can be diseased when advanced liver disease is present.[114] During preoperative evaluation, the history of liver disease should be evaluated because of the concern that the transplant did not necessarily cure the original disease or its associated problems. After transplant, hepatitis may still be a factor, as may cardiovascular disease which is commonly associated with hepatitis C. Cardiomyopathy is common in patients with alcoholic liver disease and slightly less common in those with hemochromatosis and Wilson's disease. Decreased hepatic function is not necessarily present; however, there is a very real possibility that the disease is systemic (e.g., hepatitis) and there is a continued risk of transmission to medical personnel. The transplant procedure also requires the administration of large quantities of blood products to the recipient, further exposing the patient to infectious agents. Immunosuppression causes the patient to be uniquely susceptible to such viruses as cytomegalovirus (CMV), hepatitis viruses, and human immunodeficiency virus (HIV).[115] Liver function is usually normal. Acute toxicity of cyclosporine is usually reflected by an increase in bilirubin and a rise in transaminases (SGOT, SGPT); however, these findings would not necessarily differ from those for hepatitis. A degree of compromised renal function can be expected from the cyclosporine, and serum creatinine levels have been shown to underestimate the degree of renal dysfunction.[115] Drug metabolism shows a reduced level of enzyme activity, reflected by altered steroid metabolism.[116]

Advanced liver disease exhibits striking circulatory changes characterized by an elevated cardiac index, decreased total peripheral resistance, and decreased arterial–mixed venous oxygen content difference. There is a rapid normalization of this hyperdynamic state after transplantation if the allograft exhibits good function. If the transplanted liver does not function well, these dynamics may remain or even worsen. Denervation and vasoderegulation of the grafted liver should at least be considered in the postoperative period, although it is not known how long the denervation continues. Denervation has been shown to increase the responsiveness of the blood vessels to almost any kind of stimulation. The increase in vasoreactivity appears to extend to all vasoactive agents, including a possibly exaggerated response to dopamine. Alpha stimulation constricts splanchnic vessels in all species and beta-blocking agents may also hamper splanchnic flow influenced by denervation. Neosynephrine may be preferred over norepinephrine to avoid hepatic congestion, and the agents of choice for control of hypertension seem to be hydralazine and nifedipine.[112]

The anesthetic management of these patients should incorporate all of the known pertinent preexisting disease states as well as the problems predicted on the basis of the patient's current condition. Vasoactive agents should be administered cautiously as the period during which the liver remains denervated is unknown. Agents such as enflurane should probably be avoided because of likely renal compromise. If liver function and hemodynamics are normal, these recipients can be treated as essentially normal immunosuppressed patients.

| In memory of Martin E. Mann, MD, without whom this chapter would not have been accomplished. |

REFERENCES

1. Haag BW, Stuart FP. The organ donor: Brain death, selection criteria, supply and demand. In: Flye MW, ed. *Principles of organ transplantation.* Philadelphia: WB Saunders; 1989:176–193.
2. Bart KJ, Macon EJ, Whittier FC, Baldwin RJ, Blount JH. Cadaveric kidneys for transplantation. A paradox of shortage in the face of plenty. *Transplantation.* 1981;31:379–382.

3. Benoit G, Spira A, Nicoulet I, Moukarzel M. Presumed consent law: Results of its application/outcome from an epidemiologic survey. *Transplant Proc.* 1990;22:320–322.

4. Roels L, Vanrenterghem Y, Waer M, Gruwez J, Michielsen P. Effect of a presumed content law on organ retrieval in Belgium. *Transplant Proc.* 1990;22:2078–2079.

5. Norton DJ, Nathan HM, Hamilton BT, et al. Current practices of determining brain death in potential organ donors. *Transplant Proc.* 1990;22:308–310.

6. Black PM. Brain death. *N Engl J Med.* 1978;299:338–44, 393–401.

7. Payen DM, Lamer C, Pilorget A, Moreau T, Beloucif S, Echter E. Evaluation of pulsed doppler common carotid blood flow as a noninvasive method for brain death diagnosis: A prospective study. *Anesthesiology.* 1990;72:222–229.

8. Williams GM, Ferree D, Bollinger RR, LeFor WM. Reasons why kidneys removed for transplantation are not transplanted in the United States. *Transplantation.* 1984;38:691–694.

9. Youngner SJ. Organ retrieval: Can we ignore the dark side? *Transplantation.* 1990;22:1014–1015.

10. Robertson KM, Cook DR. Perioperative management for the multiorgan donor. *Anesth Analg.* 1990;70:546–556.

11. Baum VC. Anesthesia for heart and heart–lung transplantation. In: Kapoor AS, Laks H, Schroeder J, Yacoub M, eds. *Cardiomyopathies and cardiopulmonary transplantation.* New York: McGraw-Hill; 1990:217–235.

12. Downman CBB, McSwiney BA. Reflexes elicited by visceral stimulation in acute spinal animal. *J Physiol.* 1946;105:80–94.

13. Jorgensen EO. Spinal man after brain death. The unilateral extension pronation reflex of the upper limb as an indication of brain death. *Acta Neurochirurg.* 1973;28:259–273.

14. Wetzel RC, Setzer N, Stiff JL, Rogers MC. Hemodynamic responses in brain dead organ donor patients. *Anesth Analg.* 1985;64:125–128.

15. Ciliberti BJ, Goldfein J, Rovenstine EA. Hypertension during anesthesia in patients with spinal cord injuries. *Anesthesiology.* 1954;15:273–279.

16. Johnson B, Thomason R, Pallares V, Sadove MS. Autonomic hyperreflexia. A review. *Milit Med.* 1975;140:345–349.

17. Naftchi NE, Wooten GF, Lowman EW, Axelrod J. Relationship between serum dopamine–beta-hydroxylase activity, catecholamine metabolism, and hemodynamic changes during paroxysmal hypertension in quadriplegia. *Circ Res.* 1974;35:850–860.

18. Koller J, Wieser C, Gottardis M, et al. Thyroid hormones and their impact on the hemodynamic and metabolic stability of organ donors and on kidney graft function after transplantation. *Transplant Proc.* 1990;22:355–357.

19. Mariot J, Jacob F, Voltz C, Perrier JF, Strub P. Hormonal therapy in human brain-dead potential organ donors. Comparative study. *Anesthesiology.* 1990;73:A246.

20. Novitzky D, Cooper DKC, Reichart B. Hemodynamic and metabolic responses to hormonal therapy in brain-dead potential organ donors. *Transplantation.* 1987;43:852–854.

21. Debelak L, Pollak R, Rechard C. Arginine vasopressin versus desmopressin for the treatment of diabetes insipidus in the brain dead donor. *Transplant Proc.* 1990;22:351–352.

22. Newsome Jr HH. Vasopressin: Deficiency, excess and the syndrome of inappropriate antidiuretic hormone secretion. *Nephron.* 1979;23:125–129.

23. Howlett TA, Keogh AM, Perry L, Touzel R, Rees LH. Anterior and posterior pituitary function in brain-stem-dead donors. A possible role for hormonal replacement therapy. *Transplantation.* 1989;47:828–834.

24. Ghosh S, Bethune DW, Hardy I, Kneeshaw J, Latimer RD, Oduro A. Management of donors for heart and heart–lung transplantation. *Anaesthesia.* 1990;45:672–675.

25. Nishimura N, Miyata Y. Cardiovascular changes in the terminal stage of disease. *Resuscitation.* 1984;12:175–180.

26. Heineman E, Bouwman E, Kort W, Marquet RL, Jeekel J. The donor transfusion phenomenon in rat kidney allograft model. *Transplant Proc.* 1987;19:1467–1469.

27. Deykin D. The clinical challenge of disseminated intravascular coagulation. *N Engl J Med.* 1970;283:636–644.

28. Miner ME, Kaufman HH, Graham SH, Haar FH, Gildenberg PL. Disseminated intravascular coagulation fibrinolytic syndrome following head injury in children: Frequency and prognostic implications. *J Pediatr.* 1982;100:687–691.

29. Kelly KJ, Outwater KM, Crone RK. Vasoactive amines in infants and children. *Clin Anaesthesiol.* 1984;2:427–442.

30. Outwater KM, Treves S, Lang P, Castaneda AR, Crone RK. Renal and hemodynamic effects of dopamine in infants following corrective cardiac surgery. *Anesthesiology.* 1984;61:A130.

31. Sobh MA, El-Din ABS, Moustafa FE, et al. A prospective randomized study of the protective effect of verapamil on ischemic renal injury in renal allotransplants. *Transplant Proc.* 1989;21:1230–1232.

32. Korb S, Albornoz G, Brems W, Ali A, Light JA. Verapamil pretreatment of hemodynamically unstable donors prevents delayed graft function post-transplant. *Transplant Proc.* 1989;21:1236–1238.

33. Murray JF, Gold P, Johnson BL Jr. The circulatory effects of hematocrit variations in normovolemic and hypervolemic dogs. *J Clin Invest.* 1963;42:1150–1159.

34. Rowley KM, Clubb KS, Smith JW, Cabin HS. Right-sided infective endocarditis as a consequence of flow directed pulmonary artery catheterization. A clinicopathological study of 55 autopsied patients. *N Engl J Med.* 1984;311:1152–1156.

35. Griepp RB, Stinson EB, Clark DA, Dong E, Shumway NE. The cardiac donor. *Surg Gynecol Obstet.* 1971;133:792–798.

36. McLeod AA, Neil-Dwyer G, Meyer CHA, Richardson PL, Cruickshank J, Bartlett J. Cardiac sequelae of acute head injury. *Br Heart J.* 1982;47:221–226.

37. Logigian EL, Ropper AH. Terminal electrocardiographic changes in brain-dead patients. *Neurology.* 1985;35:915–918.

38. Walsh CK, Krongrad E. Terminal cardiac electrical activity in pediatric patients. *Am J Cardiol.* 1983;51:557–561.

39. Turcotte JG. Conventional management of the brain-dead potential multi-organ donor. *Transplant Proc.* 1988;20(suppl 7):5–8.

40. Bennett AH, Harrison JH. Experience with living familial renal donors. *Surg Gynecol Obstet.* 1974;139:894–898.

41. Mazze RI. Anesthesia and the renal and genitourinary systems. In: Miller RD, ed. *Anesthesia.* 3rd ed. New York: Churchill Livingstone; 1990:1791–1805.

42. Mazze RI, Fujinaga M, Cousins MJ. Renal diseases. In: Katz J, Benumof JL, Kadis LB, eds. *Anesthesia and uncommon diseases.* Philadelphia: WB Saunders; 1990:537–559.

43. Gallo JA, Brown BR Jr, Newton DEF. Anaesthesia for organ transplantation. In: Nunn JF, Utting JE, Brown BR Jr, eds. *General anaesthesia.* 5th ed. London: Butterworths; 1989:868–879.

44. Bentley FR, Amin M, Garrison RN, Harty JI, Steinbock GS. The value of systemic heparinization during living donor nephrectomy. *Transplant Proc.* 1990;22:346–348.

45. Pienaar H, Schwartz I, Roncone A, Lotz Z, Hichman R. Function of kidney grafts from brain-dead donor pigs. The influence of dopamine and triiodothyronine. *Transplantation.* 1990;50:580–582.

46. Schneider A, Toledo-Pereyra LH, Zeichner WD, Allaben R, Whitten J. Effect of dopamine and pitressin on kidneys procured and harvested for transplantation. *Transplantation.* 1983;36:110–111.

47. Schulak JA, Novick AC, Sharp WV, Ford E. Donor pretreatment with lidocaine decreases incidence of early renal dysfunction in cadaver kidney transplantation. *Transplant Proc.* 1990;22:353–354.

48. Cooper JD. The lung donor: Special considerations. *Transplant Proc.* 1988;20(suppl 7):17–18.

49. Newton DE, Wesenhagen H. The role of the anaesthetist in transplantation. In: *Proceedings, VIIth European Congress of Anaesthesiology,* September 1, 1986:9.

50. Novitzky D, Wicomb WN, Cooper DKC, Rose AG, Feichart B. Prevention of myocardial injury during brain death by total cardiac sympathectomy in the Chacma baboon. *Ann Thorac Surg.* 1986;41:520–524.

51. Golberg LI. Dopamine—Clinical uses of an endogenous catecholamine. *N Engl J Med.* 1974;291:707–710.

52. Nishimura N, Sugi T. Circulatory support with sympathetic amines in brain death. *Resuscitation.* 1984;12:25–30.

53. Jamieson SW, Baldwin J, Stinson EB, et al. Clinical heart–lung transplantation. *Transplantation.* 1984;37:81–84.

54. Sorbara C, Pittarello D, Bonato R, Gallucci V, Giron GP. Right heart failure and prostaglandin E1 (PGE1) after heart transplantation. *Anesthesiology.* 1990;73:A223.

55. Yanaga K, Kakizoe S, Ikeda T, Podesta LG, Demetris AJ, Starzl TE. Procurement of liver allografts from non-heart beating donors. *Transplant Proc.* 1990;22:275–278.

56. Klintmalm GBG. The liver donor: Special considerations. *Transplant Proc.* 1988;20:9–11.

57. Scantlebury V, Gordon R, Tzakis A, et al. Childbearing after liver transplantation. *Transplantation.* 1990;49:317–321.

58. Murray JE, Merrill JP, Dammin GJ, Dealy JB, Alexandre GW, Harrison JH. Kidney transplantation in modified recipients. *Ann Surg.* 1962;156:337–355.

59. Starzl TE, Marchioro TL, Waddell WR. The reversal of rejection in human renal homografts with subsequent development of homograft tolerance. *Surg Gynecol Obstet.* 1963;117:385–395.

60. Calne RY, Rolles K, White DJG, et al. Cyclosporin A initially as the only immunosuppressant in 34 recipients of cadaveric organs: 32 kidneys, 2 pancreases, and 2 livers. *Lancet.* 1979;2:1033–1036.

61. Goldstein G, Schindler J, Sheahan M, Barnes L, Tsai H. Orthoclone OKT3 treatment of acute renal allograft rejection. *Transplant Proc.* 1985;17:129–131.

62. Norman DJ, Barry JM, Henell K, Funnell MB, Goldstein G, Bohannon L. Reversal of acute allograft rejection with monoclonal antibody. *Transplant Proc.* 1985;17:39–41.

63. Hooks MA. Immunosuppressive agents used in transplantation. In: Smith SL, ed. *Tissue and organ transplantation. Implications for professional nursing practice.* St. Louis, MO: CV Mosby; 1990:48–80.

64. Stoelting RK. *Pharmacology and physiology in anesthetic practice.* Philadelphia: JB Lippincott; 1987:480–498.

65. Vetten KB. Immunosuppressive therapy and anaesthesia. *S Afr Med J.* 1973;47:767–770.

66. Calabresi P, Parks RE Jr. Antiproliferative agents and drugs used for immunosuppression. In: Gilman AG, Goodman LS, Rall TW, Murad F, eds. *Goodman and Gilman's the pharmacological basis of therapeutics.* 7th ed. New York: Macmillan; 1985: 1247–1307.

67. Griepp RB, Stinson EB, Bieber CP, et al. Control of graft atherosclerosis in human heart transplant recipients. *Surgery.* 1977;81: 262–269.

68. Hess M, Hastillo A, Mohanakumar T, Wolfgang T, Lower RR. Accelerated atherosclerosis in cardiac transplantation: Role of cytotoxic B-cell antibodies and hyperlipidemia. *Circulation.* 1982;66(suppl II):152.

69. Hunt SA. Complications of heart transplantation. *Heart Transplant.* 1983;3:70–74.

70. Jamieson SW. Recent developments in heart and heart–lung transplantation. *Transplant Proc.* 1985;17:199–203.

71. Opelz G, Terasaki PI. Improvement of kidney-graft survival with increased numbers of blood transfusions. *N Engl J Med.* 1978;299:799–803.

72. Opelz G (for the Collaborative Transplant Study). *Transplant Proc.* 1987;19:149–152.

73. Roizen MF. Diseases of the endocrine system. In: Katz J, Benumof JL, Kadis LB, eds. *Anesthesia and uncommon diseases.* 3rd ed. Philadelphia: WB Saunders; 1990:245–292.

74. Weisenfeld S, Podolsky S, Goldsmith L, Ziff L. Adsorption of insulin to infusion bottles and tubing. *Diabetes.* 1968;17:766–771.

75. Cousins MJ. Hematoma following epidural block. *Anesthesiology.* 1972;37:263.

76. Carlier M, Squfflet J-P, Pirson Y, Gribomont B, Alexandre GPJ. Maximal hydration during anesthesia increases pulmonary arterial pressures and improves early function of human renal transplants. *Transplantation.* 1982;34:201–204.

77. Linke CL. Anaesthesia considerations for renal transplantations. In: Brown BR Jr, ed. *Anesthesia and transplantation surgery. Contemporary anesthesia practice.* Philadelphia: FA Davis; 1987: 183–231.

78. Graybar GB, Bready LL, eds. *Anesthesia for renal transplantation.* Boston: Nijhoff; 1987.

79. Orko R, Heino A, Bjorksten F, Scheinin B, Rosenberg PH. Comparison of atracurium and vecuronium in anesthesia for renal transplantation. *Acta Anaesthesiol Scand.* 1987; 31:450–453.

80. Fish KJ, Rice SA, Peterson KL. Renal function following cyclosporine and enflurane. *Anesthesiology.* 1990;73:A361.

81. Wickstrom I. Enflurane anesthesia in living donor renal transplantation. *Acta Anaesthesiol Scand.* 1981;25:263–269.

82. Rice MJ, Hjelmhaug JA, Southard JH. The effect of halothane on reperfusion injury in renal tubules after cold storage. *Transplant Proc.* 1990;22:450–451.

83. Chauvin M, Lebrault C, Levron JC, Duvaldestin P. Pharmacokinetics of alfentanil in chronic renal failure. *Anesth Analg.* 1987;66:53–56.

84. Koehntop DE, Noormohamed SE, Fletcher CV. Pharmacokinetics of alfentanil during renal transplantation in diabetic and non-diabetic patients. *Anesth Analg.* 1990;70:S112.

85. Reid PR, Thompson WL. The clinical use of dopamine in the treatment of shock. *Johns Hopkins Med J.* 1975;137:276–279.

86. Toledo-Pereyra LH, Frantzis P, Prough D, et al. Better renal function with naloxone treatment following hemorrhage and brain death. *Transplant Proc.* 1990;22:462–463.

87. Caine N, Sharples LD, English TAH, Wallwork J. Prospective study comparing quality of life before and after heart transplantation. *Transplant Proc.* 1990;22:1437–1439.

88. Demas K, Wyner J, Mihm FG, Samuels S. Anaesthesia for heart transplantation. A retrospective study and review. *Br J Anaesth.* 1986;58:1357–1364.

89. Grebenik CR, Robinson PN. Cardiac transplantation at Harefield. A review from an anaesthetist's standpoint. *Anaesthesia.* 1985;40:131–140.

90. Kanter SF, Samuels SI. Anesthesia for major operations on patients who have transplanted hearts, a review of 29 cases. *Anesthesiology.* 1977;46:65–68.

91. Samuels SI, Wyner J. Anaesthesia for surgery in a patient with a transplanted heart. *Br J Anaesth.* 1986;58:1199–1200.

92. Bricker SRW, Sugden JC. Anaesthesia for surgery in a patient with a transplanted heart. *Br J Anaesth.* 1985;57:634–637.

93. Cooper DKC, Becerra EA, Novitzky D, Ozinsky J, Horak A, Reichart B. Surgery in patients with heart transplants. Anaesthetic and operative considerations. *S Afr Med J.* 1986;70:137–142.

94. Pope SE, Stinson EB, Daughters GT, Schroeder JS, Ingels NB, Alderman EL. Exercise response of the denervated heart in long-term cardiac transplant recipients. *Am J Cardiol.* 1980;46: 213–218.

95. Leachman RD, Cokkinos DVP, Cabrera R, Leatherman LL, Rochelle DG. Response of the transplanted, denervated human heart to cardiovascular drugs. *Am J Cardiol.* 1971;27:272–276.

96. Kent KM, Cooper T. The denervated heart. A model for studying autonomic control of the heart. *N Engl J Med.* 1974; 291:1017–1021.

97. Hallman GL, Leatherman LL, Leachman RD, et al. Function of the transplanted human heart. *J Thorac Cardiovasc Surg.* 1969; 58:318–325.

98. Cannom DS, Graham AF, Harrison DC. Electrophysiological studies in the denervated transplanted human heart. Response to atrial pacing and atropine. *Circ Res.* 1973;32:268–278.

99. Mason JW, Winkle RA, Rider AK, Stinson EB, Harrison DC. The electrophysiologic effects of quinidine in the transplanted human heart. *J Clin Invest.* 1977;59:481–489.

100. Stinson EB, Griepp RB, Schroeder JS, Dong E Jr, Shumway NE. Hemodynamic observations one and two years after cardiac transplantation in man. *Circulation.* 1972;45:1183–1193.

101. Schroeder JS, Berke DK, Graham AF, Rider AK, Harrison DC. Arrhythmias after cardiac transplantation. *Am J Cardiol.* 1974; 33:604–607.

102. Romhilt DW, Doyle M, Sagar KB, et al. Prevalence and significance of arrhythmias in long-term survivors of cardiac transplantation. *Circulation.* 1982;66(suppl I):I219–I222.

103. McGregor CGA, Oyer PE, Shumway NE. Heart and heart–lung transplantation. *Prog Allergy.* 1986;38:346–365.

104. Bieber CP, Hunt SA, Schwinn DA, et al. Complications in long-term survivors of cardiac transplantation. *Transplant Proc.* 1981;13:207–211.

105. Samuels SI, Kanter SF. Anaesthesia for major surgery in a patient with a transplanted heart. *Br J Anaesth.* 1977;49:265–267.

106. Dawkins KD, Jamieson SW, Hunt SA, et al. Long-term results, hemodynamics, and complications after combined heart and lung transplantation. *Circulation.* 1985;71:919–926.

107. Jamieson SW, Dawkins KD, Burke C, et al. Late results of combined heart–lung transplantation. *Transplant Proc.* 1985; 17:212–214.

108. Burke CM, Morris AFR, Dawkins KD, et al. Late airflow obstruction in heart–lung transplantation recipients. *Heart Transplant.* 1985;4:437–439.

109. Triantafillou AN, Heerdt PM, Herbst TJ, Pond C, Despotis GJ. Bilateral single lung transplantation: Anesthetic management and intraoperative considerations. *Anesthesiology.* 1990;73:A89.

110. Land W. Kidney transplantation—State of the art. *Transplant Proc.* 1989;21:1425–1429.

111. Dulgosz BA, Bretan PN Jr, Novick AC, et al. Causes of death in kidney transplant recipients: 1970 to present. *Transplant Proc.* 1989;21:2168–2170.

112. Snyder JV. Postoperative evolution of extrahepatic organ function. *Transplant Proc.* 1989;21:3508–3510.

113. Kang YG, Gelman S. Liver transplantation. In: Gelman S, ed. *Anesthesia and organ transplantation.* Philadelphia: WB Saunders; 1987:139–185.

114. Van Thiel DH, Dindzans VJ, Gavaler JS, Tarter RE, Schade RR. Extrahepatic disease in liver transplant recipients. *Transplant Proc.* 1989;21:3478–3481.

115. Rubin RH, Tolkoff-Rubin NE. Infection: The new problem. *Transplant Proc.* 1989;21:1140–1445.

116. Venkataramanan R, Huang ML, Delamos B, et al. Steroid metabolism in liver transplant patients. *Transplant Proc.* 1989;21: 2452.

PART VI

Special Problems in Anesthesia and Critical Care

Malignant Hyperthermia

Jeanette F. Peter

Malignant hyperthermia (MH) is a rare but potentially fatal complication of anesthesia. It is an inherited condition involving the muscle. During a MH episode the skeletal muscle reacts abnormally to a triggering agent (usually an anesthetic drug) with an uncontrollable increase in muscle metabolism and heat production.

Historically, the first description of MH as a clinical syndrome appeared in 1960.[1] The case report described a 21-year-old patient about to have surgery, who was extremely concerned about the risks of general anesthesia because several of his relatives had died as a result of ether anesthesia. The young man developed MH and survived. This report of the episode characterized by fever, tachycardia, tachypnea, and cyanosis focused the awareness of anesthetists on this rare syndrome. About the same time, Britt, Locher, and Kalow became aware of a Wisconsin family in which 30 members had died in conjunction with general anesthesia.[2] The Wisconsin area subsequently provided a large gene pool for Britt and colleagues' study on the inheritance of MH.

It is likely that MH occurred prior to the sixties, but episodes were probably attributed to more commonly recognized causes of hyperthermia or misdiagnosed as "anesthetic convulsions."

The term *malignant hyperthermia* came into use because of the tremendous heat production that may occur. Body temperature may rise as much as 1C every 5 minutes.[3] The word *malignant* refers to the fulminating nature of the condition, which rapidly becomes fatal if vigorous therapy is not initiated.

INCIDENCE

Malignant hyperthermia is the most common cause of anesthetic-induced death in North America. The incidence of MH reported varies from 1 in 14,000 for children to 1 in 120,000 overall.[4] Ording suggests that MH occurs in 1 in 250,000 of all anesthetics administered, but in 1 in 50,000 if inhalational agents are combined with succinylcholine.[5] The ages recorded range from 2 months to 78 years. The highest incidence is between the ages of 3 and 30 years. All racial groups have been affected. Males are more commonly affected than females, but this statistic may reflect the greater number of males presenting for surgery related to trauma.[6] The mortality rate, originally over 70 percent, is now reported to be between 10 and 21 percent.[7] This decrease in mortality is attributed to earlier recognition and the discovery that sodium dantrolene effectively treats the MH syndrome.

Malignant hyperthermia is a pharmacogenetic disorder. The clinical manifestations follow the administration of a depolarizing muscle relaxant (usually succinylcholine) or any potent inhalational agent. Sympathomimetics and parasympatholytics increase the severity of already established reactions.

A condition similar to human MH was recognized by swine breeders in certain strains of pigs. The stresses related to slaughter caused accelerated metabolism and deterioration of the muscle of these pigs, resulting in the production of pale, soft exudative (PSE) pork. The incidence of PSE animals increased with inbreeding designed to develop fast-growing, heavily muscled pigs. Any stress to which these pigs were subjected, such as separation, weaning, shipping, fighting, coitus, and slaughter, resulted in increased metabolism, acidosis, muscle rigidity, high temperature, and death. This led to the term *porcine stress syndrome* (PSS).[8]

In 1966, Hall et al described the development of fatal hyperthermia with muscle rigidity after the administration of succinylcholine to pigs.[9] Since that time, strains of Landrace, Poland China, and Pietrain pigs have provided a suitable animal model for the systematic study of MH. Although there are some minor differences between porcine and human MH, the study of porcine MH has provided valuable information relating to the pathophysiology and clinical management of human patients with MH.

INHERITANCE

The inheritance of MH is more complicated than originally thought. MH is a complex genetic disease with phenotypic variations. The variety of malignant hyperthermic responses has led those studying the inheritance of MH to propose the possibility of several routes of genetic transmission.

If was hoped that studies of the pig model would clarify the issue of inheritance, but this has not been the case. There are reports of both autosomal dominant[10] and autosomal recessive[11] inheritance. Kalow and Britt conducted a breeding program over three generations, identifying susceptible pigs by response to halothane in vivo and by response of skeletal muscle fascicles to caffeine–halothane in vitro. The following observations were made: (1) The trait occurred in all animals of the second generation, in contradiction to earlier theories that MH is transmitted by a single recessive gene. (2) The offspring of both the second and third generations reacted like the mean of their parents, thus ruling out transmission by a single Mendelian trait (single dominant gene). (3) Five rather than three genotypes were identified, thus demonstrating inheritance involving at least two abnormal genes, each represented by two different alleles. Studies such as these have provided support for the idea of a multifactorial inheritance.[12]

In humans multifactorial inheritance has been proposed on the basis of familial studies. Investigators found patterns of inheritance (confirmed by muscle biopsy) to affect both sexes of each generation, some as autosomal dominant. Studies of other families showed multifactorial inheritance involving more than one gene. These individuals tend to be the average of their parents, with gradations of susceptibility among family members.[3] Britt and Kalow correlated the severity of MH reactions with muscle specimen contracture tests. They found that the muscle specimens of those who had the most severe clinical episodes reacted to halothane alone; the muscle of those who had less severe reactions reacted to caffeine alone but not to halothane; and in those who had the least severe MH episode, the muscle reacted to a caffeine–halothane mixture but not to either alone.[13]

Rosenberg and other investigators now support the concept of autosomal dominant inheritance by a single gene with variable penetrance.[14] Studies of large families such as that done by McPherson and Taylor, who studied 93 families in which MH occurred, document an autosomal dominant pattern.[15]

ETIOLOGY

The clinical manifestations of MH, such as increased heat production, generalized muscular rigidity, increased glycogenolysis, and severe lactic acidosis can all be explained by an abnormally raised calcium ion concentration in the cytoplasm of the muscle cell (myoplasm). To facilitate understanding this explanation, a description of the basic muscle structure and of the mechanism of muscle contraction follows.

The cell membrane of the muscle fiber is called the sarcolemma. The muscle fiber itself is composed of several thousand myofibrils, suspended in a matrix called sarcoplasm. Each myofibril has about 1500 thick filaments called myosin and about 3000 thin filaments called actin. Myosin is a protein whose molecules have long, rod-shaped

tail regions with enlarged heads that contain adenosine triphosphatase (ATPase) and actin binding sites. Cross-bridges extend along the myosin filaments and form linkages between the heads of the myosin molecules and the actin molecules. The thin filament, actin, is composed of roughly spherical molecules that form a double helix, which runs parallel to the myosin filaments.

The actin and myosin interdigitate, forming light and dark bands. The light bands, which contain only actin filaments, are called I bands. This is because they are isotropic to light (have equal refraction). The dark bands, which contain overlapping actin and myosin filaments, are called A bands (A bands are anisotropic to light, having different optical properties).

The point at which the actin filaments are attached to each other is called the Z-line or Z-membrane. Part of the actin filaments extend on either side of the Z-membrane to interdigitate with the myosin filaments. The portion between the Z-lines is called a sarcomere (Fig. 44–1).

Two other protein molecules, troponin and tropomyosin, are positioned along the actin strand. Troponin is made up of three subunits, TnT, TnI, and TnC. TnT binds strongly to tropomyosin, which covers the sites where the myosin heads bind to actin. TnI binds to actin, and TnC binds to calcium. Thus, the troponin–tropomyosin complex represses the interaction of myosin and actin and maintains the muscle in a resting state (Fig. 44–2).

In the sarcoplasm there is also an extensive endoplasmic reticular system called the sarcoplasmic reticulum (SR). The sarcoplasmic reticulum is composed of longitudinal tubules, which end in enlarged terminal cisternae and lie parallel to the myofibrils. Another tubular system, the transverse or T-tubules, runs perpendicular to the myofibrils. The T-tubules abut against two of the terminal cisternae of the sarcoplasmic reticulum. The T-tubule is open to the exterior of the cell and contains extracellular fluid that is continuous with fluid outside the cell (Fig. 44–3).

The muscle membrane is of limited permeability that varies with the functional state of the muscle. In the resting state, the electrical potential of the muscle interior is slightly negative (−60 to −80 mV) relative to the exterior. Sodium is actively pumped out and potassium is actively pumped in by reactions catalyzed by membrane ATPases. Thus, at rest the concentration of potassium within the muscle is high whereas that of sodium is low.

During relaxation, the level of calcium within the cyto-

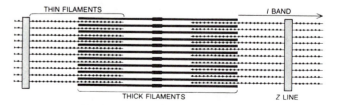

Figure 44–1. The myofibril comprises interpenetrating arrays of thin filaments composed of actin, troponin, and tropomyosin and thick filaments composed of myosin. (*Reprinted, with permission, from Cohen C. The protein switch of muscle contraction.* Sci Am. *1975;223:36–45.*)

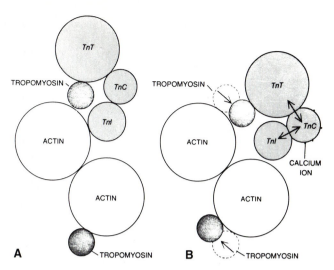

Figure 44–2. A. In the resting state the TnT subunit binds to tropomyosin and the inhibiting subunit, TnI, binds to actin. **B.** In the active state, above a critical calcium level, linkages between troponin subunits are tightened and the link between TnI and actin is weakened. Tropomyosin moves deeper into the actin groove, exposing the site at which myosin can bind. (*Reprinted, with permission, from Cohen C. The protein switch of muscle contraction. Sci Am. 1975;223:36–45.*)

plasm is low compared with that of the extracellular fluid. Calcium ions are actively extruded from the cytoplasm to the extracellular fluid across the surface membrane.

Calcium is stored in the terminal cisternae of the sarcoplasmic reticulum. The concentration of calcium within the terminal cisternae is about 1 to 3000 times that of cytoplasm. Such an enormous accumulation against a concentration gradient is brought about by reactions linked to ATP hydrolysis, catalyzed by a calcium-activated ATPase located in the terminal cisternae.

The process by which depolarization of the muscle fiber initiates contraction is called excitation–contraction coupling. The electrically excited sarcolemma is coupled to the calcium release from the sarcoplasmic reticulum. Depolarization of the cell membrane initiated by acetylcholine causes a sudden increase in the permeability of the membrane and inhibition of the membrane ATPases so that potassium ions leak out of the cell and sodium ions flow

into the cytoplasm. The electrical potential of the cell interior is then converted from being slightly negative to being slightly positive.

The wave of depolarization flows along the sarcolemma, down the transverse tubules, and across the gap junctions to the sarcoplasmic reticulum. There the current flow in some way inhibits the ATPase of the sarcoplasmic reticulum and allows the calcium ions to follow their concentration gradient, rapidly flowing out of the terminal cisternae into the cytoplasm of the muscle fiber (Fig. 44–3).

The calcium ions released by the action potential initiate muscle contraction by binding to TnC. The linkage of TnC to troponin is strengthened and the linkage of TnI to actin is weakened, allowing tropomyosin to move laterally. This movement uncovers binding sites for the myosin heads (Fig. 44–2). The heads of the cross-bridges of the myosin filaments immediately become attracted to the binding sites of the actin filaments. The cross-bridges interact with the actin filaments and pull them toward the center of the sarcomere. This interaction causes the thin filaments to slide past the thick filaments and causes shortening as the Z-lines move closer together. Force is generated and the high-energy bonds of ATP are degraded to adenosine diphosphate (ADP), releasing heat and energy (Fig. 44–3).

Once calcium is released from the cisternae and has diffused to the myofibrils, muscle contraction will continue as long as the calcium ions are present in high concentrations in the sarcoplasmic fluid; however, shortly after releasing the calcium, the sarcoplasmic reticulum begins to reaccumulate calcium ions.

A continually active calcium pump is located in the walls of the longitudinal tubules and pumps calcium ions out of the sarcoplasmic fluid back into the cisternae for storage. Therefore, except immediately after an action potential, the calcium ion concentration in the myofibrils is kept extremely low.

Once the calcium ion concentration in the sarcoplasm has been lowered sufficiently, the calcium ions dissociate from TnC. This causes tropomyosin once again to block the sites of interaction of actin and myosin and the muscle relaxes (Fig. 44–3).

In the presence of a high intracellular calcium concentration, such as occurs in MH, the myofibrils remain locked together in a persistent contraction. There is continuous and rapid production of heat as ATP is broken down by myosin

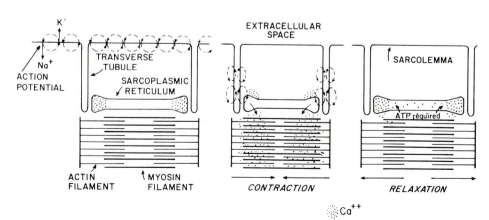

Figure 44–3. Diagrammatic representation of excitation–contraction coupling in normal skeletal muscle. (*Adapted, with permission, from Hoyle G. How is muscle turned on and off? Sci Am. 1970; 222:84–93.*)

ATPase to ADP. Excessive amounts of ADP stimulate the various metabolic pathways as ADP is rephosphorylated to form new ATP. This results in further heat production, acceleration of oxygen consumption, carbon dioxide production, and lactic acidosis. The accelerated rate of ATP production is not, however, able to keep pace with the more rapid rate of ATP breakdown. There is insufficient ATP to provide energy for the various metabolic needs of the cell membrane, which then becomes permeable to myoglobin, potassium, and muscle enzymes.

Thus, many of the known changes present in MH syndrome could be accounted for by the theory that potent inhalational anesthetic agents and muscle relaxants in some way alter the calcium-storing properties of the cellular or intracellular membrane.

PATHOPHYSIOLOGY

Skeletal Muscle Abnormalities

The exact site of the defect in the muscle cell has been the subject of a great deal of investigation. Most studies have indicated skeletal muscle as the primary defective tissue in malignant hyperthermia syndrome (MHS) subjects. Clinical indications of myopathy in MHS patients are substantiated by experimental data showing that agents that trigger MH in vivo also produce metabolic and contracture responses in MHS muscle in vitro. It has also been observed that MH muscle responds with an increased contracture when exposed to a wide variety of seemingly unrelated chemical stimuli such as halothane, caffeine, succinylcholine, potassium chloride, and the physiologic stimulus of temperature change. Such indiscriminate enhancement of the contractile response may therefore involve one of the basic regulatory mechanisms of muscle contraction.

It has been proposed that the excessive calcium present during the MH response could be due to a decreased reuptake of calcium ions by the sarcoplasmic reticulum from the myoplasm or to an increased release of calcium ions from the calcium-storing membrane of the cells, the sarcolemma, and the sarcoplasmic reticulum. Several groups have examined the reuptake of calcium by the sarcoplasmic reticulum in MHS muscle, but the results were conflicting and therefore no conclusive biochemical evidence is provided for this theory.

Accumulating evidence points to a defect in the mechanism leading to the release of calcium ions into the muscle fiber, a late step in the excitation–contraction coupling (ECC) pathway.

A very conspicuous abnormality in MH muscle is its marked sensitivity to caffeine, a drug that causes contraction of skeletal muscle by stimulating the release of calcium ions from the sarcoplasmic reticulum and by inhibiting reuptake of calcium by the sarcoplasmic reticulum. The sarcoplasmic reticulum is the focus of the current theories of malfunction during MH episodes.

It was discovered that dantrolene, a skeletal muscle relaxant, inhibited and reversed abnormal drug-induced contractures in MH muscle (Fig. 44–4). Dantrolene appears to exert its main effect by blocking the mechanism coupling depolarization of the sarcolemma membrane to calcium ion

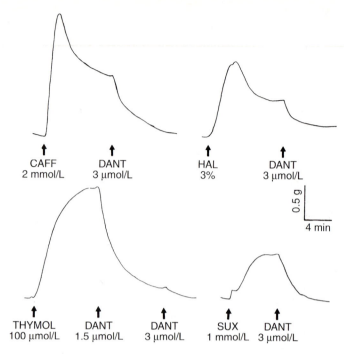

Figure 44–4. Effect of dantrolene sodium on caffeine-, halothane-, thymol-, and succinylcholine-induced contractures in malignant hyperthermia susceptible swine muscle. CAFF, caffeine; DANT, dantrolene; HAL, halothane; SUX, succinylcholine. (*Reprinted, with permission, from Okumura F, Crocker BD, Denborough MA. Br J Anaesth. 1980;52:377–383.*)

release from the sarcoplasmic reticulum, the ECC mechanism. The action of dantrolene suggests that the lesion is located at a link between the T-tubule system and the sarcoplasmic reticulum or the terminal cisternae of the sarcoplasmic reticulum, or both, and that the problem is with calcium release by the sarcoplasmic reticulum rather than calcium reuptake.

Nelson, in 1978, compared human and pig muscle metabolism and pharmacology. He found that dantrolene is effective in blocking abnormal contracture responses in both humans and the pig.[16] Nelson then traced the source of the problem in pigs to calcium channels in the membrane of the sarcoplasmic reticulum. He postulated that a defective protein combines with the anesthetic drugs to keep channels open.[17] Lopez and colleagues demonstrated increases in ionized calcium in both humans and pigs, particularly during acute MH, and they showed that dantrolene returns intracellular ionized calcium levels toward normal.[18] The clinical and laboratory data strongly suggest that the sarcoplasmic reticulum cannot control intrafibrillar concentrations of free ionized calcium and that the associated hypermetabolism is a result of compensatory stimulation of calcium pumps.

A lesion in the ECC mechanism provides a common pathophysiologic mechanism for MH inducers such as stress, depolarizing muscle relaxants, and anesthetic agents. An increased understanding of the etiology of MH has led to the realization that the most important aspect of treatment is to lower myoplasmic calcium ion content. Treatment has thus been centered around that approach.

Biochemical Changes

Although there are thousands of descriptions of MH episodes in humans, a chronologic series of events has not been reported. Clinically, certain events have been observed consistently, such as tachycardia, increased depth of ventilation, unstable blood pressure, increased body temperature, and muscle rigidity. Certain biochemical changes have been found to precede the increases in temperature and the development of rigidity so often associated with MH.

For obvious reasons, it is impossible to study MH in humans under controlled conditions. Several studies inducing MH in swine have been done to systematically collect physiologic and metabolic data. (These data are similar to findings reported during episodes of human MH.)

Blood gas changes occur within minutes of initiation of the syndrome. These are the earliest objective signs of the development of MH. In the porcine studies, the venous hydrogen ion concentration increased within 5 minutes and the arterial hydrogen ion concentration increased in 10 minutes. Gross changes in oxygen consumption and increases in carbon dioxide production indicate a massive stimulation of aerobic metabolism (Fig. 44–5). There is a two- to threefold increase in whole-body oxygen consumption and an even greater increase in carbon dioxide production so that the respiratory quotient (RQ) exceeds one. (The normal RQ is 0.8 to 1.0.) This is a result of the early development of a severe lactic acidosis with the buffering of the increase in hydrogen ions by the plasma bicarbonate. Even with the large increase in oxygen consumption and the maintenance of a mean arterial PO_2 greater than 80 mm Hg, anaerobic glycolysis and lactate production are early features of porcine MH. A sevenfold increase in the plasma lactate concentration after the severe muscle stimulation of succinylcholine did not change appreciably until the terminal stages of the syndrome.

In addition to anaerobic glycolysis and lactate production, serum potassium, magnesium, and phosphate increased significantly after 5 minutes (Fig. 44–6). This indicates a shift of these ions from the intracellular to the extracellular fluid and may be the result of an increase in the permeability of the sarcolemma membrane and the efflux of these ions from the liver. The most important changes in plasma electrolytes are the profound increases in potassium and inorganic phosphate concentrations. Although it is often assumed that the potassium is derived from the damaged striated muscle, Hall et al found that much of the potassium arises from the liver.[19] The hyperphosphatemia is probably the result of the increased rate of hydrolysis of the adenine nucleotides (ATP, ADP, and adenosine monophosphate [AMP]) within the muscle. This increase in inorganic phosphates occurred 5 to 10 minutes after the administration of halothane or succinylcholine but still prior to the clinical diagnosis of MH.

Large increases in circulating catecholamines next occur during the hyperthermic response and are associated with tachycardia, arrhythmia, and an increase in cardiac output. The ability of the animal to increase its cardiac output to meet metabolic demands in the presence of severe acidosis, hyperkalemia, and dehydration is an impressive feature of the porcine syndrome. Gronert and others have

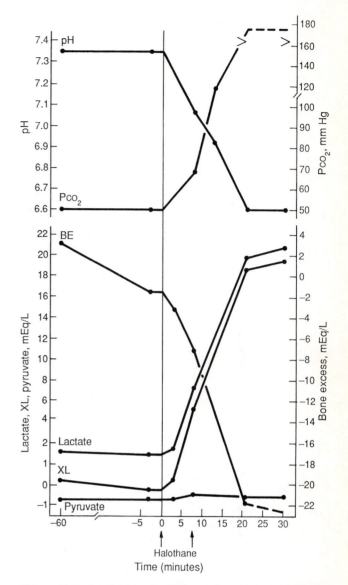

Figure 44–5. Arterial blood acid–base changes in a malignant hyperthermia susceptible Landrace pig during a malignant hyperthermia episode provoked by halothane. (*Reprinted, with permission, from Harrison GG. In Gordon RA, Britt BA, Kalow W, eds.* The international symposium on malignant hyperthermia. *Springfield, IL: Charles C Thomas; 1973:271–286.*)

shown that myocardial metabolism was normal in hyperthermic pigs, although it has been suggested that cardiomyopathy is present in some susceptible human patients.[20] Lister et al have postulated that the catecholamine stimulation of muscle metabolism is an integral part of the hyperthermic response.[21] They also demonstrated that the increase in sympathetic activity is responsible for the severe tachycardia observed in MH by preventing the tachycardia with the administration of beta-adrenergic blocking drugs to experimental pigs. They found a linear correlation between total plasma catecholamine concentration and plasma lactate concentration, providing supportive evidence for their contention that the catecholamine increase is associated with, if not directly attributable to, a product of metab-

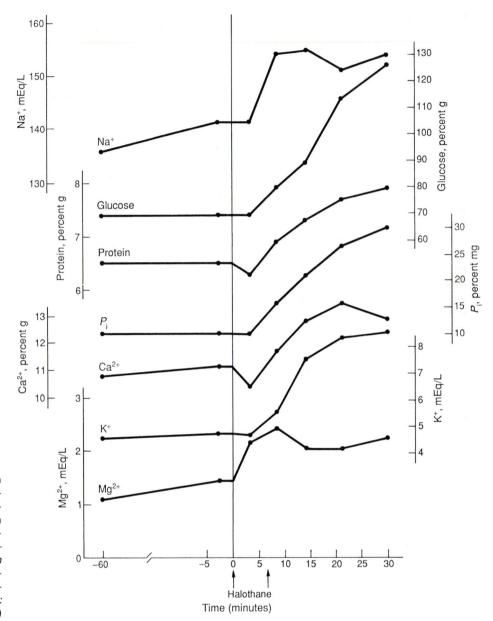

Figure 44–6. Changes in serum biochemistry determinations during a malignant hyperthermia episode in the same animal as in Figure 44–5. P_i, inorganic phosphate. (*Reprinted, with permission, from Harrison GG. In Gordon RA, Britt BA, Kulow W, eds.* The international symposium on malignant hyperthermia. *Springfield, IL: Charles C Thomas; 1973:271–286.*)

olism.[21] The metabolic and physiologic changes observed in porcine MH are essentially similar to those found after any severe muscle stimulation such as exhaustive exercise. In MH the problem arises from the subject's inability to control the severe catabolic (metabolic) state and enter a recovery phase.

Another common finding in porcine MH is hyperglycemia (Fig. 44–6). This results partly from the stimulating effects of the circulating catecholamines on hepatic glycogenolysis. Other factors contributing to the hyperglycemia include gluconeogenesis from the lactic acidosis and the inhibition of insulin secretion by the high circulating concentration of noradrenaline (Table 44–1).

An increase in heat production can be seen as early as 14 minutes after injection of succinylcholine, although the onset of hyperthermia and the temperature vary. The primary source of heat production is the skeletal muscle. The muscle

temperature may increase as rapidly as 1C per 5 minutes. Total-body oxygen consumption accounts for only 50 percent of the heat produced during MH. Remaining sources of heat include glycolysis, hydrolysis of high-energy phosphates involved in ion transport and contraction–relaxation, by neutralization of hydrogen ions, by the sodium pump enzyme system during membrane repolarization, and by free energy released but not captured as ATP during the accelerated aerobic and anaerobic metabolism that occurs during the acute episode.

Assuming that MH involves primarily a sustained increase in the intracellular concentration of calcium, considerable and continuous amounts of energy are needed to transport calcium into the sarcoplasmic reticulum and the mitochondria. The immediate sources of this energy are creatine phosphate and adenosine phosphate, which are rapidly consumed. Heat is liberated during the continued

TABLE 44–1. MAIN METABOLIC, HORMONAL, AND ELECTROLYTE CHANGES DURING PORCINE MALIGNANT HYPERTHERMIA[a]

Metabolic Changes	Hormonal Changes	Plasma Electrolyte Changes
↑ O_2 consumption ⎤ RQ > 1.0[b]	↑ ↑ ↑ Plasma noradrenaline	↑ ↑ Inorganic phosphate
↑ ↑ CO_2 production ⎦	↑ ↑ Plasma adrenaline	↑ Potassium
↓ ↓ Arterial pH	↑ ↑ Plasma glucagon	↔ Magnesium
↑ ↑ Arterial P_{CO_2}	↑ Plasma cortisol	↔ Calcium
↑ ↑ Blood lactate	↔ Plasma insulin	↓ Sodium
↑ Blood pyruvate		↓ Chloride
↑ ↑ Blood glucose		
↑ Plasma glycerol		
↔ or ↓ Plasma free fatty acids		

[a] The increases or decreases in plasma electrolyte values are relative to the observed hemoconcentration.
Reprinted, with permission, from Hall GM, Lucke JN, Lister D. Br J Anaesth. *1980;52:165–170.*

synthesis and utilization of ATP during glycolysis. The lactic acid resulting from glycolysis is transported to the liver, where part is oxidized to provide the ATP necessary to convert the remainder to glucose, again causing the liberation of much heat. Glucose synthesized in this way, and from liver glycogen, is carried to the muscle. The cycle continues and the skeletal muscle and liver operate together as a giant ATPase.

Heffron states that, contrary to earlier suggestions, it is unlikely that the heat arises from uncoupling of oxidative phosphorylation in the mitochondria of skeletal muscle.[22] Based on multiple studies, it may be concluded that mito-

chondrial respiration is not greatly impaired in MH, if at all.[23]

In normal circumstances the body maintains a relatively constant core temperature by balancing endogenous heat production against heat loss. When the metabolic rate increases, compensatory cardiovascular changes occur to increase blood flow to tissues, eliminate waste products, and assist in heat dissipation. In malignant hyperthermia, however, the high rate of heat generation and concomitant retention of heat caused by intense peripheral vasoconstriction lead to a fulminating hyperthermic syndrome.

An additional source of heat may be accelerated sub-

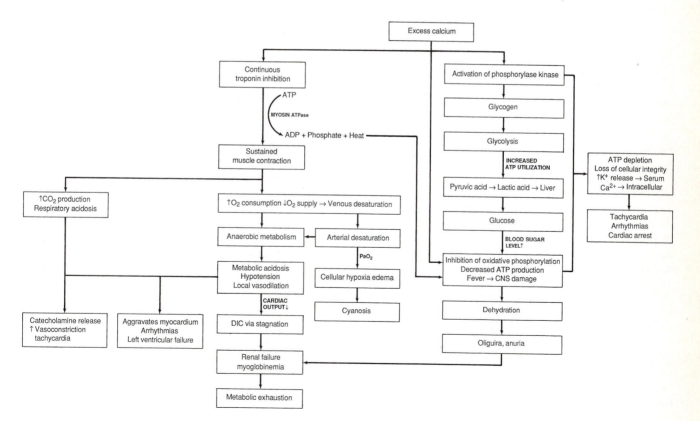

Figure 44–7. Cascade of events following excitation–contraction coupling in malignant hyperthermia muscle. ADP, adenosine diphosphate; ATP, adenosine triphosphate; CNS, central nervous system; DIC, disseminated intravascular coagulopathy.

strate cycling of glucose 6-phosphate. This is a mechanism for heat generation in muscle that has been demonstrated in pigs that developed MH. The futile cycling mechanism causes hydrolysis of ATP with rapid depletion of cellular ATP and a high output of heat and lactate. The most likely mechanism is the rupture of mitochondrial membranes and inhibition of pyruvate dehydrogenase. This leads to the formation of lactate, decreased synthesis of ATP, and decreased restitution of phosphocreatine. The release of catecholamines and an increase in membrane permeability potentiate these effects and produce rigidity, hyperthermia, and acidosis. The consequence of the inhibition of mitochondrial respiration is decreased mitochondrial synthesis of ATP. Significant decreases in ATP are seen 5 to 10 minutes before death.

Hemoconcentration occurs early in the hyperthermic response secondary to a shift of water into the intracellular space. (This is not usually seen in humans because of the massive amounts of fluid therapy generally used.)

Although tachycardia is an early sign of the onset of MH, severe arrhythmias are also common, especially after the administration of succinylcholine or in the terminal stages.

Changes in arterial pressure during MH are not consistent as both hypertension and hypotension have been reported. Blood pressure changes can occur approximately 16 minutes after the initiation of the syndrome, as can the appearance of rigidity. When metabolic changes are extreme, as in the terminal stages of MH, cardiac output and arterial pressure decrease rapidly and cardiac arrest occurs.

Lastly, venous oxygen tension progressively decreases even when 100 percent oxygen is administered. This was seen approximately 57 minutes after the initiation of the syndrome. Acute sustained increases in venous carbon dioxide are seen at the same time (Fig. 44–7).

DIAGNOSTIC CRITERIA

At present there is no simple method for detecting patients who are susceptible to MH. Therefore early recognition and treatment of the syndrome are vital for a successful outcome. MH is a disorder with a spectrum of clinical presentations ranging from the classic fulminant case to those that occur postoperatively with only mild biochemical changes. All presentations of MH are a hypermetabolic response of skeletal muscle characterized by high intracellular calcium which activates metabolic pathways that, if untreated, result in ATP depletion, acidosis, membrane destruction, and cell death. Any of the following symptoms should arouse suspicion during anesthesia unless another explanation is apparent: tachycardia, tachypnea, elevated blood pressure, rapid increase in end-tidal carbon dioxide concentration, and acidosis. Until recently, the most consistent early feature of an MH episode was tachycardia, often associated with an arrhythmia and tachypnea resulting from sympathetic nervous system stimulation secondary to hypermetabolism, hypercarbia, and hyperkalemia; however, with the end-tidal carbon dioxide analyzer now available, the earliest observable sign is a rising expired carbon dioxide tension (Table 44–2).

Muscle rigidity, the unique sign of MH, may not de-

TABLE 44–2. SIGNS AND SYMPTOMS OF MALIGNANT HYPERTHERMIA

Tachycardia (most consistent)
Tachypnea
Unstable blood pressure
Arrhythmias
Cyanosis
  Marked oxygen extraction → hypermetabolism
  Central venous desaturation
  Dark blood on surgical field
Muscle rigidity (not always present)
Profuse sweating
Mottling of the skin
Fever (late sign)

velop until late, or may be slow developing. Most typically though, rigidity begins rapidly after administration of succinylcholine and is first perceived as masseter spasm. Masseter spasm, though a seemingly common event in children, should not be taken lightly. Investigators, using the caffeine–halothane muscle contracture test, report that approximately 50 percent of patients who experience masseter muscle rigidity are diagnosed as MH susceptible.[24] Rosenberg currently recommends as management of masseter muscle rigidity either discontinuation of surgery or, at the minimum, a switch to a nontriggering anesthetic technique.[25]

Laboratory findings confirm signs of increased metabolism. Arterial blood gases demonstrate hypoxemia and severe respiratory and metabolic acidosis. Excess lactate and pyruvate begin to accumulate almost immediately, resulting in a base deficit contributing to the acidosis. Suggested limits for the diagnosis of MH are a base excess of less than – 5 mEq/L and an arterial P_{CO_2} greater than 60 torr without a reasonable explanation. Serum potassium and magnesium increase because of an increased permeability of the sarcolemma membrane. Serum phosphate increases as a result of the increased rate of hydrolysis of ATP, ADP, and AMP. Total serum calcium increases initially but later decreases precipitously. Late laboratory values are similar to the ini-

TABLE 44–3. LABORATORY FINDINGS IN MALIGNANT HYPERTHERMIA

Early	Late
Hypoxemia	Hyperglycemia
Hypercarbia	Myoglobinemia
Respiratory acidosis	Myoglobinuria
Metabolic acidosis	Elevated CPK, LDH, SGOT[a]
Hyperkalemia	Hypocalcemia
Hyperphosphatemia	Hypokalemia
Hypercalcemia	
Hypermagnesemia	

[a] CPK, creatine phosphokinase; LDH, lactic dehydrogenase; SGOT, serum glutamic–oxaloacetic transaminase.

tial values, with the addition of hyperglycemia, myoglobinemia, myoglobinuria, hypocalcemia, and an elevated creatine phosphokinase (CPK), lactic dehydrogenase (LDH), and serum glutamic–oxaloacetic transaminase (SGOT) (Table 44–3).

Fever is a later symptom. If the syndrome occurs after surgery has begun, an early sign may be the rapid heating of the anesthesia tubing and soda lime canister, or the surgeon may note that the patient's organs feel hot to the touch. The patient also may display peripheral mottling, diaphoresis, and cyanosis. In particular, when the temperature is rising and there are signs of muscle stiffness and acidosis, the diagnosis is established and treatment must be instituted.

MANAGEMENT

Malignant hyperthermia can have a varied pattern of severity and symptomatology. MH is triggered in relation to the susceptibility of the individual and to the concentration and duration of administration of the triggering agent. In many situations the full-blown, unmistakable picture of MH is not present. A tachycardia, occasionally with arrhythmias, accompanied by a gradual increase in temperature may not be impressive if the surgical procedure is brief. Some drugs, such as barbiturates and nondepolarizing muscle relaxants, appear to slow the development of MH so that termination of the anesthetic may be sufficient therapy. The simple, yet important, treatment for rigidity after administration of succinylcholine is to terminate the anesthetic. The anesthetist must be alert to these abnormalities and obtain arterial and venous blood studies to document the hypermetabolism present with an MH episode.

Gronert suggests the following as diagnostic of MH: arterial blood P_{CO_2} greater than 60 torr and rising, mixed venous blood P_{CO_2} greater than 90 torr and rising, base excess less than –5 mEq/L and falling, and a temperature increase of at least 1C per 15 minutes.[3] Once the diagnosis is confirmed, rapid vigorous therapy is necessary if the patient is to survive.

Symptomatic therapy should begin immediately and dantrolene should be given as soon as possible. Dantrolene is a hydantoin derivative, representative of a class of muscle relaxants that act directly on the skeletal muscles, inhibiting calcium release without affecting uptake (see Appendix). Dantrolene is the only medication that terminates MH in pigs after the onset of the syndrome. Numerous cases have been reported confirming its effectiveness in treating human MH. Dantrolene controls the abnormal metabolic responses and the associated acid–base imbalances, ion fluxes, and sympathetic stimulation more predictably than symptomatic therapy and is the drug of choice to treat MH (Fig. 44–8). The recommended intravenous dosage for humans is 2.5 mg/kg, which may be repeated every 5 to 10 minutes up to a total dose of 10 mg/kg.

Usually one or two doses abort the reaction. If the temperature rises or if arrhythmias occur in the recovery period, dantrolene should be continued at the rate of 1 mg/kg/h until the reaction is under control.

Dantrolene is stored as a lyophilized powder that con-

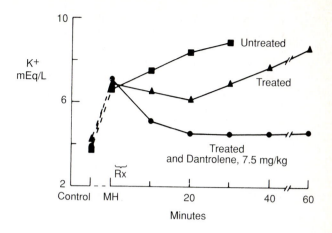

Figure 44–8. Arterial serum potassium during a malignant hyperthermia (MH) episode in swine with no treatment, with supportive treatment only, and with supportive treatment plus dantrolene. (*Reprinted, with permission, from Gronert GA, Milde JH, Theye RA:* Anesthesiology. *1976;44:488–495.*)

tains 20 mg dantrolene and 3 g of mannitol per vial. Each vial requires 60 mL of sterile water to dissolve the powder. Assistance should be obtained in mixing dantrolene, which is poorly soluble. The drug and solvents should be stored in the anesthetic area, readily available for use.

Symptomatic Therapy

In addition to the administration of dantrolene, symptomatic therapy is important for successful treatment of MH. A kit containing drugs necessary for the treatment of MH should be kept either in the operating room suite or in the recovery room and be readily available. The kit should contain 36 ampoules of dantrolene, sterile water, procainamide, bicarbonate, and other supplies needed to treat MH. Most persons experienced in the management of MH recommend using an established protocol. To deal effectively with an emergency situation, a sequence of actions such as the following patterned after the protocol recommended by the Malignant Hyperthermia Association of the United States should be defined prior to surgery and anesthesia:

1. Stop the anesthesia and surgery. Turn off all the agents except oxygen. (The patient usually will not regain consciousness until sometime postoperatively.) Change the soda lime and anesthetic tubing as soon as possible. Because of the rubber/gas solubility of the inhalational agents, some anesthetic remains in the tubing.
2. Hyperventilate with 100 percent oxygen. Hyperventilate using two to three times the minute ventilation. Hypoxemia, one of the early signs of the syndrome, will usually be corrected unless oxygen delivery has been delayed.

   Hyperventilation is often unsuccessful in lowering the P_{CO_2} to normal but must be maintained in an effort to control the severe respiratory acidosis present.
3. Give dantrolene. As soon as possible, administer

dantrolene 2.5 mg/kg intravenously. Response to dantrolene should begin within minutes. If not, repeat the dosage until the signs and symptoms are under control. Although 10 mg/kg is the recommended upper limit, more can be given as necessary as there are few significant acute side effects. The risk of myocardial depression is minimal if calcium channel blockers have not been given.

4. Cool the patient. It is necessary to institute aggressive cooling to lower the temperature. Cooling should be stopped when the temperature falls to 38.3C (101F) to prevent inadvertent hypothermia. Resume cooling if the temperature starts to rise again.

   Surface cooling by packing the patient in ice is particularly effective with small children because of their high surface area relative to body volume. In adults, iced intravenous saline (1000 mL every 10 minutes for 30 minutes) is also helpful in lowering body temperature. Additional cooling measures include iced saline lavage of the stomach, rectum, peritoneal cavity, and thorax. Gastric lavage is the quickest, most practical rapid cooling method. Cardiopulmonary bypass with a heat exchanger can be used, if available.

5. Correct the acidosis. Administer sodium bicarbonate 2 mEq/kg initially; then use the arterial blood gases as a guide for further therapy. Bicarbonate serves a dual function. It corrects the acidosis and also corrects the hyperkalemia. Increasing the pH drives potassium back into the cell.

6. Treat arrhythmias with procainamide. If arrhythmias persist after treatment of acidosis and hyperkalemia, procainamide 10 to 20 mg/kg IV can be administered over 10 minutes (1000 mg procainamide diluted in 500 mL isotonic saline). Lidocaine is *not* used because amides inhibit the transfer of calcium to the sarcoplasmic reticulum and therefore can aggravate the MH.

   Although cardiac glycosides have been used by some in the treatment of human MH without adverse effects, Britt et al, after reviewing statistical data, feel that cardiac glycosides may worsen MH by increasing myoplasmic calcium. Cardiac glycosides are currently not recommended treatment.[26]

   Calcium channel blockers have recently been studied with the expectation that abnormal calcium fluxes may be inhibited and therefore help prevent or treat MH; however, Gronert reports that the calcium antagonists appear to act earlier in the chain of activation of muscle contraction and not at the level at which MH appears to originate.[27] Thus, dantrolene remains the definitive drug for treatment of MH. Additionally, it has been demonstrated by Gallant in swine[28] and by Rubin and Zablocki in humans[29] that dantrolene and verapamil in combination can significantly depress cardiac function and can cause dangerous elevation of potassium levels. Calcium channel blockers should not be used in the acute treatment of MH.

7. Secure monitoring. Once these measures have been instituted, monitoring lines should be established to provide a guide to subsequent therapy. These include an arterial line for blood pressure, arterial blood gases, electrolytes, a Foley catheter for urine output, and a central venous pressure line.

8. Administer fluids to maintain high urine output. Massive amounts of fluids are required to prevent dehydration and to maintain a high urinary output. Initial volume loading consists of 2 to 8 mL/kg colloids and crystalloids, depending on patient response, determined by central venous pressure and urine output. A Foley catheter is mandatory. A urine output of greater than 1 mL/kg per hour prevents myoglobin from forming casts in the kidney, which can lead to renal failure. Furosemide 50 mg IV (up to four doses) and mannitol 12.5 g IV may be necessary to maintain urine output. Furosemide will also help start excretion of sodium if large amounts of sodium bicarbonate are necessary to control the acidosis.

9. Treat hyperkalemia. Standard protocol recommends giving 10 units of regular insulin in 10 mL of 50 percent dextrose and water as an intravenous bolus. This has a twofold purpose: (1) to reduce serum potassium by transferring potassium back into the cells, and (2) to provide an exogenous energy source and the transfer of glucose into the cells.

10. Provide additional therapy. Based on in vitro studies, Ellis and colleagues have recommended steroids for the treatment of human MH[30]; however, Britt and co-workers, in a retrospective review, found the mortality rate higher with steroid use in the treatment of human MH.[26] Conversely, Gronert feels that multiple factors contribute to MH-associated deaths and that steroids are probably helpful during these severe stresses.[3]

11. Observe the patient in an intensive care unit setting for at least 24 hours as recrudescence of MH may occur, particularly after a case that was difficult to treat.

Late Complications

After an acute episode, the following complications may occur.

Consumption Coagulopathy. Consumption coagulopathy, or disseminated intravascular coagulopathy (DIC), may be caused by hemolysis; increased release of tissue thromboplastins resulting from increased permeability or overt tissue damage; and shock secondary to inadequate capillary perfusion, to a defect in the red blood cell or platelet, or to some rare mechanisms related to the increased permeabilities present in fulminant MH. DIC usually occurs when the treatment has been too conservative and the patient has run markedly elevated temperatures over a prolonged period, with resultant dehydration and decreased peripheral blood flow. Various treatments reported to be useful include the administration of fresh-frozen plasma and clotting factors and heparinization.

Acute Renal Failure. Myoglobinemia and myoglobin casts in the kidney have been associated with renal failure, particularly in association with acidosis, hypovolemia, and hypotension. Therapy as previously outlined providing a high urinary output will help prevent renal damage.

Inadvertent Hypothermia. Too vigorous cooling can result in inadvertent hypothermia. This can be prevented by careful temperature monitoring and termination of cooling when the patient's temperature reaches 101F (38.3C).

Skeletal Muscle Edema and Muscle Necrosis. Sustained tetanic muscle contraction causes an increase in muscle metabolism, produces local mechanical occlusion of the blood vessels, and decreases muscle perfusion. The resultant acidosis and hypoxia produce skeletal muscle edema and ischemia leading to necrosis. When cell damage occurs, enzymes such as CPK, SGOT, and LDH are released into the circulation. Ions follow their electrochemical gradient, with potassium leaving the cell and calcium entering the cell, producing hyperkalemia and hypocalcemia.

During episodes of malignant hyperthermia, the muscle membrane wall changes in permeability, leaking various muscle constituents into the bloodstream. Myoglobulinemia and myoglobinuria result.

Neurologic Sequelae. Cerebral perfusion is essentially unchanged until the core temperature exceeds 103F; however, the cerebral metabolic rate for oxygen increases linearly with temperature. Data indicate that cerebral hypoxia will occur during hyperthermia. Thus, cerebral hypoxia and acidosis can result in sequelae such as coma, paralysis, and decerebration.

Pulmonary Edema. Pulmonary edema is usually reported after a cardiac arrest at the height of the syndrome. Treatment is the same as with other disorders.

Hyperkalemia. Hyperkalemia, caused by muscle cell damage, resolves with the return to normal temperature and stabilization of the patient. As potassium goes back into the cell, serum potassium values drop precipitously. For as long as 24 hours after MH, the patient is extremely sensitive to iatrogenic potassium administration, which may retrigger an MH episode. Potassium should therefore be given in very small amounts and only if electrocardiographic changes warrant.

Follow-up for Malignant Hyperthermia

Malignant hyperthermia is an ongoing process that may last days. Close patient monitoring is necessary even after the episode is over and must continue for 24 to 48 hours. This includes electrocardiogram, temperature, arterial line for blood pressure and blood gases, electrolytes (especially potassium, calcium), serum enzymes, coagulation studies, central venous pressure, and urine output.

Health care providers should be aware that as the initial dose of dantrolene is metabolized and excreted, retriggering can occur. Recurrences of MH have been reported up to 30 hours after the initial episode. Intravenous dantrolene has a half-life of 4 to 8 hours and should be continued for 12 to 24 hours. Oral dantrolene can be given as soon as the gastrointestinal system is functional (1 to 2 mg/kg qid for 1 to 3 days).

During the postoperative period there should be normal renal function, blood coagulation, bleeding time, and blood gases. The neurologic status must include absence of rigidity. The temperature and electrocardiogram findings must be normal. Major indications of renewed trouble are rigidity, a slow rise in potassium, and mental agitation.

Family counseling should be done during the recovery period. Families should be referred to the Malignant Hyperthermia Association of the United States (MHAUS), a voluntary nonprofit organization that provides much support and information useful to MH families. The address is MHAUS, PO Box 191, Westport, CT 06881–0191. In addition to patient support services, MHAUS provides valuable information to anesthesia providers who may have an urgent question about MH. The 24-hour hotline number is (209) 634–4917. Ask for Index Zero.

PREANESTHETIC DIAGNOSIS OF MALIGNANT HYPERTHERMIA SUSCEPTIBILITY

If it were possible to identify the MH trait preoperatively, the mortality rate could be reduced to zero. At the present time, however, no one test is inexpensive enough and noninvasive enough to use for all patients. Studies of platelet aggregation, platelet ATP depletion, and calcium uptake, the calcium ATPase test, calcium release from lymphocytes, and the monophosphorylase test all have thus far been inconclusive. Serum CPK studies are helpful in identifying the MH trait, but only when CPK is elevated in a relative of a known MH-susceptible patient.

In 1990 researchers reported finding the tentative locus of the gene for MH on chromosome 19 in humans. The gene is either identical with or close to the gene for the ryanodine receptor. The ryanodine receptor is the site on the muscle that controls the flux of calcium within the muscle.[31] If the site or locus of the genetic defect can be identified, it may be possible to detect susceptibility to MH with a simple blood test; however, a great deal of work remains to be done before this can become a reality. At present, the only certain method of detecting susceptibility is an in vitro study of muscle requiring a muscle biopsy.

The usual preoperative evaluation of susceptibility to MH consists of obtaining a personal and family history of any myopathies or a history of any unusual reaction to anesthesia and a physical examination for the existence of any clinical muscle abnormalities.

All individuals who are susceptible to MH have an underlying disease of the muscle. Muscle and connective tissue have been found to be abnormal in 67 percent of all MHS patients and in 36 percent of their first-degree relatives. Although some MHS patients are perfectly healthy, others complain of a wide range of physical abnormalities. These include short stature, club foot, webbing of the neck, ptosis, strabismus, kyphoscoliosis, lumbar lordosis, various hernias (inguinal, hiatus, umbilical), joint hypermobility, occasional repeated joint dislocations, winged scapulae, undescended testicle, calcium stones in the ureter or gallbladder, poor dental enamel, and misshapen and misplaced teeth.

Some patients exhibit skeletal muscle hypertrophy that is occasionally asymmetric. In others, the myopathy is usually subclinical, although there is some muscle atrophy, particularly in the lower parts of the thigh. MHS patients frequently complain of skeletal muscle cramps that range from mild to incapacitating, usually worse in the winter.

A variety of muscle disorders have been related to MH: Duchenne muscular dystrophy, a progressive degenerative disease of skeletal muscle; central core disease, characterized by atrophic areas in the muscle cells; Schwartz–Jampal syndrome, a myotonia-like syndrome; myotonia congenita; and King–Denborough syndrome, characterized by cryptorchidism, pectus deformity, scoliosis, and retardation. Some patients with these disorders have developed MH symptoms and signs with anesthesia.

Neuroleptic malignant syndrome (NMS) occurs in patients being treated with phenothiazines and haloperidol. It is characterized by muscle rigidity, acidosis, fever, tachycardia, and hypertension. These signs and symptoms typically develop over several hours or days and respond to both dantrolene and bromocriptine, a dopamine agonist. Although the symptoms suggest a relation to MH, some authors think NMS appears to be primarily a disorder of the dopamine receptor with secondary involvement of skeletal muscle.[14]

Although the CPK test has received much criticism because many other muscle-damaging conditions unrelated to MH can elevate the serum CPK, most experts still believe the test to be helpful in identifying families with suspected MH (Fig. 44–9). When CPK is elevated and the patient is a close relative of a known MHS individual, he or she can be considered to be susceptible. If the patient is a close relative of an MHS person but has a normal CPK on three occasions, then a muscle biopsy is necessary to determine susceptibility. The only confirmed diagnostic test, other than an unequivocal clinical episode, is the contracture response of muscle. This requires the excision of about 4 cm of thigh muscle under local anesthesia and should be performed at a center where muscle biopsies are done routinely. These tests entail exposure of the muscle to varying concentrations of caffeine and halothane. The abnormal muscle exhibits a contracture or a greater-than-normal contracture on exposure to the pharmacologic agents (Fig. 44–10).

All patients who are considered susceptible to MH should wear Medic Alert bracelets and carry cards in their wallets warning against the use of potent inhalational agents and succinylcholine. Patients and their families should be counseled as to the risks associated with exposure to triggering drugs and to excessive emotional and physical stress; however, these patients should also be reassured that when appropriate precautions are taken, anesthesia can be administered to them safely.

A problem arises in evaluating patients who do not present a clear picture of MH susceptibility. These patients may have a vague history of anesthetic problems, have muscle problems such as intermittent cramping or weakness but nothing clinically demonstrable, or a serum CPK at the upper limits of normal. The anesthetist should be aware that a majority of the patients with muscle disease are not MHS. Conversely, many MHS patients have no clinical evidence of muscle disease. There are serious implications involved in assigning the MHS label to a person or family. One must have definitive evidence before doing so. When in doubt about MH susceptibility, however, a prescribed prophylactic anesthesia routine such as the one that follows should be employed.

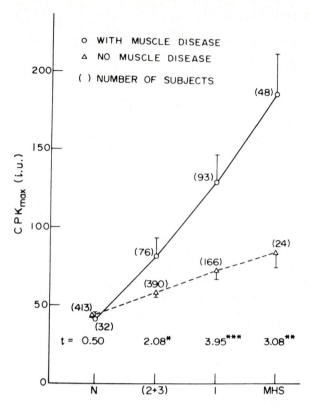

Figure 44–9. Maximum creatine phosphokinase (CPK) levels in normal (N) individuals, malignant hyperthermia susceptible (MHS) subjects, and their first-, second-, and third-degree (2 + 3) relatives. (*Reprinted, with permission, from Britt BA, Endrenyi L, Peters PL, et al. Can Anaesth Soc J. 1976;23:263–284.*)

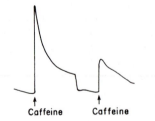

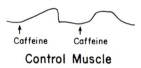

Figure 44–10. Artist's representation of the response of humans with malignant hyperthermia susceptible muscle to caffeine contrasted with the response of normal human muscle to caffeine.

PROPHYLACTIC ANESTHESIA ROUTINE FOR MALIGNANT HYPERTHERMIA SYNDROME PATIENTS

Preoperative Preparation

The patient may be admitted to the hospital preoperatively and placed on bed rest to reduce anxiety and avoid stress. During preoperative counseling the patient should be reassured about the special monitoring for MH and the treatment for MH should it develop.

Preoperative assessment should include the usual history and physical examination as well as an electrocardiogram (regardless of age), a complete blood count, serum electrolytes, liver function tests, and coagulation studies. Sedation with a barbiturate or a benzodiazepine should be given the evening before surgery.

The patient should be well premedicated in an effort to reduce anxiety and the associated catecholamine release. Phenothiazines, which may release calcium from the sarcoplasmic reticulum, should be avoided.

The role of dantrolene prophylaxis is debatable and may not be warranted if the surgery is brief or if the anesthetic is a local or regional anesthetic; however, if the surgery planned is lengthy, there are those who believe dantrolene should be administered preoperatively. Rosenberg recommends intravenous dantrolene 2.5 mg/kg over 30 minutes.[32] Allen et al have shown that oral dantrolene 5 mg/kg given 12 to 24 hours prior to surgery will achieve the same blood levels.[33] Both regimens provide effective prophylaxis for 4 to 6 hours.

Operating Room Preparation

In the operating room, routine monitoring equipment including electrocardiogram, temperature probe, cooling blanket, doppler or automatic blood pressure, pulse oximetry, capnograph, and a vapor-free anesthesia machine (no vaporizer attached) with new tubings and soda lime should be ready for use. (A previously used anesthesia machine can be purged of vapor by draining vaporizers, replacing all porous parts and the soda lime canister, and then running 100 percent oxygen through it for at least 20 minutes at 10 L per minute.) Ice, lavage tubes, and an arterial line setup should be available. All drugs and supplies mentioned in the protocol for treatment of an MH episode should be available for use.

Anesthetic Agents

Anesthetic agents and drugs that have been used safely on MHS patients include nitrous oxide, thiopental, propofol, benzodiazepines, narcotics, droperidol, pancuronium, atracurium, and vecuronium. Ketamine, anticholinesterases, and anticholinergics are probably safe to use. All potent inhalational anesthetics and depolarizing muscle relaxants should be avoided.

Spinal, epidural, regional, or local anesthesia is the technique of choice, if possible. It has been shown that all local anesthetics appear to be safe for the MH-susceptible patient. (It has not yet been proven that the amide local anesthetics will not exacerbate an ongoing episode of MH. Therefore, ester local anesthetics are used for the treatment of arrhythmias.)

An MHS patient who is having local or conduction anesthesia should be well sedated. It should also be borne in mind that stimulation during light general anesthesia could trigger an MH response as well, an additional reason for very close patient monitoring.

Episodes of MH have occurred in the postoperative period. Therefore, monitoring of the MHS patient should continue for 24 hours.

REFERENCES

1. Denborough MA, Lovell RRH. Anaesthetic deaths in a family. *Lancet.* 1960;2:45.
2. Britt BA, Locher WG, Kalow W. Hereditary aspects of malignant hyperthermia. *Can Anaesth Soc J.* 1969;16:89–98.
3. Gronert GA. Malignant hyperthermia. *Anesthesiology.* 1980;53:395–423.
4. Ellis FR, Halsall PH. Malignant hyperpyrexia. *Br J Hosp Med.* 1980;24:318–327.
5. Ording H. Incidence of malignant hyperthermia in Denmark. *Anesth Analg.* 1985;64:700–704.
6. Britt BA, Kalow W. Malignant hyperthermia: A statistical review. *Can Anaesth Soc J.* 1970;17:293–315.
7. McGuire N, Easy WR. Malignant hyperthermia during isoflurane anaesthesia. *Anaesthesia.* 1990;45:124–127.
8. Topel DG, Bickness EJ, Preston KS, et al. Porcine stress syndrome. *Mod Vet Pract.* 1968;49:40–41, 59–60.
9. Hall LW, Woolf N, Bradley JWP, et al. Unusual reaction to suxamethonium chloride. *Br Med J.* 1966;2:1305.
10. Williams CH, Lasley JH. The mode of inheritance of the fulminant hyperthermia stress syndrome in swine. In: Henschel ED, ed. *Malignant hyperthermia. Current concepts.* New York: Appleton-Century-Crofts; 1977:141–148.
11. Eikelenboom G, Minkema D, Van Eldik P, et al. Inheritance of the malignant hyperthermia syndrome in Dutch Landrace swine. In: Aldrete JA, Britt BA, eds. *Second international symposium on malignant hyperthermia.* New York: Grune & Stratton; 1978:141–146.
12. Britt BA, Kalow W, Endrenyi L. Malignant hyperthermia—Pattern of inheritance in swine. In: Aldrete JA, Britt BA, eds. *Second international symposium on malignant hyperthermia.* New York: Grune & Stratton; 1978:195–211.
13. Kalow W, Britt BA, Chan F-Y. Epidemiology and inheritance of malignant hyperthermia. *Int Anesthesiol Clin.* 1979;17:119–139.
14. Rosenberg H. Malignant hyperthermia. *ASA Annu Refresher Course Lectures Clin Update Program.* 1989;266:1–7.
15. McPherson EW, Taylor CA. The genetics of malignant hyperthermia: Evidence for heterogeneity. *Am J Med Genet.* 1982;11:273–285.
16. Nelson TE. Excitation–contraction coupling: A common etiologic pathway for malignant hyperthermic susceptible muscle. In: Aldrete JA, Britt BA, eds. *Second international symposium on malignant hyperthermia.* New York: Grune & Stratton; 1978:23–36.
17. Nelson TE. Abnormality in calcium release from skeletal sarcoplasmic reticulum of pigs susceptible to malignant hyperthermia. *J Clin Invest.* 1983;72:862–870.
18. Lopez JR, Alamo L, Caputo C, Wikinski J, Ledezma D. Intracellular ionized calcium concentration in muscles from humans with malignant hyperthermia. *Muscle Nerve.* 1985;8:355–358.
19. Hall GM, Lucke JN, Lister D. Porcine malignant hyperthermia. VII. Hepatic metabolism. *Br J Anaesth.* 1980;52:11–17.

20. Gronert GA, Mott J, Lee J. Aetiology of malignant hyperthermia. *Br J Anaesth.* 1988;60:253–267.
21. Lister D, Hall GM, Lucke JN. Porcine malignant hyperthermia. III. Adrenergic blockade. *Br J Anaesth.* 1976;48:831–837.
22. Heffron JJA. Malignant hyperthermia: Biochemical aspects of the acute episode. *Br J Anaesth.* 1988;60:274–278.
23. Ellis FR, Heffron JJA. Clinical and biochemical aspects of malignant hyperpyrexia. In: Atkinson RS, Adams AP, eds. *Recent advances in anaesthesia and analgesia.* New York: Churchill Livingstone; 1985:173–207.
24. Fletcher JE, Rosenberg H. In vitro interaction between halothane and succinylcholine in human skeletal muscle: Implications for malignant hyperthermia and masseter muscle rigidity. *Anesthesiology.* 1985;63:190–194.
25. Rosenberg H. Masseter muscle rigidity. *Communicator.* 1990;8:2.
26. Britt BA, Kwong FH-F, Endrenyi L. Management of malignant hyperthermia susceptible patients—A review. In: Henschel ED, ed. *Malignant hyperthermia. Current concepts.* New York: Appleton-Century-Crofts; 1977:63–77.
27. Gronert GA. Calcium channel blockers and therapy of malignant hyperthermia. *Communicator.* 1989;7:1–6.
28. Gallant EM. Verapamil is not a therapeutic adjunct to dantrolene in porcine malignant hyperthermia. *Anesth Analg.* 1985;64:601–606.
29. Rubin AS, Zablocki AD. Hyperkalemia, verapamil, and dantrolene. *Anesthesiology.* 1987;66:246–249.
30. Ellis FR, Clarke IMC, Applegard TN. Malignant hyperpyrexia induced by nitrous oxide and treated with dexamethasone. *Br Med J.* 1974;4:270–271.
31. McCarthy TV, Sandra Healy JM, Heffron JA, et al. Localization of the malignant hyperthermia susceptibility locus to human chromosome 19q.12–13,2. *Nature.* 1990;343:562–563.
32. Rosenberg H. Malignant hyperthermia. *ASA Annu Refresher Course Lectures Clin Update Program.* 1990;245:1–6.
33. Allen GC, Cattran CB, Peterson RG, Lanande M. Plasma levels of dantrolene following oral administration in malignant hyperthermia-susceptible patients. *Anesthesiology.* 1988;69:900–904.
34. Harrison EE. Control of malignant hyperpyrexia syndrome in MHS swine by dantrolene. *Br J Anaesth.* 1975;47:62–65.
35. Denborough MA. Current concepts of the aetiology and treatment of malignant hyperthermia. In: Aldrete JA, Britt BA, eds. *Malignant hyperthermia.* New York: Grune & Stratton; 1978:537–544.

APPENDIX: DANTROLENE SODIUM (DANTRIUM)

Dantrolene sodium, a hydantoin derivative (Fig. 44–11), is a muscle relaxant that acts specifically on skeletal muscle with no effect on cardiac or smooth muscle. It produces relaxation by acting directly on the skeletal muscle, affecting the contractile response at a site beyond the myoneural junction. Dantrolene blocks excitation–

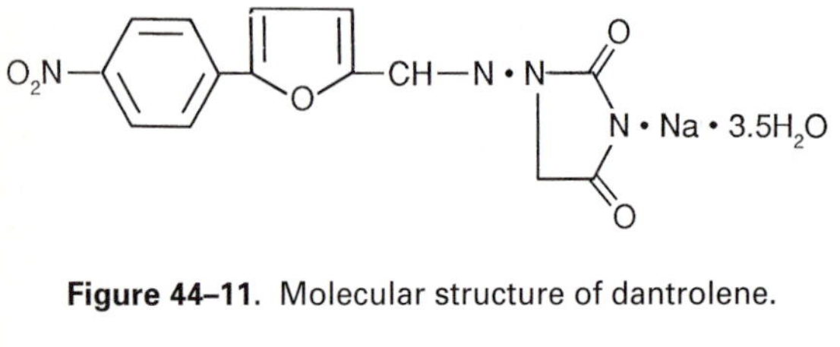

Figure 44–11. Molecular structure of dantrolene.

contraction coupling, probably by suppressing the amount of calcium ions released from the sarcoplasmic reticulum. Dantrolene selectively inhibits calcium ion release from the sarcoplasmic reticulum but does not affect sequestration of myoplasmic calcium back into the sarcoplasmic reticulum.

The half-life of intravenous dantrolene 2.5 mg/kg is approximately 12 hours. The therapeutic range at this dosage is maintained for 4 to 6 hours. Thus dantrolene should be supplemented about every 4 hours after treatment of an MH episode.

Dantrolene is metabolized by hepatic microsomal enzymes. The metabolites are excreted in the urine. Metabolic patterns are similar in adults and children. Liver dysfunction, as evidenced by blood chemistry abnormalities (liver enzyme elevation), hepatitis, seizures, and pleural diffusion with pericarditis have been reported as reactions occurring with chronic oral dantrolene use.

Clinically, dantrolene is used to control manifestations of spasticity resulting from upper motor neuron disorders, such as spinal cord injury, stroke, cerebral palsy, and multiple sclerosis.

In 1975, Harrison showed that dantrolene treatment would terminate the MH response of susceptible swine to halothane (Fig. 44–12).[34] His observations were substantiated by numerous studies of MHS swine in response to MH induced by succinylcholine and halothane and by studies of isolated swine muscle strips in which dantrolene produced relaxation of contractures induced by halothane and caffeine.

Oral dantrolene, having already been in use to treat spasticity in humans, was suggested for use as pretreatment in MHS humans. Denborough reported a study comparing the effects of several drugs including procaine, procainamide, steroids, and dantrolene on the halothane-induced contractures of human muscle in vitro. He concluded that dantrolene was the drug of choice for treating malignant hyperthermia.[35]

Harrison demonstrated that pretreatment of MHS swine with dantrolene would block the initiation of the MH response to halothane and succinylcholine.[34] Clinical reports of the effective use of dantrolene to reverse MH syndrome in humans when other supportive and drug therapies proved ineffective have established dantrolene as the drug of choice for the treatment of malignant hyperthermia. Furthermore, oral and intravenously administered dantrolene has been reported to be part of the successful prophylaxis for MH in patients with known susceptibility undergoing surgery.

In anesthetic-induced MH, evidence points to an intrinsic abnormality of the muscle tissue. In affected humans and swine, it has been postulated that "triggering agents" induce a sudden rise in myoplasmic calcium either by preventing the sarcoplasmic reticulum from accumulating calcium adequately or by accelerating its release. This rise in myoplasmic calcium ions activates the acute catabolic processes common to the MH crisis.

Dantrolene may prevent the increase in myoplasmic calcium ions and the acute catabolism within the muscle cell by interfering with the release of calcium ions

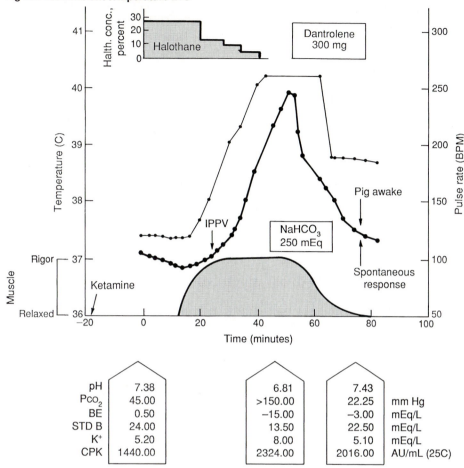

Pig No. 180 Ambient temperature 21C

pH	7.38	6.81	7.43	
Pco₂	45.00	>150.00	22.25	mm Hg
BE	0.50	−15.00	−3.00	mEq/L
STD B	24.00	13.50	22.50	mEq/L
K⁺	5.20	8.00	5.10	mEq/L
CPK	1440.00	2324.00	2016.00	AU/mL (25C)

Figure 44–12. Temperature, heart rate, and biochemical values during a malignant hyperthermia episode precipitated by halothane (HALTH) and after the administration of dantrolene in a malignant hyperthermia susceptible (MHS) pig. BE, base excess; BPM, beats per minute; CPK, creatine phosphokinase; IPPV, intermittent positive-pressure ventilation; K⁺, potassium ion; Pco₂ = pressure of carbon dioxide; STD B, standard bicarbonate. (*Reprinted, with permission, from Harrison.*[34])

from the sarcoplasmic reticulum to the myoplasm. Thus the physiologic, metabolic, and biochemical changes associated with the crisis may be attenuated or reversed.

As soon as the MH reaction is recognized, all anesthetic agents should be discontinued. An initial dantrolene intravenous dose of 2.5 mg/kg body weight should be given rapidly. Other supportive measures should also be instituted, for example, 100 percent oxygen, management of the metabolic acidosis, and institution of cooling measures. If the physiologic and metabolic abnormalities persist or reappear, this dose may be repeated up to a cumulative dose of 10 mg/kg. (Because of the high pH of the intravenous formulation, 9.5, care should be taken to prevent extravasation.)

It may be necessary to administer oral dantrolene in doses of 1 to 2 mg/kg qid for a 1- to 3-day period to prevent recurrence of the manifestations of MH.

Experience to date indicates that the dose for children is the same as for adults, with an initial intravenous dose of 2.5 mg/kg given rapidly.

Dantrolene should be available in the anesthetizing area of the operating suite and in the recovery room. It comes in ready-to-mix vials of 20 mg each. It should be reconstituted with sterile water for injection (USP) without a bacteriostatic agent. Dantrolene is incompatible with 5 percent dextrose, 0.9 percent sodium chloride, and other acidic solutions. The contents of the vial must be protected from direct light and used within 6 hours after reconstitution. The expiration date should be routinely checked before reconstitution. Dantrolene has a shelf life of 3 years.

Anesthetic Management of the Patient with Neuromuscular or Related Diseases

Lida Inge Swafford Dahm

Before the 1950s, patients with neuromuscular and spinal cord diseases were generally left at home or placed in a nursing facility to die. With the launching of the first spinal cord centers in England by Guttmann, the long-term care of these patients gradually became an art. The availability of antibiotics and the increasing knowledge of pathophysiology gave physicians the ability to extend patients' life spans into the chronic phase of the disease. Many children with birth defects or chronic debilitating disease who had previously died early in the course of their disease survived into adulthood and had an increasing number of general medical problems. Thus developed physical medicine and rehabilitation as a specialty.

With the neurologist and neurophysiologist making the diagnosis in many neuromuscularly and spinal cord-injured patients and the rehabilitation specialist designing courses of management for the subacute and chronic phases of the diseases, survival rates have increased markedly. Subsequent studies published in 1986 continue to support the trend in which overall 10-year survival for complete quadriplegic patients of all ages is 78.2 percent.[1] Recently, 12-year survival of complete quadriplegic patients shows an overall survival of 76 percent, with more significance to the anesthetist of the age differences in survival: 1–24 years, 90 percent; 25–49 years, 74 percent; and 50+ years, 26.9 percent.[1a]

Since January 1, 1991, the Texas Department of Health has begun collecting data to document the magnitude of traumatic spinal cord injuries. Thirteen key acute care hospitals and 22 inpatient rehabilitation facilities in Texas are involved.[2] The Department reported 160 traumatic spinal cord injuries from 26 (67 percent) of their 39 sentinine facilities from January through September, 1991.[2a] Treatment modalities, facilities, and costs are similar in other neuromuscular diseases. Consequently, these data may be used for delineating patient needs, which can benefit everyone with related neuromuscular problems.

GENERAL PRINCIPLES

The general principles of management of the patient with neuromuscular disease follow those for any other patient with a chronic and potentially severely disabling disease.[3-5] A good history, especially a good family history, is mandatory, as susceptible patients may have devastating complications from malignant hyperthermia and hypoglycemia. An assessment of present activity gives an idea of respiratory and cardiovascular function. Some patients may be taking as many as 20 different medications that may have both antagonizing and potentiating side effects. Many of these medications affect the autonomic nervous system as well as electrolytes and general metabolism.

An initial cardiac and respiratory baseline assessment is necessary when the patient is first seen by the surgeon. These diseases are associated with chronically progressive disabilities; thus, a return to baseline may never occur. It naturally follows that a patient whose general medical condition is worse at this time and who has had a previously difficult postoperative course will have to be managed carefully throughout the perioperative period for any subsequent surgery.

These patients may be surviving with a narrow margin of function in the neurologic, respiratory, or cardiovascular systems. They may have poor tissue turgor and peripheral vascular disease. Possibly, they have been taking steroids or other long-term medication that changes coagulability and the turgor of the vessel walls. Their neuromuscular diseases may be associated with skeletal changes so that their heads cannot be moved, or their jaws may be fixed, making intubation difficult to impossible. One can list other similar abnormalities throughout the musculoskeletal system. If surgery has been frequent, the presence of tracheostenosis or malacia should be considered, especially if there is a tracheostomy scar.

Table 45–1 is a classification of neuromuscular and related diseases.

TABLE 45–1. CLASSIFICATION OF NEUROMUSCULAR AND RELATED DISEASES

I. Neuromuscular diseases
 A. Muscular dystrophy
  1. Duchenne muscular dystrophy
  2. Central core disease
  3. Other myopathies
  4. Other muscle diseases
 B. Myoneurojunctional diseases
  1. Myasthenia gravis
  2. Myasthenic syndrome (Eaton–Lambert syndrome)
  3. Atypical plasma cholinesterase
 C. Familial periodic paralysis
II. Neural diseases
 A. Ataxias
 B. Demyelinating diseases
 C. Motor neuron diseases
 D. Others
III. Connective tissue diseases
 A. Rheumatoid arthritis
 B. Collagen diseases
 C. Granulomatous diseases
IV. Skeletal problems
 A. Scoliosis
 B. Osteogenesis imperfecta
 C. Dwarfism
 D. Other skeletal disorders
V. Spinal cord trauma
 A. Acute phase
 B. Transitional phase
 C. Chronic phase
VI. Paralysis secondary to other etiologies
 A. Tumor
 B. Infection
 C. Vascular etiology
 D. Cerebral palsy

CLASSIFICATION AND SPECIFIC CHARACTERISTICS

Neuromuscular Diseases

Duchenne Muscular Dystrophy. One of the best known of the neuromuscular diseases is Duchenne muscular dystrophy. Inheritance is through a sex-linked recessive gene, with the vast majority of patients being male. Parents of the index case may have no knowledge of the disease within their family.

The onset of muscle weakness occurs in the first decade, and the disease often progresses to death in the late teens or early twenties. A pseudohypertrophy occurs that is followed by muscular atrophy. Pulmonary function is gradually decreased severely, and there is an increase in muscle weakness that is usually associated with scoliosis.[6] The cardiopulmonary reserve is markedly reduced, which indicates to the anesthetist that these patients must be handled with care postoperatively.[7] Laboratory findings include a greatly elevated creatine phosphokinase (CPK), with electrocardiogram (ECG) and echocardiographic manifestations of ventricular dysfunction. These patients may have resting tachycardia and congestive heart failure secondary to the restrictive lung disease.

There is no specific treatment except for symptomatic care including surgery. Anesthesia may be required for muscle biopsies or orthopedic procedures early in the course of the disease. Minimal anesthetic and premedication agents should be used to avoid respiratory depression. Small doses of anticholinergics are used to minimize tachycardia. Special anesthetic considerations are directed toward the use of relaxants, because of both the muscle weakness and the susceptibility toward malignant hyperthermia.[8–10] Succinylcholine administration is contraindicated. Intubation is facilitated in these patients when they are debilitated, unless skeletal abnormalities secondary to the long-term disease might create difficulty in intubating. Awake intubation would then be advisable and a fiberoptic laryngoscope should be available. Regional anesthesia has been successfully used.[11,12]

Central Core Disease. Central core disease is associated with a weakness on exertion and an intolerance to high environmental temperatures. This is the one group of dystrophic patients who have the definite susceptibility to severe hyperkalemia, which results in ventricular fibrillation and death after small clinical doses of succinylcholine. Central core disease should be considered in any patient who reports a history of difficulties with anesthetics and multiple deaths in the family associated with either heat or exercise intolerance. Often these patients have no other prodromata of any neuromuscular disease.

Other Myopathies. Other myopathies are varieties of other muscular dystrophies, such as fascioscapulohumeral dystrophy (FSH)[13,14] and limb-girdle dystrophy, which are usually more benign than Duchenne muscular dystrophy. These dystrophies may create similar problems in anesthesia administration.[15]

Malignant hyperthermia,[16] which has overwhelming significance to the anesthetist, is considered in Chapter 44. Here, we emphasize that any patient with a history of vague or actual neuromuscular symptoms must be considered as a potential candidate for malignant hyperthermia. All of these patients must have an extensive history, physical examination, and laboratory workup.

Other Muscle Diseases. Other muscle diseases may create difficulties in anesthesia management. There are multiple disorders caused by one or more enzymatic defects in the pathways of glycogen storage and mobilization from the liver and muscle. The mucopolysaccharidoses belong to this group of inborn errors of metabolism. They are particularly associated with skeletal, heart, and liver abnormalities.[17,18] Patients with these disorders may have relatively mild symptoms or associated severe cirrhosis or congestive heart failure and, thus, early mortality. Because of the difficulty in regulating blood glucose levels, the blood sugar must be followed carefully. Preoperative intravenous fluids are needed, as fasting produces profound hypoglycemia. Administration of succinylcholine may lead to myoglobinuria; both hepatic and cardiac function may fail significantly in the perioperative period. Case reports of malignant hyperthermia have been reported in a variety of these diseases; thus triggering agents must be avoided and proper precautions taken.

Myoneurojunctional Diseases

Myasthenia Gravis. Myasthenia gravis is characterized by a fluctuating weakness that varies throughout the day and is worsened by exercise. This symptom appears to be more bothersome to the patient than the resultant fatigue. The ocular muscles generally are involved initially, and oropharyngeal weakness occurs, with difficulties in swallowing and talking when other cranial nerves are involved. At this point, both limb and neck weakness may have occurred, but only during myasthenic crisis is severe respiratory weakness observed. These patients may be classified as very mild, with almost benign symptoms, to severe, with marked bulbar symptoms and severe generalized muscle weakness. Females are affected three times more frequently than males between the ages of 10 and 40 years; after age 40, the incidence is the same in males and females.

The causative event of myasthenia gravis is unknown. Most patients have antibodies to muscle acetylcholine receptors that are not bound directly to the site that binds acetylcholine but are close to it. Because of this, binding is reduced between acetylcholine and the receptor. Involvement of the thymus gland in the disease process has led to thymectomy as the method of treatment. About 25 percent of patients may have complete remission, but those patients with a thymoma have a lower response.

The diagnosis of myasthenia gravis is made on the basis of clinical symptoms, a detailed history, and the characteristic electromyogram. Either edrophonium or neostigmine may be used as the anticholinesterase for diagnosis of the disease. The nonsurgical therapy consists of giving anticholinesterase agents, of which pyridostigmine and neostigmine, given orally, are most commonly used. The duration of action of pyridostigmine is longer and the drug has fewer side effects than does neostigmine. Patients with myasthenia gravis may also have been taking steroids.

An exacerbation of the symptoms occurs in myasthenic crisis, when severe respiratory weakness is associated with difficulty in swallowing. The increased secretions, respiratory infections, and muscle weakness produce a vicious cycle. Because of the lack of resistance to infections, respiratory support may be necessary through the crisis. A second crisis that may occur is cholinergic crisis, which can be difficult to differentiate from myasthenic crisis. Cholinergic crisis is caused by overtreatment with anticholinesterase agents, with resultant increased muscle weakness and secretions. A differential diagnosis can be made by the gradual injection of edrophonium to a maximum of 10 mg in a 70-kg patient. The patient who gets better is in a myasthenic crisis; the patient who becomes worse is in a cholinergic crisis.

The anesthetic difficulties arising are mainly those related to the muscle weakness; thus, whenever possible, the use of muscle relaxants should be avoided.[19-22] These patients may not need muscle relaxants for thymectomies. Class 2 to 4 myasthenic patients need thymectomies (class 1 patients are milder cases, and class 4 patients are the most severely affected). The need for postoperative ventilatory assistance is common.[23,24] The biggest controversy in the anesthetic management of the myasthenic patient is the use of anticholinesterase agents perioperatively. The general belief is that anticholinesterase agents should be given throughout the perioperative period to those patients who are already dependent on them. Those patients who have a relatively benign course may be watched and given the agents only as indicated.[25] Complications of anticholinesterase agents include potentiation of the vagal response and decrease in metabolism of ester local anesthetics. Also, muscle relaxation may be more difficult to produce. Patients with muscle weakness from whatever cause tolerate preoperative sedation poorly; therefore, preoperative and intraoperative depressant medications should be carefully monitored.

If the operative procedure can be performed under inhalation anesthesia alone, muscle relaxants often are not needed. The use of succinylcholine is controversial, as it has been said that myasthenics have less response to it than do normal patients. Most investigators have found that the usual intubating dose produces adequate relaxation and apparent rapid recovery; however, some patients have shown an early phase II block with an associated slow recovery. This phase II block may exist for several hours after the succinylcholine. Thus, it is better to avoid the use of muscle relaxants. There have been various attempts to decide, in the preoperative evaluation, which patients will need postoperative respiratory assistance. Generally, if the symptoms have continued for 5 or 6 years and anticholinesterases are needed, respiratory assistance postoperatively is required.

The Myasthenic Syndrome (Eaton–Lambert Syndrome). The myasthenic syndrome is associated with carcinoma, and these patients' symptoms mimic the symptoms of myasthenia gravis except that they improve with activity. Although the bronchus is the most common site of the carcinoma (especially oat cell tumor), there may be thoracic tumors of the prostate, breast, stomach, or rectum. At times, the weakness may occur 1 or 2 years before the diagnosis of carcinoma is made. Interestingly, removal of the tumor does not affect the weakness.[26]

Electromyography shows a reverse picture to that of myasthenia gravis. Although there is a reduced muscle response to single-nerve stimulation, tetanic stimulation shows a progressive increase in muscle strength as the frequency in duration of the stimulation is increased. These patients are extremely sensitive to nondepolarizing and depolarizing muscle relaxants, and weakness may last many days after their use. Thus, muscle relaxants are to be avoided.

Atypical Plasma Cholinesterase. Patients with atypical plasma cholinesterase appear normal except for a history of profound and prolonged muscle relaxation after succinylcholine. Normal patients have muscular paralysis approximately 2 to 5 minutes after administration of 1 mg/kg succinylcholine, as the drug is hydrolyzed by plasma cholinesterase. Occasionally, a patient has an abnormal plasma cholinesterase that does not have the same rate of hydrolysis as the normal cholinesterase. A local anesthetic inhibits the enzyme activities in the plasma of the patients. The percentage inhibition by dibucaine of the original hydrolysis is called the dibucaine number, or DN. The patient with normal enzymes has a DN greater than 80, the heterozygous patient has a DN of approximately 60, and a true homozygous patient with atypical plasma cholinesterase has a DN below 40.

Patients with severe liver disease, malnutrition, burns, glycophosphate poisoning, or other debilitating conditions may also have lower plasma cholinesterase activity. Both pyridophosphate eyedrops and irradiation lessen activity. The most common incidence is during the latter trimester of pregnancy, when, generally, careful monitoring of muscle relaxant doses is required. Patients with a prolonged response to succinylcholine should be ventilated until adequate recovery of the myoneural junction occurs. Normally, pharmacologic intervention is not needed; the patient simply must be provided respiratory assistance and monitored carefully.

Familial Periodic Paralysis. There are three distinct types of familial periodic paralysis—hypokalemic, hyperkalemic, and normokalemic—although certain characteristics are similar in all three. Generally, there is an autosomal dominant inheritance pattern. These patients may have attacks of quadriplegia that are related to the serum potassium level. The most common cause of death during these attacks is respiratory failure, often resulting from aspiration pneumonitis or infection. Cardiac failure and shock have also been reported.

In patients with the hypokalemic form of familial periodic paralysis, attacks may be increased by eating a heavy meal; therefore, patients must abstain from eating such a meal the day before surgery. Potassium levels should be carefully managed. No matter what procedures are to be performed, the electrocardiogram (ECG) should be closely monitored, as arrhythmias are common in this condition.[27-30] A Swan–Ganz catheter or central venous pressure monitor should be used in symptomatic patients, because cardiac failure is also a problem. There is controversy in the literature about the use of muscle relaxants; thus, it may be advisable not to administer them.

Patients with the hyperkalemic form of periodic paralysis have acute attacks unrelated to high-carbohydrate meals.[31] In fact, the attacks occur more often when the patients are hungry and may also be related to exercise. In general, attacks last for a shorter period than in patients with hypokalemia. There is an outpouring of potassium from the muscles, and treatment of the hyperkalemic form is with insulin and glucose therapy. This type of treatment might precipitate an attack in hypokalemic patients.

Hyperkalemic patients are generally treated with diuretics, whereas hypokalemic patients are administered potassium supplementation. All of these patients, including those with normokalemia, must have their serum electrolytes carefully monitored throughout the perioperative period as anesthetic problems occur mainly through small deviations in potassium levels, which may cause paralysis anytime in the perioperative period.

Neural Diseases

Ataxias, Demyelinating Diseases, and Other Diseases. The most prominent of the ataxias, Friedreich's ataxia, is a progressive disease associated with widespread conductive defects that strike in the teenage period. The patient develops nystagmus and severe cardiac arrhythmias. The ECG must be carefully monitored throughout surgery, and cardiotoxic agents should be avoided if at all possible.[32] These patients have a certain degree of muscle weakness and respiratory insufficiency during the latter stages of the disease, and therefore, respiratory depression and excess sedative agents should be avoided.

Ataxias and athetosis from other conditions have been associated with an inappropriate response to atropine. In these patients, smaller doses of atropine are used than normally given to avoid a mild febrile response with oral temperatures of 38 to 39C. An increased incidence of malignant hyperthermia has been reported in Friedreich's ataxia and in cerebral palsy patients with ataxia and athetosis.

Multiple sclerosis is the most common of the demyelinating diseases. It is associated with exacerbations and remissions and typically occurs in three distinct forms: (1) rapidly progressive or malignant form, (2) a slowly progressing form with exacerbations and incomplete remissions over a long period, and (3) a relatively benign form that is very slowly progressive and is not associated with a shortened life span. There are very few patients who have one attack and then apparently are cured with no subsequent attacks. The disease is associated with an exacerbation of weakness, visual symptoms, and numbness from paresthesias. Euphoria is general, and depression may occur. The patients are often given both steroids and adrenocorticotropin, so they may require an increased amount of steroids at the time of anesthesia and surgery. Routinely, these are necessary if either drug is given within 3 months of surgery. Spinal anesthesia is contraindicated because of the nature of the disease and the resultant medicolegal implications. Temperature must be monitored carefully, as the onset of an infection or pyrexia may produce new symptoms. There have been reports of an exacerbation of attacks after anesthesia and surgery. In general, these exacerbations are shorter in duration and do not lead to permanent changes when compared with the expected exacerbation, which can signal a more progressive downhill course.

Motor Neuron Diseases. These diseases include hereditary illnesses such as Werdnig–Hoffman and Kugelberg–Welander syndromes, which affect the anterior horn cells; the onset of symptoms may occur at birth or later in infancy and childhood. The later the onset, the milder the form of the hereditary manifestations. Other diseases are progressive muscular atrophy, primary bulbar palsy, and amyotrophic lateral sclerosis. There are no specific recommendations for anesthetic management. Instead, emphasis is on maintaining good respiratory function throughout the perioperative period in a weakened patient. Muscle relaxants may not be required and should be used sparingly as many patients are floppy secondary to their lower motor neuron involvement. In addition to the usual acute and chronic needs, progressive skeletal abnormalities occur that require surgery. With attention to detail these patients tolerate procedures well.

Patients with Down syndrome have an increased sensitivity to atropine, and thus slightly lower dosages than normal are administered. Neurofibromatosis is associated with increased bleeding when the neurofibromata are surgically excised, particularly during scoliosis corrections when the neurofibromatous lesion is in the vertebral spine.

Connective Tissue Diseases

Rheumatoid Arthritis. Patients with rheumatoid arthritis may be children or adults at the time of onset. Children with rheumatoid arthritis (Still's disease) are often taking steroids as well as experiencing all of the pubertal changes occurring during growth. These patients progress in their disease and develop severe skeletal deformities. Intubation is particularly difficult, as very often the chin rests on the sternum, and they generally have compromised cardiorespiratory function.

Adult patients with rheumatoid arthritis may have less severe skeletal deformities than do children. They are chronically ill, undernourished, and anemic, and most are polyarticular, with the small joints of the hand and foot affected. These patients may have lung involvement, with a diffuse infiltrate producing restriction and loss of compliance. One finds in both adults and children a markedly decreased ventilatory ability and low reserve as a result of the restrictive lung disease. Both pediatric and adult patients may have heart involvement in the valve leaflets, rings, myocardium, and endocardium, as well as the most common problem, amyloidosis, which involves the kidneys. Such patients may progress to renal failure, or the excretion of any drugs administered may be diminished. The most common finding is anemia of chronic disease, which is characteristic of patients with rheumatoid arthritis. This is usually not severe but is resistant to iron therapy.

Often, rheumatoid arthritis patients have been taking acetylsalicylic acid, phenylbutazone, endomethizine, or steroids. Many of the newer nonsteroidal anti-inflammatory drugs have also been used in rheumatoid arthritis.[33,34] One must be aware of the increased incidence of gastric disturbance and occult gastrointestinal bleeding, particularly if the hemoglobin is below 10 g.

Another disease with a similar pathology is ankylosing spondylitis, which involves particularly the sacroiliac joint and other end joints of the spine and hips, rather than the neck. There is significant impairment of rotating motion and a limitation of bending. These patients may have a solid ridge of bone along the lumbar spine, making diagnostic spinal tap impossible. Because they may have been taking steroids or other drugs, a careful history and significant preoperative check for mobility of the jaw and other joints must be performed. These patients generally have surgery for corrective orthopedic procedures and for complications of corticosteroid therapy, as well as ordinary surgical procedures such as appendectomy. Airway and respiratory management must be handled carefully and they should be intubated before administration of anesthesia. In general, an awake intubation with a fiberoptic laryngoscope or bronchoscope is safer than is intubation after anesthesia induction. When blood loss is expected, one must be particularly concerned about both anemia and a decreased platelet function secondary to steroidal or other therapy.

Collagen Diseases. The collagen diseases include systemic lupus erythematosus, scleroderma, polyarteritis nodosa,

and dermatomyositis. Each of these diseases is discussed briefly, followed by a discussion of the general anesthetic management.[35,36]

Systemic lupus erythematosus may be associated with pericarditis and other cardiac abnormalities as well as pleurisy. When a pericardial friction rub is present, the disease resembles rheumatic fever. There are multiple clinical problems occurring throughout the lungs and nervous system that may be associated with dysphagia, hemiplegia, and polyneuritis. The clinical course may be prolonged and characterized by exacerbations and remissions. This course may be induced by such drugs as hydralazine and isoniazid. Steroids are often used and this must be considered in the perioperative period.

Scleroderma is associated with a brawny edema in the hands, feet, and face, followed by a second stage of a waxy, smooth, and tight skin. Secondary contractures occur and may make opening the mouth extremely difficult. Dysphagia, pulmonary complications, and a significant loss of weight with weakness, fever, and joint pain occur. Cardiac involvement can result from fibrosis and can produce heart failure in association with pulmonary hypertension. Renal complications are also seen. Again, steroids are often used.

Patients with polyarteritis nodosa are particularly susceptible to chronic and acute respiratory infections. Although early signs of fever and tenderness occur more frequently in the extremities, respiratory and renal symptoms appear as well; in fact, respiratory lesions may precede the other findings. Long remissions have resulted from steroid therapy, although no cures are reported.

Another collagen disease is dermatomyositis, which affects the skin plus the muscle fibers, which become vacuolated and degenerated. This is rare and is extremely painful. Diplopia, dyspnea, and impaired sphincter control may be present; however, unlike the other collagen diseases, the lungs are generally not involved. When pulmonary symptoms do occur, they are related to the weakness, with resulting aspiration and respiratory insufficiency.

The anesthetist should consider a probable history of steroid therapy in all of these patients. Perioperative supplementation is often necessary. The presence of renal disease, which may affect renal function, should be ascertained as should cardiopulmonary status. Tightening of the skin around the mouth in the patient with scleroderma means that regional anesthesia is generally preferred over general anesthesia, with immediate access to a fiberoptic laryngoscope and other standard emergency equipment and drugs, including a cricothyrotomy set. Epinephrine in the regional anesthetic is contraindicated, however, as Raynaud's phenomenon exists. Because blood flow may be reduced in collagen diseases, determining blood pressure in the normal way can be difficult, and direct arterial monitoring would be advisable. In patients with polyarteritis nodosa, hypertension secondary to the renal disease may be present and should be considered, so that relative hypotension does not occur, with its concomitant cerebral and cardiac problems. In dermatomyositis patients, the muscle weakness may obviate the need for muscle relaxants. A myasthenic response has been demonstrated in some of the latter patients, although this is not a consistent finding. Whenever relaxation is necessary, a small test dose should be used first.

Not only must careful attention be given to the cardiorespiratory and renal systems, but the changing and vague neurologic signs and symptoms can also be frustrating to the clinician who is attempting to obtain a concise history and physical examination. The contractures resulting from skeletal, skin, and muscle deformities should be documented well before surgery.

Granulomatous Diseases. Granulomatous diseases are considered a relatively rare group of clinical symptoms varying from a pure arthritis to diseases incorporating large vessels and granulomatous lesions in many areas. All are chronic with insidious onset at varying times of life. Most of them are associated with a pulmonary infection which may easily continue to widespread consolidation.

The most important of these diseases is Wegener's granulomatosis, which is generally a triad of necrotizing giant cell granulomatosis of the upper respiratory tract and lungs, widespread vasculitis of the small arteries and veins, and focal glomerulonephritis. It progresses with gradual involvement of all the other systems and must be distinguished from tuberculosis, sarcoidosis, and mycotic infections. Of particular note is the severity of radiologic findings and the pulmonary symptoms. Symptomatic control occurs with steroids, but the disease is always fatal.

Sarcoidosis is more benign. It is a systemic granulomatous disease with spontaneous incomplete remissions in the early stages and with a slowly progressive course when the disease persists. Particularly involved are the lungs, lymph nodes, and other reticuloendothelial tissue. The disease appears to resemble tuberculosis, but the tubercle or granuloma does not result in caseation and necrosis. Instead, healing takes place by fibrosis with scar formation. Patients are characterized by severe involvement of the tissues with very few symptoms, and they are generally treated with steroids. They may also have lesions in the heart, especially in the valves, as well as in other organs of the body, but these are not as common as the lung lesions. The anesthetist is most concerned with the heart and lung findings.[37,38]

Skeletal Problems

Scoliosis. Neuromuscular diseases can result in a curvature of the spine known as scoliosis. Idiopathic scoliosis occurs during the developmental phase, particularly in young girls going through puberty. The potential exists for marked changes in respiratory and cardiovascular function when the scoliotic curve becomes severe. This may evolve when idiopathic scoliosis is left untreated for many years or after other diseases, especially such paralyzing diseases as polio

and quadriplegia, in which the deformed spine and thoracic cage produce severe restrictive pulmonary disease. These patients need to be carefully evaluated preoperatively to assess their cardiopulmonary reserve. When the reserve is markedly decreased, they must be considered for respiratory care before correction of the scoliotic curve. This may even require such assistive ventilatory efforts as a tank respirator. Those patients with scoliotic curves greater than 110 degrees should be treated in centers particularly equipped to deal with multifaceted problems, where there are surgeons who can perform rapid and relatively bloodless surgery. Careful consideration of detail and cooperation in surgical and anesthetic management can make this possible.[39–41] (Refer also to Chapter 38, Anesthesia for Orthopedic Surgery.)

An association between idiopathic scoliosis and malignant hyperthermia has been questioned but has not been notable in centers dealing specifically with scoliosis. It can thus be assumed that these patients, as any patients, have the potential for malignant hyperthermia, but scoliosis is not a condition necessarily associated with it. Patients with primary neuromuscular disease, rather than idiopathic scoliosis, have an increased incidence of malignant hyperthermia.

The anesthetic management of patients with scoliosis has been simplified since the measurement of somatosensory evoked potentials became clinically possible. This allows monitoring of sensory conduction from the lower extremities through the cerebral cortex throughout surgery. For this monitoring, it is necessary that the patients not be deeply anesthetized with halothane, isoflurane, or enflurane, which would muffle the somatosensory evoked response. Anesthesia may easily be accomplished with moderate doses of isoflurane and controlled ventilation. Careful attention to blood loss throughout the operative procedure is important.[42] Autologous blood is preferred to bank blood. When blood replacement of more than two units is required, warmed blood is better to avoid hypothermia. The rapidity of the surgical technique is directly related to the blood loss (Table 45–2).[43] Table 45–2 relates to the Harrington rod technique. The Cotrel-Dubousset technique takes about 30 minutes longer and is associated with approximately 150 to 200 mL of increased blood loss when performed by the same surgeons reported in Table 45–2 (Erwin W. Personal communication, 1991).

Osteogenesis Imperfecta. Osteogenesis imperfecta is a disease in which the bone matrix is not properly laid down, resulting in weakened bones with repetitive fractures. When these patients need surgical correction, there is increased difficulty in positioning them, and the potential exists for new

TABLE 45–2. RELATIONSHIP OF BLOOD LOSS TO TOTAL PROCEDURE TIME IN 1726 IDIOPATHIC SCOLIOSIS PATIENTS OVER A 10-YEAR PERIOD

	Age (Years)	Total Time of Procedure (minutes)	Blood Loss (mL)	Transfusion (mL)
Average	17.98[a]	116.49	754.40	494.00
Standard deviation	9.09	47.23	458.37	529.39

[a] Range: 2 to 74 years.
Reprinted, with permission, from Dahm et al.[43]

fractures in the course of operative and postoperative management. Other abnormalities associated with this disease include hyperthermia, hyperhidrosis, easy bruisability, and bleeding, with associated platelet cell dysfunction, kyphoscoliosis, cor pulmonale, and congenital heart disease, which may have valvular components. The kyphoscoliosis may cause severe restrictive pulmonary dysfunction which can complicate the preexisting cardiac problems.

Anesthetic management should include careful positioning, being aware that even mandibular fractures are a hazard. When face mask or laryngoscopy is performed, attention must be paid to the vulnerability of the mandible. The patient is positioned and moved with care. The increased bleeding tendency indicates that transfusions should be considered early in the course of surgery if bleeding is significant. Hyperthermia requires that the temperature is carefully monitored throughout the perioperative period, and when the patient is febrile, elective surgery should definitely be postponed. This is not malignant hyperthermia, and controversy exists as to the appropriateness of dantrolene.[44-46] A cooling blanket should always be available for use. Anticholinergic drugs should be accessible but must be used with caution. One technique is to give the drug intravenously in small doses immediately before it is needed, such as before induction when intubation is planned and inhalation agents are to be used. Because of cardiopulmonary problems with kyphoscoliosis, careful cardiac and pulmonary evaluations are necessary both preoperatively and throughout the perioperative period.

Dwarfism. Many types of dwarfism exist; in all, 55 syndromes have been described. Some major abnormalities are atlantoaxial instability, spinal stenosis, airway and facial abnormalities, thoracic dystrophy, kyphoscoliosis or lordosis, congenital heart disease, and hydrocephaly (and, possibly, associated mild retardation or seizure disorders). One or a combination of these may be present.[47]

The variety of vertebral abnormalities should be carefully evaluated before elective surgery, with appropriate treatment when possible. The perioperative anesthetic management should be directed toward potential difficulties in airway management. Patients may have hyperplasia of the mandible, micrognathia, or a relatively fixed jaw, creating difficulty in visualization at the time of intubation. Both the thoracic dystrophic syndrome, with a small, narrow, contracted chest cage, and kyphoscoliosis are associated with restrictive lung disease and must be considered preoperatively. Any of the congenital cardiac lesions are possible, although patent ductus arteriosus, atrial septal defects, and coarctation of the aorta are more common. Central nervous system involvement usually manifests as hydrocephalus, seizure disorders, and mental retardation.

Seizure disorders may be treated preoperatively with the medications patients are currently taking. Benzodiazepines or barbiturates may be beneficial with follow-up barbiturate anesthesia. Special guidelines for anesthetic management include avoidance, if feasible, of regional anesthesia when neurologic deficits are evident; however, regional anesthesia is indicated in some of these instances.[48] When there is paralysis or spinal stenosis, the potential for autonomic dysreflexia should be considered, and appropri-

ate alpha and beta blockers available. Cardiopulmonary status must be consistently monitored. There are no particular contraindications to any anesthetic agent as long as precise technique is used and the patency and safety of the airway are maintained.

Other Skeletal Disorders. Other diseases in this category include craniofacial dysostoses, Paget's disease of the bone, and fibrous dysplasia. Throughout these conditions, careful positioning of the patient is mandatory. Lesions may involve the vertebral column with secondary neurologic disability. The airway must be studied preoperatively because of abnormalities in the facial bones, mandible, and neck. No particular drugs are recommended or contraindicated, except airway control and ability to intubate prior to using muscle relaxants. Regional techniques are indicated only when no skeletal lesions are present at the site of needle insertion. This avoids penetration of known lesions, with attendant bleeding or neurologic deficits. In addition, these patients may have endocrine abnormalities, which also may be associated with increased bleeding. Thus, adequate blood should be available for replacement and an extensive endocrine workup may be needed. Any associated neurologic disability must be documented before the administration of anesthesia. Again, when spinal cord injury has occurred, autonomic dysreflexia is possible throughout the perioperative period.

Spinal Cord Trauma

Etiology and Diagnosis. The etiology of spinal cord trauma is primarily motor vehicle accidents; sports injuries, such as diving, are the second most frequent cause.[49] Diagnosis must be made at the site of injury. Neuropathologists have demonstrated that inappropriate handling of these patients can increase the severity of the lesion, provoke new lesions, and convert a temporary insult into permanent paralysis. This increased awareness of potential spinal cord pathology includes the evaluation in the emergency room for isolated or multiple trauma and follow-up management during the perioperative period. The patients' necks and trunks must be maintained in a neutral position with appropriate traction throughout the period of instability. The technique used in endotracheal intubation is especially important. Most trauma centers prefer intubation with the fiberoptic bronchoscope to avoid extension or flexion of the cervical vertebrae and the resultant iatrogenic increase in injury.

There are three phases in the progression after spinal cord injury: spinal shock, transitional phase (which may slowly evolve into the third phase), and the chronic phase with a neurologically impaired patient. The plasticity of the central nervous system forces the body to constantly react to a changing neurologic status until function is recovered or the lesion is stabilized. The specialty of neurology has two components intertwined with this phenomenon. Neurophysiology involves evaluation of the function of the nervous system. Restorative neurology is involved in using to the best possible level any remaining function existing after an insult. These combine to improve the outcome and quality of life of affected patients. Another purpose of neurophysiology is to evaluate the nervous system below the level of the primary or highest lesion. Secondary or incomplete lesions may have occurred at the time of injury or later, and may not be diagnosed until the neurologic system has partially stabilized. The patient may complain of aberrant sensations, pain, or other phenomena in areas not thought to be clinically innervated. Neurophysiologic evaluation through somatosensory evoked potentials, polyelectromyography, and electrospinograms can trace whether conduction occurs from the cerebral cortex through the central nervous system to the periphery and vice versa. These techniques plus an excellent history and neurologic examination are the tools for diagnosing the status of the evolving phases. They are also useful for determining if complete transection of the spinal cord is present, and thus if the prognosis of return of function is nil. This enables the patient and physicians to plan accordingly.

Acute Phase. Spinal shock is the period from the first few hours after injury to 1 to 6 weeks later. It is characterized as an areflexic and atonic stage, with loss of sphincter control, paralytic ileus, areflexic bladder, and loss of normal tendon reflexes. A specific danger is cardiopulmonary instability, with marked hypoxia and hypotension occurring with slight changes in position. Postural hypotension exists when the patient is placed in any degree of tilt; slowly, as the systems adapt to the paralyzed state, the presence of postural hypotension is lessened. This is aided through gradual progression on a tilt board until 90 degrees is reached. Patients may need to be treated with ephedrine or other similar agents to increase their tolerance of the more erect position. The duration of spinal shock depends on the severity of the spinal cord injury. The quadriplegic patient with a complete lesion has the longest phase; the individual with a temporary deficit has the most rapid progression.

The spinal cord-injured patient is poikilothermic below the level of the lesion and thus is at risk for hypothermia and resultant metabolic acidosis. Body temperature must be protected throughout surgery and the perioperative period because, distal to the lesion, the body reaches a temperature similar to that of the environment as it lacks the adaptive mechanisms of the intact neurologic system. Stress ulcers throughout the gastrointestinal tract and fluid and electrolyte imbalance may occur secondary to endogenous steroid release and exogenous steroids given therapeutically. There is an increased incidence of thromboembolic phenomena; heparin and other anticoagulants are often prescribed for weeks to months, depending on the severity of the thrombosis or pulmonary embolus.

The marked susceptibility to hyperkalemia after succinylcholine administration is the critical characteristic dictating one aspect of the anesthetic management. After severe neurologic injury, burns, or massive trauma, the entire muscle acts as a myoneural junction in the area below the lesion. When a depolarizing muscle relaxant is given, there is a massive exodus of potassium from the entire muscle belly. The efflux of potassium into the central circulation causes hyperkalemia, with serum potassium levels as high as 11 to 13 mg percent. As the serum potassium progresses toward 7 to 8 mg percent, severe arrhythmias occur, with eventual ventricular fibrillation and death. Thus, succinyl-

choline is absolutely contraindicated in these patients. Presently atracurium, vecuronium, or pancuronium, nondepolarizing relaxants with an onset of action of 2 to 3 minutes, are the muscle relaxants of choice. For rapid-sequence induction after preoxygenation and application of cricoid pressure, atracurium may safely be used as follows. One sixth of the intubating dose (in mg/kg body weight) is given. After 60 seconds, the induction dose of thiopental or another agent is administered, and the remaining five sixths of atracurium is given. After another 60 seconds, during which cricoid pressure is maintained and oxygen is administered passively, the patient is intubated. Just as the effects of the spinal cord injury vary markedly from person to person, susceptibility to succinylcholine varies and extends throughout the transitional phase. It may continue into the chronic phase as well, particularly when symptoms or signs are changing. Thus, safety dictates succinylcholine not be used in these patients.

Transitional Phase. The transitional phase is marked either by a return to the normal status in which neurologic recovery progresses or by adaptation to the paralyzed state. Abnormal sensations such as tingling may be interpreted by the patient as pain; however, this is not necessarily pain and may signal the beginning of the return of sensation and motor function, if they are to return. Cardiac condition stabilizes, with bradycardia remaining. It must be remembered that these patients are often athletic young men and women who have basically a slow heart rate. The onset of spinal cord injury just potentiates this, and heart rates of 50 to 60 beats per minute are common.

Autonomic dysreflexia is an unopposed massive sympathetic response or mass reflex response that occurs below the site of injury. It occurs in patients with a cervical or high thoracic lesion and virtually is never seen in patients paralyzed below T-8. Autonomic dysreflexia may occur after any condition resulting in quadriplegia or high paraplegia. It is characterized by severe and extremely rapid hypertension, with associated sweating and bradycardia. The bradycardia may be transient, lasting only a couple of minutes until it progresses to tachycardia, which is associated with cephalgia as the hypertension increases. The massive sympathetic outflow can lead to severe arrhythmias as well as central nervous system problems such as convulsions and cerebrovascular accidents.[50] The preferred therapy is immediate administration of 5 mg phentolamine intravenously if the blood pressure cannot be corrected rapidly by mechanical means. The most common cause is bladder or bowel distension; thus, simply emptying the bladder may correct the problem. Two surgical conditions in which autonomic dysreflexia occurs are transurethral procedures and plastic surgery on ischial and sacral ulcers. As the perisacral or perineal tissues are approached, there is an autonomic response similar to the response to a full bladder, with the possible development of autonomic dysreflexia. Local anesthetic supplementation to the anesthetic used can avoid this problem (as will spinal or epidural anesthesia). Arrhythmias may be treated with intravenous lidocaine 1 mg/kg, which may be repeated in 5 minutes if the arrhythmias recur or continue. If this treatment fails, propranolol may be necessary (0.4 mg IV is the standard adult dose). Headaches may be treated with either a barbiturate such as thiopental (in small doses of 50 to 100 mg) or a benzodiazepine such as midazolam (1 to 3 mg IV) or diazepam (5 mg IV). All of these dosages are appropriate for an adult patient. Autonomic dysreflexia is one of the worst effects of quadriplegia and must be constantly considered in surgery. The condition lasts throughout life and may appear suddenly many years after injury.

Respiratory adaptation is most profound in the high quadriplegic patient, who is without voluntary intercostal function. In the usual patient with C5–6 quadriplegia, the diaphragm alone can account for approximately 1000 to 2000 mL of vital capacity. This is down from the 3000 to 4000 mL preinjury. Development of the accessory muscles of respiration over several weeks postinjury can gradually increase the vital capacity to 2500 to 3000 mL and can assist in the development of a cough mechanism.

As autonomic dysreflexia may result from obstipation, the bowel program must be carefully monitored. Regularity in habits, fluid management, and stool softeners are needed. Attention to diet and elimination is vital perioperatively. In many patients, sphincter tone is increased, and male patients may need transurethral resection of the bladder neck or of the prostate or external sphincterotomy to allow complete bladder emptying. When stasis occurs and the bladder continues to have a high postvoiding residuum, a potential exists for reflux and subsequent degeneration of the upper tracts as well as constant bladder infections. The latter can be the nidus for other localized infections or for septicemia. Chronic renal disease is a prime cause of death. Intermittent catheterization has prevented many of the problems associated with chronic indwelling catheters. To avoid autonomic dysreflexia, spinal or epidural anesthesia is the anesthesia of choice in transurethral surgery.

Throughout the transitional period, the patient may have aberrant sensations and develop spasms. Clonus may occur after minor sensory stimuli. Physical therapy and medication are necessary to avoid contractures, which may be painful and interfere with the quality of life, including the use of remaining function. Skin infections may occur through stasis and as a result of the irritation caused by spasticity and both developing and fixed contractures. Patients must turn frequently from side to side and avoid prolonged sitting to decrease the probability of skin irritation and subsequent ulceration. As much as 50 g of protein a day may be lost from a single deep ulcer. This is associated with anemia, generalized wasting, and cachexia.

Chronic Phase. After 18 months, the chronic phase of spinal cord injury is generally reached. The exaggerated reflexes can still occur, but have usually stabilized. Reflexes now are related to the altered neuronal spasticity of the reenervated neurons. The reflexes and functions are without the inhibitory, regulatory impulses from the brain. The mass reflexes may continue and autonomic dysreflexia may already exist or develop. Plantar stimulation may evoke violent withdrawal of the lower extremities, and clonus may continue after minor sensory stimuli.

The neurologic condition is usually stable. If the patient's neurologic function begins to degenerate, secondary complications must be considered. One of these is syringomyelia, or a cyst within the spinal canal. This cyst can produce a fresh neurologic injury with the transitional signs of spinal cord damage. The cardiorespiratory condition is generally stable. Patients who have had high lesions may have difficulty with the cough mechanism and chronic pulmonary problems may occur. These must be evaluated carefully preoperatively, and infections must be treated vigorously. Some patients are prophylactically treated with intermittent positive-pressure breathing at home to avoid atelectasis and resultant pulmonary infections. The bowel and bladder regimens are stabilized to decrease the incidence of distension. Skin infections are still a concern, as are the anemia of chronic disease and potentially progressive cachexia. The opposite, morbid obesity, may occur in the patient with an uncontrolled appetite. This compounds the care required and the associated problems are magnified accordingly.

Multiple drugs are used to reduce spasticity. Dantrolene, baclofen, and diazepam are the three most common systemic agents. Regional techniques such as motor endpoint injections with 40 percent alcohol and peripheral nerve injections with 6 percent aqueous phenol, may be employed under neurophysiologic control (a Teflon-coated needle and a precise, quantitative nerve stimulator). If there are massive spasms and contractures after 18 months, the potential for phenol/glycerin, alcohol, radiofrequency, or other agents for rhizotomies should be considered in patients with complete spinal cord lesions.[51] Patients may complain of pain from spasticity or aberrant sensations. The former is treated as above, as long as residual function is not compromised unnecessarily. The latter requires extensive counseling of the patient and possibly behavior modification techniques so that the patient may adequately cope with the problem. The plasticity of the nervous system means that the various surgical techniques used to cut the nerves are generally only temporarily effective, if at all, as the pain may recur in months to years. The exception is the absolute alcohol rhizotomy, which cauterizes the spinal cord and creates a permanent lesion.

The spinal cord injury may be associated with a head injury that occurs at the time of trauma or subsequently as part of an associated cardiopulmonary catastrophe. Any severe hypoxic episodes may result in brainstem lesions. Conversely, one must constantly consider that an unconscious patient may have an associated spinal cord injury, as well as head trauma. Careful continuous evaluation must be made of the changing neurologic status throughout the phases. The spine must be stabilized at all times whenever instability is suspected.

The cauda equina syndrome, which occurs from a lesion to the lower end of the spinal conus medullaris and the nerves as they leave the spinal cord, is a lower motor neuron lesion. It is associated with flaccidity rather than spasticity and may occur alone or in addition to the upper motor neuron lesion at the time of the primary injury. As noted, approximately 10 percent or more of patients have these associated secondary spinal cord traumas. Cauda equina syndrome may be apparent early in the postinjury course or later when signs and symptoms of a mixed lesion occur with the presence of both upper and lower motor neuron components.

Paralysis Secondary to Other Etiologies

Tumor. Any malignant tumor may metastasize to the spinal cord or associated areas. Tumors of the breast, lung, and prostate are especially prevalent. Both benign and malignant tumors can develop in the spinal cord itself as well as in surrounding tissues. As the spinal cord is a relatively closed space, tumors may produce varying signs from progressive neurologic defects to sudden severe symptomatology. After neurologic and diagnostic imaging techniques are completed, a surgical diagnosis is generally needed. Emergency decompression may be required. Perioperatively the patient must be treated as any other person with an unstable spine, and the affected areas supported throughout the induction and remaining surgical period. Often radiotherapy is used either before or after neurosurgery; thus, patients have the potential to develop all the secondary complications of radiation therapy, as well as those from any associated chemotherapy. Pathologic fractures may occur from either the lesion, the radiotherapy, or both.

Infection. The most common infection involving the spinal cord is tuberculosis, with the resultant paraplegia. Rarely does quadriplegia occur, as lesions are most often in the thoracic and thoracolumbar spine. The patient may develop either acute- or insidious-onset paraplegia without evidence of pulmonary tuberculosis. The disease progresses by hematologic spread to the vertebral column and spinal cord from the lungs. In giving any anesthetic the anesthetist must assume the presence of pulmonary tuberculosis. Other spinal infections including meningitis present acutely, with symptoms and signs of infection progressing rapidly and often with a prodromal respiratory illness or sore throat. All may be associated with residual disability, depending on the severity of the infection, the response to antimicrobial agents, and the amount of residual scarring and impairment. In children, subsequent growth and development may be affected with paralysis and scoliosis present.

Vascular Lesions. The artery of Adamkiewicz is the main supply to the anterior portion of the cord at the T-8 level. After cardiac and aortic surgery there may be hypotension or hypoxia of the cord secondary to perioperative inadequate blood supply. The patient may awaken with partial or complete paraplegia which may be transient or permanent. This paraplegia may occur secondary to trauma or to hypotension from any cause, especially in a patient with peripheral vascular disease and compromised circulation.

Cerebral Palsy. The manifestations of cerebral palsy are multifaceted depending on the etiology, the severity of the lesion, and the amount of residual damage. Generally, the syndromes have been grouped into four categories: spastic, athetoid or dyskinetic, ataxic, and mixed forms. The diagnosis may not be definitive until the second year of life, and must be distinguished from progressive neurologic diseases and tumors. Scoliosis, paraplegia, quadriplegia, and other neurologic and orthopedic problems can occur. Increased sensitivity to atropine, with a mild febrile response and oral temperatures of 38 to 39C, and increased incidence of malignant hyperthermia have both been implied in cerebral palsy

patients with ataxia and athetosis. Otherwise, simply careful anesthetic management is required as with any patient, and attention is paid to each of the presenting problems.

ANESTHETIC MANAGEMENT

Preoperative Evaluation

Table 45–3 lists the various requirements in the preoperative evaluation. As stated, a detailed history including a functional history of capabilities and exercise tolerance (to whatever level), is probably the most important factor, followed by a physical examination including a detailed neurologic assessment. The numbers and types of medications and their interactions in the autonomic nervous system may be overwhelming. The chronic nature of the disabilities provokes greater drug interactions throughout the patient.

Emergency surgery often allows only an evaluation with appropriate laboratory and other diagnostic studies. For elective surgery, these patients should be in the optimal condition preoperatively, even if it means postponing surgery for weeks. This is particularly true for kyphoscoliosis surgery, in which the patient may be maintained for a period with respiratory assistance. When the patient is considered able to tolerate both surgery and postoperative treatment, surgery is performed.

Anesthetic Techniques

No specific technique is invariably safe. Extensive monitoring of pulse, pulse oximetry, blood pressure, respiration (including end-tidal carbon dioxide, as appropriate), temperature, and the electrocardiogram is mandatory whenever monitored anesthesia care, regional anesthesia, or general anesthesia is contemplated. Such monitoring is necessary for any patient. Other monitors, such as pulmonary artery and central venous catheters, direct arterial measurements, neurophysiologic monitoring, and echocardiography, are used as conditions dictate.

TABLE 45–3. PREOPERATIVE EVALUATION FOR PROPER ASSESSMENT OF PATIENT STATUS IN PATIENTS WITH NEUROMUSCULAR DISEASES

1. Complete history and physical examination (especially drug history, neurologic and neurophysiologic examination [where indicated], study of neck mobility, and exercise tolerance)
2. Anteroposterior and lateral chest x-ray, skeletal x-ray
3. Complete blood count, urinalysis, prothrombin time, partial thromboplastin time, arterial blood gas analysis (where indicated)
4. Where indicated, creatinine clearance, electrolytes, creatine phosphokinase, liver function tests, sedimentation rate, dibucaine number, occult blood in stools, drug analysis
5. Pulmonary function tests
6. Electrocardiogram, echocardiogram (where indicated)
7. Computerized axial tomography scan, magnetic resonance imaging, or myelogram in patients with myelodysplasia or other indications

Anesthesia may be induced either through inhalation or by intravenous agents or regional techniques. There are three absolute contraindications: (1) In the period after massive trauma, burns, or spinal cord injury, succinylcholine is absolutely contraindicated to avoid severe hyperkalemia which generally results in severe cardiac arrhythmias and, potentially, death. (2) The use of muscle relaxants or deep anesthesia is contraindicated in patients in whom an airway cannot be established. These agents are avoided until an adequate airway is obtained. Endotracheal intubation is often performed in an awake patient with a fiberoptic bronchoscope and local anesthesia. (3) Sufficient case reports have associated neuromuscular diseases of a variety of etiologies with malignant hyperthermia, so that any person with a family history of unusual neuromuscular symptoms or disease should be considered susceptible to malignant hyperthermia. Triggering agents should be avoided in these patients as well as in the known susceptible patients listed above.

As the cardiorespiratory system is often compromised, low-dose premedications and anesthetic agents are advisable. If the patient is taking ganglionic, alpha, or beta blockers or steroids, appropriate therapy must be used throughout the perioperative period. Steady-state anesthesia is maintained, avoiding any major shifts in vital signs including temperature. The compromised respiratory system is a constant challenge, often requiring controlled ventilation and continuous assessment of pulse oximetry and end-tidal carbon dioxide.

Even a short time in one position in the hypothermic, acidotic, or hypotensive state for a neuromuscularly compromised patient can lead to pressure necrosis of the skin with resultant tissue breakdown. Thus, careful positioning of the entire body is mandatory with appropriate padding and restraints. Emergence from anesthesia is deliberate to avoid cardiopulmonary depression or compromise, and ample time is spent in the postanesthesia area with full monitoring, either in the recovery room or in the intensive care unit, as appropriate.

Postoperative Care

Cardiopulmonary monitoring should continue as long as pain or depressant medications are required and as long as the patient is unstable in this regard. Ventilatory assistance and intermittent positive-pressure breathing is often needed.

The quadriplegic patient is said to have a 10 percent decrease in total body water compared with an intact person; there is an approximate 5 percent decrease in paraplegic patients, depending on the level of the lesion, from whatever etiology. When such patients are NPO (nothing by mouth) before surgery, they may be in a markedly dehydrated state. This is a consideration not only in the preoperative period (as an intravenous line may be started 12 to 24 hours before surgery for appropriate hydration) and operative period, when the anesthetist is carefully observing the patient, but also in the postoperative period when less precise monitoring and control may exist. Unexplained hypotension, hypoxia, or acidosis may occur then with resultant tissue breakdown and secondary problems, especially if renal disease exists. This is possible whether monitored anesthesia care, regional anesthesia, or general anesthesia is used. No matter what is done in surgery or anesthesia, the neuromuscular condition must be carefully assessed perioperatively to verify that no extension of the neurologic lesion and no decrease in function have occurred.

Specific Problems

The infant and young child with neuromuscular disease have all of the combined associated problems of pediatrics and neurology. Both maternal drug intake and disease are pertinent. Gestational age and body weight determine fluid and electrolyte replacement and drug dosages.

Geriatric patients may have the primary lesion of the neuromuscular system in addition to the associated cardiac and respiratory problems of their age and general condition. They may have a lack of reserve in one or all bodily systems.

Specific Techniques

1. Hypothermia is not indicated in the patient with acute spinal cord injury. Although hypothermia is used frequently in neurosurgery for aneurysms or similar conditions, its use here is controversial and not recommended.
2. Controlled hypotension may be used in extensive operations in patients with intact neurologic systems. When vascular damage or injury to the cord has occurred or the patient is neurologically unstable, controlled hypotension is to be avoided.
3. Extracorporeal circulation may be used to correct whatever condition or abnormality may be present, and pertinent guidelines should be followed. With all of the above conditions, cardiopulmonary reserve should be assessed and considered perioperatively.

SUMMARY

The diagnosis and management of neuromuscular disease are in their infancy. Genetic studies and treatment are changing the approach to hereditary disease. Recent studies of normal and abnormal metabolism and function of the nervous system indicate a complexity of hormonal interactions. Anesthetic management must consider the basic pathology and functional reserve of the patient coupled with the benefit of the contemplated surgery. When it is believed that the induction and management of anesthesia cannot be performed safely, either the patient should be transferred to a center where it can be done or the surgery should be postponed until the patient is in better condition. Whenever this is not possible, a full disclosure of the risks and potential benefits should be made to both the patient and the family so that a prudent and complete informed consent is possible. At all times, strict attention to detail is mandatory.

REFERENCES

1. Stover SL, ed. *Spinal cord injury: The facts and figures.* Birmingham: University of Alabama; 1986:57–59.

1a. DeVivo MJ, Stover SL, Black KJ. Prognostic factors for 12-year survival after spinal cord injury. *Arch Phys Med Rehabil.* 1992;73:156–162.

2. Zane DF, Preece MJ. *Texas Preventable Disease News.* Injury Control Program, Epidemiological Division, Texas Department of Health. January 26,1991;51:1.

2a. Reported traumatic spinal cord injuries in Texas (January–September, 1991). Injury Control Program, Epidemiology Division, Texas Department of Health. Houston, Texas. October 28, 1991.

3. Katz J, Benumof J, Kadis LB. *Anesthesia and uncommon diseases. Pathophysiologic and clinical correlations.* 2nd ed. Philadelphia: WB Saunders; 1981.

4. Stehling L, Zauder HL. *Anesthetic implications of congenital anomalies in children.* New York: Appleton-Century-Crofts; 1980.

5. Jones HR Jr, Netter FH, Trench AH. *Diseases of the peripheral motor–sensory unit. Clinical Symposia.* Summit, NJ: Ciba-Geigy; 1985;37:1–32.

6. Milne B, Rosales JK. Anaesthetic considerations in patients with muscular dystrophy undergoing spinal fusion and Harrington rod insertion. *Can Anaesth Soc J.* 1982;29:250–254.

7. Smith CL, Bush GH. Anaesthesia and progressive muscular dystrophy. *Br J Anaesth.* 1985;57:1113–1118.

8. Wang JM, Stanley TH. Duchenne muscular dystrophy and malignant hyperthermia—Two case reports. *Can Anaesth Soc J.* 1986;33:492–497.

9. Sethna NF, Rockoff MA, Worthen HM, Rosnow JM. Anesthesia-related complications in children with Duchenne muscular dystrophy. *Anesthesiology.* 1988;68:462–465.

10. Larsen UT, Juhl B, Hein-Sorensen O, Olivarius BF. Complications during anaesthesia in patients with Duchenne's muscular dystrophy (a retrospective study). *Can J Anaesth.* 1989;36:418–422.

11. Murat I, Esteve C, Montay G, Delleur MM, Gaudiche O, Saint-Maurice C. Pharmacokinetics and cardiovascular effects of bupivacaine during epidural anesthesia in children with Duchenne muscular dystrophy. *Anesthesiology.* 1987;67:249–252.

12. Hody JL. Regional anesthesia in myopathic children. *Acta Anaesth Belg.* 1988;39(suppl 2):209–213.

13. Dresner DL, Ali HH. Anaesthetic management of a patient with facioscapulohumeral muscular dystrophy. *Br J Anaesth.* 1989;62:331–334.

14. Goldberg MH, McNeish L, Clarizzio L. Correction of facial-skeletal deformities in two patients with facio-scapulo-humeral muscular dystrophy. *J Oral Maxillofac Surg.* 1989;47:996–999.

15. Karhunen U. Serum creatine kinase levels after succinylcholine in children with "muscle, eye, and brain disease." *Can J Anaesth.* 1988;35:90–92.

16. Nalda Felipe MA, Gottman S, Khambatta HJ. *Malignant hyperthermia: Current concepts.* Englewood, NJ: Normed Verlag; 1989.

17. Sjogren P, Pedersen T, Steinmetz H. Mucopolysaccharidoses and anaesthetic risks. *Acta Anaesthesiol Scand.* 1987;31:214–218.

18. Defalque RJ. Anesthesia for a patient with Kufs' disease. *Anesthesiology.* 1990;73:1041–1042.

19. Redfern N, McQuillan PJ, Conacher ID, Pearson DT. Anaesthesia for trans-sternal thymectomy in myasthenia gravis. *Ann R Coll Surg Engl.* 1987;69:289–292.

20. Rowbottom SJ. Isoflurane for thymectomy in myasthenia gravis. *Anaesth Intensive Care.* 1989;17:444–447.

21. Smith CE, Donali F, Bevan DR. Cumulative dose–response curves for atracurium in patients with myasthenia gravis. *Can J Anaesth.* 1989;36:402–406.

22. Nilsson E, Muller K. Neuromuscular effects of isoflurane in patients with myasthenia gravis. *Acta Anaesthesiol Scand.* 1990;34:126–131.

23. Gracey DR, Divertie MB, Howard FM Jr, Spencer-Payne W. Postoperative respiratory care after transsternal thymectomy in myasthenia gravis. A 3-year experience in 53 patients. *Chest.* 1984;86:67–71.

24. Eisenkraft JB, Papatestas AE, Kahn CH, Mora CT, Fagerstrom R, Genkins G. Predicting the need for postoperative mechanical ventilation in myasthenia gravis. *Anesthesiology.* 1986;65:79–82.

25. Herz BL. Colonic anastomotic disruption in myasthenia gravis. Report of two cases. *J Dis Colon Rectum.* 1987;30:809–811.

26. Lambert EH, Rooke ED. Myasthenic state and lung cancer. In: Brain RL, Norris FH, eds. *Remote effects of cancer on the nervous system.* New York: Grune & Stratton; 1965:67.

27. Melnick B, Chang JL, Larson CE, Bedger RC. Hypokalemic familial periodic paralysis. *Anesthesiology.* 1983;58:263–265.

28. Feurstein V. [Report on familial paroxysmal hypokalaemic paralysis in relation to postoperative intensive care.] *Anaesthesist.* 1980;29:632–634.

29. Rooney RT, Shanahan EC, Sun T, Nally B. Atracurium and hypokalemic familial periodic paralysis. *Anesth Analg.* 1988;67:782–783.

30. Lema G, Urzua J, Moran S, Canessa R. Successful anesthetic management of a patient with hypokalemic familial periodic paralysis undergoing cardiac surgery. *Anesthesiology.* 1991;74:373–375.

31. Aarons JJ, Moon RE, Camporesi EM. General anesthesia and hyperkalemic periodic paralysis. *Anesthesiology.* 1989;71:303–304.

32. Kubal K, Pasricha SH, Bhargava M. Spinal anesthesia in a patient with Friedreich's ataxia. *Anesth Analg.* 1991;72:257–258.

33. Roelofse JA, Shipton EA. Anaesthesia in connective tissue disorders. *South Afr Med J.* 1985;67:336–339.

34. Dillman JB. Safe use of succinylcholine during repeated anesthetics in a patient treated with cyclophosphamide. *Anesth Analg.* 1987;66:351–353.

35. Naclerios S, Bassetta P, Sorgente F, et al. The Ehlers–Danlos syndrome and its surgical implications. *Clin Ther.* 1990;132:235–248.

36. Eriksson P, Boman K, Jacobsson B, Olofsson BO. Cardiac arrhythmias in familial amyloid polyneuropathy during anesthesia. *Acta Anaesthesiol Scand.* 1986;30:317–320.

37. Vaghadia H. Facial paresis after general anesthesia. Report of an unusual case: Heerfordt's syndrome. *Anesthesiology.* 1986;64:513–514.

38. Thomas DW, Mason RA. Complete heart block during anaesthesia in a patient with sarcoidosis. *Anaesthesia.* 1988;43:578–580.

39. Stenqvist O, Sigurdsson J. The anaesthetic management of a patient with familial dysautonomia. *Anaesthesia.* 1982;37:929–932.

40. Gibbons PA, Lee IS. Scoliosis and anesthesia. *Int Anesth Clin.* 1985;23:149–161.

41. Diaz JH, Lockhart CH. Postoperative quadriplegia after spinal fusion for scoliosis with intraoperative awakening. *Anesth Analg.* 1987;66:1039–1042.

42. Phillips WA, Hensinger RN. Control of blood loss during scoliosis surgery. *Clin Orthop.* 1988;229:88–93.

43. Dahm LS, Dickson JH, Harrison GH. Peri-operative and anesthetic management of the patient with scoliosis. *Anesth Rev.* 1982;9:3–20.

44. Libman RH. Anesthetic considerations for the patient with osteogenesis imperfecta. *Clin Orthop.* 1981;159:123–125.

45. Ryan CA, Al-Ghambi AS, Gayle M, Finer NN. Osteogenesis imperfecta and hyperthermia. *Anesth Analg.* 1989;68:811–814.

46. Masuda Y, Harada Y, Honma E, Ichimiya T, Namiki A. Anesthetic management of a patient with osteogenesis imperfecta. *Jpn J Anesth.* 1990;39:383–387.

47. Berkowitz ID, Raja SN, Bender KS, Kopits SE. Dwarfs: Pathophysiology and anesthetic implications. *Anesthesiology.* 1990;73:739–759.

48. Wardall GJ, Frame WT. Extradural anaesthesia for caesarean section in achondroplasia. *Br J Anaesth.* 1990;64:367–370.

49. Albin MS, ed. *Acute spinal cord injury. Critical care clinics.* Philadelphia: WB Saunders; Especially Babinski MJ. Anesthetic considerations in the patient with acute spinal cord injury. 1987;3:619–636.

50. Schonwald G, Fish KJ, Perkash I. Cardiovascular complications during anesthesia in chronic spinal cord injured patients. *Anesthesiology.* 1981;55:550–558.

51. Muller H, Sarges R, Jouaux J, Runte W, Lampante L. Intraoperative suppression of spasticity using intrathecal baclofen. *Anaesthetist.* 1990;39:22–25.

Care of the Cancer Patient

Hollis E. Bivens

Anesthesia for the patient undergoing cancer surgery is no different from that administered to patients having other types of surgery. Techniques and methods are, of necessity, those used for other types of surgery. The difference lies in the overall condition of the patient. The effects of previous surgery, chemotherapy, and radiotherapy, as well as various disease states, alter the patient's response to anesthesia.

PREOPERATIVE EVALUATION

History and Physical Examination

As required for any diagnostic evaluation, a thorough history and physical examination are of utmost importance. A history of cardiac disease including date of infarct, surgery, medication, and electrocardiographic changes is particularly significant. Consultation with a cardiologist who is familiar with the side effects of chemotherapeutic agents, radiation, and extent of surgery is necessary in all patients with abnormal heart functions. A cardiologist who visits the operating room frequently and is familiar with the implications of anesthesia, surgery, current techniques, and problems of perioperative care will be knowledgeable as to how the patient will respond to the planned procedures. Patients who obviously cannot survive surgery may be directed toward other therapeutic modalities. Cardiac disease in the cancer patient should be controlled to the greatest extent possible before anesthesia induction.[1] The patient taking cardiac medication should be stabilized and continued on the appropriate dosage throughout the operative period.

Alcoholic patients frequently have hypertension, anemia, cardiac disease, cirrhosis, malnutrition, and dehydration in addition to cancer. Lesions of the alimentary tract may interfere with the patient's ability to eat (Figs. 46–1, 46–2, and 46–3). A program of hyperalimentation may be required to correct protein and electrolyte imbalances. Lesions of the lips (Fig. 46–4), buccal mucosa, tongue, gingiva, pharynx, trachea, and lungs are associated not only with smoking but also with alcohol abuse. In these patients,

it is not unusual to elicit a history of Guillain-Barré syndrome or acute intermittent porphyria that will directly influence the selection of anesthetic agents.

Environmental history may be of significance in patient evaluation as there is an increased incidence of cancer in patients exposed to environmental irritants. Exposure to various chemicals, nuclear radiation, sunlight, dust, and other agents may create conditions that affect the response to anesthesia. These conditions include liver and kidney damage, serum cholinesterase deficiency, anemia, and pulmonary lesions. Physical examination may reveal both unsuspected and grossly obvious variations or abnormalities that would interfere with placement of intravenous catheters, intraarterial catheters, endotracheal tubes, nasogastric tubes, electrocardiogram (ECG) electrodes, temperature monitors, and other equipment (Figs. 46–5 and 46–6).

Laboratory Examination

The laboratory examination should include, at the minimum, a sequential multiple-analyzer battery (serum glutamic–pyruvic transaminase, bilirubin, creatinine, albumin, total protein, glucose, and blood urea nitrogen determinations), a coagulation profile (which includes prothrombin time and partial thromboplastin time), measurement of hematocrit and hemoglobin, and urinalysis. In any patient taking antihypertensive medication, diuretics, cardiac medication, anticancer agents, or other medications, there may be a marked variation in serum electrolytes, especially potassium. Because these values may change within a few hours and electrolyte concentrations exert profound influence on myocardial function and drug action, the examination should be performed within 48 hours before anesthesia induction. This allows time for some corrective measures to be taken if they are necessary.

Obviously, liver function studies and enzymes are significant when a hepatic tumor or other disease produces abnormal values. Coagulation studies may indicate that bleeding problems should be anticipated during surgery or that anticoagulants are being administered and not recognized. Hematocrit and hemoglobin values must be correlated with

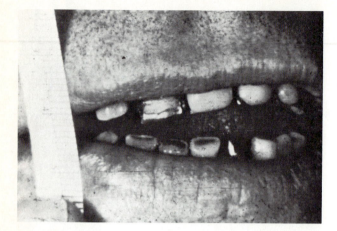

Figure 46–1. Lesion of the temporomandibular joint restricts oral opening to less than 1 cm.

the patient's clinical status. Low values may indicate a need for preoperative transfusions, early replacement of blood loss, or, if chronically low, careful monitoring of blood loss and minimal replacement.

Radiologic Examination

Radiologic examination frequently offers a synopsis of the extent of metastatic disease, allowing prior planning for surgery as a part of the overall plan of therapy or as the primary mode of treatment. Intracranial lesions require meticulous anesthetic management to prevent wide fluctuations in intracranial pressure. Chest roentgenograms may show evidence of intrathoracic tumors with obstruction, pulmonary effusion, pericardial effusion, or atelectasis that will have a direct effect on the administration of anesthesia. Bone lesions or pathologic fractures found on radiologic examination require careful patient movement and positioning.

As previously mentioned, complete cardiac evaluation is mandatory in all patients with a history of cardiovascular disease.[2] Cardiac evaluation should begin with a standard

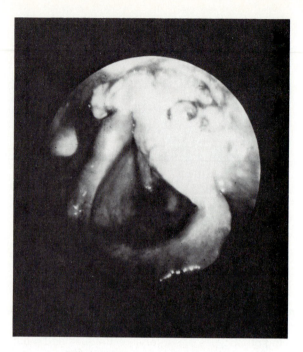

Figure 46–3. Lesion of the glottis.

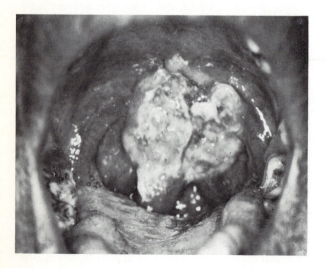

Figure 46–4. Nasal and lip lesion.

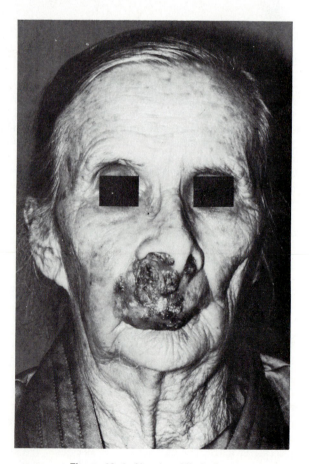

Figure 46–2. Lesion of the hard palate.

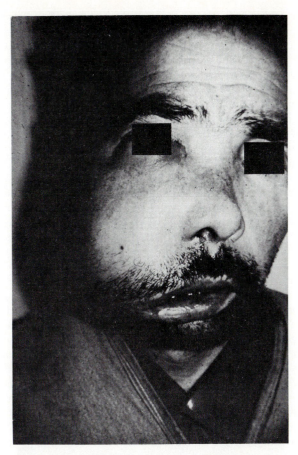

Figure 46–5. Maxillary lesion distorts entire airway.

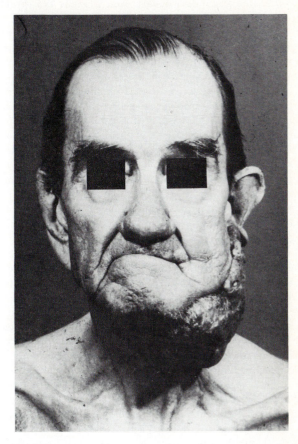

Figure 46–6. Lesion of the neck and mandible obstructs airway.

12-lead ECG in these patients as well as in all patients older than 40 years of age.

Pulmonary disease in the cancer patient is not confined to a primary or metastatic tumor. Emphysema, chronic obstructive pulmonary disease, bronchitis, previous surgery, previous infection, and chemotherapy may produce varying degrees of respiratory insufficiency. Pulmonary function studies provide an indication of the patient's ability to withstand the planned procedure, particularly if thoracic surgery is necessary. The additional data available from catheterization of the right side of the heart are required in those patients with recent myocardial infarction, respiratory failure requiring positive end-expiratory pressure (PEEP) greater than 15 cm H_2O, and sepsis. In such patients, a pulmonary artery catheter should be used throughout the operative procedure.

Medication History

A thorough medication history may be very significant in the perioperative care of the cancer patient. Drugs unlikely to be used in the noncancer population must be identified.[3–12] Chemotherapy with doxorubicin (Adriamycin) may produce cardiotoxic effects such as (1) early ECG abnormalities with multiple variations and (2) cumulative, dose-dependent, drug-induced cardiomyopathy. Most of the ECG changes are transient and revert to the original pat-

terns within 1 to 2 months of discontinuation of treatment. Cumulative, dose dependent, drug-induced cardiomyopathy produces congestive heart failure in patients receiving a cumulative dose of more than 550 mg/m^2 surface area and has also been reported at lower doses. Patients with evidence of doxorubicin cardiotoxicity must be managed carefully, using central venous pressure, blood pressure, and urinary output to monitor appropriate fluid administration. Patients with severe alteration of left ventricular function or in whom massive blood loss is anticipated should have a pulmonary artery catheter inserted preoperatively.[13]

Daunorubicin induces cardiomyopathy similar to that produced by doxorubicin; however, this is not amenable to early detection. The time from cessation of therapy to manifestation of cardiomyopathy varies from 2 to 1348 days, with the range usually 3 to 6 months after the first dose.[14]

Bleomycin is frequently used in the therapy of testicular carcinoma and may produce pulmonary fibrosis, predisposing the patient to development of acute adult respiratory distress syndrome (ARDS) postoperatively. The tissue damage produced in the lung by bleomycin is very similar to that seen in oxygen toxicity.[15] Attention must be given to the maintenance of adequate blood gas values and oxygen saturation. This may require the administration of oxygen in concentrations of 30 to 100 percent. There is some evidence in the literature that oxygen concentration is not a factor in the respiratory failure seen in some bleomycin-treated patients.

Cisplatin, another frequently used agent, produces a persistent decrease in glomerular filtration rate and may precipitate irreversible renal failure. There are some reports of possible cardiotoxicity from its use.

Plasma cholinesterase (pseudocholinesterase) enzyme activity is known to be depressed in the presence of cyclophosphamide (Cytoxan), a drug frequently used in the treatment of both neoplastic and nonneoplastic diseases. This enzyme inhibition may significantly prolong the duration of succinylcholine neuromuscular blocking action with extended periods of respiratory depression. Those who administer anesthesia to patients who have received cyclophosphamide therapy should be aware of its effects on succinylcholine action and provide proper neuromuscular monitoring.[16,17]

Cyclophosphamide, usually given in doses of 1 to 3 mg/kg per day or 10 to 15 mg/kg per week, has the major toxic effect of bone marrow depression. Also, in some patients, high-dose regimens of 120 to 240 mg/kg given over 1 to 4 days have resulted in severe hemorrhagic cardiac necrosis.[18] Some patients develop angina following the use of 5-fluorouracil (5-FU). Most reports indicate mild or no ECG changes and the changes that were noted disappeared within a few hours of onset.[19]

Most chemotherapeutic agents given intravenously produce fibrosis of the vessels used, sometimes making it very difficult to locate a patent usable vein.[20] Painful dysesthesia is manifested by symmetric polyneuropathy with doses required to achieve an antineoplastic affect with the vinca alkaloids such as vincristine and vinblastine. The presence of this peripheral neuropathy might contraindicate the use of reginal anesthesia techniques.[21]

Patients with cancer are also susceptible to other diseases that require chronic drug therapy. The patient's condition and therapeutic dosage level should be stabilized to the degree possible before administration of anesthesia. Diabetics requiring insulin must be monitored carefully with urine and blood sugar testing and possibly arterial blood gas and electrolyte determinations. Crystalline insulin may be given intravenously during the procedure if necessary. Administration of a solution of 5 percent dextrose in water containing 15 units of crystalline insulin, at a rate of 60 to 100 mL/h, is a basic technique for control. Long-acting or intermediate-acting forms of insulin should not be given on the morning of surgery.

Steroid dosages should be increased during the perioperative period, with careful reduction in the postoperative phase. Cardiac glycosides, antihypertensives, diuretics, antiarrhythmics, and similar agents must be evaluated individually. Digitalis preparations should be continued with serum potassium level monitoring. Diuretics and antihypertensive agents should be continued until the morning of surgery. The early-morning dose should not be omitted even though the patient is NPO (nothing by mouth). This is especially true if the patient is on an agent with a short therapeutic life, for example, clonidine. Beta-adrenergic blocking agents (propranolol) should be given the morning of surgery. The morning dose, or later doses if the patient is to be a late case, should be given as scheduled. Nitroglycerin paste applied to the skin before transport to the operating suite is very helpful in patients who have angina.

Monoamine oxidase inhibitors should be discontinued 2 to 3 weeks before anesthesia administration because of the variable effects of their interaction with anesthetic agents; this might not apply to some psychiatric patients. Although it is not necessary to discontinue α-methyldopa, blood bank personnel should be aware of its use when a type and cross-match are requested. Many patients using this drug show a positive direct Coombs test.

Because of underlying infection, immunosuppression from chemotherapy and radiation, and the extent of surgery, prophylactic antibiotics are used frequently. The possibility of interaction between drugs used during anesthesia and certain of these agents makes awareness of the specific antibiotics significant.

The type and location of the patient's lesion plus the effects of radiation and chemotherapy frequently cause severe malnutrition and dehydration. Obviously, such conditions can produce drastic alterations in hepatic, renal, and cardiovascular functions. The patient's response to anesthetic agents will be exaggerated. Hyperalimentation, blood component therapy, and fluid replacement should be instituted as far in advance of anesthesia administration as possible.

Drug-induced secondary anemia, leukopenia, and thrombocytopenia; pancytopenia from bone marrow metastases; anemia from gastrointestinal bleeding, hemolysis, or defective iron utilization in chronic disease; effects of increasing age; underlying, low-grade infection; and, particularly, recent myocardial infarction must also be considered when assessing the patient's overall condition before anesthesia induction and surgery.

ANESTHESIA

Selection of the anesthetic should be related to the patient's overall condition, although the agent itself is not a major consideration in anesthetic management.[22] Patients with abnormal liver function are not generally given halogenated agents. Inhalation agents should be considered in those patients who have chronic obstructive pulmonary disease. (At The University of Texas M. D. Anderson Cancer Center, approximately 95 percent of anesthetics are administered with a balanced narcotic–muscle relaxation–inhalation agent technique.) Although isoflurane is the primary inhalation agent used, halothane can be used for pediatric patients. Enflurane is no longer used because of its renal effects. Nitrous oxide is used sparingly. Compressed air is often used with oxygen and the volatile agents. Regional anesthesia, when appropriate, should always be considered.

Most cancer surgery is considered to be of a radical nature, and management of radical surgery patients requires continuous evaluation of alterations in the patient's condition. Continuous monitoring of the ECG, blood pressure, respiration, delivered oxygen concentration, tidal/minute volume, end-tidal carbon dioxide, pulse oximetry, heart rate, heart sounds, blood loss, degree of muscle relaxation, and temperature is recommended in every patient. In those patients with cardiovascular abnormalities, pulmonary disease, renal disease, hepatic dysfunction, metabolic disorders, massive blood loss, and other conditions, it may be necessary to routinely monitor urinary output, central venous pressure, direct arterial pressure, cardiac output, arterial blood gases, serum electrolytes, urine and blood glucose, and coagulation parameters. Routine electroencephalographic monitoring is practiced in some institutions for major vascular, intracranial, and other procedures.

As in any procedure, adequate ventilation must be maintained. A volume ventilator should be used in any procedure lasting longer than 30 minutes. Proper positioning and placement of support rolls aid ventilation.

Heating and cooling units should be used to maintain body temperature in all patients. Warm irrigating solutions, intravenous solutions, blood, and control of room temperature also assist in maintaining adequate patient temperature. Heating and humidification of inspired gases have proven to be particularly advantageous in maintaining body temperature.

Because of the altered physiologic condition of many cancer patients, it is important to position the patient properly, use adequate padding at pressure points, avoid excessive pressure when moving the patient, protect the eyes, and place protective barriers to prevent excess stretching, compression, and pressure on nerve and blood vessels from equipment or personnel during the procedure. Various arm, leg, chest, and head supports assist in proper positioning. Careful placement of the electrosurgery unit grounding pad is necessary to avoid excess pressure, burns, or cardiac effects. Positioning of the patient and equipment should be considered the responsibility of the entire operating team.

Large-bore intravenous catheters are mandatory during radical surgical procedures. Cannulation of the internal jugular or subclavian vein for monitoring central venous pressure or administering fluids, or both, should be considered in most patients.

Although the admonition to administer anesthesia gently should be applied to every patient, it is particularly appropriate for cancer patients as they are generally in poor physiologic condition and are highly susceptible to anesthetic agents. Their responses may be exaggerated and difficult to control. Slow induction progressing to an adequate depth of anesthesia for intubation and surgery is important to avoid stress and its effects on the patient. Constant communication and cooperation must be maintained between members of the operating team, the laboratory, and the blood bank. Changes in ventilation, circulation, and stimulation should be discussed and planned for in advance. Unexpected, abrupt changes must be communicated immediately. Fluid and blood replacement is based on blood loss, intravascular volume, urinary output, central venous pressure, arterial blood pressure, and the specific procedure being performed.

To meet the need for continuous assessment of anesthetic administration, muscle relaxation, monitoring equipment data, laboratory examination results, and administration of blood components and fluids, more than one person must be available to manage a patient undergoing radical cancer surgery. During critical times of rapid blood replacement, severe alterations in cardiovascular stability, or

changes in electrolyte and coagulation parameters, an anesthesia care team made up of several members may be required. A sufficient number of anesthesiology staff should be available in the operating suite constantly to assist with complex cases.

Reversal of narcotic and muscle relaxant effects must be monitored with the peripheral nerve stimulator and respirometer. If it is necessary to maintain assisted or controlled ventilation in the postoperative period, antagonism of these agents is undesirable. There must be satisfactory muscle strength and tidal volume if the patient is to be extubated in the operating room. Supplemental oxygen and pulse oximetry should be provided during transport from the operating room to the postanesthesia care unit (PACU) for all patients who receive general anesthesia or regional anesthesia. Assisted ventilation by use of an Ambu bag with oxygen supplement may be necessary during transport. Continuous arterial blood pressure and ECG monitoring may be performed with a battery-powered portable monitor. Portable suction devices are also available. Heating and cooling units with warm blankets should be used during the immediate recovery period.

Routine care in the recovery room should include monitoring of ECG, blood pressure, heart rate, respiratory rate and volume, temperature, peripheral oxygen saturation, urine output, rate of fluid administration, and administration of humidified oxygen. Monitoring of central venous pressure, direct arterial pressure, and Swan–Ganz catheter pressures and mechanical respiratory assistance may also be necessary. The patient's condition and care must be followed by personnel familiar with his or her status throughout the entire recovery phase and for at least 24 hours postoperatively.

SPECIAL CONSIDERATIONS

Cancer patients are highly susceptible to infection because of the immunosuppressive effects of radiation, chemotherapy, and frequently malnourishment.[23] Therefore, all equipment and supplies used must be sterilized or cleaned as completely as possible. All invasive items must be sterile, and most of these items, such as endotracheal tubes, breathing circuits, intravascular catheters, intravenous fluid administration sets, blood filters, pressure transducer lines and units, suction catheters, nasogastric tubes, esophageal stethoscopes, temperature probes, and regional block trays, are disposable. Double-lumen endobronchial tubes, armored endotracheal tubes, and preformed, specialized tracheostomy tubes are also available in disposable form, and their use should be considered. Reusable items, such as ventilator bellows, forceps, and laryngoscope blades, should be sterilized, preferably by ethylene oxide gas sterilization.

Adequate aeration of absorbent material must be accomplished before reuse. Fiberoptic laryngoscopes and bronchoscopes should be cold sterilized. Blood pressure cuffs and laryngoscope handles should be thoroughly cleaned after each use. Ventilators, warming blankets and units, anesthesia machines, monitoring units, tables, and other equipment should be cleaned after each case.

The use of Bain and Mapleson D disposable breathing

circuits should be considered in pediatric patients and some adult patients where nonrebreathing techniques are advisable. Use of the laser in the trachea poses a major risk of fire in the airway. Any endotracheal tube used must be either nonflammable or protected against ignition.[24,25]

The appropriate use of various blood components is obviously determined by their availability, rapport with the blood bank, and the time required for transportation to the operating room. Packed red blood cells diluted with saline are generally given as replacement for blood loss. Fresh whole blood may be required in some cases. All blood should be warmed before administration. Fresh-frozen plasma should be used as necessary. Plasma expanders such as plasma protein fraction and hetastarch may be useful. Intravenous fluids given throughout the procedure, such as Plasmosol and Ringer's lactate, should be regulated by the patient's needs and not given on a purely routine basis.

Patients with rare blood types, those for whom blood is not readily available, or those who will not accept blood transfusions because of religious or other beliefs may benefit from the use of a blood cell separator or cell saver.[26] This machine is normally used in blood banks for the collection of platelets and white blood cells from donors. The blood cell separator allows blood to be removed from the body at one rate and simultaneously returned at another. The reservoir of red cells so formed is kept in constant contact with the body through a closed loop (Fig. 46–7) and returned as needed.

As in all operating rooms, waste gases should be evacuated to protect the operating team. Gases should be removed from the adjustable pressure-limiting (APL) valve of the anesthesia machine and ventilator by an exhaust system separate from the vacuum used at the operating table. Air exchange within the room should be great enough to remove gases expelled when the machine is disconnected from the patient for a short time, for example, during intubation. Frequent inspection of all connections with collection and analysis of air samples at various locations must be made to maintain an atmosphere free of waste gases.

The normal body temperature of pediatric patients is more difficult to maintain compared with that of adults. It is frequently necessary to warm and humidify the operating room in addition to using a warming blanket on the operating table. For infants, use of an infrared warming unit may be advisable.

Although standardization of equipment, supplies, and location is not restricted to cancer centers, such standardization is important in large operating suites. Standard equipment throughout the suite allows parts and modules to be interchanged. The specification of locations for supplies and equipment in each room reduces confusion when personnel assignments are changed and especially during emergency situations when time for obtaining supplies is critical. Familiarity with equipment throughout the operating suite is important in total patient care.

Regional perfusion with chemotherapeutic agents for nonmetastatic lesions is usually performed in patients in whom an early diagnosis has been made. This technique allows much higher doses of the agent to be applied directly to the tumor than can be tolerated by whole-body administration.

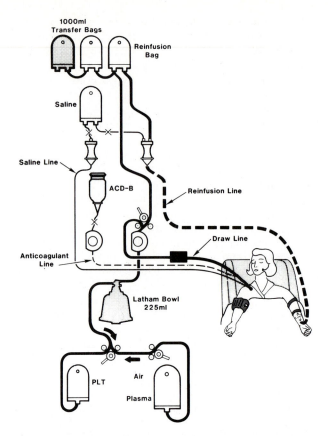

Figure 46–7. Diagram of the path used to draw, store, and reinfuse blood. ACD-B, acid–citrate–dextrose formula B; PLT, platelets.

Intraoperative radiotherapy (IORT), a specialized, direct technique for treating deep-seated cancers with doses of radiation higher than can safely be achieved by external-beam irradiation alone, is now being administered in several institutions. An electron beam-generating linear accelerator in a specially constructed central operating room with appropriate remote-controlled television cameras and anesthesia monitoring equipment administers IORT for patients with advanced gastrointestinal malignancies. One advantage of a linear accelerator is the high dose rate resulting in treatment times of only 2 to 3 minutes during which the patient is unattended inside the operating room but monitored remotely. Various treatment protocols have been established using preoperative external-beam radiotherapy with concomitant continuous-infusion systemic chemotherapy followed by electron beam intraoperative radiotherapy (EB-IORT). Preliminary experience indicates that the boost of EB-IORT has the potential to improve local control and possibly survival for patients with pancreatic and locally advanced colorectal cancer[27,28] (Rich T. Personal communication, 1991).

Subarachnoid alcohol block and celiac plexus alcohol block for control of intractable pain in advanced malignant disease should be considered in some patients with pancreatic neoplasm and other intraabdominal metastases.[29] Alcohol blocks provide long-lasting relief without the need for frequent injections. Nerve blocks with local anesthetics are very useful as diagnostic aids and for temporary relief of pain. These procedures carry a minimal risk of mortality and complications and can be performed in debilitated patients.

Patients with cancer are a special group with unique characteristics and needs. All therapy, including anesthesia for surgery and specific nerve blocks for pain relief, must be structured to meet the individual patient's needs.

The author acknowledges the contributions of Rebecca S. Williams and Rodney C. Lester to this chapter.

REFERENCES

1. DeVita V, Hellwan S, Rosenberg S, eds. *Cancer: Principles and practice of oncology.* 2nd ed. Philadelphia: JB Lippincott; 1985.
2. Ewer M, Ali M. Surgical treatment of the cancer patient: Preoperative assessment and perioperative medical management. *Surg Oncol.* 1990;44:185–190.
3. Selvin BL. Cancer chemotherapy: Implication for the anesthesiologist. *Anesth Analg.* 1981;60(6):425–434. Review Article.
4. Desiderio DP. Cancer chemotherapy: Complications and interactions with anesthesia. *Hosp Formul.* 1990;25:176–185.
5. Chung F. Cancer, chemotherapy and anaesthesia. *Can Anaesth Soc J.* 1982;29(4):364–371.
6. deCunha MF. Immunopathological and clinical correlates in immunocompromised patients. *Anesth Today.* 1990;1(3):1–6.
7. Walton B. Anesthesia, surgery and immunology. *Anaesthesia.* 1978;33:322–348. Review Article.
8. Marsoni S, Witter R. Clinical development of anticancer agents—A National Cancer Institute perspective. *Cancer Treat Rep.* 1980;68:77.
9. Eyee H, Ward J. Control of cancer chemotherapy-induced nausea and vomiting. *Cancer.* 1984;54(suppl 1):2642–2648.
10. Laszlo J, ed. *Antiemetics and cancer chemotherapy.* Baltimore: Williams & Wilkins; 1983.
11. Seigel L, Lougo D. The control of chemotherapy-induced emesis. *Ann Intern Med.* 1981;95:352–359.
12. Carlon G. Anesthetic management of the immunocompromised cancer patient. *Anesth Today.* 1990;1(3):7–9.
13. Von Hoff D, Layard M, Basa P, et al. Risk factors for doxorubicin-induced congestive heart failure. *Ann Intern Med.* 1979; 91:710–717.
14. Von Hoff D, Rozensweig M, Layard M, et al. Daunomycin-induced cardiotoxicity in children and adults: A review of 220 cases. *Am J Med.* 1977;62:200–208.
15. LaMantia KR, Glick JH, Marshall BE. Supplemental oxygen does not cause respiratory failure in bleomycin-treated surgical patients. *Anesthesiology.* 1984;60:65–67.
16. Gurman G. Prolonged apnea after succinylcholine in a case treated with cytostatics for cancer. *Anesth Analg.* 1972;51: 761–765.
17. Dillman J. Safe use of succinylcholine during repeated anesthetics in a patient treated with cyclophosphamide. *Anesth Analg.* 1987;66:351–352.
18. Slavin R, Millan J, Mullins G. Pathology of high-dose intermittent cyclophosphamide therapy. *Hum Pathol.* 1975;6:693–709.
19. Dent R, McCall I. 5-Fluorouracil and angina. *Lancet.* 1975;1: 347–348. 1975.
20. Hirsh J, Conlon P. Implementing guidelines for managing extravasation of antineoplastics. *Am J Hosp Pharm.* 1983;40: 1516–1579.
21. Payne R. Postchemotherapy and postradiation syndromes. In: Foley KN, ed. *Management of cancer pain.* New York: Memorial Sloan Kettering Cancer Center; 1985:73–93.
22. Howland W, Gondiner P. Physiologic management of the cancer patient during surgery. *Curr Probl Cancer.* 1978;3:1–50.
23. Huffman L. Cross contamination during anesthesia: A serious threat to the immunocompromised patient. *Anesth Today.* 1990; 1(3):14–17.
24. Kirby R, ed. Laser-resistant endotracheal tubes and wraps. *Technol Anesth.* 1990;11(3).
25. Garry B, Bivens H. Anesthetic technique for safe laser use in surgery. *Semin Surg Oncol.* 1990;6:184–188.
26. Warfield M, ed. Routine machine solves the problem of transfusions for Jehovah's Witnesses. *Newsletter of the University of Texas System Cancer Center M. D. Anderson Hospital and Tumor Institute.* 1981;26:2.
27. Rich T. Intraoperative radiotherapy. *Radiother Oncol.* 1986;6: 207–221.
28. Rich T. Protracted continuous 5-FU infusion with concomitant radiation therapy: Results and indications. In: Rotman M, Rosenthal CJ, eds. *Concomitant infusion chemotherapy and radiation.* New York: Springer-Verlag; 1991.
29. Chiu W. Diagnostic and therapeutic nerve block for cancer pain. *Cancer Bull.* 1981;33:93–98.

Postoperative Care of the Surgical Patient

Cecil B. Drain

Anesthesia nursing care of the surgical patient conceptually begins in the preoperative phase, moves into the intraoperative phase, and ends after the postoperative phase. During each phase it is of utmost importance that appropriate, informed anesthesia nursing care is used to facilitate positive outcomes for the surgical patient. Anesthesia care in the postanesthesia care unit (PACU) has far-reaching implications as to whether the patient will survive even the best administered anesthetic. The role of the nurse anesthetist in the PACU is one of collaboration. The nurse anesthetist has expertise that can enhance the quality of nursing care administered in the PACU.

Postanesthesia nurses (PANs) are professional nurses who are well versed in postanesthesia and critical care nursing. Ideally the nurse : patient ratio in the PACU should be 1:1. PACU nursing is a recognized clinical specialty. The nurse anesthetist can collaborate with the PAN on many administrative matters and provide expert input into the clinical process in the PACU. This chapter discusses the basic care of the patient emerging from anesthesia and includes a complete discussion of common postoperative problems such as hypoxemia, hypercarbia, airway obstruction, hypotension, hypertension, hypothermia, pain, and nausea and vomiting.

POSTANESTHESIA CARE: ADMISSION PHASE

Postanesthesia care of the patient recovering from anesthesia is a critical part of the total anesthetic experience. It is imperative that the PAN and the nurse anesthetist collaborate during the admission phase to facilitate a positive surgical and anesthetic experience for the surgical patient.

Postanesthesia Report

Ideally, the surgeon and the nurse anesthetist should accompany the patient to the PACU, where the nurse anesthetist should give the following information to the PAN[1]:

1. Patient's name, sex, age, hospital number, height and weight, and native language including communication handicaps, if any
2. Surgical procedure, including the name(s) of the surgeon(s), complications, and surgical and anesthesia times
3. Anesthetic technique and all agents used for the procedure including preoperative medication and reversal agents
4. Intraoperative course including vital signs, estimated blood loss, urine output, fluid therapy, and monitoring techniques (e.g., laboratory and radiologic studies) used during the procedure
5. Previous medical history including American Society of Anesthesiologists (ASA) physical status, baseline vital signs, medications, mental status, drug addiction history, allergies, and any other disease processes that would have an impact on the postanesthesia care

Postoperative management should be elaborated on. Areas of concentration should include oxygen therapy, breathing exercises, airway care, pain management, diagnostic tests, and, if indicated, mechanical ventilation. The anesthetist and PAN should mutually determine the postanesthesia recovery score.

Postanesthesia Recovery Score

At the completion of the postanesthesia report, the PAN and the nurse anesthetist should conduct an assessment of the patient to determine the postanesthesia recovery score (PARS).[2] This score aids both the PAN and the anesthetist in a collaborative effort to determine the focus of postanesthesia care and potential postoperative problems and to develop discharge criteria for the patient.

The PARS should be initiated when the patient is admitted to the PACU. Jointly, the nurse anesthetist and the PAN who will be providing direct nursing care to the patient conduct the PARS assessment. The nursing assessment using the PARS system should be repeated every 15 minutes by the same PAN to verify the patient's improvement or deterioration. The five primary areas of assessment in the PARS are activity, respiration, circulation, consciousness, and color. A PACU patient can receive 0, 1, or 2 points in each area of assessment, with 2 being the best score. A total score of 10 indicates that the patient is in the best possible condition, scores of 8 or 9 are considered safe, and a score of 7 or less is considered unsafe (Fig. 47–1). More specifically, the PARS system consists of the following criteria.[2]

Activity. Muscular activity is assessed by observing the patient's ability to move his or her limbs either spontaneously or on command. If the patient is able to move all four extremities, a score of 2 is given, if only two extremities can be moved, the score is 1, and if none of the extremities can be moved, a score of 0 is given. This evaluation is of particular importance when assessing patients who have received subarachnoid, epidural, brachial plexus, or Bier blocks.

Respiration. If the patient can deep breathe or perform the sustained maximal inspiration maneuver, can freely cough, and has normal respiratory rate and depth, a score of 2 is given. If the respiratory effort is labored or limited or if dyspnea is present, a score of 1 is given. If no spontaneous respiratory activity is evident and the condition necessitates ventilator or assisted respiration, the patient receives a score of 0.

Circulation. Because circulation is probably the most difficult to evaluate by a simple sign, blood pressure evaluated by comparing the reading derived in the PACU with the baseline preanesthetic systolic blood pressure value is used. When the systolic arterial blood pressure is within plus or minus 20 percent of the preanesthetic baseline level, the patient receives a score of 2. If the systolic blood pressure is within plus or minus 21 to 50 percent of the same control level, a score of 1 is given. When the PACU systolic arterial blood pressure is plus or minus 51 percent or more from the baseline reading, a score of 0 is given.

Consciousness. If the PACU patient is fully alert, as evidenced by the ability to answer questions, a score of 2 is given. If the patient is aroused only when called by name, a score of 1 is given. A score of 0 is given when the patient does not respond to auditory stimulation. For this particular assessment parameter, painful stimulation should not be used because even decerebrated patients may react to the stimulus. In addition, in such patients, it is difficult to develop a consistent, reliable, practical method of assessment.

Color. Patients who have an obviously normal or pink skin color are given a score of 2. In patients in whom normal pigmentation of the skin prevents an accurate evaluation, the color of the oral mucosa should be assessed. If there is any alteration from the normal pink appearance that is not obvious cyanosis, the patient receives a score of 1; this includes pale, dusky, or blotchy discolorations as well as jaundice. When frank cyanosis is present, a score of 0 is given.

Postanesthesia Monitoring and Orders

The standards of care for the monitoring of the postanesthesia patient have been established by the American Society of Post Anesthesia Nurses (ASPAN).[2] Use of mechanical monitoring devices in the PACU is of the same magnitude as for any patient in a critical care setting. Consequently, all patients must be constantly monitored via a continuous cardiac monitor and a blood pressure monitor; oxygen saturation and pulse via pulse oximetry and body temperature are also monitored. Along with this, the patient's level of consciousness must be monitored. All vital signs should be documented, at the minimum, every 15 minutes. Following the assessment process, a short form can be used to document the appropriate patient data. In many hospitals, the routine postanesthesia orders are in a standardized format. These orders are usually countersigned by an anesthesiologist or the surgeon (Fig. 47–2).

Name _____ Age ____ Sex ____ Date _____
Arrival Time to PACU _____ Discharge Time from PACU _____
Type of Surgery _____ Surgeon _____
_____ Analgesics Administered in PACU
Anesthetic Agents & Drugs _____ Agent   Dosage Route   Time Given
_____ ____ ____ ____ _____
_____ ____ ____ ____ _____
Preoperative History _____ ____ ____ ____ _____
_____ ____ ____ ____ _____
Preoperative Vital Signs
BP ___ / ___   P ___   R ___   PAR Score at Admission _____
Temp _____   O$_2$ Saturation _____ %   PAR Score at Discharge _____

Figure 47–1. Chart for detailing the postanesthesia recovery score (PARS).

1. Administer oxygen at ___ L/min per ___ Mask ___ Cannula

2. Vital signs q 5 minutes for first 15 minutes then q 10 minutes

3. Continue IV from OR at ___ mL/h

4. Medications:
   a. Robinul 0.2–0.4 mg IV bolus if cardiac rate is less than ___ .
   b. Lidocaine 50 mg IV bolus stat for development of PVCs > 6 per minute.
   c. Ventricular tachycardia or bigeminy; call anesthesia.
   d. _____ IV for pain.

5. Endotracheal tube care
   a. Suction prn.
   b. Administer oxygen mist per T-tube with a F_{IO_2} of _____ .
   c. May be extubated when PARS criteria of _____ is met.
   d. Obtain ABGs _____ minutes following admission to PACU.

6. Notify anesthesia if:
   a. Blood pressure < _____ or > _____
   b. Respiration   < _____ or > _____
   c. Heart rate   < _____ or > _____
   d. Oxygen saturation < _____

Figure 47–2. Routine postoperative orders to be completed in the postanesthesia care unit (PACU). ABGs, arterial blood gases; OR, operating room; PVCs, premature ventricular contractions; PARS, postanesthesia recovery score. (*Adapted, with permission, from Orkin L, Shapiro G. Admission assessment and general monitoring. In: Frost E, Andrews I, eds.* Recovery room care. Int Anesthesiol Clin. *1983;21:5. Boston: Little, Brown; 1983.*)

POSTANESTHESIA CARE: INTERMEDIATE PHASE

Maintenance of Physiologic Parameters

Respiratory System. Pulmonary complications are the single leading cause of morbidity and mortality in the postoperative period.[3] An incidence of 4.5 to 76 percent (average of 11 percent) for pulmonary complications after abdominal operations has been reported. Most research has shown that the incidence of postoperative complications is highest after upper abdominal and thoracic surgery.

Atelectasis, or collapses of the alveoli, is a common postoperative pulmonary complication. Atelectasis accounts for more than 90 percent of postoperative pulmonary complications.[3] Normally, adults breathe regularly and rhythmically and spontaneously perform a maximal inspiration or sigh every 5 to 10 minutes.[4] During anesthesia and in the immediate postoperative period, sighless respirations occur. With this absence of the spontaneous deep breaths with an inspiratory hold, lung compliance decreases, resulting in lower alveolar volume. As these lung volumes decrease in the immediate postoperative period, transpulmonary pressure decreases. Without periodic lung hyperinflations with inspiratory holds (sigh), the surfactant may not be allowed to form an appropriate layer about the terminal bronchioles and alveoli. Ultimately, the surfactant becomes bunched. Inappropriate surfactant function increases surface tension within the alveoli, which causes a higher lung recoil, or a stiff lung. One of the lung volumes reduced in the postoperative period is the functional residual capacity (FRC). When the FRC decreases into the closing capacity (CC) range, the airways leading to dependent lung zones may be effectively closed throughout the respiratory cycle. Ultimately, atelectasis, hypoxemia, and pneumonia can result.[5]

To reverse the events that lead to reduction of the FRC, the patient should be encouraged to perform a sustained maximal inspiration (SMI) maneuver.[3] In this respiratory maneuver, the patient is encouraged to take a deep inspiration and, at the peak of inspiration, to hold the inspired air for 3 seconds, then to exhale the air. The volume excursion and inspiratory hold attained by the use of an incentive spirometer are similar to those obtained with the SMI maneuver. This maneuver will increase the patient's lung volumes and, consequently, will reinflate the collapsed alveoli. The SMI is believed to increase alveolar inflation time and volume, increase lung compliance, and allow the surfactant to layer out, thus promoting an increase in lung volumes, specifically the FRC, with the end result being a decrease in the amount of atelectasis and hypoxemia.

Anesthesia, surgery, immobility and the absence of an adequate cough maneuver are some factors that cause the patient to retain secretions. Research indicates that the forced expiratory volume in 1 second (FEV_1) is reduced in the immediate postoperative period.[3] It is important for the postanesthesia nurse to initiate the cough maneuver when the patient arrives in the PACU. The cascade cough is the most effective cough maneuver that can be used because the patient has a low FEV_1 in the immediate postoperative period.

To perform the cascade cough maneuver, the patient should be taught to take a slow deep inspiration, which will increase the lung volume and open the airways via a tethering effect, allowing air to pass beyond the secretions. At the peak of inspiration, the patient is encouraged to perform multiple "mini" coughs at succeeding lower lung volumes. With each "mini" cough during exhalation, the length of the airways undergoing dynamic compression increases, thus enhancing secretion clearance effectiveness. Patients with pulmonary pathology that includes a history of retained secretions benefit from chest percussion and postural drainage to enhance the movement of secretions to larger airways, where they can be removed by the cascade cough maneuver.

The original regimen of turn–cough–deep breathe has been significantly modified. Clinical research demonstrates that the SMI maneuver and the cascade cough are more effective in reducing the incidence of postoperative complications. Repositioning of the patient every 15 minutes during the immediate postoperative period aids in better matching of ventilation to perfusion ($\dot{V}/\dot{Q}$), and secretion clearance continues to be an important part of this regimen. Hence, the *modified stir-up regimen* consisting of turn–cascade cough–SMI should be used on every patient recovering from anesthesia in the PACU.[2]

Cardiovascular System. The main anesthetic consideration in regard to the cardiovascular system in the immediate postoperative period is maintenance of the patient's cardiac output.[6] The cardiac output (CO) is determined by the heart's effectiveness as a pump and the resistance to blood flow that occurs, mainly in the arteries. The systolic blood pressure reflects the amount of blood ejected during each left ventricular contraction, the speed of blood ejection, and the resistance of the aorta to blood flow. The diastolic pressure occupies about two thirds of the cardiac cycle and represents the rate at which the pressure in the aorta falls.

The methods of determining systolic and diastolic blood pressures are direct and indirect.[7] The direct method is an invasive technique that uses cannulation of an artery. The direct method is the most accurate way to determine blood pressure, but it carries a higher morbidity than does the indirect method. The indirect method is noninvasive and includes sphygmomanometry, ultrasonic detection, or photoelectric or manual palpation techniques. The sphygmomanometric method produces blood pressure values similar to those obtained by direct measurement of intraarterial pressures, especially when the pressure is within the range 100 to 160 torr. Above 160 torr, indirect measurements tend to underestimate true systolic pressure. Below 100 torr, overestimation occurs.[7] Doppler or ultrasound devices are more accurate than standard sphygmomanometers in the hypotensive patient.

The rate of cardiac contraction also serves to determine the cardiac output. Bradycardia may reduce cardiac output; however, the slow rate does not inhibit coronary artery filling time. Thus, the major clinical problem with bradycardia is reduced cardiac output. Tachycardia, besides increasing the cardiac oxygen demand, reduces the diastolic time needed for appropriate filling of the coronary arteries, and if severe, cardiac output may become ineffectual.

Cardiac arrhythmias, specifically supraventricular arrhythmias, also reduce the heart's effectiveness as a pump. This is because cardiac arrhythmias can reduce the rate and force of contraction.

In the PACU, alterations in cardiac output can and do occur. They may be caused by hypovolemia resulting from such processes as dehydration, hemorrhage, and positive airway pressure. Cardiac dysfunction as a result of ischemia or the depressant effects of anesthetic drugs and decreased peripheral vascular resistance as a result of sepsis and anesthetic drugs also produce alterations in cardiac output.

Bradycardia and arrhythmias can be caused by hypoxemia, excess anticholinesterase drugs, or pain. Tachycardia can result from hypovolemia, fever, shock, anxiety, hypoxemia, anticholinergic drugs, or pain.

Because many cardiovascular parameters of blood pressure, pulse, and electrical activities of the heart are affected by anesthesia and surgery, constant surveillance of the cardiovascular system is mandatory in the PACU. Monitoring equipment for the ASA Class I or II patients should include continuous ECG, pulse oximetry, blood

pressure measurement by cuff, and chest auscultation. If there is any difficulty in hearing the Korotkoff or heart sounds, a Doppler or ultrasound indirect blood pressure device should be used. The Swan–Ganz pulmonary arterial catheter can be added to the monitoring armamentarium for patients of ASA Class III or higher. This method of monitoring enables the postanesthesia nurse to assess the cardiac output, peripheral vascular resistance, and blood volume of the patient. In such a patient, urinary output should be monitored to provide an index of renal perfusion and overall adequacy of cardiac perfusion.

The postanesthesia blood pressure and pulse readings should be compared with the baseline readings taken preoperatively to determine their significance. Interventions for hypotension should include the administration of oxygen and the institution of the previously described modified stir-up regimen to help eliminate the anesthetic gases and thus accelerate the emergence process. If indicated, the rate of intravenous fluid therapy should be increased, and the legs should be elevated. It should be noted that patients recovering from spinal or epidural anesthesia who experience hypotension in the PACU usually resolve their hypotensive episode when these interventions are performed. If the hypotension is still not resolved, direct and indirect vasoactive agents may be administered.[8]

Bradycardia may be treated by the vigorous use of the modified stir-up regimen and oxygen. If the bradycardia is due to anticholinesterase drugs, atropine or glycopyrrolate (Robinul) should be titrated intravenously to raise the heart rate to an acceptable level. It should be noted that glycopyrrolate is the preferred drug in the awake PACU patient because it does not cross the blood–brain barrier.[9] Finally, if the bradycardia is due to arrhythmias, the arrhythmia should be identified, documented, and treated vigorously.

In general, the patient with previously normal cardiac function can tolerate tachycardia up to 160 beats per minute without deleterious sequelae. Tachycardia is a very important postoperative sign and should be aggressively evaluated and resolved in all patients. The first intervention for tachycardia is oxygen administration. If an underlying problem, such as hypovolemia, shock, fever, hypoxemia, or excess anticholinergic drug, is not present, the tachycardia is usually due to anxiety or pain. At that point, a narcotic agonist is indicated. Should the tachycardia persist, a beta-2 agonist should be considered.[9]

Common Problems in the Postanesthesia Care Unit

Hypoxemia. Hypoxemia, which is deficient oxygenation of the blood, is a relatively common entity that occurs in the PACU. Some possible causes of postoperative hypoxemia are a low inspired oxygen concentration, ventilation–perfusion mismatching ($\dot{V}/\dot{Q}$), hypoventilation, increased oxygen consumption, decreased cardiac output, or shunt.[10]

The clinical signs of hypoxemia include hypertension, hypotension, tachycardia, bradycardia, cardiac arrhythmias, restlessness, diaphoresis, dyspnea, and tachypnea. Cyanosis, which is defined as 5 g of reduced hemoglobin, is not a reliable sign of hypoxemia; however, an oxygen saturation below 90 percent is an excellent quantitative symptom of hypoxemia. Central nervous system symptoms of hypoxemia should be evaluated in the context of such other causes as pain, full bladder, and disorientation and restlessness caused by postoperative excitement and somnolence.

Therapy for the hypoxemia patient begins with a positive assessment of hypoxemia. Objective assessment using arterial blood gases with a PaO_2 of less than 60 torr or an oxygen saturation via a pulse oximeter of less than 90 percent indicates the presence of hypoxemia. Because anesthesia, surgery, and narcotics depress respiratory mechanics and response to carbon dioxide, room air is insufficient for all patients recovering from general anesthesia. The same holds true for regional anesthesia in which any type of sedation was used. Along with this, high spinal or epidural anesthetics produce a reduced ventilatory effort with resultant hypoxemia. Another justification for an increased inspired oxygen concentration is that many patients in the PACU may shiver, have a fever, or be in disoriented or restless states. Consequently, the initial intervention to relieve hypoxemia is an increased FIO_2. Also, the patient may require interventions that are designed specifically to combat the particular cause of the hypoxemia. Patients suffering from ventilation–perfusion mismatching, hypoventilation, and shunt will respond to a vigorous modified stir-up regimen along with chest physiotherapy.[2] Patients who demonstrate possible increased oxygen consumption by shivering should be warmed to near-normal body core temperature. Patients demonstrating emergence excitement from general anesthesia will have an increased oxygen consumption. This phenomenon occurs frequently after scopolamine premedication. Intravenous physostigmine 1 to 3 mg usually reverses the scopolamine-induced delirium and ultimately reverses the hypoxemia.

Hypercapnia. Elevated carbon dioxide tensions can and do occur in the immediate postoperative period. Many factors contribute to the development of hypercapnia, including a depressed central response to carbon dioxide, inadequate muscular forces to move air, oversedation, or an increase in metabolic rate.[10]

The pathophysiology leading to hypercapnia is centered on ventilation–perfusion mismatch and a blunting of the carbon dioxide response in the respiratory center of the brain.[4] This is particularly important in the PACU when patients experience emergence excitement, shivering, or hyperthermia, all of which increase the metabolic rate and ultimately carbon dioxide production. Because of the residual effects of anesthesia, the central response to carbon dioxide is blunted; consequently, carbon dioxide cannot be adequately removed, leading to carbon dioxide retention or hypercapnia.

Assessment of hypercarbia may be difficult because of possible depression of other physiologic systems. The only definitive determinant of hypercarbia is direct blood gas analysis; however, objective signs of hypercarbia include low tidal volume and rapid respiratory rate, tachycardia, hypertension, and sternal retractions. Many hypercapnic patients subjectively demonstrate restlessness, confusion, lassitude, and somnolence.

Preventive interventions for patients with hypercarbia include aggressive use of the modified stir-up regimen. If the patient continues to demonstrate objective and subjective signs of hypercarbia, reversal of the effects of anesthesia should be considered. If the residual anesthesia is due to narcotic depression, naloxone (Narcan), an opiate receptor antagonist, should be used. Because of the unpredictable duration of action of naloxone, careful titration to effect and close monitoring are mandated. Also, titration to effect can be used should further administration of naloxone be required. It must be remembered that naloxone does not reverse the respiratory depressant effects of barbiturates and tranquilizers. If the patient does not respond to the dose of naloxone, mechanical support of ventilation may be required.

Nalbuphine (Nubain), which is chemically related to both naloxone and the potent narcotic agonist oxymorphone, has been studied in the PACU for its agonist–antagonist properties. Clinically, it has been demonstrated that 5 mg of nalbuphine administered intravenously to a patient who has narcotic respiratory depression will reverse much of the respiratory depression, yet the patient will remain analgesic.[9]

If the residual effects of anesthesia are due to inadequate skeletal muscle relaxant reversal, the patient should be evaluated for inadequate neuromuscular function. Tests to determine if neuromuscular function is depressed are the head lift, hand grip strength, vital capacity of 10 to 15 mL/kg, and inspiratory force of at least -20 to -25 cm H_2O. The best method of determining neuromuscular function is with the peripheral nerve stimulator, especially in patients with altered central nervous system function. If the assessment determines that a competitive neuromuscular blockade exists, an anticholinesterase such as neostigmine (0.07 mg/kg) and an anticholinergic such as glycopyrrolate (0.015 mg/kg) should be administered intravenously.[9] Improvement in neuromuscular function should be observed within 2 to 5 minutes of injection of the reversal drug.

Airway Obstruction. Obstruction of the upper airway, which is considered to be an extrathoracic obstruction, may be caused by obstruction of the pharynx by the relaxed soft tissue or by partial or complete laryngospasm. An extrathoracic airway obstruction can be reliably assessed. As the patient inspires, stridor can be auscultated over the partially obstructed area. Inspiratory stridor occurs because the airway pressure is more negative than atmospheric pressure during inspiration. During expiration, less stridor is heard because the airway pressure is greater than atmospheric pressure. Certainly, if complete obstruction occurs, auscultation will reveal an absence of breath sounds and sternal retractions will be observed.

As the patient is emerging from anesthesia in the PACU, the tongue may be relaxed and can occlude the pharynx, especially when the head is flexed while the patient is supine. Intervention for this type of airway obstruction begins with hyperextension of the head. If the obstruction continues, the angle of the jaw should be lifted to move the tongue off the posterior pharynx. If more interventions are required, especially in the obtunded patient, an oral or nasal airway can be inserted; however, if the airway obstruction is due to masseter spasm and the jaws are clenched tightly, a nasal airway or nasotracheal tube placed into the nasopharynx should relieve the obstructed airway.

Laryngospasm, or adduction of the vocal cords, is commonly caused by secretions or manipulation of the vocal cords. Laryngospasm can be partial or complete.[2] Partial laryngospasm is due to a partial adduction of the vocal cords. On assessment of the patient having a partial laryngospasm, inspiratory stridor over the larynx will be heard. Physiologically, this occurs because the obstruction is extrathoracic. The recommended intervention for a partial laryngospasm is the administration of 100 percent oxygen under positive pressure using a bag–valve–mask system. High inflation pressures should be avoided, and the rate of ventilation should be timed to the patient's own rate. As the obstruction improves, careful oral suctioning should be performed to prevent further laryngospasm.

Complete laryngospasm is characterized by complete adduction of the vocal cords resulting in an absence of ventilation to the point of hypoxemia. On auscultation, no breath sounds are heard and the patient exhibits the characteristic rocking motion in the lower abdominal area. At this point, a small dose of a rapid-acting depolarizing skeletal muscle relaxant (e.g., succinylcholine 0.5 to 1.0 mg/kg)[6] should be administered intravenously. Within 30 to 45 seconds postinjection, the vocal cords will begin to abduct. The patient should be ventilated gently via a bag–valve–mask system using 100 percent oxygen. Once the succinylcholine is administered, the anesthetist should be prepared to perform an endotracheal intubation if the patient cannot be ventilated adequately or if regurgitation and aspiration of stomach contents are imminent. Finally, cricoid pressure should be applied before and during intubation if the risk of aspiration is high.

In postintubation patients, especially in the pediatric age group, laryngeal edema and trauma may occur. These are significant obstructions of the extrathoracic airways because the narrowest portion of the larynx in the pediatric age group is the cricoid ring.[4] If untreated, this pathophysiologic process can progress to complete obstruction of the airway. This obstruction is extrathoracic, and inspiratory stridor is heard audibly or by auscultation. To differentiate between partial laryngospasm and laryngeal edema, 100 percent oxygen is administered via a bag–valve–mask system; the obstruction will progressively worsen if laryngeal edema is present, whereas if the patient is experiencing a partial laryngeal spasm, the stridor will be reduced and ventilatory function will improve. The assessment to differentiate between laryngeal spasm and edema should be carried out rapidly. Once laryngeal edema is determined as the cause of the airway obstruction, the patient should be placed in an upright position and administered humidified oxygen along with some nebulized racemic epinephrine. Dexamethasone should be administered intravenously to enhance the actions of the racemic epinephrine and to reduce the inflammation of the larynx.[6]

In a younger patient, laryngeal edema can progress rapidly to complete obstruction. Hence, equipment for both an oral intubation and emergency laryngotomy should be available. Oral tracheal intubation should be attempted first. If this is unsuccessful, a cricothyroidotomy should be performed by incising the cricothyroid membrane and inserting a tracheostomy tube or endotracheal tube into the airway.[6]

Hypotension. One of the more common problems in the immediate postoperative period is hypotension, which requires immediate corrective action. If the hypotension is allowed to progress, severe damage can occur to the brain, the heart, and the kidneys. Because of the high metabolic activity in these organs, any sustained abnormal decrease in the perfusion pressure can result in ischemia or infarction.

In the PACU, many situations can lead to hypotension. Hypotension can be caused by decreased cardiac output or decreased peripheral resistance. The decreased cardiac output can be a result of hypovolemia. Hypovolemia can result from excess fluid loss or inadequate fluid replacement. If the patient is being mechanically ventilated, positive airway pressure, especially positive end-expiratory pressure (PEEP), can cause hypotension. This positive pressure will, if in excess, inhibit the preload and reduce the cardiac output. Many anesthetic drugs, including halothane, isoflurane, enflurane, desflurane, sevoflurane, fentanyl, morphine, and meperidine, can cause myocardial depression to varying degrees, resulting in a reduced cardiac output. Finally, patients who have cardiac dysfunction, such as valvular disease, ischemia, and infarction, may have a reduced cardiac output.

Decreased peripheral resistance can result from several causes. Anaphylaxis and sepsis reduce peripheral resistance. The anesthetic drugs noted as causes of decreased cardiac output also decrease the peripheral resistance.

Assessment for hypotension should begin with reaffirmation of the measurement. A blood pressure cuff improperly placed or of the wrong size will result in errors in blood pressure measurement. More specifically, blood pressure cuffs that are too large yield falsely low readings. It must be remembered that the cuff width should equal approximately two thirds of the arm circumference.[7] Also, if arterial transducer measurement is being used, calibration of the monitor should be validated by a cuff or Doppler blood pressure measurement on the same arm in which the radial artery was cannulated. Improper calibration, dampening caused by air bubbles, and catheter obstruction also lead to inappropriately low blood pressure readings. Rapid bedside clinical assessment should include level of consciousness to detect brain ischemia resulting from reduced cardiac output. If urine output is less than 0.5 mL/kg per hour, hypovolemia or inadequate cardiac output is the most likely cause of the hypotension.

Once the assessment reveals the existence of hypotension, assessment of the possible cause(s) of the hypotension should be implemented. The assessment should focus on checking for continued blood loss, adequate blood replacement intraoperatively or postoperatively, myocardial ischemia or infarction through ECG confirmation, pneumothorax, cardiac tamponade, and evidence of sepsis or adverse drug effects.

Interventions to return the patient to the normotensive state may include administration of oxygen, fluid infusion, reversal of the depressant effects of the anesthetics, and treatment of arrhythmias or bradycardia. The first intervention should be the administration of oxygen to ensure tissue oxygenation. If the patient is hypovolemic, depending on the degree of loss, blood or blood products or crystalloid solutions should be administered promptly. The type of fluid chosen may not be as crucial as adequate replacement in a timely manner with any fluid. An intravenous bolus of crystalloid solution of 300 to 500 mL should be considered as the first-line intervention for hypotension.[6] Naloxone should be administered if it is determined that a narcotic is the cause of the hypotension. Vasopressors, especially those with positive inotropic action, can be used occasionally to raise the blood pressure and prevent coronary hypoperfusion. If the etiology of the hypotension is decreased peripheral resistance, vasopressors that are agonists on the alpha-1 receptors should be administered.

Many patients arrive in the PACU with excess vagal tone, which results in bradycardia and hypotension. This is especially true of patients with distended bladders or those in severe pain. Anticholinergic drugs, such as atropine (0.2 to 0.4 mg) and glycopyrrolate (0.1 to 0.2 mg) given intravenously will reverse the increased vagal effects. Finally, if the hypotension is due to excess positive airway pressure, a reduction in PEEP is required along with administration of fluids.

Hypertension. One of the more common sequelae in the immediate postoperative period is hypertension. The elevated blood pressure in the PACU is usually due to pain, hypercapnia, hypoxemia, or excessive fluids administered intraoperatively. About 50 percent of the patients who demonstrate hypertension in the PACU have a history of hypertension preoperatively. Consequently, the report to the postanesthesia nurse should include information on the patient's hypertension if it exists.

Assessment of the patient who is experiencing hypertension in the PACU should include hypothermia, pain, respiratory, and volume status. All patients with hypertension in the PACU should be aggressively treated with the modified stir-up regimen. If pain is present, appropriate medications should be administered. If hypothermia is present, it should be appropriately treated as discussed later in this chapter. If the systolic or diastolic pressure is 20 to 30 percent above the preoperative resting values or the patient complains of headache, ocular changes, or angina along with ST segment depression, antihypertensive treatment should commence.

Most patients can be treated with short-acting antihypertensive drugs. Beta-blocking drugs such as propranolol, labetalol, and esmolol are effective in treating hypertension in the PACU. Propranolol is effective in treating hypertension in patients who were on beta blockers preoperatively. This drug is administered intravenously in 0.5- to 1.0-mg increments until a reduction in blood pressure is demonstrated. Labetalol can be titrated to effect using an initial dose of 0.25 mg/kg and increasing the dose to 0.5 mg/kg up to 1.0 mg/kg every 10 to 15 minutes via the intravenous route.[9] Esmolol, an ultrashort-acting beta blocker, can be used to treat both hypertension and tachycardia. Because of its short half-life of 9 minutes, it is usually given in a loading dose of 500 µg/kg and then followed by a continuous infusion at rates of 25 to 300 µg/kg per minute.[9] Other drugs that can be used in the treatment of postoperative hypertension include hydralazine, nitroprusside, nifedipine, clonidine, and trimethaphan.

Postoperative Hypothermia. Hypothermia usually occurs during anesthesia and surgery. Consequently, hypothermia is a common syndrome in the immediate postoperative period. Hypothermia exists when a patient's core temperature is below her or his set point or when it is less than 36C. The thermal set point is defined in the anterior hypothalamus and normally is 37.1C.[11] Heat generation occurs by increasing the metabolic rate and shivering. Heat dissipation takes place by increasing blood flow to the skin, which is ultimately lost to the environment by radiation, conduction, and convection. Sweating and evaporation enhance heat loss. Finally, of particular importance to anesthesia and postoperative care, heat is lost via evaporation of water from the respiratory tract.

During the intraoperative anesthesia phase, many factors contribute to the development of hypothermia. The state of unconsciousness results in immobility and removal of the behavioral protection against the cold. The thermal regulating center in the anterior hypothalamus is depressed along with all the autoregulatory mechanisms. There is an autonomic and accompanying motor blockade that impairs heat-generating mechanisms. Cooling also occurs when the patient inspires unheated, dry anesthetic gases. In addition, the operating room is cold (18 to 21C) and the patient's skin is wet in many exposed areas.

Central temperature should be monitored using sites such as the nasopharynx, skin, esophagus, rectum, and tympanic membrane. The temperature measured in the tympanic membrane or nasopharynx estimates brain temperature. Esophageal temperature approximates myocardial temperature. Studies demonstrate the greatest precision and accuracy of temperature measurements in the urinary bladder, nasopharynx, and esophagus. Axillary, great toe, and forehead temperatures do not appear to be as accurate when compared with the previously stated sites. The disposable liquid-crystal temperature monitor only reflects a trend as studies indicate a lack of correlation between skin and central temperatures. Consequently, clinicians should not assume that changes in skin surface temperatures reliably indicate central temperature.[11]

On arrival in the PACU, a patient usually is hypothermic. Studies indicate that 60 percent of the patients have temperatures less than 36C, and 13 percent, temperatures less than 35C. If allowed to progress, the patient can experience delayed awakening and inadequate peripheral blood flow leading to thrombosis and hypoxemia.

Treatment of hypothermia in the PACU requires, first, assessment of the degree of temperature loss. If the temperature is between 36 and 37C, the patient can simply be covered with warmed blankets and heat lamps can be used to keep the patient adequately warm. If the patient's temperature is less than 36C, rapid rewarming is required to decrease the possible complications of hypothermia and decrease the postanesthesia recovery time. Rewarming prevents the thermoregulatory responses to cold such as shivering that increase the patient's discomfort and metabolic activity. It is suggested that a skin surface warming device such as the Bair Hugger be placed on the patient. In patients with a normal metabolic rate, a setting of "low" or "medium" increases the mean body temperature at about 1C per hour. A "high" setting increases the mean body temperature about 1.5C per hour.[11] Other methods of rewarming are thermal mattresses, fluid and blood warming, and environmental warming.

Postoperative Nausea and Vomiting. Among the most difficult and dangerous problems that occur in the PACU are postoperative nausea and vomiting. Although the incidence of this syndrome occurring in the PACU is low, about 5 percent (range 2 to 70 percent), it is considered a grave concern because of the problems of airway management. In addition, studies indicate that the incidence of nausea and vomiting is higher in women than in men. Other factors that excite this reflex are a history of motion sickness; surgical procedures involving the eye, ear, and mouth; and certain narcotics such as morphine. Anesthetic agents that have been studied in this area and are associated with a significant incidence of nausea and vomiting are nitrous oxide, isoflurane, and etomidate.[8]

The vomiting center is located in the medulla of the brain. It is activated by afferent impulses from the pharynx, stomach, or other portions of the gastrointestinal tract to the chemoreceptor trigger zone (CTZ) in the medulla.[4] Certainly, anesthetic gases, blood, and mucus can initiate this reflex. Also, the vomiting center can be excited by impulses received from other portions of the brain. For example, anesthetic agents and narcotics sensitize the vestibular apparatus, the center of balance. Consequently, one of the principal causes of nausea and vomiting is movement of the patient during transfer or even during repositioning. Other activators of this reflex are increased intracranial pressure, dehydration, and electrolyte imbalance. A patient experiencing nausea should be encouraged to cough and perform the SMI maneuver. Oxygen in a high concentration should be administered. A patient who begins to vomit actively should assume a head down and lateral position. Oral suctioning should be instituted if the patient is not able to control the airway completely. Rapid assessment of the patient's respiratory status should be made during and after the vomiting episode. This is done by auscultation of the chest bilaterally, listening for adventitious sounds. The pulse oximeter should be used to ensure that oxygen saturation does not fall below 90 percent. If the patient is experiencing a low oxygen saturation and adventitious sounds, aspiration should be suspected and the appropriate therapy instituted.

Pharmacologic methods of reducing the incidence of nausea and vomiting include the use of metoclopramide (Reglan) preoperatively in the dose range 5 to 20 mg, orally, intramuscularly, or intravenously. Metoclopramide enhances the action of acetylcholine (ACh) at the muscarinic synapses and in the central nervous system to antagonize dopamine.[9] This latter action is responsible for its antiemetic effect. Another drug that has a profound antiemetic effect is droperidol (Inapsine). This drug can be given preoperatively to patients who are anticipated to experience a high incidence of nausea and vomiting. The preoperative dose of this drug is 0.01 to 0.02 mg/kg via the intramuscular or in-

travenous route of administration.[9] Postoperatively, droperidol can be administered to treat the syndrome once it has commenced. Titration of this drug can begin with a dose of 0.02 mg/kg intravenously. It should be remembered that droperidol can cause oversedation, circulatory depression, and activation of the extrapyramidal system.

Postoperative Pain. Acute pain is an unpleasant sensation and emotional experience usually caused by damage to tissue or by noxious stimuli.[2] Pain receptors, called *nociceptors*, are located mainly in the skin, blood vessels, subcutaneous tissue, fascia, periosteum, and viscera, and are stimulated by noxious stimuli. Nociceptors act as transducers and convert the painful stimulus into impulses that are transmitted along peripheral fibers to the central nervous system. The degree of nociceptor input from the periphery to the central nervous system is influenced by temperature, sympathetic function, vasculature, and the chemical environment.

In the immediate postoperative period, even as the effects of anesthesia disappear, tissue injury continues, and liberation of pain-producing substances continues. These greatly reduce the high threshold of the nociceptors, leading to the production of pain. Moreover, stimulation of the cut ends of nerves further contributes to pain perception. For example, patients who have had thoracic surgery experience pain from the summation of sensory input from three sites of tissue injury: the skin, the deep somatic structures, and the involved viscera.

On reaching the central nervous system, the pain stimulus activates highly complex interactions among neural systems, psychologic factors, and cultural factors. These interactions of the sensory, motivational, and cognitive processes affect the motor system and initiate psychodynamic mechanisms that are translated physiologically into the affective responses characteristic of acute pain.

By activating the sympathoadrenal system, pain accelerates the cardiovascular system as observed by the parameters of pulse and blood pressure. If the patient has a significant degree of cardiovascular dysfunction, the pain should be lessened with appropriate intervention. It has been suggested that pain, especially at upper abdominal and thoracic surgical sites, will decrease or in fact eliminate the normal sighing (yawn) mechanism.[4] The absence of an appropriate sigh leads to reduced lung volumes and, ultimately, to the atelectasis/pneumonia sequela. Again, appropriate pain relief in these patients may reduce the incidence of atelectasis and pneumonia postoperatively.

Assessment of postoperative pain includes both behavioral and physiologic clues. Pain usually elicits an increased response by the sympathetic nervous system, which in turn produces a large amount of catecholamines, causes tachycardia, increases cardiac output, increases peripheral resistance, and ultimately increases blood pressure. Other assessment parameters of excessive sympathoadrenal activity resulting from acute pain include respiratory changes, excessive perspiration, changes in skin color, nausea, and vomiting. Other objective and subjective findings include generalized or local muscle tension or rigidity, writhing, unusual postures, knees drawn up to abdomen, restlessness, rubbing, and scratching. Finally, pain may affect the behavioral affect of the patient, so that the patient in acute pain may be irritable, depressed, or withdrawn or have behavioral reverses, such as hostility in an ordinarily quiet person.

Once the assessment has been made and it has been determined that the patient is indeed experiencing acute postoperative pain, certain interventions are suggested. If the patient has received an inhalational anesthetic, such as isoflurane, enflurane, or halothane, and demonstrates signs and symptoms of acute pain, postoperative pain relief by the use of narcotic agonists should be instituted early in the postanesthetic period. Similarly, patients receiving a nitrous oxide–narcotic technique should be medicated early in the immediate postoperative period if the intraoperative narcotics were of short duration of action. If narcotics such as sufentanil, meperidine, and morphine were used intraoperatively, the PACU patient should be administered narcotic agonists with caution to avoid respiratory depression as a result of the synergistic actions of the intraoperative and postoperative narcotic agonists. Finally, if the PACU patient was administered droperidol intraoperatively or preoperatively, great caution should be used because narcotic agonists as well as barbiturates are significantly potentiated by this butyrophenone tranquilizer. Therefore, the usual dosage of narcotic agonists should be reduced by one third to one half during the first 8 to 10 hours postoperatively.[2] A complete discussion of pain management can be found in Chapter 48.

POSTANESTHESIA CARE: DISCHARGE PHASE

Patient Teaching and Follow-Up

On the patient's arrival in the PACU, nursing interventions are focused on the modified stir-up regimen and monitoring of the patient's physiologic parameters. Many studies indicate that lung volumes, particularly in patients who have had upper abdominal or thoracic surgery, remained decreased from 5 to 7 days postoperatively.[2] Hence, the patient should be educated to continue performing the SMI maneuver with or without the use of an incentive spirometer long into the postoperative phase. Accompanying this, the cascade cough and early ambulation should be emphasized to facilitate secretion clearance and better ventilation–perfusion matching.

Follow-up should include postoperative visits by the anesthetist to all patients who were in the PACU. The focus of the postoperative assessment should be on the patient's cardiorespiratory status. Again, those patients who were ASA Class III or higher or who had upper abdominal or cardiothoracic surgery should be visited until postoperative day 7 to ensure adequate return of cardiopulmonary function.

Discharge Criteria

The use of the PARS system to score patients who are recovering from anesthesia is helpful in setting up criteria for discharge from the PACU. On arrival in the PACU, a patient's PARS may be 7 or 8. After an appropriate amount of time, allowing for metabolism and excretion of the anesthetic agents, the PARS may be 9 or 10, at which point the patient can be discharged from the PACU. Many factors determine readiness for discharge; however, the major areas to assess prior to discharge are the patient's general condition; cardiorespiratory function including specifically maintenance of a patent airway and a normal electrocardiogram; renal function (> 30 mL/h); pain relief; and laboratory data. The use of regional anesthesia, the patient's prior condition, and the use of inhalational or intravenous anesthesia all have a significant impact on the decision to discharge the patient. Finally, discharge of a patient who has been medicated with a narcotic agonist in the PACU should be delayed for 30 minutes postadministration of the drug so that the effects of the drug can be fully evaluated.

Discharging patients from the PACU can be the responsibility of the patient's principal physician, the physician director of the PACU, the CRNA, or an anesthesiologist. The nurse or physician anesthetist who administered the anesthesia intraoperatively should be consulted during the discharge phase to enhance the decision-making process and thus facilitate an improved outcome for the surgical patient.

REFERENCES

1. Frost E, Andrews I. Recovery room care. *Int Anesthesiol Clin.* 1983:21(1).
2. Drain C. *Textbook of postanesthesia nursing.* 3rd ed. Philadelphia: WB Saunders; 1992.
3. Drain C. Comparison of two inspiratory maneuvers on increasing lung volumes in postoperative upper abdominal surgical patients. *AANA J.* 1984;52:379–388.
4. Guyton A. *Textbook of medical physiology.* 8th ed. Philadelphia: WB Saunders; 1991.
5. Katz J, Benumof J, Kadis L. *Anesthesia and uncommon diseases.* 3rd ed. Philadelphia: WB Saunders; 1990.
6. Miller RD. *Anesthesia.* 3rd ed. New York: Churchill Livingstone; 1990.
7. Lake C. *Clinical monitoring.* Philadelphia: WB Saunders; 1990.
8. Barash P, Cullen B, Stoelting R. *Clinical anesthesia.* Philadelphia: JB Lippincott; 1989.
9. Stoelting R. *Pharmacology & physiology in anesthetic practice.* 2nd ed. Philadelphia: JB Lippincott; 1991.
10. Levitsky M. *Pulmonary physiology.* 3rd ed. New York: McGraw-Hill; 1991.
11. Flacke J, Flacke W. Inadvertent hypothermia: Frequent, insidious, and often serious. *Semin Anesth.* 1983;2(3):183–196.

Pain Management

Margaret Faut-Callahan and Jeanne F. Slack

The phenomenon of pain has been studied for hundreds of years, yet today it remains a major health issue. It is estimated that over 50 million Americans are disabled annually because of a pain problem.[1] Hospitalized patients report significant levels of pain associated with various diagnoses, including postsurgical, oncologic, and medical.[2–7] Pediatric patients are often found to be in pain. No single group seems to be immune from the occurrence of pain and the limited management of the symptoms.

Nurse anesthetists must familiarize themselves with the latest information and issues in pain management. For the surgical patient, it is often the nurse anesthetist who initiates the pain management plan of care. Proper assessment, application of current theories in pain management, development and evaluation of the care plan, and additional intervention are all within the realms of current nurse anesthesia practice.

The nurse anesthetist is often in the best position to assess the preoperative and intraoperative patient response to pain and the stress of surgery. On the basis of this assessment, the postoperative pain management plan is developed, incorporating all strategies in the management of pain, including pharmacologic and non-pharmacologic interventions. Developing a patient-centered approach for the management of pain provides the best mechanisms for rapid resolution of patient discomfort. Pain management is not limited to patients with acute pain. Patients often present for surgery with chronic, unrelated pain conditions that must also be evaluated. Further, nurse anesthetists are often found in pain centers providing needed pain assessment and management services.

CONCEPTUAL MODEL

Recognizing the interaction among the patient, the care providers, and the delivery system is essential in the development of an adequate pain management plan. One model

identifies the interaction between nociception, pain experience, and pain behaviors.[8] A modification of that model is depicted in Figure 48–1 which describes a systems response. This alteration highlights the need to evaluate how the success or failure of a systems response impacts on the patient.

Edwards identifies many issues related to the failure of providers to administer or of patients to obtain adequate postoperative analgesia.[9] He categorizes the issues relative to the responsibility of health care professionals, patients and families, and system and administrators (Table 48–1). It is clear that the opportunity for inappropriate pain management is an obvious and complex issue.

THEORIES OF PAIN

Many theories of pain have been studied over the years. Specificity theory was developed over two centuries ago and proposed that pain travels from a specific pain receptor to a pain center in the brain. Pattern theory encompasses several areas—peripheral pattern theory, sensory interaction theory, and central summation theory. The most well-known theory of pain was proposed by Melzack and Wall.[10] It is the gate-control theory and suggests that peripheral nerve fibers carrying painful stimuli to the spinal cord may be modulated at the spinal cord level, in the dorsal horn, where gates open to permit pain impulses to ascend toward the brain. If the gates close, pain impulses do not reach the brain. This theory was instrumental in identifying a mechanism that would support the role of emotions or past experiences in the meaning of pain. It was believed that higher central nervous system functions, such as anxiety, could influence the opening or closing of the gates.

The parallel processing model of pain further integrates the physiologic, cognitive, and emotional aspects of pain.[11] It was proposed that the physiologic and emotional properties of pain traveled through different nerve fibers. Further, it was believed that the pain experience could easily be explained at three levels. Level 1 involved neural encoding of the stimuli and created the awareness of the pain. Level 2 involved neural encoding of the stimuli with past experi-

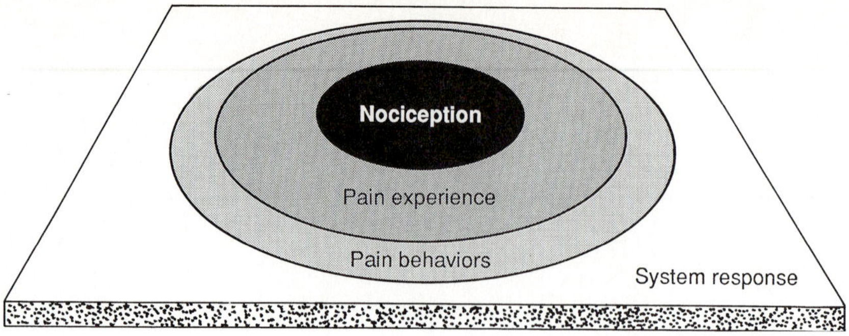

Figure 48–1. Conceptual model highlighting the interaction between nociception, pain experience, and pain behaviors on the part of the patient and the health care system's pain management response. (*Adapted, with permission, from Loeser J, Egan.*[8])

ences. Level 3 incorporated the person's beliefs about pain into the experience.

DEFINITIONS OF PAIN

Reluctance to explore beyond the boundaries of some early theories may have contributed to limited understanding of the phenomenon of pain. In 1979, however, the International Association for the Study of Pain developed a definition of pain that has provided new direction.[12] Accordingly, pain is an unpleasant sensory and emotional experience associated with actual or potential tissue damage, or described in terms of such damage. McCaffery further provides a definition of pain as "whatever the experiencing person says it is, existing whenever he says it does."[13] These definitions remind us that the caregiver is in a position of *believing* the patient and then intervening.

These definitions support the belief that pain has both physiologic and behavioral components and that pain is a complex phenomenon for which simplistic strategies for understanding and treating it are no longer appropriate. All dimensions of the pain experience are important and must be evaluated and managed.

PHYSIOLOGIC PRINCIPLES

The subjective experience of pain is the result of tissue injury. From the time of injury through the painful experience, there are many complex chemical and electrical events. Fields defines the processes involved as transduction, transmission, modulation, and perception.[13] Transduction is the process by which a noxious stimulus results in electrical activity in the sensory nerve endings. Transmission is a more complex phenomenon comprising three components: peripheral sensory nerves, relay neurons from the spinal cord to the brainstem and thalamus, and reciprocal connections between the thalamus and the cortex (Fig. 48–2). The third process, modulation, is defined as the

---

TABLE 48–1. BARRIERS TO APPROPRIATE POSTOPERATIVE PAIN MANAGEMENT

	Deficits in Knowledge/Skill	Resultant Attitude	Inappropriate Resultant Behavior
Health care professionals	Anatomy, physiology, psychology of postop pain	"The pain well"	Therapy as needed; too little, too infrequently
	Pharmacology of opioid drugs	Fear of physiologic fallout	
	Understanding how to assess pain and response to therapy	"It doesn't make any difference"	
	Knowledge of spectrum of existing drugs	Conventional approaches	Wrong drug; wrong route of administration
	Understanding existing modern pain therapy technology, including advantages/disadvantages of patient-controlled analgesia, etc.	Patients cannot determine own needs or self-medicate safely	Therapy determined by patient's ability to convince staff of sincerity: the adversarial stance
Patients and families	Knowledge of availability of modern pain control	Expect pain around a procedure; should not burden staff	Grin and bear it
	Understanding of "signals" and language to make the system respond to pain control needs	Staff are cruel, uncaring; do not understand—the ENEMY	Cajole, argue, demand: the adversarial approach
System and administrator	Knowledge of role of pain control in marketing services	Pain management team/equipment too expensive	Stonewall requests for personnel/equipment
	Knowledge of potential for reduction of surgical complications/length of stay versus expense of providing service	Service is "unnecessary"	Stonewall requests for payment

Reprinted, with permission, from Edwards[9(p527)] and from Elsevier Science Publishing Co., Inc. Copyright 1990 by the U.S. Cancer Pain Relief Committee.

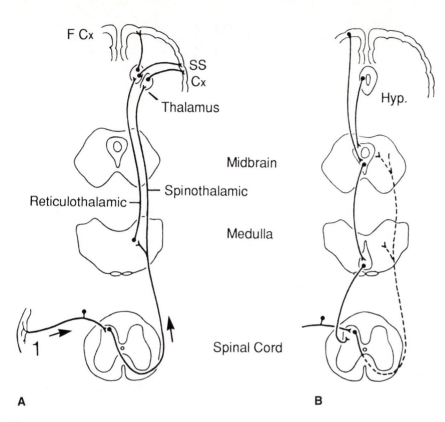

Figure 48–2. Nerve pathways of pain transmission and pain modulation. **A.** Pain transmission pathways involve peripheral sensory nerves, relay neurons from the spinal cord to the brainstem and thalamus, and reciprocal connections between the thalamus and cortex. **B.** Modulation occurs when a pathway (indicated by the broken line) within the central nervous system inhibits pain transmission at the level of the spinal cord. HYP, hypothalamus; F Cx, frontal cortex; SS Cx, somatosensory cortex. (*Reprinted, with permission, from Fields.*[13(p6)])

neural activity that leads to the control of pain transmission neurons (see Fig. 48–2). Modulation occurs because a specific pathway within the central nervous system, which inhibits pain transmission at the level of the spinal cord, can be activated by stress or analgesic drugs. The exact mechanism of the final process, perception, is yet unclear, but involves a subjective correlate that produces the perception of pain.[13]

Nociception, or the recognition of a painful stimulus, is a highly complex response. Nociceptors are primary afferent nerves that respond to noxious stimuli. The primary afferent nociceptors function in the transduction and transmission processes. Stimuli can be in the form of chemical, mechanical, or thermal energy. This stimulus is converted to an electrochemical impulse in the primary afferent neurons.

Transduction is thought to be mediated by pain-producing substances formed by cells damaged by the noxious stimuli. The nociceptors are activated by these substances which may be formed by at least three mechanisms: (1) the substance leaks out of damaged cells, (2) it is synthesized locally by enzymes from substances released by the damage, or (3) it may be released by the nociceptor itself.[13] Substances that have been identified are histamine, potassium, acetylcholine, serotonin, adenosine triphosphate, and bradykinin. Metabolic products of arachidonic acid, prostaglandins, and leukotrienes have also been found in areas of tissue damage.

Substance P, an 11-amino-acid polypeptide found in unmyelinated primary afferent fibers, is released when the fibers are activated and may actually enhance nociception. Pain-sensitive tissues have been found to be rich in substance P-containing afferent nerves. Substance P is known to cause vasodilation, produce edema, and stimulate the release of histamine.[13]

Transmission is the process by which the information is directed to the central nervous system. It is in the central nervous system that the sensation of pain is produced. Several things happen once the stimulus is transmitted to the brain; for example, the withdrawal reflexes may activate or subjective perception may occur.

The peripheral response to pain through the primary afferent nociceptors provides needed information to the spinal cord dorsal horn in the central nervous system. Cells within the dorsal horn are categorized as projection neurons, excitatory interneurons, and inhibitory interneurons. Projection neurons relay nociceptive information to higher brain centers. Excitatory interneurons relay information to projection neurons, other interneurons, or motor neurons. Inhibitory interneurons assist in the control of nociceptive transmission.

The transmission of a pain impulse is a complex electrical and chemical phenomenon. The major pathways that facilitate the transmission of a painful stimulus are depicted in Figure 48–2. Interventions developed to mediate the noxious stimulus are the foundation for successful pain management.

BEHAVIORAL COMPONENTS OF PAIN MANAGEMENT AND EFFECTS OF UNRELIEVED PAIN

There is now convincing evidence that unrelieved pain may result not only in harmful physiologic responses, but also in harmful psychologic effects.[14,15] Evidence of shortened hospital stay, decreased morbidity and mortality, and increased patient satisfaction has been reported in association with effective relief of pain.[16,17]

Pain, especially severe pain, can cause a number of changes in an individual's behavior, including increased self-absorption, withdrawal from interpersonal contact, and increased sensitivity to external stimuli such as light and sound. Emotional processes are central to the experience and expression of pain. In fact, signs of emotional distress such as fear and anxiety are frequently the most recognizable evidence that a patient is experiencing pain. Although Craig and Prkachin identified anxiety, fear, and depression as the most common emotional concomitants of pain, other emotions including anger, aggression, guilt, and subservience may be observed.[18]

Unrelieved severe pain can lead to depression and a feeling of helplessness as patients experience a loss of control over their environment. If the source of pain persists and is perceived as uncontrollable, high levels of anxiety can be precipitated.[19] In a few cases, the inability to cope with pain may create an acute psychotic reaction.[20]

Unrelieved acute pain is one of the important factors contributing to the development of delirium in the intensive care unit, which can be further exacerbated by related sleeplessness.[21] A vicious circle of pain, anxiety, fear, helplessness, and sleep deprivation occurs if pain persists unrelieved for several days.

In both the clinical setting and the laboratory, individual differences in responsiveness to noxious stimuli are documented. Clinical observations by Beecher of wounded soldiers constituted the first clear description of individual differences in pain response to injury.[22] Beecher reported that 65 percent of soldiers who were severely wounded in battle felt little or no pain. This phenomenon was attributed to the positive meaning of the pain experience: being wounded meant the soldier would be sent home. Civilian surgical teams have reported similar findings of decreased pain response after surgery on patients in developing countries because the opportunity to have corrective surgery is viewed by the patients in a very positive sense. In a study of patients in an emergency unit, 30 percent did not feel pain at the time of injury and some did not experience pain for several hours after the injury; Melzack et al concluded that the link between injury and pain is highly variable and dependent on the circumstances surrounding the injury.[23]

There is now considerable evidence that much of the variance in pain response is due to psychologic factors.[24] Anxiety has been shown to be fostered by the anticipation of an unpleasant experience.[25] Uncertainty enhances anxiety. Pain that escalates because of anxiety is likely to be reduced when information is given that reduces the uncertainty regarding questions of concern. A number of studies have demonstrated that measures that reduce anxiety have an important bearing on the acute pain experienced by patients and the need for analgesia.[26,27]

Another important area of study has been the interaction between coping style and the control the patient has over the situation. Patients who anticipate that they will have some control over stressful stimuli experience less anxiety.[28–30] Some of the effectiveness of patient-controlled analgesia (PCA) is attributed to the sense of control that is fostered when the patient knows that he or she can administer analgesia on demand.[19]

Fear of the unknown and fear of death are probably the most intense emotions a person can experience. Circumstances associated with acute postoperative pain and trauma are most likely to aggravate such fears. Fear of the unknown produced by hospitalization and the possibility of disability, loss of life, loss of freedom, and separation from one's family are all very real stressors for patients.[21,31] Further, the anxiety experienced by family members is often transferred directly to the patient and serves to reinforce fear and anxiety. In a detailed analysis of the variance in pain response, Peck identified a number of psychologic factors that can affect the individual's response to pain including fear and anxiety, meaning of pain, observable learning, perceived control of events, coping style, cultural differences, and attention/distraction.[20]

Recent studies of pain relief suggest that the initial experience with pain management may be an important determinant of future relief.[32,33] The patient's expectations may be conditional with the first experience. Therefore, if pain relief is inadequate, a negative expectation could adversely affect later pain control efforts. This has important implications for clinicians to provide adequate analgesia as quickly as possible to convey the expectation that pain control measures will continue to be effective.

FACTORS THAT INFLUENCE THE EFFICACY OF PAIN MANAGEMENT

Clinicians' attitudes, institutional priorities, and factors associated with the patient can influence clinical decisions about pain management. A number of variables affect the clinician's decision to order or administer analgesia to patients. Studies of pain management have identified that no specific group of health care providers consistently accepts responsibility for pain relief.[34,35] This has serious implications for patients because adequate analgesia must be ordered and administered to patients in a timely fashion.

One variable that influences clinicians' medication practices is the ability to accurately assess the level of pain intensity and intervene effectively to manage the patient's pain. If pain is assessed inadequately or too infrequently, relief may be inadequate. To effectively manage pain, one must understand what the experience of pain is like for the patient and accurately assess the intensity of pain. Specific issues related to measurement and assessment of pain are discussed later in this chapter.

In a study of 255 adult and pediatric patients, the clinician's stated goal for complete pain relief was not significantly related to the amount of analgesic administered or to the level of pain relief reported by the patients.[36] This lack of relationship between clinician attitudes and actual clinical practice requires further study to determine why it exists.

The clinician's perception of the severity of a patient's illness has also been reported to affect the selection of analgesic regimen. Higher pain levels are reported to be attributed to patients with objective signs of pathophysiologic disruption.[37] Yet, it is widely accepted by pain experts that physical pathology alone is not necessarily related to the amount of pain reported by an individual.[23] This finding has implications for the patient with chronic pain, who may or may not exhibit obvious pathophysiologic alterations. The pain management of the chronic pain patient may be a different type and quality from that provided the acute pain patient.

In 1973, Marks and Sachar suggested that inadequate administration of analgesia may occur because health care professionals have incorrect pharmacologic information about various analgesics and an excessive and unrealistic concern about addiction.[4] In 1980 Cohen stated that undermedication may be the result of caregivers' lack of the basic knowledge necessary to manage pain effectively. Further, Cohen found clinicians to be overly concerned with the possibility of addiction in their patients. They often lacked knowledge of the physiologic action of analgesics.[3] Review of both medical and nursing curriculums and textbooks reveals that very little formal instruction is provided about the management of pain. Even less information is provided about pharmacologic principles and use of analgesics. This inadequate knowledge base has probably contributed to misconceptions about pain and to ineffective use of pharmacologic and nonpharmacologic interventions for pain relief.

The use of narcotics for the control of pain is often associated with concerns about addiction and respiratory depression.[38] The tendency on the part of clinicians to select nontherapeutic doses of narcotic analgesics is most likely influenced by an overestimation of the incidence of narcotic addiction.[3,4,38] In a study by Porter and Jick only 4 of 11,882 patients became addicted during hospitalization.[39]

The fear of side effects such as respiratory depression is also unwarranted unless a toxic dose of the narcotic is administered. In one study, clinicians erroneously attributed analgesia rather than uncontrolled pain to be the cause of respiratory changes on the day after surgery.[3] In another study of 134 surgical patients, patients receiving effective epidural analgesia in the early postoperative phase demonstrated significantly better postoperative recovery in relation to respiratory and ambulatory parameters than patients reporting inadequate pain relief.[40] Effective analgesia may be an important "overlooked" factor in the overall efforts of the health care system to decrease the length of patients' hospitalization.

Interestingly, clinicians continue to administer medications such as digoxin to patients without apparent concern even though there is a potential for serious side effects. Clearly, an individual's pharmacologic knowledge and attitudes about narcotics can contribute to ineffective pain management.

Further complicating pain management decisions is the patient's belief about pain and analgesia which influences the patient's expression of pain and desire for pain relief. For example, if the patient believes that pain builds character, this may influence pain behavior.[41] Patients do not always report pain accurately. Patients may minimize the intensity of pain to avoid receiving medications, either out of fear of injections or out of concern about anticipated side effects. One study reported that 17 percent of patients were believed to have minimized their pain.[42]

Many patients who experience moderate to severe pain wait to ask for pain relief until the pain becomes unbearable. In a study of 259 patients, over two thirds of the patients would wait until they were in severe pain before requesting analgesia or not ask at all, expecting the clinician to know that they were experiencing pain. Furthermore, 75

percent of the patients expected that when analgesics were requested, they would be administered immediately.[43] This lag time between patient request and clinician response contributes significantly to ineffective pain management.

Some patients fail to verbalize pain needs because of the attitude expressed verbally or nonverbally by their health care providers. The patient is already feeling dependent and threatened by the strange hospital environment and may be hesitant to ask for pain relief. In some cases patients are inconsistent in verbal reports of pain. A patient may complain of unrelieved pain to the nurse, but when questioned by a physician, the patient will deny having any pain. Such contradictions in patient communication can contribute to inadequate pain relief. Patients may also be concerned about potential side effects associated with analgesics. Side effects such as drowsiness, nausea, itching, and constipation are often identified as the reasons patients refuse or limit the use of narcotic analgesics.

Clinical decision making should be based not only on the behavior exhibited by the patient but also on the pathophysiologic disruption. The clinician should consider what alterations have occurred in the patient's anatomic and physiologic integrity such as tissue anoxia, incisional repair, and fractures that require pain control.

Patient traits can also influence clinical decisions about pain management. Individuals learn to express pain in ways particular to their cultural group.[44] Therefore, the ethnic background of the patient may influence the assessment and management of pain. Other studies have demonstrated that the practitioner's beliefs about ethnic differences influences analgesic administration practices.[45] Studies of health care providers' perceptions of pain in hypothetical cases demonstrated that greater pain was inferred for Jewish and Hispanic patients in comparison to black, Asian, Mediterranean, and white patients.[46] Greater pain was also inferred for low-socioeconomic-status patients in comparison to moderate- or high-socioeconomic-status patients.

Although studies of the effect of gender on decision making related to pain management have been contradictory, age of the patient does influence pain management practices. In general, younger children and geriatric patients are prescribed and administered fewer analgesics because of the fear of side effects and myths about the patient's ability to feel pain and the misinterpretation of patient behavior.[47,48]

What information do clinicians use to evaluate whether a patient is in pain or not? In an observational study of decision making related to pain, Hammond observed 165 cues exhibited by patients and 17 responses to the cues by the health care providers.[49] Clinicians must attend to a wide variation in cues and possible responses when deciding (1) if a patient is in pain, (2) how much pain, (3) whether to provide analgesia, (4) how much to medicate, and (5) what other adjuvant interventions can enhance or potentiate the overall effect of the analgesic regimen.

Clinicians are usually the individuals implicated in poor pain management, but the patient also shares some responsibility. The patient is not a passive recipient of care and should be encouraged to participate in pain control measures. The clinician, however, must consider the patient's individual coping style and ability to use various pain relief measures.

Another factor that influences the efficacy of pain management is the expectations of the health care setting. Consideration of the impact of the health care organization has not been the focus of pain management research; however, the setting within which pain is managed can be a factor. For example, in the intensive care unit the primary focus is the management of the complex physiologic and technologic needs of the patient. Patient needs that are not life threatening, such as the need for analgesia, are not a priority. In emergency units, pain is useful for formulating the diagnosis, so analgesia may not be provided.

Other institutional factors that influence pain management include the ability of the organization to recruit and retain permanent staff. Inadequate and inconsistent care providers can further decrease accountability for providing pain relief. The changing health care reimbursement practice that restricts hospital admission of patients to the morning of major surgery is another variable that may influence the efficacy of pain management. The implication of this practice is that little or no opportunity is provided for the patient to learn various methods of pain control. The trend toward increased outpatient surgery places increasing importance on the patient's ability to understand and effectively use both pharmacologic and nonpharmacologic pain intervention techniques. As health care reimbursement and quality-of-care reviews become more focused on the outcomes experienced by patients, effective pain relief will gain increasing importance in relation to the overall recovery of the patient.

PAIN ASSESSMENT

Pain is a multidimensional phenomenon in which intensity, quality, meaning, and impact must be considered as part of the assessment. Pain and its management cannot be separated from the individual who experiences the pain. Reporting of pain requires an interaction between caregiver and patient, and depends to some extent on the relationship between the staff and patient.

If patients could always tell clinicians that they hurt and clinicians could accept the patient's report as fact, the assessment and management of pain would be significantly less complex; however, as discussed previously in this chapter, a number of variables influence the efficacy of pain management. In the clinical setting, accurate assessment and reliable pain measurement are essential for monitoring

fluctuations in the patient's pain levels and for evaluating the efficacy of pain relief therapies.

Just as methods of managing pain may vary, similarly, methods for pain assessment may also vary depending on whether the pain is acute or chronic. In the case of chronic pain, measures of behavioral functioning, coping style, and emotional state are important in the overall assessment of the patient's pain. The McGill Pain Questionnaire has greatly facilitated the assessment of the qualities of the pain experienced.[50] It provides intensity-graded scales of word descriptors that assess the sensory, affective, and evaluative aspects of the pain experience. The instrument has content and construct validity and is sensitive to the effects of different therapies of pain. The McGill Pain instrument is frequently used to measure clinical pain and patient response to treatment trials. The limitation of this instrument is that it is complex and time consuming.

To assist the clinician in identifying appropriate pain control strategies with the patient, a pain history should be obtained that considers the (1) previous experience(s) with pain and the impact of the current pain event; (2) patient knowledge and understanding of opioid and other sedative drugs; (3) history of drug usage or abuse, if any; (4) previous side effects that may have been experienced with certain drugs; and (5) the patient's coping style with stressful situations or pain (e.g., Does the patient want information and active involvement in pain control, or does the patient become more anxious and prefer a pain control approach that does not require active participation, such as is necessary with patient-controlled analgesia?).

Pain Rating Scales

Although the multidimensional nature of pain has been widely accepted, the most common approach to pain estimation continues to be unidimensional, in the form of self-report scales on which the patient is asked to rate one dimension of his or her pain, most often its intensity.[51] Such unidimensional rating scales fall into three main categories: the visual analog scale (VAS), the graphic rating scale (GRS), and the numerical rating scale (NRS).

Visual Analog Scale. The visual analog scale (VAS) consists of a 10-cm line with endpoint descriptors beyond the stops at either end (Fig. 48–3). The VAS is useful for patients with limited language skills because the choice points are

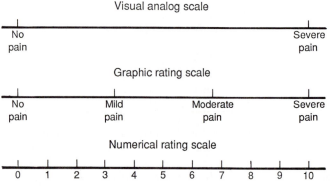

Figure 48–3. Self-reporting scales used by patients to estimate one dimension (usually intensity) of pain experience. Visual analog scale, graphic rating scale, and numerical scale are shown, each offering its own relative advantages and disadvantages (see text).

not labeled. The VAS has also been shown to be sensitive to medication effects over time and to behavioral indicators of pain.[52]

Graphic Rating Scale. A graphic rating scale is a straight-line continuum with from four to seven verbal descriptors placed in ascending order of severity at equal intervals along the line (see Fig. 48–3). This scale is usually intended for assessing the intensity of pain, so descriptors such as "none," "mild," "moderate," "severe," and "unbearable" are used.

Numerical Rating Scale. The numerical rating scale consists of a straight-line continuum numbered 0 to 10 or 0 to 100 (see Fig. 48–3). Anchor points at the two ends are usually "no pain" and "worst pain." The numerical rating scale is a self-report scale that permits more definable choices than the graphic rating scale and increases the sensitivity of the instrument.[52]

Pain Assessment in Children

Assessment of pain in children will vary depending on the child's ability to communicate verbally. For the preverbal child or for the child who is reluctant to admit pain, assessment of pain requires observations of physiologic signs and nonverbal behavior. The clinician must assess the pain associated with the procedures and pathologic processes and be especially alert to changes in the child's responses. Children, like adults, may deny pain or refuse analgesia.

Reliable and valid tools are available for assessment of pain in children. Graphic rating scales are often used to assess pain in children with cartoon facial scale being one of the most frequently used rating scales.[53] However, children are sometimes able to communicate more effectively through their drawings than they are able to do verbally. Pain drawings usually convey much more information about the child's perception of pain than other pain assessment methods.

Limitations of Pain Assessment Tools

For research purposes, the self-report rating scales provide no basis for assigning numerical values to categories and using parametric statistics in analyzing the data. Studies have found that the word and numerical categories do not represent successive identical steps in pain intensity. Attachment of a numerical value to each word category descriptor means that the numerical scores are ordinal or rank-ordered scores so that nonparametric statistics are the appropriate level of analysis.[54] The self-report scale scores obtained, however, are often treated as interval or ratio level scaling in the absence of evidence that respondents have interpreted the self-report numbers as equal increments.[51] All of the self-report scales are notable for clarity and simplicity. The scales are versatile, can be adapted to different cognitive levels, and are practical for use in a variety of clinical settings.

A limitation of the unidimensional approach to pain measurement is that the patient's pain rating is likely to be influenced by the patient's affective state and all of the other components that contribute to the pain event. The oversim-

plification of the pain experience that occurs when one mark on a line represents the patient's pain has been criticized.[55] Because the self-report scales cannot assess the diverse qualities of the pain experience, a comprehensive pain history is most useful for determining effective pain control strategies for the individual patient.

To ensure accurate pain measurement, the clinician should review the pain measurement tool with the patient and indicate how frequently the patient will be asked to report pain intensity. The patient should understand the relationship between the pain rating score and pain control measures. It is essential that both the patient and the staff using the pain measurement tool be fully familiar with the scale.

In summary, there are numerous methods of assessing pain, but generally the quantification of pain should be systematic and simple, and obtained at appropriate intervals. There should be consistency in interpretation and communication of pain ratings. Accurate assessment enables the clinician to have a clearer understanding of the patient's pain experience and a means of evaluating the effectiveness of pain relief measures and the patient's response.

PHARMACOLOGIC INTERVENTION

Pharmacologic intervention remains the mainstay of pain management. It is an obligation of the health care team to attend to and alleviate the pain as rapidly and as completely as possible. The strategy selected depends on many factors including the type, the intensity, and the expected duration of pain. A variety of analgesics are currently in use for the management of pain.

Opioid Analgesics

The opioid analgesics are commonly used to relieve pain. Opioids frequently used are listed in Table 48–2. Morphine was first purified by Serturner in 1806. Since that time, morphine and morphinelike drugs have become the foundation of analgesic therapy. Morphine works in the central nervous system to block painful stimuli. Morphine influences mu opiate receptors which are located in the brainstem modulating nuclei and the dorsal horn of the spinal cord. Specifically, it activates pain-modulating neurons that inhibit transmission from the primary nociceptor to the dorsal horn. Morphine also has a direct action at the spinal cord. It is known that opiate receptors and endogenous opioids are present at these sites. Morphine, then, works similarly to the endogenous opiates. Evidence of the specificity seen with opioid analgesia is the fact that no other analgesic works with such direct and limited effect as do the opioids. Opioids cause very little effect on other central nervous system function.

Other morphinelike drugs work in a similar manner. They produce analgesia through the same central nervous system mechanism. All have different degrees of potency, but in equianalgesic dosages, if tolerated by the patient, a similar level of analgesia is achieved. Morphine and morphinelike substances also produce similar side effects. These include mood changes, nausea and vomiting, sedation, mental clouding, respiratory depression, cough suppression, and pupillary constriction. In addition to these central

TABLE 48–2. OPIOIDS COMMONLY USED FOR ACUTE SEVERE PAIN

	Equianalgesic Initial IM Dose (mg)	Average Duration of Effect	Approximate Oral: Parenteral Ratio	Approximate Plasma t½ (h)
Morphine	10	4.5	1:6	3
Meperidine (Demerol)	75	3	1:4	3.5
Hydromorphone (Dilaudid)	1.5	4.5	1:5	2.5
Methadone (Dolophine)	10	4.5[a]	1:2	24
Codeine	130	4.5	1:2	3
Levorphanol (Levo-Dromoran)	2	4.5	1:2	14

[a] This may depend on the type of pain problem. A recent study indicates that a single dose of methadone can provide analgesia lasting 12 to 24 hours.
Reprinted, with permission, from Fields.[13(p256)]

effects, peripheral effects include decreased gastrointestinal motility, increased biliary duct pressure, pruritus, histamine release, and urinary retention.

Prolonged use of morphine and morphinelike substances has been linked to undesirable drug or disease interaction (Table 48–3). Caution must be exercised when dealing with patients with these types of conditions or on these drugs.

When managing pain problems, the most efficacious approach to pain management includes the use of opioids employing a frontload approach, that is, rapid development of a serum analgesic level. One such scheme for determining appropriate dosages of analgesics is present in Table 48–4.

Nonopioid Analgesics

Other types of drugs are also used in the management of pain. Aspirin, acetaminophen, and other nonsteroidal anti-inflammatory drugs (NSAIDs) are the most commonly used analgesics. Aspirin has been used since the turn of the century and is quite effective in the management of mild to moderate pain. Taylor and Curran reported that 60 percent of all Americans used aspirin to relieve mild pain.[56]

Aspirin and the nonsteroidal anti-inflammatory agents (Table 48–5) do not work in the central nervous system like the morphinelike substances. Instead, these drugs work in the periphery, decreasing the inflammatory response to tissue damage that accompanies the onset of pain. They act to inhibit cyclooxygenase, which catabolizes arachidonic acid into prostaglandins. Prostaglandins induce inflammation and activate peripheral nociceptors. Thus, any drugs that interfere with this mechanism should also be effective in the treatment of peripheral pain and pain associated with inflammation. Side effects of these drugs include decreased platelet aggregation and prolonged bleeding time, as well as gastric irritation.

Epidural Analgesia

The use of epidural analgesia for the control of postoperative pain, especially in the critically ill, is growing in popularity. The first spinal anesthetics were reported in 1899 and the first epidural anesthetics were reported in 1901. Cleland first demonstrated the effectiveness of epidural analgesia in early postoperative ambulation in patients undergoing extensive abdominal surgery. In 1956, Dawkins reported the use of continuous epidural analgesia with local anesthetics for postoperative pain.[57] In the 1980s, several studies demonstrated the use of epidural narcotics as a means of managing postoperative pain, with decreased total dosage of narcotics and fewer central depressant effects.[58,59]

Epidural analgesia occurs when a drug crosses the epidural space into the cerebrospinal fluid and diffuses into

TABLE 48–3 UNDESIRABLE DRUG OR DISEASE INTERACTIONS OF NARCOTIC-TYPE ANALGESICS

Drug	Interaction	Result
Meperidine	Cirrhosis	↑ Bioavailability and ↓ clearance = accumulation
Pentazocine	Cirrhosis	↑ Bioavailability and ↓ clearance = accumulation
Propoxyphene	Cirrhosis	↑ Bioavailability and ↓ clearance = accumulation
Meperidine	Renal failure	↑ Normeperidine, a toxic metabolite = accumulation
Propoxyphene	Renal failure	↑ Norporpoxyphene, a toxic metabolite = accumulation
Morphine	Age > 50 years	↓ Clearance = accumulation
Meperidine	Phenytoin	↑ Biotransformation = faster elimination
Methadone	Rifampin	↑ Biotransformation = faster elimination
Meperidine	Monoamine oxidase inhibitors	Excitation, hyperpyrexia, and convulsions
Any narcotic	Alcohol or other central nervous system depressants	Enhanced depressant effects

Reprinted, with permission, from Inturrisi CE. Role of opioid analgesics. Am J Med. 1984;77(suppl 3A):33.

TABLE 48–4. GUIDELINES FOR FRONTLOADING INTRAVENOUS ANALGESICS[a]

Drug	Total Frontload Dose (mg/kg)	Increments	Cautions
Morphine	0.08–0.12	0.03 mg/kg q10 min	Histamine effects; nausea; bilary colic; reduce dose for elderly
Meperidine	1.0–1.5	0.30 mg/kg q 10 min	Reduce dose or change drug for impaired renal function
Codeine	0.5–1.0	One third of total q15 min	Nausea
Methadone	0.08–0.12	0.03 mg/kg q15 min	Do not administer maintenance dose after analgesia achieved; accumulation; sedation
Levorphanol	0.02	50–75 µg/kg q15 min	Similar to methadone
Hydromorphone	0.02	25–50 µg/kg q10 min	Similar to morphine
Pentazocine	0.5–1.0	One-half of total q15 min	Psychomimetic effects; may cause withdrawal in narcotic-dependent patients
Nalbuphine	0.08–0.15	0.03 mg/kg	Less psychomimetic effects than pentazocine; sedation
Butorphanol	0.02–0.04	0.01 mg/kg q10 min	Sedation; psychomimetic effects similar to those of nalbuphine
Buprenorphine	≤ 0.2	One fourth of total q10 min	Long-acting like methadone, levorphanol; may precipitate withdrawal in narcotic-dependent patient; safe to give subcutaneous maintenance dose after analgesia—different from methadone

[a] A scheme for front loading the opioids most commonly used in postoperative pain treatment.
Reprinted, with permission, from Edwards[9(p530)] and from Elsevier Science Publishing Co., Inc. Copyright 1990 by the U.S. Cancer Pain Relief Committee.

the dorsal horn of the spinal cord (Fig. 48–4). The drug then binds with the opioid receptors in the dorsal horn, preventing the release of substance P, an excitatory transmitter, and thus preventing the transmission of the painful stimuli.

A second mechanism of action occurs when drugs are administered into the epidural space. Uptake of drugs by the epidural vasculature increase the plasma concentration, which is similar to the normal uptake and distribution of drugs given systemically (Fig. 48–5). Another pharmacologic action that must be recognized in the administration of epidural analgesia is the lipid solubility of the drugs administered. Fentanyl, meperidine, and sufentanil are highly lipid soluble, resulting in rapid absorption and rapid onset of drug action.

Duration of drug action is also affected by the lipid solubility of the drug. The greater the lipid solubility, the more likely the drug is to be absorbed by the epidural fat, limiting the degree to which the drug spreads within the epidural space and resulting in decreased duration of action. The opposite is true for drugs with low lipid solubility. These drugs are not absorbed which results in a higher concentration in the cerebrospinal fluid, with the possibility of cephalad spread. The degree to which the drug is absorbed by the epidural vasculature and diffuses into the cerebrospinal fluid determines the duration of drug effect.

Local anesthetics are used in a variety of ways in the management of pain: local infiltration, topical application, and major nerve blocks. Local anesthetics commonly used and specific characteristics are found in Table 48–6. Local anesthetic effect is both dose and concentration dependent. The site of action is at the nerve ending and the degree of blockade is determined by the concentration of the drug at the site.

Narcotics used for epidural analgesia are depicted in Table 48–7. Dosage, onset, and duration of drug action are shown. Wang et al were the first to report success with the use of preservative-free morphine.[60] Fentanyl has also been used in the control of postoperative pain via the epidural route.[61] In addition to narcotics and local anesthetics used alone, combination protocols have been studied in an at-

TABLE 48–5. COMMON NONOPIOID ANALGESIC AGENTS

Drug	Peak effect (h)	Plasma t½ (h)	Average Analgesic Dose (mg)	Dose Interval (hours)
Aspirin	2.0	4–6[a]	625	4–6
Diflunisal	2.5	10	500	10
Ibuprofen	1.5	3	400	4–6
Naproxen	3.0	12	250	12
Fenoprofen	2.0	2.5	200	4–6
Acetaminophen	1.0	2.0	500	3–5

[a] For active metabolite, salicylic acid.
Reprinted, with permission, from Fields.[13(p256)]

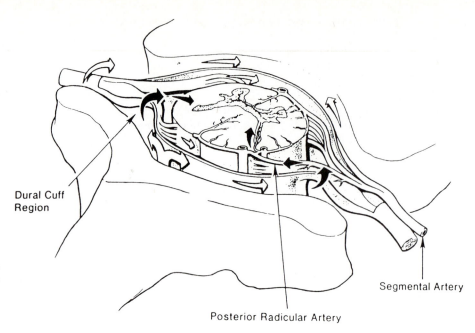

Figure 48–4. Cross section of spinal cord and epidural space. Opioid spread in epidural space is depicted by white arrows, and spread into cerebrospinal fluid and spinal cord is depicted by black arrows. In the dural cuff region, the posterior radicular spinal artery is readily accessible to opioid, and this artery directly supplies the dorsal horn region of the spinal cord. (*Reprinted, with permission, from Cousins MJ, Bridenbaugh PO. Acute and chronic pain: Use of spinal opioids. In: Cousins MJ, Bridenbaugh PO, eds.* Neural blockade in clinical anesthesia and management of pain. *Philadelphia: JB Lippincott; 1988:983.*)

tempt to determine the best drug regimen. A comparison of narcotic and local anesthetic action is found in Table 48–8.

Controversy over the optimal drugs to use via the epidural route waged through the early 1980s. Graham et al showed that although both epidural morphine and bupivicaine were effective, epidural morphine provided greater duration of analgesia with fewer side effects.[62] One year later, Modig and Paalzow reported that epidural analgesia with bupivicaine produced a more profound analgesia than epidural morphine with concomitant motor blockade[16]; however, epidural analgesia with morphine was not associated with motor or sympathetic blockade or loss of sensation. Finally, Torda and Pybus found that epidural bupivicaine produced greater intensity of analgesia but for a shorter duration than epidural morphine.[63] As conflicting as these initial reports were, the search for best use of the epidural route was underway.

Because of the problems associated with the use of local anesthetics in the epidural space for continued pain management and the discovery of opiate receptors in the substantia gelatinosa, the use of narcotics via the epidural route has increased in popularity and use for the management of pain after most types of surgery. Further, epidural analgesia provides effective postoperative pain relief with few side effects such as sedation and respiratory depression. In addition, analgesia is attained with lower total dosages than

with other conventional forms of drug administration, including intravenous, intramuscular, and patient-controlled analgesia.[64]

Patient-Controlled Analgesia

A valuable addition in the area of pain management has been the development of patient-controlled analgesia (PCA) devices. First introduced in the United States in the early 1980s, PCA has found wide acceptance from both patients and health care providers. This technique has been associated with better pain control, lower dosages of narcotic, and fewer narcotic-associated side effects.[65]

Patients control the amount and timing of drug administration as their need indicates within preset limits. Most PCA devices use digital electronics to regulate the dose of narcotic delivered via an intravenous route. A lockout mechanism prevents overadministration of the narcotic.

PCA decreases the long delays that often occur when the nurse must administer the narcotic. In addition, the use of the intravenous route facilitates the uptake and distribution of the drug. Pharmacokinetic theory suggests that a loading dose promotes the maintenance of a steady plasma level. The initial loading dose is typically administered by the nurse, as this may vary considerably from patient to patient. Graves et al reported fewer postoperative complica-

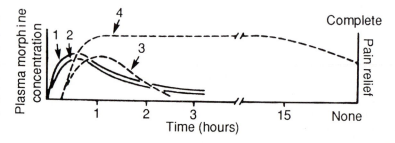

Figure 48–5. Relationship between plasma levels of epidurally and intramuscularly administered morphine and duration of analgesia. **1.** Epidural morphine plasma level. **2.** Intramuscular morphine plasma level. **3.** Intramuscular morphine analgesia. **4.** Epidural morphine analgesia. (*Reprinted, with permission, from Covino BG, Scott DB. Handbook of epidural anaesthesia and analgesia. Orlando, FL: Grune Stratton; 1985:78.*)

TABLE 48–6. CLINICAL CHARACTERISTICS AND DOSAGES OF LOCAL ANESTHETICS

	Procaine (Novocaine)	2-Chloroprocaine (Nesacaine)	Lidocaine (Xylocaine)	Mepivacaine (Carbocaine)	Prilocaine (Citanest)	Tetracaine (Pontocaine)	Bupivacaine (Marcaine)	Etidocaine (Duranest)
Latency (speed of onset)	Moderate	Fast	Fast	Moderate	Moderate	Very slow	Fast	Very fast
Penetration (diffusibility)	Moderate	Marked	Marked	Moderate	Moderate	Poor	Moderate	Moderate
Duration	Short	Very short	Moderate	Moderate	Moderate	Long	Long	Long
Optimal concentration (%)								
Infiltration	0.5	0.5	0.25	0.25	0.25	0.05	0.05	0.1
Spinal nerve and plexus block	1.5–2	1.0–2	0.5–1.0	0.5–1.0	0.5–1.0	0.1–0.25	0.25–0.5	0.5–1.0
Maximum amount (mg/kg)	12	15	6	6	6	2	2	2

Reprinted, with permission, from Wall PD, Melzack R. Textbook of pain. New York: Churchill Livingstone; 1989:726.

TABLE 48–7. EPIDURAL OPIOIDS: LATENCY AND DURATION OF POSTOPERATIVE ANALGESIA

Drug	Bolus Dose (mg)	Detectable Onset[a] (min)	Complete Pain Relief[a]	Duration[a] (h)
Morphine	5	23.5 ± 6	37 ± 6	18.1 + 8
Methadone	5	12.5 ± 2	17 ± 3	7.2 ± 4.6
Fentanyl	0.1	4–10	20	2.6–4
Meperidine	30–100	5–10	12–30	6.6 ± 3.3
Diamorphine	6	5	15	12.4 ± 6.5

[a] Values are means ± standard deviations or ranges.
Adapted, with permission, from Cousins MJ, Mather LE. Intrathecal and epidural administration of opioids. Anesthesiology. 1984;61:276.

TABLE 48–8. EFFECTS OF LOCAL EPIDURAL ANESTHETICS AND NARCOTICS

	Local Anesthetics	Narcotics
Quality of blockade		
Sympathetic blockade	Yes, dose dependent	None
Locomotion blockade	Slight to complete, dose dependent	None
Sensory blockade	All modalities, dose dependent	Mainly pain
Vascular uptake	Dose dependent and reduced by adrenalin 1:200,000	
Possible to limit segmental blockade	Yes	Yes, but may spread rostrally
Tachyphylaxis	Yes	Yes
Duration of action	Short	Short or very prolonged, depending on agent
Side effects		
Central respiratory depression	No	Yes, dose dependent
Peripheral respiratory depression	Yes, if respiratory muscles are involved	No
Urinary retention	Yes, relatively short	Yes, may be very prolonged
Pruritus	No	Yes
Nausea and vomiting	No	Yes

Reprinted, with permission, from Wall PD, Melzack R. Textbook of pain. New York: Churchill Livingstone; 1988:746.

tions when PCA was used.[65] This was presumed to be the result of the decreased level of sedation with this type of drug regimen.

NONPHARMACOLOGIC INTERVENTION

Nonpharmacologic mechanisms for the control of pain have been viewed with both enthusiasm and indifference, and should be used as adjuncts in the management of pain, rather than the sole approach. Areas that require further consideration are transcutaneous electrical nerve stimulation, relaxation and guided imagery, biofeedback, and hypnosis.

Transcutaneous Electrical Nerve Stimulation

Transcutaneous electrical nerve stimulation (TENS) has been shown effective in postoperative pain management.[66] TENS has also been shown to be effective for pain associated with arthritis, cancer, and trauma. The mechanism of action has been associated with activation of the large-diameter myelinated primary afferents which exert an inhibitory effect on the dorsal horn pain transmission neurons. It is hypothesized that stimulation of such nerve fibers would then alleviate pain. Although TENS is easy to use, patients must be cooperative and willing to work with this pain management modality. Patient education and continued surveillance of the use of the instrument are required.

Relaxation and Guided Imagery

Relaxation and guided imagery focus the patient's attention away from the pain or unpleasant experience. Patients are often instructed to meditate, count, repeat a word, or focus on parts of the body. In this regard, imagery can be used as distraction or as a method of relaxation. The use of imagery and relaxation requires the patient to make a commitment to the use and practice of this technique. Daake and Gueldner demonstrated a significant decrease in the amount of analgesics used and the patient's perception of pain with the use of guided imagery.[67] These techniques should be used in combination with pharmacologic interventions in the total pain management plan.

Biofeedback

Biofeedback has been used in various clinical settings for the relief of pain. Essential to the use of biofeedback is the ability to provide measurable physiologic parameters for the patient to use as a benchmark. Such measurements have included skin temperature, pulse rate, blood pressure, muscle activity, and electroencephalographic activity. Biofeedback has been used most commonly in the treatment of headache and stress-related syndromes.

Hypnosis

Hypnosis is one of the oldest methods used to decrease pain. It requires the cooperation of the patient and confidence in the therapist. Orne and Dinges claim that it is the manipulation of the patient's attention away from the pain.

Hypnosis has been reported to alleviate many types of acute and chronic pain.[68] Nonpharmacologic techniques in the management of pain should be considered as an adjunct to traditional therapy and when other pain management regimens do not completely control the patient's pain.

QUALITY ASSURANCE ISSUES AND PAIN MANAGEMENT

Pain is easier to prevent than it is to manage once it has become established. Therefore, beginning at the time of the initial encounter with the patient, the nurse anesthetist should encourage the patient to participate in pain control. The anesthetist should explain to the patient that pain can adversely effect the recovery process or an existing condition. The aim of pain management is to prevent significant pain from the onset. The patient must understand that dosages of analgesia may need to be increased or adjunctive therapies, such as relaxation and TENS, may be needed to provide effective pain management.

Documentation of the efficacy of pain control measures is essential for quality pain control. A recent study of 100 surgical patients indicates that documentation of pain is incomplete and infrequent.[35] Documentation is important for effective communication between the patient and health care providers. Without accurate and complete documentation, health care professionals cannot follow a consistent and appropriate plan of care to provide pain control. Documentation is also important for evaluating effectiveness of pain control strategies. Without evaluation, the nurse anesthetist may continue to use ineffective methods or insufficient analgesia for pain management. Furthermore, inconsistent and inadequate documentation of pain assessment or effectiveness of interventions could potentially be viewed to constitute a deviation from acceptable clinical practice.

Individuals who are responsible for patient care in health care organizations should evaluate their own process of pain management. Established standards of care and an organized process by which pain is acknowledged, assessed, effectively managed, and reassessed are essential. A pain care program that is sporadic and depends on patients' or families' demands for analgesia "as needed" is likely to result in intervals of inadequate pain relief and to foster the patient's anxiety, loss of control, and fatigue.

THE FUTURE IN THE MANAGEMENT OF PAIN

Over the past 20 years, researchers have commented about poor pain management in health care institutions.[3,4,41] Yet despite new technologies such as epidural analgesics, patient-controlled analgesia, and new medications, patients remain in pain. Attention should be given to how physicians and nurses make critical decisions about selecting methods of pain control and the amounts of analgesic medications ordered and administered. Much of the research on pain has focused on health care providers' beliefs and values about medicating patients in pain, but few research studies have investigated medication decisions of either physicians and nurses, as key players in the undertreatment of patients' pain. The development of a clinical decision-making model would be useful for identifying effective strategies for decreasing faulty judgments about pain management. Unfortunately, the recognition of ineffective practices in pain management has not led educators to improve the knowledge and clinical pain management skills of practitioners. Both clinicians and patients must be educated about the various options for pain control and the need for systematic assessment of interventions. Patients must understand the importance of effective pain control in the overall recovery process.

Effective pain management should begin with a comprehensive plan. The nurse anesthetist must be in the position, both by education and by conviction, to be an integral part of the planning, implementation, and evaluation process. This requires additional knowledge, skill, and patience, all of which are essential components of the nurse anesthetist role.

REFERENCES

1. Bonica JJ. Pain research and therapy: Past and current status and future needs. In: Ng LKY, Bonica JJ, eds. *Pain, discomfort and humanitarian care.* Amsterdam: Elsevier; 1980:1–46.
2. Donovan M, Dillon P, McGuire L. Incidence and characteristics of pain in a sample of medical–surgical in-patients. *Pain.* 1987; 30:69–78.
3. Cohen F. Post surgical pain relief: Patients' status and nurses' medication choices. *Pain.* 1980;9:265–274.
4. Marks RM, Sachar EJ. Undertreatment of medical patients with narcotic analgesics. *Ann Intern Med.* 1973;78:173–181.
5. Mather L, Mackie J. The incidence of postoperative pain in children. *Pain.* 1981;15:271–282.
6. Foley KM. The treatment of cancer pain. *N Engl J Med.* 1985;313(2):84–95.
7. Sriwatanakul K, Weiss OP, Alloza JL. Analysis of narcotic usage in the treatment of postoperative pain. *JAMA.* 1983;250: 926–929.
8. Loeser J, Egan D, eds. *Managing the chronic pain patient: Theory and practice at the University of Washington Multidisciplinary Pain Center.* New York: Raven Press; 1989.
9. Edwards WT. Optimizing opioid treatment of postoperative pain. *J Pain Symptom Manage.* 1990;5:S24–S37.
10. Melzack R, Wall PD. Pain mechanisms: A new theory. *Science.* 1965;150:971–979.
11. Leventhal H, Everhart D. Emotion, pain and physical illness. In: Izard CE, ed. *Emotions and psychopathology.* New York: Plenum Press; 1979.
12. Mersky H. Pain terms: A list with definitions and notes on usage—Recommended by the IASP Subcommittee on Taxonomy. *Pain.* 1979;6:249–252.
13. Fields HL. *Pain.* New York: McGraw-Hill; 1987.
14. Kehlet H. Modification of responses to surgery by neural blockade: Clinical applications. In: Cousins MJ, Bridenbaugh PO, eds. *Neural blockade in clinical anesthesia and management of pain.* 2nd ed. Philadelphia: JB Lippincott; 1988:145–188.
15. Yeager MP, Glass DD, Neff RK, Brinck-Johnsen T. Epidural anesthesia and analgesia in high risk surgical patients. *Anesthesiology.* 1987;66:729–736.
16. Modig J, Paalzow L. A comparison of epidural morphine and epidural bupivicaine for postoperative pain relief. *Acta Anaesth Scand.* 1981;25:437–441.
17. Cullen ML, Staren ED, El-Ganzouri A, Logas WG. Ivankovitch AD, Economou SE. Continuous epidural infusions for analgesia after major abdominal operations: A randomized, prospective, double-blind study. *Surgery.* 1985;98:718–728.

18. Craig KD, Prkachin KM. Non-verbal measures of pain. In: Melzack R, ed. *Pain measurement and assessment.* New York: Raven Press; 1982:173–179.
19. Johnson LR, Magnani B, Chan V, Ferrante MF. Modifiers of patient-controlled analgesia efficacy: Locus of control. *Pain.* 1989;39:17–22.
20. Peck C. Psychological factors in acute pain management. In: Cousins MJ, Phillips GD, eds. *Acute pain management.* Edinburgh: Churchill Livingstone; 1986:251–274.
21. Cousins MJ, Phillips GD. *Acute pain management.* New York: Churchill Livingstone; 1986:61–78.
22. Beecher HK. Relationship of significance of wound to the pain experienced. *JAMA.* 1956;161:1613.
23. Melzack R, Wall PD, Ty TC. Acute pain in the emergency clinic: Latency of onset and descriptor patterns. *Pain.* 1982;14:33.
24. Averill JR. Personal control over aversive stimuli and its relationship to stress. *Psychol Bull.* 1973;80:286–303.
25. Hodges WF, Spielberger CD. The effects of threat of shock on heart rate for subjects who differ in manifest anxiety and fear of shock. *Psychophysiology.* 1966;2:287.
26. Fortin F, Kirovac S. A randomized controlled trial of preoperative patient education. *Educ J Nurs Stud.* 1976;13:11.
27. Chapman CR, Cox GB. Anxiety, pain and depression surrounding elective surgery: A multivariate comparison of abdominal surgery patients with kidney donors and recipients. *J Psychosomat Res.* 1977;21:7.
28. Mandler G, Watson DC. Anxiety and the interruption of behavior. In: Speilberger CD, ed. *Anxiety and behavior.* New York: Academic Press; 1966.
29. Andrew J. Recovery from surgery with and without preparation instruction for three coping styles. *J Pers Soc Psychol.* 1970;15:233.
30. Ball TS, Vogler RE. Uncertain pain and the pain of uncertainty. *Percept Motor Skills.* 1977;3:1195.
31. Johnson M. Anxiety in surgical patients. *Psychol Med.* 1980; 10:145.
32. Craig K. Social modeling influences: Pain in context. In: Sternbach RA, ed. *The psychology of pain,* 2nd ed. New York: Raven Press; 1986:73–109.
33. Graffam CR, Johnson A. A comparison of two relaxation strategies for the relief of pain and its distress. *J Pain Symptom Manage.* 1987;2:229.
34. Sofaer B. Pain management through nursing education. In: Coop L, ed. *Recent advances in nursing: Perspectives on pain.* London: Churchill Livingstone; 1985.
35. Faut M, Paice J, Mahon S. Factors associated with the adequacy of pain control in hospitalized surgical patients. In: *Proceedings of the 13th Annual Midwest Nursing Research Society Conference, Cincinnati;* 1989:214.
36. Donovan M, Slack J, Faut M, et al. Factors associated with inadequate management of pain. In: *American Pain Society, Eighth Annual Scientific Meeting, Phoenix;* 1989.
37. Burgess A. Children's drawings as indication of sexual trauma. *Perspect Psychiatry.* 1981;19:50–58.
38. Jaffee J. Drug addiction and drug abuse. In: Goodman LS, Gilman AG, eds. *Pharmacologic basis of therapeutics.* New York: MacMillan; 1980:522–573.
39. Porter J, Jick H. Addiction rare in patients treated with narcotics. *N Engl J Med.* 1980;302:123.
40. Slack JF, Faut-Callahan ME. Efficacy of continuous epidural analgesia and the implications for patient care in the early postoperative phase. *Nurse Anesth.* 1990;1:79–89.
41. Weis DJ, Sriwatanakul K, Alloza J, Weintraub M, Lasagna L. Attitudes of patients, housestaff, and nurses toward postoperative analgesic care. *Anesth Analg.* 1983;62:70–74.
42. Lander J. Fallacies and phobias about addiction and pain. *Pain.* 1990;42:15–22.

43. Owen H, McMillan V, Rogowski D. Pain management and patient expectations. *Pain.* 1990;41:303–307.

44. Zborowski M. Cultural components in responses to pain. *J Soc Issues.* 1952;8:16–30.

45. Von Baeyer C, Johnson M, McMillan M. Consequences of nonverbal experience of pain: Patient distress and observer concern. *Soc Sci Med.* 1984;19:1319–1324.

46. Davitz J, Davitz L. *Inferences of patient's pain and psychological distress: Studies of nursing behaviors.* New York: Springer; 1981.

47. Faherty B, Grier M. Analgesic medication for elderly people postsurgery. *Nurs Res.* 1984;33:369–372.

48. Hargreaves SA. *Implementing TENS to control postoperative pain.* Edmonton, Alberta: University of Alberta; 1987. Master's thesis.

49. Hammond KR. Clinical inference in nursing: Analyzing cognitive tasks representative of nursing problems. *Nurs Res.* 1966; 15:134–138.

50. Melzack R. The McGill pain questionnaire: Major properties and scoring methods. *Pain.* 1975;1:275–299.

51. Syrjala KL, Chapman CR. Measurement of clinical pain: A review and integration of research findings. In: Benedetti C, Chapman CR, Moricca G, eds. *Advances in pain research and therapy.* New York: Livingstone Press; 1984:71–101.

52. Abu-Saad H, Holzemer WL. Measuring self-assessment of pain. *Issues Compr Pediatr Nurs.* 1981;5:337–349.

53. McGrath PA, de Veber LL, Hearn MT. Multidimensional pain assessment in children. In: Fields HL, Dubner R, Cervro F, eds. *Advances in pain research and therapy.* New York: Raven Press; 1985;9:387–393.

54. Heft MW, Parker SR. An experimental basis for revising the graphic rating scale for pain. *Pain.* 1984;19:153–161.

55. Gracely RH. Pain measurement in man. In: Bonica JJ, ed. *Pain, discomfort and humanitarian care.* Amsterdam: Elsevier/North-Holland; 1980:111.

56. Taylor H, Curran NH. *The Nuprin pain report.* New York: Louis Harris and Associates; 1985.

57. Dawkins CJM. Relief of postoperative pain by continuous epidural drip. In: *Proceedings of the Fourth Congress, Scandinavia Society of Anesthesiologists, Helsinki;* 1956:77.

58. Lang E, Theiss D, Reiss W, Sommer V. Epidural morphine for postoperative analgesia: A double-blind study. *Anesth Analg.* 1982;61:236–240.

59. Soliman JE, Safwat AM. Successful management of an elderly patient with multiple trauma. *J Trauma.* 1985;25(8):806–807.

60. Wang JK, Nauss LA, Thomas JE. Pain relief by intrathecally applied morphine in man. *Anesthesiology.* 1979;50:149–151.

61. Nautly J, Datta S, Ostheimer G. Epidural fentanyl for post cesarean delivery pain management. *Anesthesiology.* 1985;63: 694–698.

62. Graham JL, King R, McCaughey W. Postoperative pain relief using epidural morphine. *Anaesthesia.* 1980;35:158–160.

63. Torda TA, Pybus DA. Comparison of four narcotic analgesics for extradural analgesia. *Br J Anaesth.* 1982;54:291.

64. Wermaling DP, Foster TS, Rapp RP. Evaluation of a disposable, nonelectric patient controlled analgesia device for postoperative pain. *Clin Pharmacol.* 1987;6:307–314.

65. Graves DA, Foster TS, Batenhorst RS, et al. Patient controlled analgesia. *Ann Intern Med.* 1983;99:360–366.

66. Cooperman AM, Hall B, Mikalacki K, Hardy R, Sadar E. Use of transcutaneous electrical stimulation in the control of postoperative pain—Results of a prospective, randomized, controlled study. *Am J Surg.* 1977;133:185–187.

67. Daake D, Gueldner S. Imagery instruction and the control of postsurgical pain. *Appl Nurs Res.* 1989;2(3):114–120.

68. Orne MT, Dinges DF. Hypnosis. In: Wall PD, Melzak R, eds. *Textbook of pain.* Edinburgh: Churchill Livingstone; 1989: 1021–1031.

Index

Page numbers followed by *t* and *f* indicate tables and figures, respectively.

Page numbers followed by *t* and *f* indicate tables and figures, respectively.

Page numbers followed by *t* and *f* indicate tables and figures, respectively.

Page numbers followed by *t* and *f* indicate tables and figures, respectively.

Page numbers followed by *t* and *f* indicate tables and figures, respectively.

Page numbers followed by *t* and *f* indicate tables and figures, respectively.

Page numbers followed by *t* and *f* indicate tables and figures, respectively.

Page numbers followed by *t* and *f* indicate tables and figures, respectively.

Page numbers followed by *t* and *f* indicate tables and figures, respectively.

Page numbers followed by *t* and *f* indicate tables and figures, respectively.

Page numbers followed by *t* and *f* indicate tables and figures, respectively.

Page numbers followed by *t* and *f* indicate tables and figures, respectively.

Page numbers followed by *t* and *f* indicate tables and figures, respectively.

Page numbers followed by *t* and *f* indicate tables and figures, respectively.

Page numbers followed by *t* and *f* indicate tables and figures, respectively.

Page numbers followed by *t* and *f* indicate tables and figures, respectively.

Page numbers followed by *t* and *f* indicate tables and figures, respectively.

Page numbers followed by *t* and *f* indicate tables and figures, respectively.

Page numbers followed by *t* and *f* indicate tables and figures, respectively.

Page numbers followed by *t* and *f* indicate tables and figures, respectively.

White tube, 697
Whole blood, 302
  citrated, composition of, 303t
  clinical indications for, 303t
  composition of, 303t
  decreasing the use of, 309
Winton, Sophie Gran, 6
Wolff-Parkinson-White syndrome, 732, 732f
  epicardial mapping in, 732, 733f
  mechanisms of tachycardia in, 732, 733f
Wood, Alexander, 456
Work, 57
  measurement of, 65
Work hours, irregular, detrimental effects of, 167

Work practice recommendations, 170t
World War I, nurse anesthetist service in, 6–7

X
Xanthine(s), perioperative management of, 239
Xenon
  atomic number of, 58t
  atomic weight of, 58t
  symbol for, 58t
  used to measure cerebral blood flow, 680
X-ray therapy, for orthopedic patients, 651
Xylocaine. *See also* Lidocaine
  in outpatient anesthesia, 596

Y
Ytterbium, 58t
Yttrium, 58t

Z
Z-band, 361
Zidovudine, prophylaxis, for health care workers, 166
Zinc, 58t
Zirconium, 58t
Z-line(s), 776–777
Z-membrane, 776
Zwitterion, 90